# CLINICAL IMMUNOLOGY

# CLINICAL IMMUNOLOGY

Edited by

**NIMA REZAEI**

Professor of Clinical Immunology, Research Center for Immunodeficiencies, Children's Medical Center and Department of Immunology, School of Medicine, Tehran University of Medical Sciences, Iran; Network of Immunity in Infection, Malignancy and Autoimmunity (NIIMA), Universal Scientific Education and Research Network (USERN), Tehran, Iran

ELSEVIER

ACADEMIC PRESS

An imprint of Elsevier

elsevier.com/books-and-journals

Academic Press is an imprint of Elsevier
125 London Wall, London EC2Y 5AS, United Kingdom
525 B Street, Suite 1650, San Diego, CA 92101, United States
50 Hampshire Street, 5th Floor, Cambridge, MA 02139, United States
The Boulevard, Langford Lane, Kidlington, Oxford OX5 1GB, United Kingdom



ISBN: 978-0-12-818006-8

For Information on all Academic Press publications visit our website at
https://www.elsevier.com/books-and-journals

*Publisher:* Stacy Masucci
*Acquisitions Editor:* Linda Versteeg-Buschman
*Editorial Project Manager:* Sam W. Young
*Production Project Manager:* Sreejith Viswanathan
*Cover Designer:* Greg Harris
Cover design image by: Dr. Yousef Fattahi

Typeset by Aptara, New Delhi, India

This book would not have been possible without the continuous encouragement by my family. I wish to dedicate it to my daughters, Ariana and Arnika, with the hope that increasing the knowledge will lead to health to all and provide a brighter future for next generations. Whatever I have learnt, comes from my mentors. This book is therefore dedicated also to all of them, but most importantly to the patients and their families whose continuous support has guided me during all these years.

# CONTENTS

# Contributors

**Melina Farshbafnadi**
School of Medicine, Tehran University of Medical Sciences, Tehran, Iran; Cancer Immunology Project (CIP), Universal Scientific Education and Research Network (USERN), Tehran, Iran

**Sara Harsini**
Research Center for Immunodeficiencies, Children's Medical Center, Tehran University of Medical Sciences, Tehran, Iran; Association of Nuclear Medicine and Molecular Imaging (ANMMI), Universal Scientific Education and Research Network (USERN), Tehran, Iran; BC Cancer, Vancouver, BC, Canada

**Mahsa Keshavarz-Fathi**
School of Medicine, Tehran University of Medical Sciences, Tehran, Iran; Cancer Immunology Project (CIP), Universal Scientific Education and Research Network (USERN), Tehran, Iran; Research Center for Immunodeficiencies, Children's Medical Center, Tehran University of Medical Sciences, Tehran, Iran

**Amin Pastaki Khoshbin**
School of Medicine, Tehran University of Medical Sciences, Tehran, Iran; Cancer Immunology Project (CIP), Universal Scientific Education and Research Network (USERN), Tehran, Iran

**Farimah Masoumi**
School of Medicine, Tonekabon Branch, Islamic Azad University, Tonekabon, Iran

**Elaheh Nasrollahzadeh**
Cancer Immunology Project (CIP), Universal Scientific Education and Research Network (USERN), Tehran, Iran; School of Medicine, Guilan University of Medical Sciences, Rasht, Iran

**Ali Nowroozi**
School of Medicine, Tehran University of Medical Sciences, Tehran, Iran; Cancer Immunology Project (CIP), Universal Scientific Education and Research Network (USERN), Tehran, Iran

**Parmida sadat Pezeshki**
School of Medicine, Tehran University of Medical Sciences, Tehran, Iran; Cancer Immunology Project (CIP), Universal Scientific Education and Research Network (USERN), Tehran, Iran; Network of Immunity in Infection, Malignancy and Autoimmunity (NIIMA), Universal Scientific Education and Research Network (USERN), Tehran, Iran

**Sepideh Razi**
Cancer Immunology Project (CIP), Universal Scientific Education and Research Network (USERN), Tehran, Iran; School of Medicine, Iran University of Medical Sciences, Tehran, Iran; Research Center for Immunodeficiencies, Children's Medical Center, Tehran University of Medical Sciences, Tehran, Iran

**Nima Rezaei**
Research Center for Immunodeficiencies, Children's Medical Center, Tehran University of Medical Sciences, Tehran, Iran; Network of Immunity in Infection, Malignancy and Autoimmunity (NIIMA), Universal Scientific Education and Research Network (USERN), Tehran, Iran; Department of Immunology, School of Medicine, Tehran University of Medical Sciences, Tehran, Iran

**Mona Sadeghalvad**
Department of Immunology, School of Medicine, Tehran University of Medical Sciences, Tehran, Iran; Research Center for Immunodeficiencies, Children's Medical Center, Tehran University of Medical Sciences, Tehran, Iran; Network of Immunity in Infection, Malignancy and Autoimmunity (NIIMA), Universal Scientific Education and Research Network (USERN), Tehran, Iran

**Kiarash Saleki**
Student Research Committee, Babol University of Medical Sciences, Babol, Iran; USERN Office, Babol University of Medical Sciences, Babol, Iran

**Pouya Mahdavi Sharif**
School of Medicine, Tehran University of Medical Sciences, Tehran, Iran; Cancer Immunology Project (CIP), Universal Scientific Education and Research Network (USERN), Tehran, Iran

**Samaneh Zoghi**
Ludwig Boltzmann Institute for Rare and Undiagnosed Diseases (LBI-RUD), Vienna, Austria; St. Anna Children's Cancer Research Institute (CCRI), Vienna, Austria; CeMM Research Center for Molecular Medicine of the Austrian Academy of Sciences, Vienna, Austria; Network of Immunity in Infection, Malignancy and Autoimmunity (NIIMA), Universal Scientific Education and Research Network (USERN), Vienna, Austria

# Preface

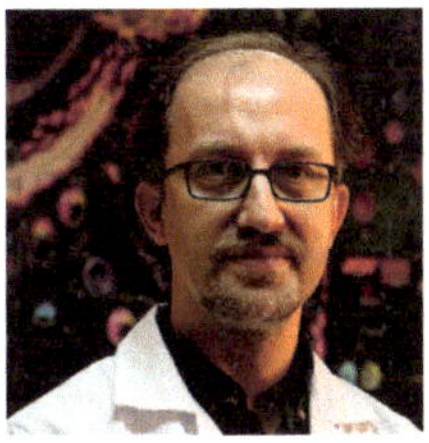

Imagine that you are an ancient being and probably a distant ancestor of all mammals. Your life relies on an elementary defense system. If you are attacked by a parasite or microbe, you stop it from harming you by releasing phagocytic cells or producing and unleashing chemicals against it. Now, imagine that during evolution, you become a more sophisticated being, and soon you realize that you need a more complex defense system in order to protect you against all pathogens. Also, this defense system must not invade your own tissues or harm your cohabitants. This defense system is called "Immune system." The immune system is one of the most incredible systems of the human body. It is made up of a vast network of cells, chemicals, tissues, and organs that protects our body from pathogenic invaders such as bacteria, fungi, viruses, and parasites, and it can keep a memory of the invaders to defend the host from any further encounters. In addition, the immune system plays a key role in the pathogenesis of cancer and controlling the growth of cancer cells. Various immunotherapeutic approaches have been approved for cancer treatment, and some of them, namely immune checkpoint inhibitors for solid tumors and CAR T-cell therapy for hematologic malignancies, are breakthroughs in cancer treatment. Any aberration from normal function of the immune system leads to the development of immune system disorders, which can be characterized by abnormally low activity or overactivity of the immune system. Immunodeficiencies are a group of immune system diseases in which the host is incapable of responding to the pathogens, properly and in a protective fashion, and they are divided into primary and secondary based on genetic and environmental causes of the disease, respectively. Any functional, developmental, proliferative, or differentiation defect of one or more components of the immune system results in the development of immunodeficiencies. Other types of immune system disorders, including autoimmune diseases and allergies, are characterized by activation of the immune system in the absence of any pathogens or tumor, or activation of innate immune response and releasing of inflammatory mediators without any evidence of an antigen-immune response in the case of autoimmune diseases or development of unfavorable immune responses against allergens in the case of allergies. Besides the development of immune system diseases, as a result of abnormal immune responses, these inappropriate responses can also lead to the rejection of the transplanted cells, tissues, and organs. Transplantation is a procedure in which cells, tissues, or organs of an individual are replaced by those of another individual or the same person. The immune system, which is designed to defend the host against foreign antigens, may act against the transplanted cells, tissue, or organ and cause rejection.

In this book, after an introduction to the immune system (Chapter 1), the definition, epidemiology, pathogenesis, clinical features, diagnosis, and treatment of allergic diseases, including asthma, allergic rhinitis, allergic conjunctivitis, urticaria and angioedema, atopic dermatitis, and allergic contact dermatitis, food allergy and gastrointestinal syndromes, drug allergy, and anaphylaxis are discussed (Chapter 2). Afterward, the immune cells and immune responses, which are involved in autoimmune reaction, initiation, and facilitation of autoimmunity, human multisystem autoimmune diseases, and some more common system-specific autoimmune diseases, are reviewed (Chapter 3). This book discusses the interaction between the immune system and transformed cells and provides an updated review on the application of immunotherapy for different cancer types, combination therapy, and immunoediting after other therapeutic approaches (Chapter 4). Then, it presents the types of immunodeficiency diseases, their possible diagnosis, and treatment (Chapter 5). Also, the definition and epidemiology, molecular mechanisms, diagnosis, and treatment of infectious diseases (Chapter 6) and different types of transplantations, the immunopathogenesis of transplantation, the process of matching the donor and the recipient, pretransplantation conditioning, and complications after transplant, and ways to manage them (Chapter 7) are reviewed in this book.

I hope that this book will be welcomed by basic scientists and clinicians who wish to extend their knowledge in the field of clinical immunology.

Nima Rezaei, MD, PhD

# Acknowledgment

I would like to express my gratitude to the Editorial Assistant of this book, Dr. Sepideh Razi. With no doubt, the book would not have been completed without her contribution. Indeed, I am so thankful to Dr. Yousef Fatahi for his contribution in designing the book cover and a few illustrations for some chapters.

*Nima Rezaei, MD, PhD*

# CHAPTER 1

# The immune system

**Samaneh Zoghi**[a,b,c,d], **Farimah Masoumi**[e], **Nima Rezaei**[f,g,h]
[a]Ludwig Boltzmann Institute for Rare and Undiagnosed Diseases (LBI-RUD), Vienna, Austria
[b]St. Anna Children's Cancer Research Institute (CCRI), Vienna, Austria
[c]CeMM Research Center for Molecular Medicine of the Austrian Academy of Sciences, Vienna, Austria
[d]Network of Immunity in Infection, Malignancy and Autoimmunity (NIIMA), Universal Scientific Education and Research Network (USERN), Vienna, Austria
[e]School of Medicine, Tonekabon Branch, Islamic Azad University, Tonekabon, Iran
[f]Research Center for Immunodeficiencies, Children's Medical Center, Tehran University of Medical Sciences, Tehran, Iran
[g]Network of Immunity in Infection, Malignancy and Autoimmunity (NIIMA), Universal Scientific Education and Research Network (USERN), Tehran, Iran
[h]Department of Immunology, School of Medicine, Tehran University of Medical Sciences, Tehran, Iran

## Introduction

The Human immune system has two major components of Innate (natural) and adaptive (specific) immunity. Both compartments work together to protect the host against disease-causing agents, which we are exposed to continuously.[1] While even metazoans have innate immunity, adaptive immunity is specific to vertebrates.[2] The cells and components of each of these immune systems are explained in the following sections.

Although the function of the immune system is to defend against infectious agents, non-infectious agents can also elicit an immune response.[3] This process can injure tissues and cause diseases such as allergy and autoimmunity. In this chapter, we are going to explain the principles and functions of the human immune system briefly.

The main characteristics and drivers of the innate and adaptive immune systems are summarized in Table 1.1.[4] In summary, innate immunity is the first and fast responder against pathogens (in a few hours to days), which recognize some common molecular patterns that are presented exclusively in microorganisms, and its function is non-specific. In contrast, the adaptive immune system reacts specifically to each antigen, and therefore, it takes longer after the infection (days to weeks) for this type of immunity to function. Antigens are microbial or nonmicrobial agents that can elicit an immune response. A very important characteristic of the immune system is to differentiate self-antigens from non-self, and any deviation from this capability can cause a pathogenic complication.[4]

## Humoral and cellular immunity

The adaptive immune system divides into two types: humoral and cellular immunity. Both are highly cooperating to defend the host against a wide range of infectious agents.[5] Humoral immunity refers to antibody molecules that are secreted to the blood

*Clinical Immunology*
DOI: https://doi.org/10.1016/B978-0-12-818006-8.00005-0

**Table 1.1** Major characteristic of Innate and adaptive immunity.

| | Innate immunity | Adaptive immunity |
|---|---|---|
| **Reacts to** | Common pathogenic determinants | Any microbial and nonmicrobial antigen |
| **Diversity of reactions** | Restricted | Very diverse due to specificity |
| **Memory** | No | Yes |
| **Differentiation of self from foreign antigen** | Yes | Yes |
| **Cellular components** | Macrophages, neutrophils, NK cells, and DCs | Lymphocytes |
| **Proteins** | Blood proteins such as the complement system and lectins | Antibodies |
| **Other components** | Skin and mucosal barriers | Tissue-resident lymphocytes and antibodies |

NK, Natural killer; DCs, Dendritic cells.

or mucosa by B lymphocytes. Antibodies are very important proteins in defense against extra-cellular pathogenic agents such as microbes and their toxins. They can neutralize the toxins and specifically recognize the microbes and flag them to be phagocytosed by phagocytic cells.[4]

Cellular immunity refers to another type of defense mechanism that is mainly conducted by T lymphocytes against intracellular pathogens, where they cannot be accessed by antibodies. In this situation, T cells function to kill the infected cell, directly by the help of cytotoxic T cells or indirectly by activation of macrophages and neutrophils to stop the spread of infection.[1,4]

## Lymphocytes and their specific receptors

B lymphocytes (B cells) and T lymphocytes (T cells) are major cellular components of the adaptive immune system. These cells can recognize antigens specifically, which occurs through their specific receptors. We will explain in the following sections the generation of these receptors with high diversity. B and T Lymphocytes present as different and distinct clones, which are the population of cells that express the same receptor with similar specificity, and each clone is unique.[6] Lymphocytes differentiate in the primary lymphoid organs, and they circulate in the blood and lymphoid organs while they are mature. However, they considered naïve cells before an antigen encounter. After recognition of their specific antigen, which they express the specific receptor against, these cells undergo several changes through signal transduction and intracellular signaling pathways, and they become an effector lymphocyte. We will further explain in the following sections how the process of lymphocyte activation takes place in B and T cells. The specific receptor on the surface of B cell is called B cell receptor (BCR), which is the same as antibody molecule, but a membrane-bound form of it. T cell receptor (TCR) is the specific receptor expressed on the surface of a T cell. Both BCR and TCR molecules have clonal differentiation and distribution.[7] We will explain more about these receptors in the T cell and B cell development sections. As mentioned in Table 1.1, an important characteristic of TCR and BCR molecules is their diversity, which enables the adaptive immune system to recognize $10^7$ to $10^9$ different antigens.

## Memory

One of the key aspects of the adaptive immune system is the ability to keep a memory of the infection and to be able to recall it much faster in the next encounter. Therefore, lymphocytes undergo changes such as growing in number and transforming from an effector cell to a memory cell, which is a very long-lived cell. The first exposure of an immune cell to its specific antigen is called the primary immune response, which also primes lymphocytes and prepares them for memory cell formation. The second encounter of memory cells with the specific antigen is called the secondary immune response, which is not only faster but also more extensive than the primary immune response.[8]

## Self-tolerance

Non-reactivity to self-antigens is a fundamental aspect of the immune system, which guarantees a successful and effective defense against foreign intruders without harming the self-tissues. This non-responsiveness of the immune system is called tolerance. Tolerance mechanisms are explained in the tolerance section, but in summary, all the self-reactive clones of lymphocytes are being eliminated or suppressed to become tolerant against self-antigens. Defects in the tolerance mechanisms and loss of self-reactivity causes autoimmunity.[9]

## Cells of the immune system

The function of the immune system is coordinated by a variety of cells, playing role in the innate and adaptive immune responses (Fig. 1.1). Most of these cells are white blood cells that arise from pluripotent hematopoietic stem cells in bone marrow.[10] Hematopoietic stem cells differentiate into two lineage precursors: common myeloid progenitor (CMP) and common lymphoid progenitor (CLP). Most of the innate immune system cells, including macrophages, granulocytes (such as neutrophils, eosinophils, and basophils), mast cells, and dendritic cells (DCs), differentiate from CMP. In contrast, specialized cells of the adaptive immune response, including B and T lymphocytes, generate from CLP.[11] Most of the immune system cells are found in the blood,

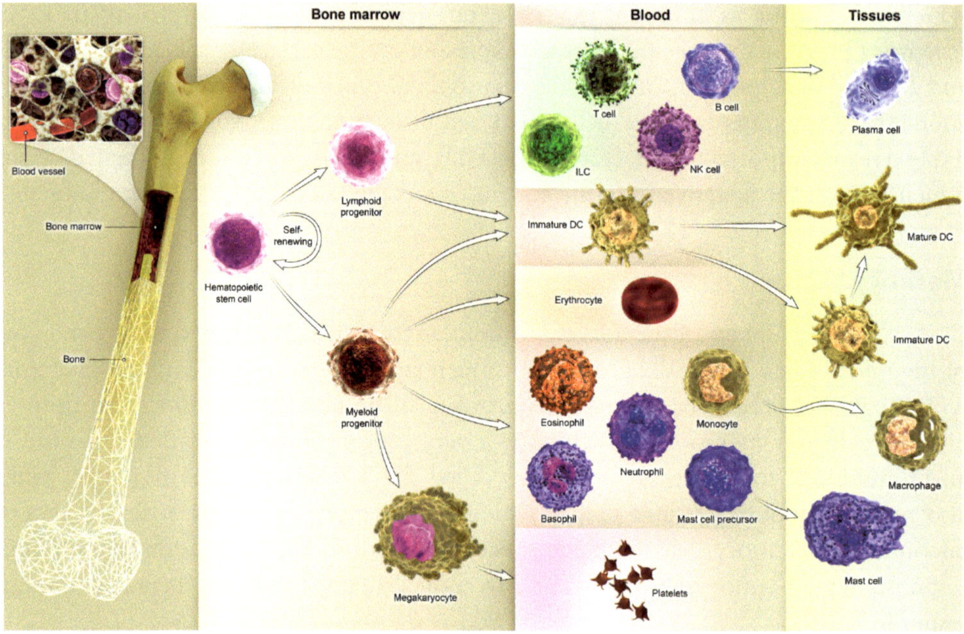


**Fig. 1.1** ***Almost all cells of the immune system cells arise from a pluripotent hematopoietic stem cell in the bone marrow.*** Hematopoietic stem cells divide into common lymphoid progenitor (CLP) and common myeloid progenitor (CMP), which gives rise to the lymphoid and myeloid lineage, respectively.

as we see their frequency in Table 1.2, but immune responses to antigens take place in lymphoid tissues.[12]

## Granulocytes

Based on morphologic differences, polymorphonuclear leukocytes or granulocytes include neutrophils, eosinophils, and basophils. Neutrophils are the most frequent granulocytes of the blood circulation, and together with monocytes/macrophages perform phagocytosis in host defense.[13] The process of phagocytosis includes entering the site of infection, capturing microorganisms or products of necrotic cells using innate immune system receptors, and ingesting and killing microorganisms within specialized cytoplasmic vacuoles called phagolysosomes.[14] Neutrophils have a short lifespan, but

**Table 1.2** Normal White Blood Cells Percentage.

| | |
|---|---|
| Neutrophils | 40–60 percent |
| Lymphocytes | 20–40 percent |
| Monocytes | 2–8 percent |
| Eosinophils | 1–4 percent |
| Basophils | <1 percent |

their response to pathogens is relatively rapid due to their cytoskeletal movements and enzymatic activity in pathogen destruction. Neutrophils also produce antimicrobial peptides that kill extracellular microbes.[15] Eosinophils contain granules mainly with basic proteins that are toxic for helminths. These cells also can be found in mucosal tissues.[16] Although mast cells derive from different bone marrow precursors, blood basophils have morphological and structural similarities to tissue mast cells. Moreover, mast cells and basophils have an important role in defense against parasites by degranulation of their biological mediators. With a similar mechanism, these cells bind to allergens through high affinity immunoglobulin (Ig) E specific FC receptor (FcεR) and mediate allergic reactions.[17]

## Monocytes/macrophages

Monocytes and macrophages are recognized as mononuclear phagocytes. Monocytes derive from bone marrow precursors and circulate in the blood, but when they migrate into tissues, they mature into macrophages and are called inflammatory macrophages. Besides, there are long-lived tissue-resident macrophages in different tissues that have developed during fetal development, like Kupffer cells in the liver or alveolar macrophages in the lung.[18]

Based on the functional aspect, there are two main groups of monocytes: the most well-known type are inflammatory or classic monocytes, which have phagocytic activity and produce inflammatory mediators, and can quickly migrate to sites of infection or tissue injury. There are also nonclassical monocytes that mainly take part in tissue repair.[19] Similarly, macrophages can gain different functional abilities and are divided into two groups: M1 macrophages, which are classically activated and mainly take part in phagocytosis, and M2 macrophages, which are alternatively activated and have tissue repair properties. Skewing toward M1 or M2 subtypes depends on cytokine milieu and activating stimuli that these cells are exposed to them.[20]

The major function of macrophages is phagocytosis and the killing of ingested microorganisms. Macrophages also ingest apoptotic cells, including neutrophils, that die at the sites of infection.[21] Through phagocytosis, macrophages are stimulated by microbial products and produce different cytokines that enhance the recruitment of monocytes and other leukocytes into the site of infection. Furthermore, phagocytized microbes are presented to lymphocytes as the antigen-presenting capacity of macrophages and activate T lymphocytes during a cellular immune response.[22]

## Antigen-presenting cells

Antigen-presenting cells (APCs) are a diverse group of immune system cells that are specialized for the presentation of antigens to lymphocytes, particularly T cells. Among APCs, there are monocytes, macrophages, B lymphocytes, cutaneous Langerhans cells, and most importantly, DCs.[23]

The main feature of APCs are the expression of class I and class II major histocompatibility complex (MHC) molecules for the presentation of antigenic peptides to cluster of differentiation (CD)8+ and CD4+ T cells, respectively, as well as other co-stimulatory molecules such as B7-1 (CD80), B7-2 (CD86), required for T cell activation. APCs capture and present antigens, along with providing cytokines that induce specific responses in cells to which they are presenting antigens.[24]

Different APCs uptake antigens and drive their specific effector functions, for example, monocytes and macrophages phagocyte opsonized antigens, and present them to T cells in the cellular immune response. T cells produce cytokines when become activated that help phagocytes to kill the ingested microorganisms.[25]

B cells antigenic presenting capacity for T cells seems to provide a mutual benefit for both sides during the humoral immune response. B cells capture antigens by their BCRs through endocytosis and present them to specific T cells by their surface MHC molecules. T cells activated by B cells also produce cytokines necessary for antibody production and B cell differentiation.[26]

## Dendritic cells (DCs)

DCs are professional APCs that efficiently sense and capture microbial antigens in innate immune responses and display them as peptides to T cells resulting in T cells activation leading to the development of adaptive immune responses and thus, linking two arms of immune response together. In comparison to monocytes/macrophages, these cells have lesser phagocytic capacity, but due to the expression of a wide range of innate immune response receptors, including toll-like receptors (TLRs), they recognize microbial molecules and become activated.[27] Following activation, these cells produce cytokines that recruit and activate innate cells at the infection sites. The innate immune response itself enhances the ability of DCs to migrate to and activate T cells during antigen presentation.[28]

DCs are recognized by having membranous projections and are divided into two main functional distinctive populations. Most DCs arise from bone marrow myeloid precursors and are commonly distributed in lymphoid tissues and mucosal epithelium. These DCs are called classical DCs and have the most potency in capturing protein antigens entered from epithelial barriers and stimulating strong T cell responses. A group of these populations is called Langerhans cells, which are located in the *epi*thelial layer of skin and sense microbial antigens entered through cutaneous barriers. Similarly, resident DCs are found in lymphoid and nonlymphoid tissues that sample antigens of their residence and potently exert CD4+ T cell responses.[29] The second group of DCs, Plasmacytoid DCs, are involved in innate anti-viral defense and production of type I interferon (IFN) in response to viruses. These cells develop from bone marrow precursors and normally are found in blood.[30] There is also a third population of DCs called follicular dendritic cells (FDCs). These cells are not derived from bone marrow precursors and do not present antigens to T cells. However, they are involved in B cell activation during the humoral immune response.[31]

## Lymphocytes

Based on differences in cell surface markers, there are four categories of lymphocytes, including T, B, NK (natural killer), and NKT (natural killer T) cells.[32] All lymphocytes differentiate from CLP cells in the bone marrow and are morphologically similar. B and T lymphocytes have a pivotal role in specific antigen recognition by expression of clonally distributed cell surface receptors with single specificity for each antigenic determinant. So, millions of clones of B and T cells can respond to their specific antigens using their unique BCRs (Ig receptor) and TCRs, respectively.[12]

B lymphocytes originate and become mature in the bone marrow. Follicular B cells, B-1 cells, and marginal zone B (MZB) cells are the main classes of B cells. Follicular B cells (B-2) have the most frequency and are found in the follicles of lymphoid organs and blood. They express a diverse set of Ig receptors and are differentiated to high affinity antibody-producing cells upon activation. B-2 cells differentiate into memory B cells after infection, which results in host protection against repeated exposure to the same antigen.[33] B-1 and MZB cells express less diverse Ig receptors and produce natural antibodies (mainly IgM) with limited diversity.[34]

T lymphocytes are divided into two main groups of helper (CD4+) and cytotoxic (CD8+) cells. TCRs expressed on lymphocytes are consisted of either $\alpha$ and $\beta$ chains ($\alpha\beta$ T cells) or $\gamma$ and $\delta$ chains ($\gamma\delta$ T cells). $\alpha\beta$ helper T cells mainly release cytokines upon antigen recognition and activation, which also help other cells such as other T cells, B cells, and macrophages in cellular and humoral immune responses while cytotoxic T cells mostly kill virus-infected cells and cancerous cells.[35] Regulatory T cells (Tregs) are the third group of CD4+ $\alpha\beta$ T cells, which are involved in immune response suppression.[36] Moreover, NKT cells, $\gamma\delta$ T cells, and mucosa-associated invariant T (MAIT) cells are a smaller group of T cells, which carry receptors with limited diversity. NKT cells exhibit both NK-like cytotoxicity and antigen-specific T-cell responsiveness.[37,38]

Lymphocytes are functionally inactive when they just become mature in generative lymphoid organs and are called naïve lymphocytes. After maturation, they migrate to secondary lymphoid tissues, where they first recognize their specific antigens and go through changes in phenotype and function. Subsequent to activation and proliferation, lymphocytes differentiate into effector cells, which eradicate antigens. Also, a small number of activated lymphocytes differentiate to memory cells, which then mediate rapid and enhanced responses in secondary exposures to specific antigens.[39]

NK cells originate from lymphoid precursors in the bone marrow and are categorized as effector cells of the innate immune response. NK cells do not express clonally distributed TCRs and are important in the early elimination of virus-infected and damaged cells. Therefore, they are known as counterparts for cytotoxic T lymphocytes (CTLs) in adaptive immune response.[40]

## Primary lymphoid organs

Primary lymphoid organs or generative lymphoid organs, including bone marrow and thymus, are the site of maturation of B cells and T cells, respectively. In fact, growth factors necessary for the early stages of lymphocyte development and also self-antigens required for selection and maturation of non-self-reactive lymphocytes are provided in primary lymphoid organs.[41]

B lymphocytes partially mature in the bone marrow and complete their final stages of maturation in the spleen, where they recognize specific antigens for the first time.[11] Bone marrow is also the main site of hematopoiesis-production of all blood cells after birth. As mentioned earlier, red blood cells, granulocytes, monocytes, DCs, mast cells, platelets, B and T lymphocytes, and innate lymphoid cells (ILCs) all originate from a common hematopoietic stem cell in the bone marrow.[10] Stromal cells and hematopoietic stem cells are located in specific niches in the bone marrow providing contact-dependent signals and growth factors required for hematopoiesis.[42] Hematopoietic stem cells are self-renewing cells that give rise to two multipotent precursors, CMP and CLP. CMP then generates mature red blood cells, platelets, granulocytes (neutrophils, eosinophils, and basophils), and the main part of DCs. CLP gives rise to T cells, B cells, and ILC lineages. The generation of blood cells from bone marrow precursors is stimulated by a group of cytokines called colony-stimulating factors (CSFs).[32]

Besides hematopoiesis, bone marrow is also populated by long-lived plasma cells, which are activated in secondary lymphoid tissues and migrate to bone marrow.[43]

T lymphocytes mature in the thymus and then enter the circulation and migrate to secondary lymphoid organs where they develop an immune response to their specific antigens.[44] The thymus is located in the anterior mediastinum and is the main site of T cells maturation from fetal developmental stages until puberty, and after that, the thymus undergoes hypertrophy. The thymus is a bilobed organ, each lobe is divided into multiple lobules by fibrous septa, and each lobule consists of a cortex and a medulla.[45] T cell precursors are called thymocytes and migrate to the thymus from bone marrow. Thymocytes start their maturation in the cortex and migrate toward the medulla as they mature. There are thymic cortical epithelial cells in the cortex, which secrete interleukin (IL)−7, a cytokine necessary for the early development of T cells. The medulla is less populated with thymocytes in comparison with the cortex. DCs, macrophages, and thymic medullary epithelial cells are found in the medulla and are crucial for the maturation and selection of non-self-reactive T cells that finally leave the thymus and migrate toward secondary lymphoid organs. A chromosomal deletion that causes failure of thymus development results in DeGeorge syndrome in patients, and these patients lack T cells. We will describe DeGeorge syndrome in detail later as a primary immunodeficiency.[46]

## Secondary lymphoid organs

Secondary lymphoid organs or peripheral lymphoid tissues, including the spleen, lymph nodes, and mucosal-associated lymphoid tissues (MALT), are the sites of recognition and initiation of the immune response toward foreign antigens. Furthermore, APCs, B cells, and T cells are located in the distinct anatomic location in secondary lymphoid tissues. Transportation of foreign antigens to these sites guarantees the generation and development of specific adaptive immune response.[47]

Lymph nodes are a part of the lymphatic system, which also includes lymphatic vessels that collect interstitial fluid or lymph (including invaded microbes in case of infections) from all vascularized tissues and discharge it into their draining lymph nodes. Lymph collected from all over the human body is finally released to a large lymphatic vessel called the thoracic duct. Lymph from the thoracic duct is discharged into the superior vena cava, thus returning the lymph to the blood.[48]

Lymph nodes are capsular tissues, which are located along lymphatic vessels throughout the body. Microbial antigens entered through epithelial surfaces are entered lymph nodes through afferent lymphatic vessels as a free form or captured by DCs. Each lymph node consists of a cortex and a medulla. B cells and FDCs mainly are located in the follicles in the cortex, whereas DCs and T cells mainly migrate to paracortical regions below follicles. This anatomic isolation of cells is mediated by the secretion of special cytokines called chemokines from lymph node stromal cells, which binds to their specific ligands on B and T cells and direct their migration. This anatomic segregation ensures B and T cells, which are located near their stimulating APCs, FDCs, and DCs, respectively.[49]

It is also important to note that lymphoid tissue-inducer cells (a type of ILCs) stimulate the development of secondary lymphoid tissues by secretion of cytokines known as lymphotoxins.[50]

Spleen is another capsular secondary lymphoid organ, which mainly functions as a site for initiation of the adaptive immune response against microbial antigens entered through blood. Spleen has an important role in the removal of aging and damaged blood cells, immune complexes, and opsonized microbes by splenic macrophages. Spleen is divided into red pulp and white pulp. Red pulp consists of blood-filled vascular sinusoids, and white pulp is a lymphocyte rich region with similar B cells and T cells anatomic segregation to lymph nodes. B cells are mainly located in follicles, whereas T cells reside in regions near artery branches called periarteriolar lymphoid sheaths (PALS). The space between red and white pulp is called marginal zone, which is a region of specialized cells (especially MZB cells) surrounding the marginal sinus.[51]

Besides lymph nodes and spleen, non-capsulated lymphoid structures are found in almost all epithelial barriers like skin, gastrointestinal mucosa, and bronchial mucosa. These skin-associated lymphoid tissues (SALT) and mucosa-associated lymphoid tissues (MALTs) respond to a variety of microbes entered through the skin and mucosal barriers. These tissues contain diffusely distributed innate and immune cells, which recognize and initiate adaptive immune responses toward pathogens while maintaining tolerance against a wide range of commensal microorganisms found in epithelial barriers.[52,53]

## Innate immunity

The innate immune system, as it can be inferred from its name, refers to immediate pre-existing defense mechanisms that combat microbes upon their invasion to host. It is the eldest and first line of defense against microbes. Activation of the innate immune response against microorganisms also provides signals necessary for activation of specific adaptive immune responses even if the innate immune response is not able to eradicate invaded microbes on its own. An important function of innate immunity is defending the body against pathogens at the epithelial barriers such as the skin and the gastrointestinal and respiratory tracts by maintaining the physical integrity of barriers and the production of antimicrobial peptides. Moreover, the innate immune response has an important role in tissue repair through the removal of damaged or dead cells mediated by macrophages.[54]

As mentioned, activation of the innate immune response itself can determine the nature of the adaptive immune response, since innate immune system components react differently to each microbe, which results in activation of the proper and optimum adaptive immune response against each microorganism. One of the protective procedures of innate immune response is inflammation, which results in leukocytes and soluble molecule infiltration to the original site of infection or injured tissues. Another key feature of innate immune reaction is antiviral defense, which leads to the elimination of virus-infected cells by the production of antiviral cytokines such as type I IFNs and activation of NK cells. The innate immune response includes different cell types and soluble molecules, which will be discussed briefly here.[55]

## Recognition of microbes in the context of innate immune system

Cells of the innate immune system recognize a limited set of molecular structures (in comparison with a broad diversity of antigens recognized by receptors of the adaptive immune system) that are expressed either by microbes or by damaged and dead host cells. These structures are called pathogen-associated molecular patterns (PAMPs) and damage-associated molecular patterns (DAMPs), respectively. Some examples of PAMPs include microbial nucleic acids such as viral double-stranded RNA, bacterial unmethylated CpG DNA sequences, and bacterial cell wall structures such as lipopolysaccharide (LPS) in gram-negative bacteria or lipoteichoic acid in gram-positive bacteria. Most

PAMPs are structures necessary for microbes' normal life cycles and normally are not expressed by mammalian cells.[56]

Various groups of molecules in the body are able to sense PAMPs and DAMPs, known as pattern recognition receptors (PRRs). These molecules can be categorized into two main groups: cell-associated molecules expressed on the cell membrane or in the cytosol and also soluble molecules, which are found in serum. Some important families of cell-associated PRRs include TLRs, NOD-like receptors (NLRs), and C-type lectin receptors (CLRs). Macrophages and DCs express a wide variety of these receptors, which help them to recognize and ingest microbes and damaged cells and also to initiate signaling cascades, which result in inflammatory response and production of antiviral cytokines.[57]

## Cellular component of innate immunity

Perhaps the most important cells of the innate immune system are located in epithelial barriers, which form physical and chemical defense mechanisms against environmental microbes. In fact, epithelial cells bind tightly together, making a continuous layer, which prevents microbe entrance at the skin and mucosal surfaces of the gastrointestinal, respiratory, and genitourinary tracts. In the skin, keratinocytes at the outer layer of the epidermis can block the passage of microbes from the surface. Production of mucin by mucosal epithelial cells interrupts by microbe colonization at mucosal tissues. Epithelial cells and some other leukocytes produce antimicrobial peptides such as defensins and cathelicidin, which are toxic for a broad range of microorganisms.[58,59]

Moreover, epithelium contains a special type of lymphocytes with limited diversity called intraepithelial lymphocytes (IELs). Although still main proportion of human T lymphocytes carries $\alpha\beta$ TCRs, the frequency of $\gamma\delta$ T lymphocytes is higher among IELs in comparison to other tissues. IELs have cytotoxic properties, and they can recognize a small group of microbial structures and also have the ability to produce cytokines and activate phagocytes.[60]

If microbes cross the epithelial barriers, then phagocytes such as neutrophils and macrophages are responsible for microbe ingestion and initiation of the inflammatory response.[61]

Furthermore, DCs express a broad range of PRRs, including different TLRs and cytoplasmic PRRs, which leads to efficient recognition of various PAMPs and DAMPs expressed by microbes. DCs become activated upon engagement of their recognizing receptors and produce cytokines that promote leukocyte infiltration to the infection site. These properties of DCs result in the activation of T cell response in a way that efficiently eliminates microbes. Indeed, the nature of microbe determines naïve T cell differentiation toward a distinct T helper (Th) subgroup, efficient in combating relative microbe type.[62]

Another group of innate immune system cells, which arise from common lymphoid precursor lineage, are called ILCs that lack clonally distributed TCRs but resemble lymphocytes. These cells are tissue residents of epithelial barriers that can play a substantial role in the early response against microbes that cross the barriers.[63] There are three different types of ILCs called ILC1, ILC2, and ILC3, which express transcription factors and produce cytokines similar to Th1, Th2, and Th17 CD4+ T cell subsets, respectively. These cells are activated by cytokines in the context of innate immune response and then produce distinct cytokines when become activated, and therefore, they can take part in different pathways of host defense against distinct types of pathogens. ILC1 cells produce IFN-γ and are important for defense against intracellular microbes. ILC2s produce IL-5, IL-9, and IL-13 and have a role in defense against helminthic parasites. Also, ILC2s may contribute to the development of allergic diseases. ILC3s produce IL-22 and/or IL-17 and participate in the defense against extracellular fungi and bacteria and also help in preserving the integrity of epithelial surfaces.[64]

NK cells are considered as type one ILCs, which produce IFN-γ and exert cytotoxic properties against cells infected with viruses, intracellular bacteria, and also cancerous cells. Human NK cells are mainly found in the blood, spleen, and liver. NK cells are considered as counterparts for CTLs in innate immunity so that they kill their target before activation of the adaptive immune response. Also, they have the ability to produce IFN-γ once become activated, which enhances the phagocytosis capacity of macrophages during the adaptive immune response. These cells can be recognized by surface CD56 and CD16 expression.[65] NK cells do not express clonally distributed receptors, whereas they express a range of germline-encoded activating and inhibiting receptors, which help NK cells distinguish between healthy cells versus infected cells. NK activating receptors include killer cell immunoglobulin-like receptors (KIRs), CD16, and NKG2D receptor, the latter recognizes ligands on infected cells such as MHC-like molecules expressed by virus-infected cells.[66] NK cells inhibiting receptors such as some KIR family receptors and NKG2A receptor recognize class I MHC molecules expressed by normal cells, so delivering inhibiting signals to NK cells that regulate their activation. While almost all nucleated cells express class I MHC molecules, virus-infected cells or malignant cells fail to produce and express these molecules on their surface, resulting in a lack of inhibiting receptor engagement by NK cells, and thus, activation of cytotoxic response through activating receptors. In fact, the consequence of signals delivered by activating and inhibiting receptors to NK cells determines the final fate of NK cell response. If NK cells become activated, they release granules containing perforin and granzymes similar to CTLs. Perforin becomes polymerized on the target cell surface, which results in making holes through that granzymes then enter and initiate a sequence of signaling events resulting in target cell apoptosis.[67]

## Humoral components of innate immunity

Besides the cellular component of innate immunity, there are soluble mediators, which exist in blood circulation and extracellular fluids and are important in innate host defense against pathogens that enter these sites. These soluble mediators, including complement system, pentraxins, collectins, and ficolins, are referred to as humoral components of innate immunity similar to antibodies and B cell response, which is mentioned as the humoral immune response in adaptive immunity.[68]

The complement system includes plasma proteins and also complement receptors and regulators on the immune system cell surface. Complement proteins activation is based on proteolytic cascades so that when one of the inactive complement system proteins becomes activated through enzymatic changes, cleaves and activates the next protein. This results in cascade activation and amplification in the number of proteins that are produced. Final products induce the effector function of the complement system, which includes target cell lysis, inflammation, and reinforcement of phagocytosis by the generation of opsonins.[69]

The complement system can be activated through classic, alternative, and lectin pathways. Classic pathway, as it can be inferred from its name, is the first discovered pathway and can be activated by antibodies bound to microbial surface. The initiator protein in this pathway is called C1q, which binds to the antibody-antigen complex and results in cascade activation of the complement system. As C1q can be activated by antibodies, the classic pathway is also considered an important effector mechanism of the humoral branch of adaptive immunity. When C1q binds to antigen-bound antibodies, two serine proteases C1 molecule complex called C1r, and C1s become activated and start the cleavage and activation of other complement proteins involved in proteolytic cascade activation.[70]

The alternative pathway is initiated by C3 complement protein cleavage and activation. In normal status, C3 is constitutively becomes activated in serum and binds to cell surfaces, but the presence of complement system regulators at the surface of host cells inhibits activation of the alternative pathway and prevents self-damage. On microbial surfaces, due to the lack of regulatory molecules, C3 can directly become activated and initiate the alternative pathway of complement system activation.[71]

The lectin pathway of the complement system is activated by binding a member of the collectin family called mannose-binding lectin (MBL) to mannose residues on microbial glycoproteins and glycolipids. MBL structurally is similar to the C1q component of the complement system. When MBL binds to microbes, two proteases called mannose-associated serine protease (MASP)1 and MASP2, which are similar to the C1r and C1s molecules in C1 component, become activated and start downstream proteolytic pathway similar to the classic pathway.[72]

Recognition of microbes by any of the three mentioned pathways results in the generation of an important complex called C3-convertase, which cleaves C3 to two molecules, C3a and C3b. C3b is the bigger component and binds to the microbial surface and other components of the complement system, which form C5-convertase. C5-convertase, as it can be inferred from its name, cleaves C5 to C5a and C5b. The bigger part, C5b, remains attached to the microbial surface and then binds to C6, C7,

C8, and C9, which form a complex molecule called membrane attack complex (MAC). MAC makes a hole in the cell membrane and results in cell lysis at the site of complement activation.[73]

C3b also serves as an opsonin and has a receptor on phagocytes, which in this way, promotes phagocytosis. Small components of complement proteins such as C3a and C5a are known as anaphylatoxin, which promotes inflammation by increasing the permeability of vessels, degranulation of mast cells, and also recruitment of leukocytes to the site of infection.[12]

Deficiencies in the complement system components cause different immunodeficiency diseases and syndromes. For example, lack of C3 results in higher susceptibility to bacterial infections. Also, deficiencies in MAC complex components increase the risk of special infections such as infection with Neisseria bacteria.[32]

There is another group of soluble molecules belonging to the pentraxin family, which can recognize different microbial structures and activate the complement system through binding to the C1q molecule. C reactive protein (CRP), Pentraxin3 (PTX3), and serum amyloid P (SAP) are members of the pentraxin family. Perhaps one of the most important proteins in this family is CRP, which is also known as an acute phase protein. CRP is very low in the plasma of healthy individuals, but during infections, it can be produced by hepatocytes (induced by pro-inflammatory cytokines such as IL-1 and IL-6), and its concentration can reach up to 1000-fold in patients' serum. PTX3 is also considered an acute phase protein, which is mainly produced by DCs and macrophages and is activated by TLR ligands or tumor necrosis factor (TNF) cytokine. PTX3 can recognize various microbial structures and activates the complement classic pathway.[74]

Collectin family of soluble molecules in the innate immunity include MBL and pulmonary surfactant proteins SP-A and SP-D. As mentioned earlier, MBL is structurally similar to the C1q molecule. MBL recognizes mannose and fucose carbohydrates on microbial surfaces and activates the complement system through the lectin pathway. SP-A and SP-D are among the surfactants, which are found in the alveoli of the lungs and reduce the surface tension of the alveolar fluid so that maintain the alveolar ability during respiratory expansion. In addition, SP-A and SP-D have an important role as innate immunity effector molecules, and they can bind to microbes and act as opsonins and therefore, they can facilitate phagocytosis by alveolar macrophages.[75]

## Major histocompatibility complex (MHC) and antigen presentation

T cells can only recognize antigens that are previously processed and presented on the surface of other cells, and they cannot recognize soluble antigens, unlike B cells, which are able to recognize soluble and extracellular antibodies.[76]

Antigens are presented on the surface of specialized proteins called MHC molecules to CD4+ and CD8+ T cells. There are two different types of these molecules, each specifically presents antigen to one particular T cell type, and this ability ensures the activation of the correct immune response against antigens. Some MHC molecules present the internalized antigens to T CD4+ cells, while others present antigens that are produced inside the cell to CD8+ T cells. In this section, we briefly describe the structure and function of these molecules and their critical role in the immune response.

T cells can mostly recognize short peptides that are displayed by MHC molecules, unlike B cells that are able to recognize protein and non-protein antigens without MHCs. T cells learn to recognize antigen only on the surface of MHCs during their maturation process, which ensures the MHC restriction of mature T cells. MHC molecules are highly polymorphic among different individuals, which can influence the T cell capability of recognizing different antigens. This is one of the reasons why people respond differently to a certain infection, while it recovers fast in one person, it can get severe in the other. There are two main classes of MHC molecules expressed on human cells. Class IMHC, which consists of A, B, and C molecules, are expressed on all nucleated cells of humans, while class II molecules, which consist of DR, DP, and DQ subgroups, are only expressed by APCs.

The process of displaying antigen by MHC to T cells is called antigen presentation and the professional cells having this function are APCs.[77] Different cell types in humans, such as DCs, macrophages, and B cells, have APC functions, while DCs are considered the most specialized APCs. We should also know that professional APCs are the cells that constitutively express MHC molecules, but there are some cell types such as vascular endothelial and epithelial cells that MHC expression is inducible on them under specific circumstances. Please note that when we use the term APCs, we mostly mean the cells that express MHC class II

All human nucleated cells express MHC I. Therefore, there is no need for such a term when we talk about MHC I. This means that all nucleated cells are able to present peptides to CD8+ T cells. Here, by peptides, we mostly mean virus and tumoral peptides, which can infect or occur in every nucleated cell, and they can be presented to CD8+ cytotoxic cells to eliminate them.

## The phenomenon of MHC restriction

As mentioned before, T cells can only recognize an antigenic peptide, which is presented in the cleft of the MHC molecule. The TCR recognizes both the peptide and MHC molecule that presents the peptide. During the T cell maturation process, T cells are educated to recognize antigens in form of a complex with self MHC molecules.[78]

## MHC structure

In humans, the MHC genes are located in a large segment of DNA (about 3500 kgbases) on the short arm of chromosome 6. The set of MHC alleles, which is located on each chromosome, is called an MHC haplotype.[79]

MHCs are among molecules known as Ig superfamily, which means they have an Ig-like structure. In MHC class I, only one polypeptide chain, and in MHC class II, both polypeptide chains are Ig-like, each of which consists of an extracellular, a transmembrane, and an intracellular domain. The extracellular domain contains the peptide-binding cleft (or MHC groove), where antigenic peptides can bind. Therefore, the cleft of MHC is highly polymorphic.

### *MHC I structure*

MHC I consists of one Ig-like polymorphic α-chain plus non-polymorphic β2-microglobulin, which is not encoded by the MHC genes. These two chains are linked noncovalently. α-chain consists of 3 domains (α1, α2, and α3) (Fig. 1.2), where the MHC groove is formed by α1 and α2 domains and binds to small peptides of 8–11 amino acids. The MHC groove is closed in MHCI, and therefore, it cannot accommodate larger peptides. We will later explain the processing procedure that converts proteins to small peptides, which are suitable for the MHC groove. α1 and α2 domains are polymorphic to be able to bind to antigenic peptides, whereas the α3 domain has a conserved and non-polymorphic amino acid sequence and it contains the CD8 binding site. A complete MHC I molecule contains α chain, β2-microglobulin, and antigenic peptide, and this trimeric complex is stable to express on the cell surface.[80] Each heterozygous individual expresses six different MHC class I molecules, two inherited alleles from *HLA-A*, *B*, and *C*.

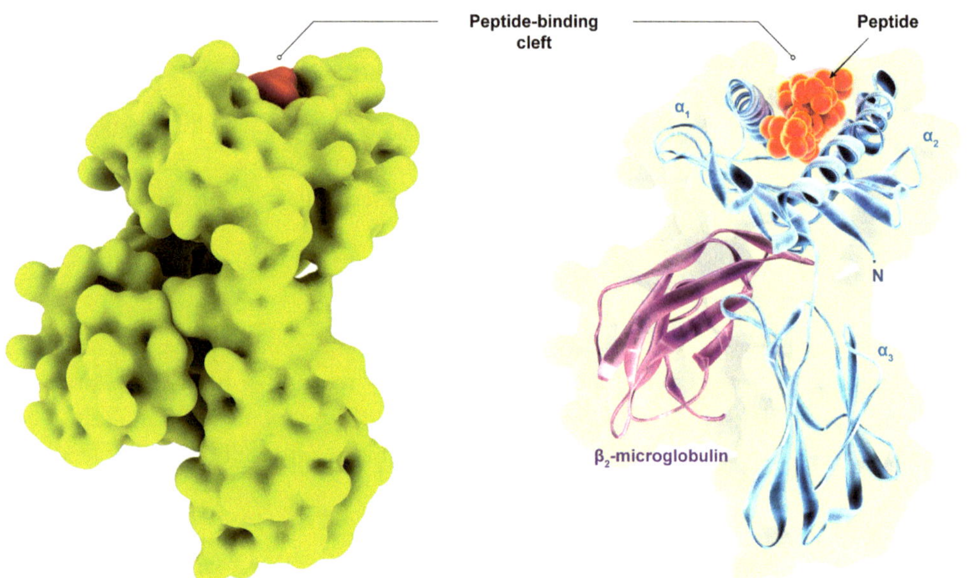


**Fig. 1.2** ***Structure of MHC class I molecule.*** Consisted of a polymorphic α chain and nonpolymorphic β2-microglobulin (β2m), noncovalently attached together.

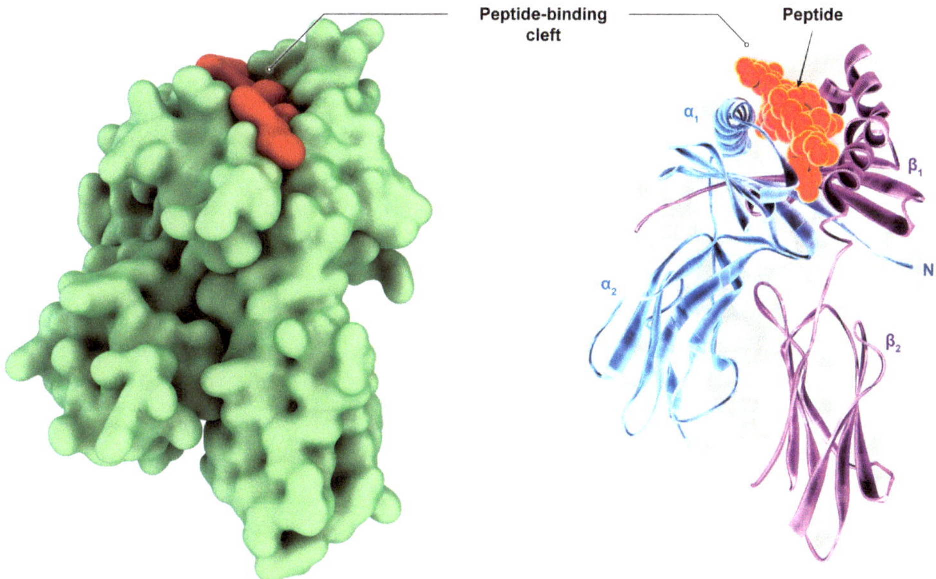


**Fig. 1.3** ***Structure of MHC class II molecule.*** Consisted of a polymorphic α chain and a polymorphic β chain, noncovalently attached together.

### *MHC II structure*

MHC II consists of two Ig-like polymorphic (α and β) chains, which are noncovalently bonded (Fig. 1.3).[81] The groove of MHC II is formed by α1 and β1 domains and binds to peptides of up to 30 amino acids (optimally 12–16 residues) as it has open ends. α1 and β1 domains are polymorphic, with a higher polymorphism in the β chain. Both α2 and β2 domains have conserved and non-polymorphic amino acid sequences and contribute to binding to CD4. Similar to what was mentioned in MHCI, here also a complete MHC II molecular structure contains α and β chains plus antigenic peptide, which is stable to be expressed on the cell surface. Each heterozygous individual expresses six to eight different MHC class II molecules, two inherited alleles from *HLA-DQ*, *DP*, and two or four alleles of *HLA-DR*

It is important to know that each MHC I or II molecule can bind to many different peptides (both self and foreign), and that is how few MHC molecules of each individual can present an enormous number of antigenic peptides. To increase the chance of interaction with the specific T cells, the MHC-peptide complexes have a long half-life, which means they can stay on the cell surface for days. Not all MHC-peptides of the cell surface should bear the same peptide to be able to activate specific T cells, and a fraction of them (about 100 similar complexes) are enough to do so.

## MHC presentation

Most of the proteins are bigger than being able to fit on the MHC cleft. Therefore, during the process of antigen processing, they cleaved with proteases upon internalization. Later on, the cleaved peptides are loaded on the MHC molecules and move to the cell surface to be displayed to T cells.

Cytosolic proteins are displayed on the surface of MHCI, while extracellular proteins are presented on MHC II molecules after internalization.

### *MHC I processing and presentation pathway*

Viral proteins, which are synthesized in the infected cell and any bacterial protein that is inserted or transported to the cell cytosol, can enter MHC I pathway (Fig. 1.4).[82] Other proteins such as endosomal proteins that escaped from the endosome, tumoral proteins, and endoplasmic reticulum (ER) misfolded proteins are other sources of antigenic peptides of the MHC I pathway. All such proteins degrade in the proteasome and are recognized by CD8+ T cells.

Proteases are protease complexes in the cytosol in a cylindrical shape with two inner β rings and two α rings on the sides. Each of the rings contains seven subunits where three of them are catalytic sites. Proteasome recognize their target protein by a flag, which is a chain of a small peptide called ubiquitin. Proteasomes can cleave the ubiquitinated proteins into short peptides, which can be later on transferred to ER by a specific transporter. IFN-γ can enhance proteasome activity, and therefore, promote the MHC I presentation process.[83] There is a specialized transporter in the ER membrane called transporter associated with antigen processing (TAP), which transports the cleaved products of the proteasome to ER in an adenosine triphosphate (ATP) manner. In the lumen

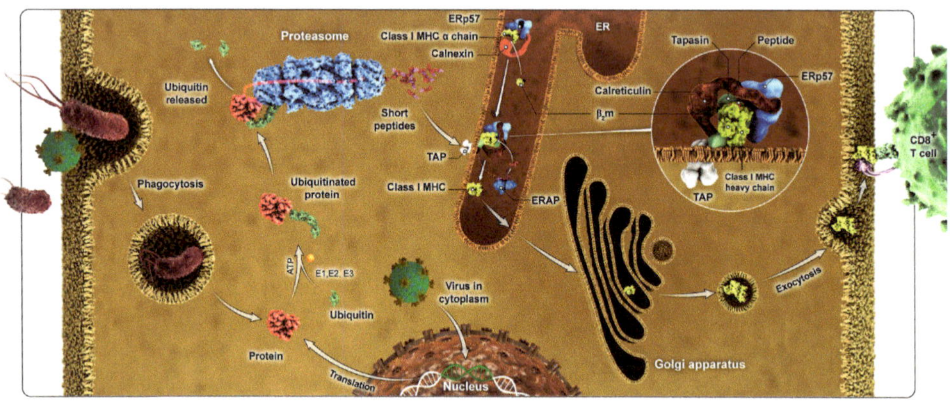


**Fig. 1.4** ***MHC class I antigen processing and presentation.*** The pathway is explained in the text. Proteasome proteolysis antigenic proteins in the cytosol, then they enter the ER via TAP and land on the MHCI groove. ER, endoplasmic reticulum; ERAP, Endoplasmic reticulum-associated peptidase; β2m, β2-microglobulin; TAP, transporter associated with antigen processing; Ub, ubiquitin.

of ER, TAP is associated with tapasin, an MHC chaperon molecule. Thus, the peptides can bind to empty and freshly synthesized MHC I molecules in ER. If the antigenic peptide in the ER does not have a proper size, ER-resident aminopeptidase (ERAP) trims it in the ER. When MHC I is loaded with a peptide, it can exit the ER and be expressed to the cell surface through ER-Golgi-exocytic vesicles. The cleft of MHC II molecules is blocked by a protein called invariant chain ($I_i$) in the ER. Therefore, mentioned antigenic peptides cannot assemble to MHCII

### *MHC II processing and presentation pathway*

Extracellular proteins that internalize the cell by phagocytosis, endocytosis, or pinocytosis by an APC enter the MHC II pathway (Fig. 1.5).[84] In fact, these proteins are cleaved by lysosomal proteases such as cathepsins in the late endosome, following the fusion of lysosomes to endosomes. In addition to extracellular proteins, every endocytosed protein that enters this pathway can be either a cell surface protein or a cytosolic protein taken up by autophagy. Each APC cell type expresses specific receptors to internalize antigens, such as Fc receptors and complement receptors on DCs and macrophages, and surface Ig receptors on B cells.[85]

The α and β chains of the MHC class II molecule are synthesized in ER and assembled by ER chaperones such as calnexin. As mentioned earlier, $I_i$ blocks the cleft of MHCII, and this trimeric protein can attach to three MHC II molecules at the same time. Additionally, $I_i$ directs MHC II molecules to the late endosome and lysosome, where they can find suitable antigenic peptides to present. In the late endosomes, $I_i$ is degraded by proteases, and only a small part of it remains in the MHC cleft, which is called class II-associated $I_i$ peptide (CLIP). The replacement of CLIP with

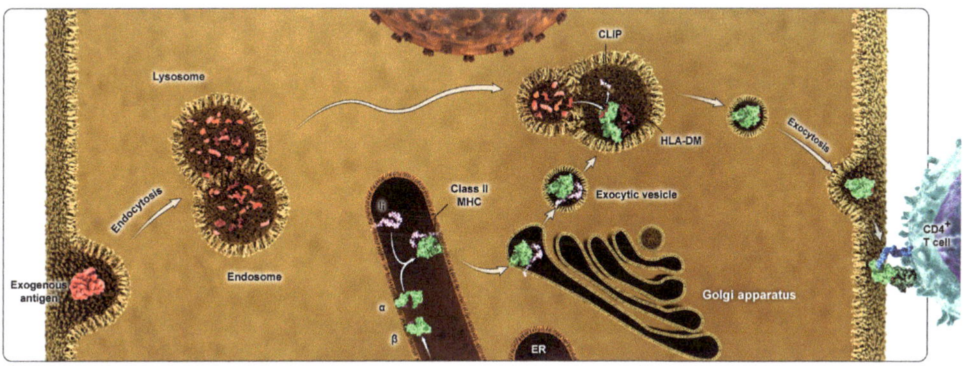


**Fig. 1.5** ***MHC class II antigen processing and presentation.*** The pathway is explained in the text. The endosome containing the antigenic protein first fuses to the lysosome and then to the MHC II containing vesicles, and finally, the antigenic peptide lands on the MHC groove. CLIP, class II-associated invariant chain peptide; ER, endoplasmic reticulum; Ii, invariant chain.

antigenic peptide occurs with the help of HLA-DM, a structurally similar molecule to MHCIIHLA-DM is encoded by *MHC* genes, although it is not polymorphic as MHC molecules. HLA-DM functions in exchanging CLIP with antigenic peptides, preferentially the ones that have a high affinity for MHC II. The MHC II cleft is open. Therefore, larger peptides can attach to it and trim further by the endosome proteases to reach the optimum size of 10–30 amino acids.

Once MHC-peptide complexes are stable, their containing vesicles fuse to the cell membrane, and they will be expressed on the cell surface, being recognizable by T cells.

## Cross-presentation

This is a process when an antigenic peptide enters the cell cytosol from endosomes and presents to the CD8+ T cells. Normally, extracellular antigens are expressed on MHCII, as mentioned in the previous section, but some cells such as DCs have the ability to present such antigens on MHC I to CD8+ cells. This process is called cross-presentation. For instance, DCs can uptake a tumor cell or a virus-infected cell and present another cell's antigen to CD8+ T cells. This process is required to initiate an effective immune response by a professional APC against viral and tumor antigens.[86]

The MHC processing and presentation pathway is adapted to the type of response, which is needed for different antigens. CD4+ T cells activate following the MHC II pathway and increase the phagocytosis capacity of macrophages and provide help for B cells to produce antibodies, both of which are required for an immune response to extracellular antigens. CD8+ T cells activate following MHC I pathway and kill the virus-infected or tumor cells.

As described earlier, MHC genes are polymorphic, and each individual has a different set of these molecules. Therefore, people respond differently to a specific antigen, and this is based on how well their MHC molecules can bind and present this particular antigen. This also shows why people are responding differently to vaccines and why they are allergic to different things. Also, having different MHC molecules on the cells is a confining factor for organ transplantation between humans.

Most of what we mentioned in this season was about protein antigens. We should also mention here the term, Immunodominant epitope, which is an epitope from a protein antigen that can better bind, and therefore, better present to T cells and consequently can stimulate a stronger immune response.

Glycolipid antigens can be presented by CD1, a non-classic MHC molecule, and this complex is recognized by NKT cells. NKT cells are a type of NK cells that also express TCRs with very limited diversity.

Most of T cells in humans express a TCR molecule, which is consisted of one $\alpha$ and one $\beta$ chain (will be discussed later), but there is also a small population of T cells with a $\gamma\delta$ TCR chains. These cells are called $\gamma\delta$ T cells, and they are not MHC-restricted, unlike αβ T cells. These cells are able to recognize not only protein antigens but also lipids, phosphorylated molecules, and alkylamines.

## B lymphocytes

As mentioned at the beginning of this chapter, B lymphocytes are major cells of the adaptive immune system. They are antibody-producing cells, which highlights their major role in the humoral immune system as well. Here we begin the section with B cell development and the structure and formation of BCRs, and then we continue with how these cells get activated, and we will end the section with the function of these cells.

## B lymphocyte development

The first place for B cell development is the fetal liver, and the development takes place in the bone marrow after birth. In the bone marrow, B cells develop from their precursors to the immature state. This consists of pro B to pre B and then Pre B to immature B cell transformation. We will briefly explain the process in this section. Ig rearrangement starts at the early stages of B cell development in bone marrow, which is triggered by the expression of recombination activating gene 1 and 2 (Rag1/Rag2 ) recombinases. Pre B cells are the first cells to express a pre-BCR, which has the rearranged heavy chain of Ig and the surrogate light chain. Immature B cells express the full rearranged membrane-bound Igs (i.e., BCR) before they exit bone marrow. The final differentiation steps of immature B to mature B cells occurs majorly in the spleen. Finally, mature B cells home in follicles of secondary lymphoid organs and wait there to meet their specific antigen.

As mentioned, Ig rearrangement is an important checkpoint in the developmental steps of B cells, and it ensures the diversity of Ig repertoire. To have a better understanding of Ig rearrangement events, we should briefly explain the structure and encoding genes of Ig molecules. A human antibody molecule consists of two heavy and two light chains. There are four different types of the heavy chain (μ in IgM, γ in IgG, α in IgA, and ε in IgE), each of which, including one variable ($V_H$) and several constant ($C_H1$, $C_H2$, $C_H3$, …) domains encoding by *IgH* gene loci on chromosome 14. There are two different types of Ig light chains (κ and λ), which are consisted of one variable and one constant domain structurally similar to the heavy chains. κ gene is on chromosome 2, while λ is on chromosome 22. κ to λ usage ratio is 2 to 1. Therefore, most Ig molecules contain a κ light chain in humans.

*IgH* genes are segmented and contain several variable (V), diversity (D), and joining (J) segments, while *Ig*κ and *Ig*λ genes contain only V and J segments. During the arrangement process, one of each V, D (if exists), and J segments will be randomly selected and linked together to build the variable domain of Ig chains. This process is called V(D)J recombination, and the responsible enzymes are called V(D)J recombinases or Rag-1/Rag-2. *RAG* genes are expressed only during the development of B and T lymphocytes, and mutations in these genes cause severe combined immunodeficiency (SCID) with a lack of B and T cells. Artemis is another enzyme involved in V(D)J recombination, and mutations in Artemis cause SCID, as well. The diversity of Ig and TCR is not only the result of a random combination of the gene segments but also the consequence of junctional diversity. Junctional diversity includes the deletion or addition of nucleotides in the junction of gene segments with the help of enzymes such as Artemis and terminal deoxynucleotidyl transferase (TdT) to add P and N nucleotide in the junctions. It should be mentioned that the diversity mechanisms result in 107 different clones of Ig and TCR in humans, and also, they lead to many nonfunctional receptors that will be deleted later during the selection processes.[87,88]

Ig recombination starts at the pro B stage, where Rag1/Rag2 and TdT enzymes are expressed, and the VDJ rearrangement of the IgH chain takes place. After VDJ rearrangement and the forming of variable domain, a Cμ (constant region of μ heavy chain) segment attaches to VDJ, and a full messenger ribonucleic acid (mRNA) of the heavy chain will be translated to protein. Allelic exclusion is a phenomenon that allows only one of the two inherited alleles to encode the heavy chain in each B cell clone, and this leads to an identical heavy chain in all cells of a clone. Expression of μ heavy chain turns the pro B to pre B cell stage, and these cells express preliminary BCRs on their surface, including the heavy chain plus two other proteins called surrogate of light chain, λ5, and V pre B. These two are non-variable and have a similar structure to Ig light chain. The expression of pre BCR is considered as a checkpoint in B cell development.[89] A protein tyrosine kinase called Bruton's tyrosine kinase (Btk) is activated downstream of pre BCR, and its following signals lead to pre B cells survival, proliferation and certification to transform to the later stages. Mutations in the *BTK* gene cause X-linked agammaglobulinemia (XLA) and B cell maturation failure in humans. Pre BCR signals also trigger the VJ rearrangement of the Igκ light chain in a similar way to the heavy chain. The rearrangement always starts from the κ chain, and it goes to the λ chain only if it was not successful. This phenomenon is called light chain isotype exclusion. As a result of this phenomenon, each clone of B cells can only express the κ or λ light chain.

When B cells express a full IgM on their surface, they transform into immature B cells. A successful rearrangement, therefore, is considered as the license for the positive selection of immature B cells. Only under these circumstances, immature B cells receive survival signals from the BCR tonic signaling. self-reactive immature B cells that strongly recognize a self-peptide in the bone marrow get another chance to change the specificity of their receptor in a process called receptor editing.[90] Rag1/Rag2 can be transiently expressed in this stage once more, and the autoreactive immature B cells can perform another round of Ig light chain rearrangement to change the specificity of the B cell clone and save it from deletion. If receptor editing will not be successful, the clone will negatively select and die by apoptosis.

## B cell subsets

Most B cells are derived from bone marrow and are called B-2 cells. After exiting the bone marrow, they become transitional B cells till they move to the spleen. In the spleen, they can develop into either MZB cells or follicular B cells. B-1 cells are another subset of B cells that develop from the fetal liver. The majority of B cells are follicular B cells that express surface IgM and IgD with the same antigen specificity (i.e., identical variable section and different constant region). Therefore, Mature recirculating B cells are IgM+ and IgD+, and they receive survival signals through the BCR tonic signaling while they are naïve. Additionally, the B cell-activating factor of the TNF family (BAFF) cytokine, through its ligand APRIL, provides further survival and maturation signals for B cells. Naïve B cells recirculate from lymph node to blood and back to find their specific antigens. Otherwise, they die after a few months.

MZB cells were primarily found in the marginal sinus of the spleen, but they exist in human lymph nodes, as well. They only express IgM (not IgD) BCRs with a limited diversity plus a high level of CD21. B1 cells differentiate into short-lived IgM-producing plasma cells in response to blood-borne microbes.[91]

B1 cells develop from the fetal liver and have very limited diversity compared to follicular B cells, and in mice, they express CD5.[92] They respond to common microbial polysaccharide and lipid antigens and secrete IgM in response to them. It is believed that the antibodies against ABO blood group antigens are also produced by B1 cells.

## B cell activation

Mature naïve B cells home to secondary lymphoid organs to find and recognize their specific antigen through their BCR. As we mentioned before, B cells can recognize intact (not processed) antigens via different routes in lymph nodes. B cells respond to protein antigens in a T cell-dependent manner, and they can also respond to polysaccharide antigens independently. BCR complex (membrane Ig plus Igα and Igβ proteins) functions in antigen recognition and the following signal transduction. Complement receptor 2 or CD21 expresses on the surface of follicular B cells and MZB cells and plays as a co-receptor to facilitate B cell activation. The ligand of complement receptor 2 is the C3d fragment of complement that attaches to the microbial antigens following complement activation. TLRs can also enhance B cell activation by recognizing their ligands on microbial antigens. Human B cells express TLR-5, 7, and 9.

Myeloid cells such as DCs and macrophages can also enhance B cell response to antigens by capturing and carrying antigens to the lymphatic follicles, where B cells are. Myeloid cells promote B cell activation by producing cytokines such as BAFF and indirectly through activation of Th cells.

B cells require BCR cross-linking to initiate the response. T cell-independent antigens such as polysaccharides easily cross-link BCRs because they are usually multivalent.

Protein antigens, however, are not multivalent, and B cells require the help of T cells to respond effectively to these antigens.

Both naïve T and naïve B cells encounter the protein antigen in the T cell zone and follicle of lymph nodes, respectively. As mentioned before, DCs process and present the antigen on the surface of MHC molecules to T cells. The same antigen can be recognized by naïve B cells without processing and presentation. When both T and B are activated, they move toward the follicle edge to meet each other, and this happens by changes in the expression of chemokine receptors. Upon activation, T cells downregulate C—C chemokine receptor (CCR)7 and upregulate C-X-C chemokine receptor (CXCR)5, which is a receptor for chemokine (C-X-C motif) ligand (CXCL)13 and is highly expressed in follicles. B cells, on the other hand, downregulate CXCR5 and upregulate CCR7, which allows them to move toward the T cell zone, where there is a high level of CCL19 and CCL21. In this interaction, B cells can again present the antigen to T cells and receive T cell help instead and differentiate into antibody-producing plasma cells. T cells express CD40 ligand (CD40L) (CD154) upon activation, which interacts with CD40 on the B cells and stimulates B cells proliferation and differentiation into plasma cells through activation of nuclear factor kappa B (NF-κB) and activator protein-1 (AP-1) transcription factors. Mutations in the *CD40L* gene result in defective antibody production (isotype switching and affinity maturation) and a disease called X-linked hyper IgM syndrome (XHIGM).

The germinal center is a very important location, where critical events take place for the production of long-lived plasma cells, high affinity antibodies, and memory B cells. Germinal center forms in lymphoid follicles about 4 to 7 days after T-B interaction. Activated B cells start to proliferate in the dark zone of the germinal center, and they are called centroblasts in this step. Later, they turn into centrocytes in the light zone of the germinal center, where they interact with T follicular helper (Tfh) cells and FDCs. after T-B interaction, some of the activated T cells turn into Tfh cells with high expression of CXCR5, programmed cell death protein (PD)−1, inducible co-stimulator (ICOS), and IL-21.[93] FDCs have an important role in the selection of B cells in germinal center reactions. These cells express Fc receptors and complement receptors, which capture and display antigens. They are not APCs, but they just hold the antigens to select B cells with high affinity BCRs (Ig). These B cells that express high affinity Igs for the antigens will survive and differentiate into plasma cells. Plasma cells leave the germinal center and home in the bone marrow, and memory B cells recirculate. B cells undergo somatic hypermutation of Ig variable genes in the germinal center. This happens by point mutations in the regions called complementarity-determining regions (CDRs), and the enzyme activation-induced deaminase (AID) plays a role in this process. AID changes some of the C nucleotides to U and U changes to T in replication or will be excised by another enzyme called Uracil N-glycosylase (UNG), and later the error-prone DNA repair enzymes can substitute the U with any nucleotide. As a result of somatic hypermutation, the Ig V segment changes, and later, the B cells, which produce the highest affinity antibodies, will selectively survive in the lymphoid follicle. This phenomenon is called affinity maturation, and CD40-CD40L interaction together with FDCs are essential for it.[94]

As mentioned above, B cells have IgM and IgD receptors, but later in their differentiation process, they can produce other classes of antibodies such as IgG, IgA, and IgE. This happens by changing the constant region of Ig in response to different cytokines, and it is called isotype switching. Class switching is generally dependent on the nature of the antigen, which the antibody is producing against. For many bacteria and viruses, the primary IgM will be switched to IgG in the immune response, and this is stimulated by IFN-$\gamma$. Igs can switch to IgE in response to helminths and Th2 type cytokines. When the antibody is needed in the mucosal areas, it switches to IgA, and transforming growth factor (TGF)-$\beta$, BAFF, and APRIL stimulate this transformation. Again CD40-CD40L interaction is essential for isotype switching because the signaling through this interaction results in the expression of AID in B cells and the subsequent so-called switch recombination. Switch regions are specific GC-rich nucleotide sequences that locate in the intron between J and C segments, i.e., before every C region, and they can be recognized by AID. The result of this process is the replacement of the C$\mu$ region with any other constant region with the VDJ segment remaining unchanged on the DNA level. Isotype switching makes B cells more efficient responders by having the appropriate class of antibodies.[94]

## Plasma cell differentiation

Once the B cells get activated, they either transform to plasma cells or memory B cells in the germinal center.[95] To become a plasma cell, B cells must undergo structural changes required to be an antibody-producing factory. For example, they grow in size and develop their secretory system (ER) in addition to no longer expressing surface Ig as a result of transforming the Ig molecule to the secretory form. Plasma cells can be short or long-lived. Short-lived plasma cells are generally developed in response to T cell-independent antigens such as polysaccharides. These cells are also developing in the early stages of T cell-dependent response, but the major type of plasma cells in response to protein antigens are long-lived plasma cells. They survive by receiving signals through their receptor BCMA, which is another ligand for BAFF. These cells are then later home in the bone marrow and produce the specific Igs for years.

Non-protein antigens like polysaccharides can also elicit antibody response and differentiation of plasma cells, which generally produce low affinity antibodies with no or very limited isotype switching to IgG and IgA. As mentioned before, these are mostly B1 cells and MZB cells.

## Memory B cell

Memory cell formation is a critical characteristic of the immune system, and it is required to defend the same pathogen faster and more efficiently in a second encounter.

Memory B cells are formed during the germinal center events, where they express antiapoptotic protein such as B-cell lymphoma protein (BCL)−2 that allows them to live for a long time. They normally recirculate between blood and lymphoid organs. Successful vaccines are the ones that can trigger the differentiation of memory cells.[96]

## Effector functions of antibodies

In addition to different classes of antibodies, some antibodies like IgG and IgA have a few subclasses that are slightly different in their structure and also in their function. In humans, IgG has 4 subclasses of IgG1 to IgG4, and IgA has IgA1 and IgA2 subclasses. Several cells of the immune system express Fc receptors, which enable them to capture immune complexes.

Neutralization: One of the main functions of antibodies is to recognize the microbial antigen or toxin and neutralize them in order to prevent them from binding or entering the host cells and causing infection. This is the function of the variable segment of antibodies. IgG is mainly neutralizing the antigens in the blood, while IgA does this function on mucosal surfaces.[97,98]

Opsonization and phagocytosis: Some classes of antibodies (mostly IgG1 and IgG3) recognize the antigen through the variable segment and facilitate phagocytosis of antigen through Fc-Fc receptor interaction on phagocytic cells. When antibody molecules cover an antigen, this is called opsonization. Macrophages and neutrophils will recognize the opsonized antigen, and they ingest and kill it intracellularly. Some complement system products such as C3b can also opsonize and facilitate the uptake of antigens.[99]

Antibody-dependent cell-mediated cytotoxicity (ADCC): This is another important function of antibodies. NK cells express the Fc receptor for IgG, and they can recognize antibody-coated cells, which results in NK cell degranulation and killing of the target cells.

IgG antibodies can pass through the placenta to the fetus. Therefore, maternal antibodies are the major defense mechanism of neonates. Other classes of antibodies like IgM and IgG1, IgG2, and IgG3 have the ability to activate the so-called classic pathway of the complement system.

Mast cells and eosinophils express Fc receptor for IgE and it can trigger mast cell degranulation and eosinophil mediated defense against helminths. IgA antibodies are crucial for mucosal immunity. IgA antibodies are secreted to the lumen of respiratory and GI tracts and neutralize the microbial antigens in the first encounter location.

## T lymphocytes

T cells are one of the two major players of the adaptive immune system. They are the drivers of cell-mediated immunity, and their help is also essential for antibody production against protein antigens.[100] Antibodies can only neutralize or opsonize the extracellular antigens, and therefore, are accessible. There are plenty of other antigens that can survive in the cells, and they are considered intracellular pathogens, and T cells can eliminate the infected or tumoral cells.

T cells have two different classes based on their surface markers, CD4+ and CD8+ T cells, with CD4+ T cells being twice more frequent than CD8+ T cells in humans. CD4+ T cells are mainly helping B cells in addition to producing phagocytosis stimulating cytokines, while CD8+ T cells have the major role in defense against intracellular and tumoral antigens.[101]

## T cell development

T cell development is partially similar to B cells, which means they first develop in the fetal liver, and the precursors are moved to the bone marrow after birth. The maturation of T cells takes place in the thymus, which is a specialized primary lymphoid organ for this process. The thymus shrinks by age, and this results in decreased thymic output with aging. The multipotent progenitors of T cells home to the outer cortex of the thymus, and they are called thymocytes.[102] This migration is led by chemokines and chemokine receptors. Progenitors of T cells express CCR9, while the thymic cortex has a high concentration of CCL25, the ligand for CCR9. T cells acquire αβ or γδ TCR in the cortex, and the αβ TCR+ cells further acquire CD4+ and CD8+ on their way to thymus medulla. Again, the movement of thymocytes from cortex to medulla is according to the chemokine gradient. High levels of CCL19 and CCL21 are expressed in the thymic medulla, while T cells express CCR7, which is the receptor for CCL19 and CCL21. T cells become either CD4+ or CD8+ after exiting the thymus, and they follow the gradient of sphingosine 1 phosphate to the blood while they express the sphingosine 1 phosphate receptor.

TCR rearrangement in T cell development starts with γδ TCR, and it continues later with rearrangement of αβ TCR. The expression of CD4 and CD8 markers on T cells are also considered as a checkpoint for T cell development. All thymocytes are double negative for CD4 and CD8 markers upon their arrival to the thymus, and they are considered pro T cells. Rag1 and Rag2 are expressed in this stage to initiate TCR rearrangement within the TCR β gene segment. Similar to the rearrangement steps in B cells, initially, a Dβ segment attaches to Jβ, and later the Vβ segment connects to DJβ, and finally, the constant segment completes the TCR β gene for transcription. Only the cells that successfully rearrange and express the β chain are allowed to continue the further developmental process. When thymocytes express so-called pre-TCR, which consists of TCR β chain plus pre-Tα, they are known as pre T cells. It should be mentioned that the pre TCR expresses as a complex together with CD3 and ζ proteins. The signals mediated by pre-TCR result in proliferation and survival of pre T cells, and they trigger further rearrangement of TCR α genes. These signals also lead to allelic exclusion in TCR β genes. Pre T cells change their surface markers, and they change to double-positive thymocytes for CD4 and CD8 markers. They express αβ TCR for the first time and undergo positive selection at the double-positive stage. TCR α chain lacks D segments and has no allelic exclusion, which allows both alleles to rearrange. Therefore, T cells can express two α chains with a similar β chain. Positive selection ensures the survival of the T cells that can recognize antigenic peptides in the groove of self MHC molecules. Otherwise, the T cell will die in the thymus and will not be able to continue the maturation process.

The final step of T cell maturation is the lineage-fate decision and becoming single positive for either CD4 and CD8 surface markers and enter the thymus medulla and later leave there to secondary lymphoid organs.[103] CD4+ T cells are able to recognize antigen in self MHCII, while CD8+ T cells recognize it in self MHC I. Negative selection is happening in the single positive stage, which ensures the elimination of the T cell clones with high affinity against self-peptides (self-reactive). They either die by apoptosis or differentiate to Tregs to minimize self-reactivity of T cells as a mechanism of central tolerance. We will discuss the tolerance mechanisms later in this chapter. The APCs in the thymus (i.e., thymic epithelial cells) express self-proteins that are widely expressed in human tissues. Additionally, they express autoimmune regulator (AIRE), which is a nuclear protein inducing the expression of tissue-specific antigens in the thymus. Mutation in *AIRE* results in autoimmune polyendocrine syndrome.

The differentiation of γδ T cells happens prior to αβ T cells as mentioned before. In other words, if the rearrangement of γ and δ gene segments is taking place successfully before β chain rearrangement (in 10 percent of the time), the cell will differentiate to the γδ T cell. γδ T cells have less diversity compared to αβ T cells.[104]

## T cell activation

Naïve T cells get activated in the secondary lymphoid organs by APCs, mainly DCs, the professional and most potent APC for naïve T cell activation. DCs are located in the T cell zone of lymph nodes, and they present many antigens at the same time. When T cells recognize their specific antigen, they become activated, proliferate, produce cytokine, and differentiate to effector or memory T cells. After activation, T cells can perform their effector functions in the peripheral tissues (discussed later). According to the nature and location of antigen, DCs can either present the antigen on MHC I and activate naïve CD8+ T cells or present on MHC II and activate naïve CD4+ T cells. Other APCs such as B cells and macrophages can present the antigen to activated T cells. The first signal for the activation of T cells is always the antigen itself. T cells not only recognize peptide-MHC but also have other surface receptors and co-receptors that participate in this interaction.[105] The second signal, which is required for full activation of T cells, is provided by co-stimulatory molecules on APCs. B7-1 (CD80) and B7-2 (CD86) are the most famous co-stimulators on activated APCs, and they interact with CD28 on T cells to provide the second signal.[106] B7 is not expressed, or very lowly expressed on resting APCs, and only after stimulation by microbial antigens, it upregulates. Activated CD4+ T cells can also induce the expression of B7 on APCs via CD40-CD40L interaction. The expression of CD40L increases upon T cell activation, which is important for T cell effector functions. The stimulation of T cells with self-antigens is generally happening by the low level of B7-CD28 signal, which is more regulatory rather than activating, and it is important for the maintenance of T cell tolerance.[107]

The first and the second signal (TCR and CD28 signaling) result in activation of PI3 and Akt kinases in addition to PLC and MAP kinases and ultimately results in T cell survival, proliferation, production of cytokines, and differentiation to effector and memory cells. The effector and memory cells are less dependent on the second signal, and therefore, they can activate with other APCs.

Both B7 and CD28 have other family members with different functions. CD28 family consists of ICOS (CD278), cytotoxic T lymphocyte-associated protein (CTLA)−4 (CD152), and PD-1. ICOS is important for germinal center events, TfH development, and the production of antibodies. CTLA-4 and PD-1 have an inhibitory function and are important for the limiting phase of the immune response. These two receptors have a role in T cell tolerance, as well, and dysregulation in their expression results in autoimmune disorders. The ligands of the mentioned receptors are ICOSL, B7, and programmed death ligand (PD-L)1, respectively. Blocking of B7:CD28 interaction by CTLA-4-Ig is an approved therapy for transplant rejection and rheumatoid arthritis. CTLA-4-Ig has the extracellular domain of CTLA-4, and its intracellular domain is Fc of human IgG. CTLA-4 has a higher affinity for B7 compared to CD28. Therefore, it is used for the B7:CD28 blockade. Antibodies against CTLA-4 and PD-1 are being used in cancer immunotherapy because they can block the inhibitory function of these molecules.[108]

Upon activation of T cells, the surface expression of CD69, CD25, and CD40L increases. Following the increase of CD69, the sphingosine 1-phosphate receptor decreases, and this mediates the release of T cells from the lymphoid organs. Sphingosine 1-phosphate has a high concentration in the lymphoid organs, and naïve T cells highly express sphingosine 1-phosphate receptor, which attracts these cells to the primary lymphoid organs. CD25 or the α chain of IL-2 receptor upregulates upon T cell activation, and this allows T cell to respond to IL-2 (T cell growth, differentiation, and survival factor). Other cytokine receptors in addition to adhesion molecules (integrins such as lymphocyte function-associated antigen (LFA)−1 and very late antigen (VLA)−4, and selectins such as CD62L) also upregulate during the process of T cell activation with the aim of helping T cells to perform their effector functions and to migrate to different tissues.[109]

IL-2 is the main T cell growth factor, and the transcription from the IL-2 gene, in addition to the expression of its receptor, is induced after the activation of naïve T cells. IL-2 induces antiapoptotic proteins such as BCL-2. It also promotes the cell cycle through activation of mammalian target of rapamycin (mTOR) signaling.[110] Other cytokines such as IFN-γ and IL-4 production are also influenced and enhanced by IL-2. Tregs constitutively express IL-2 receptors because IL-2 is essential for the survival and function of these cells. IL-2 also drives T cell clonal expansion to 1000 and up to 50,000 folds for the antigen-specific CD4+ and CD8+ T cells, respectively. Effector T cells produce other cytokines and influence other cells such as B cells and macrophages during the immune response.

Another crucial part of a T cell activation process is the formation of memory T cells, which guarantee a long-term immunity against an antigen. The process of memory T cell formation is not fully understood, but we know that a proportion of T cells turn into memory cells, which can remain lifelong and express high levels of anti-apoptotic proteins. The memory formation makes immunization via vaccines feasible because these cells can respond faster and to a greater state against antigens compared to naïve T cells. It is believed that the frequency of memory T cells against particular antigens is higher than that of the specific naïve cells. Memory cells have the ability of self-renewing in the absence of antigen and upon reinfection, they can rapidly migrate to the infectious tissue and respond in a few days. IL-7 is a critical cytokine for the survival of memory cells and memory T cells express IL-7 receptor (CD127). Therefore, CD127 is a memory cell surface marker. Other markers of memory T cells include CD45RO and CD27. Recently, the memory cell population has been divided into two categories of central memory (TCM) and effector memory (TEM) based on their residence location and their function. TCMs home to the lymph nodes because they express CCR7, and CD62L and they maintain a reservoir of the memory cells. They have low effector function. On the other hand, TEMs do not express homing markers, and they serve as the memory cells that rapidly turn into effector T cells in the tissues, and they produce cytokines like IFN-γ.[111]

T cell activation is declined after the elimination of antigens. This is in part the result of the lack of stimuli, which leads to less IL-2 availability, and declined expression of antiapoptotic proteins. Consequently, the activated cells die and attenuate the immune response. As mentioned earlier, a few receptors such as PD-1 and CTLA-4 are also expressed later on the activated T cells, and they help limit the immune response.

## CD4+ T cells effector functions

CD4+ T cells recognize phagocytosed antigens presented with APCs. Phagocytic cells such as macrophages, as a part of innate immunity, can phagocyte microbial antigens and kill them. However, many bacterial antigens can resist this process and survive in the phagocytic vesicles. Fortunately, phagocytic cells express MHC II molecules, and they can process and present microbial antigens to T cells. CD4+ T cells express ligands (such as CD40L), and they produce cytokines upon activation. Therefore, they enhance the function of phagocytes. CD4+ T cells have different subsets with different cytokine production capabilities, and we are going to briefly explain different subsets of CD4+ T cells in this chapter.

The main subsets of T CD4+ effector cells are Th1, Th2, and Th17 cells. These cells activate in response to different types of pathogens, and the secreted cytokines from APCs drive their differentiation in the lymphoid organs. Each subset produces different cytokines and expresses different transcription factors. In addition to the mentioned subsets, Tregs are yet another subset of CD4+ T cells, which have more regulatory properties rather than activating, and they are crucial for the maintenance of tolerance against self-antigens.[112,113]

Th1 cells: The main pathogens that elicit Th1 response are intracellular pathogens (bacteria or virus) that survive inside phagocytes. Th1 differentiation happens when DCs, macrophages, or NK cells secrete IL-12, IL-18, and IFN-γ in response to the mentioned pathogens. Th1 cells majorly produce IFN-γ, which stimulates further Th1 differentiation and prevents Th2 and Th17 differentiation. T-bet, signal transducer and activator of transcription (STAT)1, and STAT4 are Th1 specific transcription factors, and they are induced by antigen plus cytokine. IFN-γ induces STAT1 and T-bet, while IL-12 induces STAT4. T-bet and STAT4 transcription factors increase IFN-γ production in a positive loop manner.[114] Th1 cells have a distinct pattern of homing as they express CXCR3 and CCR5, which attract them to the site of infection. The cells of the innate immunity produce chemokines in response to the infectious agents in the tissues to attract T cells. Th1 cells migrate to the sites of inflammation by expressing ligands for E and P selectin.

Th1 cells activate macrophages (classic activation of macrophage or M1 macrophages) to kill the microbial antigens by IFN-γ secretion in addition to CD40-CD40L interaction. Macrophages enhance their ability to phagocyte and to destroy the antigen, in addition to antigen-presenting ability in the presence of IFN-γ. IFN-γ not only promotes Th1 and prevents Th2 and Th17 differentiation but also drives class switching of B cells toward IgG production and prevents switching to IgE.

Th1 cells also produce TNF to recruit other leukocytes and IL-10, which suppresses the immune response by inhibiting DCs and macrophages.

Th2 cells: Unlike Th1, Th2 cells do not enhance phagocytosis, but they activate eosinophils and mast cells to mediate allergic reactions and to defend the host against helminths. Therefore, Th2 cells differentiate in response to allergens and helminthic pathogens. IL-4 is known as the major cytokine that mediates differentiation to Th2. However, other cytokines such as IL-25, IL-33, and thymic stromal lymphopoietin can also mediate Th2 differentiation. Mast cells and Th2 cells are both sources of IL-4, while other mentioned cytokines are produced from damaged tissue cells. GATA3 and STAT6 are Th2 specific transcription factors, which are induced following TCR signals and IL-4. Induction of GATA3 results in transcription of Th-2 specific cytokines, including IL-4, IL-5, and IL-13, while suppressing IL-12 receptor and consequently Th1 differentiation.[115] IL-4 mediates class switching to IgE antibody, and in a positive loop, stimulates further differentiation to Th2 cells. IL-13 can also have a role in switching to IgE. IL-4 and IL-13 both can activate macrophages through the alternative pathway, which is different from the activation of macrophages through IFN-γ. By alternative activation, macrophages (which are called M2 macrophages) not only have an anti-inflammatory function but also produce enzymes for tissue repair. Therefore, Th2 cells stimulate M2 macrophage activation and suppress M1 macrophage activation. IL-4 and IL-13 also have an important role in mucus secretion in the airways and peristalsis in the gastrointestinal tract. Through these cytokines, Th2 cells have a role in defense mechanisms at mucosal barriers.

IL-5 activates mature eosinophils and also stimulates the differentiation of these cells. Eosinophils express receptors for the Fc fraction of IgE, and via this receptor, they can recognize helminths that are covered with IgE, and they can kill them. Th2 cells express CCR3, CCR4, and CCR8 for their tissue migration.

Th17 cells: Th17 cells mainly have a role in the neutrophil recruitment (neutrophilic inflammation) to the infection site. These cells activate against certain extracellular bacterial and fungal infections, and they have roles in inflammatory and autoimmune diseases. Th17 cells differentiate in response to secreted IL-6, IL-1, and IL-23 from DCs. While the first two cytokines are important for Th17 differentiation, IL-23 is believed to be functional later when Th17 cells proliferate. TGF-β is another important cytokine for the differentiation of Th17 cells. Differentiation to Th1 and Th2 suppresses Th17, and therefore, IFN-γ and IL-4 both have suppressor functions for Th17 differentiation.[116]

The key transcription factors of Th17 cells consist of retinoic acid receptor-related orphan receptor gamma t (RORγt) and STAT3, which are activated by TGF-β and IL-6. Th17 cells produce IL-17 and IL-22 and express CCR6. IL-17 family consists of IL-17A to F, and the main known function of them is performed by IL-17A. This cytokine is inflammatory as it recruits neutrophils, and to some extent monocytes, and stimulates defensin production, which is a natural antimicrobe. IL-22 has also a similar role but mainly in the epithelial surfaces, where it stimulates inflammation in addition to the production of antimicrobial substances to maintain the integrity of the epithelial barrier.

Another cytokine produced by Th17 cells is IL-21, which has an autocrine function to amplify Th17 differentiation apart from its role in Tfh cell generation, B cell activation in the germinal center, and CD8+ T and NK cells activation.

Defective Th17 differentiation results in recurrent fungal and bacterial infections, mainly in the skin (like chronic mucocutaneous candidiasis). This happens due to mutation in STAT3, and the disease is called hyper IgE syndrome or Job syndrome. Th17 has been shown to have a role in many inflammatory diseases such as multiple sclerosis, psoriasis, inflammatory bowel disease, and rheumatoid arthritis. Inhibition of Th17 is considered as a therapeutic approach for the mentioned diseases.

## CD8+ T cells effector functions

The main role of these cells is cell cytotoxicity, which includes the killing of virus-infected cells (having virus in their cytosol), bacteria-infected cells (when the bacteria have escaped from the endosome to the cytosol), and tumor cells.[117] Therefore, these cells are crucial for the eradication of the infection source. When naïve CD8+ T cells recognize antigen presented by DCs in the groove of MHC I and co-stimulatory molecules (like B7) in the lymphoid organs, they differentiate to effector CTLs. The differentiation process arm CTLs with cytolytic granules containing perforin and granzymes in addition to IFN-γ production, while the expression of their encoding genes happens during differentiation. At the molecular level, T-bet and eomesodermin drive the transcription of lytic granule genes.[118]

DCs are the most potent APCs for stimulation of naïve CD8+ T cells, and a fraction of DCs can present MHC I pathway-specific antigens by so-called cross-presentation. Most virus-infected or tumoral cells are not necessarily DCs but rather tissue cells. In this situation, DCs uptake the whole cell, and by transferring the antigens from the endosome to cytosol, they can present their antigens by MHC I. Recent investigations show that CD4+ T cells are also important for a successful CTL differentiation, especially when the antigen was not able to elicit a strong innate immune reaction. The evidence to this finding is a defective CTL response in the human immunodeficiency virus (HIV) infected patients, where HIV mainly targets CD4+ T cells. The help of CD4+ T cells could be either through cytokine secretion (such as IL-2 and IL-21) or through activation of DCs by CD40-CD40L interaction. Another source of IL-2 is CD8+ T cells. IL-2 is important for the differentiation and proliferation of CTLs in addition to the generation of memory CD8+ T cells.[119] Other important cytokines for CTL differentiation are IL-12, type I IFNs, and IL-21. IL-15 is believed to be important for the survival of memory CD8+ T cells.

Activated CTLs migrate to the site of infection, where they recognize the target cells by their specific TCRs. CD8 as the co-receptor and LFA-1 contribute to this encounter, where LFA-1 (adhesion molecule) binds to intercellular adhesion molecule (ICAM)−1 and helps the formation of a synapse with the target cell. This process allows CTL to specifically kill its target cell by secreting the granule toxic contents to the synapse area without harming the adjacent non-infected cells. However, as the infected cells are destroyed, CTL function can lead to tissue injury and be responsible for the immunopathogenesis of viral infections such as hepatitis B and C. CTLs are important players of tumor immunity and acute graft rejection, as well.[120]

The CTL (and NK cell) granule contents are mainly granzymes and perforin. Perforin is a cytolytic membrane pore-forming protein, which is similar to the complement C9 subunit. Granzymes are serine proteases cutting proteins after aspartate residues, and granzyme B seems to be the most important of all granzymes for CTL cytotoxicity. Perforin makes the pore for granzyme B to enter through and cleave various proteins such as caspase-3 and stimulate the mitochondrial pathway of apoptosis in the target cells.[121] CTLs express Fas ligand (FasL), and they can kill their target cell by interacting with CD40 followed by caspase activation and apoptosis. One of the other important roles of CD8+ T cells is the activation of macrophages together with Th1 cells through secretion of IFN-γ. CTLs also secrete IL-17, and therefore, they have an important role in inflammation and inflammatory diseases. Mutation in perforin results in hemophagocytic lymphohistiocytosis (HLH), where CTLs are unable to kill their target cells, but they recurrently produce IFN-γ, which leads to overactivated macrophages that ingest red blood cells.

T cell exhaustion is a term, which refers to a gradual deterioration of CTL response as a result of chronic antigen encounters. CTLs express inhibitory markers such as PD-1 in this situation, and they become inactive. This has been seen in chronic viral infection and cancer.[122]

## γδ T cells

Less than 5 percent of the T cells have a TCR consisting of γδ chains. Their characteristics are limited to TCR diversity, and they are resident in certain tissues such as epithelium, and it is believed that they have TCR specificity only for the common pathogens of these tissues. About 10 percent of intraepithelial lymphocytes in humans are γδ T cells. They are not restricted to MHC, and they do not need antigen processing by APCs to recognize their antigens. γδ T cells recognize protein and nonprotein antigens such as lipids commonly found in microbes presented by nonclassical MHCI-like molecules. The role of these cells is not completely clear yet, but they are able to kill infected cells and produce cytokines such as IL-17.[123]

## NKT cells

These cells are also developing in the thymus, and they express both markers of NK cells (like CD56), and they express the TCR. The TCR consists of αβ chains with very limited diversity. A fraction of these cells can be characterized by their specific α chain in humans, Vα24-Jα18, and they are called iNKT cells (i for invariant). The TCR of NKT cells recognizes lipid antigens presented with CD1, and they secrete IL-4 and IFN-γ. It is believed that these cells might have roles in both innate and adaptive immunity, especially against the microbes containing lipid antigens, such as mycobacteria.[124]

## MAIT cells

These cells are mucosa-associated invariant T cells, which express invariant TCR αβ called Vα7.2-Jα33. They recognize some fungal and bacterial riboflavin metabolites presented by MHC class I-related protein 1 (MR1). These cells are mostly CD8+ and are activated by cytokines such as IL-12 and IL-18. They are capable of producing inflammatory cytokines such as TNF and IFN-γ. About half of the MAIT cell population resides in the liver. Therefore, it is believed that these cells defend us from the microbial flora of the intestine.[125]

## Mechanisms of tolerance

Immunologic tolerance is referred to immune system unresponsiveness against an antigen, which is induced by previous exposure to that antigen in a specific condition. In fact, our immune system responds to foreign antigens while remains are unresponsive against self-antigens. This self-non-self-discrimination feature of the immune system results in tolerance or unresponsiveness against safe antigens. Failure in tolerance mechanisms leads to immune reaction towards autologous antigens, which may cause autoimmune diseases.[126] The reason underlying the production of autoreactive B and T lymphocytes in the body is that antigen-specific receptors are generated by randomized recombination of different gene segments during lymphocyte development. So, some B and T cell clones carry autoreactive antigen receptors, which express high affinity receptors for self-antigens. These self-reacting clones should be recognized and removed by tolerance mechanisms to prevent autoreactive reactions.[127] Tolerance mechanisms sense and remove self-reacting lymphocytes at two main levels: central and peripheral tolerance. During central tolerance, recognition of self-antigens by developing lymphocytes in central or generative lymphoid tissues (bone marrow and thymus) with high affinity results in autoreactive lymphocyte elimination. This phenomenon ensures the production of naïve mature lymphocytes, which do not react with self-antigens. However, if for any reason, a clone of self-reactive lymphocytes escapes the central tolerance and enters the blood circulation, peripheral tolerance mechanisms prevent activation of these lymphocytes, which may damage self-tissues. Induction of tolerance in lymphocytes is acquired by recognition of specific antigens using BCRs or TCRs.[128]

Central and peripheral immunologic tolerance is induced by different mechanisms in T and B cells.

## T cell tolerance

T cells have a prominent role in the induction and maintenance of tolerance towards self-antigens. In fact, the majority of pathologic autoinflammatory reactions are due to the lack of helper CD4+ T cell tolerance, which also mediates the production of autoantibodies. T cell tolerance is mediated at two levels of central and peripheral tolerance.[129] As a result of central T cell tolerance, developing immature T cells, which recognize MHC self-antigen complexes presented by APCs with high affinity, are eliminated or deleted by apoptosis. This process is called clonal deletion or negative selection and ensures matured T cell repertoire, which exit thymus to peripheral tissues, do not respond to self-antigens, which are found in the thymus during T cells development. Negative selection takes place in the cortex and medulla of the thymus, which deletes double-positive and single-positive T cells that strongly respond to self-antigens, respectively. Negative selection assures mature lymphocytes that leave the thymus to the periphery do not respond to antigens, which are presented in the thymus by thymic epithelial cells.[130] Expression of self-antigens from peripheral tissues in the thymus is under control of a transcription factor called AIRE, which is mainly expressed by medullary thymic epithelial cells.[131] In fact, expression of self-antigens by medullary thymic epithelial cells in the thymus is dependent on AIRE, so that mutation in the *AIRE* gene results in multi-organ autoimmune disease called autoimmune polyendocrine syndrome type 1. In autoimmune polyendocrine syndrome type 1, autoreactive T and B cells are activated and injure different organs, including parathyroids, adrenals, and pancreatic islets.[132] We will discuss autoimmune disease later in detail. Although the vast majority of self-reacting lymphocytes are deleted through negative selection. Some of these cells are differentiated to Tregs in the thymus, which then induce tolerance against other self-reacting T lymphocytes that escape central tolerance and enter the periphery.[133] In fact, central tolerance is not flawless, and there are self-antigen reacting T cells, which escape clonal deletion and leave the thymus to blood circulation. Peripheral tolerance mechanisms are responsible for T cell tolerance against tissue-specific self-antigens (mainly those that are not found in the thymus) in peripheral tissues.[134] Mechanisms of T cell peripheral tolerance include inducing anergy, suppression by Tregs, and deletion.[135] Anergy or functional unresponsiveness occurs when CD4+ T cells recognize antigens in the absence of a second signal or co-stimulation. We know that lymphocytes need two signals for full activation. The first signal is provided through antigen recognition, while the second signal is delivered when co-stimulatory molecules on APCs (such as B7-1 and B7-2 molecules) bind to their ligand (CD28) on CD4+ T cells. The expression of co-stimulatory molecules on APCs is dependent on the activation of the innate immune response, which normally happens in the presence of foreign antigens. Self-antigens are continuously presented to self-reactive T cells in the absence of innate immunity and the expression of co-stimulatory molecules. Thus, self-reactive T cells become anergic and do not differentiate into effector T cells.[136] Another mechanism, which leads to T cell anergy is regulation by inhibitory receptors. Engagement of inhibitory molecules from CD28 family receptors (mainly CTLA-4 and PD-1) on T cells to B7 family molecules on APCs inhibits T cell activation.[137] CTLA-4 is expressed on activated T cells as well as Tregs and is an important molecule in self-tolerance. Polymorphisms in the *CTLA-4* gene are associated with several autoimmune diseases such as type 1 diabetes and Graves' disease. Both CTLA-4 and CD28 bind the same ligands, B7-1 (CD80) and B7-2 (CD86), but the affinity of CTLA-4 for B7 is considerably higher than CD28. So, when CTLA-4 is expressed on self-reactive T cells or Tregs, it competes for binding to B7 molecules on APCs and results in their internalization and digestion. Thus, the amount of B7 molecules on APCs to provide co-stimulation through CD28 is reduced. Recall that the level of B7 molecules on resting APCs expressing self-antigens is rather limited. So, low affinity CD28 molecules do not engage B7 molecules in this condition.[138] Another inhibitory receptor from the CD28 family is PD-1. PD-1 is expressed on activated T cells, and its ligands, PD-L1, and PD-L2 are found on APCs. PD-1 expression is increased on T cells when there is continuous antigen stimulation, such as in the case of self-antigens, tumors, and chronic infections. This molecule has an important role in maintaining self-tolerance in T cells, especially when exposure to antigen is prolonged.[139]

It has been shown that CTLA-4 and PD-1 molecules block T cells activation as checkpoints in the immune response, which has led to the idea of activation of T cell response by reducing these checkpoints, which is called Immune checkpoint blockade. For example, the blockade of CTLA-4 using anti-CTLA-4 antibody has reinforced anti-tumor immunity and is approved for the treatment of advanced melanoma and other cancers. Checkpoint blockade targeting PD-1 and its ligands has shown even more efficacy and less toxicity than that of anti-CTLA-4 in several cancers.[140]

Suppression by Tregs is another mechanism of peripheral T cell tolerance. Tregs are a subset of CD4+ T cells, which also express a high level of IL-2 receptor α chain (CD25) and the FoxP3 transcription factor.[141] Mutation in the *FoxP3* gene results in Tregs deficiency and causes a rare autoimmune disease called immune dysregulation, polyendocrinopathy, enteropathy, X-linked syndrome (IPEX). Autoimmune manifestation in this syndrome shows Tregs importance in maintaining self-tolerance.[142] As mentioned, CD4+ CD25+ FoxP3+ Tregs are the main group with suppressive activity. They also express high levels of CTLA-4 molecule, which helps them regulate self-responding T cells. These Tregs are generated in two sites. Natural or thymic regulatory T cells (tTregs) are generated as a result of self-antigen recognition by developing CD4+ T cells in the thymus, while Induced or peripheral regulatory T cells (pTregs) are generated when mature CD4+ T cells recognize self-antigens in the absence of innate immune response in peripheral lymphoid organs. TGF-β and IL-2 are important cytokines for the generation and maintenance of Tregs.[143]

Tregs suppress immune responses at induction of T cell activation or effector phase of T cell responses by different mechanisms. Tregs also have the ability to suppress B cells and NK cells. Tregs produce inhibitory cytokines such as TGF-β and IL-10.[144]

TGF-β is produced by Tregs and activated macrophages. This cytokine inhibits proliferation and effector functions of T cells and also inhibits macrophage activation. TGF-β is an important differentiation cytokine in Tregs development, and together with IL-1 and IL-6, promotes Th17 subset differentiation. Moreover, TGF-β is an important cytokine in tissue repair at the final stages of inflammatory reactions.[145]

IL-10 is another inhibitory cytokine and is produced by Tregs, activated macrophages, DCs, and some B cells. This cytokine inhibits macrophages and DCs through different mechanisms. IL-10 prevents the production of IL-12 by macrophages and DCs. IL-12 itself is an important cytokine to promote IFN-γ secretion, which plays an important role in innate and adaptive cell-mediated immune reactions.

IL-10 prevents expressions of co-stimulatory and MHC II molecules on APCs. Thus, it inhibits T cell activation.[146]

Tregs also decrease the B7 molecules expressed on APCs through the expression of CTLA-4, and therefore, reduce the stimulating property of APCs. Besides, these cells express a high level of IL-2 receptor (CD25) and consume IL-2 cytokine in the environment. So, other T cells become deprived of IL-2, which is also necessary for their proliferation.[141]

As mentioned earlier, Tregs have substantial a role in self-tolerance, as we see defects in Tregs or resistance of effector cells to suppressor effects of these cells contributes to the pathogenesis of different autoimmune and inflammatory diseases, including inflammatory bowel disease, type 1 diabetes, multiple sclerosis, and allergic disorders. In addition to the role of Tregs in the control of autoimmunity, there is also evidence stating that Tregs present in different tissues such as skin, muscles, and lungs promote tissue repair and help to maintain tissue integrity after inflammatory reactions. Moreover, Tregs have been shown to be crucial for preserving tolerance against the fetus and preventing abortion.[147]

Deletion by apoptotic cell death or activation-induced cell death (AICD) is the third mechanism of peripheral T cell tolerance. In fact, recognition of self-antigen by high affinity or repeated exposure of T cell with self-antigens results in cell death through two different pathways, which will be described later in this chapter.[148]

## B cell tolerance

While T cell tolerance is important for unresponsiveness to thymus-dependent self-antigens (peptides), B cell tolerance has a prominent role in maintaining tolerance against thymus-independent self-antigens, such as polysaccharides and lipids. Also, B cell tolerance is important to prevent the production of autoantibodies. Similar to T cells, B cell tolerance involves central and peripheral tolerance.[149] Developing immature B cells, which recognize self-antigens, either with high or low affinity in the bone marrow, go through central B cell tolerance mechanisms, including receptor editing, deletion, and anergy. When developing B cells recognize self-antigens with high affinity, they change their specificity or become deleted. Receptor editing happens with immature B cells when they recognize self-antigens that are in high concentration in the bone marrow, and it usually results in BCR cross-linking, which delivers a strong signal to cells. As a result, RAG enzymes become reactivated and repeat another VJ recombination in the Igκ light chain gene locus. So, a new Ig light chain is expressed, creating a BCR with a new specificity. If newly generated BCR is not productive, VJ recombination may be repeated at λ light chain loci that is why the majority of B cells with λ BCR may have undergone receptor editing during their maturation.[150] If receptor editing does not result in the production of non-self-reactive BCRs, B cells may undergo deletion. Sometimes developing B cells in the bone marrow recognize self-antigens with low affinity (such as soluble self-antigens that do not cross-link different surface BCRs), which results in B cells anergy. Anergic B cells that leave the bone marrow are functionally unresponsive due to loss of surface BCRs or antigen receptor signaling blockade.[151]

Self-reactive mature B cells that leave the bone marrow to peripheral tissues should be controlled by peripheral tolerance. B cell peripheral tolerance prevents mature B lymphocytes to respond against self-antigens in peripheral tissues by anergy, deletion, and regulation.[152] If mature B cells recognize self-antigens in the absence of specific Th cells assistance or co-stimulatory molecules that are produced as a result of the innate immune response, they become anergic. These anergic self-reactive B cells are repeatedly stimulated by self-antigens but do not receive enough growth factors that are needed for their survival. Also, self-reactive B cells that recognize self-antigens with high affinity in peripheral tissues may be deleted by apoptosis. Another mechanism of peripheral B cell tolerance is regulation. Some B cells that recognize self-antigens with second signal co-stimulation in peripheral tissues become regulated through the engagement of regulatory receptors such as CD22 and FCγRIIB.[153]

## Apoptosis

Program cell death or apoptosis is mediated through intrinsic or extrinsic pathways.[154] The main proteins that are involved in the intrinsic (mitochondrial) pathway are BCL-2 family proteins. Both pro-apoptotic and anti-apoptotic proteins are found in this family. When cells are under stress (i.e., lack of growth factor, DNA damage, some receptor signaling such as recognition of self-antigens with high affinity by immature lymphocytes), stress sensors of the BCL-2 family such as Bim molecules in lymphocytes become activated and bind to other pro-apoptotic proteins of this family. These activated proteins increase mitochondrial permeability. As a result, cytochrome c leaks to the cytosol and activates caspase proteins, which cause cell death. In this pathway, cytochrome c together with APAF-1 protein activates caspase-9, which activates other caspase proteins and results in DNA fragmentation and apoptotic death. The extrinsic pathway is directly mediated by death receptors and their ligands. Most of these receptors belong to the TNF receptor family members and bind to their ligands from TNF family molecules. Perhaps the most important pair involved in the apoptotic deletion of self-reactive T cells are Fas death receptors that engage FasL from the TNF family. When surface Fas binds to FasL on another cell (or itself), caspase-8 becomes activated, which activates other downstream caspases and results in apoptotic cell death. Apoptosis with either pathway results in changes such as the formation of membrane blebs, fragmentation of nucleus, and generation of apoptotic bodies. Phagocytes recognize these changes and engulf apoptotic cells without generation of inflammation.[12,155]

Clonal deletion is an important mechanism in both B and T cells tolerance. As an example, T cells that recognize self-antigens with high affinity in the thymus or peripheral tissues activate Bim molecule and die by intrinsic pathway but normal cells receive signals from growth factors or TCRs that activate anti-apoptotic proteins such as BCL-2, which promotes cell survival and prevents apoptosis. But T cells that are at repeated exposure to self-antigens express Fas and FasL molecules concurrently and engagement of these molecules leads to the activation of extrinsic pathway and cell death.[148]

## References


1. Paul WE. *Fundamental Immunology*. 2012.
2. Boehm T, Swann JB. Origin and evolution of adaptive immunity. *Annu Rev Anim Biosci*. 2014;2:259–283.
3. Marshall JS, Warrington R, Watson W, Kim HL. An introduction to immunology and immunopathology. *Allergy, asthma, and clinical immunology: official journal of the Canadian Society of Allergy and Clinical Immunology*. 2018;14(Suppl 2):49.
4. Abul K, Abbas AHL, Pillai S. *Cellular and Molecular Immunology*. 9th ed. Philadelphia: Elsevier; 2018.
5. Silverstein AM. Cellular versus humoral immunology: a century-long dispute. *Nat. Immunol.* 2003;4(5):425–428.
6. Cohn M, Mitchison NA, Paul WE, Silverstein AM, Talmage DW, Weigert M. Reflections on the clonal-selection theory. *Nat. Rev. Immunol.* 2007;7(10):823–830.
7. Nielsen SCA, Boyd SD. Human adaptive immune receptor repertoire analysis-Past, present, and future. *Immunol. Rev*. 2018;284(1):9–23.
8. Pradeu T, Du Pasquier L. Immunological memory: what's in a name? *Immunol. Rev*. 2018;283(1): 7–20.
9. Jiang H, Chess L. How the immune system achieves self-nonself discrimination during adaptive immunity. *Adv. Immunol.* 2009;102:95–133.
10. Kawamoto H, Katsura Y. A new paradigm for hematopoietic cell lineages: revision of the classical concept of the myeloid–lymphoid dichotomy. *Trends Immunol.* 2009;30(5):193–200.
11. Lai AY, Kondo M. T and B lymphocyte differentiation from hematopoietic stem cell. *Seminars in Immunology*: Elsevier; 2008.
12. Abbas AK, Pillai S. *Cellular and Molecular Immunology, 9e*. Philadelphia, PA: Elsevier Saunders. 2012.
13. Hidalgo A, Chilvers ER, Summers C, Koenderman L. The neutrophil life cycle. *Trends Immunol.* 2019;40(7):584–597.
14. Gordon S. Phagocytosis: an immunobiologic process. *Immunity*. 2016;44(3):463–475.
15. Lawrence SM, Corriden R, Nizet V. How neutrophils meet their end. *Trends Immunol.* 2020;41(6):531–544.
16. Kita H. Eosinophils: multifaceted biological properties and roles in health and disease. *Immunol. Rev*. 2011;242(1):161–177.
17. Galli SJ, Gaudenzio N, Tsai M. Mast cells in inflammation and disease: recent progress and ongoing concerns. *Annu. Rev. Immunol.* 2020;38:49–77.
18. Geissmann F, Manz MG, Jung S, Sieweke MH, Merad M, Ley K. Development of monocytes, macrophages, and dendritic cells. *Science*. 2010;327(5966):656–661.
19. Guilliams M, Ginhoux F, Jakubzick C, Naik SH, Onai N, Schraml BU, et al. Dendritic cells, monocytes and macrophages: a unified nomenclature based on ontogeny. *Nat. Rev. Immunol.* 2014;14(8):571–578.
20. Murray PJ, Wynn TA. Protective and pathogenic functions of macrophage subsets. *Nat. Rev. Immunol.* 2011;11(11):723–737.
21. Greenlee-Wacker MC. Clearance of apoptotic neutrophils and resolution of inflammation. *Immunol. Rev*. 2016;273(1):357–370.
22. Parkin J, Cohen B. An overview of the immune system. *Lancet North Am. Ed.* 2001;357(9270):1777–1789.
23. Kashem SW, Haniffa M, Kaplan DH. Antigen-presenting cells in the skin. *Annu. Rev. Immunol.* 2017;35:469–499.
24. Merad M, Sathe P, Helft J, Miller J, Mortha A. The dendritic cell lineage: ontogeny and function of dendritic cells and their subsets in the steady state and the inflamed setting. *Annu. Rev. Immunol.* 2013;31:563–604.

25. Luciani C, Hager FT, Cerovic V, Lelouard H. Dendritic cell functions in the inductive and effector sites of intestinal immunity. *Mucosal Immunol.* 2021:1–11.
26. Ghosh D, Jiang W, Mukhopadhyay D, Mellins ED. New insights into B cells as antigen presenting cells. *Curr. Opin. Immunol.* 2021;70:129–137.
27. Mildner A, Jung S. Development and function of dendritic cell subsets. *Immunity*. 2014;40(5):642–656.
28. Lee HK, Iwasaki A. Innate control of adaptive immunity: dendritic cells and beyond. *Seminars in immunology*. 2007.
29. Banchereau J, Steinman RM. Dendritic cells and the control of immunity. *Nature*. 1998;392(6673): 245–252.
30. Shortman K, Sathe P, Vremec D, Naik S, O'Keeffe M. Plasmacytoid dendritic cell development. *Adv. Immunol.* 2013;120:105–126.
31. Heesters BA, Myers RC, Carroll MC. Follicular dendritic cells: dynamic antigen libraries. *Nat. Rev. Immunol.* 2014;14(7):495–504.
32. Murphy K, Weaver C Janeway's immunobiology: garland science. 2016.
33. LeBien TW, Tedder TF. B lymphocytes: how they develop and function. *Blood, The Journal of the American Society of Hematology*. 2008;112(5):1570–1580.
34. Wang Y, Liu J, Burrows PD, Wang J-Y B cell development and maturation. B Cells in Immunity and Tolerance. 2020:1-22.
35. Fabbri M, Smart C, lymphocytes Pa RT. *Int. J. Biochem. Cell Biol.* 2003;35(7):1004–1008.
36. Apostolou I, Sarukhan A, Klein L, von Boehmer H. Origin of regulatory T cells with known specificity for antigen. *Nat. Immunol.* 2002;3(8):756–763.
37. Godfrey DI, MacDonald HR, Kronenberg M, Smyth MJ, Van Kaer L. NKT cells: what's in a name? *Nat. Rev. Immunol.* 2004;4(3):231–237.
38. Garner LC, Klenerman P, Provine NM. Insights into mucosal-associated invariant T cell biology from studies of invariant natural killer T cells. *Front. Immunol.* 2018;9:1478.
39. Mackay CR. Homing of naive, memory and effector lymphocytes. *Curr. Opin. Immunol.* 1993;5(3):423–427.
40. Geiger TL, Sun JC. Development and maturation of natural killer cells. *Curr. Opin. Immunol.* 2016;39:82–89.
41. Boehm T, Bleul CC. The evolutionary history of lymphoid organs. *Nat. Immunol.* 2007;8(2):131–135.
42. Zhao E, Xu H, Wang L, Kryczek I, Wu K, Hu Y, et al. Bone marrow and the control of immunity. *Cell. Mol. Immunol.* 2012;9(1):11–19.
43. Chu VT, Berek C. The establishment of the plasma cell survival niche in the bone marrow. *Immunol. Rev.* 2013;251(1):177–188.
44. Spits H. Development of αβ T cells in the human thymus. *Nat. Rev. Immunol.* 2002;2(10):760–772.
45. Boehm T. Thymus development and function. *Curr. Opin. Immunol.* 2008;20(2):178–184.
46. Kumar BV, Connors TJ, Farber DL. Human T cell development, localization, and function throughout life. *Immunity*. 2018;48(2):202–213.
47. TD R, Carragher DM, Rangel-Moreno J. Development of secondary lymphoid organs. *Annu. Rev. Immunol.* 2008;26:627–650.
48. Swartz MA. The physiology of the lymphatic system. *Adv. Drug Deliv. Rev.* 2001;50(1–2):3–20.
49. Girard J-P, Moussion C, Förster R. HEVs, lymphatics and homeostatic immune cell trafficking in lymph nodes. *Nat. Rev. Immunol.* 2012;12(11):762–773.
50. Bar-Ephraïm YE, Mebius RE. Innate lymphoid cells in secondary lymphoid organs. *Immunol. Rev.* 2016;271(1):185–199.
51. Mebius RE, Kraal G. Structure and function of the spleen. *Nat. Rev. Immunol.* 2005;5(8):606–616.
52. Van de Pavert SA, Mebius RE. New insights into the development of lymphoid tissues. *Nat. Rev. Immunol.* 2010;10(9):664–674.
53. Mörbe UM, Jørgensen PB, Fenton TM, von Burg N, Riis LB, Spencer J, et al. Human gut-associated lymphoid tissues (GALT); diversity, structure, and function. *Mucosal Immunol.* 2021:1–10.
54. Medzhitov R, Janeway Jr C. Innate immune recognition: mechanisms and pathways. *Immunol. Rev.* 2000;173:89–97.
55. Iwasaki A, Medzhitov R. Control of adaptive immunity by the innate immune system. *Nat. Immunol.* 2015;16(4):343–353.

56. Akira S, Uematsu S, Takeuchi O. Pathogen recognition and innate immunity. *Cell*. 2006;124(4):783–801.
57. Jeannin P, Jaillon S, Delneste Y. Pattern recognition receptors in the immune response against dying cells. *Curr. Opin. Immunol*. 2008;20(5):530–537.
58. Riera Romo M, Pérez-Martínez D, Castillo Ferrer C. Innate immunity in vertebrates: an overview. *Immunology*. 2016;148(2):125–139.
59. Whitsett JA, Alenghat T. Respiratory epithelial cells orchestrate pulmonary innate immunity. *Nat. Immunol*. 2015;16(1):27–35.
60. Hayday A, Theodoridis E, Ramsburg E, Shires J. Intraepithelial lymphocytes: exploring the Third Way in immunology. *Nat. Immunol*. 2001;2(11):997–1003.
61. Dale DC, Boxer L, Liles WC. The phagocytes: neutrophils and monocytes. *Blood*. 2008;112(4):935–945.
62. Gordon S. Pattern recognition receptors: doubling up for the innate immune response. *Cell*. 2002;111(7):927–930.
63. Sonnenberg GF, Artis D. Innate lymphoid cells in the initiation, regulation and resolution of inflammation. *Nat. Med*. 2015;21(7):698–708.
64. Juelke K, Romagnani C. Differentiation of human innate lymphoid cells (ILCs). *Curr. Opin. Immunol*. 2016;38:75–85.
65. Vivier E, Tomasello E, Baratin M, Walzer T, Ugolini S. Functions of natural killer cells. *Nat. Immunol*. 2008;9(5):503–510.
66. Lanier LL. NK cell recognition. *Annu. Rev. Immunol*. 2005;23:225–274.
67. Caligiuri MA. Human natural killer cells. *Blood, The Journal of the American Society of Hematology*. 2008;112(3):461–469.
68. Holmskov U, Thiel S, Jensenius JC. Collectins and ficolins: humoral lectins of the innate immune defense. *Annu. Rev. Immunol*. 2003;21(1):547–578.
69. CA J J, Travers P, Walport M, Shlomchik MJ. The complement system and innate immunity, *Immunobiology: The Immune System in Health and Disease*. 5th edition: Garland Science. 2001.
70. Merle NS, Noe R, Halbwachs-Mecarelli L, Fremeaux-Bacchi V, Roumenina LT. Complement system part II: role in immunity. *Front. Immunol*. 2015;6:257.
71. Rother K, Till GO. *The Complement System*: Springer Science & Business Media. 2012.
72. Garred P, Genster N, Pilely K, Bayarri-Olmos R, Rosbjerg A, Ma YJ, et al. A journey through the lectin pathway of complement—MBL and beyond. *Immunol. Rev*. 2016;274(1):74–97.
73. Muller-Eberhard HJ. The membrane attack complex of complement. *Annu. Rev. Immunol*. 1986;4(1):503–528.
74. Bottazzi B, Doni A, Garlanda C, Mantovani A. An integrated view of humoral innate immunity: pentraxins as a paradigm. *Annu. Rev. Immunol*. 2009;28:157–183.
75. van de Wetering JK, van Golde LM, Batenburg JJ. Collectins: players of the innate immune system. *Eur. J. Biochem*. 2004;271(7):1229–1249.
76. Long EO. Antigen processing for presentation to CD4+ T cells. *New Biol*. 1992;4(4):274–282.
77. Blum JS, Wearsch PA. Cresswell P. Pathways of antigen processing. *Annu. Rev. Immunol*. 2013;31: 443–473.
78. Rossjohn J, Gras S, Miles JJ, Turner SJ, Godfrey DI, McCluskey J. T cell antigen receptor recognition of antigen-presenting molecules. *Annu. Rev. Immunol*. 2015;33:169–200.
79. Horton R, Wilming L, Rand V, Lovering RC, Bruford EA, Khodiyar VK, et al. Gene map of the extended human MHC. *Nat. Rev. Genet*. 2004;5(12):889–899.
80. Bjorkman PJ, Saper MA, Samraoui B, Bennett WS, Strominger JL, Wiley DC. Structure of the human class I histocompatibility antigen, HLA-A2. *Nature*. 1987;329(6139):506–512.
81. Monaco JJ. Structure and function of genes in the MHC class II region. *Curr. Opin. Immunol*. 1993;5(1):17–20.
82. Maffei A, Papadopoulos K, Harris PE. MHC class I antigen processing pathways. *Hum. Immunol*. 1997;54(2):91–103.
83. Basler M, Kirk CJ, Groettrup M. The immunoproteasome in antigen processing and other immunological functions. *Curr. Opin. Immunol*. 2013;25(1):74–80.
84. Malnati MS, Marti M, LaVaute T, Jaraquemada D, Biddison W, DeMars R, et al. Processing pathways for presentation of cytosolic antigen to MHC class II-restricted T cells. *Nature*. 1992;357(6380): 702–704.

85. Roche PA, Furuta K. The ins and outs of MHC class II-mediated antigen processing and presentation. *Nat. Rev. Immunol.* 2015;15(4):203–216.
86. Rock KL, Shen L. Cross-presentation: underlying mechanisms and role in immune surveillance. *Immunol. Rev.* 2005;207:166–183.
87. Jung D, Giallourakis C, Mostoslavsky R, Alt FW. Mechanism and control of V(D)J recombination at the immunoglobulin heavy chain locus. *Annu. Rev. Immunol.* 2006;24:541–570.
88. Johnson K, Reddy KL, Singh H. Molecular pathways and mechanisms regulating the recombination of immunoglobulin genes during B-lymphocyte development. *Adv. Exp. Med. Biol.* 2009;650: 133–147.
89. Clark MR, Mandal M, Ochiai K, Singh H. Orchestrating B cell lymphopoiesis through interplay of IL-7 receptor and pre-B cell receptor signalling. *Nat. Rev. Immunol.* 2014;14(2):69–80.
90. Nemazee D. Receptor editing in lymphocyte development and central tolerance. *Nat. Rev. Immunol.* 2006;6(10):728–740.
91. Cerutti A, Cols M, Puga I. Marginal zone B cells: virtues of innate-like antibody-producing lymphocytes. *Nat. Rev. Immunol.* 2013;13(2):118–132.
92. Montecino-Rodriguez E, Dorshkind K. B-1 B cell development in the fetus and adult. *Immunity*. 2012;36(1):13–21.
93. Crotty S. T follicular helper cell differentiation, function, and roles in disease. *Immunity*. 2014;41(4):529–542.
94. Hwang JK, Alt FW, Yeap LS. Related Mechanisms of Antibody Somatic Hypermutation and Class Switch Recombination. *Microbiol Spectr.* 2015;3(1) Mdna3-0037-2014.
95. Nutt SL, Hodgkin PD, Tarlinton DM, Corcoran LM. The generation of antibody-secreting plasma cells. *Nat. Rev. Immunol.* 2015;15(3):160–171.
96. Kurosaki T, Kometani K, Ise W. Memory B cells. *Nat. Rev. Immunol.* 2015;15(3):149–159.
97. Burton DR, Hangartner L. Broadly Neutralizing Antibodies to HIV and Their Role in Vaccine Design. *Annu. Rev. Immunol.* 2016;34:635–659.
98. Corti D, Lanzavecchia A. Broadly neutralizing antiviral antibodies. *Annu. Rev. Immunol.* 2013;31: 705–742.
99. Tofte RW, Peterson PK, Schmeling D, Bracke J, Kim Y, Quie PG. Opsonization of four Bacteroides species: role of the classical complement pathway and immunoglobulin. *Infect. Immun.* 1980;27(3): 784–792.
100. Crotty S. A brief history of T cell help to B cells. *Nat. Rev. Immunol.* 2015;15(3):185–189.
101. Taniuchi I, Ellmeier W. Transcriptional and epigenetic regulation of CD4/CD8 lineage choice. *Adv. Immunol.* 2011;110:71–110.
102. Carpenter AC, Bosselut R. Decision checkpoints in the thymus. *Nat. Immunol.* 2010;11(8):666–673.
103. Singer A, Adoro S, Park JH. Lineage fate and intense debate: myths, models and mechanisms of CD4-versus CD8-lineage choice. *Nat. Rev. Immunol.* 2008;8(10):788–801.
104. Morath A, Schamel WW. αβ and γδ T cell receptors: similar but different. *J. Leukoc. Biol.* 2020;107(6):1045–1055.
105. Lenschow DJ, Walunas TL, Bluestone JA. CD28/B7 system of T cell costimulation. *Annu. Rev. Immunol.* 1996;14:233–258.
106. Acuto O, Michel F. CD28-mediated co-stimulation: a quantitative support for TCR signalling. *Nat. Rev. Immunol.* 2003;3(12):939–951.
107. Harris NL, Ronchese F. The role of B7 costimulation in T-cell immunity. *Immunol. Cell Biol.* 1999;77(4):304–311.
108. Schildberg FA, Klein SR, Freeman GJ, Sharpe AH. Coinhibitory Pathways in the B7-CD28 Ligand-Receptor Family. *Immunity*. 2016;44(5):955–972.
109. Worbs T, Förster R. T cell migration dynamics within lymph nodes during steady state: an overview of extracellular and intracellular factors influencing the basal intranodal T cell motility. *Curr. Top. Microbiol. Immunol.* 2009;334:71–105.
110. Zoncu R, Efeyan A, Sabatini DM. mTOR: from growth signal integration to cancer, diabetes and ageing. *Nat. Rev. Mol. Cell Biol.* 2011;12(1):21–35.
111. Sallusto F, Geginat J, Lanzavecchia A. Central memory and effector memory T cell subsets: function, generation, and maintenance. *Annu. Rev. Immunol.* 2004;22:745–763.

112. Zhu J, Yamane H, Paul WE. Differentiation of effector CD4 T cell populations (*). *Annu. Rev. Immunol.* 2010;28:445–489.
113. Zhou L, Chong MM, Littman DR. Plasticity of CD4+ T cell lineage differentiation. *Immunity.* 2009;30(5):646–655.
114. Mullen AC, High FA, Hutchins AS, Lee HW, Villarino AV, Livingston DM, et al. Role of T-bet in commitment of TH1 cells before IL-12-dependent selection. *Science (New York, NY).* 2001;292(5523):1907–1910.
115. Usui T, Nishikomori R, Kitani A, Strober W. GATA-3 suppresses Th1 development by downregulation of Stat4 and not through effects on IL-12Rbeta2 chain or T-bet. *Immunity.* 2003;18(3):415–428.
116. Lee YK, Mukasa R, Hatton RD, Weaver CT. Developmental plasticity of Th17 and Treg cells. *Curr. Opin. Immunol.* 2009;21(3):274–280.
117. Williams MA, Bevan MJ. Effector and memory CTL differentiation. *Annu. Rev. Immunol.* 2007;25:171–192.
118. Pearce EL, Mullen AC, Martins GA, Krawczyk CM, Hutchins AS, Zediak VP, et al. Control of effector CD8+ T cell function by the transcription factor Eomesodermin. *Science.* 2003;302(5647):1041–1043 (New York, NY).
119. Pipkin ME, Sacks JA, Cruz-Guilloty F, Lichtenheld MG, Bevan MJ, Rao A. Interleukin-2 and inflammation induce distinct transcriptional programs that promote the differentiation of effector cytolytic T cells. *Immunity.* 2010;32(1):79–90.
120. Kaech SM, Cui W. Transcriptional control of effector and memory CD8+ T cell differentiation. *Nat. Rev. Immunol.* 2012;12(11):749–761.
121. Voskoboinik I, Whisstock JC, Trapani JA. Perforin and granzymes: function, dysfunction and human pathology. *Nat. Rev. Immunol.* 2015;15(6):388–400.
122. Wherry EJ, Kurachi M. Molecular and cellular insights into T cell exhaustion. *Nat. Rev. Immunol.* 2015;15(8):486–499.
123. Chien YH, Meyer C, Bonneville M. γδ T cells: first line of defense and beyond. *Annu. Rev. Immunol.* 2014;32:121–155.
124. Godfrey DI, Stankovic S, Baxter AG. Raising the NKT cell family. *Nat. Immunol.* 2010;11(3): 197–206.
125. Godfrey DI, Koay HF, McCluskey J, Gherardin NA. The biology and functional importance of MAIT cells. *Nat. Immunol.* 2019;20(9):1110–1128.
126. Schwartz RH. Historical overview of immunological tolerance. *Cold Spring Harb. Perspect. Biol.* 2012;4(4):a006908.
127. Von Boehmer H, Melchers F. Checkpoints in lymphocyte development and autoimmune disease. *Nat. Immunol.* 2010;11(1):14–20.
128. Mathis D, Benoist C. Back to central tolerance. *Immunity.* 2004;20(5):509–516.
129. Stritesky GL, Jameson SC, Hogquist KA. Selection of self-reactive T cells in the thymus. *Annu. Rev. Immunol.* 2012;30:95–114.
130. Starr TK, Jameson SC, Hogquist KA. Positive and negative selection of T cells. *Annu. Rev. Immunol.* 2003;21(1):139–176.
131. Anderson MS, Su MA. AIRE expands: new roles in immune tolerance and beyond. *Nat. Rev. Immunol.* 2016;16(4):247–258.
132. Mathis D, Aire Be C. *Annu. Rev. Immunol.* 2009;27:287–312.
133. Hsieh C-S, Lee H-M, Lio C-WJ. Selection of regulatory T cells in the thymus. *Nat. Rev. Immunol.* 2012;12(3):157–167.
134. Redmond WL, Sherman LA. Peripheral tolerance of CD8 T lymphocytes. *Immunity.* 2005;22(3): 275–284.
135. Mueller DL. Mechanisms maintaining peripheral tolerance. *Nat. Immunol.* 2010;11(1):21–27.
136. Baxter AG, Hodgkin PD. Activation rules: the two-signal theories of immune activation. *Nat. Rev. Immunol.* 2002;2(6):439–446.
137. Schildberg FA, Klein SR, Freeman GJ, Sharpe AH. Coinhibitory pathways in the B7-CD28 ligand-receptor family. *Immunity.* 2016;44(5):955–972.
138. Walker LS, Sansom DM. The emerging role of CTLA4 as a cell-extrinsic regulator of T cell responses. *Nat. Rev. Immunol.* 2011;11(12):852–863.

139. Okazaki T, Chikuma S, Iwai Y, Fagarasan S, Honjo T. A rheostat for immune responses: the unique properties of PD-1 and their advantages for clinical application. *Nat. Immunol.* 2013;14(12):1212–1218.
140. Wei SC, Duffy CR, Allison JP. Fundamental mechanisms of immune checkpoint blockade therapy. *Cancer Discov.* 2018;8(9):1069–1086.
141. Bilate AM, Lafaille JJ. Induced CD4+ Foxp3+ regulatory T cells in immune tolerance. *Annu. Rev. Immunol.* 2012;30:733–758.
142. Gambineri E, Torgerson TR, Ochs HD. Immune dysregulation, polyendocrinopathy, enteropathy, and X-linked inheritance (IPEX), a syndrome of systemic autoimmunity caused by mutations of FOXP3, a critical regulator of T-cell homeostasis. *Curr. Opin. Rheumatol.* 2003;15(4):430–435.
143. Ohkura N, Kitagawa Y, Sakaguchi S. Development and maintenance of regulatory T cells. *Immunity.* 2013;38(3):414–423.
144. Chaudhry A, Rudensky AY. Control of inflammation by integration of environmental cues by regulatory T cells. *J. Clin. Invest.* 2013;123(3):939–944.
145. Letterio JJ, Roberts AB. Regulation of immune responses by TGF-β. *Annu. Rev. Immunol.* 1998;16(1):137–161.
146. Mosser DM, Zhang X. Interleukin-10: new perspectives on an old cytokine. *Immunol. Rev.* 2008;226(1):205–218.
147. Wing K, Sakaguchi S. Regulatory T cells exert checks and balances on self tolerance and autoimmunity. *Nat. Immunol.* 2010;11(1):7–13.
148. Strasser A, Puthalakath H, O'reilly LA, Bouillet P. What do we know about the mechanisms of elimination of autoreactive T and B cells and what challenges remain. *Immunol. Cell Biol.* 2008;86(1):57–66.
149. Meffre E, Wardemann H. B-cell tolerance checkpoints in health and autoimmunity. *Curr. Opin. Immunol.* 2008;20(6):632–638.
150. Pelanda R, Torres RM. Receptor editing for better or for worse. *Curr. Opin. Immunol.* 2006;18(2):184–190.
151. Nemazee D. Mechanisms of central tolerance for B cells. *Nat. Rev. Immunol.* 2017;17(5):281–294.
152. Fagarasan S, Honjo T. T-Independent immune response: new aspects of B cell biology. *Science.* 2000;290(5489):89–92.
153. Wardemann H, Nussenzweig MC. B-cell self-tolerance in humans. *Adv. Immunol.* 2007;95:83–110.
154. Rathmell JC, Thompson CB. Pathways of apoptosis in lymphocyte development, homeostasis, and disease. *Cell.* 2002;109(2):S97–S107.
155. Kashyap D, Garg VK, Goel N. Intrinsic and extrinsic pathways of apoptosis: role in cancer development and prognosis. *Adv Protein Chem Struct Biol.* 2021;125:73–120.

# CHAPTER 2

# Asthma and Allergy

**Parmida sadat Pezeshki[a,b,c], Ali Nowroozi[a,b], Sepideh Razi[b,d,e], Nima Rezaei[c,e,f]**
[a]School of Medicine, Tehran University of Medical Sciences, Tehran, Iran
[b]Cancer Immunology Project (CIP), Universal Scientific Education and Research Network (USERN), Tehran, Iran
[c]Network of Immunity in Infection, Malignancy and Autoimmunity (NIIMA), Universal Scientific Education and Research Network (USERN), Tehran, Iran
[d]School of Medicine, Iran University of Medical Sciences, Tehran, Iran
[e]Research Center for Immunodeficiencies, Children's Medical Center, Tehran University of Medical Sciences, Tehran, Iran
[f]Department of Immunology, School of Medicine, Tehran University of Medical Sciences, Tehran, Iran

## Introduction

In the nineteenth century, Louis Pasteur et al. introduced a new system named the immune system, which its duty is to protect the body against microorganisms. However, the industrial revolution of Europe and the United States and the use of vaccines and novel injectable drugs resulted in new disorders and reactions which were unknown to physicians.[1] In 1906, a pediatrician named Clemens von Pirquet published an article entitled "Allergie". In this article, he stated that the encounter of the body to a substance leads to antibody production, which can modify the subject's reaction to the substance, and he named it allergy, which comes from Greek words allos and ergia meaning different or other and action or energy, respectively. He mentioned that these changes in subject reaction to the substance could be either protective, which the subject does not show any signs and symptoms after exposure (i.e., actual immune response), or harmful, which the subject develops signs and symptoms of an illness (i.e., hypersensitivity), and he included the patients with asthma, urticaria and hay fever, and subjects who show the unusual immune reaction to antisera and vaccines in this form of the immune response.[2]

Although scientists were interested in studying allergy, its underlying causes were mostly unknown until the 1960s. In that decade, Ishizaka[3] and Johannson[4] independently identified immunoglobulin (Ig)E from the serum of cases with allergy. This discovery showed the molecular cause of the allergy, and it became a basis for more clinical researches.

Allergic diseases are characterized by unfavorable immune responses against allergens, which leads to the development of clinical signs and symptoms of allergy, and they remain a challenge for scientists. According to recent studies, the prevalence of allergic diseases is increasing not only in developed countries but also in developing countries. It is estimated that 25 percent of the population suffers from allergic diseases, which could affect the quality of life and result in a substantial economic burden.[5] Several hypotheses have been proposed to explain the increased prevalence of allergic disorders, such as the hygiene hypothesis, and biodiversity hypothesis or microflora hypothesis.[6,7] According

*Clinical Immunology*
DOI: https://doi.org/10.1016/B978-0-12-818006-8.00002-5

to the hygiene hypothesis, due to lifestyle changes, the incidence of infectious diseases decreased among people, which is correlated with an increased prevalence of allergic and autoimmune diseases. The microflora hypothesis declares that dysbiosis that happens early in life leads to immune dysregulation, which could increase the susceptibility to allergic diseases.

This chapter aims to review the definition, epidemiology, clinical features, diagnosis and treatment of asthma, allergic rhinitis, allergic conjunctivitis, urticaria and angioedema, atopic dermatitis, and allergic contact dermatitis, food allergy and gastrointestinal syndromes, drug allergy, and anaphylaxis.

## Asthma

### Definition and classifications

Asthma (also called bronchial asthma) is an extremely heterogeneous condition, usually associated with chronic inflammation of airways.[8-10] Inflammation-induced swelling and edema result in the narrowing of the airways, which in turn causes breathing difficulties. Therefore, asthma is considered an obstructive pulmonary disease.

Asthma presents in different manners (i.e., phenotypes). A common classification is dividing asthma into allergic (atopic) and non-allergic asthma. Allergic asthma is the most common phenotype[11] and is characterized by high levels of IgE (the hallmark of allergic asthma) and a high number of type 2 T helper (Th) cells as a reaction to certain allergens.[11,12] Atopic asthma most frequently occurs in the younger population, and the development of asthma in older age is usually indicative of other sub-types. Non-allergic asthma is further divided into different phenotypes (e.g., smoking-related, obesity-related, and exercise-induced asthma).[12,13] Late-onset eosinophilic asthma is a type of non-allergic asthma, involving high Th2 and eosinophil counts but low IgE levels. Compared with allergic asthma, it is more severe, presents in the older population, and is usually resistant to steroid treatment.[13]

Another method of subtyping asthma is based on the dominant immune cell population rather than clinical features (i.e., endotypes). This classification, introduced in 1999,[14] divided asthma into Th2-high and Th2-low endotypes. In Th2-high asthma, type 2 inflammatory pathways (described later on in this chapter) result in eosinophilic inflammation, while in Th2-low asthma, other cells such as neutrophils are involved.[15] Assessment of Th2-mediated inflammation laboratory features is commonly done by sputum analysis,[15] and sputum eosinophilia is the most prominent characteristic.[16]

### Epidemiology and risk factors

Asthma is relatively common.[9] Approximately 3.5 percent of people are already diagnosed with the disease, and more than 40 million people are diagnosed each year globally.[17] Asthma is more frequent in children, as 36 percent of new cases are below five years of age.[17] Moreover, females are at a higher risk of developing asthma than males (Odds Ratio (OR), 1.06).[17]

Due to similarities between mucosal linings of the respiratory tract and some other sites such as the middle ear, nasal cavity, and lower airways, and their similar chronic inflammation patterns,[18] some mucosal diseases are common in patients with asthma. The two most common conditions that co-exist with asthma are allergic rhinitis and sinusitis, with a prevalence of 73–79 percent among asthmatic patients.[19,20]

If a person develops asthma during childhood, it might resolve later in life but could also persist through adulthood.[16] As a multi-factorial disease,[21] several risk factors have been identified for asthma development and the chance of persisting through adulthood, including genetics, gender, exposure to tobacco, specific types of respiratory and gastrointestinal tract microbiome, and air pollutions.[16,21-24] If atopy is present in a child, there is a 4 to 20 fold increase in the chance of developing allergic asthma.[25,26] Recently, stress (both before and after birth) has also been suggested as a potential risk factor for asthma development.[27] According to some studies, severe viral respiratory infections in childhood might also increase the risk of asthma development.[28] However, frequent exposure to microbes in childhood is thought to reduce asthma incidence by training the body to produce a less severe response to foreign agents such as allergens (i.e., hygiene hypothesis).[22-24] A study on murine showed that microbial exposure reduces inflammation caused by allergies via interleukin (IL)−10-associated inhibitory pathways.[29]

## Etiology and pathogenesis

### *Etiology*

Asthma is a result of a wide range of interactions between the respiratory system and the immune system, many of which are still unknown. Multiple biological, environmental, and genetic elements contribute to asthma development.

### Genetics

Genetics seems to have an essential role in asthma development, with an estimated heritability of 35–95 percent.[30] Multiple gene loci are thought to affect the chance of asthma development, including protein folding genes (e.g., ORMDL3 and GSDBM), atopy genes (e.g., IL-4, FCR1A, and CYF1P2), and epithelial genes (e.g., IRAKIM, toll-like receptor (TLR)-associated genes, and GSTP1).[31,32]

### Epigenetics

DNA methylation, histone modifications, and mitochondrial RNA modifications are all examples of epigenetic changes, which lead to gene expression regulation in the absence of DNA sequence alteration. Epigenetic changes are associated with inflammatory disturbances. DNA methylation, which is related to tobacco smoke exposure, could inhibit the transcription of anti-inflammatory factors.[32,33] Histone modification, on the other hand, acts by modifying T cell profiles.[32]

## Viral infections

It has been reported that if an infant experiences a severe infection with the respiratory syncytial virus, there is a 20 percent chance of developing asthma in the future.[34]

### *Pathogenesis*

The pathophysiology of asthma comprises numerous complex mechanisms and their components, of which the most significant ones are discussed below.

## Inflammation

As stated earlier, inflammation of the airways is the cornerstone of asthma pathogenesis. Although there are several mechanisms responsible for airway inflammation,[35] Th2-mediated inflammation (i.e., type 2 inflammation) is the predominant pathway.[16] In allergic asthma, the inflammation is induced by allergic sensitization.[36] Type 2 inflammation, which is responsible for the manifestations of many atopic diseases,[32] comprises activation of a variety of immune cells such as Th2 cells, basophils, mast cells, and plasma cells along with the production of specific substances, namely IL-4, IL-5, and IL-13.[11,37] These cytokines are responsible for naïve T cell to Th2 differentiation, eosinophil maturation and its release into the circulation, and proliferation of epithelial cells and IgE producing B lymphocytes, respectively.[38-40] Eosinophils are also maintained and activated by the granulocyte-macrophage colony-stimulating factor (GM-CSF). In vitro studies show that GM-CSF could provoke eosinophil activation when incubated with adhesion molecules such as vascular cell adhesion molecule (VCAM)−1 and intracellular adhesion molecule (ICAM)−1, even when IL-5 is not present (i.e., the VCAM-1/CC chemokines/GM-CSF pathway).[41] The role of each of the mentioned elements in producing asthma clinical manifestations will be described later in this chapter.

In some non-allergic cases, especially neutrophilic asthma, a disruption in the innate immune system results in activation of an IL-17-mediated pathway involving Th1 and Th17 cells, consequently initiating the inflammation.[11] Neutrophils are recruited into the lungs as a result of IL-17 production. Furthermore, IL-17 results in airway hyperresponsiveness (AHR) in patients with non-allergic asthma.[11] In patients with severe neutrophilic asthma, elevated levels of interferon (IFN)-γ and tumor necrosis factor (TNF)-α levels are observed,[42] both contributing to inflammation and AHR.[43,44] Also, it has been reported that high IFN-γ levels, along with low secretory leukocyte protease inhibitor (SLPI) titers are a sign of severe asthma.[45]

Eosinophilic non-allergic asthma is another non-atopic asthma variant. This phenotype usually has a late-onset, presents severely, and is resistant to high dose steroid therapy.[11,46] Type 2 innate lymphoid cells (ILCs) are crucial in developing eosinophilic non-allergic asthma[11] and, the Th2 pathway is absent in this phenotype. However, ILC2s precipitate eosinophil recruitment via IL-5 and IL-13 production, which is stimulated by the release of prostaglandin (PG)D2, IL-33, IL-25, and thymic stromal lymphopoietin (TSLP) as a result of epithelial injury. Air pollutants and microorganisms are two common causes of epithelial damage in these patients.[11,36] Additionally, levels of lipoxin A4, which is a suppressor of eosinophil-induced inflammation, are reduced in eosinophilic non-allergic asthma, which is another contributing factor.[47]

All of the mechanisms mentioned above and phenotypes might overlap and lead to a mixed pattern of granulocytic inflammation or change from one phenotype to another over time.[36]

## Tissue remodeling

The pathological changes that happen during asthma and asthma attacks in airways are called tissue remodeling. (Histologically, airways are mostly modified during exacerbations and are only minimally changed in between them.).[32,48] In the mucosal layer, hyperplasia of the epithelium and goblet cell metaplasia (resulting in mucus hypersecretion) occur (goblet cell metaplasia is not present in Th2-low endotypes).[49,50] It has been reported that changes in the mucosal layer are correlated with asthma severity.[51] In the submucosal layer, smooth muscles undergo hypertrophic changes, collagen deposition occurs, and large mucous glands are increased, leading to narrowing of the airways and increased mucus production.[37] Moreover, the thickening of the basement membrane is visible in asthmatic patients, probably due to myofibroblasts' activity.[52] However, its exact pathophysiology is not yet fully understood, and it seems to be unrelated to levels of Th2 cytokines.[53]

## IgE

Atopic asthma is initiated by exposure to an allergen in a susceptible individual. When the allergen enters the body, it is received by the immune system, mainly Th2 cells, and subsequently, a cascade of immune responses starts.[11] IgEs produced by plasma cells attaches to surfaces of basophils, mast cells, and eosinophils, acting as a receptor for the allergen in future encounters. Polycyclic aromatic hydrocarbons that are found in air pollutants could also lead to increased IgE production.[54] Upon re-entry, the allergen binds to its specific IgE, which causes the release of substances such as leukotrienes from cytoplasmic granules of the mentioned cells. These mediators act on their target cells and produce clinical manifestations of asthma such as AHR and mucus secretion (i.e., type 1 hypersensitivity).[48] IgE also plays many other roles in asthma development,[11] such as amplifying allergen-based Th2 activation,[55] directly activating eosinophils, inducing the release of granular substances,[56] and promoting cytokine release from airway smooth muscles, which the latter triggers airway remodeling by inducing the contraction and proliferation of the smooth muscles.[57]

### Mast cells

Mast cells play a significant role in asthma development, mainly by producing and releasing proteases (e.g., growth factors and tryptase).[11] These substances induce smooth muscle changes, hypersecretion of mucus, and tissue remodeling in airways.[58] Moreover, in severe asthma cases, mast cells produce high amounts of PGD2.[59] PGD2, in turn, attaches to its receptors (D prostanoid and Th2 chemoattractant receptor-homologous molecule (CRTH2)) on Th2 cells and leading to the development of asthma manifestations such as airway inflammation and airway obstruction.[60,61] Although mast cells are increased in non-allergic asthma, they are more abundant and more active in the allergic phenotype.[62,63]

### Eosinophils

Similar to mast cells, eosinophils participate in the development of asthma by releasing specific substances including leukotrienes, major basic protein (MBP), eosinophil peroxidase (EPO), eosinophil cationic protein (ECP), eosinophil-derived neurotoxin (EDN), transforming growth factor (TGF)-β and IL-5.[64] In patients with asthma, the number of eosinophils is not only elevated in circulation but also it is increased in airway tissue, which is an important factor in the pathogenesis of bronchial asthma.[65] Eosinophil recruitment and maintenance is mainly caused by Th2 cells and leukotrienes.[11,66] Th2 lymphocytes produce IL-4 and IL-13 that increase endothelial expression ofVCAM-1. VCAM-1 mediates eosinophils' adhesion to the endothelium.[67] After adhesion, leukotrienes, especially leukotriene D4, cause the migration of eosinophils through the endothelium into the tissue and, later on, the release of cytoplasmic protein-containing granules from eosinophils.[68] Leukotrienes are also involved in airway remodeling (e.g., increase in smooth muscle mass)[69] together with TGF-β. Another possible role of eosinophils in asthma's pathogenesis is by promoting AHR that is most likely induced by MBPs.[70] However, some studies indicate that eosinophilic inflammation in the airways is not correlated with AHR.[71-73]

### Epithelium

Because of the physiologic changes in asthmatic patients, the airway epithelium's function differs from that of the normal population. In patients with allergic asthma, airway epithelial cells release TSLP, IL-25, and IL-33 secondary to epithelial damage.[74] Large amounts of TSLP in the lungs results in AHR[74] and IL-25 and IL-33 production that leads to an increase in type 2 inflammatory cytokines (e.g., IL-4, IL-5, and IL-13).[75] IL-4 and IL-13 further damage the epithelium,[76] and the cycle is repeated. Additionally, epithelial damage causes ciliary dysfunction that, in turn, leads to pulmonary malfunction and AHR.[77]

## Clinical features

Asthma symptoms are mainly related to obstruction of airways.[32] Due to pathological mechanisms described above, AHR and airway remodeling occur, resulting in the airways' tightening.

### History

The most prominent asthma symptoms are dyspnea, wheezing, chest tightness, cough, and airway obstruction.[9,10] There is usually more than one symptom present in typical asthma cases, and symptoms are worsened at night or early morning. Although the underlying inflammatory process is thought to be continuous,[32] symptoms might not always present but rather appear intermittently. Episodes of acute at relatively severe symptom presentations are called asthma exacerbations (or attacks), which are variable in degree and time. These characteristics are extremely valuable in diagnosing asthma. It is noteworthy that the frequency of exacerbations is not correlated with their intensity.[20] Certain factors trigger asthma attacks, such as viral infections, weather, exercising, atopic encounters, tobacco smoke, and chemical irritant stimuli.[9,32,78] Approximately 50 percent of asthma cases experience at least one exacerbation annually, and patients younger than 18 years old, children with reduced FEV1, females, and black race (compared to white) experience asthma attacks more frequently.[32,79]

Wheezing in children could be categorized into three groups: 1) transient early wheezing, which resolves within the first 3 to 5 years of life and is independent of family history or atopy, 2) non-atopic wheezing, which persists into adolescence and is a result of viral respiratory infections until the age of 3 rather than allergic sensitization, and 3) atopic wheezing, which is IgE mediated as related to AHR.[80] In one-third of asthmatic children who present wheezing among their symptoms, wheezing continues through adulthood. Risk factors for wheezing persistence and relapse include atopic sensitivity, female sex, and smoking.[80]

Apart from the cardinal symptoms mentioned above, early-onset allergic asthma is often accompanied by eczema, rhinitis, food allergy, or coughing and wheezing during viral respiratory diseases. A family history of asthma might also be present.[36] Allergic rhinitis is seen in both allergic and non-allergic asthma cases. Nearly 80 percent of all asthmatic patients also have allergic rhinitis.[81]

### Clinical findings

Airflow obstruction is one of the main characteristics of asthma,[32] howbeit, the constriction is reversible to some degree (except in a portion of severe cases),[82] either by the cessation of the attack or medical treatment. The reversible nature of the airway obstruction is crucial in the diagnosis of asthma.[32] Hyperinflation of lungs and thoracic hyperexpansion as a consequence of airflow obstruction is evident upon physical examination and imaging.[20] In thoracic CT imaging of severe asthmatic patients, bronchiectasis and thickening of the bronchial walls are evident, with a higher prevalence of bronchiectasis in smokers.[83]

In severe and especially fatal asthma exacerbation cases, mucus clearing is impaired, and mucus plugs form in the airways.[16]

Due to its atopic nature, skin prick test or specific IgE testing is positive in patients with allergic asthma.[84]

## Diagnosis

The diagnosis of asthma is made based on a detailed history, clinical testing of airflow obstruction, and exclusion of other diagnoses.[9,10] Testing usually includes lung function tests (i.e., spirometry or peak expiratory flow (PEF)), with forced expiratory volume in 1 s (FEV1) and FEV1/FVC (forced vital capacity) being the main determinants of expiratory airflow obstruction. An FEV1/FVC ratio above 0.75–0.80 in adults and 0.9 in children is considered normal.[85] Due to the intermittent nature of asthma symptoms, pulmonary evaluation is more beneficial during or after attacks.[36] Decreased FEV1 and FEV1/FVC ratio, along with clinical symptoms, are suggestive of asthma (sole reduction of FEV1 is not sufficient as it is common in many other pulmonary diseases). To further strengthen the diagnosis of asthma, a test that is indicative of variability in airway obstruction is required. The test may either increase or reduce FEV1 after specific challenges, and if FEV1 is altered by a reasonable degree, it reflects the presence of variable airflow limitation. Tests that result in elevated FEV1 include bronchodilator reversibility test and anti-inflammatory trial test. On the other hand, exercise challenge test and bronchial challenge test (by methacholine or histamine) are expected to reduce FEV1. If FEV1 greatly varies between visits or PEF is highly inconsistent over two weeks, it could also be in favor of asthma.[9] For children under six in whom asthma symptoms are frequently associated with viral infections and spirometry is unreliable, a corticosteroid and bronchodilator trial helps establish the diagnosis.[86] It is best if diagnostic procedures are initiated before corticosteroid administration, although many patients happen to be on controller medications based on the initial diagnosis of asthma in primary care. In such cases, patients must be classified and tested according to symptoms and airflow obstruction severity.[9]

## Differential diagnosis

Differential diagnoses of asthma include but are not limited to foreign body aspiration, chronic obstructive pulmonary disease (COPD), gastroesophageal reflux disease (GERD), cystic fibrosis, and other cough-producing etiologies.[10,20] Cough-producing inflammatory diseases such as allergic rhinitis and sinusitis should differentially diagnosed from asthma. The absence of wheezing, no early morning symptoms, and resistance to asthma treatment, in addition to other allergic rhinitis futures such as nasal blockage and sneezing, make the diagnosis of asthma unlikely.[87]

GERD is one of the most common etiologies of chronic cough, and in some cases, could also result in wheezing. A careful history and relation of symptoms to nutritional habits help distinguish asthma from GERD.[87]

Symptoms starting from early infancy suggest a genetic disorder such as cystic fibrosis, primary ciliary dyskinesia (PCD), and immunodeficiency diseases.[88] In patients with PCD, recurrent respiratory infections alter the physiology of the lungs. Additionally, mucus hypersecretion and some pathophysiological changes occur that are also present in asthma, such as smooth muscle hypertrophy. The result of these alterations is an obstructive pattern in spirometry, which is also a sign of asthma. Therefore, many of PCD cases are incorrectly diagnosed as chronic asthma, which turns out to be refractory to classic asthma treatments. If PCD remains undiagnosed, frequent infections will inevitably lead to bronchiectasis and, therefore, must be ruled out. Measurement of nasal nitric oxide is an acceptable screening method for PCD, in which levels of nasal nitric oxide are significantly reduced compared with healthy individuals.[88,89]

Cystic fibrosis and diffuse bronchiectasis could produce chronic coughs, and sputum hyperproduction differentiates them from asthma.[88] Another prominent sign of cystic fibrosis is recurrent infections, further strengthening the diagnosis. The diagnosis of cystic fibrosis can be confirmed by a sweat chloride test.[87]

If antibiotic therapy is turning out to be effective in a patient with a chronic wet cough, the diagnosis is most likely protracted bacterial bronchitis (PBB).[88] Similar to PCD, untreated PBB might also cause bronchiectasis in children.

Physical examination revealing one-sided thoracic sounds, together with an acute onset of respiratory symptoms, points towards foreign body aspiration.[88]

Preschool children with very few episodes of wheezing or dry coughs should not be hastily diagnosed with asthma but rather questioned about other symptoms, presumably revealing upper respiratory tract infection. These symptoms are likely to disappear at school age.[88]

## Treatment

In the treatment of asthma, the aim is to reduce symptoms and unfavorable outcomes. The therapeutic course of asthma is continuous and requires persistent follow-up, assessment, and modification.[9] Two basic principles apply when selecting appropriate asthma treatment for a patient: controlling current symptoms and preventing future adverse events. While single-drug therapy with short-acting beta-agonists (SABAs) was previously recommended for patients with few symptoms, SABA monotherapy is no longer advised in adolescents and adults, according to the Global Initiative for Asthma (GINA) guidelines.[9] Therefore, inhaled corticosteroids (ICS) are now the mainstay of treatment in all patients over the age of 11. Corticosteroids reduce inflammation in respiratory tissues and inhibit mucus hypersecretion. Additionally, they have little side-effects (especially when inhaled), and on the other hand, numerous advantages. Corticosteroids reduce symptom occurrence, the frequency of exacerbations, and mortality and increase the quality of life in asthmatic patients.[10,90-92] Thus, it is most beneficial if corticosteroids are initiated at the time of diagnosis, as delaying steroid treatment leads to diminished lung function and the requirement of higher doses in the future.[9,93-95]

Determinants for treatment-of-choice in an asthma case are symptom frequency, and less importantly, symptom severity (Table 2.1). GINA guidelines treatment recommendations for children (age 6–11) are slightly different from those of adolescents and

**Table 2.1** GINA initial pharmacological treatment recommendations for patients with asthma (age ≥6).

| | | Disease severity | | | |
|---|---|---|---|---|---|
| | | Infrequent symptoms and no risk of exacerbation | Symptoms' occurrence ≥ twice a month but not on most days | Symptoms on most days causing trouble or night-time awakening ≥once a week; particularly if the patient has any risk factors for exacerbation | Severe symptoms or presenting with acute exacerbation |
| **Age group** | >11 | Low dose ICS–formoterol when needed | Controller low dose ICS + SABA when needed<br>Or<br>Low dose ICS–formoterol when needed | Controller low dose ICS–LABA + ICS–formoterol or SABA when needed<br>Or<br>Controller medium–dose ICS + SABA when needed | Controller high dose ICS<br>Or<br>Controller medium–dose ICS–LABA<br>Oral corticosteroids may also be considered |
| | 6–11 | SABA when needed | Controller low dose ICS + SABA when needed | Controller low dose ICS-LABA + SABA when needed<br>Or<br>Controller medium-dose ICS + SABA when needed | Controller medium-dose ICS-LABA + SABA when needed<br>Oral corticosteroids may also be considered |

GINA, Global Initiative for Asthma; ICS, Inhaled corticosteroid; SABA, Short-acting beta-agonist; LABA, Long-acting beta-agonist; LAMA, long-acting muscarinic antagonist; LTRA, leukotriene receptor antagonist.

adults (age >11).[9] For example, as previously mentioned, SABA monotherapy is not recommended in patients >11 years old. However, children age 6–11 with minimal symptoms could be treated with as needed SABA alone.

Generally, asthma medications are classified into two categories: a) controller treatments, which must be taken routinely to prevent future symptoms and exacerbations, and b) symptom relievers, taken when needed. According to GINA guidelines, ICS-formoterol (formoterol is a long-acting beta-agonist (LABA),) and SABAs are the advised symptom relievers in patients above and below 11 years of age, respectively.

Both before and after initiating treatment, disease status, represented by symptoms and lung function, must be recorded. Medications might be stepped-up or stepped-down according to the patient's response.

### *GINA guidelines*

#### Patients >11 years old

For a patient with very few symptom occurrences and no risk of exacerbations, low dose ICS-LABA (usually ICS-formoterol) when needed has been suggested. If the patient has symptoms or needs to use symptom reliever twice a month or more, controller low dose ICS plus as needed SABA or as needed low dose ICS-formoterol is recommended.[9] If symptoms are frequent or wake the patient up once a week or more, particularly if the patient has any risk factors for asthma exacerbation, low dose ICS-LABA for maintenance plus ICS-formoterol or SABA as needed is an effective treatment. Controller medium-dose ICS plus SABA, when needed, is also an alternative approach.[9] Severe asthma symptoms or presenting with acute exacerbation urges treatment with high dose ICS or medium-dose ICS-LABA, and even oral corticosteroids on a case-by-case basis.[9]

#### Patients between 6 and 11 years old

While ICS-formoterol is the recommended symptom reliever in older patients, SABAs are preferred in children. In children with infrequent symptoms (<2 symptoms per month), the physician may either prescribe no maintenance treatment or low dose ICS as the controller. Children who experience symptoms or require reliever more than twice per month but not on most days are recommended to be controlled by low dose ICS combined with as needed SABA. Presentation of troublesome symptoms on most days, or at least one night-time awakening per week because of symptoms, especially if accompanied by risk factors, requires treatment with controller low dose ICS-LABA or medium-dose ICS, plus reliever SABA. At last, in cases with most severe symptoms, treatment comprises controller medium-dose ICS-LABA, as needed SABA, and for selected patients, oral corticosteroids.[9]

### *Novel therapies*

Other than bronchodilators and steroids that have been the classic treatment options for asthma, newly developed drugs are under development, targeting specific cytokine pathways and molecules involved in asthmatic inflammatory processes (e.g., IL-4, IL-5, IL-13, and IL-17 pathways).[69] However, all are yet to be approved, except Omalizumab, an anti-IgE monoclonal antibody approved as an alternative option for refractory atopic asthma.[69]

### *Non-pharmacological treatments*

Patients with asthma are encouraged to stop tobacco usage, engage in physical activities, and avoid or limit exposure to allergens.[9] Subcutaneous or sublingual immunotherapy (SCIT and SLIT, respectively) for allergies might be helpful in selected cases, especially in those with co-existent rhinoconjunctivitis.[9]

### *Severe and difficult to treat asthma cases*

Further evaluation is required if a patient is still experiencing symptoms or is only controlled under the most aggressive treatments. It is estimated that 5 percent–10 percent of all asthma cases are severe.[96] The most severe cases often have a mixed eosinophilic-neutrophilic pattern in sputum cytology.[97] As a preliminary evaluation, it must be confirmed that the patient is, in fact, a severe asthma case, as 12 percent–30 percent of patients do not have severe asthma, and another etiology is causing their symptoms.[98,99] A detailed medication history must be taken to ensure proper usage of the given medicine. Studies show that 32 percent–56 percent of patients do not take their medicine properly.[96] If any underlying comorbidities are present, which might contribute to a worsened asthma degree, they must be controlled or treated. Finally, if no other measures succeed, the patient must be referred for asthma phenotyping, which provides a more informative insight into the disease. Consequently, more phenotype-specific therapies could be implemented, resulting in better control of the condition.[9] Severe asthma cases are frequently referred to as "corticosteroid resistant", which is not completely true, and 89 percent of cases respond to corticosteroids to some extent.[100] It has been reported that treatment with intramuscular triamcinolone can reduce sputum eosinophilia and improve FEV1 in patients with severe asthma.[101,102] Furthermore, novel therapies, including anti-IgEs and anti-interleukins, are being developed and studied in terms of effectiveness, which have the potential to replace traditional therapies in the treatment of severe asthma cases.[96]

### *Management of asthma exacerbations*

After confirmation of an asthma exacerbation, severity must be determined. In mild to moderate exacerbations, the patient can talk in phrases and has increased respiratory rate but is not agitated. Slight tachycardia might also be present, and O2 saturation is 90 percent–95 percent. Severe attacks are characterized by a very high respiratory rate (>30), a heart rate of >120 bpm, and O2 saturation of <90 percent. The patient is usually able to talk in words, but not phrases, is agitated, and uses accessory respiratory muscles. PEF may decrease to ≤50 percent of predicted value or personal best. Drowsiness, confusion, and silent chest indicate a life-threatening condition, and the patient should be promptly transferred to the intensive care unit.[9]

SABA must be administered for every patient with mild to moderate exacerbation and could also be considered in more severe attacks, although evidence is weak for these cases. Dosage and frequency may be altered after at least one hour of treatment, depending on the patient's response.[9]

Oral corticosteroid must be administered for all patients experiencing exacerbations, except for extremely mild attacks. Oral corticosteroid initiation is especially valuable in patients with deteriorating conditions and those who have increased their medication before presenting. Due to the similar effectiveness of oral and intravenous routes and a higher risk of complications when administering intravenously, oral corticosteroids are preferred and must be continued for a few days.[9] If oral corticosteroid is unavailable, the high-dose inhaled corticosteroid is a reasonable alternative, which reduces hospitalization if administered within one hour after the presentation.[9]

$O_2$ saturation must be kept under 96 percent (93 percent−95 percent) to prevent hypercapnia and respiratory failure. Even in settings where pulse oximetry is unavailable, oxygen therapy should be applied. In such scenarios, the patient must be monitored for worsening status and deterioration. Furthermore, titrated oxygen is a superior choice to 100 percent oxygen, as it has proven to be less fatal and more beneficial in terms of outcomes.[9]

Symptoms and respiratory function should be monitored regularly and closely. An FEV1 or PEF of 60 percent−80 percent of predicted or personal best, along with symptom improvement, indicates a favorable clinical response, and the patient might be considered for discharge.[9]

## Allergic rhinitis

### Definition

Rhinitis is the inflammation of the nasal mucosal membrane, characterized by the presence of a minimum of two nasal symptoms (e.g., rhinorrhea, blockage, sneezing, and itching).[103,104] Allergic rhinitis results from an IgE mediated response to an allergen.[103] Depending on how a patient encounters the allergen, allergic rhinitis could be classified into seasonal (i.e., hay fever, in which pollens act as allergens), perennial (in which allergens are persistent throughout the year, such as dust mites), and episodic (in which the patient sporadically encounters the allergen, such as a pet of another person) phenotypes.[105,106] However, this classification is not accurate enough, as many perennial cases may not present symptoms all year long, or in some highly sensitive patients, even minimal levels of pollen in the air might cause atopic symptoms. Therefore, since 2001, allergic rhinitis and its impact on asthma (ARIA) guidelines recommend categorizing allergic rhinitis based on symptom duration and frequency into intermittent and persistent allergic rhinitis. Persistent allergic rhinitis is defined as the presence of symptoms for at least four weeks in a row and at least five days per week. If symptoms do not occur for four consecutive weeks or happen only four days or less, the patient is classified into the intermittent allergic rhinitis group.[106] The systemic atopic process causing allergic rhinitis is also related to other allergic diseases such as asthma, allergic conjunctivitis, and rhinosinusitis.[103]

### Epidemiology and risk factors

Allergic rhinitis is the most prevalent allergic condition in the United States.[104] It is estimated that 10 percent to 40 percent of people have allergic rhinitis,[104,107] and its prevalence has been growing throughout the years, and given the fact that many cases do not seek treatment from a physician and are self-treated, actual numbers are expected to be higher than the ones reported.[104]

In 80 percent of allergic rhinitis cases, symptom presentation starts before 20 years of age.[104] Allergic rhinitis affects adult men and women equally, although, in children, it is more frequent in boys.[108]

Family history and genetics are two important risk factors for allergic rhinitis development,[109] with ORs for positive family history reaching as high as 6 in some studies.[110] Allergic rhinitis is highly associated with asthma. Studies show that 50–85 percent of asthma patients have AR, and on the other hand, allergic rhinitis cases are six times more likely to have asthma.[104,111] Additionally, alcohol drinkers and smokers are at a higher chance of being diagnosed with allergic rhinitis.[109] Moreover, the presence of dust mites, fungi, mold, and some other allergens have also been associated with a higher allergic rhinitis prevalence.[109]

## Pathogenesis

Allergic rhinitis is the result of a typical atopic reaction.[104] Initially, dendritic cells located in the mucosal membrane of the nasal cavity catch the inhaled allergens and present them to naïve helper T (Th0) cells. This interaction precipitates Th0 differentiation into type Th2 lymphocytes.[112] Th2-mediated inflammation induces a cascade of events, including secretion of multiple cytokines such as IL-4, IL-15 and, IL-13, which are the hallmarks of Th2 response. IL-4 triggers IgE production by lymphocytes and plasma cells, while IL-5 is responsible for recruiting and maintaining the eosinophil population. IgEs then, in turn, attach to the surface of basophils and mast cells, now acting as receptors for the allergen. Upon allergen attachment to the now receptor-acting IgEs, substances such as histamine, leukotrienes, PGs, and tumor necrosis factors are released, contributing to the manifestation of early symptoms (e.g., sneezing, rhinorrhea, and itching) by increasing mucus secretion, vascular permeability, and smooth muscle contraction.[112] Following activation of basophils and mast cells, other immune cells such as macrophages, eosinophils, and neutrophils migrate to the nasal region, giving rise to the late phase of the inflammatory reaction, which occurs 4–6 h after initial exposure to the allergen and includes further production of inflammatory mediators.[113,114] The most prominent symptom of the late phase reaction is nasal blockage.[114]

## Clinical features

A family history of atopic diseases might be present in patients with allergic rhinitis.[109] The most common allergic rhinitis symptoms include nasal blockage, rhinorrhea, sneezing, and nasal itching.[104] If itchy and watery eyes are present, it is due to allergic conjunctivitis, which is commonly associated with allergic rhinitis.[104] Symptoms usually start within minutes of exposure to the allergen and last for hours. Nasal obstruction and hypersensitivity, postnasal discharge, and hyposmia are among the late-phase symptoms.[114] While adolescents and adults are capable of clearing their nasal cavity from secretions by blowing their nose, younger children usually try to do it by coughing, snorting, or sniffing.[104]

Vasodilator agents produced in the nasal cavity, resulting in congestion and might cause venous dilation in the periorbital region, manifesting as allergic shiners.[104]

## Diagnosis

Allergic rhinitis is speculated in any patient with typical allergic symptoms (e.g., sneezing, rhinorrhea, nasal obstruction, and nasal itching), especially if at least two symptoms are present for an hour on most days.[115] Accordingly, a thorough history is invaluable in diagnosing AR. Identifying a possible allergen responsible for the symptoms or a positive family history further guides us towards diagnosing allergic rhinitis.[104] Smokes, fumes, and some chemical substances are among agents that might be assumed as allergens. However, their irritant nature is more dominant than their allergic characteristics and generally are not associated with allergic rhinitis.[105] Many other atopic conditions tend to co-exist with AR, such as asthma and allergic conjunctivitis. The presence of these conditions raises the possibility of allergic rhinitis co-existence.[104]

Erythematous epithelium and swollen turbinates might be found upon physical examination of the nasal cavity.[104] In suspected cases with nasal blockage, alternative etiologies for nasal obstruction such as nasal polyps could be identified, ruling out allergic rhinitis as the diagnosis.[104] In some patients, the eustachian tube might be partially blocked due to swelling of the nasal mucosa, manifesting in tympanic membrane dysfunction detected by pneumatic otoscopy, although otoscopic studies are generally normal in allergic rhinitis patients.[104,116]

While some studies suggest confirmation of diagnosis with allergy testing,[103,114] others believe that testing is not required in all cases, but only for patients resistant to empiric treatment and target therapy candidates(105). Two common means of allergy testing are skin testing (either via skin prick test or intradermal test) and serum-specific IgE level measurement.[104]

Rhinitis has numerous sub-types, and all should be kept in mind when investigating for allergic rhinitis. Allergic conjunctivitis is a key factor in differentiating allergic rhinitis from other rhinitis subtypes.[114] Moreover, positive allergy tests are indicative of allergic rhinitis.[114]

## Differential diagnosis

The most common etiology of non-allergic rhinitis is non-allergic rhinopathy (71 percent of non-allergic rhinitis cases). Another name for this condition is vasomotor rhinitis. However, inflammation does not play a major role in its pathogenesis (although neurosensory irregularities do), and therefore, non-allergic rhinopathy is the preferred term. Non-allergic rhinopathy is a chronic disease and mainly manifests by rhinorrhea. Other symptoms include nasal congestion, postnasal drip, and cough. Nevertheless, non-allergic rhinopathy is a diagnosis of exclusion and is suspected when other conditions that could cause the same symptoms, such as chronic rhinosinusitis, infectious rhinitis, and anatomical abnormalities, are ruled out.[107,117]

Occupational rhinitis is another differential diagnosis of allergic rhinitis. It could be allergic or non-allergic and is related to workplace exposure.[114] A history of recent systemic medication is suggestive of drug-induced rhinitis.[107] Patients who have used topical intranasal decongestants for a long period are at risk of developing rhinitis medicamentosa, characterized by typical rhinitis symptoms along with chronic nasal blockage and poor shrinkage of nasal mucosa on physical examination.[107,118] Infectious rhinitis could have a viral (up to 98 percent of cases in children) or bacterial etiology and are not routinely associated with nasal itching or sneezing. Also, cervical lymphadenopathy and pharyngitis are suggestive of an infectious cause.[119]

Viral upper respiratory infections are among differential diagnoses of AR, although unlike AR, patients with viral upper respiratory infections are likely to develop fever or myalgia.[105]

Systemic rheumatologic diseases such as granulomatosis with polyangiitis, eosinophilic granulomatosis with polyangiitis (i.e., Churg-Strauss syndrome), sarcoidosis, and systemic lupus erythematosus could present with upper respiratory and sinonasal symptoms. Recurrent epistaxis, disruption of the nasal septum, pain over the dorsum of the nose, crusting, and anosmia are key sinonasal features that could differentiate granulomatosis with polyangiitis from AR. Sinonasal characteristics of eosinophilic granulomatosis with polyangiitis include chronic rhinosinusitis with polyps and anosmia. Sarcoidosis rarely affects the upper respiratory tract, and when it does, nasal symptoms are nonspecific, such as epistaxis, nasal pain, and anosmia.[107]

Epistaxis, headaches, and unilateral nasal symptoms such as unilateral nasal blockage and unilateral rhinorrhea should raise suspicion for alternative etiologies, such as cerebrospinal fluid rhinorrhea, sinonasal tumors, and chronic rhinosinusitis.[105]

According to British Society of Allergy and Clinical Immunology guidelines, red flag symptoms indicating a more serious etiology which may need referral should be considered, including bloody purulent discharge, epistaxis, pain, and nasal obstruction, rhinitis, crusting, nasal deformity as a result of the perforated septum, nasal pain, and stuffiness.[120,121]

## Treatment

Treating allergic rhinitis mainly relies on prevention and symptom relief, as no definite cure has yet been found (similar to many other allergic diseases).[104] The basic step in controlling allergic rhinitis is to minimize exposure to allergens, which cause the symptoms. Reducing indoor humidity to prevent mites' growth, spending less time outdoors in pollen seasons, and avoiding pets might be helpful in some patients.[104]

Antihistamines are among the most prescribed medications for allergic diseases, including AR. Both first-generation (e.g., diphenhydramine) and newer (e.g., cetirizine, fexofenadine) antihistamines have seemingly similar efficacies, although the former exhibit higher rates of the central nervous system (CNS) and cardiac side effects, and according to some experts, are no longer recommended.[103,104,122,123] Additionally, novel antihistamines have a higher affinity for H1 receptors,[105] the group of histamine receptors that play a major role in allergic rhinitis pathogenesis. Even though intranasal antihistamines act more rapidly than the oral variations, they both have similar efficacy in relieving each and every symptom, except nasal congestion, for which nasal antihistamines are more effective.[124]

Intranasal corticosteroids (INCSs) are the most beneficial agents in treating AR, as they have shown to be superior to antihistamines, anti-leukotrienes, and a combination of antihistamines and anti-leukotrienes in palliating every symptom, with the highest efficacy in relieving nasal obstruction.[105,125-127] As described above, nasal inflammation is the mainstay of allergic rhinitis pathogenesis. Therefore, anti-inflammatory drugs such as corticosteroids are reasonable therapeutic options as first-line treatments for AR, especially for patients with mild to moderate persistent symptoms.[104] For cases with moderate to severe disease, a combination of INCSs and antihistamines could be effective.[128] Systemic corticosteroids must not be used as routine therapy but rather as relievers in patients with the most drastic symptoms.[103]

Cleansing nasal cavities with isotonic saline has proven to reduce symptoms by almost 30 percent, either as nasal sprays or high-volume irrigation.[129] Furthermore, saline douching increases the efficacy of INCSs.[130]

Inhibiting leukotriene activity with leukotriene receptor antagonists has been studied in patients with AR. Although these groups of medications have superior efficacy compared with placebo, they turned out to be non-superior to antihistamines and inferior to intranasal corticosteroids.[131,132] As a result, leukotriene receptor antagonists are considered second or third-line treatment for allergic rhinitis.[104,133]

While the above-mentioned therapeutic options mainly contribute to symptom relief, allergy immunotherapy (AIT) targets the disease more fundamentally and manipulates the immune system's reaction to allergens. This treatment is recommended in cases that desired results are not achieved via pharmacotherapy.[133] Throughout the treatment course (which might take years to complete), the body is forced to encounter gradually increasing doses of the allergen (administered either subcutaneously or sublingually), causing a steadily developing tolerance against the atopic agent. It has been shown that AIT could be effective against pollens and dust mites, while patients with sensitivity to molds and animal danders are less likely to benefit from this therapy.[104,116] Nonetheless, whether AIT should be performed for all patients and whether it is cost-effective remain matters of debate.[134]

## Allergic conjunctivitis

### Definition

Ocular allergy, also called allergic conjunctivitis, is a common immunological disorder that affects the ocular surface. The most common type of allergic conjunctivitis is seasonal allergic conjunctivitis (SAC), which is not a very serious condition and does not affect the patients' sight, but it could cause discomfort in individuals during the fall and spring. Patients with perennial allergic conjunctivitis (PAC), which is another type of allergic conjunctivitis, suffer from some symptoms during the year. However, they can experience seasonal exacerbations. Other types of ocular allergy named atopic keratoconjunctivitis (AKC) and vernal keratoconjunctivitis (VKC) can lead to more severe symptoms such as corneal ulceration, ptosis, keratoconus, conjunctival scarring, and visual loss.[135]

## Epidemiology

Allergic conjunctivitis is estimated to affect between 15 percent to 40 percent of the population.[136] This disease's prevalence has been possibly underestimated because it is a comorbid condition of asthma and rhinitis. Additionally, it may be challenging to diagnose allergic conjunctivitis due to some similarities between this disorder's symptoms and other ocular diseases.[135]

## Pathogenesis

Allergic conjunctivitis is initiated by exposure to an allergen in a susceptible individual. The Th2 cells produce pro-inflammatory cytokines, such as IL-3, IL-4, IL-5, and IL-13, which could activate B cells to release IgE. IgE attaches to the membrane of mast cells. Upon re-entry of the allergens, they bind to the specific IgE that results in degranulation of mast cells and the release of histamine, tryptase, leukotrienes, and PGs (i.e., type 1 hypersensitivity). The release of these mediators leads to different symptoms, including redness, pruritus, chemosis, tearing, and papillary reaction. This early phase of allergic reaction starts immediately after exposure to the allergens and could last 20–30 min. After a few hours, the late phase of allergic response happens by infiltration of inflammatory cells, such as lymphocytes, neutrophils, eosinophils, and basophils to the epithelium that could increase the risk of tissue damage.[137]

## Clinical features

Pruritus is the most common symptom of this disorder. Other signs and symptoms of allergic conjunctivitis include redness, tearing, gritty sensation, swelling, discharge, and blurring of vision. Additionally, in severe cases, photophobia could also be present.[138,139]

It is necessary to ask the patients about the signs and symptoms of other allergic diseases like asthma, allergic rhinitis, and atopic dermatitis because ocular allergies are a frequent comorbid condition with other allergic disorders. Additionally, a positive family history of allergic diseases could increase the risk of developing allergic conjunctivitis. Asking about the use of medications and history of exposure to the allergens such as pollens, pests, and pets is also important.[137] In physical examination, papillae might be seen in the limbal conjunctiva of the eye, which could result in cobblestoning

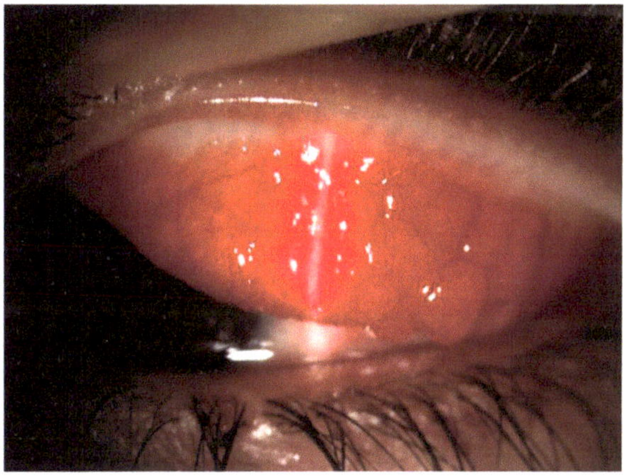

**Fig. 2.1** ***Cobble stone appearance in a patient with vernal keratoconjunctivitis.***[376]

(Fig. 2.1) and limbal lesions named Horner-Trantas dots (Fig. 2.2) that are collections of eosinophils and epithelial debris. These dots are usually correlated with chronic types of allergic conjunctivitis, such as AKC and VKC.[139]

## Diagnosis

The diagnosis of allergic conjunctivitis is clinical. However, several laboratory tests can be used to support the diagnosis. Skin prick test is an inexpensive test that has a high sensitivity for the diagnosis of patients with allergies. If this test is contraindicated or its results are inconclusive, serum-specific IgE measurements can be used.[137]

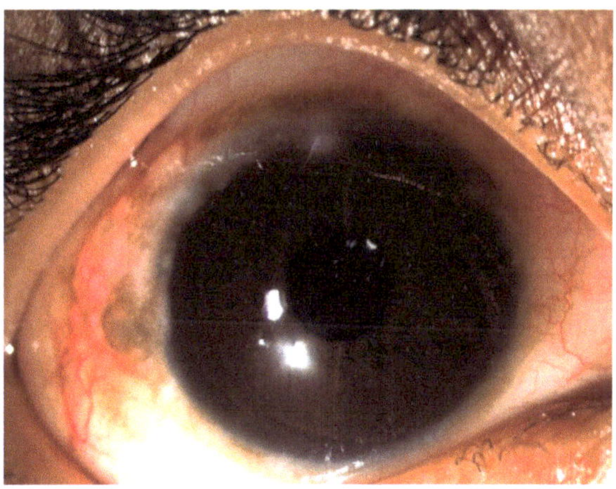

**Fig. 2.2** ***Horner-Trantas dots in a patient with vernal keratoconjunctivitis.***[376]

## Treatment

Patients with ocular allergies are recommended to reduce their exposure to allergens by following these recommendations: 1) using sunglasses which can act as a barrier to allergens 2) using eyelid cleaners that can help to wash away the allergens 3) avoiding unnecessary exposure to pollens by keeping the windows shut and spending less time outdoors 4) reducing contact with animals 5) avoidance of rubbing eyes 6) using hypoallergenic covers for bedding 7) washing the bedding in hot water.[135]

Topical antihistamines have been extensively used for the treatment of allergic conjunctivitis. These agents can immediately relieve the itching and the redness of the eye by blocking histamine, inhibiting eosinophil migration, and stabilizing the mast cells.[140] However, they can have some side effects, such as local irritation.[141]

Mast cell stabilizers prevent degranulation of mast cells and release of preformed histamine and other chemotactic factors. They can inhibit both the early and late phases of ocular allergic responses. Mast cell stabilizers decrease itching, irritation, and hyperemia of the eye, and in order to provide their best effect, these agents should be used prophylactically before exposure to the allergens.[139,142]

Topical decongestants can help reduce the redness, chemosis, and hyperemia by the mechanism of vasoconstriction. However, long-term use of these agents is not suggested due to their side effects, including burning and stinging upon instillation, mydriasis, and rebound hyperemia or conjunctivitis medicamentosa.[143] It has been reported that combination therapy using antihistamines with decongestants has been more effective than using either of them alone. However, this combination can increase the risk of decongestant side effects, and their prolonged use is not recommended.[143]

Topical non-steroidal anti-inflammatory drugs (NSAIDs) are not used as first-line therapy for allergic conjunctivitis, but they can be prescribed as additive therapy. These agents reduce the symptoms of discomfort, such as pruritus, by inhibiting the cyclooxygenase pathway and PG production.[144] NSAIDs' side effects include irritation upon instillation that could reduce patient adherence and rarely corneal perforation.[145]

Topical corticosteroids are effective in the treatment of both acute and chronic phases of allergic conjunctivitis, and they can relieve the ocular symptoms and signs of all phases by their immunosuppressive and anti-inflammatory properties. However, topical corticosteroids have some side effects, such as secondary infection, cataract formation, increasing intraocular pressure (IOP), delayed wound healing; and triggering glaucoma. Therefore, they are recommended to be prescribed for uncontrolled and more severe cases of ocular allergies and are not suggested for long-term use.[139]

Allergen-specific immunotherapy (SIT) is an effective therapy for patients with allergic conjunctivitis. The goal of this treatment is to generate immune tolerance to specific allergens. In this approach, increasing doses of allergens are delivered via sublingual immunotherapy (SLIT) or subcutaneous immunotherapy (SCIT) route, which leads to the induction of Th1 immune responses and inhibition of Th2 immune responses. Additionally, immunotherapy induces regulatory T cells (Tregs), which can decrease Th2 immune responses.[146] The side effects of this form of therapy, including anaphylaxis, can occur. Therefore, the patients should receive SLIT or SCIT in places where medical staff is trained to treat these reactions.[144]

## Urticaria and angioedema

## Definition and classification

### Definition

Urticaria is a medical condition that affects 10 percent–20 percent of the population in their lifetime, identified by the development of wheals (hives), described as edema in the upper layers of skin, angioedema, or both (Fig. 2.3).[147,148]

Heinrich Quincke first described angioedema in 1882. It is a medical condition, resulted from the release of vasoactive mediators and increased vascular permeability, and subsequent localized and non-pitting edema in the deeper layers (dermal, subcutaneous, mucosal, or submucosal) of skin, gastrointestinal tract, or upper respiratory system.[149] Angioedema is mediated by bradykinin secretion or histamine, or other inflammatory agents released from mast cells. The latter type is more frequent and mostly occurs as a manifestation of urticaria. Bradykinin mediated angioedema- also named primary angioedema- has an either hereditary or acquired basis, mostly resulted from the defect of C1 inhibitor (C1-INH). Moreover, it is not usually associated with urticaria.[150]

### Classification

Urticaria is classified based on the duration of symptoms and also triggers and causes of the disease. Recurrence of wheels -with or without angioedema- for less than six weeks is referred to as acute urticaria, and more than six weeks is referred to as chronic

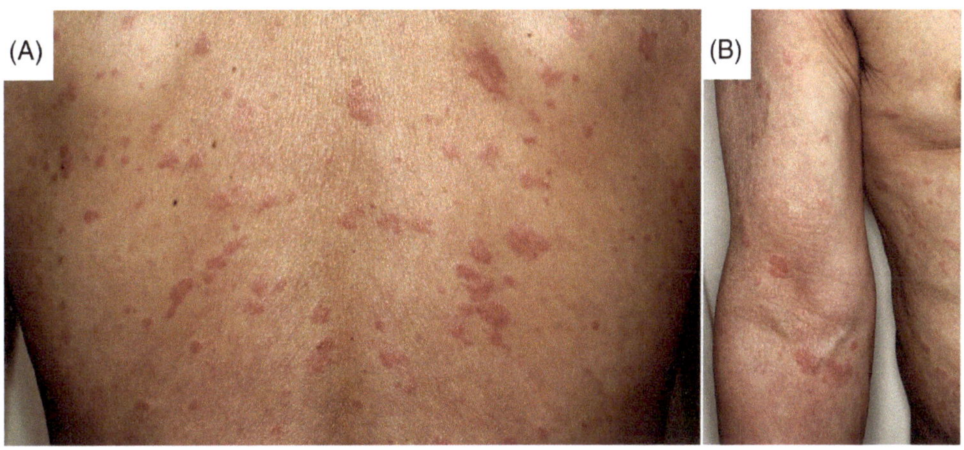


**Fig. 2.3** ***Urticaria on the trunk (A) and upper limb (B).***[377]

urticaria. Chronic urticaria is either chronic spontaneous urticaria (CSU) or chronic inducible urticaria (CIndU).[151]

### Acute urticaria

Acute urticaria is determined by the repeated occurrence of spontaneous wheals, with or without angioedema, for less than six weeks. The disease is mostly triggered by infections in the upper respiratory tract, drug reactions, and food intolerance.

### Chronic spontaneous urticaria (CSU)

In CSU, the lesions appear spontaneously, and they are not induced by an external trigger. Food or drug intolerance, activation of the coagulation cascade, genetic disposition, or autoimmunity can initiate the histamine release from mast cells and trigger the symptoms. About 30 percent–40 percent of these cases produce autoantibodies, which are IgGs against IgE receptors FcεRIa or IgE antibodies. Obesity and higher body mass index (BMI), malignancies, anxiety, dissociative and somatoform disorders, immunosuppressive drug administration, and chronic use of systemic corticosteroids are among risk factors for developing CSU.[152-154]

### Chronic inducible urticaria (CInU)

In this subtype of urticaria, the symptoms are induced by a specific trigger, and they are limited to the area of stimulus exposure. Moreover, the signs and symptoms mostly last less than 2 h. Based on the type of stimulus, CInU is identified as physical urticaria or non-physical urticaria. Aquagenic, cholinergic (stimulated by the sudden increase in body core temperature), cold, contact, delayed pressure, heat, solar, and dermatographism urticaria are categorized as the subtypes of CInU.[151]

According to the European Academy of Allergy and Clinical Immunology, four types of acquired and three types of hereditary angioedema have been identified.[155] By classifying and identifying different types of Angioedema on the basis of etiology and pathophysiology, treatment administration would be more successful.

### Acquired angioedema (AAE)

**Idiopathic histaminergic acquired angioedema (IH-AAE)** Idiopathic histaminergic acquired angioedema (IH-AAE) is the most prevalent form of angioedema. Most of the non-hereditary angioedema cases are responsive to antihistamine treatment, suggesting a role for histamine secretion from the mast cells and basophil cells. The histamine-secretion implies an allergic cause for this disease.

**Idiopathic non-histaminergic acquired angioedema (InH-AAE)** This term refers to a non-hereditary type of angioedema that is unresponsive to antihistamine treatment. This is the least defined group of angioedema cases. However, most of the acquired, antihistamine unresponsive cases were reported to be associated with a high bradykinin level. Sometimes the term "bradykinin-mediated" is used to refer to this type of angioedema. However, the scientific evidence for an increased bradykinin concentration is not yet enough. Also, the role of other vasoactive mediators, such as cysteinyl leukotrienes, PGs, and platelet-activating factor, should be considered.

**Acquired angioedema related to angiotensin-converting enzyme inhibitors (ACEI-AAE)** Angiotensin-converting enzyme (ACE) is involved in bradykinin breakdown. The inhibition of ACE results in elevated levels of bradykinin and subsequent "bradykinin mediated" angioedema. The variability of proteins involved in bradykinin degradation is associated with a higher risk of ACEI-AAE, which reinforce bradykinin mediated basis for this type of angioedema.

### Acquired angioedema with C1 inhibitor deficiency (C1-INH-AAE)

Angioedema patients with C1-INH deficiency, which has no mutation in the gene coding C1 inhibitor (SERPING1) and no family history of angioedema are categorized in this group. Consumption of C1-INH and other components of the classical complement system may cause the release of bradykinin. Attachment of autoantibodies against C1-INH or low-grade lymphoproliferative disorders may result in its loss of function and C1-INH-AAE.

### Hereditary angioedema (HAE)

**Hereditary angioedema with C1 inhibitor deficiency (C1-INH—HAE)** Mutations in one of the two alleles of the C1 inhibitor coding gene (SERPING1) result in C1-INH—HAE. Mutations may lead to two phenotypes of reduced plasma levels of C1-INH (type I) or normal levels of dysfunctional C1-INH (type II), which results in the facilitated release of bradykinin, the main mediator of C1-INH—HAE. Therefore, patients with hereditary angioedema do not respond to conventional angioedema treatments like antihistamines, corticosteroids, and adrenaline therapy.

**Hereditary angioedema with normal C1 inhibitor and factor XII mutation (FXII-HAE) and of unknown origin (U-HAE)** In this category, the plasma level and function of the C1-INH is normal. However, the family history of angioedema recurrence suggests a hereditary basis for this type. Investigations suggest some mutations in the coagulant F12 gene locus. However, in some cases with a family history of angioedema and normal C1-INH levels, genetic defects have not been detected. The term Hereditary angioedema with normal C1-INH and factor XII mutation (FXII-HAE) refers to the patients with mutations in the F12 locus, and the term Hereditary angioedema with normal C1-INH of unknown origin (U-HAE) is used to refer to the patients with no genetic defect detected.

## Epidemiology

The lifetime prevalence of urticaria depends on age, gender, and nationality. The lifetime prevalence of all types of urticaria was reported to be 8.8 percent in a cross-sectional study.[156] The estimated global lifetime prevalence is 1.6 percent−8.4 percent, and the point prevalence is reported between 0.1–3.4 for chronic urticaria. Latin America and Asia had the highest, and North America had the lowest point prevalence estimate of chronic urticaria, and women were reported to have a slightly higher point prevalence than men.[157]

According to a systematic study, the prevalence of ACEI-AAE was estimated to be between 7 and 26 in 100,000, C1-INH—HAE between 1.1 and 1.6 per 100,000, and C1-INH-AAE was estimated to be 0.15 per 100,000.[158] The ACEI-AAE is estimated to be the most prevalent non-allergic angioedema with an occurrence in the 0.1 percent−0.7 percent of ACE inhibitor drug recipients.[159]

## Etiology and pathogenesis

Infection is the most common cause of acute urticaria. Allergens and pseudo-allergens can also trigger acute urticaria, such as medication and foods. Approximately in 50 percent of cases with acute urticaria, no specific trigger has been identified.[160,161] Chronic urticaria, in most cases, has an autoimmune basis. As autoimmune diseases such as hypo/hyperthyroidism, celiac disease, systemic lupus erythematosus, rheumatoid arthritis, and type 1 diabetes are reported to be more prevalent, especially in women with chronic urticaria.[162,163] The IgG autoantibodies against IgE or IgE receptor on mast cells is detected in these patients. The binding of these IgGs to their targets activates mast cells and results in excessive histamine release.[164]

The key molecule in the HAE and C1-INH-AAE is the C1-INH molecule. C1-INH plays a role not only in the complement system, in which it inhibits activated C1r and C1s but also in the bradykinin-forming cascade. C1-INH inhibits the autoactivation of the XII factor, and subsequently, the activation and the digestion of prekallikrein to kallikrein. Kallikrein itself can activate the remaining FXII,[165] and then the digestion of high molecular weight kininogen to bradykinin. Bradykinin then interacts with its constitutively expressed G-protein coupled B-2 receptor and causes vasodilation and an increase in vascular permeability.[166,167] Although FXII activation is a stage in this cascade, an in vitro study has shown that the bradykinin formation can happen in an independent pathway from FXII activation. As prekallikrein can itself bind to the high molecular weight kininogen and produce bradykinin. C1-INH can inhibit the autoactivation of this complex, too.[168] Therefore, in the case of FXII-HAE and C1-INH—HAE, bradykinin is produced in the cascade.

In HAE type I and II, the plasma level, or the function of C1-INH protein is reduced due to a dominant mutation on its gene SERPING1. C1-INH replacement, inhibition of plasma kallikrein, or blockade of the bradykinin B-2 receptor are the treatment options for this disease. As mentioned before, there is another type of HAE with normal C1-INH expression. A mutation in the FXII gene is detected in 30 percent of these patients. Although the function of C1-INH in inhibiting activated C1 in the complement system is normal in these cases, some in vitro studies showed a 40 percent−60 percent of the normal activity of C1-INH in inhibiting FXII and kallikrein.[169,170] However, the etiology of this FXII- and U-HAE should be further investigated.

## Diagnosis

The diagnosis of urticaria mostly relies on examining clinical signs and symptoms, such as wheals and angioedema skin lesions. Also, the clinical history of lesions' recurrence, timing, site and distribution, potential stimulus, and family and medication history are needed.[171]

If the angioedema's recurrence is without wheals, angioedema should be diagnosed as a disease of its own, and the diagnosis should specify the angioedema subtype.

Low levels of C4 and normal levels of C3 support the diagnosis. Quantitative and functional measurements of the C1 esterase inhibitor activity confirm the diagnosis. Low levels of C1q suggest the diagnosis of acquired C1 esterase inhibitor deficiency.[172]

HAE is diagnosed by measuring the antigen plasma level and function of C1-INH.[173] The function of C1-INH is one of the most important clinical parameters in HAE and C1-INH-AAE diagnosis.[174] C4 complement protein level is also measured as a screen test for HAE.[175] However, there are some evidence that a normal C4 plasma level would not exclude the possibility of HAE, and the C1-INH function is a more promising diagnostic technic.[176] The measurement of function and levels of C1-INH can lead to C1-INH-AAE diagnosis. Additionally, normal C3 levels and low levels of C4 help the diagnosis, and low levels of C1q propose the C1-INH-AAE diagnosis.[172] The plasma level of complement system proteins in ACEI-AAE is usually normal. Therefore, the diagnosis is based on the observation of ACE inhibitor medication and subsequent development of angioedema without urticaria. However, the measurement of C1-INH levels are suggested in ACEI-AAE as taking ACE inhibitors may provoke or unmask HAE or other subtypes of AAE.[161]

## Differential diagnosis

A differential diagnosis is essential for a disease like angioedema with such diverse clinical manifestations. As before said, two main pathways are resulting in angioedema, allergic pathway by mast cell activation and histamine excessive release and non-allergic pathway by the bradykinin production. In allergic angioedema, the skin lesions appear and also resolve rapidly, while in non-allergic type, it takes hours for the lesions to appear, and it takes days to resolve. Allergic angioedema can appear at any age, while in non-allergic angioedema, the symptoms appear mostly in the 4th decade for acquired, 6th decade for ACE inhibitor-related acquired, and 1–2nd decade for hereditary angioedema. In allergic angioedema, the lesions mostly appear in the face and neck. Also, there is a high possibility of lesion appearance in the upper respiratory tract and subsequent asphyxiation.[177] In fact, asphyxiation is the main reason for the high rate mortality of 30 percent–50 percent in HAE cases due to improper diagnosis and intervention.[178]

## Treatment

The first step in urticaria management is to control symptoms by avoiding potential triggering factors.[153] Avoidance from anti-inflammatory drugs, heat, tight clothing, pseudo-allergens such as food additives, and spices are needed.[171] In the cases of acute urticaria, antihistamine therapy can be effective in most cases.[171] Due to the autoimmune and histamine-mediated basis of chronic urticaria, current clinically available treatments for chronic urticaria are mostly second-generation, non-sedating antihistamines as first-line therapy and omalizumab (an anti-IgE antibody) as second-line therapy in patients refractory to antihistamines.[151] The mechanism of action of omalizumab is likely to bind to the free IgE and subsequently reduce the IgE receptor FcεRI on the mast cells, and basophils surface, thus reducing mast cell activity, reversing basopenia, and lowering the activity of IgG autoantibodies against FcεRI and IgE.[179] The updosing of second-generation, non-sedating, non-impairing antihistamine agents has also been suggested to be used as second-line therapy. As in a meta-analysis study, 63.2 percent of non-responding CSU patients to first-line therapy responded to antihistamine updosing.[180] Cyclosporin, an inhibitor of histamine release from mast cells and basophils, has also been used to treat conventional-therapy resistant patients, especially in idiopathic or severe cases of chronic urticaria.[181] In the cases of severe acute or chronic urticaria, a short course of oral corticosteroid therapy might also be required.[182]

The treatment for histamine-mediated angioedema is similar to the therapies used in urticaria. In the cases of HAE or non-histamine-mediated angioedema, known as bradykinin-mediated angioedema, the treatment is categorized into three courses: treatment of acute attacks, short-term prophylactic treatment, and long-term prophylactic treatment. The treatment of acute attacks aims to reduce the severity and duration of an attack at the moment, while prophylactic treatment aims to prevent the occurrence or reduce the severity and duration of angioedema attacks generally (long-term), or in the time of expecting stress, or increased risk of angioedema, such as dental surgery and intubation (short-term).[183] Replacement of C1-INH in patients can be a helpful acute treatment. Berinert and Ruconest, which are plasma-derived and recombinant C1-INH, respectively, are administered intravenously as a treatment for angioedema. In patients who are non-responsive to C1-INH replacement, Icatibant or Ecallantide are used as a second-line treatment, which is a bradykinin receptor blocker and a plasma kallikrein inhibitor, respectively. In prophylactic treatment, C1-INH replacement is also used. Berinert and Cinryze are given during the anticipated high-risk procedure.

Androgen therapy, such as Danazol, can be administered in cases of short prophylactic treatment. Tranexamic acid, an antifibrinolytic agent, is also used in pregnant women, children, and patients who cannot tolerate androgens. For long-term prophylactic treatment, plasma-derived C1-INH, and Lanadelumab, which is a monoclonal antibody against plasma kallikrein, are suggested as first-line therapy.[173]

## Atopic dermatitis and allergic contact dermatitis

### Definition of atopic dermatitis

Atopic dermatitis also named atopic eczema, Besnier's prurigo, or infantile eczema, is a common chronic relapsing inflammation in the skin with pruritic and exanthematous lesions. Lesions mostly occur in skin fold areas like the eyelid, neck, forehead, hands, and feet. Atopy is referred to as the inherited production of IgE against a low number of environmental antigens, such as pollen, house dust mites, and specific foods. As an allergic reaction and IgE excessive production are absent in about half of the patients, atopic dermatitis is not a definitive medical term.[184]

### History of atopic dermatitis

The term "eczema" was developed by Willan and Bateman for defining the condition of "an eruption of minute vesicles, non-contagious, crowded together; and which from the absorption of fluid they contain form into thin flakes or crusts. This eruption is generally the effect of irritation, whether internally or externally applied".[185] The term "eczema" comes from a Greek word meaning "eruption". The introduction of the term Atopic dermatitis goes back to 1933 when Fred Wise (1881–1950) and Marion Sulzberger (1895–1983) used the term to define infantile eczema, which occurs mostly in the face and flexural fold areas and in people with a familial history of atopic disorders.[186]

In 1967, Gunnar Johansson (1911–1998) and Hans Bennich discovered the function and structure of IgE protein[187] and its elevated plasma levels association with asthma.[188] The association between elevated IgE levels and atopic dermatitis were discovered later, and in 1978, Bruno Wüthrich proposed an important role for IgE in the etiology and pathogenesis of atopic dermatitis rather than a simple association.[185] However, the exact pathogenesis of atopic dermatitis is yet to be investigated. In 1980, Jon Hanifin and Georg Rajka proposed the first systematic diagnostic approach for atopic dermatitis.[189]

### Epidemiology and risk factors of atopic dermatitis

The prevalence of the disease is variable in different regions. The prevalence of up to 20 percent has been reported in Russia, while in Finland, a prevalence of only 4.3 percent has been reported.[190] Another global study reported the prevalence of atopic dermatitis ranging from 0.9 percent in India to 22.5 percent in Ecuador, with higher values in Asia and Latin America, and from 0.2 percent in China to 24.6 percent in Columbia, with the higher values in Africa and Latin America for the 13 to 14 age group.[191] Also, there is an increasing incidence of atopic dermatitis, both in developed and developing countries.[192] Therefore, the efficient management and prevention of the disease should be highly considered and studied to reduce the probable burden of the disease in the following years. The incidence is not different between males and females. There is a seasonal variation of more primarily severe symptoms in winter. There is usually a family history of either atopic dermatitis, asthma, or seasonal allergic rhinitis.[190]

Atopic dermatitis occurs in all age groups. However, it is more prevalent in children, with the onset, usually in 2 or 3 months of age.[190] Approximately 10 percent−20 percent of children are affected by this disease, and half of them would be put into remission in adulthood.[193] Less than 10 percent of adults are affected by Atopic dermatitis,[194] of which 25 percent has an adult-onset disease.[195]

Family history, mutations in the filaggrin (FLG) gene, and some environmental factors may play a role as risk factors in atopic dermatitis. Family history is known to be the most vital risk factor for atopic dermatitis. The risk of developing atopic dermatitis in children with one or two parents with atopic dermatitis is 1.5 fold and 3–5 fold higher, compared to children with no family history of atopic dermatitis.[196] Mutations in the FLG gene have been associated with a higher risk of developing atopic dermatitis, more severity of the disease, and a higher possibility of concomitant asthma, especially in patients of European ancestry.[197] Also, some environmental factors such as exposure to cats from a young age may be a diagnostic risk of atopic dermatitis in people with this mutation. Some environmental factors such as living in urban areas or dry climate, lower exposure to pathogens, and frequent exposure to antibiotics at young ages have been associated with a higher risk of atopic dermatitis.[196]

## Etiology and pathogenesis of atopic dermatitis

It has been hypothesized that atopic dermatitis pathogenesis has an immunological basis. As the elevated levels of IgE production, activated mast cells, eosinophils, and IL-4, and downregulated levels of IFN-γ is associated with disease development. IL-4 is a cytokine secreted from Th2 cells and can attenuate the B cells' IgE production and further mast cell activity. Therefore, Th2 hyper-activation (type 2 immune response) may be the underlying immunological basis of atopic dermatitis. Moreover, the downregulation of IFN-γ, which is secreted from Th1 and inhibits Ig production, suggests Th1 hypo-activation, which has a synergic effect in the disease pathogenesis.[190]

Some mutations in the FLG gene encoding Filaggrin protein, which is an important protein forming the skin barrier, have been detected that is associated with atopic dermatitis and more severe clinical features.[198,199] Filaggrin controls the composition of cells in the skin's granular layer and the aggregation of keratin filaments into compact bundles. Filaggrin metabolites moisturize the skin and improve its pH. Filaggrin deficiency leads to increased penetration of allergens and also micro-organisms colonization in the skin. The loss-of-function mutations in the FLG gene increase the risk of atopic dermatitis development by impairing the skin barrier. Other genetic, epigenetic, and immunologic factors can affect skin barrier integrity via affecting filaggrin or other proteins expression and function. Other than loss-of-function mutations, Intragenic copy number variations and epigenetic modifications on the FLG gene has been associated with atopic dermatitis development. Moreover, lack of humidity and lower temperatures can decrease filaggrin levels, as it is hydrolyzed in a dry environment. This can explain the localized pattern of atopic dermatitis lesions, which are seen mostly in the areas exposed to the air like cheeks and hands. Also, skin irritants, high pH, physical damage, and prolonged use of topical corticosteroids can decrease filaggrin level by increasing its degradation or decreasing its expression. Therefore, this may explain the reason why environmental factors, such as climate, bathing procedure, and chemicals, can highly affect atopic dermatitis, and also why only 20–30 percent of patients with atopic dermatitis have a "loss-of-function" mutation in their FLG gene.[200]

TSLP has an important role in atopic dermatitis pathogenesis. It is mostly produced by epidermal keratinocytes, and its production is triggered by both environmental allergens and immunological agents such as pro-inflammatory and Th2 cytokines and IgE. TSLP can induce Th2 cells, and it has been reported that the expression of TSLP is increased in the skin lesions of patients with atopic dermatitis. Additionally, there is evidence of omega-6 fatty acid deficiency in patients with atopic dermatitis. The role of omega-6 FA deficiency in the pathogenesis might be because of the inadequate PGE1 and PGE2 production, which are major metabolites of omega-6 FA. Studies have shown that PGE1 and PGE2 can suppress IgE production. In a study on mouse models of atopic dermatitis, the blocking of PG synthesis by indomethacin enhanced the type 2 immune response in the skin of the mice and increased IgE, IL-33, and TSLP plasma level, and IL-4-producing CD45+TCRb1+ cell numbers. The study results proposed an anti-inflammatory role for PGE2-EP2 by downregulating TSLP expression and, thus, type 2 immunity inhibition.[201-203]

## Clinical features of atopic dermatitis

The most common clinical features of atopic dermatitis are pruritus, lichenification, xerosis, flexural involvement, influenced by environmental and emotional factors, early onset of disease, and worsening of itch with sweating. Although most of these clinical features are among the most common features, they are partly related to ethnicity and age. Atopic dermatitis is usually acute in infants, and it mostly affects the extensor surfaces of the limbs and the face. It can also affect the trunk, but the napkin area is generally spared. From the age of 2 onwards, patients present with polymorphous manifestations of atopic dermatitis, mostly on flexural folds. In adolescents and adults, excoriated and lichenified plaques at eyelids, ankles, wrists, and flexures can be seen. It can also involve the scalp, upper trunk, and shoulders (Fig. 2.4). It has been reported that the signs and

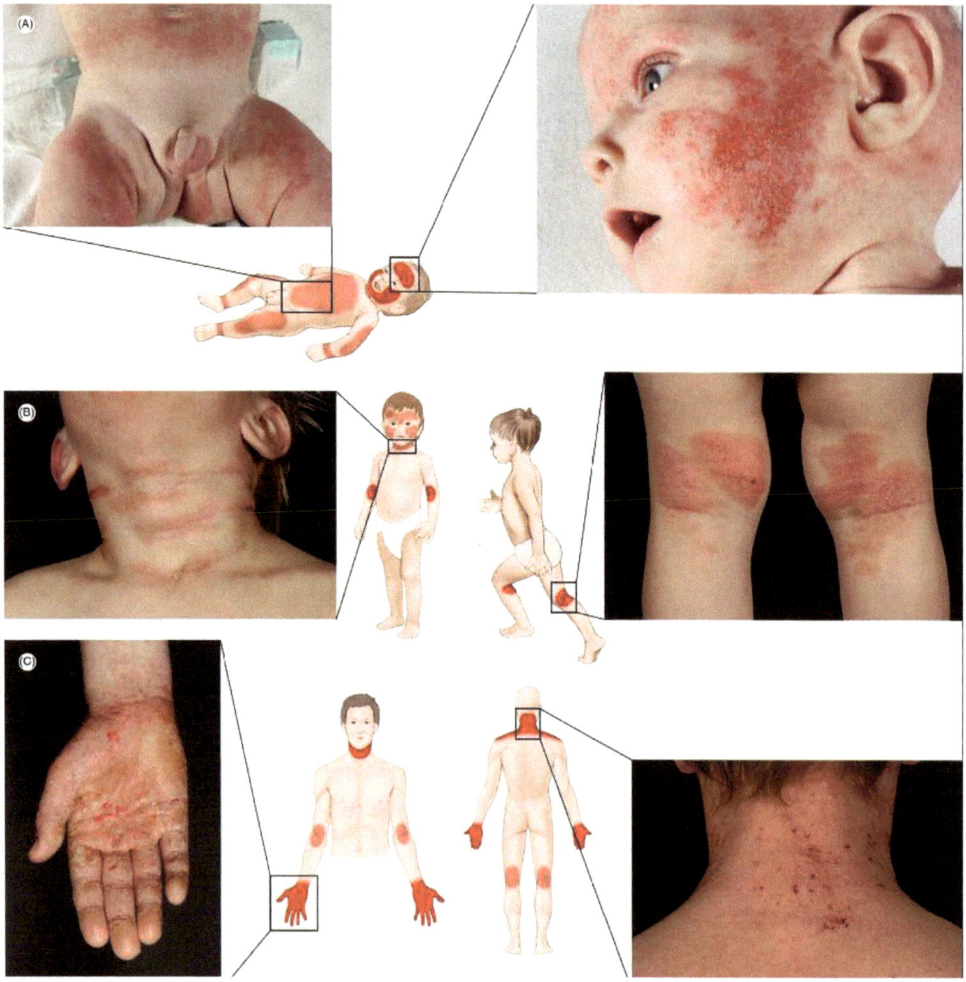


**Fig. 2.4** ***Atopic dermatitis at different ages.*** (A) An infant with face, extensor surfaces of the limbs, and trunk involvement. The napkin area is spared. (B) Atopic dermatitis mostly affects flexural folds in children. (C) In adolescents and adults, excoriated and lichenified plaques at eyelids, ankles, wrists, and flexures can be seen. It can also involve the scalp, upper trunk, and shoulders.[378]

symptoms of adult-onset atopic dermatitis are generally milder than child-onset atopic dermatitis. However, the prevalence of foot dermatitis is higher among adults. The mild sign and symptoms of adult-onset atopic dermatitis may pose a challenge to the diagnosis of this disease from other adults' skin conditions.[195,204,205]

## Diagnosis of atopic dermatitis

As said before in the history of the atopic dermatitis section, Hanifin and Rajka proposed the first diagnostic criteria for atopic dermatitis based on clinical features and some objective tests such as IgE plasma level measurement and skin prick test. The diagnostic criteria had 4 major features: pruritus, characteristic morphology and distribution, chronicity of lesions, and personal or family history of atopy (asthma, allergic rhinitis, atopic dermatitis), and 23 minor features, such as hand or foot dermatitis, cheilitis, elevated levels of IgE, xerosis, immediate (type I) skin reactivity, or onset at a young age. The presence of 3 major and 3 minor features was essential for atopic dermatitis diagnosis.[189] However, some other studies pointed out that the criteria are mostly used for white, hospital-based cases of atopic dermatitis and are not applicable to all ages, genders, and ethnicities.[206,207] Moreover, some of the major features like the personal or family history of atopy, were not identified as significant as some minor features like xerosis in these criteria.[208]

Williams et al. developed one of the most validated diagnostic approaches in 1994. The study was performed with 31 criteria, 13 historical and 18 clinical and physical criteria. They excluded the invasive tests like prick test or IgE plasma level measurement. They chose 120 cases with atopic dermatitis and 102 hospital-control with skin diseases other than atopic dermatitis and also population-controls with complaints unrelated to skin complexities. Their observers were blinded for the primary diagnosis. At the end of the study, six criteria were the best discriminators for atopic dermatitis diagnosis from other skin diseases, including the history of flexural involvement, onset under the age of 2, history of an itchy rash, personal history of asthma, history of dry skin, and visible flexural dermatitis.[207] All the criteria except for flexural dermatitis were historical features. This emphasizes the role of historical features in atopic dermatitis, as the physical clinical features may be heterogeneous among atopic dermatitis patients.

There are several guidelines developed for atopic dermatitis diagnosis, mostly in children. From the most widely used guidelines, we can mention "Atopic eczema in under 12: diagnosis and management" by the national institute for health and care excellence published in 2007,[209] and the American Academy of Dermatology guideline published in 2013.[210] These guidelines try to discriminate against other similar skin conditions such as Allergic contact dermatitis or seborrheic dermatitis, which are prevalent skin diseases, especially in infants, and may even overlap with atopic dermatitis in these patients.

## Differential diagnosis of atopic dermatitis

Atopic dermatitis is a common skin condition. However, the diverse morphology of the clinical manifestation may pose a challenge to the diagnosis of atopic dermatitis. Psoriasis, allergic contact dermatitis, molluscum dermatitis, tinea corporis, mycosis fungoides, dermatomyositis, pityriasis lichenoides chronica, Langerhans cell histiocytosis, polymorphous light eruption, actinic prurigo, and nutritional deficiency are among the skin conditions that should be differentially diagnosed from atopic dermatitis.[211]

## Treatment of atopic dermatitis

As the skin barrier defects are one of the significant factors in atopic dermatitis incidence, the first step in efficient atopic dermatitis management is proper skin hydration and bathing practice. Bathing in lukewarm water may hydrate the skin and decrease the irritants and germ on the skin surface. However, applying moisturizers, emollients, or other topical medications is crucial to avoid trans-epidermal water loss after bathing. A meta-analysis study investigating the efficacy of non-pharmacological moisturizers in atopic dermatitis treatment has shown a higher efficacy in moisturizers, which contain two or more active agents rather than single-agent moisturizers, and also glycyrrhetinic acid, vitis vinifera, hyaluronic acid, telmesteine, and shea butter were beneficial substances in moisturizers for atopic dermatitis treatment.[212] Emollient therapy is suggested to have a protective role in preventing atopic dermatitis. In a study, the full-body emollient application from 3 weeks to 6 months after birth reduced the relative risk of atopic dermatitis by 50 percent.[213]

Topical corticosteroids are the first-line therapy for acute flares and exacerbations. They are also usually prescribed for patients with refractory atopic dermatitis after basic skincare and are more efficient than moisturizers in treating atopic dermatitis.[214] They are available in different strengths, from low potency (class 7 is the least potent) to high potency (class 1 is the most potent). Low and medium potency topical corticosteroids are prescribed for mild and moderate-severe acute flares.[215] Wet Wrap Therapy (WWT) is also used besides topical corticosteroid therapy to boost corticosteroids' effect in refractory moderate-severe cases.[216] The topical corticosteroids are administered, followed by wrapping two-layer of cotton clothing or bandages (the first layer is wet with warm water, and the outside layer is dry). WWT facilitates the penetration of topical medication into the skin layers and subsequently increases medications' efficacy by a very low cost.[217] However, applying mid-higher potency topical corticosteroid therapy with WWT should be considered, as the facilitated penetration may increase the risk of topical corticosteroid therapy adverse events such as skin atrophy, hypopigmentation, telangiectasia, acneiform lesions, striae, and perioral dermatitis.[218]

Other approved drug group for atopic dermatitis is calcineurin inhibitors. Calcineurin is a highly conserved eukaryotic Ca-calmodulin dependent serine/threonine phosphatase.[219] Calcineurin plays an important role in lymphocyte activation and cytokine secretion by activating the NFAT family transcription factors. Calcineurin inhibitors are immunosuppressive drugs that inhibit the cytokine secretion either by inhibiting calcineurin function or its interactions with NFAT.[220] Two topical calcineurin inhibitors, tacrolimus ointment, and pimecrolimus cream, are approved for atopic dermatitis treatment. In children, the efficacy of tacrolimus 0.03 percent or 0.1 percent and also pimecrolimus 1 percent for treating atopic dermatitis was shown to be better than vehicles and other conventional therapies, and with no significant difference in the adverse events.[221,222] There is a fear of using corticosteroids due to the concerns about their adverse events, so caregivers and patients refuse to continue their treatment with topical corticosteroids for a longer period. Studies show that therapy with calcineurin inhibitor significantly reduces the need for topical corticosteroid therapy in the case of acute flares.[222,223] Moreover, calcineurin inhibitors' efficacy is reported to be the same as topical corticosteroids in atopic dermatitis treatment.[223] Also, another anti-inflammatory agent, crisaborole 2 percent topical ointment, which is a phosphodiesterase- 4 inhibitor, is approved for atopic dermatitis treatment in children older than two years with mild to moderate atopic dermatitis.[224,225]

The therapeutic advantage of human umbilical cord blood-derived mesenchymal stem cells (hUCB-MSCs) in moderate-severe atopic dermatitis treatment has been investigated in both preclinical and clinical studies.[226,227] It is shown that nucleotide-binding oligomerization domain 2 (NOD2)-activated hUCB- MSCs can inhibit both the migration and degranulation of mast cells by NOD2-cyclooxygenase-2 signaling pathway, higher PGE2 production, and IL-4 induced TGF-β1 production.[226] The clinical study also showed a dose-dependent improvement in atopic dermatitis manifestations after hUCB-MSCs infusion. The IgE plasma level and eosinophil counts were also decreased, and no severe adverse event was observed.[227] These data may suggest hUCB-MSCs subcutaneous infusion as a safe and efficient therapy for atopic dermatitis patients.

In the refractory or unresponsive cases to topical corticosteroids and other conventional therapies, ultraviolet phototherapy and immunosuppressive agents can be applied. Short-term phototherapy with narrow-band ultraviolet B is reported to have not only immunosuppressive effects but also it can have anti-bacterial effects and improve skin integrity.[215] Nonspecific immunosuppressive agents such as cyclosporine, azathioprine, methotrexate, and mycophenolate mofetil are administered off-label (except for cyclosporine) for the treatment of refractory or persistent cases of severe atopic dermatitis. These drugs are mostly used for short-time treatment because of causing potential toxicities and side effects. Cyclosporine is the only approved and also is the most efficient immunosuppressor agent that has been used as second-line therapy for short-term treatment of patients with atopic dermatitis. However, its long-term administration is restricted because of adverse events.[196] Also, the usage of dupilumab as a biologic agent was approved in 2017 as a treatment for chronic moderate-severe atopic dermatitis. Dupilumab is a humanized monoclonal antibody against the IL-4 receptor on the cells of the immune system. It inhibits the function of IL-4 and IL-13, which further results in the inhibition of Th2 differentiation and IgE production. Biological agents are more targeted than other non-specific immuno-suppressants. Understanding specific immunological mechanisms underlying atopic dermatitis can help explore new biological targets and find efficient therapeutic agents.[196,228]

In conclusion, avoiding irritants (such as soaps, detergents, scratchy clothing), proper skincare (i.e., emollients, moisturizers) and regular bathing, topical corticosteroid, anti-calcineurin therapy, and adjunctive therapies, like WWT, ultraviolet phototherapy, immunosuppressive agents and monoclonal antibodies such as dupilumab can help patients to control and reduce the frequency of severe flares.

## Definition of allergic contact dermatitis

Allergic contact dermatitis is a relatively common inflammatory skin condition. Clinical manifestations of allergic contact dermatitis are pruritus, erythema, vesicles, itching, and scales, which can be an acute, subacute, or chronic disorder. It accounts for 20 percent of contact dermatitis cases (the remaining 80 percent is mostly irritant contact dermatitis). The morphological manifestations of the irritant and allergic contact dermatitis are similar. However, they are different in etiology and pathophysiology. Irritant contact dermatitis is a result of direct damage to the skin without an immune-mediated reaction. However, allergic contact dermatitis is a type 4-mediated hypersensitivity response of the immune system to a specific allergen about 48 h after allergen exposure. The most important allergens are metal (nickel, cobalt, and gold), antibiotics (such as neomycin and bacitracin), topical medications (such as estrogen and testosterone transdermal therapeutic systems and local anesthetics),[229] food preservatives, cosmetics, and personal care products (Fig. 2.5).[230] Contact dermatitis is the fifth most prevalent and eighth skin disease with most costs in the United States.[231]

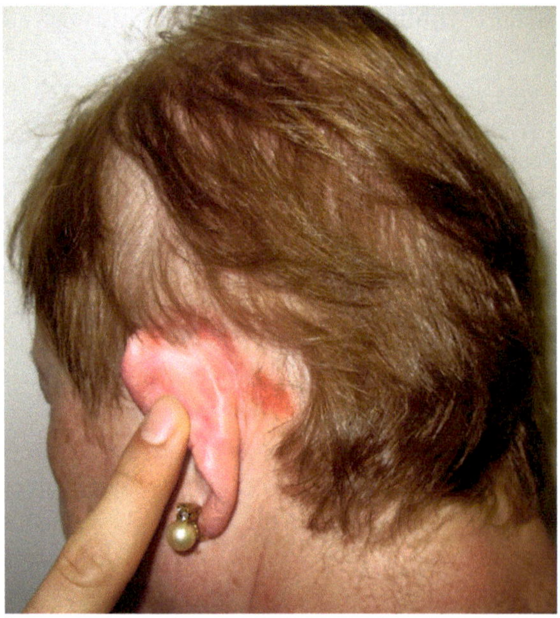

**Fig. 2.5** ***Allergic contact dermatitis caused by temple tip.***[379]

## Epidemiology of allergic contact dermatitis

Allergic contact dermatitis has about 20 percent average prevalence in all age groups and a two-fold prevalence in women compared to men.[232] The higher prevalence can be because of the difference in exposure to certain allergens, such as cosmetics. For example, in the case of nickel allergy, women are more exposed to the allergen because of wearing jewelry. The prevalence of allergic contact dermatitis is lower among children and young adults (16.5 percent).[233] It has been reported that allergic contact dermatitis, along with irritant contact dermatitis, is among the most prevalent occupational skin disorders and can highly affect the performance of workers.[230]

## Pathogenesis of allergic contact dermatitis

As said before, allergic contact dermatitis is a type4-mediated hypersensitivity reaction resulting from the allergen-specific T cells reaction to the allergen exposure. In the first stage, which is sensitization, the allergen that is mostly a hapten (a low-weight molecule that is conjugated with a larger molecule such as a protein and can induce an immune response) is recognized as a foreign antigen and engulfed by epidermal or dermal dendritic cells and Langerhans cells. The antigen-presenting cells (APCs) then migrate to the skin lymph nodes to evoke the naïve T cells priming. The naïve T cells can recognize the newly introduced antigen, differentiate, expand, proliferate, and form colonies of effector and memory allergen-specific T cells. Then, in the next episode of allergen re-exposure, the allergen-specific T cell colonies proliferate and are recruited to the skin. There, the APCs such as Langerhans cells, dendritic cells, and probably keratinocytes activate the T cells by presenting the allergen through their major histocompatibility complex (MHC) II. The APCs also release cytokines that can downregulate the inhibitory signal of Tregs and polarize the T cells to differentiate into helper 1, 2, or 17 or CD8+ cytotoxic T cells. The allergen-specific T cells then elicit an immune response, which results in the clinical signs and symptoms of allergic contact dermatitis.[230]

Studies showed that in non-allergic patients compared to patients with allergic contact dermatitis, the allergen-specific T cells' proliferation is inhibited by Tregs through secretion of immune-inhibitory cytokines such as IL-10. Also, in patients with allergic contact dermatitis to nickel, both nickel hapten-specific CD4+, and CD8+ T cells were present while in the non-allergic patients, only nickel hapten-specific CD4+ T cells were found, which secreted higher IL-10 and lower IFN-$\gamma$ compared to nickel hapten-specific CD4+ T cells in patients with allergic contact dermatitis to nickel.[234] Later, another study suggested that both hapten-specific naïve and effector CD4+ cells are inhibited by regulatory CD4+ CD25+ T cells in non-allergic people. The T cells expressing cutaneous lymphocyte-associated Ag (CLA) had a stronger inhibitory effect on effector T cells and inhibit them in a cell-to-cell manner rather than by cytokine production, and in the absence of these Tregs, the hapten-specific T cells could proliferate.[235] In another study, the level of TGF-$\beta$ produced by Tregs in patients with allergic contact dermatitis was significantly lower than controls. However, the number of CD4+ CD25+ and CD4+ CD25 high Tregs was elevated in patients. The development of allergic contact dermatitis despite the increased number of Tregs may suggest the association of defected Tregs with allergic contact dermatitis pathogenesis.[236]

## Clinical features of allergic contact dermatitis

There are different phases of skin lesions in allergic contact dermatitis. The first phase is the erythematous phase characterized by erythema and edema, and then the madidans phase with papules, several vesicles, erosions, and moistening. Crusts characterize the next stage, and then in the squamous stage, a horny layer of skin appears after skin repair. Blistering and swelling may also happen in severe cases. The most perceptible symptom of allergic contact dermatitis is the itching. Skin lesions are initially limited to the contact site with well-defined edges but, they may spread symmetrically in the next stages as one of the most important signs to differentiate the irritant contact dermatitis from allergic contact dermatitis is the allergic contact dermatitis lesions' more spreading from the contact area. Also, the onset of the irritant contact dermatitis is more rapid than the allergic contact dermatitis, as the lesions in acute allergic contact dermatitis appear about 24–48 h after contact with the hapten.[237]

The allergic contact dermatitis skin lesions may persist and develop into chronic allergic contact dermatitis. The clinical features of chronic allergic contact dermatitis are lichenification, fissures, pigmentation, pruritus, and skin lesions with a symmetric pattern, distant spread, and less sharp borders.[237,238]

## Diagnosis of allergic contact dermatitis

For diagnosis of allergic contact dermatitis, history taking, complete physical examination, and diagnostic tests are required. A clinician should ask questions regarding chronology of the symptoms, personal and family history of atopic diseases, allergies, or other skin conditions. Also, occupation and hobbies, usage of cosmetics, skincare products, or any suspicious agent, and intake of topic and systemic medications should be inquired.[239] In physical examination, the identification of the type and also the distribution of skin lesions can be helpful. For example, the distribution of lesions on the eyelid, face, neck, or hands may suggest cosmetics or skincare products as the culprit agents.[230]

Patch testing is the gold-standard test for the diagnosis of allergic contact dermatitis. A base-line list of relevant allergens, with their suitable vehicle and concentration, should be tested in any patient with acute or chronic allergic contact dermatitis and also in patients with atopic dermatitis, especially those who are unresponsive to treatments and suspected to developing allergic contact dermatitis.[240] In some cases, in which the result for patch testing is negative despite a suggestive primary diagnosis, repeated open application tests could be performed. In this test, the suspected allergens are applied daily for about 2 weeks until a positive result is yielded.[239]

## Treatment of allergic contact dermatitis

The most important step in allergic contact dermatitis treatment is to identify the offending allergen and avoid them. As many allergic contact dermatitis causing allergens are present in the chemical nomenclature of daily products, the avoidance might be difficult for the patients. There are some digital tools such as SkinSAFE (www. SkinSafeProducts. com, HER Inc./Mayo Clinic) and CAMP (Contact Allergen Management Program, www. ContactDerm.org) that provide the patients and health providers a list of safe to use products. Also, surveillance on the ingredients and potentially allergic agents in the products besides population-based epidemiological studies can result in some efficient regulatory interventions such as the ban of preservative methyldibromo glutaronitrile (MDGN) from cosmetics in European Union countries.[241]

Topical corticosteroids can be used as a treatment for allergic contact dermatitis. However, degradation products of corticosteroids can cause allergic contact dermatitis themselves, and it should be considered in the cases of no-response or worsened manifestation after topical corticosteroid therapy.[229] The delayed allergic contact dermatitis due to corticosteroid therapy is mostly mediated by betamethasone-17-valerate, tixocortol pivalate, dexamethasone 21 phosphate disodium, triamcinolone acetonide, budesonide, and alclomethasone dipropionate.[242]

## Food allergy and gastrointestinal syndromes

### Definition

Food allergies are one of the most prevalent non-communicable diseases, especially among children, which are caused by specific immunologic reactions to food.[243] In guidelines by the United States National Institutes of Allergy and Infectious Diseases (NIAID), food allergy is defined as "adverse health effect arising from a specific immune response that occurs reproducibly on exposure to a given food".[244] The immune response can be IgE mediated or non-IgE mediated or the combination of both. Food allergy is different from the term "food intolerances", which result in non-immune related adverse events.

IgE mediated food allergy is associated with the onset of acute symptoms after about minutes to 2 h after allergen exposure.[245] Despite the efforts to prevent allergic reactions via eliminating the food allergens from the diet of affected patients, unintended exposure to allergens still can cause severe allergic reactions and anaphylaxis. Hence, some consistent rules in the food industry are needed to label allergens in the products to reduce the disease burden. The accidental exposure to the allergen and the subsequent limitation in patients' and their families' social life are among the factors affecting the patients' health-related quality of life.[246]

In IgE mediated food allergy, there is an initial step IgE sensitization, in which the allergen-specific B cells differentiate and proliferate into IgE producing plasma cells.

The IgE antibodies are then localized on the surface of mast cells and blood basophils. In some cases, sensitization occurs without signs and symptoms of food allergy in the exposure to that specific food allergen. Therefore, it is important to consider that the sensitization of the immune system alone cannot define the food allergy. Food allergy symptoms occur after sensitization, where the re-exposure of the food allergen to the immune system, and engagement of the allergen with its membrane-bound IgEs on mast cells and basophils, results in the excessive release of histamine and other allergic mediators.[244]

Enterocolitis, proctocolitis, and enteropathy are among the syndromes of non-IgE mediated food allergy, which is mainly cell-mediated. Although most of the food allergy reactions are IgE mediated, non-IgE mediated food allergies are usually because of immunological reactions without IgE production, such as eosinophilic inflammation of the gastrointestinal tract.[244] It primarily affects infants with symptoms like vomiting, diarrhea, abdominal cramps, and occasionally blood in the stool and poor weight gain. Eosinophilic esophagitis and atopic dermatitis are among the food allergies with mixed etiologies, both IgE and non-IgE mediated food allergies.[245]

Food allergens are mostly proteins with a 5–100 kDa molecular weight,[247] but rarely they are chemical haptens.[244] Most of the food allergens can elicit an immune response in cooked or raw, or even digested form, but the allergens that are primarily in the fruits and vegetables usually cannot cause the reaction in the cooked form. Additionally, most of the food allergen proteins can lead to an allergic reaction even when they are inhaled. The cross-reactivity between food and inhalant allergens can also happen and cause various mild to severe symptoms.[248] Cross-reactivity is a circumstance when the antibodies can react with not only their specified antigen but also the similar antigens and initiate an immune response.[244] There is cross-reactivity between allergens in different foods, for example, between chicken and fish parvalbumins[249] or among crustaceans.[250] One of the syndromes, which is caused by the cross-reactivity between the allergens in pollens and the allergens in raw fruits, vegetables, or nuts, is the "oral allergy syndrome" or "pollen-food allergy syndrome". The reaction happens while eating fresh fruit because of prior sensitization to an inhalant pollen allergen. It is usually associated with mild and transient pruritus and/or angioedema limited to the oral cavity and oropharynx.[251]

The most common food allergens are found in egg, milk, peanut, tree nuts, fish, crustacean and molluscan shellfish, wheat, soy, celery, mustard, sesame, and lupine in the United States and Europe.[244,247] Food oils can have less allergenicity if the proteins are removed in food processing.[244]

## Epidemiology and risk factors

There are many challenges to determine the prevalence of food allergy because of the variations in food allergy definition, inconsistent study designs, and an over-estimation in patients' self-report studies. Moreover, with more than 170 foods reported to cause an allergy, studies only focus on a limited number of allergic foods.[244] The prevalence of food allergy in the United States is estimated to be 5 percent in adults and 8 percent in children, and it is reported to be increased in the last years.[252] Another American study showed the prevalence of food allergy in children to be 6.53 percent. It was a self-report population-based survey (the National Health and Nutrition Examination Survey [NHANES]), so the slightly higher reported prevalence maybe because of the self-report. Milk (1.94 percent), peanut (1.16 percent), and shellfish (0.87 percent) were the most allergic foods in this study.[253] In other developed countries, the food allergy prevalence was reported to be similar to United States estimates.[253]

There are many risk factors for food allergy. The family history of atopic diseases is an important risk factor, as the history of atopic disease in an immediate family member enhance the risk of food allergy by 40 percent, and the history in 2 immediate family members increases its risk by 80 percent compared to children without atopic disease family history. Ethnicity and sex are also associated with the increased risk of developing food allergy as it has been demonstrated that Asians and non-Hispanic ethnicities and male sex in children are at higher risk. Additionally, environmental factors, such as having older siblings or pets, can decrease the risk of food allergy.[253,254]

## Etiology and pathogenesis

In IgE mediated food allergy, the OX40L+ dendritic cells in the presence of inflammatory cytokines such as IL-25, IL-33, and TSLP recognize the food allergen as an invading pathogen. Then, they migrate to the lymph nodes and stimulate the release of inflammatory cytokines. By presenting the allergen through their MHC II complex and the cross-talk of OX40L on the dendritic cells and OX40 on the naïve T cells, the differentiation of naïve T cells into food-specific Th2 T cells are promoted.[255] The Th2 sensitization results in the B cells' stimulation to produce allergen-specific IgEs, which then will be attached to the FCε receptors of mast cells and basophils. After the sensitization to the food allergen, the re-exposure to the allergen results in the binding of the IgE to its FCε receptors on the surface of mast cells and basophils and the rapid onset of allergic reactions through excessive release of allergic mediators such as histamine, proteases like tryptase, platelet-activating factor, PGs, leukotrienes, TNF-α and proteoglycans, which can cause vasodilation, increased vascular permeability, recruitment of allergic inflammatory cells, and enhancement of inflammatory cytokine release. Histamine has a key role in the allergic reaction and can lead to vasodilation, an increase in vascular permeability and cardiac output, and glandular secretion. It also induces the most severe symptom of food allergy that is anaphylaxis, through its H1 and H2 receptors. Platelet-activating factor is another important mediator of anaphylaxis, which is a bronchoconstrictor and can increase vascular permeability.[256,257]

Besides dendritic cells and Th2 cells, type 2 innate lymphoid cells are reported to have a crucial role in the allergic state by secreting inflammatory cytokines, suppressing

Tregs, and promoting the function of mast cells.[258] Th2 cells secrete IL-5 and IL-13, which promote the differentiation of the inflammatory effector cells: eosinophils and basophils, and IL-4, which promotes B cells' production of the IgE. There is also a suggested role for Th9 cells to promote growth, survival, and accumulation of the mast cells during the allergic reaction.[259]

The integrity of the epithelial membrane plays an important role in the pathogenesis of food allergy. Allergens or other antigens can normally cross the membranes with facilitated mechanisms such as active transport via epithelial cells, para-cellular transport, villous microfold cells (M cells), trans-epithelial dendrite (a subset of specialized dendritic cells), and goblet cells.[260] The latter has shown to play an important role in transporting soluble low-weight antigens to the underlying lamina properia. The preferential antigen delivery and the exposure of luminal antigens to the tolerogenic dendritic cells through goblet cells can lead to food tolerance.[261,262] The term "food tolerance" is defined as when "an individual is symptom-free after consumption of the food or upon oral food challenge weeks, months, or even years after the cessation of treatment".[244] The mechanism underlying food tolerance is poorly investigated. However, there is a potential role for tolerogenic CD103+ dendritic cells in the non-activated state, which present and process the allergen.[263] CX3CR1+ macrophages can also engulf the antigen and produce IL-10 that is an anti-inflammatory cytokine.[264] There is evidence of increased intestinal inflammation in the goblet cell deficiency,[265] which can partially be because of the impaired antigen delivery to tolerogenic CD103+ dendritic cells. The CD103+ dendritic cells migrate and transport the antigen to the nearest lymph node. There, in the presence of secreted TGF-β, IL-10, and retinoic acid, the dendritic cells promote the differentiation and proliferation of the Foxp3+ Tregs, which further migrate to the lamina properia of the intestine and, via its inhibitory receptors, prevent the function of effector Th2 T cells, eosinophils, basophils, and mast cells, and consequently a decrease in IgE production and histamine release.[266] It has been reported that in the presence of anti-inflammatory cytokines (i.e., IL-10 and TGF-β), the B cells are switched to produce IgA rather than IgE. The food allergen-specific IgA level has been associated with food tolerance and desensitization to a food allergen.[267]

There are many proposed models for the etiology of food allergy and other allergic syndromes, including hygiene hypothesis, dual allergen exposure hypothesis, and vitamin D hypothesis, which are the most widely accepted ones. The hygiene hypothesis claims that the presence of persistent infections in childhood can lead to induction and activation of regulatory and anti-inflammatory pathways that further reduces the risk of allergies. The hypothesis is backed by the evidence of the increased prevalence of allergies in recent years, especially in the developed world. There are other ideas supporting this hypothesis, such as the early bacterial and viral infections before the maturation of the immune system push toward a dominant Th1 based immune response and not a

Th2 response. However, some early Th2 inducing infection, such as helminth infection, is also negatively associated with allergy.[268]

The dual-allergen (or early) exposure hypothesis claims that avoiding a specific allergic food from childhood cannot prevent sensitization and further allergic reactions as the infant is still exposed to similar respiratory or cutaneous allergens in the environment. It is based on the observation of a higher incidence of food allergy among infants with atopic dermatitis. Additionally, this hypothesis proposes that early oral exposure to food allergens can induce immune tolerance.[269] The vitamin D hypothesis was proposed in 1999 when scientists identified a correlation between vitamin D level and allergic symptoms. It was first claimed that higher vitamin D plasma level is associated with a higher prevalence of allergy in developed countries. However, sufficient data rejected this idea, and conversely implied a negative correlation between vitamin D level and particularly maternal vitamin D intake during pregnancy and lactation, and allergy prevalence.[270-274]

## Clinical features

The onset of symptoms in IgE mediated food allergy is rapid, diverse, and can involve almost all of the body systems, but mostly affecting the skin, respiratory, gastrointestinal, cardiovascular, and neurological systems. The diversity of clinical manifestations reflects the complexity of several reactions between the food protein, immune system, gastrointestinal tract, and other involved organs. One of the most severe symptoms of food allergy is anaphylaxis, which is a severe allergic reaction. It mostly has a rapid onset and is the most frequent cause of death in food allergy.[275]

Skin is the most frequently affected organ in the food allergy, which is present in about 70–80 percent of patients with positive oral food challenges.[276-278] Urticaria, angioedema, flushing, pruritus, and erythematous morbilliform rash are among the IgE mediated skin manifestations, and contact dermatitis, and dermatitis herpetiformis are among the cell-mediated reactions. Atopic dermatitis is a manifestation mediated by both IgE and cellular reactions.[279] Urticaria and angioedema are supposed to be some of the most frequent symptoms and skin manifestations in the food allergy. However, the prevalence may occasionally differ according to the region or the type of food. Acute urticaria is more associated with the IgE-mediated immune response to food than chronic urticaria. It may happen by the entrance of the food through the gastrointestinal route or the topical contact with the food allergen. The latter is named contact urticaria. The contact urticaria occurs rather instantly, while the acute urticaria resulting from the gastrointestinal entrance of the food protein usually occurs within 2 h.[279]

Ocular symptoms of food allergy, including conjunctivitis, itching, lacrimation, redness, and periorbital edema, could be present. The respiratory manifestations of the food allergy can range from mild to severe and also can involve both the upper and lower respiratory systems. They are mostly followed by other systematic reactions, but they can happen solely, too.[280] Rubbing, or sniffing of the nose, nasal congestion, rhinorrhea, throat tightness, throat pain, increased occurrence of dry cough, hoarseness, expiratory or inspiratory wheezing, and in severe forms stridor followed by complete obstruction of the airway are among the potential respiratory symptoms. There is a higher probability of asthmatic reactions in the exposure to steam or vapor of cooking foods or inhalation of food allergens. Also, asthmatic symptoms of food allergy should be suspected in cases with a history of refractory asthma, atopic dermatitis, gastroesophageal reflux, and food allergy.[280,281]

The IgE mediated gastrointestinal manifestations are itchiness in the oropharynx and oral cavity, nausea, vomiting, diarrhea, and abdominal cramps. The symptoms may occur within 2 h, as other IgE mediated food allergy symptoms. Other more serious, lower gastrointestinal tract symptoms such as bloody stool, weight loss, and failure to thrive, and constipation are mostly because of non-IgE mediated food allergy.[280]

Cardiovascular and also neurological manifestations have the most severe consequences. Hypotension, vascular collapse, tachycardia and arrhythmia, dizziness, unconsciousness, and changes in mental status are the most frequent cardiovascular and neurological symptoms. They mostly happen alongside the other skin or respiratory manifestations.[280,281]

## Diagnosis

Diagnosis of IgE mediated food allergy includes investigating a history of classic allergic symptoms, physical exam, elimination diets, and the evidence of food-specific IgE by a skin-prick or a serum IgE testing.[282]

The oral food challenge is currently the gold standard for the diagnosis of food allergy. When the results of skin-prick or serum IgE tests are negative during the elimination diet, or there are discrepancies between the results, an oral food challenge can help with the diagnosis.[281] Moreover, the initiation or continuation of a food elimination diet should not be determined only by the serum IgE results but also by the oral food challenge results, especially in children with atopic dermatitis.[278]

There are some cases with positive test results in serum IgE or skin prick tests that have food tolerance, or there are some patients with food allergy whose test results are negative. Therefore, in order to avoid misdiagnosis, it is better to use a combination of diagnostic tests in a specific order. For instance, the history leading to test operation and the test results leading to the decision of whether an oral food challenge is needed or not.[282] In a study with 100 allergic and 100 tolerant infants to peanut, only 26 percent of allergic infants had a positive serum IgE test result (15 kUA/L or greater), and 65 percent needed a positive oral food challenge to confirm the diagnosis. In the skin prick test, only 57 percent of patients had a confirmed diagnosis (8 mm or greater), and 35 percent needed a further oral food challenge for the diagnosis confirmation. This study suggested a combinatory approach of Ara h2 (a dominant allergen in peanut) IgE test, which has the same specificity as the whole peanut plasma serum IgE but a higher sensitivity (60 percent vs. 26 percent), after the whole peanut plasma serum IgE test to reduce the number of needed oral food challenge by almost two-third (95 vs. 32). Ara h2 serum IgE test in the infants with 3 to 7 mm of skin prick test also reduced the number of needed oral food challenge test by more than a half.[283]

Molecular or component-resolved diagnostics (CRD) tests and the basophil activation test have also shown promising results for diagnosing patients with food allergy. Intradermal tests, atopy patch tests, measurement of the total plasma IgE level, IgG4 testing, and applied kinesiology are among the diagnostic tests that are not currently recommended for routine cases of food allergy.[282]

Although the sensitivity and specificity of tests and the threshold values are assessed for tests like serum IgE or skin prick test, it is important to consider that the values may be different according to age,[284] race, geographical region,[285] and even method of the test operation.[286]

## Treatment

The pillar of food allergy treatment is to avoid the allergen in the diet. In breastfed infants, the maternal elimination diet may be necessary. In infants who are not exclusively breastfed, extensively hydrolyzed, amino acid-based, or other specific formulas can be included in the diet.[287] However, the treatment reliance on dietary elimination may impair the growth and weight gaining of infants. For example, in cow milk allergy, the intact proteins of cow milk should be eliminated, and in the case of inadequate diet substitution, the infants would face severe growth problems.[288]

An adequately supplemented elimination diet, with counseling of a physician and dietary specialist, would not only affect children's growth and weight gaining[289] but also it can improve growth indices, stool consistency, regurgitation, and other symptoms related to food allergy.[290]

The whey or casein-based extensively hydrolyzed formula (EHF) is used regularly to treat cow milk allergy patients. In these formulas, the intact cow milk proteins are hydrolyzed into smaller peptides (MW below 1500 Da) through enzymatic reactions. There is a diversity in the composition of different EHFs. Therefore, they may differ in hypoallergenicity, adverse events, nutritional value, and taste.[291] Usually, infants with cow milk allergy can tolerate lactose. However, in some infants, enteropathy and intestinal damage from allergic reactions may result in secondary lactose intolerance. Moreover, the lactose from cow milk might be contaminated with residual cow milk protein allergens and cause allergy in some hypersensitive infants.[287] These groups of allergic infants may benefit from a lactose-free or low-lactose EHF. However, in infants with normal digestive and absorption functions, lactose might even act as a prebiotic agent and improve the healthy microbiota and metabolites.[292] It has been reported that the administration of probiotic Lactobacillus rhamnosus GG (LGG) added to a casein-based EHF in children with cow milk allergy can reduce the risk of development of other allergic manifestations in life and also can decrease the functional gastrointestinal disorders.[293] The combination therapy can also increase the tolerability rate in these children.[294] The trace amount of allergens in EHF may trigger an allergic reaction, but it can also induce food tolerance. The latter data suggest that the administration of probiotic LGG added to casein-based EHF can promote tolerability rather than allergic reactions.

For most of the infants with cow milk allergy, EHF can lead to the complete resolution of the symptoms. However, in cases of hypersensitive or severe food allergy or malabsorptive enteropathy, amino acid-based formula (AAF) administration is suggested. AAF provides amino acids instead of intact proteins or small peptides.[287] Hence, as protein allergens are completely absent in AAF, it cannot induce food tolerance.[295] Meyer et al. provided a practical guideline of the situations in which amino acid-based formula can benefit the cow milk allergy patients or is necessary for their treatment. The suggested conditions are incomplete symptoms' resolution on EHF, growth deficiency or inadequate weight gain, several food groups eliminated from the diet, severe complex gastrointestinal food allergies, eosinophilic esophagitis, food protein-induced enterocolitis syndrome, severe eczema, and symptoms occurrence in breast-fed infants.[296]

Food allergy can tremendously affect patients and their family lifestyles in many aspects. Besides the fact that providing a special diet for allergy patients can be expensive, patients need dietary counseling to select suitable manufactured food products and also need to be educated to read the food labels. Since 2006, the Food Allergen Labeling and Consumer Protection Act (FALCPA) set a rule that food manufacturing companies have to put precautionary statements regarding the presence of the eight major allergens: milk, egg, soy, wheat, tree nuts, peanut, crustacean shellfish, and fish on their products. Although labeling would be helpful to guide the patients in selecting the suitable product, educating them regarding the statements on the labels is necessary as some statements may lead to misunderstanding.[281]

Eating out in restaurants and also in schools can be a big challenge for food allergy patients. Strategies to raise awareness and information of restaurant managers and workers regarding food allergy and its restrictions can help them provide and recommend safe food products to their allergic customers. A study showed that about 10 percent of food workers had this misunderstanding about food allergies that a small amount of allergen cannot provoke an allergic reaction in patients. This lack of information can be potentially dangerous. Also, strategies in schools to provide allergen-free Tables can reduce the risk of food allergy reactions in schools and affect allergic children's quality of life as children spend most hours of the day in school.[281,297]

Another therapeutic option for food allergy patients is introducing trace amounts of allergen and stepwise up-dosing through a specific period of time. The antigen can be delivered through oral, sublingual, or epicutaneous routes, named Oral immunotherapy (OIT), sublingual immunotherapy (SLIT), and Epicutaneous immunotherapy (EPIT), respectively. OIT is reported to be more effective in increasing the threshold of tolerable dosing and desensitization. However, the rate of systematic and local adverse reactions is also higher in OIT compared to EPIT and SLIT.[298] Currently, combination therapy of OIT and omalizumab, which is an anti-IgE monoclonal antibody, is suggested to enhance the efficacy of the treatment.[299] Omalizumab attaches to the IgE and inhibits IgE binding to its FcεRI receptor on the mast cells and basophils.[300] Another potential therapeutic approach uses omalizumab-IgE complexes to neutralize the circulating allergens in blood and inhibit their engagement with membrane-bound IgEs on mast cells and basophils.[301]

Managing anaphylaxis, as the most severe clinical manifestation of food allergy, should be highly considered in patients with food allergy. Intramuscular epinephrine administration is efficient in improving the symptoms promptly. Epinephrine maintains the blood pressure by its vasoconstricting effect and dilates the respiratory tract to improve respiration. Carrying epinephrine auto-injectors for patients with a positive test for food allergen-specific IgE and a history of a previous anaphylactic reaction is suggested, as delayed epinephrine injection increases the rate of hospitalization and also the risk of death due to anaphylaxis.[281,282] Also, as the second-line treatment, H1-antihistamines alone, or with H2-antihistamines, and also glucocorticoids can be administered to improve the blood pressure and heart rate in an anaphylactic reaction.[281]

## Prevention

As there is an increasing trend in the prevalence of food allergy, many studies prioritize effective approaches to prevent food allergy by reducing exposure to risk factors or other methods. The methods are mostly based on the etiologic hypotheses of food allergy, including hygiene hypothesis, dual allergen exposure hypothesis, and vitamin D hypothesis. The primary prevention methods seek to reduce the probability of an infant's sensitization and antibody production against a certain antigen, while the secondary prevention methods focus on reducing the incidence of allergic reactions in already sensitized infants and/or infants with other atopic disorders.[291]

Breastfeeding plays an important role in the prevention of food allergy. It provides the required energy, essential nutrients, maternal antibodies, and growth factors for the infant. In a meta-analysis studying the effect of breastfeeding in infants with or without a family history of atopic disorders, exclusive breastfeeding during the first 3 months of infancy was shown to be a protective factor for atopic dermatitis in children with a positive family history, but not in children without the family history.[302] Other studies also implied the association of exclusive breastfeeding in early infancy with a lower incidence of allergic asthma and allergic rhinitis during childhood.[303,304] Although exclusive breastfeeding has been known as a protective factor against allergic disorders in childhood, its effect is still controversial, and some studies failed to prove its role as a protective factor.[305]

The earlier prevention approaches were mostly based on the avoidance of allergic food and exclusive breastfeeding in the primary months after birth and late introduction of potentially allergic foods, such as the introduction of any complementary solid food after 6 months, dairy products after 1 year, egg after 2 years and peanut, nuts, and seafood after three years.[306] However, recent studies suggest that the early introduction of solid foods within 4–6 months after birth can reduce the incidence of allergic reactions in childhood, especially in high-risk groups such as infants with a positive family history.[307,308] A study on more than 2000 infants in Australia showed that early introduction of the cooked egg within 4–6 months was associated with a lower risk of developing egg allergy compared to the introduction in 10–12 months and after 12 months. The study also failed to imply an association between breastfeeding duration and the time of other solid food introduction with the probability of developing egg allergy.[309] The results of this study declared that avoiding early exposure to food antigens may be the reason for the growing incidence of food allergy in the past decades. Another study demonstrated that early oral exposure to egg might lower the risk of development of egg allergy in infants with eczema.[310] Additionally, the early peanut introduction to high-risk infants is proposed as a validated preventive approach to prevent peanut allergy in infants with a high risk of allergy development. In a study of 4–11 months-old infants with allergy to egg, severe eczema, or both, the avoidance of peanut significantly increased the risk of developing peanut allergy both in the sensitized and non-sensitized groups.[311] Another randomized control trial showed a significantly negative association of rates of developing the allergy to peanut and egg within the age of 1 to 3 years (in the per-protocol analysis but not in the intention-to-treat analysis), with the early introduction (6 months old) of these foods. However, the early introduction of cow's milk, sesame, whitefish, and wheat had not a crucial effect on allergy development.[312] It should be considered that there is a need for more backing data regarding the early introduction of allergens. The dosing, introduction of multiple food antigens, and the safety of this approach should be thoroughly investigated.

The composition of intestinal microbial flora and also the early exposure to bacterial, viral, and parasite pathogens have a pivotal role in the maturation of the immune system and its deviation toward a Th2 response.[268,313,314] The primary composition of intestinal microbiota in the neonatal and infant periods can tremendously affect childhood health by competitive colonization, immune system modulation, uptake and distribution of resources, or by influencing physiological development in these primary periods.[315] There is evidence of differences in the early intestinal microbial flora and metabolites composition in allergic and non-allergic infants.[316] Infants with atopic disorders usually have less diversity in their bacterial flora compared to non-allergic infants. So, these evidences propose that modifying the bacterial flora and increasing its diversity, for example, by administrating probiotics or prebiotics, can be implemented as preventive and also therapeutic approaches. In the study of Wopereis et al., a partially hydrolyzed protein formula supplemented with nondigestible oligosaccharides (prebiotics) could improve the intestinal microbiota in the taxa diversity, pH, and metabolites in the high-risk infants for allergy and consequently prevent atopic dermatitis in this group.[316] In another study, the 6-month supplementation of oral LGG improved the diversity and metabolites composition of the intestinal microbiome in the high-risk infants for allergy. There were also fatty acids in their fecal sample, which induced the Tregs ex vivo. However, 6 months after supplementation cessation, the metabolic profile was changed, and the level of LGG in the microbiota was decreased, suggesting that the remodeling was not permanent.[315] The mother's gut microbiota and breast milk microbiota can also highly affect the infant's microbiota composition. Breastfeeding can improve the combination of microbial flora in the intestine by inducing the growth of Bifidobacteria.[317] The Bifidobacteria can further improve the mucosal homeostasis and increase the tolerance in the intestinal mucosa via interaction with Tregs and TLRs.[313]

Among other preventing approaches is vitamin uptake during pregnancy and lactation. Vitamin D deficiency is getting more prevalent around the world as its concentration is so low in the food. It is an important immunomodulatory agent in the human body, and an optimal >50nmol/L plasma level of 25-hydroxyvitamin D is needed in infants, children, adults, and during pregnancy and lactation.[318] Low levels of vitamin D in children and adolescents have been associated with atopic disorders.[319] Studies show that increased uptake of vitamin D in pregnant mothers can lower the risk of allergic rhinitis, asthma, and wheezing in their children.[271,272,274] However, another study reported that a high level of vitamin D in maternal and cord blood increases the risk of sensitization and food allergy within the first two years of life. They also observed a negative correlation between high vitamin D levels in cord blood and the number of Tregs.[320] The role of vitamin D in preventing or inducing food allergy and other allergic disorders has remained unresolved. However, it is proposed that vitamin D may play a dual-dose dependent role in preventing food allergy, with both low and high levels increasing the risk of allergy development.[321] Therefore, further studies are needed to identify the adequate dose of vitamin D to prevent food allergy in different individuals regarding sex, atopic history, etc.

## Drug allergy

### Definition

Side effects or adverse drug reactions can happen after the administration of almost all drug types. However, the frequency of these adverse reactions may differ for different drug types. For example, antibiotics and antiepileptics can cause drug allergies frequently.[322] The drug-induced adverse reactions are classified into two A and B types due to their underlying etiology. Type A drug reactions are associated with predictable, almost common, dose-dependent reactions, which are related to the pharmacologic action of the drug. On the other hand, type B (or off-target) drug reactions are unpredictable, uncommon, not dose-dependent, and mostly mediated by immunologic or allergic adverse reactions.[322,323] Drug allergy or drug hypersensitivity is categorized as a type B adverse drug reaction. The clinical manifestations of drug allergies can range from mild symptoms such as skin rash to much more severe symptoms such as severe cutaneous adverse reactions and anaphylaxis.

## Epidemiology and risk factors

Adverse drug reactions are the chief complaint of about 3 percent to 6 percent of all hospital admissions, and 10 percent−15 percent of hospitalized patients experience it. Most of these adverse reactions (80 percent) are identified as "type A" reactions. Therefore, drug allergies and other non-immune mediated adverse drug reactions (pseudo-allergic reactions) account for 15 percent−20 percent of these adverse reactions. Cutaneous manifestations are reported as the most prevalent symptom in hospital-based studies.[324] Also, drug-induced anaphylaxis as the most severe manifestation of drug allergy has an estimated incidence of 0.04 percent to 3.1 percent and a mortality rate of 0.65 percent.[325] Severe cutaneous adverse drug reactions are rare symptoms of drug allergy with an incidence of 2–7/million every year for Stevens-Johnson syndrome (SJS) and toxic epidermal necrolysis (TEN). However, the mortality rates for these manifestations are significantly high (5 percent−10 percent for SJS, 30 percent for SJS/TEN, and 50 percent for TEN).[326]

Several factors related to the patients' characteristics, or the drug itself, may cause drug allergy. The drug's chemical structure and ability to trigger immune system reactions, the drug administration route, the dosage regimen, and the frequency of exposure are considered drug-related risk factors. There is a higher probability of causing a drug allergy by drugs with a higher molecular weight like insulin or drugs that can act as a hapten (i.e., small molecules that can bind to certain proteins in the body and act as an allergen) such as Penicillin. These drugs can trigger the immune system and cause an allergic adverse reaction. Drug administration through intravenous, intramuscular, or topical routes may cause a higher risk of drug allergy compared to oral administration. Moreover, the patients who take a certain number of doses over a prolonged period of time are at a higher risk of developing drug allergy compared to patients who receive an equal amount at a single dose.[327]

The other risk factors which are mostly host-related are gender, age, comorbidities and viral infections, and genetics. Women are reported to be more affected by allergic reactions to drugs.[327,328] Also, drug allergies are less reported in children compared to adults. However, this could be as a result of higher usage and predisposition to drugs in adults, and subsequently higher rates of drug sensitization and allergy in the adults, and it is still unclear that adults are more vulnerable to the development of drug allergy than children.[324] Patients with chronic viral infections such as *human immunodeficiency virus*

(*HIV*), *Epstein-Barr virus* (*EBV*), or *herpes simplex virus* (*HSV*) infections may have higher rates of drug allergy.[327] Recent studies sought to find some genetic biomarkers of drug allergy in patients. For example, certain Human Leukocyte Antigen (HLA) class I alleles (HLA-B*15:02, HLA-A*31:01, and HLA- A*24:02) are reported to increase the risk of cutaneous adverse drug reactions caused by Aromatic antiepileptic drugs.[329] Also, some other specific HLA alleles (HLA-B*27:05, HLA-B*38:02, and HLA-DRB1 × 08:03) are reported to be associated with agranulocytosis induced by some anti-thyroid drugs.[330] Thus, screening for these alleles is recommended in some populations with a higher frequency of these alleles. Identifying certain allergy biomarkers would help physicians prescribe appropriate medications and reduce the economic and clinical disease burden of drug allergy and hypersensitivity by rendering the "unpredictable" type B drug reactions predictable.

## Etiology and pathogenesis

Drugs can cause drug allergy via different mechanisms. These immune-mediated allergic reactions are categorized into 4 types according to Gell and Coombs classification. IgE mediated drug hypersensitivity (type I), IgG and IgM mediated cytotoxicity (type II), complex immune reaction (type III), and T-cell mediated drug hypersensitivity (type IV) are defined as the main mechanisms underlying drug allergy.[331] Type I, II, and III are antibody-mediated, leading to acute symptoms, while type IV cell-mediated reactions lead to delayed adverse reactions. Type I and IV reactions are more common than type II and III.[332]

Most of the drugs have a low molecular weight. Thus, they are not immunogen per se. However, they can act as haptens, or their metabolites can act as haptens (which, in this case, the drug is called prohapten). Haptens are small molecules (<1000 Da) that can covalently bind to proteins and cause unwanted immunogenicity. Another proposed mechanism is that drugs may reversibly bind to immune receptors such as T cell receptor (TCR) or HLA molecules on immune cells and trigger an immune reaction.[322,332]

The early studies on hypersensitive reactions induced by β-lactam antibiotics led to the introduction of the hapten concept in drug allergy. A study to identify the pattern of flucloxacillin (a synthetic penicillin) conjugation to the albumin protein by mass spectrometry showed that flucloxacillin only binds to 10 specific Lysine residues, two of them (Lys 190 and Lys212) were the most reactive and bound promptly to flucloxacillin in vivo. However, the in vitro experiments have shown that flucloxacillin could bind to both N-acetyl lysine and N-acetyl cysteine methyl esters.[333] The restricted, dose- and time-dependent pattern of albumin and flucloxacillin conjugation provides specific targets to study the allergenicity of hapten-protein conjugation in hypersensitive patients.

After the first exposure to hapten-protein complexes, complexes are engulfed by APCs. The APCs then migrate to relevant lymph nodes and present the allergens through their HLA to the naïve T cells. Then the antigen-specific T cells recognize the presented complex and proliferate to antigen-specific effector and memory T cells. These antigen-specific T cells are then transported to the tissues and can initiate an adaptive immune response following the re-exposure to the hapten-protein complex. The activated Th2 cells can also stimulate B cell differentiation to produce IgE, while Th1 cells enhance IgG and IgM production.[332] Also, sensitization can happen as a result of cross-reactivity between similar antigens. For example, IgEs specific for galactose-α−1,3-galactose, which is found in cetuximab (a chimeric mouse-human IgG1 monoclonal antibody) and also ABO blood group, were present in the pretreatment samples of 68 percent of patients with cetuximab induced allergic reaction. The study results suggest that in more than half of these patients, the sensitization to cetuximab results from cross-reactivity. However, in 1 out of 51 patients without an allergic reaction to cetuximab, the antibodies were present, suggesting that, in some cases, sensitization may not lead to allergy.[334] The presence of IgE against galactose-α−1,3-galactose can be used as a predictive biomarker of anaphylaxis in patients. Weiss et al.[335] screened 60 patients for this antibody before starting medication with cetuximab. The negative predictive value was 100 percent, and no patient with a negative result for the screening test went through anaphylaxis.

Two pathways have been proposed in forming an immune-mediated allergic response: activation of T cells through antigen recognition by their TCR, and detecting a "maturation signal" by antigen detecting dendritic cells and further formation of a co-stimulatory signal, which further stimulate the T cells activation.[322] Dendritic cells can detect the drug-related oxidative stress, and also some "stress sensor" proteins' modification, namely maturation signals. Thus, dendritic cells can produce a stress response and activate other innate immune response elements before inducing the allergen-specific T cells activation. The dendritic cells' maturation occurs in a hapten dose-dependent manner. In lower levels of hapten exposure, dendritic cells are partially activated, and when dendritic cells are exposed to higher levels of hapten, the drug-induced death of other cells in the tissue leads to complete activation of dendritic cells. Concomitant diseases such as HIV infection and cystic fibrosis might accelerate this step.[322]

The intact chemical structure of some drugs cannot act as haptens, but the normal metabolic processing and bio-activation in the cells through drug-metabolizing enzymes can result in metabolites, which can haptenate proteins. These drugs are called prohaptens. For example, in Jenkins et al. study, not only flucloxacillin but also its metabolite 5-hydroxymethyl flucloxacillin could covalently bind and modify the serum albumins on the same Lysine residues and causes more severe adverse reactions.[333]

Sulfamethoxazole is another example of prohapten drugs. The parent drug (sulfamethoxazole) cannot bind to the serum proteins and cause allergy by itself. However, it can be "bio-activated" to a hapten through two steps. Sulfamethoxazole is first metabolized to sulfamethoxazole hydroxylamine in the liver. Sulfamethoxazole hydroxylamine can then be oxidized into nitroso of sulfamethoxazole. Both metabolite intermediates can bind to a range of serum and also membrane-bound proteins and produce several different hapten-protein conjugate allergens.[336]

Most drugs are formulated to bind to a certain protein receptor or enzyme and alter its function. The term pharmacophore is defined as "an ensemble of steric and electronic features that is necessary to ensure the optimal supramolecular interactions with a specific biological target and to trigger (or block) its biological response." by the International Union of Pure and Applied Chemistry (IUPAC).[337] Although drugs' pharmacophore is specified to bind to a certain target molecule in the body, some immune receptors may have ligand binding sites similar to the target protein of a drug. The diversity and heterogeneity of protein receptors on the T cells may increase the risk of drugs' cross-interaction with TCRs and, subsequently, activation of T cells. This mechanism of T cell activation by direct interaction of drug molecules with immune receptors is called the p-i concept (pharmacologic interactions of drugs with immune receptors).[338] As the non-covalent interactions are more labile compared to covalent conjugation in the hapten-protein complexes, this mechanism may only stimulate a response in pre-activated T cells. Similar to hapten induced responses, chronic viral infections, oxidative stress pathways, or drug-induced death of other cells in the tissue can reinforce the T cells response.[322]

## Clinical features

The IgE-mediated reactions occur promptly after drug administration, and symptoms appear in seconds (in parental administration) or minutes (in oral administration) after taking the medication. The primary symptoms are usually rashes, eruptions, and itching in hands, foot, axial and genital area, and also redness in the face and thorax. These initial symptoms may not be serious by themselves. However, they can indicate upcoming severe symptoms such as anaphylaxis. Thus, they should be taken seriously. The following symptoms are generalized urticaria within 10–15 min, swelling in tongue and larynx, acute bronchospasm with dyspnea and chest tightness, and periorbital and perioral edema.[338]

The T cell-mediated (type IV immune reactions) symptoms occur mostly in the skin. The rashes may appear between 6 h to 10 days after drug administration, so they are usually called delayed allergic reactions.[338] The skin manifestations of delayed drug adverse reactions can range from milder involvements such as maculopapular exanthema (MPE), acute generalized exanthematous pustulosis (AGEP), fixed drug eruption (FDE), and to more severe and life-threatening conditions such as SJS, TEN, and drug-induced hypersensitivity syndrome (DIHS)/drug reaction with eosinophilia and systemic symptoms (DRESS) which have a low prevalence in the population but, they cause a high disease burden and mortality rate.[326] In severe conditions, delayed allergic reactions can also affect the liver, kidney, lung, and pancreas[338] or cause systematic symptoms such as fever, lymphadenopathy, and eosinophilia.[331]

## Diagnosis

The diagnosis of drug allergy mostly relies on the patient's clinical history of allergic reactions and also, examining clinical signs and symptoms. As the skin is usually the most affected organ in drug allergy, a thorough examination of the skin is necessary.[323] In the next stages, diagnostic tests such as skin prick test or intradermal test might be necessary. History taking is the pillar of drug allergy diagnosis and guides the physicians to select suitable laboratory or diagnostic tests and stop the usage of the suspected drugs. Detailed questions regarding the current and previous medications, the onset of symptoms, characteristics and location of the symptoms, previous occurrence of similar symptoms, concurrent medications, the indication of drug usage, and other comorbidities or underlying clinical conditions should be inquired.[339]

For the diagnosis of anaphylaxis, serum total mast cell neutral serine protease tryptase of the plasma can be measured. Almost 30 min after the onset of anaphylaxis, the serum tryptase level starts to increase and remains increased for up to 6 to 8 h.[340] Hence, it has been suggested to measure the plasma level of tryptase 1–2 h after the onset of anaphylaxis.[341,342] Platelet activation factor (PAF), chymase, carboxypeptidase A3, dipeptidyl peptidase I (DPPI), basogranulin, and C—C chemokine ligand (CCL)−2 are also the emerging diagnostic biomarkers of anaphylaxis. However, tryptase measurement is still considered the gold standard for anaphylaxis diagnosis.[342]

For the diagnosis of IgE-mediated drug allergy, the level of allergen-specific IgE levels in the plasma should be measured. The positive results indicate that the patient is sensitized to that specific allergen. However, sensitization does not lead to allergic reactions in all cases. Skin tests can also be used to assess the presence of allergen-specific antibodies and the possibility of an allergic reaction after drug intake. For assessing the risk of immediate reactions, skin prick test, and intradermal test are used. However, the negative predictive value of these tests is not reassuring for most of the antibiotics (except for penicillin). Therefore, the positive results may indicate a high risk of allergic reactions, but the negative results do not definitely rule out the risk.[331] Due to the low negative predictive value, combinatory diagnostic approaches are suggested. For example, besides skin diagnostic tests, oral challenge tests are usually performed to determine the cause of the allergy. In the skin prick test, a small amount of drug in liquid or powder is applied to a small area of the forearm, and then the skin is perforated by a lancet. Also, 0.9 percent serum saline and histamine are used as negative and positive controls, respectively, and the result is compared to these controls. Positive results usually appear within 20 min. However, the symptoms that appear within 24 to 48 h may be considered as delayed positive results.[343]

Skin patch testing and delayed intradermal testing are used for the diagnosis of delayed drug reactions. Delayed intradermal testing is shown to be more sensitive than patch testing. In these tests, the drug preparations are usually applied via petrolatum or other vehicles to a small area of skin for 48 h, and then the occurrence of delayed symptoms is investigated for the next 48 to 96 h.[331] The delayed skin tests should be performed at least 4 weeks after discontinuation of corticosteroids and other immunosuppressant agents and 4–6 weeks after the occurrence of acute symptoms to reduce the risk of false-positive, false-negative, or systemic reactions.[343]

## Specific drugs

### *Non-Steroidal anti-inflammatory drugs (NSAIDs)*

Allergy to NSAIDs is the second most prevalent allergy after antibiotics. About 1.9 percent of adults have experienced an allergic reaction to this drug type, and about 29 percent of drug allergy complaints are because of NSAIDs.[344] Also, by causing 48.7 percent−57.8 percent of drug-induced anaphylaxis, they are the most frequent cause of this phenomenon. The incidence of anaphylaxis is usually accompanied by asthma, rhinosinusitis, and nasal polyps in adults.[325]

The reactions of NAISD-induced allergy are classified into 5 groups. The most common type is Aspirin-exacerbated respiratory disease (AERD). It is an acquired syndrome which its symptoms, including persistent nasal congestion, nasal polyposis, and rhinitis, mostly begin during early adulthood, and it is continued by other manifestations, which include asthma and hypersensitivity to COX-1 inhibitors. AERD is mostly accompanied by acute respiratory manifestations such as rhinorrhea, acute nasal congestion, bronchoconstriction, chest tightness, and ocular erythema. It affects both the upper and lower respiratory tract within 30 to 120 min after drug intake. Also, some other non-respiratory symptoms, such as abdominal cramps and diarrhea, nausea, and skin eruptions, may happen in some of the patients.[344]

Multiple NSAID-exacerbated urticaria/angioedema occurs in 12 percent−30 percent of patients with chronic urticaria, followed by COX-1 inhibitors intake. The symptoms are mostly cutaneous and appear within minutes after drug administration. The reaction is not considered as IgE-mediated. It seems that the underlying immune defect in patients with chronic urticaria triggers the degranulation of mast cells and subsequent allergic reaction.[344] In multiple NSAID-induced urticaria/angioedema in otherwise asymptomatic patients, patients with no history of urticaria or angioedema develop cutaneous symptoms within 1–6 h of the intake of any COX-1 inhibitor drug. Single NSAID-induced anaphylactic reactions happen without cross-reactivity between different COX-1 inhibitor drugs. It may cause urticaria, angioedema, and/or anaphylaxis within a short period of time. All four reaction types were acute. However, in some cases, NSAIDs can lead to delayed reactions, such as fixed drug eruptions, SJS/TEN, MPE, AGEP, DRESS, and contact dermatitis (by topical NSAIDs).[344]

### *β-Lactam antibiotics*

β-Lactam antibiotics, including penicillins and cephalosporins, are widely used antibiotics. About 8 percent and 1 percent of adults in the United States population have once had an allergic reaction to penicillins and cephalosporins, respectively.[345] After NSAIDs, β-Lactam antibiotics are the most frequent cause of anaphylaxis and are the culprit drug in 75 percent of deaths because of anaphylaxis.[325]

Acute allergic reactions are mediated by IgE antibodies, which are present in the body as a result of previous sensitization, and IgG mediates delayed reactions within 7–10 days after the first exposure to the drug and 1–2 days after the re-exposure.[346] Patients with β-Lactam antibiotics-induced allergy could experience the immediate type of immune reaction, and usually, more than one system is affected, and only a slight percentage of the patients develops urticaria and/or angioedema alone. Delayed type of immune response can also happen, which can lead to MPE, AGEP, DRESS, FDE, SJS, TEN, and serum sickness-like symptoms.[347] In the diagnosis of β-Lactam antibiotics-induced allergic reaction, history taking plays an important role. Diagnostic tests and desensitization should not be performed in patients with a history of severe cutaneous adverse drug reactions and other delayed systemic symptoms. The oral challenge test is the gold standard for diagnosing IgE-mediated and acute symptoms of penicillin allergy. However, skin diagnostic tests are also performed to confirm tolerance or hypersensitivity to this drug class.[345]

Cross-reactivity is a relatively common phenomenon between penicillins, cephalosporins, and carbapenems. They all share a β-Lactam ring in their chemical structure. However, cross-reactivity may be due to similar side chains in penicillins and especially first-generation cephalosporins. So, cephalosporin administration is applicable in patients with penicillin allergy as long as the side chains are not similar. It is reported that patients with an allergy to penicillin develop a higher risk of allergy even to other drug types. Thus, medications should be prescribed with more caution in this group of patients.[348]

### Angiotensin-converting enzyme inhibitors (ACE-I)

Angiotensin-converting enzyme inhibitors (ACE-I) is widely used as an anti-hypertensive drug. However, 0.1 percent–0.7 percent of patients taking ACE-I develop ACE-I-induced angioedema. The inhibition of ACE stops the degradation of bradykinin and subsequently increases its plasma level. Bradykinin then causes vasodilation, increased vascular permeability, and further development of angioedema. Patients with a history of ACE-I-induced angioedema should not be tested or challenged for these drugs, as severe symptoms in this high-risk group of patients may happen.[349]

### Radiocontrast media (RCM)

Radiocontrast Media (RCM) are substances used to enhance the contrast of X-ray-based imaging. The prevalence of allergic reactions to RCM is reported to range between 0.7 percent–3 percent for non-ionic RCM and 3.8 percent to 12.7 percent for monomeric ionic RCM.[350] By introducing the non-ionic RCMs, the rate of anaphylaxis and other severe adverse reactions has tremendously decreased from 12.1 percent to about 0.04 percent.[325] Older age, previous allergic reaction to RCM, previous frequent exposure to RCM, and history of atopy and asthma have been associated with higher risks of developing allergic reactions.[325,351] The reactions are classified as immediate and delayed forms. The immediate reactions can be mediated by sensitization and subsequent IgE production, or mediated by tryptase, bradykinin, or other vasoactive agents' secretion via the direct effect of RCM on mast cells, and causing anaphylaxis-like symptoms. The delayed reactions are mostly manifested by MPE and are triggered by T cell-mediated response.[351]

### *Biological drugs*

The use of biological immune modulators to treat cancer and inflammatory diseases is getting more and more widespread. These biological drugs, also called biological agents or biological modifiers, are mostly cytokines, monoclonal antibodies, or soluble receptors that affect the function of the immune system. These agents are proteins with higher molecular weights than conventional drugs, thus they may have more immunogenicity and their metabolism pathways are different. Because of the structural and functional differences of biological drugs, allergy mechanisms to this type of drugs are often distinct from Gell and Coombs classification. Uncontrolled doses of cytokines or other regulatory molecules can lead to high-dose reactions such as capillary leak syndrome, immunodeficiency, autoimmunity, or allergic reactions. Also, cross-reaction can happen when a molecule affects off-target cells. The adverse reactions can be both cell or antibody-mediated. Moreover, these agents can cause non-immunological effects like depression.[339]

## Treatment

The first step of drug allergy treatment is to stop the intake of culprit medications and treat the symptoms. For mild rashes and eruptions, the administration of antihistamines may relieve itching. Systemic steroid therapy is necessary for those patients with a progressive rash with other severe or prolonged symptoms such as fever, nausea, and arthralgia. The patients with severe cutaneous adverse drug reactions may need a prolonged period of systemic steroid therapy.[331] Administration of epinephrine as first-line therapy and β2-agonists and glucocorticoids as second-line therapy should be considered for the treatment of patients with anaphylaxis.[325]

When a certain medication is necessary, and there is a high risk of allergy to that certain drug, desensitization approaches may be applicable. A temporary clinical tolerance may be achieved when increasing doses of a culprit drug are administered at specific intervals. The desensitization approach is not attempted in all patients with a history of severe cutaneous adverse reactions, except for patients with mild and uncomplicated exanthems and fixed drug eruptions. Due to the high risk of adverse reactions, the procedure must be done under strict precautions and when there is no effective alternative for the culprit drug. Thus, the pros and cons of applying desensitization therapy should be thoroughly examined before starting the treatment.[331,352]

## Anaphylaxis

### Definition

Second National Institute of Allergy and Infectious Diseases (NIAID)/Food Allergy and Anaphylaxis Network (FAAN) symposium in 2005 defined anaphylaxis as a severe, potentially life-threatening, hyperacute systemic allergic response to an allergen.[353] Other definitions of anaphylaxis by other entities such as the World Health Organization (WHO) are either derived from or more or less similar to the one mentioned, all emphasizing its sudden onset, seriousness, and its capacity to be fatal.[354] In the clinical setting, anaphylaxis is defined and identified by a set of signs and symptoms,[353,355] which will be discussed later.

Anaphylactic reactions could be divided into uniphasic (most common), biphasic, and protracted (persistent) types. In a patient with uniphasic anaphylaxis, symptoms appear and resolve quickly and do not recur afterward. On the other hand, in a biphasic reaction, the patient experiences a second wave of symptoms several hours after the first, even though there has been no external trigger. Persistent anaphylaxis is rare and might even take weeks to disappear.[356-358]

### Epidemiology and risk factors

It is estimated that 0.05 percent to 2 percent of people experience an anaphylactic reaction at least once in their lifetime,[359] and it seems to be more common among children and adolescents.[359] According to a survey in the United States, 1.6 percent to 5.1 percent of adults reported a "probable" or "very likely" history of anaphylaxis.[360]

Foods, medication, and insects are the most common causes of anaphylaxis.[361] In the last 20 years, food anaphylaxis has become two times more frequent than it was before. Some genetic studies have indicated that this phenomenon is, to some degree, due to newly emerged allergens consequent to novel processing methods used in the food industry.[362,363]

With current treatment options, fatal anaphylaxis is very rare, with a prevalence of 0.69 per million people in the United States.[364] The most frequent known types of anaphylaxis causing death are medication (contributing to over 50 percent of the cases), venom, and food anaphylaxes.[364] However, in outpatient settings, food anaphylaxis death is more common than any other type.[364]

The most important risk factor for anaphylaxis development is atopy. Furthermore, numerous elements result in a greater risk of serious complications in a patient experiencing an anaphylactic reaction, such as age, medications, and comorbid diseases (e.g., asthma and other pulmonary diseases).[365] Additionally, the use of drugs that reduce blood pressure, such as β-blockers, ACE-Is, and diuretics, leads to a higher chance of hypotension or shock during an anaphylactic reaction. β-blockers can also increase the risk of bronchospasm.[362]

## Pathogenesis

Like most other allergic reactions, anaphylaxis follows a type 1 IgE and Th2-mediated hypersensitivity pathway. When an antigen that the patient is sensitive to is detected by the immune system (mainly Th2 cells and B lymphocytes), plasma cells start producing vast amounts of antigen-specific IgE. These Igs attach to the surface of basophils and mast cells and capture the antigens upon reentry, precipitating degranulation of mast cells and basophils.[356,362] However, in some cases, the release of substances from basophils and mast cells is not IgE dependent but rather affected by other factors such as IgG immune complexes, drugs, or radiocontrast agents.[356]

Basophils and mast cells release several types of mediators upon degranulation, such as leukotrienes, cytokines (e.g., TNF-α, IL-4, IL-5), histamine, and growth factors. These substances cause the recruitment of immune cells, resulting in the continuation of the inflammatory cascade,[356,366] as well as smooth muscle contraction and increased vascular permeability, leading to hypotensive shock and bronchoconstriction.[362]

In some cases, cardiogenic, hypovolemic, and distributive shock mechanisms come together and cause a severe hypotensive state (i.e., anaphylactic shock). Increased permeability of capillaries and vasodilation caused by cytokines and substances released through the inflammatory cascade, increase third space fluid accumulation and reduce venous return and consequently preload and cardiac output, especially in an upright position (i.e., empty heart syndrome). While in some less severe cases, the heart might be able to compensate for the loss of blood pressure to some degree by increasing pulse rate (i.e., tachycardia), in others, hypotension persists, and no improvement is observed.[356]

## Clinical features

Anaphylaxis has the potential to involve almost any system in the human body.[356] Life-threatening complications arise from cardiovascular and pulmonary systems involvement (i.e., shock and obstruction of airways).[356]

The involvement of the skin and mucosal surfaces is present in 80 percent−90 percent of anaphylaxis cases. Manifestations may include urticaria, angioedema in airways, which might lead to obstruction of airways, pruritus, and flushing.[356]

60 percent to 70 percent of patients experience respiratory complications such as laryngeal edema presenting as vocal changes, wheezing, coughing, rhinitis, dyspnea, and chest tightness. If not appropriately treated, hypoxia, respiratory failure, and death might occur in severe cases.[356,362]

Cardiovascular involvement, an extremely serious and fatal consequence of anaphylaxis, has an incidence of 40 percent–50 percent. Vasodilation and myocardial damage may cause hypotension or shock, urinary or fecal incontinence, reduced cardiac output, myocardial ischemia, arrhythmia, and cardiac arrest.[356]

The involvement of the gastrointestinal system, which is seen in 40 percent–50 percent of cases, might result in nausea, vomiting, diarrhea, and intestinal edema, causing dehydration, hypovolemia, or abdominal pain.[356]

In less than 15 percent of cases, anaphylaxis precipitates neurological injuries such as dizziness, confusion, headaches, or even more serious events such as syncope and seizure.[356]

It is especially important in infants to recognize all signs and symptoms of an anaphylactic reaction, as some clinical features of anaphylaxis are quite common in the everyday life of an infant, such as flushing, dysphonia, and spitting after nutrition.[362,367]

## Diagnosis

The diagnosis of anaphylaxis is mainly symptomatic and must be performed promptly. A diagnosis of anaphylaxis is highly likely in either of these scenarios: 1) acute mucocutaneous manifestations + acute respiratory symptoms, or hypotension or end-organ damage 2) development of two or more of the following symptoms immediately after exposure to a likely allergen: mucocutaneous symptoms, acute respiratory symptoms, persistent gastrointestinal symptoms, hypotension or end-organ damage, 3) hypotension (systolic blood pressure $< 90$ mmHg or reduced more than 30 percent from baseline) after exposure to a known allergen.[353,361]

Measuring plasma tryptase and histamine levels (two of the mediators released during the inflammatory process) might reveal an anaphylactic reaction if measured within minutes (for histamine) or hours (for tryptase) of symptom onset. However, laboratory confirmation is unnecessary for clinical diagnosis and initiation of treatment, and serology tests are generally used for retrospective verification of the diagnosis.[356,368,369]

## Differential diagnosis

Many conditions could be considered as differential diagnoses of anaphylaxis include asthma, flushing syndromes, syncope, anxiety attack, and vocal cord dysfunction. Severe asthma exacerbations present symptoms similar to those of anaphylaxis, such as wheezing and dyspnea. However, skin symptoms and serious cardiovascular events are uncommon in asthma. Isolated angioedema (not associated with urticaria) might resemble anaphylaxis, involves a bradykinin-mediated mechanism, and is usually a result of the use of drugs such as ACE-Is and dipeptidyl peptidase 4 (DPP4) inhibitors, hereditary angioedema, lymphoproliferative diseases, or monoclonal gammopathy of unknown significance.[361,370,371] Screening of bradykinin-mediated angioedema is done by measuring the C4 and C1-INH levels.[361]

## Treatment

Intramuscular epinephrine shot in the anterolateral surface of the thigh is the treatment of choice for anaphylaxis and must be administered as soon as possible. Epinephrine acts on sympathetic receptors, causing vasoconstriction and bronchodilation, therefore restoring blood pressure and airflow. Injections could be performed either by commercial syringes with autoinjectors or by manually drawing up from an epinephrine vial.[361] If needed, injections could be repeated every 3 to 5 min.[367] Intramuscular injection is preferred to intravenous injection, as the latter carries the risk of several side effects (e.g., arrhythmia) and dosing errors,[361] except for cases who do not respond to intramuscular epinephrine and fluid replacement.[353] No contradictions have been declared for epinephrine administration in anaphylaxis.

Antihistamines cannot be used instead of epinephrine in the treatment of anaphylaxis due to their slow onset of action, although they can be advantageous in relieving dramatic symptoms such as pruritus and urticaria.[353]

Once primary results have been obtained from epinephrine injection, adjunctive recovery measures must be taken into action to reduce the sequela, most notably adverse effects of hypotension and respiratory malfunction.[367] Supine leg raise, which increases venous return and preload, along with intravenous fluid resuscitation, and in selected cases, vasopressor administration, mitigate hypotension in patients.[372] Oxygen therapy must be applied conservatively (to reduce the chance of hyperoxia-induced paradoxical tissue hypoxia) in patients with respiratory symptoms or hypoxia.[373] In patients with an oropharyngeal obstruction or laryngeal edema, intubation is recommended.[356,361] Short-acting β agonists might be administered for patients with dyspnea, wheeze, or hypoxia, with or without short-acting muscarinic receptor antagonists.[361] Corticosteroids may reduce the chance of a biphasic reaction, although their effects are yet to be proven statistically.[361] In cases with refractory anaphylaxis, epinephrine infusion might be necessary. Patients with refractory anaphylaxis who are also taking β-blocker medications, may benefit from glucagon therapy, which could help with chronotropy and inotropy.[374,375] All patients are required to have epinephrine autoinjector pens at their disposal, preferably at all times, after being discharged from the hospital. Additionally, patients must be referred to an allergist for further workup and examinations.[361]

## References


1. Igea JM. The history of the idea of allergy. *Allergy*. 2013;68(8):966–973.
2. von Pirquet C. Allergie. *Munch Med Wochenschr*. 1906;30:1457–1458.
3. Ishizaka K, Ishizaka T, Hornbrook MM. Physico-chemical properties of human reaginic antibody. IV. Presence of a unique immunoglobulin as a carrier of reaginic activity. *Journal of immunology (Baltimore, Md: 1950)*. 1966;97(1):75–85.
4. Bennich H, Johansson SGO, Killander J. Studies on a new class of human immunoglobulins: II Chemical and physical properties editor *Gammaglobulins Structure and Control of Biosynthesis Stockholm*: Almqvist & Wiksell; 1967:199–205.

5. Wang J, Wu J, Lai H. Allergic disease epidemiology *Allergy Bioinformatics*: Springer; 2015:15–41.
6. Okada H, Kuhn C, Feillet H, Bach JF. The 'hygiene hypothesis' for autoimmune and allergic diseases: an update. *Clinical and experimental immunology*. 2010;160(1):1–9.
7. Stiemsma LT, Turvey SE. Asthma and the microbiome: defining the critical window in early life. *Allergy, asthma, and clinical immunology: official journal of the Canadian Society of Allergy and Clinical Immunology*. 2017;13:3.
8. American Academy of Allergy AaI. Asthma Overview [Available from: https://www.aaaai.org/conditions-and-treatments/asthma.
9. Global Initiative for Asthma. Global Strategy for Asthma Management and Prevention (2020 update) 2020, Available from: https://ginasthma.org/wp-content/uploads/2020/06/GINA-2020-report_20_06_04-1-wms.pdf.
10. Nakamura Y, Tamaoki J, Nagase H, Yamaguchi M, Horiguchi T, Hozawa S, et al. Japanese guidelines for adult asthma 2020. *Allergology International*. 2020.
11. Boonpiyathad T, Sözener ZC, Satitsuksanoa P, Akdis CA. Immunologic mechanisms in asthma. *Semin Immunol*. 2019;46:101333.
12. Froidure A, Mouthuy J, Durham SR, Chanez P, Sibille Y, Pilette C. Asthma phenotypes and IgE responses. *European Respiratory Journal*. 2016;47(1):304.
13. Kuruvilla ME, Lee FE-H, Lee GB. Understanding Asthma Phenotypes, Endotypes, and Mechanisms of Disease. *Clin Rev Allergy Immunol*. 2019;56(2):219–233.
14. Wenzel SE, Schwartz LB, Langmack EL, Halliday JL, Trudeau JB, Gibbs RL, et al. Evidence That Severe Asthma Can Be Divided Pathologically into Two Inflammatory Subtypes with Distinct Physiologic and Clinical Characteristics. *American Journal of Respiratory and Critical Care Medicine*. 1999;160(3):1001–1008.
15. Svenningsen S, Nair P. Asthma Endotypes and an Overview of Targeted Therapy for Asthma. *Front Med (Lausanne)*. 2017;4:158.
16. Russell RJ, Brightling C. Pathogenesis of asthma: implications for precision medicine. *Clin Sci (Lond)*. 2017;131(14):1723–1735.
17. Mattiuzzi C, Lippi G. Worldwide asthma epidemiology: insights from the Global Health Data Exchange database. *International Forum of Allergy & Rhinology*. 2020;10(1):75–80.
18. Bachert C, Vignola AM, Gevaert P, Leynaert B, Van Cauwenberge P, Bousquet J. Allergic rhinitis, rhinosinusitis, and asthma: one airway disease. *Immunology and Allergy Clinics of North America*. 2004;24(1):19–43.
19. Dixon AE, Kaminsky DA, Holbrook JT, Wise RA, Shade DM, Irvin CG. Allergic Rhinitis and Sinusitis in Asthma: differential Effects on Symptoms and Pulmonary Function. *Chest*. 2006;130(2):429–435.
20. Maslan J, Mims JW. What is asthma? Pathophysiology, demographics, and health care costs. *Otolaryngol Clin North Am*. 2014;47(1):13–22.
21. Dharmage SC, Perret JL. Custovic A. Epidemiology of Asthma in Children and Adults. *Frontiers in Pediatrics*. 2019;7(246).
22. Stern J, Pier J, Litonjua AA. Asthma epidemiology and risk factors. *Seminars in Immunopathology*. 2020;42(1):5–15.
23. Moraes TJ, Sears MR, Subbarao P. *Epidemiology of Asthma and Influence of Ethnicity. Semin Respir Crit Care Med*. 2018;39(01):003–011.
24. Kuruvilla ME, Vanijcharoenkarn K, Shih JA. Lee FE-H. Epidemiology and risk factors for asthma. *Respiratory Medicine*. 2019;149:16–22.
25. Sporik R, Holgate ST, Platts-Mills TA, Cogswell JJ. Exposure to house-dust mite allergen (Der p I) and the development of asthma in childhood. A prospective study. *N Engl J Med*. 1990;323(8):502–507.
26. Illi S, von Mutius E, Lau S, Niggemann B, Grüber C, Wahn U. Perennial allergen sensitisation early in life and chronic asthma in children: a birth cohort study. *Lancet*. 2006;368(9537):763–770.
27. Wong KO, Hunter Rowe B, Douwes J, Senthilselvan A. Asthma and Wheezing Are Associated with Depression and Anxiety in Adults: an Analysis from 54 Countries. *Pulmonary Medicine*. 2013;2013:929028.
28. Jackson DJ, Gangnon RE, Evans MD, Roberg KA, Anderson EL, Pappas TE, et al. Wheezing rhinovirus illnesses in early life predict asthma development in high-risk children. *American Journal of Respiratory and Critical Care Medicine*. 2008;178(7):667–672.

29. Navarro S, Cossalter G, Chiavaroli C, Kanda A, Fleury S, Lazzari A, et al. The oral administration of bacterial extracts prevents asthma via the recruitment of regulatory T cells to the airways. *Mucosal Immunology*. 2011;4(1):53–65.
30. Ober C, Yao T-C. The genetics of asthma and allergic disease: a 21st century perspective. *Immunol Rev*. 2011;242(1):10–30.
31. Moffatt MF, Gut IG, Demenais F, Strachan DP, Bouzigon E, Heath S, et al. A large-scale, consortium-based genomewide association study of asthma. *N Engl J Med*. 2010;363(13):1211–1221.
32. Mims JW. Asthma: definitions and pathophysiology. *International Forum of Allergy & Rhinology*. 2015;5(S1):S2–S6.
33. Breton CV, Siegmund KD, Joubert BR, Wang X, Qui W, Carey V, et al. Prenatal tobacco smoke exposure is associated with childhood DNA CpG methylation. *PLoS One*. 2014;9(6):e99716.
34. Szabo SM, Levy AR, Gooch KL, Bradt P, Wijaya H, Mitchell I. Elevated risk of asthma after hospitalization for respiratory syncytial virus infection in infancy. *Paediatr Respir Rev*. 2013;13(Suppl 2):S9–15.
35. Page C, O'Shaughnessy B, Barnes P. Pathogenesis of COPD and Asthma. *Handb Exp Pharmacol*. 2017;237:1–21.
36. Papi A, Brightling C, Pedersen SE, Reddel HK. Asthma. *The Lancet*. 2018;391(10122):783–800.
37. Fahy JV. Type 2 inflammation in asthma–present in most, absent in many. *Nat Rev Immunol*. 2015;15(1):57–65.
38. Russkamp D, Aguilar-Pimentel A, Alessandrini F, Gailus-Durner V, Fuchs H, Ohnmacht C, et al. IL-4 receptor α blockade prevents sensitization and alters acute and long-lasting effects of allergen-specific immunotherapy of murine allergic asthma. *Allergy*. 2019;74(8):1549–1560.
39. Hassani M, Koenderman L. Immunological and hematological effects of IL-5(Rα)-targeted therapy: an overview. *Allergy*. 2018;73(10):1979–1988.
40. Mitamura Y, Nunomura S, Nanri Y, Ogawa M, Yoshihara T, Masuoka M, et al. The IL-13/periostin/IL-24 pathway causes epidermal barrier dysfunction in allergic skin inflammation. *Allergy*. 2018;73(9):1881–1891.
41. Nagata M, Sedgwick JB, Kita H, Busse WW. Granulocyte Macrophage Colony-stimulating Factor Augments ICAM-1 and VCAM-1 Activation of Eosinophil Function. *American Journal of Respiratory Cell and Molecular Biology*. 1998;19(1):158–166.
42. Berry MA, Hargadon B, Shelley M, Parker D, Shaw DE, Green RH, et al. Evidence of a role of tumor necrosis factor alpha in refractory asthma. *N Engl J Med*. 2006;354(7):697–708.
43. Lee B-J, Moon H-G, Shin T-S, Jeon SG, Lee E-Y, Gho YS, et al. Protective effects of basic fibroblast growth factor in the development of emphysema induced by interferon-γ. *Experimental & Molecular Medicine*. 2011;43(4):169–178.
44. Thomas PS, Yates DH, Barnes PJ. Tumor necrosis factor-alpha increases airway responsiveness and sputum neutrophilia in normal human subjects. *American Journal of Respiratory and Critical Care Medicine*. 1995;152(1):76–80.
45. Raundhal M, Morse C, Khare A, Oriss TB, Milosevic J, Trudeau J, et al. High IFN-γ and low SLPI mark severe asthma in mice and humans. *J Clin Invest*. 2015;125(8):3037–3050.
46. Brusselle GG, Maes T, Bracke KR. Eosinophils in the Spotlight: eosinophilic airway inflammation in nonallergic asthma. *Nature Medicine*. 2013;19(8):977–979.
47. Barnig C, Cernadas M, Dutile S, Liu X, Perrella MA, Kazani S, et al. Lipoxin A<sub>4</sub> Regulates Natural Killer Cell and Type 2 Innate Lymphoid Cell Activation in Asthma. *Science Translational Medicine*. 2013;5(174):174ra26.
48. Barrios RJ, Kheradmand F, Batts L, DB Corry. Asthma: pathology and pathophysiology. *Arch Pathol Lab Med*. 2006;130(4):447–451.
49. Cohn L, Homer RJ, Marinov A, Rankin J, Bottomly K. Induction of airway mucus production By T helper 2 (Th2) cells: a critical role for interleukin 4 in cell recruitment but not mucus production. *J Exp Med*. 1997;186(10):1737–1747.
50. Lee JJ, McGarry MP, Farmer SC, Denzler KL, Larson KA, Carrigan PE, et al. Interleukin-5 expression in the lung epithelium of transgenic mice leads to pulmonary changes pathognomonic of asthma. *J Exp Med*. 1997;185(12):2143–2156.
51. Stinson SE, Amrani Y, Brightling CE. D prostanoid receptor 2 (chemoattractant receptor-homologous molecule expressed on TH2 cells) protein expression in asthmatic patients and its effects on bronchial epithelial cells. *J Allergy Clin Immunol*. 2015;135(2):395–406.

52. Gizycki MJ, Adelroth E, Rogers AV, O'Byrne PM, Jeffery PK. Myofibroblast involvement in the allergen-induced late response in mild atopic asthma. *Am J Respir Cell Mol Biol*. 1997;16(6):664–673.
53. Bossley CJ, Fleming L, Gupta A, Regamey N, Frith J, Oates T, et al. Pediatric severe asthma is characterized by eosinophilia and remodeling without T(H)2 cytokines. *J Allergy Clin Immunol*. 2012;129(4):974–982 e13.
54. Tsien A, Diaz-Sanchez D, Ma J, Saxon A. The organic component of diesel exhaust particles and phenanthrene, a major polyaromatic hydrocarbon constituent, enhances IgE production by IgE-secreting EBV-transformed human B cells in vitro. *Toxicol Appl Pharmacol*. 1997;142(2):256–263.
55. Khan SH, Grayson MH. Cross-linking IgE augments human conventional dendritic cell production of CC chemokine ligand 28. *Journal of Allergy and Clinical Immunology*. 2010;125(1):265–267.
56. Matucci A, Vultaggio A, Maggi E, Kasujee I. Is IgE or eosinophils the key player in allergic asthma pathogenesis? Are we asking the right question? *Respiratory Research*. 2018;19(1):113.
57. Ferreira DS, Carvalho-Pinto RM, Gregório MG, Annoni R, Teles AM, Buttignol M, et al. Airway pathology in severe asthma is related to airflow obstruction but not symptom control. *Allergy*. 2018;73(3):635–643.
58. Amin K. The role of mast cells in allergic inflammation. *Respiratory Medicine*. 2012;106(1):9–14.
59. Fajt ML, Gelhaus SL, Freeman B, Uvalle CE, Trudeau JB, Holguin F, et al. Prostaglandin $D_2$ pathway upregulation: relation to asthma severity, control, and TH2 inflammation. *J Allergy Clin Immunol*. 2013;131(6):1504–1512.
60. Barnes N, Pavord I, Chuchalin A, Bell J, Hunter M, Lewis T, et al. A randomized, double-blind, placebo-controlled study of the CRTH2 antagonist OC000459 in moderate persistent asthma. *Clin Exp Allergy*. 2012;42(1):38–48.
61. Domingo C, Palomares O, Sandham DA, Erpenbeck VJ, Altman P. The prostaglandin D2 receptor 2 pathway in asthma: a key player in airway inflammation. *Respiratory Research*. 2018;19(1):189.
62. Amin K, LÚDvÍKsdÓTtir D, Janson C, Nettelbladt O, BjÖRnsson E, Roomans GM, et al. Inflammation and Structural Changes in the Airways of Patients with Atopic and Nonatopic Asthma. *American Journal of Respiratory and Critical Care Medicine*. 2000;162(6):2295–2301.
63. Bradding P, Brightling C. Mast cell infiltration of airway smooth muscle in asthma. *Respiratory Medicine*. 2007;101(5):1045.
64. Nakagome K, Nagata M. Involvement and Possible Role of Eosinophils in Asthma Exacerbation. *Front Immunol*. 2018;9:2220.
65. Terl M, Sedlák V, Cap P, Dvořáková R, Kašák V, Kočí T, et al. Asthma management: a new phenotype-based approach using presence of eosinophilia and allergy. *Allergy*. 2017;72(9):1279–1287.
66. Laitinen LA, Haahtela T, Vilkka V, Lee TH, Spur BW. Leukotriene E4 and granulocytic infiltration into asthmatic airways. *The Lancet*. 1993;341(8851):989–990.
67. Nagata M, Sedgwick JB, Vrtis R, Busse WW. Endothelial cells upregulate eosinophil superoxide generation via VCAM-1 expression. *Clin Exp Allergy*. 1999;29(4):550–561.
68. Saito K, Nagata M, Kikuchi I, Sakamoto Y. Leukotriene D4 and eosinophil transendothelial migration, superoxide generation, and degranulation via β2 integrin. *Annals of Allergy, Asthma & Immunology*. 2004;93(6):594–600.
69. Olin JT, Wechsler ME. Asthma: pathogenesis and novel drugs for treatment. *Bmj*. 2014;349:g5517.
70. Wong DT, Elovic A, Matossian K, Nagura N, McBride J, Chou MY, et al. Eosinophils from patients with blood eosinophilia express transforming growth factor beta 1. *Blood*. 1991;78(10):2702–2707.
71. Crimi E, Spanevello A, Neri M, Ind PW, Rossi GA, Brusasco V. Dissociation between Airway Inflammation and Airway Hyperresponsiveness in Allergic Asthma. *American Journal of Respiratory and Critical Care Medicine*. 1998;157(1):4–9.
72. Wilson NM, James A, Uasuf C, Payne DN, Hablas H, Agrofioti C, et al. Asthma severity and inflammation markers in children. *Pediatric Allergy and Immunology*. 2001;12(3):125–132.
73. Djukanović R, Wilson SJ, Kraft M, Jarjour NN, Steel M, Chung KF, et al. Effects of Treatment with Anti-immunoglobulin E Antibody Omalizumab on Airway Inflammation in Allergic Asthma. *American Journal of Respiratory and Critical Care Medicine*. 2004;170(6):583–593.
74. Licona-Limón P, Kim LK, Palm NW, Flavell RA. TH2, allergy and group 2 innate lymphoid cells. *Nature Immunology*. 2013;14(6):536–542.
75. Roan F, Obata-Ninomiya K, Ziegler SF. Epithelial cell–derived cytokines: more than just signaling the alarm. *The Journal of Clinical Investigation*. 2019;129(4):1441–1451.

76. Saatian B, Rezaee F, Desando S, Emo J, Chapman T, Knowlden S, et al. Interleukin-4 and interleukin-13 cause barrier dysfunction in human airway epithelial cells. *Tissue Barriers*. 2013;1(2):e24333.
77. Thomas B, Rutman A, Hirst RA, Haldar P, Wardlaw AJ, Bankart J, et al. Ciliary dysfunction and ultrastructural abnormalities are features of severe asthma. *J Allergy Clin Immunol*. 2010;126(4):722–729 e2.
78. Levy ML, Fletcher M, Price DB, Hausen T, Halbert RJ, Yawn BP. International Primary Care Respiratory Group (IPCRG) Guidelines: diagnosis of respiratory diseases in primary care. *Prim Care Respir J*. 2006;15(1):20–34.
79. Fuhlbrigge AL, Kitch BT, Paltiel AD, Kuntz KM, Neumann PJ, Dockery DW, et al. FEV1 is associated with risk of asthma attacks in a pediatric population. *Journal of Allergy and Clinical Immunology*. 2001;107(1):61–67.
80. Stein RT, Martinez FD. Asthma phenotypes in childhood: lessons from an epidemiological approach. *Paediatr Respir Rev*. 2004;5(2):155–161.
81. Boulet LP, Boulay M. Asthma-related comorbidities. *Expert Rev Respir Med*. 2011;5(3):377–393.
82. Benayoun L, Druilhe A, Dombret M-C, Aubier M, Pretolani M. Airway Structural Alterations Selectively Associated with Severe Asthma. *American Journal of Respiratory and Critical Care Medicine*. 2003;167(10):1360–1368.
83. Gupta S, Siddiqui S, Haldar P, Raj JV, Entwisle JJ, Wardlaw AJ, et al. Qualitative analysis of high-resolution CT scans in severe asthma. *Chest*. 2009;136(6):1521–1528.
84. Handoyo S, Rosenwasser LJ. Asthma phenotypes. *Current Allergy and Asthma Reports*. 2009;9(6): 439–445.
85. Quanjer PH, Stanojevic S, Cole TJ, Baur X, Hall GL, Culver BH, et al. Multi-ethnic reference values for spirometry for the 3–95-yr age range: the global lung function 2012 Eqs. *European Respiratory Journal*. 2012;40(6):1324.
86. Quirt J, Hildebrand KJ, Mazza J, Noya F, Kim H. Asthma. *Allergy, Asthma & Clinical Immunology*. 2018;14(2):50.
87. Ramamurthy MB. Asthma Mimickers: approach to Differential Diagnosis. *The Indian Journal of Pediatrics*. 2018;85(8):667–672.
88. Ullmann N, Mirra V, Di Marco A, Pavone M, Porcaro F, Negro V, et al. Asthma: differential Diagnosis and Comorbidities. *Frontiers in pediatrics*. 2018;6:276.
89. Marthin JK, Nielsen KG. Choice of nasal nitric oxide technique as first-line test for primary ciliary dyskinesia. *Eur Respir J*. 2011;37(3):559–565.
90. Juniper EF, Kline PA, Vanzieleghem MA, Ramsdale EH, O'Byrne PM, Hargreave FE. Effect of Long-term Treatment with an Inhaled Corticosteroid (Budesonide) on Airway Hyperresponsiveness and Clinical Asthma in Nonsteroid-dependent Asthmatics. *American Review of Respiratory Disease*. 1990;142(4):832–836.
91. Sullivan SD, Buxton M, Andersson LF, Lamm CJ, Liljas B, Chen YZ, et al. Cost-effectiveness analysis of early intervention with budesonide in mild persistent asthma. *Journal of Allergy and Clinical Immunology*. 2003;112(6):1229–1236.
92. Pauwels RA, Löfdahl CG, Postma DS, Tattersfield AE, O'Byrne P, Barnes PJ, et al. Effect of inhaled formoterol and budesonide on exacerbations of asthma. Formoterol and Corticosteroids Establishing Therapy (FACET) International Study Group. *N Engl J Med*. 1997;337(20):1405–1411.
93. Busse WW, Pedersen S, Pauwels RA, Tan WC, Chen YZ, Lamm CJ, et al. The Inhaled Steroid Treatment As Regular Therapy in Early Asthma (START) study 5-year follow-up: effectiveness of early intervention with budesonide in mild persistent asthma. *J Allergy Clin Immunol*. 2008;121(5):1167–1174.
94. Selroos O, Pietinalho A, Löfroos AB, Riska H. Effect of early vs late intervention with inhaled corticosteroids in asthma. *Chest*. 1995;108(5):1228–1234.
95. Selroos O. Effect of disease duration on dose-response of inhaled budesonide in asthma. *Respir Med*. 2008;102(7):1065–1072.
96. Chung KF, Wenzel SE, Brozek JL, Bush A, Castro M, Sterk PJ, et al. International ERS/ATS guidelines on definition, evaluation and treatment of severe asthma. *European Respiratory Journal*. 2014;43(2):343.
97. Hastie AT, Moore WC, Meyers DA, Vestal PL, Li H, Peters SP, et al. Analyses of asthma severity phenotypes and inflammatory proteins in subjects stratified by sputum granulocytes. *J Allergy Clin Immunol*. 2010;125(5):1028–1036 e13.
98. Robinson DS, Campbell DA, Durham SR, Pfeffer J, Barnes PJ, Chung KF. Systematic assessment of difficult-to-treat asthma. *European Respiratory Journal*. 2003;22(3):478.

99. Aaron SD, Vandemheen KL, Boulet l-P, McIvor RA, FitzGerald JM, Hernandez P, et al. Overdiagnosis of asthma in obese and nonobese adults. *Canadian Medical Association Journal*. 2008;179(11):1121.
100. Bossley CJ, Saglani S, Kavanagh C, Payne DNR, Wilson N, Tsartsali L, et al. Corticosteroid responsiveness and clinical characteristics in childhood difficult asthma. *European Respiratory Journal*. 2009;34(5):1052.
101. ten Brinke A, Zwinderman AH, Sterk PJ, Rabe KF, Bel EH. Refractory" eosinophilic airway inflammation in severe asthma: effect of parenteral corticosteroids. *Am J Respir Crit Care Med*. 2004;170(6):601–605.
102. Ogirala RG, Aldrich TK, Prezant DJ, Sinnett MJ, Enden JB, Williams Jr MH. High-dose intramuscular triamcinolone in severe, chronic, life-threatening asthma. *N Engl J Med*. 1991;324(9):585–589.
103. Scadding GK. Optimal management of allergic rhinitis. *Arch Dis Child*. 2015;100(6):576–582.
104. Kakli HA, Riley TD. Allergic Rhinitis. *Prim Care*. 2016;43(3):465–475.
105. Seidman MD, Gurgel RK, Lin SY, Schwartz SR, Baroody FM, Bonner JR, et al. Clinical practice guideline: allergic rhinitis. *Otolaryngol Head Neck Surg*. 2015;152(1 Suppl):S1–43.
106. Brożek JL, Bousquet J, Agache I, Agarwal A, Bachert C, Bosnic-Anticevich S, et al. Allergic Rhinitis and its Impact on Asthma (ARIA) guidelines-2016 revision. *J Allergy Clin Immunol*. 2017;140(4): 950–958.
107. Wise SK, Lin SY, Toskala E, Orlandi RR, Akdis CA, Alt JA, et al. International Consensus Statement on Allergy and Rhinology: allergic Rhinitis. *International forum of allergy & rhinology*. 2018;8(2): 108–352.
108. Bousquet J, Van Cauwenberge P, Khaltaev N. Allergic rhinitis and its impact on asthma. *J Allergy Clin Immunol*. 2001;108(5 Suppl):S147–S334.
109. Chong SN, Chew FT. Epidemiology of allergic rhinitis and associated risk factors in Asia. *World Allergy Organ J*. 2018;11(1):17.
110. Alsowaidi S, Abdulle A, Shehab A, Zuberbier T, Bernsen R. Allergic rhinitis: prevalence and possible risk factors in a Gulf Arab population. *Allergy*. 2010;65(2):208–212.
111. Leynaert B, Neukirch C, Kony S, Guénégou A, Bousquet J, Aubier M, et al. Association between asthma and rhinitis according to atopic sensitization in a population-based study. *J Allergy Clin Immunol*. 2004;113(1):86–93.
112. Bernstein DI, Schwartz G, Bernstein JA. Allergic Rhinitis: mechanisms and Treatment. *Immunology and Allergy Clinics of North America*. 2016;36(2):261–278.
113. Weber RW. Allergic Rhinitis. *Primary Care: Clinics in Office Practice*. 2008;35(1):1–10.
114. Greiner AN, Hellings PW, Rotiroti G, Scadding GK. Allergic rhinitis. *Lancet*. 2011;378(9809): 2112–2122.
115. Min Y-G. The Pathophysiology, Diagnosis and Treatment of Allergic Rhinitis. *Allergy Asthma Immunol Res*. 2010;2(2):65–76.
116. Small P, Kim H. Allergic rhinitis. *Allergy, Asthma & Clinical Immunology*. 2011;7(1):S3.
117. Kaliner MA, Baraniuk JN, Benninger M, Bernstein JA, Lieberman P, Meltzer EO, et al. Consensus Definition of Nonallergic Rhinopathy, Previously Referred to as Vasomotor Rhinitis, Nonallergic Rhinitis, and/or Idiopathic Rhinitis. *World Allergy Organ J*. 2009;2(6):119–120.
118. Ramey JT, Bailen E, Lockey RF. Rhinitis medicamentosa. *J Investig Allergol Clin Immunol*. 2006;16(3):148–155.
119. Quillen DM, Feller DB. Diagnosing rhinitis: allergic vs. nonallergic. *Am Fam Physician*. 2006;73(9): 1583–1590.
120. Angier E, Willington J, Scadding G, Holmes S, Walker SBritish Society for Allergy & Clinical Immunology (BSACI) Standards of Care Committee. Management of allergic and non-allergic rhinitis: a primary care summary of the BSACI guideline. *Prim Care Respir J*. 2010;19(3):217–222.
121. Scadding GK, Kariyawasam HH, Scadding G, Mirakian R, Buckley RJ, Dixon T, et al. BSACI guideline for the diagnosis and management of allergic and non-allergic rhinitis (Revised Edition 2017; First edition 2007). *Clin Exp Allergy*. 2017;47(7):856–889.
122. Spangler DL, Brunton S. Efficacy and central nervous system impairment of newer-generation prescription antihistamines in seasonal allergic rhinitis. *South Med J*. 2006;99(6):593–599.
123. Church MK, Maurer M, Simons FE, Bindslev-Jensen C, van Cauwenberge P, Bousquet J, et al. Risk of first-generation H(1)-antihistamines: a GA(2)LEN position paper. *Allergy*. 2010;65(4):459–466.

124. Berger W, Hampel Jr F, Bernstein J, Shah S, Sacks H, Meltzer EO. Impact of azelastine nasal spray on symptoms and quality of life compared with cetirizine oral tablets in patients with seasonal allergic rhinitis. *Ann Allergy Asthma Immunol*. 2006;97(3):375–381.
125. Weiner JM, Abramson MJ, Puy RM. Intranasal corticosteroids versus oral H1 receptor antagonists in allergic rhinitis: systematic review of randomised controlled trials. *Bmj*. 1998;317(7173):1624–1629.
126. Yáñez A, Rodrigo GJ. Intranasal corticosteroids versus topical H1 receptor antagonists for the treatment of allergic rhinitis: a systematic review with meta-analysis. *Ann Allergy Asthma Immunol*. 2002;89(5):479–484.
127. Weinstein SF. Combination therapy in the treatment of allergic rhinitis. *Allergy Asthma Proc*. 2002;23(1):1–3.
128. Simons FE, Simons KJ. Histamine and H1-antihistamines: celebrating a century of progress. *J Allergy Clin Immunol*. 2011;128(6):1139–1150 e4.
129. Hermelingmeier KE, Weber RK, Hellmich M, Heubach CP, Mösges R. Nasal Irrigation as an Adjunctive Treatment in Allergic Rhinitis: a Systematic Review and Meta-analysis. *American Journal of Rhinology & Allergy*. 2012;26(5):e119–ee25.
130. Li H, Sha Q, Zuo K, Jiang H, Cheng L, Shi J, et al. Nasal saline irrigation facilitates control of allergic rhinitis by topical steroid in children. *ORL J Otorhinolaryngol Relat Spec*. 2009;71(1):50–55.
131. Grainger J, Drake-Lee A. Montelukast in allergic rhinitis: a systematic review and meta-analysis. *Clinical Otolaryngology*. 2006;31(5):360–367.
132. Wilson AM, O'Byrne PM, Parameswaran K. Leukotriene receptor antagonists for allergic rhinitis: a systematic review and meta-analysis. *Am J Med*. 2004;116(5):338–344.
133. Roberts G, Xatzipsalti M, Borrego LM, Custovic A, Halken S, Hellings PW, et al. Paediatric rhinitis: position paper of the European Academy of Allergy and Clinical Immunology. *Allergy*. 2013;68(9):1102–1116.
134. Hoyte FCL, Nelson HS. Recent advances in allergic rhinitis. *F1000Res*. 2018;7 F1000 Faculty Rev-333.
135. O'Brien TP. Allergic conjunctivitis: an update on diagnosis and management. *Current opinion in allergy and clinical immunology*. 2013;13(5):543–549.
136. Rosario N, Bielory L. Epidemiology of allergic conjunctivitis. *Current opinion in allergy and clinical immunology*. 2011;11(5):471–476.
137. Dupuis P, Prokopich CL, Hynes A, Kim H. A contemporary look at allergic conjunctivitis. Allergy, asthma, and clinical immunology: official journal of the Canadian Society of. *Allergy and Clinical Immunology*. 2020;16:5.
138. Bielory L. Allergic and immunologic disorders of the eye. Part II: ocular allergy. *J Allergy Clin Immunol*. 2000;106(6):1019–1032.
139. Bielory L, Delgado L, Katelaris CH, Leonardi A, Rosario N, Vichyanoud P. ICON: diagnosis and management of allergic conjunctivitis. *Ann Allergy Asthma Immunol*. 2020;124(2):118–134.
140. Raizman M., Luchs J., Shovlin J.P., Wolf R., editors. Ocular Allergy: a Scientific Review and Expert Case Debate2013.
141. Leonardi S, Marchese G, Marseglia GL, La Rosa M. Montelukast in allergic diseases beyond asthma. *Allergy Asthma Proc*. 2007;28(3):287–291.
142. Butrus S, Portela R. Ocular allergy: diagnosis and treatment. *Ophthalmology clinics of North America*. 2005;18(4):485–492 v.
143. Abelson MB, Paradis A, George MA, Smith LM, Maguire L, Burns R. Effects of Vasocon-A in the allergen challenge model of acute allergic conjunctivitis. *Archives of ophthalmology (Chicago, Ill: 1960)*. 1990;108(4):520–524.
144. Kari O, Saari KM. Updates in the treatment of ocular allergies. *Journal of asthma and allergy*. 2010;3:149–158.
145. Guidera AC, Luchs JI, Udell IJ. Keratitis, ulceration, and perforation associated with topical nonsteroidal anti-inflammatory drugs. *Ophthalmology*. 2001;108(5):936–944.
146. Broide DH. Immunomodulation of allergic disease. *Annu Rev Med*. 2009;60:279–291.
147. Leznoff A. Urticaria and angioedema. *Asian Pac J Allergy Immunol*. 1984;2(2):272–278.
148. Fineman SM. Urticaria and angioedema: a practical approach. *South Med J*. 1980;73(7):915–919.
149. Greaves M, Lawlor F. Angioedema: manifestations and management. *Journal of the American Academy of Dermatology*. 1991;25(1 Pt 2):155–161 discussion 61-5.

150. Ciaccio CE. Angioedema: an overview and update. *Missouri medicine*. 2011;108(5):354–357.
151. Radonjic-Hoesli S, Hofmeier KS, Micaletto S, Schmid-Grendelmeier P, Bircher A, Simon D. Urticaria and Angioedema: an Update on Classification and Pathogenesis. *Clin Rev Allergy Immunol*. 2018;54(1):88–101.
152. Zbiciak-Nylec M, Wcisło-Dziadecka D, Kasprzyk M, Kulig A, Laszczak J, Noworyta M, et al. Overweight and obesity may play a role in the pathogenesis of chronic spontaneous urticaria. *Clinical and experimental dermatology*. 2018;43(5):525–528.
153. Lapi F, Cassano N, Pegoraro V, Cataldo N, Heiman F, Cricelli I, et al. Epidemiology of chronic spontaneous urticaria: results from a nationwide, population-based study in Italy. *The British journal of dermatology*. 2016;174(5):996–1004.
154. Hide M, Francis DM, Grattan CE, Hakimi J, Kochan JP, Greaves MW. Autoantibodies against the high-affinity IgE receptor as a cause of histamine release in chronic urticaria. *N Engl J Med*. 1993;328(22):1599–1604.
155. Cicardi M, Aberer W, Banerji A, Bas M, Bernstein JA, Bork K, et al. Classification, diagnosis, and approach to treatment for angioedema: consensus report from the Hereditary Angioedema International Working Group. *Allergy*. 2014;69(5):602–616.
156. Zuberbier T, Balke M, Worm M, Edenharter G, Maurer M. Epidemiology of urticaria: a representative cross-sectional population survey. *Clinical and experimental dermatology*. 2010;35(8):869–873.
157. Fricke J, Ávila G, Keller T, Weller K, Lau S, Maurer M, et al. Prevalence of chronic urticaria in children and adults across the globe: systematic review with meta-analysis. *Allergy*. 2020;75(2):423–432.
158. Aygören-Pürsün E, Magerl M, Maetzel A, Maurer M. Epidemiology of Bradykinin-mediated angioedema: a systematic investigation of epidemiological studies. *Orphanet Journal of Rare Diseases*. 2018;13(1):73.
159. Sobotková M. Angiotensin-converting enzyme inhibitor-induced angioedema: epidemiology, pathogenesis and management. *Vnitrni lekarstvi*. 2018;64(10):928–933.
160. Frigas E, Park MA. Acute urticaria and angioedema: diagnostic and treatment considerations. *American journal of clinical dermatology*. 2009;10(4):239–250.
161. Kanani A, Betschel SD, Warrington R. Urticaria and angioedema. *Allergy, Asthma & Clinical Immunology*. 2018;14(2):59.
162. Leznoff A, Josse RG, Denburg J, Dolovich J. Association of chronic urticaria and angioedema with thyroid autoimmunity. *Archives of dermatology*. 1983;119(8):636–640.
163. Confino-Cohen R, Chodick G, Shalev V, Leshno M, Kimhi O, Goldberg A. Chronic urticaria and autoimmunity: associations found in a large population study. *J Allergy Clin Immunol*. 2012;129(5):1307–1313.
164. Kaplan AP, Greaves M. Pathogenesis of chronic urticaria. *Clin Exp Allergy*. 2009;39(6):777–787.
165. Kaplan AP, Ghebrehiwet B. The plasma bradykinin-forming pathways and its interrelationships with complement. *Molecular immunology*. 2010;47(13):2161–2169.
166. Golias C, Charalabopoulos A, Stagikas D, Charalabopoulos K, Batistatou A. The kinin system–bradykinin: biological effects and clinical implications. Multiple role of the kinin system–bradykinin. *Hippokratia*. 2007;11(3):124–128.
167. Hall JM. Bradykinin receptors. *General pharmacology*. 1997;28(1):1–6.
168. Joseph K, Tholanikunnel BG, Bygum A, Ghebrehiwet B, Kaplan AP. Factor XII-independent activation of the bradykinin-forming cascade: implications for the pathogenesis of hereditary angioedema types I and II. *J Allergy Clin Immunol*. 2013;132(2):470–475.
169. Kaplan AP, Joseph K. Pathogenic mechanisms of bradykinin mediated diseases: dysregulation of an innate inflammatory pathway. *Advances in immunology*. 2014;121:41–89.
170. Banday AZ, Kaur A, Jindal AK, Rawat A, Singh S. An update on the genetics and pathogenesis of hereditary angioedema. *Genes & Diseases*. 2020;7(1):75–83.
171. Bernstein JA, Lang DM, Khan DA, Craig T, Dreyfus D, Hsieh F, et al. The diagnosis and management of acute and chronic urticaria: 2014 update. *J Allergy Clin Immunol*. 2014;133(5):1270–1277.
172. Markovic SN, Inwards DJ, Frigas EA, Phyliky RP. Acquired C1 esterase inhibitor deficiency. *Annals of internal medicine*. 2000;132(2):144–150.
173. Betschel S, Badiou J, Binkley K, Borici-Mazi R, Hébert J, Kanani A, et al. The International/Canadian Hereditary Angioedema Guideline. *Allergy, asthma, and clinical immunology: official journal of the Canadian Society of Allergy and Clinical Immunology*. 2019;15:72.

174. Wagenaar-Bos IG, Drouet C, Aygören-Pursun E, Bork K, Bucher C, Bygum A, et al. Functional C1-inhibitor diagnostics in hereditary angioedema: assay evaluation and recommendations. *Journal of immunological methods*. 2008;338(1–2):14–20.
175. Gompels MM, Lock RJ, Morgan JE, Osborne J, Brown A, Virgo PF. A multicentre evaluation of the diagnostic efficiency of serological investigations for C1 inhibitor deficiency. *Journal of clinical pathology*. 2002;55(2):145–147.
176. Tarzi MD, Hickey A, Förster T, Mohammadi M, Longhurst HJ. An evaluation of tests used for the diagnosis and monitoring of C1 inhibitor deficiency: normal serum C4 does not exclude hereditary angio-oedema. *Clinical and experimental immunology*. 2007;149(3):513–516.
177. Bova M, De Feo G, Parente R, De Pasquale T, Gravante C, Pucci S, et al. Hereditary and Acquired Angioedema: heterogeneity of Pathogenesis and Clinical Phenotypes. *International archives of allergy and immunology*. 2018;175(3):126–135.
178. Farkas H. Management of upper airway edema caused by hereditary angioedema. *Allergy, asthma, and clinical immunology: official journal of the Canadian Society of Allergy and Clinical Immunology*. 2010;6(1):19.
179. Kaplan AP, Giménez-Arnau AM, Saini SS. Mechanisms of action that contribute to efficacy of omalizumab in chronic spontaneous urticaria. *Allergy*. 2017;72(4):519–533.
180. Guillén-Aguinaga S, Jáuregui Presa I, Aguinaga-Ontoso E, Guillén-Grima F, Ferrer M. Updosing nonsedating antihistamines in patients with chronic spontaneous urticaria: a systematic review and meta-analysis. *The British journal of dermatology*. 2016;175(6):1153–1165.
181. Godse KV. Cyclosporine in chronic idiopathic urticaria with positive autologous serum skin test. *Indian journal of dermatology*. 2008;53(2):101–102.
182. Godse KV. Severe chronic urticaria treated with oral mini-pulse steroid therapy. *Indian journal of dermatology*. 2010;55(4):402–403.
183. Bowen T, Cicardi M, Farkas H, Bork K, Longhurst HJ, Zuraw B, et al. International consensus algorithm for the diagnosis, therapy and management of hereditary angioedema. *Allergy, asthma, and clinical immunology: official journal of the Canadian Society of Allergy and Clinical Immunology*. 2010;6(1):24.
184. Thomsen SF. Atopic Dermatitis: natural Histor y. *Diagnosis, and Treatment. ISRN Allergy*. 2014;2014:354250.
185. Kramer ON, Strom MA, Ladizinski B, Lio PA. The history of atopic dermatitis. *Clinics in dermatology*. 2017;35(4):344–348.
186. Wise F, Sulzberger M. *The 1933 Year Book of Dermatology and Syphilology*: Chicago: Year Book Publishers Inc; 1933.
187. Johansson SG, Bennich H. Immunological studies of an atypical (myeloma) immunoglobulin. *Immunology*. 1967;13(4):381–394.
188. Johansson SG. Raised levels of a new immunoglobulin class (IgND) in asthma. *Lancet*. 1967;2(7523):951–953.
189. Hanifin J, Rajka G. Diagnostic features of atopic dermatitis. *Acta Derm Venereol (Stockh)*. 1980;92 (suppl. 44):7.
190. Knoell KA, Greer KE. Atopic dermatitis. *Pediatrics in review*. 1999;20(2):46–51 quiz 2.
191. Odhiambo JA, Williams HC, TO Clayton, Robertson CF, Asher MI. Global variations in prevalence of eczema symptoms in children from ISAAC Phase Three. *J Allergy Clin Immunol*. 2009;124(6):1251–1258 e23.
192. Williams H, Stewart A, von Mutius E, Cookson W, Anderson HR. Is eczema really on the increase worldwide? *J Allergy Clin Immunol*. 2008;121(4):947–954 e15.
193. Berke R, Singh A, Guralnick M. Atopic dermatitis: an overview. *Am Fam Physician*. 2012;86(1):35–42.
194. Silverberg JI. Public Health Burden and Epidemiology of Atopic Dermatitis. *Dermatologic clinics*. 2017;35(3):283–289.
195. Lee HH, Patel KR, Singam V, Rastogi S, Silverberg JI. A systematic review and meta-analysis of the prevalence and phenotype of adult-onset atopic dermatitis. *Journal of the American Academy of Dermatology*. 2019;80(6):1526–1532 e7.
196. Torres T, Ferreira EO, Gonçalo M, Mendes-Bastos P, Selores M, Filipe P. Update on Atopic Dermatitis. *Acta medica portuguesa*. 2019;32(9):606–613.
197. Peng W, Novak N. Pathogenesis of atopic dermatitis. *Clin Exp Allergy*. 2015;45(3):566–574.
198. Giwercman C, Lerbaek A, Bisgaard H, Menné T. Classification of atopic hand eczema and the filaggrin mutations. *Contact dermatitis*. 2008;59(5):257–260.

199. Meng L, Wang L, Tang H, Tang X, Jiang X, Zhao J, et al. Filaggrin gene mutation c.3321delA is associated with various clinical features of atopic dermatitis in the Chinese Han population. *PLoS One*. 2014;9(5):e98235.
200. Thyssen JP, Kezic S. Causes of epidermal filaggrin reduction and their role in the pathogenesis of atopic dermatitis. *J Allergy Clin Immunol*. 2014;134(4):792–799.
201. Sawada Y, Honda T, Nakamizo S, Nakajima S, Nonomura Y, Otsuka A, et al. Prostaglandin E(2) (PGE(2))-EP2 signaling negatively regulates murine atopic dermatitis-like skin inflammation by suppressing thymic stromal lymphopoietin expression. *J Allergy Clin Immunol*. 2019;144(5):1265–1273 e9.
202. Takai T. TSLP expression: cellular sources, triggers, and regulatory mechanisms. *Allergology international: official journal of the Japanese Society of Allergology*. 2012;61(1):3–17.
203. Melnik B, Plewig G. Are disturbances of omega-6-fatty acid metabolism involved in the pathogenesis of atopic dermatitis? *Acta dermato-venereologica Supplementum*. 1992;176:77–85.
204. Yew YW, Thyssen JP. Silverberg JI. A systematic review and meta-analysis of the regional and age-related differences in atopic dermatitis clinical characteristics. *Journal of the American Academy of Dermatology*. 2019;80(2):390–401.
205. Weidinger S, Novak N. Atopic dermatitis. *The Lancet*. 2016;387(10023):1109–1122.
206. Schultz Larsen F, Hanifin JM. Secular change in the occurrence of atopic dermatitis. *Acta dermato-venereologica Supplementum*. 1992;176:7–12.
207. Williams HC, Burney PG, Hay RJ, Archer CB, Shipley MJ, Hunter JJ, et al. The U.K. Working Party's Diagnostic Criteria for Atopic Dermatitis. I. Derivation of a minimum set of discriminators for atopic dermatitis. *The British journal of dermatology*. 1994;131(3):383–396.
208. Diepgen TL, Fartasch M. Recent epidemiological and genetic studies in atopic dermatitis. *Acta dermato-venereologica Supplementum*. 1992;176:13–18.
209. 1 Guidance | Atopic eczema in under 12s: diagnosis and management | Guidance | NICE. 2007.
210. Eichenfield LF, Tom WL, Chamlin SL, Feldman SR, Hanifin JM, Simpson EL, et al. Guidelines of care for the management of atopic dermatitis: section 1. Diagnosis and assessment of atopic dermatitis. *Journal of the American Academy of Dermatology*. 2014;70(2):338–351.
211. Barrett M, Luu M. Differential Diagnosis of Atopic Dermatitis. *Immunol Allergy Clin North Am*. 2017;37(1):11–34.
212. Micali G, Paternò V, Cannarella R, Dinotta F, Lacarrubba F. Evidence-based treatment of atopic dermatitis with topical moisturizers. Giornale italiano di dermatologia e venereologia: organo ufficiale. *Societa italiana di dermatologia e sifilografia*. 2018;153(3):396–402.
213. Simpson EL, Chalmers JR, Hanifin JM, Thomas KS, Cork MJ, McLean WH, et al. Emollient enhancement of the skin barrier from birth offers effective atopic dermatitis prevention. *J Allergy Clin Immunol*. 2014;134(4):818–823.
214. Fishbein AB, Mueller K, Lor J, Smith P, Paller AS, Kaat A. Systematic Review and Meta-analysis Comparing Topical Corticosteroids With Vehicle/Moisturizer in Childhood Atopic Dermatitis. *Journal of pediatric nursing*. 2019;47:36–43.
215. Waldman AR, Ahluwalia J, Udkoff J, Borok JF, Eichenfield LF. Atopic Dermatitis. *Pediatrics in review*. 2018;39(4):180–193.
216. Wollenberg A, Barbarot S, Bieber T, Christen-Zaech S, Deleuran M, Fink-Wagner A, et al. Consensus-based European guidelines for treatment of atopic eczema (atopic dermatitis) in adults and children: part I. *Journal of the European Academy of Dermatology and Venereology: JEADV*. 2018;32(5):657–682.
217. Nicol NH, Boguniewicz M. Wet Wrap Therapy in Moderate to Severe Atopic Dermatitis. *Immunol Allergy Clin North Am*. 2017;37(1):123–139.
218. Chong M, Fonacier L. Treatment of Eczema: corticosteroids and Beyond. *Clinical reviews in allergy & immunology*. 2016;51(3):249–262.
219. Rusnak F, Mertz P. Calcineurin: form and function. *Physiological reviews*. 2000;80(4):1483–1521.
220. Martínez-Martínez S, Redondo JM. Inhibitors of the calcineurin/NFAT pathway. *Curr Med Chem*. 2004;11(8):997–1007.
221. Huang X, Xu B. Efficacy and Safety of Tacrolimus versus Pimecrolimus for the Treatment of Atopic Dermatitis in Children: a Network Meta-Analysis. *Dermatology (Basel, Switzerland)*. 2015;231(1):41–49.
222. Wahn U, Bos JD, Goodfield M, Caputo R, Papp K, Manjra A, et al. Efficacy and safety of pimecrolimus cream in the long-term management of atopic dermatitis in children. *Pediatrics*. 2002;110 (1 Pt 1):e2.

223. Sigurgeirsson B, Boznanski A, Todd G, Vertruyen A, Schuttelaar M-LA, Zhu X, et al. Safety and Efficacy of Pimecrolimus in Atopic Dermatitis: a 5-Year Randomized Trial. *Pediatrics*. 2015;135(4):597–606.
224. Cheape AC, Murrell DF. 2 percent Crisaborole topical ointment for the treatment of mild-to-moderate atopic dermatitis. *Expert review of clinical immunology*. 2017;13(5):415–423.
225. Yang H, Wang J, Zhang X, Zhang Y, Qin ZL, Wang H, et al. Application of Topical Phosphodiesterase 4 Inhibitors in Mild to Moderate Atopic Dermatitis: a Systematic Review and Meta-analysis. *JAMA dermatology*. 2019;155(5):585–593.
226. Kim HS, Yun JW, Shin TH, Lee SH, Lee BC, Yu KR, et al. Human umbilical cord blood mesenchymal stem cell-derived PGE2 and TGF-β1 alleviate atopic dermatitis by reducing mast cell degranulation. *Stem cells (Dayton, Ohio)*. 2015;33(4):1254–1266.
227. Kim HS, Lee JH, Roh KH, Jun HJ, Kang KS, Kim TY. Clinical Trial of Human Umbilical Cord Blood-Derived Stem Cells for the Treatment of Moderate-to-Severe Atopic Dermatitis: phase I/IIa Studies. *Stem cells (Dayton, Ohio)*. 2017;35(1):248–255.
228. Chun PIF, Lehman H. Current and Future Monoclonal Antibodies in the Treatment of Atopic Dermatitis. *Clin Rev Allergy Immunol*. 2020;59(2):208–219.
229. Nguyen HL, Yiannias JA. Contact Dermatitis to Medications and Skin Products. *Clin Rev Allergy Immunol*. 2019;56(1):41–59.
230. Nassau S, Fonacier L. Allergic Contact Dermatitis. *The Medical clinics of North America*. 2020;104(1):61–76.
231. Lim HW, Collins SAB, Resneck Jr JS, Bolognia JL, Hodge JA, Rohrer TA, et al. The burden of skin disease in the United States. *Journal of the American Academy of Dermatology*. 2017;76(5):958–972 e2.
232. Thyssen JP, Linneberg A, Menné T, Johansen JD. The epidemiology of contact allergy in the general population–prevalence and main findings. *Contact dermatitis*. 2007;57(5):287–299.
233. Alinaghi F, Bennike NH, Egeberg A, Thyssen JP, Johansen JD. Prevalence of contact allergy in the general population: a systematic review and meta-analysis. *Contact dermatitis*. 2019;80(2):77–85.
234. Cavani A, Mei D, Guerra E, Corinti S, Giani M, Pirrotta L, et al. Patients with allergic contact dermatitis to nickel and nonallergic individuals display different nickel-specific T cell responses. Evidence for the presence of effector CD8+ and regulatory CD4+ T cells. *The Journal of investigative dermatology*. 1998;111(4):621–628.
235. Cavani A, Nasorri F, Ottaviani C, Sebastiani S, De Pità O, Girolomoni G. Human CD25+ regulatory T cells maintain immune tolerance to nickel in healthy, nonallergic individuals. *Journal of immunology (Baltimore, Md: 1950)*. 2003;171(11):5760–5768.
236. Reduta T, Stasiak-Barmuta A, Laudańska H. CD4+CD25+ and CD4+CD2+high regulatory T cells in disseminated and localized forms of allergic contact dermatitis: relation to specific cytokines. *Folia histochemica et cytobiologica*. 2011;49(2):255–262.
237. Novak-Bilić G, Vučić M, Japundžić I, Meštrović-Štefekov J, Stanić-Duktaj S, Lugović-Mihić L. Irritant and Allergic Contact Dermatitis - Skin Lesion Characteristics. *Acta clinica Croatica*. 2018;57(4):713–720.
238. Nosbaum A, Vocanson M, Rozieres A, Hennino A, Nicolas JF. Allergic and irritant contact dermatitis. *European journal of dermatology: EJD*. 2009;19(4):325–332.
239. de Waard-van der Spek FB, Darsow U, Mortz CG, Orton D, Worm M, Muraro A, et al. EAACI position paper for practical patch testing in allergic contact dermatitis in children. *Pediatric allergy and immunology: official publication of the European Society of Pediatric Allergy and Immunology*. 2015;26(7):598–606.
240. Fonacier L. A Practical Guide to Patch Testing. *The journal of allergy and clinical immunology in practice*. 2015;3(5):669–675.
241. Johansen JD, Veien N, Laurberg G, Avnstorp C, Kaaber K, Andersen KE, et al. Decreasing trends in methyldibromo glutaronitrile contact allergy–following regulatory intervention. *Contact dermatitis*. 2008;59(1):48–51.
242. Gönül M, Gül U. Detection of contact hypersensitivity to corticosteroids in allergic contact dermatitis patients who do not respond to topical corticosteroids. *Contact dermatitis*. 2005;53(2):67–70.
243. Sicherer SH. Epidemiology of food allergy. *J Allergy Clin Immunol*. 2011;127(3):594–602.
244. Boyce JA, Assa'ad A, Burks AW, Jones SM, Sampson HA, Wood RA, et al. Guidelines for the Diagnosis and Management of Food Allergy in the United States: summary of the NIAID-Sponsored Expert Panel Report. *J Allergy Clin Immunol*. 2010;126(6):1105–1118.

245. Burks AW, Tang M, Sicherer S, Muraro A, Eigenmann PA, Ebisawa M, et al. ICON: food allergy. *J Allergy Clin Immunol*. 2012;129(4):906–920.
246. Stensgaard A, Bindslev-Jensen C, Nielsen D, Munch M, DunnGalvin A. Quality of life in childhood, adolescence and adult food allergy: patient and parent perspectives. *Clinical & Experimental Allergy*. 2017;47(4):530–539.
247. Matsuo H, Yokooji T, Taogoshi T. Common food allergens and their IgE-binding epitopes. *Allergology International*. 2015;64(4):332–343.
248. Werfel T, Asero R, Ballmer-Weber BK, Beyer K, Enrique E, Knulst AC, et al. Position paper of the EAACI: food allergy due to immunological cross-reactions with common inhalant allergens. *Allergy*. 2015;70(9):1079–1090.
249. Kuehn A, Codreanu-Morel F, Lehners-Weber C, Doyen V, Gomez-André SA, Bienvenu F, et al. Cross-reactivity to fish and chicken meat - a new clinical syndrome. *Allergy*. 2016;71(12):1772–1781.
250. Leung PS, Chow WK, Duffey S, Kwan HS, Gershwin ME, Chu KH. IgE reactivity against a cross-reactive allergen in crustacea and mollusca: evidence for tropomyosin as the common allergen. *J Allergy Clin Immunol*. 1996;98(5 Pt 1):954–961.
251. Price A, Ramachandran S, Smith GP, Stevenson ML, Pomeranz MK, Cohen DE. Oral allergy syndrome (pollen-food allergy syndrome). *Dermatitis: contact, atopic, occupational, drug*. 2015;26(2):78–88.
252. Sicherer SH, Sampson HA. Food allergy: epidemiology, pathogenesis, diagnosis, and treatment. *J Allergy Clin Immunol*. 2014;133(2):291–307 quiz 8.
253. Savage J, Johns CB. Food allergy: epidemiology and natural history. *Immunol Allergy Clin North Am*. 2015;35(1):45–59.
254. Koplin JJ, Allen KJ, Gurrin LC, Peters RL, Lowe AJ, Tang ML, et al. The impact of family history of allergy on risk of food allergy: a population-based study of infants. *International journal of environmental research and public health*. 2013;10(11):5364–5377.
255. Blázquez AB, Berin MC. Gastrointestinal dendritic cells promote Th2 skewing via OX40L. *Journal of immunology (Baltimore, Md: 1950)*. 2008;180(7):4441–4450.
256. Galli SJ, Tsai M. IgE and mast cells in allergic disease. *Nat Med*. 2012;18(5):693–704.
257. Peavy RD, Metcalfe DD. Understanding the mechanisms of anaphylaxis. *Current opinion in allergy and clinical immunology*. 2008;8(4):310–315.
258. Noval Rivas M, Burton OT, Oettgen HC, Chatila T. IL-4 production by group 2 innate lymphoid cells promotes food allergy by blocking regulatory T-cell function. *J Allergy Clin Immunol*. 2016;138(3):801–811 e9.
259. Sehra S, Yao W, Nguyen ET, Glosson-Byers NL, Akhtar N, Zhou B, et al. TH9 cells are required for tissue mast cell accumulation during allergic inflammation. *J Allergy Clin Immunol*. 2015;136(2): 433–440 e1.
260. Miller MJ, Knoop KA, Newberry RD. Mind the GAPs: insights into intestinal epithelial barrier maintenance and luminal antigen delivery. *Mucosal Immunol*. 2014;7(3):452–454.
261. McDole JR, Wheeler LW, McDonald KG, Wang B, Konjufca V, Knoop KA, et al. Goblet cells deliver luminal antigen to CD103+ dendritic cells in the small intestine. *Nature*. 2012;483(7389):345–349.
262. Johansson MEV, Hansson GC. Immunological aspects of intestinal mucus and mucins. *Nature Reviews Immunology*. 2016;16(10):639–649.
263. Scott CL, Aumeunier AM, Mowat AM. Intestinal CD103+ dendritic cells: master regulators of tolerance? *Trends in immunology*. 2011;32(9):412–419.
264. Steinbach EC, Plevy SE. The role of macrophages and dendritic cells in the initiation of inflammation in IBD. *Inflammatory bowel diseases*. 2014;20(1):166–175.
265. Eri RD, Adams RJ, Tran TV, Tong H, Das I, Roche DK, et al. An intestinal epithelial defect conferring ER stress results in inflammation involving both innate and adaptive immunity. *Mucosal Immunol*. 2011;4(3):354–364.
266. Coombes JL, Siddiqui KR, Arancibia-Cárcamo CV, Hall J, Sun CM, Belkaid Y, et al. A functionally specialized population of mucosal CD103+ DCs induces Foxp3+ regulatory T cells via a TGF-beta and retinoic acid-dependent mechanism. *J Exp Med*. 2007;204(8):1757–1764.
267. Sugimoto M, Kamemura N, Nagao M, Irahara M, Kagami S, Fujisawa T, et al. Differential response in allergen-specific IgE, IgGs, and IgA levels for predicting outcome of oral immunotherapy. *Pediatric allergy and immunology: official publication of the European Society of Pediatric Allergy and Immunology*. 2016;27(3):276–282.

268. Yazdanbakhsh M, Kremsner PG, van Ree R. Allergy, parasites, and the hygiene hypothesis. *Science (New York, NY)*. 2002;296(5567):490–494.
269. Lack G. Early exposure hypothesis: where are we now? *Clin Transl Allergy*. 2011;1(Suppl 1):S71.
270. Wjst M, Dold S. Genes, factor X, and allergens: what causes allergic diseases? *Allergy*. 1999;54(7): 757–759.
271. Camargo Jr CA, Rifas-Shiman SL, Litonjua AA, Rich-Edwards JW, Weiss ST, Gold DR, et al. Maternal intake of vitamin D during pregnancy and risk of recurrent wheeze in children at 3 y of age. *The American Journal of Clinical Nutrition*. 2007;85(3):788–795.
272. Devereux G, Litonjua AA, Turner SW, Craig LC, McNeill G, Martindale S, et al. Maternal vitamin D intake during pregnancy and early childhood wheezing. *The American journal of clinical nutrition*. 2007;85(3):853–859.
273. Miyake Y, Tanaka K, Okubo H, Sasaki S, Arakawa M. Maternal consumption of dairy products, calcium, and vitamin D during pregnancy and infantile allergic disorders. *Ann Allergy Asthma Immunol*. 2014;113(1):82–87.
274. Erkkola M, Kaila M, Nwaru BI, Kronberg-Kippilä C, Ahonen S, Nevalainen J, et al. Maternal vitamin D intake during pregnancy is inversely associated with asthma and allergic rhinitis in 5-year-old children. *Clin Exp Allergy*. 2009;39(6):875–882.
275. Cianferoni A, Muraro A. Food-induced anaphylaxis. *Immunol Allergy Clin North Am*. 2012;32(1): 165–195.
276. Mankad VS, Williams LW, Lee LA, LaBelle GS, Anstrom KJ, Burks AW. Safety of open food challenges in the office setting. *Ann Allergy Asthma Immunol*. 2008;100(5):469–474.
277. Thalayasingam M, Loo EX, Tan MM, Bever HV, Shek LP. A review of oral food challenges in children presenting to a single tertiary centre with perceived or true food allergies. *Singapore medical journal*. 2015;56(11):622–625.
278. Fleischer DM, Bock SA, Spears GC, Wilson CG, Miyazawa NK, Gleason MC, et al. Oral food challenges in children with a diagnosis of food allergy. *The Journal of pediatrics*. 2011;158(4):578–583 e1.
279. Tam JS. Cutaneous Manifestation of Food Allergy. *Immunol Allergy Clin North Am*. 2017;37(1): 217–231.
280. Ho MH, Wong WH, Chang C. Clinical spectrum of food allergies: a comprehensive review. *Clin Rev Allergy Immunol*. 2014;46(3):225–240.
281. Anvari S, Miller J, Yeh CY, Davis CM. IgE-Mediated Food Allergy. *Clin Rev Allergy Immunol*. 2019;57(2):244–260.
282. Sicherer SH, Sampson HA. Food allergy: a review and update on epidemiology, pathogenesis, diagnosis, prevention, and management. *J Allergy Clin Immunol*. 2018;141(1):41–58.
283. Dang TD, Tang M, Choo S, Licciardi PV, Koplin JJ, Martin PE, et al. Increasing the accuracy of peanut allergy diagnosis by using Ara h 2. *J Allergy Clin Immunol*. 2012;129(4):1056–1063.
284. Komata T, Söderström L, Borres MP, Tachimoto H, Ebisawa M. The predictive relationship of food-specific serum IgE concentrations to challenge outcomes for egg and milk varies by patient age. *J Allergy Clin Immunol*. 2007;119(5):1272–1274.
285. Lieberman JA, Glaumann S, Batelson S, Borres MP, Sampson HA, Nilsson C. The utility of peanut components in the diagnosis of IgE-mediated peanut allergy among distinct populations. *The journal of allergy and clinical immunology In practice*. 2013;1(1):75–82.
286. Santos AF, Brough HA. Making the Most of In Vitro Tests to Diagnose Food Allergy. *The journal of allergy and clinical immunology In practice*. 2017;5(2):237–248.
287. Høst A, Koletzko B, Dreborg S, Muraro A, Wahn U, Aggett P, et al. Dietary products used in infants for treatment and prevention of food allergy. Joint Statement of the European Society for Paediatric Allergology and Clinical Immunology (ESPACI) Committee on Hypoallergenic Formulas and the European Society for Paediatric Gastroenterology. *Hepatology and Nutrition (ESPGHAN) Committee on Nutrition. Arch Dis Child*. 1999;81(1):80–84.
288. Isolauri E, Sütas Y, Salo MK, Isosomppi R, Kaila M. Elimination diet in cow's milk allergy: risk for impaired growth in young children. *The Journal of pediatrics*. 1998;132(6):1004–1009.
289. Berry MJ, Adams J, Voutilainen H, Feustel PJ, Celestin J, Järvinen KM. Impact of elimination diets on growth and nutritional status in children with multiple food allergies. *Pediatric allergy and immunology: official publication of the European Society of Pediatric Allergy and Immunology*. 2015;26(2):133–138.

290. Dupont C, Bradatan E, Soulaines P, Nocerino R, Berni-Canani R. Tolerance and growth in children with cow's milk allergy fed a thickened extensively hydrolyzed casein-based formula. *BMC pediatrics*. 2016;16:96.
291. Heine RG. Food Allergy Prevention and Treatment by Targeted Nutrition. *Annals of nutrition & metabolism*. 2018;72(Suppl 3):33–45.
292. Francavilla R, Calasso M, Calace L, Siragusa S, Ndagijimana M, Vernocchi P, et al. Effect of lactose on gut microbiota and metabolome of infants with cow's milk allergy. *Pediatric allergy and immunology: official publication of the European Society of Pediatric Allergy and Immunology*. 2012;23(5):420–427.
293. Nocerino R, Di Costanzo M, Bedogni G, Cosenza L, Maddalena Y, Di Scala C, et al. Dietary Treatment with Extensively Hydrolyzed Casein Formula Containing the Probiotic Lactobacillus rhamnosus GG Prevents the Occurrence of Functional Gastrointestinal Disorders in Children with Cow's Milk Allergy. *The Journal of pediatrics*. 2019;213:137–142 e2.
294. Berni Canani R, Di Costanzo M, Bedogni G, Amoroso A, Cosenza L, Di Scala C, et al. Extensively hydrolyzed casein formula containing Lactobacillus rhamnosus GG reduces the occurrence of other allergic manifestations in children with cow's milk allergy: 3-year randomized controlled trial. *J Allergy Clin Immunol*. 2017;139(6):1906–1913 e4.
295. Nowak-Węgrzyn A, Chatchatee P. Mechanisms of Tolerance Induction. *Annals of Nutrition and Metabolism*. 2017;70(suppl 2):7–24.
296. Meyer R, Groetch M, Venter C. When Should Infants with Cow's Milk Protein Allergy Use an Amino Acid Formula? A Practical Guide. *The journal of allergy and clinical immunology In practice*. 2018;6(2):383–399.
297. Radke TJ, Brown LG, Hoover ER, Faw BV, Reimann D, Wong MR, et al. Food Allergy Knowledge and Attitudes of Restaurant Managers and Staff: an EHS-Net Study. *Journal of food protection*. 2016;79(9):1588–1598.
298. Nurmatov U, Dhami S, Arasi S, Pajno GB, Fernandez-Rivas M, Muraro A, et al. Allergen immunotherapy for IgE-mediated food allergy: a systematic review and meta-analysis. *Allergy*. 2017;72(8):1133–1147.
299. Langlois A, Lavergne M-H, Leroux H, Killer K, Azzano P, Paradis L, et al. Protocol for a double-blind, randomized controlled trial on the dose-related efficacy of omalizumab in multi-food oral immunotherapy. *Allergy, Asthma & Clinical Immunology*. 2020;16(1):25.
300. Eggel A, Baravalle G, Hobi G, Kim B, Buschor P, Forrer P, et al. Accelerated dissociation of IgE-FcεRI complexes by disruptive inhibitors actively desensitizes allergic effector cells. *J Allergy Clin Immunol*. 2014;133(6):1709–1719 e8.
301. Chang TW. The pharmacological basis of anti-IgE therapy. *Nature biotechnology*. 2000;18(2):157–162.
302. Gdalevich M, Mimouni D, David M, Mimouni M. Breast-feeding and the onset of atopic dermatitis in childhood: a systematic review and meta-analysis of prospective studies. *Journal of the American Academy of Dermatology*. 2001;45(4):520–527.
303. Mimouni Bloch A, Mimouni D, Mimouni M, Gdalevich M. Does breastfeeding protect against allergic rhinitis during childhood? A meta-analysis of prospective studies. *Acta paediatrica (Oslo, Norway: 1992)*. 2002;91(3):275–279.
304. Gdalevich M, Mimouni D, Mimouni M. Breast-feeding and the risk of bronchial asthma in childhood: a systematic review with meta-analysis of prospective studies. *The Journal of pediatrics*. 2001;139(2):261–266.
305. Yang YW, Tsai CL, Lu CY. Exclusive breastfeeding and incident atopic dermatitis in childhood: a systematic review and meta-analysis of prospective cohort studies. *The British journal of dermatology*. 2009;161(2):373–383.
306. Fiocchi A, Assa'ad A, Bahna S. Food allergy and the introduction of solid foods to infants: a consensus document. Adverse Reactions to Foods Committee, American College of Allergy, Asthma and Immunology. *Ann Allergy Asthma Immunol*. 2006;97(1):10–20 quiz 1, 77.
307. Fewtrell M, Bronsky J, Campoy C, Domellöf M, Embleton N, Fidler Mis N, et al. Complementary Feeding: a Position Paper by the European Society for Paediatric Gastroenterology, Hepatology, and Nutrition (ESPGHAN) Committee on Nutrition. *Journal of pediatric gastroenterology and nutrition*. 2017;64(1):119–132.
308. Kleinman RE. American Academy of Pediatrics recommendations for complementary feeding. *Pediatrics*. 2000;106(Supplement 4).

309. Koplin JJ, Osborne NJ, Wake M, Martin PE, Gurrin LC, Robinson MN, et al. Can early introduction of egg prevent egg allergy in infants? A population-based study. *J Allergy Clin Immunol.* 2010;126(4):807–813.
310. Palmer DJ, Metcalfe J, Makrides M, Gold MS, Quinn P, West CE, et al. Early regular egg exposure in infants with eczema: a randomized controlled trial. *J Allergy Clin Immunol.* 2013;132(2) 387-92.e1.
311. Du Toit G, Roberts G, Sayre PH, Bahnson HT, Radulovic S, Santos AF, et al. Randomized trial of peanut consumption in infants at risk for peanut allergy. *N Engl J Med.* 2015;372(9):803–813.
312. Perkin MR, Logan K, Tseng A, Raji B, Ayis S, Peacock J, et al. Randomized Trial of Introduction of Allergenic Foods in Breast-Fed Infants. *N Engl J Med.* 2016;374(18):1733–1743.
313. Fritz JH, Le Bourhis L, Magalhaes JG, Philpott DJ. Innate immune recognition at the epithelial barrier drives adaptive immunity: aPCs take the back seat. *Trends in immunology.* 2008;29(1):41–49.
314. Shanahan F. The gut microbiota-a clinical perspective on lessons learned. *Nat Rev Gastroenterol Hepatol.* 2012;9(10):609–614.
315. Durack J, Kimes NE, Lin DL, Rauch M, McKean M, McCauley K, et al. Delayed gut microbiota development in high-risk for asthma infants is temporarily modifiable by Lactobacillus supplementation. *Nature communications.* 2018;9(1):707.
316. Wopereis H, Sim K, Shaw A, Warner JO, Knol J, Kroll JS. Intestinal microbiota in infants at high risk for allergy: effects of prebiotics and role in eczema development. *J Allergy Clin Immunol.* 2018;141(4):1334–1342 e5.
317. Isolauri E. Development of healthy gut microbiota early in life. *Journal of Paediatrics and Child Health.* 2012;48(s3):1–6.
318. Paxton GA, Teale GR, Nowson CA, Mason RS, McGrath JJ, Thompson MJ, et al. Vitamin D and health in pregnancy, infants, children and adolescents in Australia and New Zealand: a position statement. *The Medical journal of Australia.* 2013;198(3):142–143.
319. Hollams EM. Vitamin D and atopy and asthma phenotypes in children. *Current opinion in allergy and clinical immunology.* 2012;12(3):228–234.
320. Weisse K, Winkler S, Hirche F, Herberth G, Hinz D, Bauer M, et al. Maternal and newborn vitamin D status and its impact on food allergy development in the German LINA cohort study. *Allergy.* 2013;68(2):220–228.
321. Wjst M. Is vitamin D supplementation responsible for the allergy pandemic? *Current opinion in allergy and clinical immunology.* 2012;12(3):257–262.
322. Pichler WJ, Naisbitt DJ, Park BK. Immune pathomechanism of drug hypersensitivity reactions. *J Allergy Clin Immunol.* 2011;127(3 Suppl):S74–S81.
323. Waheed A, Hill T, Dhawan N. Drug Allergy. *Primary Care: Clinics in Office Practice.* 2016;43(3):393–400.
324. Thong BY, Tan TC. Epidemiology and risk factors for drug allergy. *British journal of clinical pharmacology.* 2011;71(5):684–700.
325. Montañez MI, Mayorga C, Bogas G, Barrionuevo E, Fernandez-Santamaria R, Martin-Serrano A, et al. Epidemiology, Mechanisms, and Diagnosis of Drug-Induced Anaphylaxis. *Front Immunol.* 2017;8:614.
326. Chung WH, Wang CW, Dao RL. Severe cutaneous adverse drug reactions. *The Journal of dermatology.* 2016;43(7):758–766.
327. Warrington R, Silviu-Dan F. Drug allergy. *Allergy, Asthma & Clinical Immunology.* 2011;7(1):S10.
328. Gomes E, Cardoso MF, Praça F, Gomes L, Mariño E, Demoly P. Self-reported drug allergy in a general adult Portuguese population. *Clin Exp Allergy.* 2004;34(10):1597–1601.
329. Mullan KA, Anderson A, Illing PT, Kwan P, Purcell AW, Mifsud NA. HLA-associated antiepileptic drug-induced cutaneous adverse reactions. *Hla.* 2019;93(6):417–435.
330. Ramsbottom KA, Carr DF, Rigden DJ, Jones AR. Informatics investigations into anti-thyroid drug induced agranulocytosis associated with multiple HLA-B alleles. *PLoS One.* 2020;15(2):e0220754.
331. Dykewicz MS, Lam JK. Drug Hypersensitivity Reactions. *The Medical clinics of North America.* 2020;104(1):109–128.
332. Schnyder B, Pichler WJ. Mechanisms of drug-induced allergy. *Mayo Clinic proceedings.* 2009;84(3):268–272.
333. Jenkins RE, Meng X, Elliott VL, Kitteringham NR, Pirmohamed M, Park BK. Characterisation of flucloxacillin and 5-hydroxymethyl flucloxacillin haptenated HSA in vitro and in vivo. *Proteomics Clinical applications.* 2009;3(6):720–729.

334. Chung CH, Mirakhur B, Chan E, Le QT, Berlin J, Morse M, et al. Cetuximab-induced anaphylaxis and IgE specific for galactose-alpha-1,3-galactose. *N Engl J Med*. 2008;358(11):1109–1117.
335. Weiss J, Grilley Olson J, Deal AM, Chera B, Weissler M, Murphy BA, et al. Using the galactose-α-1,3-galactose enzyme-linked immunosorbent assay to predict anaphylaxis in response to cetuximab. *Cancer*. 2016;122(11):1697–1701.
336. Manchanda T, Hess D, Dale L, Ferguson SG, Rieder MJ. Haptenation of sulfonamide reactive metabolites to cellular proteins. *Molecular pharmacology*. 2002;62(5):1011–1026.
337. Wermuth CG, Ganellin CR, Lindberg P, Mitscher LA. Glossary of terms used in medicinal chemistry (IUPAC Recommendations 1998). *Pure and Applied Chemistry*. 1998;70(5):1129–1143.
338. Pichler WJ, Adam J, Daubner B, Gentinetta T, Keller M, Yerly D. Drug hypersensitivity reactions: pathomechanism and clinical symptoms. *The Medical clinics of North America*. 2010;94(4):645–664 xv.
339. Khan DA, Solensky R. Drug allergy. *J Allergy Clin Immunol*. 2010;125(2 Suppl 2):S126–S137.
340. Castells M. Diagnosis and management of anaphylaxis in precision medicine. *J Allergy Clin Immunol*. 2017;140(2):321–333.
341. Schwartz LB, Metcalfe DD, Miller JS, Earl H, Sullivan T. Tryptase levels as an indicator of mast-cell activation in systemic anaphylaxis and mastocytosis. *N Engl J Med*. 1987;316(26):1622–1626.
342. Beck SC, Wilding T, Buka RJ, Baretto RL, Huissoon AP, Krishna MT. Biomarkers in Human Anaphylaxis: a Critical Appraisal of Current Evidence and Perspectives. *Front Immunol*. 2019;10:494.
343. Phillips EJ, Bigliardi P, Bircher AJ, Broyles A, Chang YS, Chung WH, et al. Controversies in drug allergy: testing for delayed reactions. *J Allergy Clin Immunol*. 2019;143(1):66–73.
344. Laidlaw TM, Cahill KN. Current Knowledge and Management of Hypersensitivity to Aspirin and NSAIDs. *The journal of allergy and clinical immunology In practice*. 2017;5(3):537–545.
345. Macy E. Penicillin and beta-lactam allergy: epidemiology and diagnosis. *Curr Allergy Asthma Rep*. 2014;14(11):476.
346. The Use of Antibiotics. A Comprehensive Review with Clinical Emphasis. *Annals of internal medicine*. 1976;84(6):763.
347. Wurpts G, Aberer W, Dickel H, Brehler R, Jakob T, Kreft B, et al. Guideline on diagnostic procedures for suspected hypersensitivity to beta-lactam antibiotics. *Allergo Journal International*. 2019;28(5):121–151.
348. Bhattacharya S. The facts about penicillin allergy: a review. *Journal of advanced pharmaceutical technology & research*. 2010;1(1):11–17.
349. Kostis WJ, Shetty M, Chowdhury YS, Kostis JB. ACE Inhibitor-Induced Angioedema: a Review. *Current hypertension reports*. 2018;20(7):55.
350. Kim MH, Park CH, Kim DI, Kim KM, Kim HK, Lim KH, et al. Surveillance of contrast-media-induced hypersensitivity reactions using signals from an electronic medical recording system. *Ann Allergy Asthma Immunol*. 2012;108(3):167–171.
351. Sánchez-Borges M, Aberer W, Brockow K, Celik GE, Cernadas J, Greenberger PA, et al. Controversies in Drug Allergy: radiographic Contrast Media. *The journal of allergy and clinical immunology In practice*. 2019;7(1):61–65.
352. Scherer K, Brockow K, Aberer W, Gooi JH, Demoly P, Romano A, et al. Desensitization in delayed drug hypersensitivity reactions – an EAACI position paper of the Drug Allergy Interest Group. *Allergy*. 2013;68(7):844–852.
353. Sampson HA, Muñoz-Furlong A, Campbell RL, Adkinson Jr NF, Bock SA, Branum A, et al. Second symposium on the definition and management of anaphylaxis: summary report–Second National Institute of Allergy and Infectious Disease/Food Allergy and Anaphylaxis Network symposium. *J Allergy Clin Immunol*. 2006;117(2):391–397.
354. Turner PJ, Worm M, Ansotegui IJ, El-Gamal Y, Rivas MF, Fineman S, et al. Time to revisit the definition and clinical criteria for anaphylaxis? *World Allergy Organ J*. 2019;12(10):100066.
355. Sampson HA, Muñoz-Furlong A, Bock SA, Schmitt C, Bass R, Chowdhury BA, et al. Symposium on the definition and management of anaphylaxis: summary report. *J Allergy Clin Immunol*. 2005;115(3):584–591.
356. LoVerde D, Iweala OI, Eginli A, Krishnaswamy G. Anaphylaxis. *Chest*. 2018;153(2):528–543.
357. Lee S, Sadosty AT, Campbell RL. Update on biphasic anaphylaxis. *Current opinion in allergy and clinical immunology*. 2016;16(4):346–351.

358. Zisa G, Riccobono F, Calamari AM, D'Antonio CD, Galimberti M. A case of protracted hypotension as unique symptom of a biphasic anaphylaxis to amoxicillin. *European annals of allergy and clinical immunology*. 2009;41(2):60–61.
359. Lieberman P, Camargo CA, Bohlke K, Jick H, Miller RL, Sheikh A, et al. Epidemiology of anaphylaxis: findings of the American College of Allergy, Asthma and Immunology Epidemiology of Anaphylaxis Working Group. *Annals of Allergy, Asthma & Immunology*. 2006;97(5):596–602.
360. Wood RA, Camargo CA, Lieberman P, Sampson HA, Schwartz LB, Zitt M, et al. Anaphylaxis in America: the prevalence and characteristics of anaphylaxis in the United States. *Journal of Allergy and Clinical Immunology*. 2014;133(2):461–467.
361. Chu DK, McCullagh DJ, Waserman S. Anaphylaxis for Internists: definition, Evaluation, and Management, with a Focus on Commonly Encountered Problems. *Medical Clinics of North America*. 2020;104(1):25–44.
362. Hernandez L, Papalia S, Pujalte GG. Anaphylaxis. *Prim Care*. 2016;43(3):477–485.
363. Koplin JJ, Mills EN, Allen KJ. Epidemiology of food allergy and food-induced anaphylaxis: is there really a Western world epidemic? *Current opinion in allergy and clinical immunology*. 2015;15(5):409–416.
364. Jerschow E, Lin RY, Scaperotti MM, McGinn AP. Fatal anaphylaxis in the United States, 1999-2010: temporal patterns and demographic associations. *J Allergy Clin Immunol*. 2014;134(6):1318–1328 e7.
365. Brown SG, Stone SF, Fatovich DM, Burrows SA, Holdgate A, Celenza A, et al. Anaphylaxis: clinical patterns, mediator release, and severity. *J Allergy Clin Immunol*. 2013;132(5):1141–1149 e5.
366. Krishnaswamy G, Ajitawi O, Chi DS. The human mast cell: an overview. *Methods Mol Biol*. 2006;315:13–34.
367. Simons FER, Ardusso LRF, Bilò MB, El-Gamal YM, Ledford DK, Ring J, et al. World Allergy Organization Guidelines for the Assessment and Management of Anaphylaxis. *World Allergy Organization Journal*. 2011;4(2):13–37.
368. Waterfield T, Dyer E, Wilson K, Boyle RJ. How to interpret mast cell tests. *Archives of disease in childhood - Education & practice edition*. 2016;101(5):246.
369. Vitte J. Human mast cell tryptase in biology and medicine. *Molecular immunology*. 2015;63(1):18–24.
370. Zanichelli A, Azin GM, Wu MA, Suffritti C, Maggioni L, Caccia S, et al. Diagnosis, Course, and Management of Angioedema in Patients With Acquired C1-Inhibitor Deficiency. *The Journal of Allergy and Clinical Immunology: In Practice*. 2017;5(5):1307–1313.
371. Maurer M, Magerl M, Ansotegui I, Aygören-Pürsün E, Betschel S, Bork K, et al. The international WAO/EAACI guideline for the management of hereditary angioedema-The 2017 revision and update. *Allergy*. 2018;73(8):1575–1596.
372. Pumphrey RSH. Fatal posture in anaphylactic shock. *Journal of Allergy and Clinical Immunology*. 2003;112(2):451–452.
373. Chu DK, Kim LHY, Young PJ, Zamiri N, Almenawer SA, Jaeschke R, et al. Mortality and morbidity in acutely ill adults treated with liberal versus conservative oxygen therapy (IOTA): a systematic review and meta-analysis. *The Lancet*. 2018;391(10131):1693–1705.
374. Zaloga GP, Delacey W, Holmboe E, Chernow B. Glucagon Reversal of Hypotension in a Case of Anaphylactoid Shock. *Annals of internal medicine*. 1986;105(1):65–66.
375. Javeed N, Javeed H, Javeed S, Moussa G, Wong P, Rezai F. Refractory anaphylactoid shock potentiated by beta-blockers. *Cathet Cardiovasc Diagn*. 1996;39(4):383–384.
376. Singhal D, Sahay P, Maharana PK, Raj N, Sharma N, Titiyal JS. Vernal Keratoconjunctivitis. Surv Ophthalmol. 2019; 64(3):289–311. 1879-3304. doi:10.1016/j.survophthal.2018.12.001.
377. Hori H, Fukuchi T. Sugawara Hitoshi Chronic urticaria with inflammation. *Eur J Intern Med*. 2021;83:84–85. doi:10.1016/j.ejim.2020.11.006.
378. Weidinger S, Novak N. Atopic dermatitis. *Lancet*. 2016;387(10023):1109–1122. doi:10.1016/S0140-6736(15)00149-X.
379. Rozas-Muñoz E, Gamé D, Serra-Baldrich E. Allergic Contact Dermatitis by Anatomical Regions: Diagnostic Clues. Actas Dermosifiliogr (Engl Ed). 2018; 109(6):485–507. 2173-5778. doi:10.1016/j.ad.2017.05.011. 29031485.

# CHAPTER 3

# Autoimmune diseases

**Sara Harsini**[a,b,c], **Nima Rezaei**[a,d,e]

[a]Research Center for Immunodeficiencies, Children's Medical Center, Tehran University of Medical Sciences, Tehran, Iran
[b]Association of Nuclear Medicine and Molecular Imaging (ANMMI), Universal Scientific Education and Research Network (USERN), Tehran, Iran
[c]BC Cancer, Vancouver, BC, Canada
[d]Network of Immunity in Infection, Malignancy and Autoimmunity (NIIMA), Universal Scientific Education and Research Network (USERN), Tehran, Iran
[e]Department of Immunology, School of Medicine, Tehran University of Medical Sciences, Tehran, Iran

## Introduction

The diverse immune system developed to fulfill the primary goal of protecting hosts against external threats to the organism. There are, nevertheless, two major areas in which aberrations from this initial function of the immune system leads to pathology, immune deficiency syndromes in which the inability of the components of the immune system to respond in a protective fashion to pathogen results in pathology, and autoimmune diseases, characterized by the activation of the immune system in the absence of an external threat. This host of diseases can be either characterized as those displaying the activation of the adaptive immune response with T and B lymphocytes responding to self-antigens in the absence of any detectable microbial assault or tumor invasion, which constitute the vast majority of diseases regarded to be of autoimmune origin, or those presenting with the activation of the innate immune system and an excess of inflammatory mediators with no evidence of an antigen-specific immune response. Hence, inflammation and tissue damage are known to appear in the absence of infection, toxin exposure, trauma or tumor growth in this category of diseases.[1] It is important to state that in some circumstances the immune activation may be triggered by infection but then persists in the absence of any detectable microbial antigen.[1,2] Notwithstanding the fact that self-reactivity is noted in many diseases of autoimmune nature, the evidence that the reactivity to self is directly responsible for tissue damage may still be lacking.

Over 80 distinct autoimmune diseases with an increasing incidence have been defined thus far.[3,4] This group of diseases comprises some organ-specific diseases and some other reflecting a variety of immunological dysfunctions involving multiple organs.[5] Although each autoimmune disease individually is thought of as being relatively uncommon, the prevalence of all autoimmune diseases is approximately 5 percent−7 percent, imposing significant effects on patients' mortality and morbidity,[6-9] with autoimmune thyroid disease and type I diabetes known as the most common of these conditions. The facts that autoreactivity is an aspect of every normal immune system and that it is a crucial

*Clinical Immunology*
DOI: https://doi.org/10.1016/B978-0-12-818006-8.00001-3

component of immune homeostasis, are important in understanding the high incidence of these diseases. Actually, the repertoire of immunocompetent lymphocytes playing role in protective immunity is chosen based on autoreactivity, as circulating B cells need to weakly interact with autoantigens in order to receive survival signals, while T cells can survive the initial steps of T cell selection as a result of the recognition of self-antigen within the antigen-binding cleft of MHC.[10–12] Furthermore, in order for the immune system not to demonstrate pathogenic autoreactivity associated with tissue damage, an active process demanding constant vigilance is required to regulate physiologic autoreactivity, as it is well understood that an overexuberant response leads to potential autoreactivity, whereas too little response can potentially lead to neglect of danger.

Autoimmune diseases can be initiated at any age with different diseases having their characteristic age of onset. There is generally an increased frequency of autoimmune diseases in women, with a female-to-male ratio mostly ranging from 10: 1 to 1: 1 in different conditions. Considering the role of genetic susceptibility and environmental factors as the key risk factors leading to loss of tolerance,[13] different incidence and prevalence of autoimmune diseases between geographical regions could be partly explained. The geoepidemiology becomes even more complex when variations in gender, ethnicity, age and other demographic factors are taken into account. Patients with one autoimmune disease are more susceptible to a second autoimmune disease.[6,8,14] In addition, there is a genetic predisposition to autoimmunity with the prevalence of autoimmune diseases being increased in first-degree relatives and monozygotic twins in almost all patients.[15] Given the possibility that the genetic traits have been selected for organisms' capacity to protect against invading pathogens,[16,17] aspects of the genetic predisposition may be shared by many different autoimmune diseases.[18,19] Moreover, it is of note that the genetic factors affecting autoreactivity have been suggested to be distinct from those involved in determining the severity of tissue damage[20] or specific organ vulnerability[16,17]; therefore, despite the similar pathways promoting autoreactivity in different individuals, they present with different autoimmune diseases.[18,21] In spite of significant advances in the diagnosis, disease classification, as well as the treatment of autoimmune diseases over the past decade, there is still a paucity of data on the etiological events leading to various incidence and prevalence amongst the autoimmune diseases.

## Immune cells and immune responses

The immunological basis of the autoimmunity has been discussed in detail in chapter 1. Herein, we shall try to provide a quick fresh look at the key concepts and mechanisms underlying the development of autoimmune disorders.

## Innate immune activation

The innate immune system is the host's immediate line of defense protecting against invading pathogens. Specific cell populations of the innate immune system are critical in bridging the gap between innate and adaptive immunity.[22] While the function of certain innate immune cells is to attack infected cells directly, others are specialized to activate the adaptive immune system and to trigger effector functions to eliminate the microorganism. The activation of the innate immune response may be the primary event involved in promoting the disease process in many, if not all, autoimmune diseases.[23] Innate immune responses exhibit broad specificity through recognition of pathogen-associated molecular patterns (PAMPs) and damage-associated molecular patterns (DAMPs) using pattern recognition receptors (PRRs)[24,25] and by binding to Fc receptors of opsonized antigens coated with complement or antibody and complement receptors. Along with the molecular mimicry of certain infectious agents associated with autoimmune diseases, containing cross-reactive antigens to a host antigen, less specific means of activation of the innate immune response can induce autoimmune disease, as well. Different mechanisms of interaction between the innate immune system with autoimmune processes, either of which or a combination of all can be involved in autoimmune diseases, have been describe:d[1] Antigen-presenting cells activated by the infectious agent, could present autoantigens in the lymph nodes or spleen and this might prime autoreactive T cells instead of inducing toleranc;e[2] Replication of infectious agents in a peripheral non-lymphoid organ promotes inflammation with the recruitment of peripheral ignorant T cells, resulting in activating priming of peripheral ignorant auto-reactive T cell;s[3] Following priming of auto-reactive T cells, innate immune response can enhance the effector phase against a target organ; and[4] Activation of the innate immune system can directly lead to host organ damage even without the involvement of adaptive immune cells. Several organ-specific and clinically important autoimmune diseases demonstrate these multiple steps, not necessarily occurring at the same time, that might lead to organ destruction and manifest autoimmune disease.[26]

Besides the primary role of the innate immune system in the etiopathogenesis of autoimmune diseases, it should be kept in mind that the innate immune system can be also activated secondarily in autoimmune disease. Tissue injury can result in the activation of innate immune cell networks[27,28] and this can lead to an autoimmune response. Extensive tissue injury culminates in the posttranslational alteration of self-antigen such that it becomes immunogenic,[29] or the presentation of normally sequestered self-antigen in a proinflammatory setting, enhanced by apoptosis of cells following tissue damage.[30-32] The release of soluble mediators (DAMPs) such as defensins, cathelicidins, HMGB1, and heat shock proteins following tissue injury can stimulate TLRs and other proinflammatory receptors to further potentiate immune activation pathways.[33] The involvement of both the innate and the adaptive immune systems in the process of autoimmune induced tissue injury is regarded as a fact.

The amplification of the inflammatory pathways can take place following the activation of dendritic cells (DCs) and other myeloid cells by immune complexes containing endogenous Toll-like receptor (TLR) ligands, such as citrullinated proteins, RNA, or DNA.[34,35] As previously suggested by murine models of diabetes, rheumatoid arthritis, systemic lupus, IBD, and more, TLR signaling, both in myeloid cells and lymphocytes, stands as a major feature of such autoimmune diseases.[36-39] Animal models have also depicted that the blockade of pathways of the innate immune system might lead to the amelioration of many autoimmune diseases and that a low threshold for the triggering of myeloid cells and differentiation of monocytes to DCs renders those models more susceptible for autoimmune disease. Additionally, some DNA and RNA sensors along with their associated adaptors and downstream signaling molecules can help regulate autoimmune responses to nucleic acids during the course of a protective immune response to viral pathogens. However, multiple functions of some of the signaling molecules involved in innate immunity make it difficult to target them for therapeutic purposes.[40,41]

Different environmental factors might also nonspecifically initiate and accelerate autoimmunity by activating the innate immune system leading to the secretion of pro-inflammatory cytokines, such as type I interferons that have been shown to be responsible for the initiation of lupus and the Koebner phenomenon in psoriasis.[42]

Other examples of the involvement of the innate immune system in autoimmune diseases are an excess accumulation of proinflammatory apoptotic debris as a result of complement deficiencies in systemic lupus erythematosus,[43-45] increased levels of type 1 interferon in first degree relatives of some patients with systemic lupus erythematosus,[46] the production of pathogenic oxidized DNA after exposure to TLR containing immune complexes as a result of atypical neutrophil cell death by NETosis in lupus,[47-51] increased inflammatory response to intestinal flora in inflammatory bowel disease (IBD) as a consequence of genetic alterations in bacterial sensing, autophagy, and endoplasmic reticulum (ER) stress pathways of the innate immune system,[52,53] and much more.

## Central and peripheral tolerance

The concept of immune tolerance is regarded as an ability of the immune system to prevent immune recognition of self.[54] The development of self-tolerance incorporates both central and peripheral mechanisms to eliminate self-reactive lymphocytes, thereby preventing the immune system from targeting self-molecules, cells or tissues. There should be a lack of stringency in the suppression of autoreactive cells for autoimmunity to develop. B and T cells normally undergo a selection process during their maturation in primary lymphoid organs, the bone marrow and thymus, respectively, so as to eliminate autoreactive cells and preserve self-tolerance.[11,55-58] Given that somatic mutation of immunoglobulin genes routinely generates autoreactivity, a second process of selection also takes place for B cells following this process.[58-62] This process, termed central tolerance, plays a crucial role in shaping immune system homeostasis. Central tolerance befalls during fetal life. After entering the thymus from the bone marrow, developing lymphocytes undergo positive selection in the thymic cortex before maturing and entering the circulation. In addition, lymphocytes with potential reactivity against self-peptides are negatively selected and removed in the thymic medulla. Similarly, B cells undergo a process of negative selection in the bone marrow and in the spleen where B cells migrate as transitional cells after exiting the bone marrow, prior to achieving immunocompetence. Immature B cells expressing surface IgM that recognizes self-antigens encountered during early maturation are deleted by a process known as clonal deletion or clonal anergy. The threshold for this negative selection is different for each individual.[63,64] Autoreactive B cells might escape elimination by receptor editing. It is still unclear whether positive selection on self-antigen is required for B cells' survival and if they need to display some degree of autoreactivity.

The process of negative selection of T and B cells mediated by engagement of the TCR or BCR in a noninflammatory setting, that occurs in the periphery as well as in primary lymphoid organs in order to eliminate autoreactive cells that do not encounter autoantigen in the thymus or bone marrow, is termed peripheral tolerance.[58,63,65,66] Despite some differences in antigen receptor signaling pathways, expression of costimulatory molecules and coreceptors, that exist between immature T or B cells and their mature counterparts, engagement of the antigen receptor is key to both central and peripheral tolerance. Mouse models of autoimmunity suggest that susceptibility to autoimmune diseases might result from a general lack of stringency in B or T-cell tolerance, while some cases might exhibit stage-specific defects.[67-70] This distinction could help establish more tailored treatment strategies based on their tolerance impairment mechanism in different subsets of patients.

Even under the strict vigilance of central and peripheral tolerance explained above, small numbers of potential self-reactive T and/or B lymphocytes can still leak out into the periphery, and this could culminate in either transient physiological autoimmunity without evidence of clinical disease or classical/pathological autoimmunity which leads to tissue damage.[71-74] Key concepts of the immune tolerance, comprising central tolerance, peripheral anergy, T regulatory cells (Tregs) and the homeostasis produced by chemokines and cytokines and their cognate receptors are discussed in detail in chapter 1.

## Adaptive immune activation and regulatory lymphocytes

The stimulation of T and B cells in the periphery requires reception of two signals, one via ligation of the antigen receptor and the other by employing a costimulatory receptor. When the critical antigen-presenting cells in primary immune response, namely, DCs, capture and present microbial antigens that bind to pattern-recognition receptors or TLRs, they transiently upregulate costimulatory molecules CD80 (B7.1) and CD86 (B7.2) and are transformed from tolerogenic to immunogenic. T cells identifying microbial peptides in either major histocompatibility complex (MHC) class I or II molecules on the immunogenic DCs will be activated. These expressed ligands activate CD28 and dramatically enhance TCR activation of phosphatidylinositol-3-kinase (PI3K)/protein kinase AKT and the transcription factor nuclear factor kappa B (NF-κB).[75,76] While still a naïve cell, T cells require a high-affinity interaction with the TCR to be activated; however, as a result of epigenetic transformations and changes in the structure of lipid rafts in the membrane facilitating rapid receptor cross-linking and less requirement for costimulatory signals, memory T cells can be activated by lower-affinity interactions. Hence, the threshold is set higher for the activation of naïve T cells by a self-peptide self-MHC complex as compared with memory T cells.[77] There is emerging evidence that the balance of transcriptional regulators expressed in each T cell and the epigenetic changes are responsible for the determination and reinforcement of T cell phenotypes, respectively. Inflammation or infection can affect T-cell function, converting T cells phenotype from protective to those intensifying inflammation, through T-cell reprogramming triggered by signals from the innate immune system.[78] The activated T cells also provide costimulatory signals to B cells facing microbial antigen.

The molecular mimicry is the state in which both a microbial peptide and a self-peptide are recognized by T cells and this could be a mechanism by which autoimmunity can be provoked by infection.[79] Mouse models of autoimmunity have suggested that the lower the stringency in the negative selection of naïve T cells, the more presence of T cells activated by foreign antigens and displaying pathogenic autoreactivity at the same time, and this phenomenon stands as a major contributor to autoimmunity. On the other hand, the cross-reactive B cells which bind both microbial antigen and self-antigen can present novel epitopes of self-antigen following their ingestion and processing and as these presented epitopes are often different from what presented by DCs, they can activate T cells with novel auto-specificities.[80-83] Therefore, the resultant expanded activated repertoire of T cells critically contribute to a cascade of autoreactivity.[84] There are data suggesting that both the molecular mimicry following activation by microbial antigen and the self-antigen can drive autoreactivity.[79,85] According to the systemic lupus erythematosus studies, an excess of apoptotic debris, modifications in the antigens they present, or altered forms of nucleic acids can activate endosomal TLRs and transform DCs from tolerogenic into an immunogenic state, activate B cells and hence lead to a lupus-like serology with antichromatin reactivity.[47,86-89]

Exhausted T cell is a CD8 T-cell phenotype characterized by programmed death (PD1) expression, which exhibits altered metabolic profile, including glucose dependence, high persistent mTOR, and increased mitochondrial depolarization and can recognize antigens but not initiate effector functions.[90] This T cell phenotype is associated with cancer, infectious disease and autoimmunity and arise as the immune response progresses from the acute phase to the chronic phase as the costimulation from CD4 T cells and antigen level wane.[91] The molecular profile of exhaustion is linked to cancer progression and the inability to clear chronic infections but it represents a better prognosis in some autoimmune diseases.[92] The administration of immune checkpoint inhibitors that antagonize key coinhibitory molecules such as CTLA4 and PD1 and activate exhausted cells as part of cancer chemotherapy has been shown to induce a broad spectrum of autoimmune diseases in a substantial number of patients. These side effects are more frequent when a combination of CTLA4 and PD1 directed therapies are used, followed by the sole administration of anti-CTLA4 and then anti-PD1 therapy. This whole situation demonstrates the trade-off between immunocompetence and autoimmunity.[93,94]

The mechanisms of action of regulatory T and B cells are another area of research interest. $CD4^+$ Tregs represent a Th cell subset that arises either early during thymic development in a manner dependent on CD28 and IL-2 in response to TCR encounter with self-antigens with an avidity lower than that needed for negative selection, or later after antigen exposure in the periphery in a manner dependent on IL-2 and TGF-β and augmented by the vitamin A metabolite retinoic acid, and helps to maintain self-tolerance and controlling immune responses.[95-97] These cells exert their regulatory function in different ways, including induction of apoptosis of effector lymphocytes, inhibition of DC function, depriving effector T cells of cytokines or essential amino acids culminating in apoptosis, or production of inhibitory cytokines. $CD4^+CD25^+$ Tregs, critical cells for sustaining peripheral self-tolerance, express Foxp3, the lineage-defining transcription factor for Tregs,[98] the expression of which is stabilized by epigenetic modifications of DNA, enhancing transcriptional availability of inhibitory cytokines while hindering access of transcription factors to DNA-encoding inflammatory cytokines,[99,100] with spontaneous mutations known to result in the development of severe, multiorgan autoimmunity in both mice and humans.[101-103] This finding supports the notion that Tregs are pivotal actors in restricting potentially autoreactive Th cells and that defective Treg function may underlie the development of certain autoimmune diseases. In vitro studies have demonstrated that Tregs regulate effector T-cell activation and expansion both by acting directly on the responding effector T cell, through direct granzyme mediated cytolysis, restricting the bioavailability of IL-2 either by decreasing IL-2 transcription or its consumption, and secretion of inhibitory cytokines IL-10 and TGF-β,[104-107] as well as indirectly, by modifying APC function, either by preventing APC maturation or by downregulating the expression of B7-1 or B7-2,[108-110] which is dependent upon Treg expression of CTLA-4, which physically removes B7-1 and B7-2 from the APC via transendocytosis following binding them.[111,112]

Type 1 regulatory T (Tr1) cells are a Th subset exerting a regulatory function mainly via the expression of expressing immunosuppressive cytokines such as TGF-β or IL-10 in the absence of Foxp3 expression[113] and can be induced by IL-27.[114-116] IL-27 activates the pivotal factors for Tr1 cell differentiation, including STAT1 and STAT3,[117] and in its exogenous form, it induces transcription of IL-21, c-Maf and inducible costimulator (ICOS), which altogether cooperate in the amplification of Tr1 cells.[113,117-119] AHR, HIF1α, IRF1, and BATF are also amongst other transcription factors involved in Tr1 cell differentiation.[120,121] Once activated, Tr1 cells facilitate suppression through both restraining cytokine production and contact-mediated lysis of effector cells. IFNγ and galectin 1, as suggested by recent studies, might stimulate DCs to produce IL-27, suggesting a potential way for therapeutic activation of Tr1 cells.[122]

There are also several checkpoints, including receptor editing, clonal deletion, anergy and prevention of the production of inflammatory cytokines and autoreactive responses by Bregs and Tregs in the periphery, to prevent autoimmunity through curtailment of the escape of autoreactive B cells to the periphery and their activation. IgM antibodies with low-affinity autoreactivity can induce opsonization of apoptotic material and noninflammatory clearance and hence, suppress immune responses.[123] Regulatory B cells (Bregs), a subset of B cells with regulatory functions, can produce potent antiinflammatory cytokines IL-10 and TGF-β, restraining the excessive inflammation associated with autoimmunity and playing an important role in the maintenance of tolerance.[124] Animal models have shown that B cell-derived IL-10 could dampen the severity of inflammation in multiple autoimmune diseases.[125,126] Bregs contribute to the maintenance of peripheral tolerance by the production of the antiinflammatory cytokines IL-10 and/or TGFβ, either directly by preventing the differentiation of Th1, Th17, and CD81 T cells or indirectly by transforming targeted effector T cells to Tregs.[125] It has been suggested that an increase in IL-10 production by Bregs follows exposure to an autoantigen and this leads to an enhanced ability to suppress autoimmune responses.[127] Cytokines including IL-1, IL-6, IL-21, and IL-35 and CD40 engagement are known as other signals inducing IL-10-producing Bregs.[128-130] Isolated Bregs fail to increase the production of IL-10 in response to CD40 ligation and to suppress the production of proinflammatory cytokines by T cells in lupus patients.[131] Interestingly, a successful B cell depleting anti-CD20 monoclonal antibody for treating some autoimmune conditions, namely, rituximab, might act through both depleting autoantibody-producing B cells and changing the balance between pathogenic and Bregs following B cell repopulation.[132,133] Please see Chapter 1 for a more in-depth discussion on the adaptive immune system and regulatory cells.

## Defective suppression of immune activation

In order to restore immune homeostasis following the stimulation of an immune response, a great proportion of the cells that have undergone clonal expansion should be eliminated and a defect in this process act as a risk factor for autoimmune diseases. Downregulation of the immune response is critical to normal homeostasis of the immune system and is mediated by different inhibitory pathways. The elimination of T and B cells usually takes place soon after their activation. Cross-linking of the BCR and FcRIIB by antigen-antibody complexes eventually leads to the downmodulation of B cell response. This can be exemplified by the FcRIIB deficiency on B cells in lupus cases, resulting in poor control of the autoantibody production.[134,135] For the T cell, this occurs, in part, by the interaction between multiple coinhibitory molecules expressed on activated T cells, such as PD1 and CTLA4, with their receptors either within lymphoid organs or in the peripheral site of inflammation.[136] Either the mutation in these molecules or their pharmacologic inhibition is associated with autoimmunity.[137-139] In some cases, defective activation-induced cell death of B and T cells modulated by Fas-Fas ligand interactions can lead to autoimmunity.[140,141]

## Tissue damage

Various effector pathways are known to be involved in tissue destruction, depending on the autoimmune disease. It is also noteworthy to mention that the mechanisms promoting autoimmune disease might differ from those propagating tissue damage. The promiscuous nature of the immune system and the commonly orchestrated immune responses implementing multiple cell populations could make the treatment of some autoimmune diseases, such as SLE, very challenging.

The autoantibodies, a common feature of autoimmune diseases,[142] not only are key components in their diagnosis and classification, but may also be involved in tissue destruction through a variety of mechanisms, including the cytotoxic destruction of cells by cell surface binding and lysis by complement activation and/or antibody-dependent cell-mediated cytotoxicity (ADCC) as the most common pathways of destruction,[143] interaction with cell surface receptors, which can both activate and block selective pathways as it happens at the level of antithyroid-stimulating hormone and anti-acetylcholine receptor for Graves' disease and myasthenia gravis, respectively, and binding to extracellular molecules, such as in the antiphospholipid antibody syndrome.[144] Autoreactive cytotoxic T cells also recognize target cells following binding of the appropriate combination of MHC I and autoantigen-derived peptides to the TCR, resulting in direct destruction of target cells through[1] activation of Fas-Fas ligand, which incites apoptosi;s[2] secretion of cytokines causing tissue injury; and[3] secretion of cytotoxic granules disintegrating cell membrane and triggering apoptosis.[2]

A body of evidence has suggested that the microenvironment and the cytokine profile of the autoreactive B and T cells and the effector cells differ between their initial site of activation, namely, secondary lymphoid organs, and the target organs in which tissue fibrosis is eventually observed.[145-147] Certain cytokines capable of inducing autoreactivity in certain occasions might preclude tissue damage in some other contexts, and vice versa, hence, there is no clear-cut distinction between their proinflammatory and anti-inflammatory properties. Considering the differential effects of the cytokines and other mediators in the immune activation and tissue destruction processes, it seems possible to therapeutically revert immune-mediated tissue destruction, even as autoreactivity goes on uninhibitedly.[148,149] Examples of such differential effects are IL-10, which exerts anti-inflammatory effects through inhibition of APCs, but act as T-cell proliferation, immunoglobulin class switching, and antibody production driver later in the disease process[150,151]; proinflammatory interferon-γ that can antagonize the differentiation of IL-17-producing T cells and hence shows anti-inflammatory features in the early stages of some autoimmune diseases[152-154]; and the TGF-β, inhibiting the initiation of autoreactivity, but accelerating tissue fibrosis later on.[155]

A major concern in autoimmune diseases is tissue fibrosis, characterized by the deposition of collagen and extracellular matrix due to the prolonged induction of myofibroblasts and failed resolution and repair, that can be triggered by several different factors, including the activation of coagulation pathways, excessive cell death, ER stress, cytokines and other immune mediators, such as TGF-β, conversion of which by either mechanical stress or chemical danger signals from a latent form to an activated profibrotic form, leading to fibroblast differentiation.[156-159] Infection, local tissue hypoxia and ongoing tissue damage with an accumulation of toxic metabolites are amongst the factors impairing the resolution of fibrosis.[157]

There are also conspicuous roles for innate immune cells in tissue damage. Neutrophils, eosinophils and mast cells can propagate tissue fibrosis. Macrophages, either recruited to the site of the lesion or being intrinsically present at the target organs, act as critical players in both the initial inflammatory process and the dead tissue clearance and tissue repair stage.[160,161]

## Initiation and facilitation of autoimmunity

### Noninfectious environmental triggers

Environmental exposures or changes in the internal environment are important triggers for the expression of autoimmunity. Accumulating evidence suggests that autoimmune diseases result from environmental exposures in genetically predisposed individuals.[162-166] Environmental agents might also have an impact on epigenetic modifications, modulated by heritable but potentially adjustable changes in chromatin structure or DNA methylation.[167,168] Autoimmune diseases, in the same manner as cancers, could be considered as multifactorial entities in which a multitude of genetic and environmental factors must interact and may need to do so in the correct order, perhaps preceding the development of the clinical disease by months to years. While certain environmental factors play a role in disease pathogenesis, some other factors seem to have a role in disease progression, severity and clinical presentation or might serve as protective factors.[169] Although the mechanisms at work in noninfectious environmental factors associated with autoimmune diseases remain poorly uncovered, it has been suggested that different pathogenic mechanisms are likely involved in the development of different syndromes.

#### *Physical activity*

Lack of exercise is associated with aggravated forms of certain autoimmune conditions in humans, including scleroderma, systemic lupus erythematosus and myositis.[170,171] Animal models have also shown that the adoption of an exercise regimen might dampen autoimmune disease activity.[172] Although the role of physical activity in autoimmunity had gained much attention, Further studies are still required for a better understanding of its impact on autoimmune diseases.

### Vitamin D

Besides the known role of vitamin D in the modulation of calcium metabolism, cellular growth, proliferation and apoptosis,[173] it has been found to have many impacts on the immune system as a natural immune modulator.[174] Decreased vitamin D levels have been confirmed in multiple autoimmune diseases, including multiple sclerosis, psoriasis, systemic lupus erythematosus, rheumatoid arthritis and vitiligo,[175-177] however, it is still not clear whether vitamin D deficiency is a cause or consequence of autoimmunity.

### Smoking

Tobacco smoke is a well-recognized risk factor for seropositive rheumatoid arthritis, Crohn's disease as well as for all combined autoimmune thyroid disease,[178,179] while the results of the studies of smoking and multiple sclerosis, Hashimoto's thyroiditis and systemic lupus erythematosus have been inconclusive.[163,180] Several pathways might be implicated in disease development. Cigarette smoke may elicit an innate immune response employing different TLR stimulating compounds it contains. Smoking can also promote the development of rheumatoid arthritis by modifying gene expression in the joint[181] and interacting with the HLA haplotype.[182] Smoking has also been associated with primary biliary cholangitis, Sjogren's syndrome and certain phenotypes of the idiopathic inflammatory myopathies.[183-185] On the contrary, a negative association has been demonstrated between smoking and the development of ulcerative colitis, indicating different roles of the chemicals in tobacco in various contexts.

### Pharmaceutical agents

The appearance of autoimmune diseases following exposure to drugs is of great interest and extensively reviewed, however, few drugs have been assessed in epidemiologic investigations and the underlying interaction of drugs with genetic and other risk factors is yet to be deciphered. Drug-related autoimmune diseases, in many circumstances, might differ from nondrug-linked diseases in terms of genetic, clinical or serologic features. Amongst more than 80 autoimmune diseases reported anecdotally to be associated with drugs, lupus-like syndromes are the most commonly recognized, characterized by autoantibodies to single-stranded DNA and histones. Drug-linked lupus differs from the non-drug-related form in the presence of autoantibodies to single-stranded DNA versus double-stranded DNA, genetic background, frequency of arthritis, neurologic and renal involvement.[186] Although such lupus-like syndromes might reverse when drugs are discontinued, there remains the likelihood that the disease persists in some cases.

### Stress

Stressful life events have been shown to predispose to the development of many autoimmune diseases. Empowering immune responses by induction of TNF-alpha, IL-1, and IL-8, and inhibition of transforming growth factor-beta production, have been suggested as possible mechanisms of how stress plays a role in autoimmune diseases.[187] There is evidence for an association between stress and Graves' disease, celiac disease, alopecia areata, lupus, type 1 diabetes, vitiligo and juvenile idiopathic arthritis.[188-191]

### *Vaccines*

Vaccination is a long-established public health measure, which might lead to immune-mediated adverse events, but this should not prevent the use of vaccination.[192] There are rare instances of autoimmune reactions and autoimmune disease that have been developed after vaccination in genetically predisposed individuals, however, only a few have been deemed to be associated with a disease, such as thrombocytopenic purpura after the measles vaccine and chronic arthritis after rubella virus vaccine, likely via the mechanisms of molecular mimicry.[193] Less is known whether vaccines can aggravate autoimmune diseases.

## Diet and gut microbiome

The role of the microbiome is being studied intensively for its impact on the regulation of immune responses and autoimmune diseases.[194-197] Being affected by genetic background, age, gender, antibiotics, dietary components, such as consumption of processed foods, intake of dietary fiber, and exposure to beneficial microbes,[198-200] diverse bacteria are identified at epithelial barriers including the skin and the gut, whereby they play a crucial role in digestion and production of essential vitamins and metabolites. Disruption of the beneficial gut commensal flora has been propounded as the driver of certain inflammatory diseases.[201,202]

Evidence has emerged suggesting a role for an altered, dysbiosis-related microbiota composition in the pathogenesis of both autoimmune and nonautoimmune inflammatory diseases, including Sjogren's syndrome, Behcet's disease, scleroderma,[203] multiple sclerosis,[204] rheumatoid arthritis,[205-207] type 1 diabetes,[208-211] Crohn's disease and ulcerative colitis,[212,213] celiac disease,[214] lupus, and others.[215] It is assumed that a combination of the absence of protective commensal species and the presence of certain bacterial species promote disease. Short-chain fatty acids (SCFAs), which are the major metabolites produced by gut commensal bacteria, as well as the omega-3 fatty acids and tryptophan catabolites are currently regarded as the leading metabolites that likely play protective roles for autoimmune and other inflammatory diseases, contributing to gut and immune homeostasis. Bacterial metabolites exert their protective, anti-inflammatory, protolerogenic actions via well-characterized receptors, transcription factors, and epigenetic mechanisms. The less dietary fiber ingested, the lower the production of SCFAs, which are probably the most important metabolites in gut homeostasis and this might underlie the development of certain autoimmune diseases as well as, allergies, asthma, Alzheimer's disease and cardiovascular disease.[216,217] Although the gut has been considered as the main site where the dietary metabolites acted on the mucosal immunity and epithelial integrity, for instance, it has been suggested that systemically distributed metabolites, such as SCFAs, might play a role in the course of macrophage/dendritic cell (DC) differentiation in the bone marrow, inflammatory responses, and lung responses.[218,219]

Apart from the profound effect of diet on the composition of gut microbiota, certain diets may take a part in the development of some autoimmune diseases.[220] Celiac disease, characterized by an immune response to ingested wheat gluten and related proteins of rye and barley, with autoantibodies acting against transglutaminase leading to intestinal inflammation, crypt hyperplasia and villous atrophy, is an example of a food-associated autoimmune disease, for which dietary intervention with a gluten-free diet stands as the main treatment modality.[221]

## Infectious triggers

Inherent genetic susceptibility and infection are equally important factors in the extremely complex and multimechanistic pathogenesis of autoimmune diseases. Microbial antigens have the potential to trigger or amplify autoreactivity through molecular mimicry, bystander activation of autoreactive cells, epitope spreading and infection-induced enhancement and maintenance of autoreactive T cells and APC signaling.[222,223] It is noteworthy that more than one possible microbial trigger might be present for some autoimmune diseases. The causal relation between microbial infection, the antimicrobial response, and autoimmune disease have been clearly verified in autoimmune conditions such as Guillain Barre´ syndrome, where antibody cross-reactivity between human gangliosides and lipopolysaccharides of C. jejuni has been depiceted, and rheumatic fever, initiated by streptococcal infection and mediated by cross-reactivity between streptococcal and cardiac myosin.[85,224-228] T cell or antibody cross-reactivity with both self and microbial antigen or microbial infection is known to precede some other autoimmune disease.[223,229,230] Epitope spreading, frequently via B cell-mediated antigen presentation, to other epitopes on the same protein or associated proteins following the initiation of response to self-antigen could be the mechanism involved in the pathogenesis of autoimmune diseases, as well.[231] Several questions are still left unresolved regarding how pathogenic challenges may interrupt immune regulation and precipitate autoimmunity.

## Genetics and epigenetics

Almost all autoimmune diseases are complex genetic traits, resulting from a combination of environmental, genetic and stochastic risk factors, each contributing a fairly small degree of risk. As genotypes at more than one different loci contribute to disease vulnerability in an indistinguishable manner, the disease phenotype is a weak predictor of the presence of a susceptibility gene. A few autoimmune diseases have been identified as monogenic in nature.[232,233] An example of a monogenic autoimmune disease is autoimmune polyendocrinopathy-candidiasis ectodermal dystrophy, a disease of multiple endocrine organs often initiated in childhood or teenage years, presenting with chronic Candida infection, autoimmune hypoparathyroidism and Addison's disease, which is a consequence of a deletion in the autoimmune regulator (AIRE) gene.[234-237] Even though the absence of the AIRE gene, which encodes a protein promoting the expression of tissue-specific genes in medullary epithelial cells in the thymus which then affects negative selection in the thymus and thus self-antigen presentation,[67,238] seems sufficient for autoimmunity, the phenotype of the consequent disease can be quite variable even within a single family. Autoimmune lymphoproliferative syndrome (ALPS), characterized by the accumulation of a polyclonal population of double-negative T cells ($CD3^{+}TCR\alpha\beta^{+}CD4^{-}CD8^{-}$), B cells and by autoantibody production, is another monogenic autoimmune disease resulting from a defect in the Fas gene.[239-242] The engagement of Fas protein, expressed on activated lymphocytes, by Fas ligand, accelerates the death of the Fas-expressing cells and hence downregulates the immune response. Immunodysregulation polyendocrinopathy enteropathy X-linked syndrome (IPEX), resulting from defective Foxp3 gene localized to Xp11.23[243] and IL2Rα deficiency, consequence of a deletion of the CD25 gene, both harboring mutations that modify the functional development of $CD4^{+}CD25^{+}$ Tregs and culminate in the loss of peripheral tolerance,[244] are other examples of monogenic autoimmune diseases affecting the bowel and endocrine organs.

The majority of autoimmune diseases are not monogenic, but rather have multiple genetic factors that play a role. For most autoimmune diseases, multiple genetic factors contribute to the disease phenotype and a summation of susceptibility and resistance loci play a role in individuals' risk of developing an autoimmune disease. Despite the identification of a number of autoimmunity associated genetic variants, mostly in non-coding regions of genes,[245-247] genome-wide association studies (GWAS) have revealed the major histocompatibility complex (MHC) locus as the polymorphic locus most closely associated with autoimmune diseases,[19] however, these results have failed to have major predictive strength. Specific HLA alleles strongly associated with autoimmune diseases have been identified in systemic lupus erythematosus (HLA class II: DR3, DR2 and DR8; HLA class III: SCIVaL, CFB, RDBP, DOM3Z, STK19C4A and C4B), type 1 diabetes (HLA class II: DQ2 and DQ8; HLA class I: HLA-A and DQB1 × 0602), autoimmune thyroid disease (HLA class II: DR3 and DR4), rheumatoid arthritis (HLA class II: DR4; HLA class III: TNF), celiac disease (HLA class II: DQ2 and DQ8) and psoriasis (HLA class I: Cw*0602, Cw1203, and HCP5).[248] GWAS have also identified genetic risk loci other than MHC, confers a modest risk for autoimmunity.[19,249]

GWAS have described several uncommon loci, associated with gene products involved in both innate and adaptive immune responses, demonstrating the occurrence of multiple autoimmune diseases within one individual and the predisposition to autoimmunity within families.[18,250] This concept is exemplified by the polymorphisms of cytotoxic T-lymphocyte associated protein 4 (CTLA4), an inhibitory costimulatory molecule present on activated T cells, which confers risk for Graves' disease, type 1 diabetes, and autoimmune hemolytic anemia,[251] as well as interferon regulatory factor 5 and transportin 3 encoding IRF5-TNPO3, which contributes to the accumulation of lymphocytes within lymphoid organs, failure of autoreactive native T cells elimination, TLR signaling, mediation of apoptosis triggered by the TNF-related apoptosis-induced ligand, development of dendritic cells, polarization of inflammatory macrophage and Th1–Th17 responses. IRF5-TNPO3 conveys risk for lupus, rheumatoid arthritis, ulcerative colitis, primary biliary cholangitis, and Sjogren's syndrome.[252] Similarly, CARD15 (NOD-2) gene plays a role in both inflammatory bowel disease and psoriasis,[253-256] and polymorphisms in tyrosine phosphatase nonreceptor type 22 (PTPN22), having a dual role and involved in the modulation of lymphocyte receptor signaling, is associated with type 1 diabetes, SLE, RA, and Graves' disease and Crohn's disease.[257] Some other gene variants shared by multiple autoimmune diseases comprise BTB and CNC homolog 2 (BACH2), chemokine C—C motif receptor 6 (CCR6), suppressor of cytokine signaling 1 (SOCS1), pseudouridylate synthase 10 (PUS10), mitogen-activated protein kinase 1 (MAPK1), RNA-binding motif protein 17 (RBM17), signal transducer and activator of transcription 4 (STAT4), thymocyte selection associated (THEMIS), intercellular adhesion molecule 3 (ICAM3), runt-related transcription factor 1 (RUNX1), IKAROS family zinc finger 3 (IKZF3), tyrosine kinase 2 (TYK2), CD80, tumor necrosis factor receptor superfamily member 14 (TNFRSF14), interleukin-12 receptor, beta 2 (IL-12RB2), RAD51 paralog B (RAD51B) and IL-12B[249,258] It should be emphasized that as the GWAS method distinguishes only prevailing polymorphisms with frequencies of between 1 percent and 5 percent within the population, the genetic risk variants recognized by this method account for only a small proportion of the overall contributing heritable risk factors of the disease.[19,245] Longitudinal cohorts are being assessed to identify Combinations of genes, predictive of the risk of disease.[259-262]

The concordance rate of 12–67 percent of autoimmune disease in monozygotic twins indicate a contribution from stochastic and environmental factors and the complementary mechanisms involved in gene regulation.[263,264] According to the studies performed, gene expression based on changes in DNA sequence or mutations is not sufficient to ultimately result in various disease phenotypes and that epigenetic deregulation affects the severity of these diseases.[265] It is also becoming evident that environmental changes can modify gene expression patterns, hence, epigenetic alterations, which might have an impact on the immune system function by changing the access of DNA regions to the transcriptional machinery through histone acetylation, DNA methylation, modifications that preclude transcription through inhibitor miRNAs, and ubiquitination or citrullination associated alterations in the intracellular protein longevity or processing, can have a potential role in the interactions between the environment and genes.[266-268] Epigenetic events are associated with loss of tolerance in certain autoimmune conditions, including hypomethylation of peptidylarginine deaminase 2 (PAD2)[269] and Src homology region 2 domain-containing phosphatase-1[270] in multiple sclerosis, histone deacetylase inhibitors in rheumatoid arthritis,[271] insulin DNA hypermethylation in type 1 diabetes,[272] acetylation of histone H4 in aquaporin 5 gene promoter in Sjogren's syndrome,[273] methylation of the CD40L promoter in primary biliary cholangitis,[274] microRNA signaling in type 1 diabetes, lupus, ulcerative colitis, multiple sclerosis, psoriasis and Sjogren's syndrome[275-277] and histone acetylation in active $CD4^+$ T cells in lupus.[278]

## Multisystem autoimmune diseases

### Systemic lupus erythematosus

#### *Definition and Epidemiology*

Systemic lupus erythematosus (SLE) is a systemic autoimmune disease with protean clinical manifestations and complex pathogenesis, more prevalent in the women of child-bearing age, resulting in significant morbidity and mortality worldwide. SLE is typically associated with antinuclear antibodies (ANA), in particular anti-double-stranded DNA (anti-dsDNA) antibodies, forming immune complexes and activating different cell types in genetically susceptible individuals, leading to multiorgan damage. Incidence rates of between almost 2 and 8 per 100,000 have been reported with differences partly due to genetics and the design of the study.[279,280] Several studies have confirmed the higher incidence and prevalence in African American, Hispanic and South Asian and Caribbean populations.[281-284]

#### *Pathogenesis*

SLE is a classical polygenic disease, with multiple genetic variants that contribute to disease susceptibility,[285-291] although it can be monogenic in nature, predominantly in younger patients. There is a high sibling recurrence ratio in SLE.[292] Early twin studies reported a monozygotic concordance rate of up to 69 percent, however, overreporting bias is suspected.[293] Deficiencies in early complement proteins from the classical pathway, such as C1q and C4, and mutations in TREX1, a DNA exonuclease,[294,295] genes involved in type I interferon production, nucleic acid sensing, clearance of self-antigen, apoptosis, and tolerance render individuals susceptible to SLE.[296] GWAS showed at least 62 loci associated with SLE, including PTPN22, STAT4, IRF5, FCRG2A, HLA-DRB1, ETS1, WDFY1, IKZF1, BLK, BANK1, and ITGAM-ITGAX.[246,297-301]

Over 100 autoantibodies have been illustrated in SLE.[302] Almost all SLE patients are positive for ANA, a diverse group of autoantibodies targeting DNA, DNA-binding proteins, histones, RNA, RNA-associated proteins, autoantibodies associated with phospholipids or cell membrane proteins, some associated with organ-specific manifestations, which present with a nuclear homogenous, nuclear centromeric, nuclear fine-speckled or nuclear coarse speckled patterns.[303] Anti-dsDNA, the most widely assayed autoantibody in SLE, as well as anti-Sm are the most specific for SLE. Free DNA, released from dying cells via apoptosis, necrosis and the development of neutrophil extracellular traps (NETosis),[304] and dsDNA antibodies combine to shape antigen-antibody complexes, deposited in organs as in the kidney and skin and eventually result in end-organ damage by complement activation and antibody-dependent cellular cytotoxicity. Dysregulation of the innate immune system and the adaptive immune system are involved in the pathogenesis of SLE.[305] Different immune cells, such as autoreactive B and T cells, dendritic cells, neutrophils, innate lymphoid cells, natural killer cells, stromal cells and tissue-resident lymphocytes are suggested to be implicated in pathogenesis. Defects in central tolerance, anergy, and peripheral tolerance in SLE occurs many years before the onset of clinical disease.[306-308]

### *Clinical features*

Various and sometimes poorly defined clinical manifestations and lupus subsets make the precise disease delineation in SLE difficult. Constitutional symptoms such as fever, weight loss, lymphadenopathy and fatigue may precede clinical diagnosis and the overt mucocutaneous, musculoskeletal, cardiac, vascular, pulmonary, renal, hematologic and neuropsychiatric manifestations and can sometimes be the most troubling and intractable for patients. Given the fact that a diagnosis can be made on the basis of three forms of mucocutaneous disease and a positive ANA, a cautious inspection of the mucus and cutaneous membranes are necessary. This group of manifestations consists of malar rash, the classical feature of lupus which can be photosensitive, bullous lupus, epidermal necrolysis, livedo reticularis, and a maculopapular lupus rash, subacute psoriaform and occasionally depigmented and telangiectatic rashes, chronic discoid rash, lupus panniculitis, chilblain lupus, oral ulcers of the tongue, palate, and buccal area, nasal ulceration, hair loss and fragile hair. Myocardial and endocardial inflammation, such as LibmanSacks endocarditis, accelerated atherosclerosis, pericarditis and pericardial effusion account for lupus cardiac manifestations with the two latter as the commonest cardiac presentations. Twenty percent of SLE patients present with Raynaud's phenomenon and may need management with nifedipine or iloprost, or sildenafil and bosentan in the case of digital ulceration. Medium-to-high titer of IgA, IgG, or IgM antiphospholipid antibody, lupus anticoagulant or positive IgA, IgG, or IgM anti-β2 glycoprotein antibody are defined as antiphospholipid syndrome and might eventually lead to thrombosis and recurrent miscarriage. Leucopenia, hemolytic anemia, thrombocytopenia, pleuritis and exudative pleural effusion are other features of SLE, which can be challenging to manage. Interstitial fibrosis and interstitial pneumonitis are amongst other SLE pulmonary manifestations. Neurological manifestations of SLE encompass a wide group including peripheral neuropathies, seizures, stroke and transient ischemic attacks, cranial nerve palsies, acute confusional states and psychosis. Musculoskeletal manifestations of SLE range from synovitis and tenderness of joints with early morning stiffness, Jaccoud's arthropathy, avascular necrosis as a complication of steroid therapy, commonly affecting the hip and tibial plateau, myalgia that may be related to medications such as statins to myositis as an uncommon feature. Lupus nephritis remains one of the most important

SLE manifestations present in up to 35 percent of patients, which can progress to end-stage renal failure in 10 percent–20 percent of patients.[309-314]

### *Treatment*

Anchor drugs in the treatment of SLE during the acute and quiescent phase are disease-modifying agents, particularly chloroquine and hydroxychloroquine (HCQ), which has demonstrated survival benefit and protection against thrombosis.[315,316] HCQ level optimization does not seem to convey added benefit.[317] Considering the risk of retinal toxicity especially in those with concomitant risk factors, including higher HCQ dose, the use of tamoxifen, longer duration of use and preexisting renal or retinal disease, a maximum daily HCQ dose of less than 5.0 mg/kg real weight has been suggested.[318] Other disease-modifying drugs, such as azathioprine, generally administered as a steroid-sparing agent, particularly in patients with renal involvement,[319] mycophenolate mofetil (MMF), used as effective induction therapy in lupus nephritis,[320,321] calcineurin Inhibitors, namely cyclosporin A, tacrolimus and voclosporin, exerting side effects such as hypertension, hirsutism and gingival hyperplasia, although being complicated to monitor, shown to be useful when significant leucopenia or other toxicities occur with mycophenolate, azathioprine, or cyclophosphamide,[322] intravenous steroids, and cyclophosphamide, which has been used as a mainstay of treatment in acute lupus nephritis.[323] Biologic agents with beneficial roles in SLE comprise rituximab, a chimeric monoclonal antibody against CD20, depleting B cells but not plasma cells, useful in renal and extrarenal SLE,[324] belimumab, reducing CD20-positive B cells, and anti-dsDNA autoantibodies, and short-lived plasmablasts through inhibition of upregulated BLyS, a key B-cell survival factor,[325] and atacicept, which is a fusion protein of the transmembrane activator and calcium modulator and cyclophilin ligand interactor (TACI) receptor with human IgG.[326] Research is underway to assess other potential agents and treatment measures such as mesenchymal stem-cell transplant,[327] plasma exchange,[328] autologous hematopoietic stem-cell transplantation (HSCT),[329] ustekinumab, a monoclonal antibody against the p40 subunit of IL-12 and IL-23,[330] janus kinase (JAK) inhibitors such as tofacitinib, epratuzumab, a monoclonal antibody targeting CD22 on B cells,[331] sifalimumab, a human monoclonal antibody binding to IFN-α,[332] rontalizumab, a human monoclonal antibody targeting all subtypes of IFN-α,[333] anifrolumab, a type I IFN receptor antagonist,[334] and bortezomib, a proteasome inhibitor.[335]

## Rheumatoid arthritis

### *Definition and Epidemiology*

Rheumatoid arthritis (RA) is the prototypic autoimmune joint disease, affecting 0.5–1 percent of the populations in the industrialized world and a higher frequency in women than men (23:1),[336-338] that might eventually impair quality of life and enormous consequences of the burden of the disease to the individual and society. It has been suggested that both genetic and environmental factors, such as adverse socioeconomic conditions,[339-341] smoking, associated with increased tumor necrosis factor and autoantibody production,[339,342-344] hormonal factors,[336] and the microbiome as an important regulator of autoimmunity,[345-347] might play an important role in the development of RA.

### Genetics and autoimmune characteristics

Various genetic associations have been found in RA, many of them in or near the genes coding for cytokines and their receptors, signal transduction molecules and costimulatory molecules,[348] mostly related to autoantibody-positive RA,[343,349] including HLA-DRB1-0401, −0404, −0405, −0408; HLA-DRB1-0101, −0102; HLA-DRB1-1001; and HLA-DRB1-1402 which together are present in about 80 percent of RA patients[350]; and non-MHC genes such as PTPN22,[351] SNPs in the complement component 5/TNF receptor-associated factor 1 (TRAF1) region at chromosome 9q33,[352] a variant allele of STAT4, located on chromosome 2q[353] together with polymorphisms in the CD40 and the TNF, alpha-induced protein 3 genes.[354] In addition, SNPs in the DCIR gene (a C-type lectin) and IRF5 are the genetic associations with seronegative RA.[355,356]

The presence of autoantibodies in the circulation and synovial fluid is the immunologic hallmark of RA, the appearance of which prior to the onset of RA is indicative of the hypothesis that the activation of the autoimmune response takes place long before clinical manifestations become evident and that the development of the disease is a multistep process with an initial trigger provoking autoimmunity.[357]

Rheumatoid factor (RF) is a family of autoantibodies directed against the Fc portion of immunoglobulin G that can be produced by B cells infiltrating the synovial membrane,[358,359] possibly exerting physiologic roles such as elimination of modified IgG and enhancement of immune complex clearance by amplifying complement binding and increasing the size of immune complex,[360,361] and was the first autoantibody ever described in RA,[362] found in up to 80 percent of RA patients. RFs can be of different isotypes, including IgM-RF, associated with significant joint damage especially at high levels (> 50 IU/mL),[363-365] IgG-RF, and IgA-RF, predictive for the development of RA and associated with worse prognosis.[366,367] RFs are not specific for RA and can occur in some other autoimmune rheumatic diseases and infections[368-371] and even in up to 5 percent of healthy individuals, in whom an up to the 26-fold increased risk of developing RA exists,[372] indicating the involvement of RF in the pathways to inflammation and joint destruction as a consequence of immune complex formation and succeeding Fc receptor binding, complement activation, and subsequent elevation of inflammatory cytokines levels.[373-375] RF levels are known to alter rapidly with changes in disease activity and diminishes following effective therapy.[376]

Another important autoantibodies in RA, anticitrullinated-protein antibodies (ACPAs), have been suggested to be somewhat more specific than RF, associated with a bad outcome, levels of which do not rapidly change with changes of disease activity or effective therapy, in contrast to RF.[376,377] RF and ACPA overlap in more than 90 percent of RA, potentiating the proinflammatory properties of immune complexes on macrophages[378] and resulting in erosive joint destruction in severe RA.[367,379] A variety of other autoantibodies, comprising autoantibodies to heterogeneous nuclear ribonucleoprotein (hnRNP) A2 (anti-RA33), occurring in 30–40 percent of RA patients,[365,380] and anti-collagen antibodies,[381,382] can also be found in RA, verifying the broad autoimmune nature of the disease. T cell-mediated autoimmunity has also been demonstrated for hnRNPA2 and collagen.[383,384] Posttranslational modifications of antibodies are yet other mechanisms to modify their effector functions and shifting toward a more proinflammatory profile, for instance.[385-387]

### *Clinical features*

As required by the 2010 ACR/EULAR classification criteria,[388] the presence of clinical synovitis (synovial involvement leading to swelling), as the main clinical characteristics of RA, in at least one joint helps diagnosing RA with the more joints affected (swollen or painful), the easier the fulfillment of the criteria. Apart from some joints, such as the distal interphalangeal joints, that are generally spared, many other joints can be involved, especially those of the fingers, wrists, toes, and knees[389] that can be painful upon motion and visibly swollen or upon clinical examination and tender to mild pressure and stiff for several hours after rest. Subchondral bone erosions, damage to cartilage and eventually completely destroyed joints can be the result of RA synovitis. The chronic inflammatory state of RA and insufficient treatment can be associated with extra-articular manifestations, including vasculitis, interstitial lung disease,[390] secondary amyloidosis, lymphoma,[391] cardiovascular disease[392] and increased mortality.[393]

### *Treatment*

The current treatment strategy for RA, based on a treat-to-target strategy, targeting remission or low disease activity, warrants cautious monitoring of the disease activity in order to promptly correct the approach when the target is not achieved. Disease-modifying antirheumatic drugs (DMARDs) are able to disrupt the inflammatory process. Combination of a conventional synthetic DMARD, methotrexate, with short-term, low dose glucocorticoids is able to achieve remission in almost 25 percent of patients at the early stages of RA.[394] When an insufficient response is reached, targeted DMARDs, either biological, such as TNF inhibitors, including infliximab, adalimumab, certolizumab pegol, etanercept, and golimumab; interleukin 6 receptor inhibitors, including tocilizumab and sarilumab; T-cell costimulation blocker, abatacept; and B-cell-directed monoclonal antibody, rituximab, or synthetic agents, such as tofacitinib, a pan-JAK inhibitor that interferes with signal transduction and cell activation triggered by IL-6, granulocyte-monocyte colony stimulating factor, interferons (type I and type II), and common γ-chain cytokines (such as IL-2 or IL-15).144; JAK 1/2 inhibitor baricitinib, can be administered, usually combined with methotrexate.[395]

## Juvenile idiopathic arthritis

### *Definition and Epidemiology*

Juvenile idiopathic arthritis (JIA) heterogeneous group of chronic arthritides of unknown etiology, lasting more than 6 weeks with the age of onset of prior to 16 years,[396,397] known as the most common chronic rheumatic condition in childhood with an incidence and prevalence varying considerably across the world according to geographic and ethnic differences. This group of diseases is characterized by the chronic inflammatory process primarily involving the synovial membrane, culminating in osteocartilaginous damage with subsequent physical functional disability. Although the debate surrounding classification is yet to be resolved, the International League of Associations for Rheumatology (ILAR) criteria[398] is currently being used to classify patients into either distinct or heterogeneous categories, including systemic JIA (sJIA), rheumatoid factor (RF) positive polyarthritis, enthesitis-related arthritis, oligoarthritis, rheumatoid factor negative polyarthritis, juvenile psoriatic arthritis (JPsA) and undifferentiated arthritis, based on laboratory and clinical findings during the first 6 months of the disease.

### *Pathogenesis*

Despite the heterogeneity of juvenile idiopathic arthritis, certain susceptibility genes have been identified, such as HLA class I (HLA A-2 and HLA B27) and HLA class II (HLADRB1 and HLA DP) alleles, as well as non-HLA candidate genes, including various cytokine genes, PTPN22, MIF, SLC11A6, and WISP3.[399-410] Considering the fact that joint inflammation in JIA is characterized by selective accumulation of activated memory T cells clustered around antigen-presenting dendritic cells in the synovium,[411-413] it is known that the autoreactive immune response is initially induced by an adaptive response against a self-antigen and soon after that, almost all the immune system play role in the immune response.[414-416] Both natural Tregs, directly derived from the thymus, and antigen-induced Tregs have been shown to be present in increased numbers in the synovial fluid and peripheral blood of patients with remitting forms of JIA, with heat shock proteins (heat shock proteins (hsp)60 and dnaJ) being the well-defined antigens.[417-421] T-helper 17 cells, characterized by the expression of transcription factor RORc and reciprocal relation with FOXP3-positive Tregs, have also been identified in the joints of JIA, playing role in the regulation of joint inflammation.[422,423] sJIA is associated with an overproduction of the proinflammatory cytokine IL-6,[424,425] a unique IL-1 signature,[426-428] and abnormal expression of IL-18, a crucial factor for the activation of natural killer cells, which is subsequently compromised in sJIA patients because of an IL-18-receptor signaling defect.[429,430] The phagocyte-specific S100 proteins, also known as myeloid-related proteins (MRPs), exerting proinflammatory effects on other immune cells and acting as endogenous activators of TLR, belong to a novel group of damage associated molecular pattern molecules (DAMP) and are regarded as biomarkers for disease and treatment response in patients with sJIA.[431-433] This can be exemplified by the increase in the serum concentration of MRP-8 (S100A8) and MRP-14 (S100A9) in patients with systemic disease, that can stand as biomarkers for the disease and as potential targets for immune treatment.[434-436]

### *Clinical features*

As stated, based on clinical criteria, JIA encompasses different forms of chronic arthritis. sJIA accounts for 10–15 percent of JIA cases and is defined by generally symmetrical and polyarticular arthritis that might be absent at onset but could emerge during disease course and systemic manifestations, such as high-spiking fever, an evanescent salmon pink skin rash characteristically occurring at fever peaks, generalized lymphadenopathy, serositis, hepatosplenomegaly, myalgias, abdominal pain, leukocytosis with neutrophilia, thrombocytosis, high C-reactive protein level, microcytic anemia, high erythrocyte sedimentation rate and dysregulated immune response involving the persistent activation of T lymphocytes and macrophages and resulting in cytokine storm, in about 5–8 percent of patients, known as macrophage activation syndrome (MAS),[437] which is characterized by the sudden onset of sustained fever, pancytopenia, hepatosplenomegaly, neurological symptoms, liver insufficiency, coagulopathy with hemorrhagic manifestations, increases level of triglycerides, low sodium levels, elevated ferritin, soluble CD163 and soluble IL-2 receptor concentrations, that might eventually lead to the development of severe multisystem involvement, if not recognized and treated in a timely manner.[438]

RF positive polyarthritis is a chronic erosive disease with poor prognosis occurring in 5 percent of JIA patients usually in late childhood or adolescence with a female predominance, characterized by the involvement of five or more joints during affecting principally wrists and the small joints of the hands and feet usually in a symmetrical pattern during the first 6 months of the disease, positive RF, the presence of rheumatoid nodules in about a third of patients, low-grade fever, lymphadenopathy, weight loss, increased levels of acute phase reactants, moderate normochromic and normocytic anemia, and positive antibodies against cyclic citrullinated peptides.

Enthesitis-related arthritis, accounting for 5–10 percent of the JIA cases with a male gender predilection, primarily affects the larger joints of the lower extremities in HLA-B27 positive patients, usually starts after the age of 6 and is generally accompanied by enthesitis, commonly at the calcaneal insertions of the Achilles tendon and of the plantar fascia and the tarsal area, and some develop hip involvement or symptomatic acute uveitis.[439,440]

Oligoarthritis is the most frequent JIA category, defined as the involvement of four or fewer joints during the first 6 months of disease and further classified as either persistent, affecting 4 or fewer joints throughout the disease course, or extended, affecting 5 or more joints after 6 months from disease onset. Except for chronic anterior uveitis, occurring in about 20–30 percent of children with oligoarthritis, extra-articular manifestations are infrequent. ANA positivity stands as a strong risk factor for developing uveitis.[441,442]

RF negative polyarthritis is the most heterogeneous JIA category, affecting 5 or more joints during the first 6 months of disease in the absence of IgM RF, with at least two distinct clinical phenotypes, one defined by overt symmetric arthritis of large and small joints initiated at school age with negative ANA, resembling adult-onset RF-negative RA; and the other is comparable to ANA positive early-onset oligoarthritis, except for the initial number of involved joints.[443]

JPsA, on the other hand, does not represent a clearly defined entity JIA category. This group is characterized by the concurrent presence of arthritis and psoriatic rash or, the presence of arthritis and two of the following: nail pitting or onycholysis, dactylitis and a family history of psoriasis in a first-degree relative, in the absence of the rash.[444,445] Patients not fulfilling the inclusion criteria of other categories are categorized as undifferentiated arthritis group.

### *Treatment*

With the improvement in JIA care and considering different therapeutic approaches according to the diverse JIA categories, remission has become an achievable target in a large proportion of patients.[446,447] Intraarticular steroid injections have been shown to play an important role in preventing deformities. MTX could be administered in patients who do not respond adequately to nonsteroidal anti-inflammatory drugs (NSAIDs) and intraarticular steroid injections,[448] and those with polyarticular JIA not responding properly to MTX could benefit from anti-TNF agents such as adalimumab (also useful in the case of JIA-associated uveitis[449]) and golimumab (humanized monoclonal antibodies to TNF-$\alpha$) and etanercept (the soluble TNF-$\alpha$ receptor).[450-452] Patients with polyarthritis resistant to TNF-$\alpha$-inhibitors can use CTLA-4 Ig, abatacept, as an approved therapeutic option.[453] Tocilizumab, an IL-6 receptor inhibitor, has shown efficacy for the treatment of patients with polyarticular JIA.[454] IL-1 and IL-6 inhibitors, including anakinra, canakinumab and tocilizumab, are the therapeutic options in steroid dependent sJIA patients.[446] Although the consumption of corticosteroid has substantially decreased with the advent of biologic treatments, they are still the best choice in the case of myocarditis, serositis, anemia and MAS, with the treatment of the latter requiring high-dose steroids and cyclosporine.

## Systemic sclerosis

### *Definition and Epidemiology*

Systemic sclerosis (SSc), or so-called scleroderma, is an autoimmune connective tissue disease with complex pathogenesis and diverse clinical manifestations, associated with substantially diminished quality of life and excess morbidity and mortality, with a pooled standardized mortality ratio (as compared with the gender and age-matched general population) of 3.53.[455] SSC has a female predominance with female-to-male ratios of between 3:1 and 9:1,[456,457] an incidence and prevalence varying notably in different geographic regions, as well as varying age of onset based on ethnicity and gender with earlier age of onset in African American population. A combination of the genetic background, stochastic and environmental factors, such as occupational silica exposure particularly in male patients and viral exposures, namely Cytomegalovirus and Epstein Barr virus, are thought to be implicated in the etiopathogenesis of SSc.[458] Along with indurated skin, showing marked patient-to-patient variability in pattern, as the distinguishing hallmark, SSc can virtually involve all organs.[459] Diffuse cutaneous SSc (dcSSc), customarily having extensive, rapidly progressive, skin induration ascending from the distal fingers to proximal extremities and the trunk, sometimes concomitant with interstitial lung disease and acute scleroderma renal crisis, and limited cutaneous SSc (lcSSc), characterized by Raynaud's phenomenon preceding other disease manifestations, are two partially overlapping subsets of SSc with distinctive natural histories.

### *Pathogenesis*

The complex pathogenesis of SSc reflects three interrelated processes, inflammation/autoimmunity,[460] microvascular disease,[459] and fibrosis, elicited by myofibroblasts and fibroblasts activated as a consequence of autoimmunity, inflammation and microvascular damage, in multiple organs.[461] SSc is a polygenic disease associated with multiple genetic susceptibility loci, although not sufficient alone for the development of the disease, but might establish a vulnerable host with autoantibody expression.[462] While the strongest disease associations have been noted on chromosome 6 in the HLA class II region, the advent of GWAS and large-scale candidate gene studies have led to the identification of robustly validated SSc susceptibility loci outside the HLA region, the majority of which are likely implicated in immune regulation.[463-468] SSc has been shown to be associated with the DRB1-11:04, DQA1-05:01, and DQB1-03:01 haplotypes and the DQB1 allele, supporting the notion that HLA class II genes mainly contribute to SSc pathogenesis through regulating autoantibody expression. Several other genetic loci shown to be associated with SSC susceptibility include TNFSF4 (OX40L), PTPN22, CD247, STAT4, BANK1, PRDM1, C8orf13/BLK, CCR6, BLK, all mainly contributing through adaptive immunity; TNFAIP3, IRAK1/MECP2 and NFKB, all acting through NFkB signaling; IRF5, IRF7, IRF8, contributing through both innate immunity and interferon pathway; IRF4, acting through interferon pathway; GRB10, acting through insulin-like growth factor; CAV1 and CSK, contributing through fibrosis; SOX5 and DNASE1L3, contributing through apoptosis; ATG5, contributing through autophagy; GSDMA, contributing through gene expression regulation, and IL12RB2, 1L12RB1 and TYK2, contributing through IL-12 pathway. The functional characterization of the contribution of the above-mentioned disease-associated genetic variants to the molecular and cellular modifications underlying clinical manifestations remains a considerable challenge.

SSc is associated with mutually exclusive and highly specific autoantibodies, standing as the best biomarkers predictive of specific organ presentations.[469,470] Roughly 96 percent of the SSc patients are ANA-positive, experiencing more vasculopathic complications, but are less likely to have GI manifestations.[471] Antitopoisomerase I antibody (anti-Scl-70) is more prevalent in Black and Asian patients and is associated with diffuse cutaneous involvement, progressive interstitial lung disease and poorer survival.[470,472-475] Anticetromere antibody, more frequent in whites, is associated with limited cutaneous involvement, cooccurrence of biliary cirrhosis, calcinosis and better survival rates.[472,475-477] Anti-U3-RNP (antifibrillarin) antibody is more common among Black and Native North American patients and is associated with pulmonary arterial hypertension and poor survival rates.[475,478,479] On the other hand, Anti-PM-Scl antibody is associated with limited cutaneous involvement, calcinosis, SSc overlap with other connective tissue diseases, and lower mortality rates.[480,481] Anti-RNA polymerase III antibody is associated with diffuse cutaneous involvement, pulmonary arterial hypertension, scleroderma renal crisis, gastric antral vascular ectasia and the contemporaneous onset of malignancy.[475,482-488]

Microangiopathy, a common early event in SSc underlying various clinical manifestations of SSc such as Raynaud's phenomenon, ischemic digital ulcers, mucocutaneous telangiectasia, scleroderma renal crisis, watermelon stomach, myocardial involvement and pulmonary arterial hypertension,[489] can be triggered by viruses, chemokines, thrombogenic microparticles, activation of the alternate complement pathways, circulating cytotoxic factors and functional autoantibodies targeting endothelial cells and phospholipids. Endothelial injury culminates in impaired secretion of prostacyclin, nitric oxide and endothelin-1, elevated level of ICAM-1, increased vascular permeability and leukocyte diapedesis through the endothelium, activation of coagulation cascades, enhanced thrombin production, dysregulated fibrinolysis, and aggregation of platelets, which produce serotonin, platelet-derived growth factor (PDGF), and thromboxane, contributing to further vascular injury. A combination of the above-mentioned processes, vascular medial hypertrophy, adventitial fibrosis, and impaired ability to repair damaged vessels, underpins progressive SSc vascular disease.

The presence of disease-specific autoantibodies, type I IFN gene signatures,[490] increased levels of IL-4, IL-6, IL-17, IL-33, CCL2, and CXCL4, familial clustering of SSc with other autoimmune diseases,[469] presence of T and B cells with oligoclonal antigen receptors, and post immunoablative hematopoietic stem-cell therapy vascular regeneration and fibrosis resolution in some SSc cases, support the notion that autoimmunity and inflammation are key players in SSc pathogenesis.

### Clinical features

SSc can involve virtually any organ. Secondary Raynaud's phenomenon is the most common extracutaneous manifestation of SSc, characterized by episodes of reversible vasoconstriction in the fingers and toes, that can be triggered by cold temperature, emotional stress and vibration. Widened capillaries, decreased capillary density, and irregular angiogenesis can be observed in this phenomenon.[460] The hallmark of SSC, distinguishing it from other connective tissue diseases, is bilateral symmetrical skin thickening. Starting in the distal extremities, skin involvement advances to proximal areas in an ascending fashion. Calcinosis cutis is common on the extremities, especially on the distal finger pads, palms, extensor surfaces of the forearms, and the olecranon and prepatellar bursae. The lesion can ulcerate, creating cutaneous ulcers on the tips of the fingers. The skin might have a salt and pepper sign due to the scarcity of pigments in the perifollicular areas, more prominent on the scalp, chest and upper back. Telangiectasias are most frequently observed on the face, buccal mucosa, lips and hands, the number of which correlates with the severity of microvascular disease and pulmonary arterial hypertension. Capillary abnormalities in the proximal nail fold of the hands are frequently noted in patients with systemic sclerosis. Microstomia, beaked nose and perioral furrows may also be detected on the face.[491] Pulmonary complications of SSc encompass interstitial lung disease, pulmonary arterial hypertension, and less common manifestations such as recurrent aspiration complicating chronic GERD, pleural reactions, chest wall fibrosis induced restrictive physiology, obliterative bronchiolitis, pulmonary hemorrhage as a result of endobronchial telangiectasia, and spontaneous pneumothorax.[492,493] Involvement of other systems are also noted in SSC patients, including the musculoskeletal, presented as frequent arthralgias, tendon friction rubs and muscle weakness; gastrointestinal, manifesting with esophageal dysmotility with esophageal reflux and dysphagia; cardiac, such as congestive heart failure as the disabling complication of pulmonary arterial hypertension; and finally scleroderma renal crisis presenting as the sudden onset of malignant hypertension and if left untreated, as renal failure.[494,495]

### *Treatment*

In light of the multisystemic nature of the SSc, treatment regimens typically include combinations of therapies affecting different aspects of the disease. Disease-modifying immunomodulatory agents such as glucocorticoids, oral and intravenously administered cyclophosphamides, mycophenolate mofetil, tocilizumab, rituximab, abatacept, extracorporeal photochemotherapy, high-dose chemotherapy followed by autologous hematopoietic stem-cell reconstitution, cyclosporine, azathioprine, plaquenil, thalidomide, and rapamycin, that are effective in other rheumatic and autoimmune diseases have generally shown only modest or no benefit in SSc.[496-498] Pirfenidone and the multikinase inhibitor nintedanib show modest benefit in patients with idiopathic pulmonary fibrosis.[499] Six to twelve months of treatment with cyclophosphamide, combined with low-dose prednisone, or mycophenolate mofetil for up to 2 years, have been shown to slow lung function reduction and delineate respiratory symptoms in SSc-associated ILD.[496] Lung transplantation can be considered in patients showing continued progression of ILD despite maximum tolerable medical therapy. Dihydropyridine calcium channel blockers, ACE inhibitors, angiotensin II receptor blockers, 5-phosphodiesterase inhibitors (e.g., sildenafil), topical nitroglycerine, intermittent IV infusions of prostanoids such as treprostinil, low-dose aspirin, dipyridamole, endothelin-1 receptor antagonists, digital sympathectomy, intradigital injections of botulinum or nerve block, and empirical long-term therapy with statins and antioxidants are different agents targeting vascular injury in order to reduce the frequency, duration, and severity of vasospastic episodes, improve ischemic ulcer healing, preclude ischemic events, and hamper the progression of obliterative vasculopathy. Despite the poor prognosis of pulmonary arterial hypertension, treatment with an oral endothelin-1 receptor antagonist such as bosentan, phosphodiesterase 5 inhibitors such as sildenafil, guanylate cyclase stimulator riociugat, selective prostacyclin receptor agonist selexipag, prostacyclin analogs such as epoprostenol or treprostinil, were shown to improve patients' outcomes to various degrees. The outcome of the scleroderma renal crisis has shown an improvement, using short-acting ACE inhibitors such as captopril, in combination with angiotensin II receptor blockers, calcium channel blockers, prostacyclins, complement pathway inhibitors such as eculizumab, endothelin-1 receptor blockers or direct renin inhibitors, in cases of persistent hypertension.

## Spondyloarthropathies

### *Definition and Epidemiology*

The spondyloarthritis (SpA) diseases comprise several related but phenotypically distinct disorders, including ankylosing spondylitis (AS), with an estimated prevalence of 0.2–0.9 percent and a male-to-female ratio of around 2:1 normally starting in the second decade of life, characterized by the presence of structural changes in the bone on X-rays, reactive arthritis (ReA), arthritis/spondylitis with inflammatory bowel disease (IBD), and arthritis/spondylitis with psoriasis. Associations with HLA-B27, shared clinical symptoms such as inflammatory back pain, and similar patterns of peripheral joint involvement with asymmetric arthritis mainly of the lower extremities, and the possibility of sacroiliitis, spondylitis, uveitis and enthesitis, are the main links between these categories.[500]

### *Genetics and autoimmune characteristics*

The susceptibility to AS has been estimated to be more than 90 percent genetically determined. MHC is regarded as the major susceptibility locus, contributing approximately 36 percent to the overall genetic risk with HLAB27 as the most relevant single factor for the pathogenesis of SpA,[501-503] and other MHC genes, such as HLA-B60 and HLA-DR1, as associated genes of minor importance. Non-MHC genes, including ERAP1, IL-23R, gene deserts 2p15 and 21q22, IL-1R2, ANTXR2, TNFSF15, TNFR1, STAT3, and TRADD have been suggested some other genetic associations of SpA.[504-509]

As suggested by the persistence of microbial antigens at the sites of inflammatory arthritis in patients with ReA, exposure of the immune system to bacteria seems important in triggering SpA.[510] The persistence of bacterial antigens in the articular spaces might result in the pathological priming of T cells cross-reacting to the autologous antigens. A relative lack of Th1-cytokines, such as TNFα and IFNγ, which are crucial for the effective elimination of the ReA-associated bacteria, appears to be relevant for the occurrence and persistence of ReA, while Th2 cytokines, such as IL-4, or antiinflammatory cytokines, such as IL-10, inhibiting effective elimination of ReA-associated bacteria possibly by down-regulation of the Th1-cytokines, were found relatively upregulated in ReA.[511-513] The positive association between IBD and SpA[514] could be partly explained by the hypothesis that leakage in the gut mucosa as a consequence of the related inflammation presumably allows the interaction of the immune system with the normal gut bacteria, indicating a link between the gut and its microbiota and pathogenesis of axial SpA.[515,516] The triggers and cellular sources of pathogenic cytokine secretion are poorly delineated in AS. An increased percentage of IL-17A$^+$ cells, mostly of myeloid origin, demonstrated in the subchondral bone marrow of facet joints in patients with AS[517] as well as the IL-17-expressing mononuclear and polymorphonuclear, synovial cell infiltrates found in inflamed peripheral joints of SpA patients,[518] suggest the contribution of innate immune cells towards pathogenic IL-17 production in AS. Increased numbers of IL-23$^+$ cells were also shown within bone marrow cells, particularly cells of myeloid origin, in facet joints from AS patients.[519] IL-23 is induced during the unfolded protein response triggered by protein misfolding. In addition, stimulation of innate cells with triggers of unfolded protein response leads to increased LPS-induced production of the inflammatory cytokines, specially IFNβ and IL-23.[520]

### *Clinical features*

Axial SpA presents with inflammatory back pain characterized by morning stiffness as the leading clinical symptom, mostly starting with sacroiliitis and then proceeding to spondylitis, spondylodiscitis, arthritis of the small intervertebral joints, spinal ankylosis as a reaction to the inflammation, limiting spinal mobility, as well as extraspinal manifestations such as peripheral asymmetric arthritis predominantly of the lower limbs, enthesitis and relapsing uveitis. Sacroiliitis, presenting with active inflammation and/or structural damage on MRI or X-ray, together with laboratory results, such as HLA-B27 and increased CRP also aids diagnosis of axial SpA.[521,522] Clinical manifestations compatible with SpA, including oligoarthritis of the lower extremities and/or spinal inflammation, are present in up to 50 percent of the patients with psoriatic arthritis, and these show HLA-B27 positivity in about 25 percent to 60 percent of cases. Almost 10–20 percent of the patients with IBD manifest with arthritis, usually as transient peripheral arthritis of the lower limbs. ReA occurs after a few days up to 46 weeks of a preceding infection of the urogenital tract with Chlamydia trachomatis or of the gut with enterobacteria, such as Campylobacter jejuni, Salmonella, Yersinia, or Shigella,[523] manifesting as peripheral oligoarthritis, and less commonly polyarthritis, inflammatory back pain, enthesitis, or conjunctivitis/uveitis, and is usually positive for HLA-B27 in 30 percent to 60 percent of the cases. Laboratory evidence of the previous or present bacterial infections is also crucial for making a diagnosis.[524]

### *Treatment*

Despite the limited effectiveness of disease-modifying antirheumatic drugs and corticosteroids only in patients with predominant peripheral arthritis, NSAIDs and physiotherapy have been shown as effective modes of treatment over the last few decades. There is also supporting evidence suggesting the role of anti-TNFα blockers, including both monoclonal anti-TNFα antibody infliximab and soluble TNF-receptor construct etanercept, and the IL-17 inhibitor secukinumab in the treatment of patients with AS, however, these results are yet to be further investigated.[525-530]

## Sjogren's disease

### *Definition*

Sjogren's syndrome (SS) is the second most common autoimmune disease, after rheumatoid arthritis, with a great deal of clinical variability, and depending upon how this syndrome is defined, it might even turn out to be more prevalent than rheumatoid arthritis. SS, characterized by lymphocytic infiltration of the exocrine glands and other organs in association with the production of various autoantibodies, might occur either as a primary syndrome or as a secondary syndrome in association with other autoimmune diseases, such as SLE, myositis, RA, SSc, and primary biliary cirrhosis.[531-533]

### *Immune characteristics*

A shift in Th1/Th2 cytokine balance in favor of Th1 responses,[534] the expansion of IL-17 producing Th17 cells, the secretion of IL-22 by a subset of NK cells and Th17 cells,[535] induction of plasminogen activator system by IFNg,[536] IL-7 and its receptor (IL-7Ra),[537] and the impaired balance between Th17/T regulatory cells with a predominance of Th17 cells are known to provoke local inflammation and injury in SS.[538,539] Increased numbers of B-cell population $CD21^{-}$/low, enriched in autoreactive clones, have been detected in and the presence of macrophages in the histopathological lesion has been shown in primary Sjogren's syndrome patients complicated by lymphoma.[540-542] Recruitment of type I IFN producing plasmacytoid dendritic cells and the activation of type I IFN/B-cell activating factor (BAFF) pathway have also been depicted in SS patients.[543] Moreover, the epithelium, acting as antigen-presenting cells actively contributing towards the development of the inflammatory context by cytokine production and recruitment of various immunocytes, has been suggested as a chief component of disease pathogenesis.[544-546] In addition, persistent activation of NFkB pathways due to impaired function of IkBa kinase and tumor necrosis factor-a induced protein-3 (TNFAIP3) have been demonstrated in Sjogren's syndrome.[547,548]

## Clinical features

Dry eyes and dry mouth are defining features of SS. Apart from these two features, a typical SS case presents with tiredness, arthralgia, mild anemia, high erythrocyte sedimentation rate, high IgG levels with positive ANA, Ro and/or La autoantibodies, and low levels of C4. Sicca symptoms include dry eyes, generally noted by patients as ocular discomfort, grittiness, contact lens intolerance and photosensitivity, red eyes, shallow erosions of the conjunctiva, xerostomia, dysphagia, dry fissured or red atrophic tongue, oral candida, dry fissured or red atrophic tongue, dental caries, parotid and submandibular gland swelling,[549] dry cough, dry nose, dry skin and vaginal dryness, causing dyspareunia.[550] Non-sicca (systemic) manifestations comprise fatigue, fibromyalgia, weight loss, anemia, fever, arthralgia, non-erosive and not deforming arthritis, myopathy, Raynaud's phenomenon, purpura, vasculitic rashes, cognitive dysfunction, depression, peripheral nervous system involvement, particularly sensory neuropathies and less commonly, mononeuritis multiplex, cranial and autonomic neuropathies,[551] upper respiratory tract and large and small airways disease, interstitial lung disease, interstitial nephritis, causing renal tubular acidosis, nephrogenic diabetes insipidus, symptomatic hypokalemia, interstitial cystitis, myocardial disease, pericarditis, dysphagia, nausea, dyspepsia, and chronic atrophic gastritis. Sjögren's syndrome is associated with autoimmune thyroid disease, celiac disease and lymphocytic interstitial pneumonitis.[552] There is a 5–10 percent lifetime risk of lymphoma in patients with Sjögren's syndrome, associated with risk factors such as lymphopenia, low C4 level, cryoglobulins, cutaneous vasculitis, persistent salivary gland enlargement, lymphadenopathy, and palpable purpura.[550]

## Treatment

The treatment of patients with SS must be individualized to the existing manifestations. As there is still no definitive cure for the SS, currently available treatments aim at palliation of symptoms, prevention of complications, treatment of extra-glandular manifestations and selection of patients for immunosuppressive therapy based on the severity, activity and extent of disease. According to the treatment recommendations published by the Sjogren's Foundation for the management of patients with SS,[553] topical fluoride, masticatory stimulation, sugar free lozenges or gums, mannitol, xylitol, secretagogues (Pilocarpine and Cevimeline), chlorhexidine mouthwash and nonfluoride remineralizing agents are recommended for the management of oral problems; artificial tears, gels, ointments, topical steroids, topical cyclosporine, punctal plugs, Pilocarpine, Cevimeline, contact lenses, topical autologous serum, permanent punctal occlusion, eyelid surgery and systemic antiinflammatory therapy are encouraged for the management of eye problems, depending on the severity of disease; exercise and dehydroepiandrosterone are strongly recommended to relieve fatigue; hydroxychloroquine, methotrexate and short and long term corticosteroids are recommended to manage musculoskeletal pain, depending on disease severity; rituximab is the only biological agent positively recommended for pulmonary disease, vasculitis, inflammatory arthritis, cryoglobulinemia, peripheral neuropathy and severe parotid swelling.[553]

The use of certain biological agents in SS have been evaluated, such agents include a soluble lymphotoxin beta receptor IgG fusion protein precluding the actions of lymphotoxin beta, Baminercept[554]; a monoclonal antibody blocking BAFF, Belimumab[555]; a soluble CTLA-4-Ig interrupting T-cell activation, Abatacept[556]; a monoclonal antibody to the IL-6 receptor to prevent the development of plasma cells; a monoclonal antibody to inducible T cell costimulator-ligand (ICOS-L) to prevent T follicular helper cells activation and subsequent secretion of high-affinity autoantibodies; a PI3K inhibitor to inhibit B- and T-cell activation; and a monoclonal antibody blocking CD 40 to prevent B-cell activation.[553] The only one with significant positive results to warrant its use is rituximab.[557-560]

## Autoimmune myopathies

### *Definition*

The autoimmune myopathies are an uncommon heterogeneous family of diseases, occurring either as distinct diseases, namely, dermatomyositis (DM), polymyositis (PM), and immune-mediated necrotizing myopathy (IMNM) or as a manifestation of other systemic autoimmune diseases such as SLE or scleroderma, all unified by autoimmune damage of skeletal muscle as their primary target.[561] Skin (in DM), cardiac muscle, lung and synovial joints are other tissues frequently affected.

### *Pathogenesis*

The autoantibodies elaborated in autoimmune myositis identifies a family of autoantigens exerting prominent functions, including gene expression,[562] DNA repair machinery,[563-565] protein translation,[566,567] posttranslational modification,[568] nuclear body formation,[569] and the exosome complex. Several autoantigens such as Ro52 and MDA5 are also elicited by interferons.[570,571] A striking association with disease subsets has been noted for myositis-specific autoantibodies. Antisynthetases (anti-Jo-1, PL-7, PL-12, EJ, OJ, KS, Ha, Zo) are frequently associated with the antisynthetase syndrome, a clinical syndrome with Raynaud's phenomenon, relatively mild myositis, mechanic's hands, inflammatory arthritis of the small joints of the hands, and ILD.[572] Anti-Mi-2, anti-melanoma differentiation-associated protein (anti-MDA5, anti-CADM140), antitranscription intermediary factor 1$\gamma$ (anti-p155), antinuclear matrix protein 2 (anti-NXP2, anti-MJ), and anti-SAE1 are associated with DM. Anti-3-hydroxy-3-methylglutaryl coenzyme A (anti-HMGCR) and Anti-SRP are the autoantibodies associated with necrotizing myopathy.[573-578] The majority of myositis autoantigens are susceptible to cleavage by the cytotoxic lymphocyte granule protease, granzyme B (GrB).[579] Moreover, several nonspecific myositis-associated antibodies seen in immune-mediated inflammatory myopathies and other connective tissue diseases have been recognized, comprising antibodies to Ro52, observed in approximately 25 percent of patients with myositis[580]; anti-Ku antibodies, described in up to 55 percent of cases of myositis/systemic sclerosis overlap syndrome with frequent joint involvement, Raynaud syndrome, and increased risk of ILD[581]; Anti-PMScl antibodies, detected in patients with myositis/systemic sclerosis overlap syndrome and associated with lung and esophageal involvement[582]; anti-U1 RNP antibodies, identified in patients with myositis, SLE, glomerulonephritis and scleroderma[583]; as well as antibodies against some other components of the ribonucleoprotein complex (RNP, U2 RNP, U4/U6 RNP, and U5 RNP).

The combination of several immunogenetic risk factors, including class-2 HLA alleles and interferon-inducible genes as well as environmental factors, have been implicated in the pathogenesis of dermatomyositis.[584,585] Given the fact that dermatomyositis muscles contain abundant interferon-secreting plasmacytoid dendritic cells,[586] the interferon overproduction has been a proposed mechanism of the pathology seen in dermatomyositis, although how this leads to the loss of capillaries and perifascicular atrophy still remains unclear. Other studies have suggested immunogenetic risk factors, such as the class-2 HLA-allele DRB1 × 08:03 to play a role in anti-SRP myopathy,[587] and DRB1 × 11:01, found in 70 percent of patients with anti–HMG-CoA reductase antibodies, as a risk factor for anti–HMG-CoA reductase myopathy.[587,588]

### *Clinical features*

The autoimmune myopathies can manifest by the subacute onset of painless weakness, principally involving proximal muscles in a symmetrical way[589-591]; involvement of striated muscle of the nasopharynx and upper esophagus resulting in tendency to aspiration, difficulty in swallowing, nasal regurgitation, and weakness of phonation in some cases; weakness of the respiratory muscles in severe cases; increased levels of creatine kinase (CK), aspartyl transaminase, alaninyl transaminase and aldolase A; irritable myopathy on electromyography; systemic inflammatory symptoms such as malaise and fever; skin involvement (in DM) characterized by the Gottron's papules on the dorsal aspect of the metacarpophalangeal and proximal interphalangeal joints, a violaceous eruption affecting the shawl area, chest, flanks, and thighs, a heliotrope rash on the face around the eyelids, and skin ulcers and palmar papules[574]; rheumatoid arthritis-like inflammatory synovitis of the small joints of the hands; and interstitial lung disease in 20–65 percent of patients.[592,593]

### *Treatment*

Treatment of this class of disorders currently focuses entirely on the modification of the immune side of the pathogenic cycle. Although clinical experience suggests efficacy with some immunosuppressive strategies, there is still little body of evidence on the efficacy of specific agents. Early anticancer therapies might be of benefit in cases with cancer as the initial immune response drivers.

## Antiphospholipid syndrome

### *Definition*

The antiphospholipid syndrome (APS) is a systemic autoimmune disease usually diagnosed following obstetric or thrombotic morbidity in patients with persistent (more than 12 weeks), high-level antiphospholipid antibodies (aPL) seropositivity and significant related morbidity and mortality.[594,595] It should be emphasized that aPL may be detected in up to 1–5 percent of the general population, usually detected transiently at low levels in healthy individuals, more frequent in older cases and in association with malignancies, infections, exposure to certain drugs and vaccinations, and will not develop APS in most cases.[595,596] APS can appear in systemic autoimmune diseases such as SLE, with a prevalence of 30–40 percent in SLE (secondary APS)[596]; though, it mostly occurs without other autoimmune manifestations (primary APS).

### *Pathogenesis*

Several genes, both the HLA loci and some unrelated to the HLA system have been shown to be associated with APS, including DRB1-04, DR7, DRw53, DQB1-0301/4, DQB1-0604/5/6/7/9, DQA1-0102, and DQA1-0301/2,[597] STAT 4,[598] 12q24.12,[599] and PTPN22[600] and valine/leucine[247] polymorphism of B2GPI.[601]

A plasma protein binding avidly to phospholipid surfaces, β2-glycoprotein I, is the main target of antiphospholipid antibodies,[602] binding of which to antiphospholipid antibodies enhances the expression of prothrombotic cellular adhesion molecules, including tissue factor and E-selectin, down-regulates the activity of the tissue factor pathway inhibitor,[603] activates complement[604,605] and suppresses activated protein C activity.[606] Monocytes and monocyte-derived microparticles also express elevated levels of tissue factor in patients with APS.[607] In addition, research demonstrates the critical role of platelets, expressing and synthesizing glycoprotein IIb/IIIa (the receptor for fibrinogen),[608] and thromboxane A2, hence playing a major role in the prothrombotic interactions between antiphospholipid antibodies and endothelial cells.[609] Annexin A2, a tissue plasminogen activator receptor, p38 mitogen-activated protein kinase (p38 MAPK) and NFκB may act as important mediators in these processes.[610-614] Complement-mediated functional disruption of the endothelium and trophoblast contributes to the antiphospholipid antibodies associated with microthrombosis and pregnancy complications.[615] Moreover, the trophoblast damage might be partly a result of antiphospholipid antibodies triggered inflammatory response mediated by the TLR4/MyD88 pathway.[616] Neutrophil activation and subsequent expression of tissue factor and the secretion of neutrophil extracellular traps (NETosis) and IL-8 are also important factors in antiphospholipid antibody–associated thrombosis.[617-619]

## Clinical features

The wide spectrum of clinical presentations of APS is characterized by single vessel or multiple vascular venous and arterial thromboses, pregnancy complications and moderate thrombocytopenia, induced by both thrombotic and immune-mediated mechanisms.[620,621] The clinical features of 1000 patients with APS, followed up for 10 years within the Euro-Phospholipid project include peripheral thrombosis (deep vein thrombosis, 38.9 percent, superficial thrombophlebitis in legs, 11.7 percent, arterial thrombosis in legs, 4.3 percent, venous thrombosis in arms, 3.4 percent, arterial thrombosis in arms, 2.7 percent, subclavian vein thrombosis, 1.8 percent, jugular vein thrombosis, 0.9 percent), neurologic manifestations (migraine, 20.2 percent, stroke, 19.8 percent, transient ischemic attack, 11.1 percent, epilepsy, 7.0 percent, multiinfarct dementia, 2.5 percent, chorea, 1.3 percent, acute encephalopathy, 1.1 percent), pulmonary manifestations (pulmonary embolism, 14.1 percent, pulmonary hypertension, 2.2 percent, pulmonary microthrombosis, 1.5 percent), cardiac manifestations (valve thickening/dysfunction, 11.6 percent, myocardial infarction, 5.5 percent, angina, 2.7 percent, myocardiopathy, 2.9 percent, vegetations, 2.7 percent, coronary bypass rethrombosis, 1.1 percent), intraabdominal manifestations (glomerular thrombosis, renal infarction, renal artery thrombosis, and renal vein thrombosis, 2.7 percent, esophageal or mesenteric ischemia, 1.5 percent, splenic infarction, 1.1 percent), cutaneous manifestations (livedo reticularis, 24.1 percent, ulcers, 5.5 percent, pseudovasculitis lesions, 3.9 percent, digital gangrene, 3.3 percent, cutaneous necrosis, 2.1 percent), osteo-articular manifestations (arthralgia, 38.7 percent, arthritis, 27.1 percent, avascular necrosis of bone, 2.4 percent), ophthalmologic manifestations (amaurosis fugax, 5.4 percent, retinal artery thrombosis, 1.5 percent), E.N.T. manifestations (nasal septum perforation, 0.9 percent), hematological manifestations (thrombocytopenia ($<$ 100,000 per μL), 29.6 percent, hemolytic anemia, 9.7 percent), obstetric manifestations (preeclampsia, 9.5 percent, eclampsia, 4.4 percent, abruptio placentae, 2.0 percent), and fetal manifestations (early fetal losses ($<$ 10 weeks), 35.4 percent, late fetal losses (=> 10 weeks), 16.9 percent, live births, 47.4 percent, prematures, 10.6 percent).[622]

## Treatment

Considering subjects' the benefits and risks of antithrombotic therapies against the risk of thrombosis, the management of APS is directed towards antithrombotic medications. Thromboprophylaxis with typical doses of low molecular weight heparin (LMWH) should be prescribed in high-risk situations, including prolonged immobilization, surgery and puerperium period, in all aPL carriers. Individuals with persistent positivity of multiple and/or high titer aPL should consider the administration of low-dose aspirin (LDA, 75–100 mg/day).[623] Oral anticoagulant therapy should be administered in cases of definite APS with a first venous thrombosis event (target INR of 2.0–3.0) and definite APS and arterial thrombosis and/or recurrent events (target INR of over 3.0). Indefinite antithrombotic therapy is also endorsed in cases of definite APS and thrombosis.[624] It has been shown that rivaroxaban, a direct anti-Xa inhibitor, might be an effective choice in APS with previous venous thromboembolism.[625] Women without previous episodes of thrombosis are commonly prescribed LMWH at prophylactic doses, or therapeutic doses in case of previous thrombotic events.[626,627] Immunosuppressive treatments might show beneficial effects in APS patients and aPL-positive cases. Examples are HCQ in SLE patients with or without aPL, primary arterial and venous thromboses prevention in aPL-positive individuals,[628] refractory APS cases[629] and women with previous thrombosis and/or ischemic placenta-mediated complications[630]; and rituximab in difficult-to-treat APS patients, in patients with hematologic and microthrombotic/microangiopathic manifestations,[626] and refractory and accelerated forms of APS resulting in multiorgan failure (catastrophic APS).[631] In the latter condition, catastrophic APS, an aggressive therapy, using anticoagulation, glucocorticoids, and plasma exchange and/or intravenous immunoglobulins[632,633] or the use of a humanized monoclonal antibody against complement protein C5, eculizumab, might be effective.[624]

## Immunoglobulin G4-related disease

### *Definition and Epidemiology*

Immunoglobulin G4-related disease (IgG4-RD) is a multiorgan immune-mediated condition, more commonly occurring in middle-aged to elderly men with a male to female ratio of approximately 3:2, which was first recognized in the pancreas.[634-636] The pancreas is only one of more than a dozen organs involved by IgG4-RD and the expanding knowledge of this disease has provided important insights into the associations of numerous conditions once considered single-organ diseases, including Riedel's thyroiditis, autoimmune pancreatitis (AIP), Küttner's tumor (bilateral submandibular gland enlargement), retroperitoneal fibrosis (RPF), and many more.[637] Considering the observations of limited repertoires of plasmablasts and a particular $CD4^+$cytotoxic T lymphocyte, IgG4-RD is regarded as an antigen-driven disease,[638,639] likely triggered by multiple antigens such as galectin-3, recently identified as a candidate antigenic driver in approximately 30 percent of IgG4-RD patients in one study.[640]

### *Pathogenesis*

Antigen-driven interactions among cells of the B lymphocyte lineage, including activated B cells and plasmablasts, at least two $CD4^+$T lymphocytes, $CD4^+$T follicular helper cells and a $CD4^+$CTL, are involved in IgG4-RD.[641] B cells and the cells of their lineage play a variety of roles in IgG4-RD,[638,642] including the production of IgG4 (mostly by short-lived plasmablasts and plasma cells) and antigen presentation to T cells. The most abundant cell observed within affected tissues is $CD4^+$ T cell. Given the fact that $CD4^+$CTLs undergo large clonal expansions, infiltrate tissues affected by the disease in large numbers, actively produce cytokines in these tissues, and diminish with rituximab-induced disease remission,[639,643] these cells have been suggested to be the as principal drivers of IgG4-RD. These cells express perforin and granzymes and demonstrate cytolytic capacity. $CD4^+$CTLs may contribute to fibrosis by multiple mechanisms, including profibrotic cytokine secretion, including interleukin IL-1β, TGF-β, and IFN-γ, and via the stimulation of apoptosis in targeted cells. It has been hypothesized that activated B cells might induce the activation of $CD4^+$CTLs at the sites of disease through antigen presentation.[641] Signaling lymphocytic activation molecule family (SLAMF7), an antigen expressed on cells of the B lymphocyte lineage and $CD4^+$CTLs in IgG4-RD,[644] acts via homotypic interactions between infiltrating B and T cells and thus plays a critical role in the IgG4-RD disease process.[645]

### *Clinical features*

IgG4-RD can manifest with lymphadenopathy, either generalized or localized adjacent to an affected organ without any predilection for any particular set of lymph nodes; lacrimal gland enlargement (dacryoadenitis) as the most common feature of ophthalmic manifestations of IgG4-RD; proptosis; inflammation and thickening of the extraocular muscles; mild-to-moderate peripheral eosinophilia and serum IgE concentration elevations; allergic rhinitis; nasal polyps; chronic sinusitis; nasal obstruction; rhinorrhea; diffuse inflammation in the pharynx, hypopharynx, and Waldeyer's ring; mass lesions in the sinuses; destructive lesions in the middle ear and facial bones; thickening of the bronchovascular bundle; pulmonary nodules; groundglass opacities; pleural thickening; interstitial lung disease; involvement of the brain parenchyma presenting as hypertrophic pachymeningitis; hypophysitis, leading to hormone deficiencies from both the anterior and posterior pituitary; peripheral nerve lesions in the area of the orbit with common involvement of the trigeminal and infraorbital nerves; tubulointerstitial nephritis (TIN), commonly accompanied by profound hypocomplementemia, that might result in subnephrotic proteinuria, renal atrophy, advanced renal dysfunction and even end-stage renal disease; membranous glomerulonephropathy; Type 1 AIP, depicting the classic histopathological findings of lymphoplasmacytic sclerosing pancreatitis, that might lead to secondary diabetes mellitus or even exocrine pancreatic failure leading to massive weight loss; IgG4-related sclerosing cholangitis and cholecystitis; IgG4-related aortitis, that can culminate in aneurysms or dissections in the thoracic aorta; coronary artery lesions, sometimes associated with aneurysm formation; chronic periaortitis; retroperitoneal fibrosis; IgG4-RD of the thyroid gland, presenting with overwhelmingly fibrotic lesions, namely, Riedel's thyroiditis; fibrosing mediastinitis; sclerosing mesenteritis; cutaneous manifestation such as erythematous papules typically affecting the head and neck; and prostatic enlargement as a result of IgG4-related prostate disease.[637]

### *Treatment*

Glucocorticoids are currently the first-line treatment for IgG4-RD, resulting in symptomatic response within 2 weeks and the elimination of clinical manifestations within

23 months; however, in many instances, disease relapse could follow the discontinuation of glucocorticoids.[646] Other potential treatment approaches are anti-CD20-targeted therapy, such as rituximab as an alternative to glucocorticoids with clinical responses of variable durations[647,648]; costimulatory blockade using abatacept, a fusion protein composed of the extracellular domain of CTL-associated protein 4 and the IgG1 constant domain, that can interfere with ligation to the costimulatory CD28 molecule on T cells after binding to CD80/86 on antigen-presenting cells, leading to disease amelioration; and elotuzumab, an immunostimulatory mAb directed against SLAMF7, which activates NK cells and leads to ADCC of the SLAMF7-expressing cellular target.[637]

## System-specific autoimmune diseases

As an in-depth explanation of all human system-specific autoimmune diseases is beyond the capacity of this chapter, a few common diseases have been chosen to be covered in this section.

### Nervous system

#### *Multiple sclerosis*

#### Definition and Epidemiology

Multiple sclerosis (MS) is a chronic autoimmune disease of the central nervous system (CNS) with a median age of 23–24 years at onset of symptoms, showing a female predominance with a 3:2 female-to-male ratio.[649,650] MS is a complex disease with several genetic and environmental contributing factors heretofore identified. Several genes, amongst which various MHC alleles as well as non-MHC candidate genes such as TNFRSF6B, RPS6KB1, SOX8, CXCR5, NFKB1, were shown convey strong evidence of association, have been implicated in the pathogenesis of this complex disease.[651,652] Besides, well defined environmental factors, in particular vitamin D, ultraviolet B light (UVB) exposure, obesity, smoking, and Epstein–Barr virus (EBV) infection, have been demonstrated.[653]

#### Immune pathogenesis

Considering the observations of an increased proportion of T cells from MS patients expressing the characteristic Th1 chemokine receptor pattern, CXCR3/CCR5; MS plaques expressing increased levels of the corresponding chemokines[654,655]; a bias toward Th1 cytokines as depicted by the analysis of cytokine mRNA in CSF from MS patients[656]; the presence of the proinflammatory cytokines TNF-α and IL-12 in the MS plaques[657,658]; and secretion of cytokines more consistent with Th1-mediated response by the MBP-reactive T cells derived from patients with MS,[659] support the hypothesis that Th1 cells may be pathogenic in MS. Besides that, Th17 cells have been suggested to have a putative role in establishing the MS phenotype. It has been shown that pathogenic Th17 cells are capable of gaining early access to the CNS.[660,661] It is hypothesized that peripherally activated Th17 cells might migrate across the blood-CSF barrier and gain access to circulating CSF through binding to adhesion molecules and chemokine receptors expressed on the choroid plexus, and can then access perivascular tissue and trigger a cascade of proinflammatory events.[662,663] Th17 cells might also increase blood-brain barrier permeability by producing IL-17 and IL-22, which subsequently leads to the facilitation of the influx of immune cells, including autoreactive Th17 cells, IFN-γ secreting Th1, γδ T cells, cytotoxic $CD8^+$ cells, B cells, and immunoglobulin-secreting plasma cells,[664] and thus creating an inflammatory environment containing infiltrates of cells that cause downstream damage of the CNS.[665] Moreover, it has been postulated that the suppressive ability of Tregs is compromised and substantially reduced in response to autoreactive T cells in patients with MS.[666] No single antigen has been demarcated in the pathogenesis of MS. However, autoantigen-specific T cells have been implicated both in healthy individuals and in patients with MS, which can contribute to myelin destruction and axonal damage in addition to secondary inflammation following activation by local APCs following their entrance into the inflamed CNS environment as described above.

Given the marked presence of oligoclonal bands and elevated intrathecal synthesis of IgG within the CSF of MS patients; increased incidence of EBV infection and its potential to prime the immune system in patients with MS; the evidence showing B-cell clones populating the meninges, which might be related to the B-cell infiltrates in MS lesions[667]; the presence of ectopic lymphoid follicles, containing proliferating B cells, plasma cells, T cells, and dendritic cells, resembling germinal centers in the meninges of SPMS patients with the corresponding diffuse meningeal inflammation[668]; and the production of proinflammatory cytokines, such as IL-6, by B cells in EAE mice,[669] B-cell involvement has been postulated to play an imperative role in MS pathogenesis.

## Clinical features

Demyelinating lesions of MS and accompanying edema, inflammation, gliosis, and axonal loss may involve any site along myelinated CNS white matter tracts, resulting in variable signs and symptoms depending on the pathways involved. MS can present with alteration or absence of sensation as a result of the involvement of spinothalamic or posterior column fibers; visual loss due to optic neuritis; limb weakness and spasticity resulting from disruption of corticospinal tracts; tremors and incoordination of gait or limbs secondary to cerebellar or spinocerebellar fiber involvement; abnormalities of cranial nerve function as a consequence of brainstem lesions[670]; and less commonly, bowel, bladder, and sexual dysfunction mainly related to disruption in spinal cord pathways[671]; as well as fatigue, depression, and cognitive changes possibly due to axonal loss.[672-674] MS can be categorized into subtypes, including radiologically isolated syndrome (RIS), commonly recognized incidentally on MRI of the brain in the absence of signs or symptoms which might develop the clinical symptoms in case of CNS inflammation, a high lesion burden, with positive oligoclonal bands (OCBs) or elevated IgG index in the cerebrospinal fluid (CSF); clinically isolated syndrome (CIS), usually occurring in young adults, characterized by the presentation of the initial episode of demyelination, typically in the form of an optic neuritis, cerebellar, or brainstem syndrome, during which neurological symptoms develop over hours to several days, last for at least 24 h to several weeks, and steadily vanish with no more than 30 days between attacks[675,676]; relapsing-remitting MS (RRMS), in patients developing further clinical episodes followed by relapses, usually presenting with complete recovery from relapses early in the course of disease and diminished recovery from relapses as the disease progresses, 40–50 percent of whom, if untreated, will stop experiencing attacks and develop a neurodegenerative progressive disease secondary to the chronic CNS inflammation, termed as secondary progressive MS (SPMS),[677] associated with markedly fewer gadolinium-enhancing lesions and decreased brain parenchymal volume[678-680]; and primary progressive MS (PPMS), occurring in approximately 15 percent of the patients, characterized by the absence of acute attacks at the onset but showing a gradual clinical decline in the form of a progressive myelopathy or a progressive cerebellar syndrome in the form of ataxia, associated with a lack of substantial response to immunotherapy.[681]

### Treatment

Immunotherapies, shown to be most effective in the RRMS, CIS, and early progressive forms of MS having an inflammatory component, are available in different administration forms, comprising infusion-based, oral, and self-injection medications. Infusion-based medications have been regarded as the most effective FDA-approved immunotherapies to date, including natalizumab (Tysabri), a monoclonal antibody acting against the very late activation antigen-4 (VLA-4), the $\alpha 4\beta 7$ integrin expressed on activated T cells and monocytes, and a ligand for VCAM expressed on CNS endothelial cells[682,683]; alemtuzumab (Lemtrada), a humanized CD52-directed monoclonal antibody resulting in depletion and repopulation of B lymphocytes and T lymphocytes[684,685]; and ocrelizumab (Ocrevus), a fully humanized monoclonal antibody targeting CD20-positive B cells approved for both RRMS and PPMS.[686,687] FDA-approved oral medications for MS consist of fingolimod (Gilenya), targeted toward lymphocyte migration out of lymph nodes due to the engagement of a G-protein-coupled receptor, $S1P_1$, present on the surface of the lymphocytes[688,689]; teriflunomide (Aubagio), the active metabolite of leflunomide, inhibiting de novo pyrimidine nucleotide synthesis and thus reducing T-cell and B-cell proliferation[690]; and dimethyl fumarate, BG-12 (Tecfidera), an oral formulation of fumaric acid, which metabolizes to monomethyl fumarate and causes activation of the nuclear factor E2-related factor-2 pathway, exerting both neuroprotective effects, reducing myelin damage in the CNS, as well as antiinflammatory effects.[691-694] The FDA-approved injection-based therapies include the β-Interferons[695]; which act on the blood-brain barrier by interfering with T-cell adhesion to the endothelium, binding

VLA-4 on T cells, inhibiting the T-cell expression of MMP, reducing T-cell activation by interfering with HLA class II and costimulatory molecules B7/CD28 and CD40: CD40L, immune deviation of Th2 over Th1 cytokine profile, or normalization of the ratio of IFN-γ Foxp3 Tregs; glatiramer acetate (Copaxone), resulting in cytokine shift from one proinflammatory to antiinflammatory and regulatory form[696]; and daclizumab.

## *Myasthenia gravis*

### Definition and Epidemiology

Myasthenia gravis (MG) is amongst the best understood human autoimmune diseases affecting all races and ages, with various predisposing factors, including genetic susceptibility markers such as MHC class I and II loci, acetylcholine receptor (AChR) alpha subunit, IgG heavy and light chains, Fc gamma receptor IIa, TAP, CTLA4, and PTPN22; certain drugs, notably penicillamine; and the molecular mimicry between AChR subunits and microbial proteins.[697-703]

### Immune characteristics

AChR antibodies belong to variable IgG subclasses, predominantly IgG1 and IgG3,[704] which bind with a high affinity and specificity to the intact receptor, predominantly to the extracellular portion of the receptor, and eventually lead to loss of AChR through three major mechanisms, including complement mediated destruction, crosslinking and accelerated degradation, and functional blockade. MuSK Abs, on the other hand, belong predominantly to the non-complement-fixing IgG4 subclass,[705] which have been demonstrated to be monovalent for a critical receptor tyrosine kinase for the formation and maintenance of the neuromuscular junction, consisting of an extracellular portion made up of three immunoglobulin-like domains and a cysteine-rich domain, namely MuSK,[706] and can hence prevent MuSK interaction with its coreceptor, LRP4, which causes the impairment of the AChR clustering pathway.[707,708] LRP4 Abs are predominantly of the IgG1 subclass and have been assumed to act through complement activation and by interrupting agrin LRP4 binding to MuSK.[709] Although not proven to have a clear role in the disease pathogenesis yet, Abs against agrin, ColQ, cortactin, and rapsyn have also been described in MG patients.[710-714]

AChR-specific $CD4^+$ T lymphocytes can be detected in both the peripheral blood and thymuses of MG patients and the observation that clinical improvement follows their removal with anti-CD4 monoclonal Abs supports their pathogenic role.[715] These lymphocytes and the cytokines they produce can affect the type of autoimmune response induced in MG. The presence of Th1, Th2, Th17, and Treg cells has been confirmed by the analysis of blood from MG patients.[716] An obvious increase in Th17 and a decrease in Tregs have been noted during the development of experimental autoimmune MG (EAMG) in rats.[717] Notwithstanding the fact that no change could be found in Treg numbers in MG subjects compared to healthy individuals in initial investigations,[718] a specific functional impairment in those Foxp3+ Tregs has been acknowledged afterward.[719]

The breakdown of central and peripheral tolerance checkpoints is a crucial factor in the pathogenesis of MG. It has been delineated that an increased frequency of autoreactive B cell receptors could be noted in patients with AChR and MuSK MG compared to the healthy controls.[720] Furthermore, both the frequency and function of Bregs were shown to be diminished in MG patients compared with the healthy individuals and were linked to disease activity.[721-723] A reduced quantity of Tregs was also shown in a recent study on AChR-MG patients.[724] In addition, abnormal production of thymus derived follicular T helper cells (ThF) might play a role in the development of MG. Follicular regulatory T (Tfr) cells, a subpopulation of Treg, have been propounded to regulate the function of ThF, responsible for B cell maturation and high affinity Ab production in germinal centers. An increased number of ThF and a decreased frequency of Tfr in the peripheral blood of MG patients have been recently shown to have an inverse correlation with the disease severity.[725]

## Clinicopathologic features

MG is an autoimmune disorder characterized by fatigable muscle weakness, usually affecting the extraocular muscles at the onset which manifests as diplopia and/or ptosis. It can remain confined to the ocular muscles (ocular MG) or progress and involve other muscle groups, commonly facial, axial, limb, bulbar, and respiratory muscles (generalized MG), the latter of which can be life-threatening. Thymic abnormalities, notably thymic hyperplasia and thymoma, are commonly observed in MG patients. The diagnosis is based on clinical presentation, serological confirmation, and/or electromyographic evidence of a defect in neurotransmission using repetitive nerve stimulation and/or single fiber electromyography.[726]

Defined serologically, MG can be categorized to five main subgroups, reflecting different age of onset, HLA association, thymic pathology,[727] and presence of antibodies against non-AChR proteins, including muscle-specific kinase (MuSK), lipoprotein receptor-related protein 4 (LRP4) and the striatal muscle intracellular proteins, titin and ryanodine receptor (RyR).[726]

Early-onset acetylcholine receptor-antibody positive MG, usually present before the age of the 50 years with a notable female predominance and is shown to be associated with HLA A1, B8, DR3, DR2, DR52, DPB1, DQB1, and DR9 in different populations.[727-730] Extraocular muscles' involvement is typically present at the onset before generalizing, whilst a proportion will remain merely ocular; the thymus is commonly hyperplastic.

Late-onset acetylcholine receptor-antibody positive MG present after 50 years of age with a male preponderance and shows a weak association with HLA B7, DR2[727] and DR4, DQw8,[731] with over half of patients having detectable Abs against titin and

RyR,[732] and 25 percent having Abs against the cytokines, interferon-α, or interleukin-12.[733] This subgroup shares clinical phenotype with early-onset form, while ocular MG might be more prevalent.[734] Contrarily to early-onset form, the thymus is generally atrophic in this group.

The coexistence of thymoma in 10 percent of the MG patients is termed as thymoma-associated MG, which can occur at any age but most common amongst the 40–60 age group without a gender predominance. Although generalized MG with detectable amounts of AChR antibodies is frequently present, ocular and seronegative cases have also been described.[735] Antibodies directed at titin and RyR are typically observed in more than 90 percent, neutralizing Abs against interferon-α in approximately 70 percent, and Abs against IL-12 in around 50 percent of the thymoma associated MG cases.[732,733,736]

MuSK antibody positive MG occurs at any age, peaking in the 30s with a female preponderance and a significant association with HLA DR14 and DQ5[737] and DRB16 and DQB5[738] in some populations, and a phenotype different than AChR-MG with noticeable ocular, bulbar, neck, and respiratory weakness[739,740] and a normal or atrophic thymus.[741,742] And lastly, the seronegative subgroup which can be present at any age and has shown associations with HLA- DR14 and DQ5, can present with mild thymitis or thymic hyperplasia in some cases. Reevaluation of the diagnosis and repeating the antibody tests should be considered after 6 to 12 months in this group of patients.[726]

### Treatment

The acetylcholinesterase inhibitors are the mainstay of symptomatic therapy in MG but the majority of cases will also require generalized immunosuppression with corticosteroids, azathioprine, mycophenolate, and immunomodulation with intravenous immunoglobulin and plasmapheresis. Thymectomy is commonly performed in early-onset MG and has recently shown beneficial effects in AChR-MG as well.[743] Newer biological agents, such as the monoclonal anti-CD20 agent, Rituximab (RTX) have demonstrated benefits in refractory cases.[744]

## *Guillain barre´ syndrome*

### Definition and Epidemiology

Substantial evidence exists for autoimmune pathogenesis in an important group of peripheral nerve diseases, including the acute inflammatory neuropathies referred to as the Guillain Barre´ syndrome (GBS) and Fisher syndrome (FS). GBS is currently the commonest cause of acute flaccid neuromuscular paralysis worldwide with an incidence increasing steadily with advancing age and male predominance (1.25:1).[745,746] The severity of GBS might vary from mild with full recovery in 10 percent of the cases, bed-ridden in 40 percent, complete paralysis with ventilatory dependence in 20 percent and death in 3.5–12 percent of the patients.[747,748] No convincing correlations have been proven between disease susceptibility or GBS subtypes and host MHC class I or class II haplotypes or genes for various components of the immune response.[749-751]

Gastroenteritis caused by C. jejuni; upper respiratory tract infection or other febrile episodes caused by cytomegalovirus, Epstein Barr virus, Mycoplasma pneumoniae, and Haemophilus influenzae; Zika virus; as well as swine flu and rabies vaccinations, have all been causatively implicated.[745,752-754]

## Autoimmune features

Molecular mimicry has been invoked as a pathogenic mechanism underlying postinfectious autoimmune AMAN and FS. AIDP may also be very similar to these disease categories in terms of the pathogenicity of autoantibodies,[1,755] as antiganglioside antibodies and their cognate antigens, gangliosides, can be depicted in patient serum and peripheral nerves, respectively. Gangliosides are sialic acid containing glycolipids enriched in the nervous system with GM1, GD1b, GD1a, and GT1b as the most copious ones. GQ1b is relatively enriched in the oculomotor cranial nerves in FS,[756,757] and GM1 and GD1a at the nodes of Ranvier and in motor nerve terminals (MNTs) in AMAN.[758,759] Antibodies to ganglioside species are polyclonal, predominantly of IgG class, particularly complement-fixing IgG1 and IgG3.[760-763] Several reports have shown antibodies against single gangliosides GM1, GM1(NeuGc), GM1b, GalNAc-GM1b, GD1a, GalNAc-GD1a, GD1b, 9–0-acetyl GD1b, GD3, GT1b, GQ1b, GQ1bα, LM1, galactocerebroside, and sulfated glucuronyl paragloboside (SGPG) in inflammatory neuropathies.[764] It has been drawn to attention that certain GBS subtypes might be correlated to serum antibodies against putative ganglioside antigens.[762,765-772] Besides, Antibodies to ganglioside complexes have been recently identified.[773,774] Such antibodies act not only through injuring intact nerve fibers to induce neuropathy but also by adversely affecting recovery by either initiating more severe neuropathic disease or impeding the nerve repair process necessary for recovery.[775,776] Antibodies binding to nerves at gangliosides and channels-enriched nodes of Ranvier, possibly resulting in the blockade or alteration of channel function.[777] Binding of antibodies and complement to nodal structures might lead to destabilization of the membrane culminating in trains of uncontrolled miniature end-plate potentials recognizable in models.[778]

Early in the course of GBS, circulating activated T cells have been depicted.[779] The predominant cells in nerves are αβT cells with CD4 and CD8 ratios similar to peripheral blood.[780] In addition, γδT cells found in GBS-affected nerves require either αβT cells or IL-2/IL-15 to proliferate and are capable of identifying nonprotein antigen and are hence candidates for responding to known carbohydrate and ganglioside antigens.[781,782] Both αβ and γδT cells might be capable of providing help to orchestrate class switching of antiganglioside antibodies to IgG1 and IgG3. Lymphocyte activation is demonstrated by increased numbers of circulating T cells bearing activation markers and elevated levels of Th1 cytokines including IFN-γ, IL-2, IL-2 receptor and TNF-α and diminished concentrations of TGF-β1,[779,783-785] homing and migration of which to the peripheral nerve are moderated by E-selectin and mucins binding L-selectin and sialyl Lewis antigens[786] and then VCAM-1 and ICAM-1, both increased early in GBS progression.[787] Chemokines play role in leukocyte recruitment localization and trafficking[788] and matrix metalloproteinases (MMPs) facilitate diapedesis through the vascular endothelium and the basal lamina, all implicated in the pathogenesis of GBS.[789,790] Macrophages, both resident and enrolled from the circulation,[786] remain the key component in perpetuating endoneurial inflammatory damage through targeting normal looking nerves and Schwann cells in experimental autoimmune neuritis (EAN) and AIDP[791,792] probably by antibody-targeted cellular cytotoxicity and complement-dependent mechanisms[793,794]; secreting a host of inflammatory mediators including MMPs, TNF-α, nitric oxide, eicosanoids, neutral proteases, lipases, and phospholipases, all contributing to nerve damage[795,796]; and directing T-cell apoptosis reducing the ongoing shifting of T-cell response toward Th2 with upregulation of IL-4,[797] TGF-β1, IL-10, and cytolysin in models of disease[798] during recovery from GBS.

## Clinicopathologic features

Diverse GBS variants have been identified thus far, including acute inflammatory demyelinating polyradiculoneuropathy (AIDP), acute motor axonal neuropathy (AMAN), acute motor and sensory neuropathy (AMSAN), Miller Fisher syndrome, acute pan-autonomic neuropathy, acute pure sensory neuropathy, acute motor conduction block neuropathy, and regional variants such as pharyngo-cervical-brachial type. AIDP constitutes more than 95 percent of the GBS cases in Europe and North America, presenting with a monophasic rapidly evolving neuropathic (sensory-)motor paralysis in two or more limbs over less than 4 weeks in a typically ascending pattern; bladder disturbance; numbness; facial weakness; tingling; pain; swallowing difficulty[747]; the autonomic disturbance with arrhythmia and fluctuating blood pressures; absent or reduced tendon reflexes; less than 50 leukocytes per μL and increased CSF in 80 percent of the cases[799]; antiganglioside antibodies in the serum detected by enzyme-linked immunosorbent assay (ELISA)[800]; slowed motor conduction velocities, delayed F-waves, and preserved compound muscle action potential (CMAP) amplitudes consistent with demyelination, with a spared sural nerve, that might be complicated by conduction failure and axonal degeneration, observed on electrophysiological studies; typically patchy multifocal perivascular T-cell infiltration with demyelination with the involvement of proximal and terminal nerve segments[801]; and blood nerve barrier (BNB) breakdown and deposition of activated complement components in some but not all cases of AIDP.[794]

AMAN is a pure motor variant of GBS[802] presenting with minimal sensory impairment and autonomic involvement; reduced CMAP amplitudes, absent F-waves with normal distal motor latencies, and conduction velocity on electrophysiological studies; absent sensory involvement[803]; as well as an antibody-mediated immune attack directed preferentially against the motor axons causing primary axonal degeneration in the absence of prominent T-cell inflammation.[793,804,805] AMSAN is a more severe form of

AMAN with similar pathology and the involvement of both sensory and motor nerve roots, a more severe course and delayed recovery.[804,806]

The Miller Fisher syndrome or FS[807] encompasses ophthalmoplegia, ataxia, and areflexia without limb weakness, and accounts for around 5 percent of GBS cases. This syndrome has been shown to be associated with preceding C. jejuni infection and can manifest with facial and bulbar weakness.[802,806]

### Treatment

The efficacy of immunotherapies in GBS is reinforced by good evidence.[808] Plasma exchange has been shown to accelerate recovery in nonambulant patients preferably started within 2 weeks of disease onset.[809] Intravenous immunoglobulin is still probably the intervention of choice, which is as effective as plasma exchange.[810] According to studies performed, there is no indication for the use of steroids in GBS. The use of complement inhibitor eculizumab and immunoadsorption of pathogenic antiganglioside antibodies in GBS has been explored, however, further, larger studies are awaited.[802,811]

## Endocrine system

### *Autoimmune thyroiditis*

### Definition

Autoimmunity constitutes above 90 percent of the non-iatrogenic hypothyroidism in iodine-sufficient countries with a peak incidence at 50–60 years of age and a female preponderance of 5–10 times, which might be due to the influence of sex steroids or skewed X chromosome inactivation.[812-814] The association of thyroiditis with other endocrinopathies as part of type 2 autoimmune polyglandular syndrome as well as the frequent presence of thyroid autoantibodies in other family members of AT patients suggest the role of underlying genetic factors, such as HLA alleles,[815] exemplified by the association of HLA-DR3 and to a lesser extent HLA-DR4 with Hashimoto's thyroiditis, and HLA-DR5 with postpartum thyroiditis; CTLA-4[816]; LPP; BACH2[817]; and MAGI3.[818] There is also a propensity for progression to AT or Graves' disease in Turner's and Down's syndromes.[819,820]

### Clinicopathologic characteristics

Several types of autoimmune thyroiditis (AT), including goitrous (Hashimoto's) thyroiditis, usually presenting with firm and painless goiter with an irregular surface, moderate-to-extensive lymphocytic infiltration and variable fibrosis, usually euthyroid at presentation, which can also manifest as subclinical thyroid failure and might eventually lead to hypothyroidism; atrophic thyroiditis (primary myxedema), typically diagnosed when hypothyroidism is apparent biochemically and clinically, with evidence of fibrosis and variable lymphocytic infiltrate in the atrophied thyroid gland[821]; juvenile thyroiditis, presenting as small goiter with moderate lymphocytic infiltrate; postpartum thyroiditis, identified with transient thyrotoxicosis and/or hypothyroidism occurring 3–6 months after delivery with small goiter and some lymphocytic infiltrate; silent thyroiditis, characterized by transient thyrotoxicosis and/or hypothyroidism with small goiter and some lymphocytic infiltrate; and focal thyroiditis, which can be progressive in some cases and occurs in 20–40 percent of autopsied thyroid specimens, associated with thyroid carcinoma, have been described. Lymphoma is known as a rare complication of AT. An abnormal thyroid ultrasound pattern is highly suggestive of AT[822] and the diagnosis can usually be made in patients having biochemical evidence of hypothyroidism as well as TG and/or TPO antibodies.

## Autoimmune features

Circulating autoantibodies against thyroglobulin (TG), a 660-kDa homodimeric glycoprotein secreted by thyroid follicular cells (TFC) and stored in the luminal colloid, and thyroid peroxidase (TPO), a 100–105-kDa apical membrane protein responsible for tyrosine iodination and coupling in the formation of thyroid hormones, can be usually identified at very high levels in most AT patients and low levels in focal thyroiditis. Other autoantibodies associated with AT consist of TSH-receptor (TSH-R) blocking antibodies (TBAb), present in approximately 20 percent of the patients with AT[823] and contributing towards hypothyroidism in some case; antibodies against Na1/I2 transporter and pendrin, occurring in 10–20 percent of the AT patients[824]; and autoantibodies against T4 and T3, found in 15–35 percent of the patients with AT.

Upregulation of an array of adhesion molecules and selectins on endothelial cells together with the expression of reciprocal adhesion molecules, including CD11a, CD18, CD29, CD49a, and CD49e, on the lymphocytes infiltrating the thyroid gland, resulting in the recruitment of lymphocytes to the thyroid gland, and this infiltrate can then produce various chemokines, including CXCL12, CXCL13, and CCL22, which can aid homing.[825] The autoimmune process can also be aggravated by the contribution of TFC towards the chemokine pool.[826] Predominant cells in the thyroid infiltrate are $CD4^+$ T cells, many of which are in the activated status.[827] There is also an increase in the number of activated HLA-$DR^+$ T cells and a reduced number of $CD8^+$ T cells in active thyroiditis.[828] AT might initiate with a pauciclonal T-cell response and then will propagate to a polyclonal T-cell response targeting various autoantigens and epitopes by the time of clinical presentation.

A T-cell epitope on TG has been recognized which can specifically bind to the MHC class II disease susceptibility HLA-DRβ1-Arg74 molecule and this might stimulate T cells and initiate an immune response that eventually involves other autoantigens, suggesting that self-tolerance may be first impaired for TG and then for TPO.[829,830] No dominant T-cell epitope has been identified for TPO and considerable heterogeneity has been noted within and between individual patients.[831] Defective Tregs activity has been suggested in both AT and Graves' patients.[832] A mixed Th1 and Th2 response has been demonstrated in Hashimoto's thyroiditis.[833] It has been propounded that the aberrant expression of MHC class II on TFC adjacent to T cells producing IFN-γ (Hamilton et al., 1991), following the appearance of a lymphocytic infiltrate, could initiate or propagate the autoimmune response by transforming the TFC into antigen-presenting cells in Hashimoto's thyroiditis and Graves' disease.[834] However, considering the fact that TFC does not express costimulatory molecules even after cytokine exposure, they are unlikely to initiate the autoimmune response.[835] Class II-expressing TFC can activate T-cell lines and clones derived from the thyroids of patients, which are not dependent on B7 costimulation.[835,836] Resistant T cells to tolerance induction and class II-expressing TFC in patients with AT may then help to propagate the autoimmune response.[837] TFC may also take part in the autoimmune process through the expression of other immunologically active molecules such as CD40 and CD56.

### Treatment

Treatment is generally straightforward, consisting of T4 replacement therapy, which might lead to the elimination of TBAb and spontaneous remission in 10 percent of the patients after several years, the permanence of which is yet to be determined.[838,839]

### *Graves' disease*

### Definition and Epidemiology

Graves' disease, characterized by the production of TSH-R-stimulating antibodies (TSAb), is the most frequent cause of hyperthyroidism with a prevalence of around 4 in 1000 and a 5–10 times female preponderance, that shares many immunological features with AT.[814,840] Future studies are still required to elucidate the relative significance of environmental factors such as stress, iodine intake, and smoking, and their interaction with each other and with genetic factors affecting the development of Graves' disease.

### Genetics and autoimmune features

There is a 20–30 percent concordance between monozygotic twins for Graves' disease, which is above 10-fold higher than for dizygotic twins[841](Brix et al., 1998). HLA-DR3 allele, polymorphisms in genes, affecting B and T cells, such as CTLA-4, FCRL3, CD25, PTPN22 and CD226; TSH-R gene; RNASET2-FGFR1OP-CCR6 region at 6q27; LPP; PRICKLE1; BACH2; FGFR1OP; MMEL1; as well as the gene encoding TG have been associated with Graves' disease.[815,817,842-846]

TSAb can occur in over 95 percent and TG and TPO autoantibodies can be detected in up to 80 percent of the patients. Thyroid cells shed the A-subunit of TSH-R, which is formed as a result of the receptor complex posttranslational processing at the hinge region, which is capable of binding to TSAb more avidly than the holoreceptor, and this plays role in the stimulation and affinity maturation of TSAb, an IgG1 subclass restricted and often $\lambda$ light chain-restricted autoantibody.[847,848] TSAb-induced activation of the TSH-R leads to increased production of cAMP, however, TSH-R antibodies might cause induction of other intracellular signaling pathways as well. There is also a group of TSH-R neutral antibodies that do not promote cAMP production but can aid thyroid cell apoptosis in vitro.[849] Reduced number of circulating $CD8^+$ T cells and increased number of $HLA\text{-}DR^+$ T cells have been demonstrated in active Graves' disease.[850] Intrathyroidal $CD4^+$ and $CD8^+$ T cells are also present in varying proportions with homing mechanisms similar to that of AT.[825] No discrete Th1 or Th2 pattern has been delineated.[851] Cytokines' production, including IL-1, IL-6, IL-8, and IL-10, some of which could be expressed by TFC, are significantly elevated. Numerous Tregs with impaired activity, partly resulting from defective plasmacytoid dendritic cell function and elevated levels of thyroid hormone,[852] are present in the thyroid in Graves' disease but are not capable of terminating disease.[853]

### Clinicopathologic characteristics

Graves' disease is associated with hypertrophy and hyperplasia of the thyroid follicles, the appearance of columnar epithelium folded into the follicular lumen, formation of new small follicles with little colloid, a variable degree of lymphocytic infiltration, the formation of germinal centers, and possibly lymphoid hyperplasia in the lymph nodes, thymus, and spleen, in the untreated state. More than 70 percent of the patients with Graves' disease have thyroid-associated ophthalmopathy (TAO), which is not exclusive to Graves' disease and might initially reveal enlarged extraocular muscles and then progress to clinically apparent eye disease in around 50 percent of the patients.[854] Around 1 percent of the patients, especially those with marked TAO, may develop thyroid dermopathy, usually presenting as pretibial myxedema.[855]

### Treatment

Treatment with antithyroid drugs, namely carbimazole, methimazole, or propylthiouracil, result in a permanent remission in around 40 percent of the patients.[856,857] Relapse is likely after antithyroid drugs in patients who smoke, those having evidence of a strong Th2 response, or younger patients with severe hyperthyroidism or a large goiter.[858,859] Subtotal thyroidectomy results in a gradual fall in most patients over a year, whereas radioiodine treatment can be followed by a rise in thyroid autoantibodies at around 3 years.[860] The elimination of autoantigens following the complete ablation of thyroid tissue leads to the disappearance of all thyroid autoantibodies.[861] TAO can be treated using supportive measures in mild cases and with corticosteroids or other immunosuppressive agents in moderate-to-severe cases.[862]

## *Autoimmune diabetes*

### Definition and Epidemiology

Autoimmune diabetes, also referred to as type 1 diabetes mellitus or insulin dependent diabetes mellitus, is a chronic immune-mediated disease of unidentified etiology and mode of inheritance characterized by insulin deficiency due to pancreatic islet beta-cell destruction with increasing blood glucose levels, leading to patient's dependence on lifelong exogenous insulin treatment.[863,864] The incidence rate of autoimmune diabetes varies considerably between countries, showing the highest incidence in Scandinavia, Europe, and North America and still lower incidence in most Asian countries. Autoimmune diabetes has undergone an increase of 3–5 percent per year in the last few decades, with a doubling time of almost 20 years.[865] Although the etiology of autoimmune diabetes is not well comprehended,[864] it is generally accepted as a hereditary disease, with the HLA class II genes as the most important susceptibility genes, accounting for approximately 50 percent of the genetic contribution to the disease.[864,866] It should be noted that high-risk genotypes vary between countries. Analyses of genetic predisposition, mainly HLA, and of standardized islet autoantibodies have made it possible to explore the pathogenesis and to predict autoimmune diabetes.[864,867,868] Autoimmune diabetes is characterized by a complex and prolonged subclinical phase, also referred to as prodrome or prediabetes, initiated by an autoimmune reaction against either insulin in HLA DR4-DQ8 children or glutamic acid decarboxylase (GAD65) in HLA DR3-DQ2 children[869-872] that can be followed by the development of more autoantibodies against either insulin (IAA), GADA, islet antigen-2 (IA-2A), or the zinc transporter 8 (ZnT8A), with asymptomatic subclinical stages lasting a month to years before the clinical onset. The cumulative risk of diabetes varies according to high antibody levels, positivity for multiple autoantibodies, age, younger age at seroconversion, and persistent positivity for IAA.[873]

## Diagnosis and classification

The diagnosis of diabetes is based on a fasting blood glucose concentration of more than 7•0 mmol/L (126 mg/dL), a random blood glucose concentration of greater than 11•1 mmol/L (200 mg/dL) accompanied by symptoms, an abnormal result from an oral glucose tolerance test (OGTT), or a glycated hemoglobin (HbA1c) concentration of more than 48 mmol/mol (6•5 percent), the latter of which is less sensitive for making a diagnosis than fasting or stimulated blood glucose measurements.[874] Abnormal glycemia must be present on two different occasions in order to make a diagnosis in the absence of symptoms. It is still uncertain whether the utility of HbA1c with or without continuous glucose monitoring is of great value to diagnose diabetes in children.[875-877] OGTT is regarded as a sensitive indicator of impaired glucose homeostasis and type 1 diabetes.[878]

Proper classification of autoimmune diabetes requires the confirmation of the presence of beta-cell autoantibodies along with elevated blood glucose.[879] More than 90 percent of patients with newly diagnosed autoimmune diabetes have measurable antibodies targeting specific β-cell proteins, comprising insulin (IAA), glutamate decarboxylase (GADA), islet antigen 2 (IA-2A), zinc transporter 8 (ZnT8A), and tetraspanin-7.[880] The classification of autoimmune diabetes updated by the American Diabetes Association includes Stage I, as the subclinical stage in which patient has developed autoimmunity with two or more islet autoantibodies, is still normoglycemic and asymptomatic with normal beta-cell function and no indication of insulitis; Stage II as the subclinical stage with dysglycemia, rising glucose levels detectable with OGTT, islet beta-cell loss, signs of insulitis during late Stage II, and the presence of two or more islet autoantibodies; and Stage III as the clinical stage with beta-cell destruction, insulin deficiency, dysglycemia, and hyperglycemia-related symptoms such as polyuria and thirst.[881] Type 1 diabetes in children commonly manifests with polyuria, polydipsia, weight loss, and diabetic keto-acidosis in approximately a third of cases.[882] Type 1 diabetes in adults might not present with the classic symptoms observed in children and can be more variable. Decreased C-peptide level is considered as a marker of severe endogenous insulin deficiency, useful to direct classification and treatment of diabetic cases examined over 3 years after clinical diagnosis; however, there is no single clinical feature to properly distinguish type 1 from non-type 1 diabetes at diagnosis.[883] The majority of patients with clinically evident autoimmune diabetes develop secondary micro- and macrovascular complications later in life.[864,881] Lifelong treatment with exogenous insulin is required for survival in these patients.

## Genetics and immune characteristics

Although not sufficient to cause the autoimmune reaction against the insulin-producing beta cells, the highest risk for type 1 diabetes is conferred by HLA-DR-DQ. It is contemplated that an etiological trigger such as a common virus infecting beta cells might lead to autoimmunity against specific autoantigens, such as insulin or GAD65, and this will be followed by the emergence of a second islet autoantibody and so on.[871] Genetic factors associated with apoptosis,[884,885] endoplasmic reticulum stress,[885,886] or autophagy,[887] account for other possible mechanisms during pathogenesis. More than 60 loci, the majority of which are related to the function of the immune system, have been identified as non-HLA genetic factors contributing to type 1 diabetes risk,[867,888-890] IL2, CD25, INS VNTR, IL18RAP, IL10, IFIH1, PTPN22, IL2RA, CTLA4, CCR5, IL27, IL7R, CD226, SH2B3, ERBB3, and CD69 to name a few. However, these are known to confer a low risk of autoimmune diabetes. Beside these genetic susceptibility loci, certain environmental factors, most importantly viral infections, as well as dietary factors such as gluten[891] and vitamin D,[892,893] have been speculated to either trigger an autoimmune response or affect the pathogenesis.[894,895]

Although there is initially no sign of reduced beta-cell function in the preclinical prodromal phase of autoimmune type 1 diabetes, it seems that a selective loss of pancreatic islet beta cells seems to occur later in the disease process, as Stage II dysglycemia is known to be associated with T cell mediated destruction and insulitis.[896,897] Impaired thymic T cell negative selection has been linked to insulin reactivity[897](Bluestone et al., 2010). Considering the fact that both negative and positive selection and Treg stimulation in the thymus are crucial for effective control of autoreactivity in peripheral tissue,[898,899] a loss of the normal regulatory immune mechanisms, as well as an imbalance between Treg cells and effector T lymphocytes, have been implicated in Stage I and II autoimmune diabetes. In a comparison made between children with multiple autoantibodies and controls, a decrease in mRNA expression levels of T-cell subtype markers has been delineated, possibly revealing exhaustion of the immune system after the potent immune activation during a lengthy autoimmune process and this might play a central role in determining the outcome of the disease.[92,900]

Four major autoantigens, namely, proinsulin, the exclusive beta cell specific antigen[901]; insulin, the main target for the T-lymphocyte attack particularly in young children[902]; GAD65, specific for beta cells but also expressed in other cells[903]; and IA-2 and the isoform IA-2β, important antigens especially in HLA-DQ8 haplotype carriers,[904] have been described in autoimmune type 1 diabetes together with an expanding list of proposed minor autoantigens,[905] including the secretory vesicle-associated proteins, chromogranin A, VAMP2 and NPY, HSP-60 and HSP-70, IGRP, Glima-38, and much more.[906] The immune reaction against these minor autoantigens reflects the fact that presentation of new antigen to inflammatory cells of the immune system culminates in the activation of new T lymphocytes, also known as antigen and epitope spreading.[898] It should be kept in mind that the precise role of T- and B-lymphocyte reactivity and autoantibodies against most of the above-mentioned autoantigens in the progression from Stage I to II and III has yet to be determined.

## Management

None of the efforts to intervene with the autoimmune process using a wide variety of immune suppressive agents have been successful to prevent the loss of beta cells and preserve residual beta-cell function long term, thus far.[907-909] Further elaboration on the diabetes management methods currently in practice is beyond the scope of this chapter and can be studied in detail elsewhere.[910]

### *Polyendocrine syndromes*

## Definition

Autoimmune polyendocrine syndromes (APS) are characterized by immune-mediated destruction of two or more endocrine glands usually accompanied by the involvement of several nonendocrine organs and tissues, divided into the ultrarare APS type 1 (APS-1), which is of monogenic nature caused by mutations in the Autoimmune Regulator (AIRE) gene, which plays a dual role in the thymus, both to foster the expression of tissue-specific antigens and to enable the generation of a specific subset of Tregs, and the prevalent APS type 2 (APS-2), associated with a complex inheritance involving certain MHC alleles and variants in a range of other genes, mostly implicated in the adaptive and innate immune system. Numerous autoantibodies, correlated with clinical components, have been identified in both conditions.

## Genetics and autoimmune features

APS-1 is inherited in an autosomal recessive manner, occurring as a defect in the AIRE gene on chromosome 21q22.3. The most frequently identified mutations are R257X in exon 6,[911,912] 967–979del13bp,[913-916] R139X,[917] R203X,[918] and Y85C.[911,913,915,916]

Recently, certain heterozygous missense mutations, mostly located in the first plant homeodomain (PHD1) (suggested to predispose for vitamin B12 deficiency/pernicious anemia and vitiligo) and in a few cases, in the SAND domain (having a propensity for autoimmune thyroid disease),[919] have been recognized, giving rise to APS-1 with dominant inheritance.[920] Additionally, some HLA alleles are deemed correlated with certain components of APS-1.[921,922]

APS-2 is a syndrome of polygenic inheritance, strongly associated with the HLA gene locus in chromosome 6p21. HLA DRB1 × 03:01 (DR3) DQA1 × 05:01 DQB1 × 02:01 (DQ2) and DRB1 × 04:01 (DR4) DQA1 × 03:01 DQB1 × 03:02 (DQ8) haplotypes have shown consistent associations with APS-2.[923-926] Conversely, the haplotypes DRB1 × 01 (DR1) DQA1 × 01:01 DQB1 × 05:01 (DQ5), DRB1 × 13:01 DQB1 × 06:03 DQA1 × 01:03, DRB1 × 13:02 DQB1 × 06:04 DQA1 × 01:02, and DRB1 × 07 DQB1 × 02:01 DQA1 × 02:01 were found to protect against Addison's disease.[927] Moreover, HLA-B8[928] has been shown to be associated with Addison's disease, while HLA-B15 was protective of the progression to overt disease.[929] Other genes located in the HLA region, such as TNF has been associated with APS-2,[923] and the 21-Hydroxylase as well as major histocompatibility complex class I chain-related MIC-A polymorphisms in exon 5, Involved in NK and T-cell activation, have demonstrated a positive association with Addison's disease.[930,931] In addition, a number of other susceptibility genes, mostly involved in immunity and inflammation, have been characterized in Addison's disease and APS-2, although they are not specific for these conditions. These genes include CTLA-4[932-934]; NALP1, involved in inflammation[935]; the programmed death ligand 1[936]; PTPN22[937,938]; the lymphocyte cell surface molecule FCRL3[939]; the class II, major histocompatibility complex transactivator[940,941]; and BACH2.[942]

Certain autoantibodies have been associated with each of the major components of APS-1 and APS-2. The main autoantigens have been identified as thyroid peroxidase, thyroglobulin, and the TSH receptor in autoimmune thyroid disease; glutamic acid decarboxylase-65 (GAD65), islet antigen-2 (IA-2), and the beta-cell-specific zinc transporter Zn8 (ZnT8) in type 1 diabetes; steroid 21-hydroxylase (P450c21 or CYP21) in Addison's disease[927,943-945]; NALP5, a protein highly expressed in the parathyroid gland, in hypoparathyroidism[946]; side-chain cleavage enzyme (P450scc or CYP11A1) and steroid 17-alpha-hydroxylase (P450c17 or CYP17) in the autoimmune involvement of gonadal tissues[947-951]; and CYP1A2 in autoimmune hepatitis in APS-1.[952] Although not proven yet, mechanisms interrupting immune tolerance to specific organs can be considered as the reason for the coexistence of certain diseases of APS. Several other organ-specific self-antigens have been identified, against which autoantibodies could be detected in APS, including aromatic L-amino acid decarboxylase in type 2 autoimmune hepatitis[953]; tryptophan hydroxylase in autoimmune enteropathy[954]; tyrosine hydroxylases in alopecia[955]; glutamic acid decarboxylase 2 (GAD2/GAD65)[956,957] and GAD1/GAD67 in

APS-1[958]; transglutaminase-4 (TGM4), a prostate-specific autoantigen[959]; and cancer testis autoantigens such as PDILT and different MAGE proteins.[960,961] The genes for many of the above-mentioned autoantigens, many of which are intracellular phosphoproteins and proteins expressed in lymphoid cells, are not AIRE-regulated.[961] Besides, APS-1 patients display autoantibodies targeting a number of interferons and interleukins, such as various isoforms of type 1 interferon alpha and omega (IFN-$\alpha$ and IFN-$\omega$), highly specific but not entirely exclusive for APS-1[962-964]; IL-17A, IL-17F, and IL-22 correlated with the presence of candidiasis[965,966]; IFN-$\lambda$1, IFN-$\lambda$−2, IFN-$\lambda$−3, IL-5, IL-6, and IL-32.[967,968] The organ-specific autoantibodies against P450c21, P450c17, and P450scc are shared between APS-1 and APS-2.[956,969,970] However, there are some differences in the expression of autoantibodies between these two syndromes, as autoantibodies to GAD65 and/or IA-2 protein are frequently observed in APS-2 patients with type 1 diabetes, while anti-GAD65 autoantibodies have been suggested to correlate to malabsorption and vitiligo in APS-1 patients.[956,961]

## Clinical features

APS-1, also referred to as polyglandular autoimmune syndrome type 1 or autoimmune polyendocrinopathy candidiasis ectodermal dystrophy has a broad spectrum of clinical presentations. The major components shaping the clinical picture include chronic mucocutaneous candidiasis (CMC), hypoparathyroidism, as the most frequent and sometimes only endocrine component in APS-1,[971] followed by Addison's disease, observed in about half of the patients.[972-974] Some minor components such as periodic fever with nail dystrophy, keratoconjunctivitis, and rash can appear earlier than these major manifestations.[975] It is now apparent that the phenotypic variability in the appearance of these main manifestations is large.[973,976] Patients can harbor about 45 different diseases, with CMC, hypoparathyroidism, periodic fever with rash, and keratitis appearing earlier in the disease course, while other manifestations commence in adult age.[975,977] Other endocrinopathies in falling frequencies are gonadal insufficiency, more common in females,[951] type 1 diabetes, autoimmune thyroid disease and hypophysitis. Patients can manifest with gastrointestinal autoimmunity, notably enteropathy with malabsorption and/or obstipation, exocrine pancreatitis, autoimmune gastritis, and hepatitis, the involvement of ectodermal structures, such as alopecia, keratoconjunctivitis, and enamel dysplasia, vitiligo and nail dystrophy, interstitial nephritis,[978] hyposplenism or splenic atrophy,[973,976] pneumonitis,[979] pure red cell aplasia,[977] hypertension and increased mineralocorticoid sensitivity,[234] retinitis,[980] lipodystrophy,[981] peripheral neuropathy,[982] ptosis,[977] metaphyseal dysplasia[983] and polyarthritis.[984]

APS-2 is classically defined as a combination of Addison's disease with autoimmune thyroid disease and/or type 1 diabetes.[985] Clinical manifestations such as vitiligo, hypergonadotropic hypogonadism, alopecia and autoimmune gastritis with or without pernicious anemia, although are less frequent compared to the major manifestations stated, are prevalent.

### Treatment

Anticandidal drugs such as amphotericin B, ketoconazole, fluconazole or itraconazole can be administered in APS-1 patients to treat used candidiasis.[986-988] Replacement therapy with hydrocortisone, cortisone acetate, and fludrocortisone (to replace aldosterone) has been efficiently used for Addison's disease. The therapy of hypoparathyroidism is aimed at providing normal calcium levels and includes calciferol sterols (vitamin D hydroxylated forms, calcitriol or calcidiol) and calcium salt preparations, preferably calcium carbonate, and possibly, recently available recombinant parathyroid hormone,[989] the efficiency and safety of which still needs to be justified. The candidate therapeutic strategies targeting the immune system include cyclosporine A, leading to temporary remission in APS-2[990]; rituximab to regain adrenocortical function in autoimmune Addison's disease[991]; anti-CD3 monoclonal drugs in type 1 diabetes; steroid and azathioprine in autoimmune hepatitis[973]; rituximab and cyclosporine A in interstitial lung disease[992]; cyclosporine A and mycophenolate mofetil to treat malabsorption[993,994]; and topical steroids and cyclosporine to induce remission in keratitis.

## Gastrointestinal system

### *Autoimmune gastritis and pernicious anemia*

### Definition and Epidemiology

Pernicious anemia is the result of advanced autoimmune gastritis, as one of the most common autoimmune diseases, which is asymptomatic in its initial stages. Pernicious anemia, although uncommon prior to the age of 30 years, represents the most frequent cause of vitamin B12 deficiency with an estimated prevalence of approximately 2 percent in Western adult populations at or over the age of 60 years and shows a racial predilection for northern Europeans.[995]

### Genetics and autoimmune features

Predisposition to pernicious anemia appears to be partly due to certain genetic factors, including HLA locus,[996] although not substantiated in other studies, NALP1,[997] specific genes in mice such as two major genes on chromosome 4, termed Gasa1 and Gasa2,[998] as well as Gasa3 on chromosome 6, and Gasa4 on chromosome 17.[999]

Autoimmune gastritis is associated with polyclonal autoantibodies predominantly of the IgG isotype to gastric parietal cells[1000] directed toward both the catalytic 100 kDa α subunit and the 6090 kDa glycoprotein β-subunit of the gastric enzyme responsible for acidification of gastric luminal contents located on specialized secretory membranes of gastric parietal cells, namely $H^+/K^+$ ATPase, resulting in depletion of $H^+/K^+$ ATPase activity from parietal cell membranes in vitro[1001-1004]; and at least two distinct antibodies against their secreted product, IF, one reacting with the binding site for vitamin B12, inhibiting the subsequent binding of IF with free vitamin; and the other reacting with an antigenic determinant remote from this site.[1005,1006]

According to human studies, a notable increase in $CD4^+$ and $CD8^+$ T cells and a six-fold increase in non-T cells have been demonstrated in the cellular infiltrate of stomachs of patients with pernicious anemia[1007,1008] and this finding is in keeping with the observations made by electron microscopy showing lymphocytes line up against the membranes of gastric parietal cells and zymogenic cells in the gastric mucosa. Moreover, $H^+/K^+$ ATPase-specific $CD4^+$ T cell clones, capable of recognizing a number of epitopes in the $H^+/K^+$ ATPase $\alpha$ and $\beta$ subunits[1009] and biased toward the production of IFN-$\gamma$ and TNF-$\alpha$ or IL-4 by some clones,[1010] most of which also display perforin or FAS-dependent cytotoxic activity, have been isolated from the gastric mucosa of patients with autoimmune gastritis. T cell immune response to the gastric $H^+/K^+$ ATPase has been shown as a necessary component for the initiation and development of autoimmune gastritis.[1011] Extensive studies on the pathways that lead to immunological tolerance to the gastric $H^+/K^+$ ATPase have suggested that the protection from gastritis is mediated almost exclusively by tolerogenic mechanisms in the local tissue environment. High avidity $H^+/K^+$ ATPase-specific T cells exit the thymus and represent the residue of a T cell repertoire that has been subjected to partial extrathymic deletion in the periphery,[1012] occurring following antigen-specific activation of $H^+/K^+$ ATPase-specific $CD4^+$ T cells in the stomach draining paragastric lymph node. Dendritic cells and $Foxp3^+$ regulatory T cells (Tregs) mediate additional mechanisms of peripheral tolerance by affecting the activation of self-reactive T cells that remain after the clonal deletion.[1012-1016]

## Clinical features

Autoimmune gastritis is silent in the early stages with the gastric lesion being predictable by immunologic markers specific for gastric autoimmunity 20–30 years before the onset of clinical manifestations.[1017] Approximately 10–15 percent of the patients with autoimmune gastritis develop pernicious anemia when stores of vitamin B12 are depleted.[1018,1019] Gastritis eventually leads the deficiency of a protein avidly binding to dietary vitamin B12, intrinsic factor (IF), which provokes vitamin B12 transport to the terminal ileum for absorption by multifunctional endocytic cubilin receptors in the ileum,[1020-1022] resulting in clinically evident vitamin B12 deficiency associated with megaloblastic anemia caused by defective DNA synthesis,[1023,1024] decreased serum pepsinogen I levels, decreased serum pepsinogen I/II ratio, and elevated serum gastrin levels,[1025-1027] and can present with palor, tiredness, sore tongue, abdominal discomfort, neuropsychiatric syndromes, such as sensory impairment, abnormal reflexes, motor impairment, spastic paraparesis, mental or psychiatric disturbances,[1028] and an increased risk of developing gastric cancer and gastric carcinoids.[1029,1030] Pernicious anemia is the consequence of insufficient IF production and not associated with gastritis or achlorhydria in childhood. Pernicious anemia occurs concomitantly with the autoimmune endocrinopathies and the antireceptor autoimmune diseases, such as insulin-dependent type 1 diabetes mellitus, primary ovarian failure, Hashimoto's thyroiditis, vitiligo, primary Addison's disease, premature graying of the hair, myasthenia gravis, primary hypoparathyroidism, thyrotoxicosis, and the Lambert-Eaton syndrome.[1031-1033]

## Treatment

Pernicious anemia is routinely treatable by vitamin B12 replacement, either with a daily intake of high-dose oral vitamin B12 tablets (1000–2000 μg) or intramuscular monthly injections, to correct hematologic manifestations and neurological complications; however, this therapy is not capable of reversing the destruction of the gastric mucosa as the underlying cause of the disease.[1034] The ectopic expression of the gastric autoantigen and treatment using Tregs has shown promise for long-term reversal of gastric lesions in mice,[1035,1036] and requires further investigations to validate the benefit in humans.

### *Autoimmune hepatitis*

## Definition and Epidemiology

Autoimmune hepatitis (AIH) is an inflammatory liver disease of unknown etiology with a female predominance (3:1 ratio), characterized by elevated transaminase and IgG levels, interface hepatitis on histology, and positive autoantibodies, the profile of which allows its classification to AIH type 1 and 2. Prompt institution of immunosuppressive treatment generally provides a mostly symptom-free long-term survival, preventing liver failure.

## Genetics and autoimmune features

Several susceptibility genes have been proposed in patients with AIH, mostly located within the HLA region, including HLA-DRB1, HLA-DR3 and DR4 loci, which are linked to susceptibility to AIH-1[1037-1041]; allelic variation within HLA-DRB1, HLA-DR3 and HLA-DR7 in AIH type 2[1042]; CTLA-4[1043]; the TNF-α gene promoter[1044]; and Fas.[1045]

Key to the diagnosis of AIH is positivity for circulating autoantibodies, ANA and SMA in AIH type 1, and anti-LKM1 and anti-LC1 in AIH type 2.[1046-1049] It should be noted, however, that these autoantibody profiles may occasionally coexist.[1046] The pathogenesis of AIH, particularly AIH-1, is not yet fully elucidated.[1050,1051] However, the existence of a few numbers of autoantigenic epitopes has been hypothesized, considering the evidence of oligoclonality of the T cell receptor repertoire among liver infiltrating T cells.[1052] On the other hand, components of cytochrome P450 2D6 (CYP2D6) have been identified as the autoantigenic epitopes recognized by both B cells and the T cell receptors of CD4 and CD8 T cells in type 2 AIH.[1050] A hypothesized theory of AIH immunopathogenesis entails trigger of AIH in genetically susceptible individuals by viral infections, such as HAV, HCV, HEV, EBV, HSV and measles,[1050,1051,1053] or exposures to drugs or xenobiotics, either as a consequence of molecular mimicry of autoantigens or through the presentation of hepatic autoantigens lying within apoptotic bodies of dying hepatocytes.[1054] Albeit the role of Treg dysfunction remains controversial, the pathogenic activities of effector T cells in both AIH-1 and 2 as a consequence of reduced number and functional capacity autoantigen-specific CD4 Tregs, which are crucial in inhibition of the autoimmune effector cell response(s),[1055-1057] has been recently suggested as a possible mechanism involved in the loss of tolerance in AIH. This highlights the need for recognizing the autoantigenic CD4 and CD8 T cell epitopes in AIH-1.[1054]

## Clinical features

Although AIH type 1 affects all ages, almost 80 percent of AIH type 1 cases are diagnosed before the age of 60 years with two peaks, one in childhood/adolescence and the other in adulthood around the age of 40 years,[1058-1060] with 40–60 percent of patients having a chronic disease course with nonspecific symptoms such as fatigue, abdominal pain, arthralgia, and nausea.[1061] AIH type 2 is rare in older ages and mainly affects children/adolescents, constituting one-third of all cases in pediatrics with a clinical course similar to AIH type 1,[1062] and young adults. Children and young might more frequently experience acute presentations compared to older patients, even presenting as fulminant hepatic failure, especially in patients with AIH type 2.[1063] Adult patients might present acutely with jaundice, arthralgia, anorexia, and fatigue, in about one-third of cases.[1064,1065] It is also not uncommon for AIH to present with a relapsing pattern as acute hepatitic episodes alternating with spontaneous clinical and biochemical improvement. Less commonly, complications of portal hypertension, such as hypersplenism or gastrointestinal bleeding, might comprise the first symptoms of AIH.

Considering the wide spectrum of presenting features, AIH should be suspected and ruled out in all patients with symptoms and signs of prolonged, relapsing, or severe liver disease in order to promptly institute the appropriate treatment. At least one-third of AIH patients manifest with cirrhosis at the time of diagnosis, demonstrating the longstanding disease process.[1058,1059] A family history of autoimmune disorders is present in almost 40 percent of AIH patients, and approximately 20 percent of both adult and pediatric patients with AIH present with autoimmune diseases or associated autoimmune characteristics, such as thyroiditis, inflammatory bowel disease, type 1 diabetes, arthritis, hemocytopenia, and vitiligo, at diagnosis or during follow-up and pediatric patients.[1066-1068]

## Treatment

Attainment of an early complete remission to prevent disease progression and to uphold it using the lowest possible dose of medications for long term are the primary aims of treatment in AIH. Except for a fulminant onset AIH with encephalopathy, AIH, irrespective of the degree of liver impairment, responds well to immunosuppressive treatment.[1060,1069] A combination of predniso(lo)ne and azathioprine has long been the mainstay of treatment for AIH.[1070,1071] Currently available second-line drugs, the advantage of some of which over standard treatment remains to be evaluated in controlled studies, include calcineurin inhibitors, cyclosporine and tacrolimus, which have been used as steroid-sparing agents to induce remission whilst avoiding high-dose steroid adverse effects[1072-1074]; budesonide, although ineffective in patients with cirrhosis,[1058,1059] possibly a valid alternative in patients at selected risk of adverse effects from prednisolone or in maintaining remission in patients who have achieved it with predniso(lo)ne[1075]; 6MP[1076] or 6- thioguanine[1077] in patients with azathioprine intolerance; mycophenolate mofetil, in difficult-to-treat cases[1072,1078,1079]; rituximab, in some cases of difficult-to-treat AIH[1080,1081]; infliximab, an anti-TNF-α agent, in treatment-resistant patients[1082-1084]; methotrexate, probably in some patients refractory or intolerant to first-line therapy[1085]; the m-TOR inhibitors sirolimus and everolimus, although mostly have disappointing results.[1086-1088] In patients presenting with fulminant hepatic failure (grades IIIV encephalopathy) unresponsive to steroids, or who progress to end-stage liver disease despite immunosuppression,[1048] liver transplantation is the treatment of choice, followed by long term prednisolone treatment at a dose higher than that generally used after liver transplantation for other conditions to prevent a recurrence. Considering the central role of loss of immunoregulation in the pathogenesis of AIH, studies are underway to restore the ability of Tregs to expand in number, with consequently enhanced function.

## Blood disorders

### *Autoimmune hemolytic anemia*

#### Definition

Autoimmune hemolytic anemia (AIHA) is a classic model of type II hypersensitivity, with autoantibody-coated RBC removed from the circulation by phagocytes of the reticuloendothelial system (RES), mainly splenic macrophages, and/or lysis by complement fixation,[1089,1090] which can be classified by the type of autoantibody and by the presence of underlying disease.[1091] AIHA is divided into primary (idiopathic), in the absence of any associated condition, or as secondary if there is a coexisting disease that may be deemed causal or has shared etiology, such as infection, immune disease neoplasia and drug-induced conditions.[1089,1090] Depending on the optimum temperature at which pathogenic autoantibodies bind RBC, they can be described as either cold, usually of Ig-M class, which is responsible for 15–20 percent of human AIHA cases,[1089] binding more avidly at 4 °C than at higher temperatures and results in intravascular hemolysis if it triggers complement to form membrane attack complexes (MAC),[1092] overcoming protective regulators on the RBC such as CD35, CD55, and CD59,[1093,1094] or can be of IgG class, namely the Donath Landsteiner (DL) hemolysins, which binds RBC if the temperature falls below 37 °C and then fix complement to elicit MAC formation and fulminant intravascular hemolysis when warmed again[1089,1095]; or warm reactive, as the most common cause of AIHA and reacting more strongly with RBC at 37 °C than at lower temperatures, mainly of the IgG class, provoking extravascular hemolysis, principally by Fc receptor (FcγR)-mediated[1090] or CR-mediated erythrophagocytosis by deposition of C3b and C3d that can strongly enhance opsonization[1096] by interacting with specific receptors including CR1 and CR3,[1097] with splenic macrophages acting as the main effectors of RBC destruction.[1090] Mixed pathogenic autoantibodies of both types can be observed in up to 7 percent of the patients.[1091]

## Genetics and immune features

Almost 60 percent of the patients with warm AIHA express the HLA-DR15 allele.[1098] It has also been depicted that a promoter haplotype correlated to decreased expression and function of the inhibitory FcγR FcγRIIb, resulting in enhanced phagocytosis of IgG-opsonized RBC and increased antibody responsiveness, renders the NZB mice susceptible to AIHA.[1099,1100] Moreover, the fact that AIHA becomes progressively more frequent with age might reflect impaired immune regulation.[1091,1101]

Many of the major red blood cell (RBC) autoantigens in AIHA have been established, including Ii blood group system of carbohydrate differentiation antigens against which cold reactive RBC autoantibodies act[1102]; the I antigen, predominant on adult RBC, as well as i expressed at low levels[1103,1104]; and Pr,[1105] all identified in CAS; P in PCH[1095]; the Rh proteins,[1106] as the most common targets in human warm AIHA; glycophorins; and RBC anion channel protein, Band 3.[1106] Investigation of pathogenic responses to such autoantigens has unraveled some mechanisms underlying the loss of self-tolerance in warm AIHA.

Autoantibodies, the complement system, phagocytes, cytotoxic $CD8^+$ T cells and NK cells performing ADCC, B and T lymphocytes including the $CD4^+$ Tregs, and cytokines are implicated in the pathogenesis of warm AIHA. Molecular mimicry of foreign antigens from exogenous infectious and noninfectious agents, such as drugs, crossreacting with RBC self-antigens, including Rh proteins, glycophorins and band 3, might conquer self tolerance and induce AIHA. Moreover, viruses may cause polyclonal activation of B lymphocytes, which can then result in the appearance of forbidden clones, which can be accompanied by lymphoproliferative disorders. Increased number of a $CD4^+$ T-helper cell subset, Th17 cells, along with an increase in the cytokine they produce, IL-17, have been shown to play a role in AIHA.[1107] Moreover, a reduced number of Tregs have been reported in patients with AIHA.[1108] The imbalance between Th1 cells, capable of eliciting cell-mediated activity, and the IL-2, IL-12, IFN-Y, and TNF-ß cytokines they produce, and Th2 cells, promoting humoral responses and secreting IL-4, IL-5, IL-6, IL-10, and IL-13, may also play a role.[1109] A reduced Th1 and a prominent Th2 profile might likely trigger the pathogenesis of AIHA.[1110,1111]

## Clinical features

The prevailing clinical features in both cold hemagglutinin disease (CAS)[1089] and warm AIHA[1090] reflect the anemia, predominantly instigating lethargy and dyspnea, pallor, icterus, hemoglobinuria massive hemolysis, cyanosis or even necrosis of the bodily extremities in CAS,[1089] recurrent bouts of anemia and hemoglobinuria due to exposure to cold in AIHA due to DL antibodies,[1089] as well as splenomegaly or hepatomegaly associated with extravascular hemolysis in warm AIHA.[1090] Besides anemia, there can be evidence of erythroid regeneration with reticulocytosis[1089,1090] or even a poor erythroid response,[1112] the latter as a consequence of either the physiological lag in enhanced RBC production following acute hemolysis, autoimmune reactions precluding RBC regeneration,[1113] or an underlying bone marrow disorder[1114]; increased bilirubin, aspartate transaminase, and lactate dehydrogenase levels as a result of hemolysis; RBC autoagglutination in cold AIHA; spherocytes in warm AIHA.

## Treatment

Currently applicable treatment strategies in cold and warm AIHA include supportive care for anemia; transfusion in life-threatening cases of anemia[1089,1090]; preventing unnecessary exposure to low temperatures in patients with pathogenic cold reactive autoantibodies[1089]; treatment of the underlying condition in cases of secondary disease; corticosteroids or cytotoxic drugs with frequently poor response in CAS[1089]; targeting B cells with the anti-CD20 monoclonal antibody rituximab[1115,1116] as an effective treatment for AIHA refractory to conventional treatments[1117] and now regarded as the first line of therapy in some centers when combined with steroids[1118]; corticosteroids, considered to be the most frequent first-line therapy for warm AIHA[1090] which act through downregulation of macrophage FcγR to increase the survival of IgG-sensitized RBC[1119] and reduction of autoantibody production[1120]; cytotoxic drugs such as cyclophosphamide or azathioprine, administered as second-line therapies; as well as splenectomy to eradicate an important site of extravascular hemolysis.[1090,1117]

### *Immune thrombocytopenia*

## Definition

Immune thrombocytopenia (ITP) is an acquired prototypic organ-specific autoimmune disorder defined by a platelet count of lower than $100 \times 10^9\ L^{-1}$ as a consequence of augmented platelet destruction and defective platelet production,[1121,1122] mediated by both antiplatelet antibodies and T cell-mediated cytotoxicity, with peak incidence during childhood and in adults greater than 60 years of age.[1123] ITP is slightly more prevalent in males in childhood and women in the 30–60 years age group.[1123,1124] The main clinical consequence of thrombocytopenia is bleeding due to impaired primary hemostasis and platelet plug formation. According to the 2010 International Working Group (IWG) consensus of ITP experts, ITP is defined as an isolated thrombocytopenia in the absence of other known conditions and secondary in about 20 percent of cases, occurring in the context of conditions associated with immune dysregulation, including infections with human immunodeficiency virus (HIV), hepatitis C virus (HCV), Helicobacter pylori, cytomegalovirus, and Varicella zoster; autoimmune disorders such as SLE, Evans syndrome and APS; lymphoproliferative disorders such as chronic lymphocytic leukemia, Hodgkin's lymphoma, non-Hodgkin's lymphoma and large granular T-lymphocyte leukemia; vaccination, particularly against measles-mumps-rubella; drugs such as Depakote, quinine and quinidine; and as a side effect of bone marrow transplantation.[1125-1127]

## Pathogenesis

Primary ITP is a heterogeneous acquired autoimmune condition presenting with thrombocytopenia as a result of a combination of different predisposing factors, including the presence of pathologic antiplatelet autoantibodies, T cell-mediated platelet destruction, and defective megakaryopoiesis.[1128-1130] Autoantibodies, predominantly IgG and less commonly IgA or IgM,[1131] are secreted against platelet surface antigens, such as components of the glycoprotein (GP) IIb/IIIa and GPIb/IX complexes and anti-GPVI.[1132,1133] Autoreactive antibodies might be secreted by B lymphocytes and plasma cells, which are present in increased number, particularly in the spleen, followed by the peripheral blood, bone marrow, and probably lymph nodes,[1134,1135] and can be recognized by phagocytes with Fcγ-receptors while bound to platelets, resulting in the antibody-mediated destruction via phagocytosis mainly occurring in the spleen.[1136,1137] Antibody binding can also induce complement-mediated platelet lysis.[1138] In addition to the production of autoreactive antibodies, increased levels of B cell activating factor (BAFF) in ITP may contribute to disease activity by rescuing autoreactive B and T cells from apoptosis and by promoting survival of long-lived splenic plasma cells.[1133,1139] Decreased number and impaired function of IL-10 producing Bregs, which play a crucial role in immune suppression through triggering the differentiation of Tregs, modulating Th1/Th2 balance, and inhibiting activation of monocytes, have also been identified in patients with ITP.[1140-1142]

T cells and dysregulation of T-cell populations also play a significant role in the pathogenesis of ITP through a variety of mechanisms. Decreased Th2 polarization and an increased Th1/Th2 ratio have been shown to have an inverse correlation with platelet count in ITP, probably by causing an increase in platelet phagocytosis.[1133,1143] In addition, $CD8^+$ cytotoxic T cells can directly lyse platelets and prevent platelet production in the bone marrow.[1144,1145] It has also been depicted that a population of autoreactive GPIIb/IIIa $CD4^+$ T cells can enhance the production of antiplatelet antibodies.[1146] Moreover, the reduced number and defective function of Tregs are implicated in the abnormal ITP immune environment.[1147]

Finally, evidence suggests that in spite of the normal or elevated number of MKs in bone marrow biopsies, the platelet production is impaired in many ITP patients,[1148] supported by evidence of abnormal apoptosis and impaired megakaryocyte growth in cell culture with ITP plasma observed by electron microscopy,[1149,1150] none or minimal elevation of serum thrombopoietin levels in patients with ITP as well as the success of the TPO receptor agonists.[1151] One other method of regulation of the number of platelets, driven by platelet clearance, is through the binding of platelets to the Ashwell-Morrell receptor (AMR) system in the liver.[1152] Under nonpathological conditions, desialylation of membrane proteins takes place as platelets age,[1153] resulting in the recognition of these platelets by the AMR and their subsequent clearance from circulation, and this, in turn, drives TPO messenger RNA production.[1154] Nevertheless, the majority of antibody-coated platelets in ITP are assumed to be depleted via FcR-mediated phagocytosis and not in the above-mentioned fashion.

## Clinical features

ITP is characterized by an isolated platelet count of less than $100 \times 10^9\ L^{-1}$ in the absence of other underlying disorders and occurs in both children and adults, both of which have similar platelet counts at diagnosis and bleeding symptoms with severe thrombocytopenia, but with likely distinctive underlying disease processes, suggested by the observation of spontaneous remission in the majority of children with ITP and the chronic nature of the disease in most adults.[1155,1156] Severe extemporaneous or posttraumatic bleeding, such as mucocutaneous, genitourinary, gynecologic, gastrointestinal, or intracranial hemorrhage (ICH), the latter of which occurs more commonly in adults, especially prevalent in patients over the age of 60 years, compared to children,[1157,1158] might occur with platelet values of less than $10 \times 10^9\ L^{-1}$ and less frequently in patients with platelets between $10 \times 10^9$ and $20 \times 10^9\ L^{-1}$.[1158,1159] Factors such as lower platelet counts, older age, prior hemorrhage, and male gender are associated with increased risk of bleeding.[1156-1158] Severe ITP is defined as having clinically significant bleeding and very low platelet counts requiring initiation of treatment, increased doses of medications, or additional therapies.[1127] Those with severe ITP or significant risk of bleeding, not responsive to splenectomy are described as refractory ITP.[1127] Besides the major concern in patients with ITP, bleeding, an increased risk of thromboembolism has also been depicted, which could be possibly attributed to enhanced platelet activation and cell derived microparticles with perhaps some contribution of treatment effect.[1160-1162]

## Treatment

Patients with a platelet count of less than $10 \times 10^9\ L^{-1}$ and most of the patients with platelet counts ranging from $10 \times 10^9$ to $30 \times 10^9\ L^{-1}$, depending on bleeding and/or bruising symptoms, medical comorbidities, and fatigue, are treated.[1163] First-line treatments all aiming at reducing autoantibody-mediated platelet destruction[1136] include steroids, IVIG, slowing platelet destruction and enhancing platelet half-life; and IV anti-D, that can be administered in RhD antigen positive patients with negative direct antiglobulin test (DAT) and intact spleens.[1164,1165] In cases that first-line treatment does not result in permanent improvement and/or clinical remission, steroids are no longer of use, and other reasonable options, such as splenectomy resulting in the achievement of a normal platelet count in around 60 percent of the patients postsurgery and maintaining a sustained response at 5 years[1166,1167]; rituximab, depleting circulating CD-20-positive antibody-producing B cells with an overall response rate of around 50–60 percent[1168,1169]; thrombopoietin receptor agonists (TPO-Ras), eltrombopag and romiplostim, which bind to the TPO receptor and trigger megakaryopoiesis and henceforth platelet production[1170]; danazol; dapsone; azathioprine; vincristine; mycophenolate mofetil; and cyclophosphamide,[1171-1175] should be considered.

## Cardiovascular system

### *Rheumatic fever and rheumatic heart disease*

### Definition and Epidemiology

Rheumatic fever (RF)/rheumatic heart disease (RHD) is the most definite example of molecular mimicry following an untreated Streptococcus pyogenes infection in children, which elicits autoimmune reactions against human tissues and present a complex network of several genes that control both innate and adaptive immune responses that predispose to the diverse clinical manifestations. The incidence of IHD is greater than 50 per 100,000 children in some developing countries and of at least 15.6 million cases and the leading cause of around 233,000 deaths/year, worldwide.[1176]

### Genetics and autoimmune features

RHD is the most serious complication of RF depending on multiple host factors, mediating a heart tissue driven autoimmune response elicited by an impaired immune response against S. pyogenes. RF/RHD is associated with several genes, some of which are related to the innate immune response, including mannan-binding lectin-2 (MBL2), TLR-2, Ficolin, FcγRIIA, MBL-associated serine protease-2 (Masp2), and macrophage inhibitory factor (MIF) genes; adaptive immune response, including HLA-DRB1, DRB3, DQB1, DQA1, and CTLA4 genes; or both the innate and adaptive immune responses, including TNF-α, IL-10, TGF-B1 and IL-1Ra genes.[1177-1194]

In view of the cross-reactions between streptococcal antigens present as a result of throat infection by S. pyogenes and human tissue proteins, predominantly heart tissue proteins in individuals with a genetic predisposition, which initiate an inflammatory process leading to intense cytokine secretion by monocytes and macrophages that in turn induce the activation of B and T lymphocytes, RF/RHD is considered as the most notable example of molecular mimicry in human pathological autoimmunity. Several Streptococcal heart tissue cross-reactive antibodies, discussed elsewhere in details,[1195-1197] also play a role in the development of the disease through activating the heart tissue valvular endothelial cells which then enhances the expression of adhesion molecules such as VCAM1, mediating cellular infiltration by neutrophils, monocytes, B and T cells[1198]; and the expression of chemokines by activated endothelial cells, stimulating the expression of integrins, selectins, and succeeding transendothelial migration of leukocytes. $CD4^+$ infiltrating T cells predominate the heart rheumatic lesions.[1199]

The development of Aschoff bodies, a granulomatous lesion consisting of macrophages, Anitschkow cells, multinucleated cells, and polymorphonuclear leukocytes, in the myocardium and/or endocardium, together with the secretion of inflammatory cytokines such as IL-1, TNFα, and IL-2, have been found in the heart tissue in patients with RHD, the latter of which is dependant on the developmental phase of the Aschoff bodies,[1200] possibly initiating and perpetuating the inflammatory process leading to heart tissue damage. Molecules such as integrins, chemokine and cytokines, namely IFNγ, IL-23, and IL-17, involved in the recruitment of T and B lymphocytes culminating in the autoimmune reactions, have been described involved with the inflammatory process in rheumatic heart lesions.[1195,1196]

### Clinical features

The major manifestations include polyarthritis, generally migratory and very painful, and as one of the earliest and most frequent disease manifestations in 60–80 percent of the patients, usually involving the peripheral large joints; carditis, the most serious manifestation of the disease, occurring a few weeks after the infection, and usually presenting as a pancarditis, mitral and aortic regurgitation (AR) caused by valvulitis, or endocarditis, which is the most severe sequel commonly resulting in chronic rheumatic heart disease (RHD); Sydenham's chorea, usually a delayed manifestation, present in 30–40 percent of patients and characterized by involuntary movements, particularly of the face and limbs, muscular weakness, disturbances of speech and gait, and voluntary movements; subcutaneous nodules and erythema marginatum, characterized by nodules on the surface of joints and skin lesions, respectively, along with the minor manifestations, comprising fever, arthralgia, prolonged PR interval, increased erythrocyte sedimentation rate, and the presence of C-reactive protein.[1201,1202]

### Treatment

Preventive and therapeutic methods currently in use include either oral antibiotic (usually penicillin) or a single injection of penicillin acute throat infections caused by group A Streptococcus bacteria for primary prevention of ARF; several years of antibiotic therapy to prevent fever and heart disease in case of acute RHD; open heart surgery to repair or replace heart valves in patients with severely damaged heart valves; antiinflammatory medications such as salicylates or corticosteroids to reduce inflammation in ARF; monthly injections of antibiotic, such as Penicillin for a period of 5 years in patients having one attack of RF or for up to 40 years in the presence of carditis; persistent use of low doses of antibiotics such as penicillin, sulfadiazine or erythromycin to avert re-occurrence of RHD in patients with RF; and the ACE inhibitors, diuretics, beta-blockers, digoxin and corticosteroids if patients develop congestive heart failure. In addition, progress is being made in developing group A streptococcal vaccines.[1203]

## Future perspectives and concluding remarks

Over the past several years, progressive advancement in our understandings of immunopathogenesis has redirected us to a more clear approach to the study of autoimmunity and has resulted in an enormous expansion of potential therapeutic targets. We have witnessed a change in our understanding of autoimmunity through the identification of different patterns of genetic polymorphisms contributing to autoimmunity risk and multiple mechanisms involved in the aberrant regulation of gene expression resulting in autoimmunity, and more remain to be identified. Identification of such gene and protein expression patterns will help to elucidate the common mechanisms of immune dysfunction among multiple autoimmune diseases and those unique to a particular disease.

Despite the development of multiple new therapeutic strategies, leading to major advances in treatment for some but not all autoimmune diseases, over the past two decades, there are still numerous knowledge gaps to be filled. The expansion of high-throughput technologies to determine such gene polymorphisms, gene expression, protein expression and epigenetic changes in different populations of patients with autoimmune diseases might provide new insights into disease pathogenesis and can suggest potential biomarkers of immune function to predict the likelihood of developing a particular autoimmune condition in individual patients, monitor disease activity even prior to the emergence of clinical symptomatology, prognosticate, improve the therapy through the establishment of new therapeutic targets and new therapeutic strategies, and characterize the response to therapy at an early time point, making timely interventions possible. Thus, the identification of such biomarkers will allow testing of therapies with the potential to prevent or cure the autoimmune disease before the ultimate tissue damage and can potentiate customization of therapy for individual patients, thereby improving efficacy and preventing avoidable toxicities and expense. Although gaining the knowledge and its translation from bench to bedside will be a time-intensive way to go through, this is the bright side we can look on.

## References


1. Rose NR, Bona C. Defining criteria for autoimmune diseases (Witebsky's postulates revisited). *Immunology today*. 1993;14(9):426–430.
2. Davidson A, Diamond B. Autoimmune diseases. *New England Journal of Medicine*. 2001;345(5):340–350.
3. Lerner A, Jeremias P, Matthias T. The world incidence and prevalence of autoimmune diseases is increasing. *Int J Celiac Dis*. 2015;3(4):151–155.
4. Patterson CC, Dahlquist GG, Gyürüs E, Green A, Soltész G, Group ES. Incidence trends for childhood type 1 diabetes in Europe during 1989–2003 and predicted new cases 2005–20: a multicentre prospective registration study. *The Lancet*. 2009;373(9680):2027–2033.
5. Yu C, Gershwin ME, Chang C. Diagnostic criteria for systemic lupus erythematosus: a critical review. *Journal of autoimmunity*. 2014;48:10–13.
6. Cooper GS, Bynum ML, Somers EC. Recent insights in the epidemiology of autoimmune diseases: improved prevalence estimates and understanding of clustering of diseases. *Journal of autoimmunity*. 2009;33(3–4):197–207.
7. Hayter SM, Cook MC. Updated assessment of the prevalence, spectrum and case definition of autoimmune disease. *Autoimmunity reviews*. 2012;11(10):754–765.
8. Jacobson DL, Gange SJ, Rose NR, Graham NM. Epidemiology and estimated population burden of selected autoimmune diseases in the United States. *Clinical immunology and immunopathology*. 1997;84(3):223–243.

9. Wang Y, Wang J, Sun Y, Wu Q, Fu Y-X. Complementary effects of TNF and lymphotoxin on the formation of germinal center and follicular dendritic cells. *The Journal of Immunology*. 2001;166(1):330–337.
10. Gu H, Tarlinton D, Müller W, Rajewsky K, Förster I. Most peripheral B cells in mice are ligand selected. *The Journal of experimental medicine*. 1991;173(6):1357–1371.
11. Vallejo AN, Davila E, Weyand CM, Goronzy JJ. Biology of T lymphocytes. *Rheumatic Disease Clinics*. 2004;30(1):135–157.
12. Nobrega A, Stransky B, Nicolas N, Coutinho A. Regeneration of natural antibody repertoire after massive ablation of lymphoid system: robust selection mechanisms preserve antigen binding specificities. *The Journal of Immunology*. 2002;169(6):2971–2978.
13. Leung PS, Wang J, Naiyanetr P, Kenny TP, Lam KS, Kurth MJ, et al. Environment and primary biliary cirrhosis: electrophilic drugs and the induction of AMA. *Journal of autoimmunity*. 2013;41:79–86.
14. Marrie RA, Reider N, Cohen J, Stuve O, Sorensen PS, Cutter G, et al. A systematic review of the incidence and prevalence of autoimmune disease in multiple sclerosis. *Multiple sclerosis journal*. 2015;21(3):282–293.
15. Wahren-Herlenius M, Dörner T. Immunopathogenic mechanisms of systemic autoimmune disease. *The Lancet*. 2013;382(9894):819–831.
16. Liu K, Li Q-Z, Delgado-Vega AM, Abelson A-K, Sánchez E, Kelly JA, et al. Kallikrein genes are associated with lupus and glomerular basement membrane–specific antibody–induced nephritis in mice and humans. *The Journal of clinical investigation*. 2009;119(4):911–923.
17. Liao L, Sindhwani R, Rojkind M, Factor S, Leinwand L, Diamond B. Antibody-mediated autoimmune myocarditis depends on genetically determined target organ sensitivity. *The Journal of experimental medicine*. 1995;181(3):1123–1131.
18. Cho JH, Gregersen PK. Genomics and the multifactorial nature of human autoimmune disease. *New England Journal of Medicine*. 2011;365(17):1612–1623.
19. Gutierrez-Arcelus M, Rich SS, Raychaudhuri S. Autoimmune diseases—Connecting risk alleles with molecular traits of the immune system. *Nature Reviews Genetics*. 2016;17(3):160.
20. Martini S, Nair V, Keller BJ, Eichinger F, Hawkins JJ, Randolph A, et al. Integrative biology identifies shared transcriptional networks in CKD. *Journal of the American Society of Nephrology*. 2014;25(11):2559–2572.
21. Cotsapas C, Voight BF, Rossin E, Lage K, Neale BM, Wallace C, et al. Pervasive sharing of genetic effects in autoimmune disease. *PLoS Genet*. 2011;7(8):e1002254.
22. Banchereau J, Briere F, Caux C, Davoust J, Lebecque S, Liu Y-J, et al. Immunobiology of dendritic cells. *Annual review of immunology*. 2000;18(1):767–811.
23. Mills KH. TLR-dependent T cell activation in autoimmunity. *Nature Reviews Immunology*. 2011;11(12):807–822.
24. Childs K., Goodbourn S. Pattern Recognition Receptors. eLS. 1-9.
25. Broz P, Monack DM. Newly described pattern recognition receptors team up against intracellular pathogens. *Nature Reviews Immunology*. 2013;13(8):551–565.
26. A two-step model for the induction of organ-specific autoimmunity. In: Limmer A, Sacher T, Alferink J, Nichterlein T, Arnold B, Hämmerling GJ, eds. *Novartis Foundation Symposium 215-Immunological Tolerance: Immunological Tolerance: Novartis Foundation Symposium*: Wiley Online Library; 2007. 215.
27. Kawai T, Akira S. Toll-like receptors and their crosstalk with other innate receptors in infection and immunity. *Immunity*. 2011;34(5):637–650.
28. Miyake Y, Yamasaki S. Sensing necrotic cells. *Self and Nonself*. 2012:144–152.
29. Doyle HA, Mamula MJ. Autoantigenesis: the evolution of protein modifications in autoimmune disease. *Current opinion in immunology*. 2012;24(1):112–118.
30. Bratton DL, Henson PM. Neutrophil clearance: when the party is over, clean-up begins. *Trends in immunology*. 2011;32(8):350–357.
31. Horwitz MS, Ilic A, Fine C, Rodriguez E, Sarvetnick N. Presented antigen from damaged pancreatic β cells activates autoreactive T cells in virus-mediated autoimmune diabetes. *The Journal of clinical investigation*. 2002;109(1):79–87.
32. Vezys V, Lefrançois L. Cutting edge: inflammatory signals drive organ-specific autoimmunity to normally cross-tolerizing endogenous antigen. *The Journal of Immunology*. 2002;169(12):6677–6680.

33. Gallo PM, Gallucci S. The dendritic cell response to classic, emerging, and homeostatic danger signals. Implications for autoimmunity. *Frontiers in immunology*. 2013;4:138.
34. Toll-like receptor driven B cell activation in the induction of systemic autoimmunity. In: Green NM, Marshak-Rothstein A, eds. Toll-like receptor driven B cell activation in the induction of systemic autoimmunity. *Seminars in immunology*. 2011.
35. Sokolove J, Zhao X, Chandra PE, Robinson WH. Immune complexes containing citrullinated fibrinogen costimulate macrophages via Toll-like receptor 4 and Fcγ receptor. *Arthritis & Rheumatism*. 2011;63(1):53–62.
36. Rivas MN, Koh YT, Chen A, Nguyen A, Lee YH, Lawson G, et al. MyD88 is critically involved in immune tolerance breakdown at environmental interfaces of Foxp3-deficient mice. *The Journal of clinical investigation*. 2012;122(5):1933–1947.
37. Pagni PP, Traub S, Demaria O, Chasson L, Alexopoulou L. Contribution of TLR7 and TLR9 signaling to the susceptibility of MyD88-deficient mice to myocarditis. *Autoimmunity*. 2010;43(4):275–287.
38. Herlands RA, Christensen SR, Sweet RA, Hershberg U, Shlomchik MJ. T cell-independent and toll-like receptor-dependent antigen-driven activation of autoreactive B cells. *Immunity*. 2008;29(2):249–260.
39. Andersson U, Tracey KJ. HMGB1 is a therapeutic target for sterile inflammation and infection. *Annual review of immunology*. 2011;29:139–162.
40. Sharma S, Campbell AM, Chan J, Schattgen SA, Orlowski GM, Nayar R, et al. Suppression of systemic autoimmunity by the innate immune adaptor STING. *Proceedings of the National Academy of Sciences*. 2015;112(7):E710–E7E7.
41. Pawaria S, Sharma S, Baum R, Nündel K, Busto P, Gravallese EM, et al. Taking the STING out of TLR-driven autoimmune diseases: good, bad, or indifferent? *Journal of leukocyte biology*. 2017;101(1):121–126.
42. Koutouzov S, Mathian A, Dalloul A. Type-I interferons and systemic lupus erythematosus. *Autoimmunity reviews*. 2006;5(8):554–562.
43. Elkon KB, Santer DM. Complement, interferon and lupus. *Current opinion in immunology*. 2012;24(6):665–670.
44. Manderson AP, Botto M, Walport MJ. The role of complement in the development of systemic lupus erythematosus. *Annu Rev Immunol*. 2004;22:431–456.
45. Macedo ACL, Isaac L. Systemic lupus erythematosus and deficiencies of early components of the complement classical pathway. *Frontiers in immunology*. 2016;7:55.
46. Niewold TB. Interferon alpha as a primary pathogenic factor in human lupus. *Journal of interferon & cytokine research*. 2011;31(12):887–892.
47. Caielli S, Athale S, Domic B, Murat E, Chandra M, Banchereau R, et al. Oxidized mitochondrial nucleoids released by neutrophils drive type I interferon production in human lupus. *Journal of Experimental Medicine*. 2016;213(5):697–713.
48. Grayson PC, Carmona-Rivera C, Xu L, Lim N, Gao Z, Asare AL, et al. Neutrophil-related gene expression and low-density granulocytes associated with disease activity and response to treatment in antineutrophil cytoplasmic antibody–associated vasculitis. *Arthritis & rheumatology*. 2015;67(7):1922–1932.
49. Villanueva E, Yalavarthi S, Berthier CC, Hodgin JB, Khandpur R, Lin AM, et al. Netting neutrophils induce endothelial damage, infiltrate tissues, and expose immunostimulatory molecules in systemic lupus erythematosus. *The Journal of Immunology*. 2011;187(1):538–552.
50. Kienhöfer D, Hahn J, Stoof J, Csepregi JZ, Reinwald C, Urbonaviciute V, et al. Experimental lupus is aggravated in mouse strains with impaired induction of neutrophil extracellular traps. *JCI insight*. 2017;2(10).
51. Jorch SK, Kubes P. An emerging role for neutrophil extracellular traps in noninfectious disease. *Nature medicine*. 2017;23(3):279–287.
52. De Souza HS, Fiocchi C. Immunopathogenesis of IBD: current state of the art. *Nature reviews Gastroenterology & hepatology*. 2016;13(1):13.
53. Stange EF, Wehkamp J. Recent advances in understanding and managing Crohn's disease. *F1000Research*. 2016;5.
54. Wang L., Wang F.-S., Chang C., Gershwin M.E. Breach of tolerance: primary biliary cirrhosis. 2014.

55. Alexandropoulos K, Danzl NM. Thymic epithelial cells: antigen presenting cells that regulate T cell repertoire and tolerance development. *Immunologic research*. 2012;54(1–3):177–190.
56. Von Boehmer H, Melchers F. Checkpoints in lymphocyte development and autoimmune disease. *Nature immunology*. 2010;11(1):14.
57. Rajewsky K. Clonal selection and learning in the antibody system. *Nature*. 1996;381(6585):751–758.
58. Goodnow CC, Vinuesa CG, Randall KL, Mackay F, Brink R. Control systems and decision making for antibody production. *Nature immunology*. 2010;11(8):681–688.
59. Brink R. The imperfect control of self-reactive germinal center B cells. *Current opinion in immunology*. 2014;28:97–101.
60. DeFranco AL. Germinal centers and autoimmune disease in humans and mice. *Immunology and cell biology*. 2016;94(10):918–924.
61. Liu Z, Davidson A. BAFF and selection of autoreactive B cells. *Trends in immunology*. 2011;32(8):388–394.
62. Shlomchik MJ. Sites and stages of autoreactive B cell activation and regulation. *Immunity*. 2008;28(1):18–28.
63. Nemazee D. Mechanisms of central tolerance for B cells. *Nature Reviews Immunology*. 2017;17(5):281.
64. Monroe JG, Bannish G, Fuentes-Panana EM, King LB, Sandel PC, Chung J, et al. Positive and negative selection during B lymphocyte development. *Immunologic research*. 2003;27(2–3):427–442.
65. The origin of DCs and capacity for immunologic tolerance in central and peripheral tissues. In: Devi KSP, Anandasabapathy N, eds. The origin of DCs and capacity for immunologic tolerance in central and peripheral tissues. *Seminars in immunopathology*. 2017.
66. Tsubata T. B-cell tolerance and autoimmunity. *F1000Research*. 2017;6.
67. Anderson MS, Su MA. Aire and T cell development. *Current opinion in immunology*. 2011;23(2):198–206.
68. Vinuesa CG, Cook MC, Angelucci C, Athanasopoulos V, Rui L, Hill KM, et al. A RING-type ubiquitin ligase family member required to repress follicular helper T cells and autoimmunity. *Nature*. 2005;435(7041):452–458.
69. Linterman MA, Rigby RJ, Wong R, Silva D, Withers D, Anderson G, et al. Roquin differentiates the specialized functions of duplicated T cell costimulatory receptor genes CD28 and ICOS. *Immunity*. 2009;30(2):228–241.
70. Seo S, Mandik-Nayak L, Erikson J. B cell anergy and systemic lupus erythematosus. *Curr Dir Autoimmun*. 2003;6:1–20.
71. Salinas GF, Braza F, Brouard S, Tak P-P, Baeten D. The role of B lymphocytes in the progression from autoimmunity to autoimmune disease. *Clinical immunology*. 2013;146(1):34–45.
72. Hang L, Nakamura RM, Tubbs R. Current concepts and advances in clinical laboratory testing for autoimmune diseases. *Critical reviews in clinical laboratory sciences*. 1997;34(3):275–311.
73. Avrameas S, Selmi C. Natural autoantibodies in the physiology and pathophysiology of the immune system. *Journal of autoimmunity*. 2013;41:46–49.
74. Panda S, Ding JL. Natural antibodies bridge innate and adaptive immunity. *The journal of immunology*. 2015;194(1):13–20.
75. Narayan P, Holt B, Tosti R, Kane LP. CARMA1 is required for Akt-mediated NF-κB activation in T cells. *Molecular and cellular biology*. 2006;26(6):2327–2336.
76. Goodnow CC. Multistep pathogenesis of autoimmune disease. *Cell*. 2007;130(1):25–35.
77. Weng N-p, Araki Y, Subedi K. The molecular basis of the memory T cell response: differential gene expression and its epigenetic regulation. *Nature Reviews Immunology*. 2012;12(4):306–315.
78. Nakayamada S, Takahashi H, Kanno Y, O'Shea JJ. Helper T cell diversity and plasticity. *Current opinion in immunology*. 2012;24(3):297–302.
79. Cusick MF, Libbey JE, Fujinami RS. Molecular mimicry as a mechanism of autoimmune disease. *Clinical reviews in allergy & immunology*. 2012;42(1):102–111.
80. Bockenstedt LK, Gee RJ, Mamula MJ. Self-peptides in the initiation of lupus autoimmunity. *The Journal of Immunology*. 1995;154(7):3516–3524.
81. Yan J, Harvey BP, Gee RJ, Shlomchik MJ, Mamula MJ. B cells drive early T cell autoimmunity in vivo prior to dendritic cell-mediated autoantigen presentation. *The Journal of Immunology*. 2006;177(7):4481–4487.

82. Sinmaz N, Nguyen T, Tea F, Dale RC, Brilot F. Mapping autoantigen epitopes: molecular insights into autoantibody-associated disorders of the nervous system. *Journal of neuroinflammation*. 2016; 13(1):219.
83. Sercarz EE, Lehmann PV, Ametani A, Benichou G, Miller A, Moudgil K. Dominance and crypticity of T cell antigenic determinants. *Annual review of immunology*. 1993;11(1):729–766.
84. Whitmire JK, Asano MS, Kaech SM, Sarkar S, Hannum LG, Shlomchik MJ, et al. Requirement of B cells for generating CD4+ T cell memory. *The Journal of Immunology*. 2009;182(4):1868–1876.
85. Cunningham MW. Autoimmunity and molecular mimicry in the pathogenesis of post-streptococcal heart disease. *Frontiers in bioscience: a journal and virtual library*. 2003;8:s533–s543.
86. Valle FM, Balada E, Ordi-Ros J, Vilardell-Tarres M. DNase 1 and systemic lupus erythematosus. *Autoimmunity Reviews*. 2008;7(5):359–363.
87. Peng Y, Elkon KB. Autoimmunity in MFG-E8–deficient mice is associated with altered trafficking and enhanced cross-presentation of apoptotic cell antigens. *The Journal of clinical investigation*. 2011;121(6):2221–2241.
88. Colonna L, Lood C, Elkon KB. Beyond apoptosis in lupus. *Current opinion in rheumatology*. 2014;26(5):459.
89. Filardy AA, Pires DR, Nunes MP, Takiya CM, Freire-de-Lima CG, Ribeiro-Gomes FL, et al. Proinflammatory clearance of apoptotic neutrophils induces an IL-12lowIL-10high regulatory phenotype in macrophages. *The Journal of Immunology*. 2010;185(4):2044–2050.
90. Bengsch B, Johnson AL, Kurachi M, Odorizzi PM, Pauken KE, Attanasio J, et al. Bioenergetic insufficiencies due to metabolic alterations regulated by the inhibitory receptor PD-1 are an early driver of CD8+ T cell exhaustion. *Immunity*. 2016;45(2):358–373.
91. McKinney EF, Smith KG. T-cell exhaustion: understanding the interface of chronic viral and autoinflammatory diseases. *Immunology and cell biology*. 2016;94(10):935–942.
92. McKinney EF, Lee JC, Jayne DR, Lyons PA, Smith KG. T-cell exhaustion, co-stimulation and clinical outcome in autoimmunity and infection. *Nature*. 2015;523(7562):612–616.
93. Day D, Hansen AR. Immune-related adverse events associated with immune checkpoint inhibitors. *BioDrugs*. 2016;30(6):571–584.
94. Cappelli LC, Gutierrez AK, Bingham III CO, AA Shah. Rheumatic and musculoskeletal immune-related adverse events due to immune checkpoint inhibitors: a systematic review of the literature. *Arthritis care & research*. 2017;69(11):1751–1763.
95. Kasper IR, Apostolidis SA, Sharabi A, Tsokos GC. Empowering Regulatory T Cells in Autoimmunity. *Trends Mol Med*. 2016;22(9):784–797.
96. Wing K, Sakaguchi S. Regulatory T cells exert checks and balances on self tolerance and autoimmunity. *Nat Immunol*. 2010;11(1):7–13.
97. Panduro M, Benoist C, Mathis D. Tissue Tregs. *Annu Rev Immunol*. 2016;34:609–633.
98. Hori S, Nomura T, Sakaguchi S. Control of regulatory T cell development by the transcription factor Foxp3. *Science*. 2003;299(5609):1057–1061.
99. Josefowicz SZ, Lu l-F, Rudensky AY. Regulatory T cells: mechanisms of differentiation and function. *Annual review of immunology*. 2012;30:531–564.
100. Hsieh C-S, Lee H-M, Lio C-WJ. Selection of regulatory T cells in the thymus. *Nature Reviews Immunology*. 2012;12(3):157–167.
101. Bennett CL, Christie J, Ramsdell F, Brunkow ME, Ferguson PJ, Whitesell L, et al. The immune dysregulation, polyendocrinopathy, enteropathy, X-linked syndrome (IPEX) is caused by mutations of FOXP3. *Nature genetics*. 2001;27(1):20–21.
102. Khattri R, Cox T, Yasayko S-A, Ramsdell F. An essential role for Scurfin in CD4+ CD25+ T regulatory cells. *Nature immunology*. 2003;4(4):337–342.
103. Wildin RS, Ramsdell F, Peake J, Faravelli F, Casanova J-L, Buist N, et al. X-linked neonatal diabetes mellitus, enteropathy and endocrinopathy syndrome is the human equivalent of mouse scurfy. *Nature genetics*. 2001;27(1):18–20.
104. Collison LW, Workman CJ, Kuo TT, Boyd K, Wang Y, Vignali KM, et al. The inhibitory cytokine IL-35 contributes to regulatory T-cell function. *Nature*. 2007;450(7169):566–569.
105. Grossman WJ, Verbsky JW, Barchet W, Colonna M, Atkinson JP, Ley TJ. Human T regulatory cells can use the perforin pathway to cause autologous target cell death. *Immunity*. 2004;21(4):589–601.

106. Thornton AM, Shevach EM. CD4+ CD25+ immunoregulatory T cells suppress polyclonal T cell activation in vitro by inhibiting interleukin 2 production. *The Journal of experimental medicine*. 1998;188(2):287–296.
107. Pandiyan P, Zheng L, Ishihara S, Reed J, Lenardo MJ. CD4+CD25+Foxp3+ regulatory T cells induce cytokine deprivation-mediated apoptosis of effector CD4+ T cells. *Nat Immunol*. 2007;8(12):1353–1362.
108. Onishi Y, Fehervari Z, Yamaguchi T, Sakaguchi S. Foxp3+ natural regulatory T cells preferentially form aggregates on dendritic cells in vitro and actively inhibit their maturation. *Proceedings of the National Academy of Sciences*. 2008;105(29):10113–10118.
109. Liang B, Workman C, Lee J, Chew C, Dale BM, Colonna L, et al. Regulatory T cells inhibit dendritic cells by lymphocyte activation gene-3 engagement of MHC class II. *The Journal of Immunology*. 2008;180(9):5916–5926.
110. Borsellino G, Kleinewietfeld M, Di Mitri D, Sternjak A, Diamantini A, Giometto R, et al. Expression of ectonucleotidase CD39 by Foxp3+ Treg cells: hydrolysis of extracellular ATP and immune suppression. *Blood, The Journal of the American Society of Hematology*. 2007;110(4):1225–1232.
111. Wing K, Onishi Y, Prieto-Martin P, Yamaguchi T, Miyara M, Fehervari Z, et al. CTLA-4 control over Foxp3+ regulatory T cell function. *Science*. 2008;322(5899):271–275.
112. Qureshi OS, Zheng Y, Nakamura K, Attridge K, Manzotti C, Schmidt EM, et al. Trans-endocytosis of CD80 and CD86: a molecular basis for the cell-extrinsic function of CTLA-4. *Science*. 2011;332(6029):600–603.
113. Type 1 regulatory T cells (Tr1) in autoimmunity. In: Pot C, Apetoh L, Kuchroo VK, eds. Type 1 regulatory T cells (Tr1) in autoimmunity. *Seminars in immunology*. 2011.
114. Meka RR, Venkatesha SH, Dudics S, Acharya B, Moudgil KD. IL-27-induced modulation of autoimmunity and its therapeutic potential. *Autoimmunity reviews*. 2015;14(12):1131–1141.
115. PI3K-Akt pathway enhances the differentiation of interleukin 27-induced type 1 regulatory T cells. In: Nagai S, Adiba-Nadya N, Tezuka H, Ohteki T, Matsuda S, Azuma M, eds. PI3K-Akt pathway enhances the differentiation of interleukin 27-induced type 1 regulatory T cells. *EUROPEAN JOURNAL OF IMMUNOLOGY*. 2019.
116. Wojno EDT, Hunter CA. New directions in the basic and translational biology of interleukin-27. *Trends in immunology*. 2012;33(2):91–97.
117. Hall AOH, Silver JS, Hunter CA. The immunobiology of IL-27. *Advances in immunology*. 2012;115:1–44.
118. Pot C, Jin H, Awasthi A, Liu SM, Lai C-Y, Madan R, et al. Cutting edge: IL-27 induces the transcription factor c-Maf, cytokine IL-21, and the costimulatory receptor ICOS that coordinately act together to promote differentiation of IL-10-producing Tr1 cells. *The Journal of Immunology*. 2009;183(2):797–801.
119. Induction of regulatory Tr1 cells and inhibition of TH17 cells by IL-27. In: Pot C, Apetoh L, Awasthi A, Kuchroo VK, eds. Induction of regulatory Tr1 cells and inhibition of TH17 cells by IL-27. *Seminars in immunology*. 2011.
120. Mascanfroni ID, Takenaka MC, Yeste A, Patel B, Wu Y, Kenison JE, et al. Metabolic control of type 1 regulatory T cell differentiation by AHR and HIF1-α. *Nature medicine*. 2015;21(6):638–646.
121. Karwacz K, Miraldi ER, Pokrovskii M, Madi A, Yosef N, Wortman I, et al. Critical role of IRF1 and BATF in forming chromatin landscape during type 1 regulatory cell differentiation. *Nature immunology*. 2017;18(4):412–421.
122. Ilarregui JM, Croci DO, Bianco GA, Toscano MA, Salatino M, Vermeulen ME, et al. Tolerogenic signals delivered by dendritic cells to T cells through a galectin-1-driven immunoregulatory circuit involving interleukin 27 and interleukin 10. *Nature immunology*. 2009;10(9):981.
123. Chen Y, Park Y-B, Patel E, Silverman GJ. IgM antibodies to apoptosis-associated determinants recruit C1q and enhance dendritic cell phagocytosis of apoptotic cells. *The Journal of Immunology*. 2009;182(10):6031–6043.
124. Mauri C, Bosma A. Immune regulatory function of B cells. *Annual review of immunology*. 2012;30:221–241.
125. Carter NA, Vasconcellos R, Rosser EC, Tulone C, Muñoz-Suano A, Kamanaka M, et al. Mice lacking endogenous IL-10–producing regulatory B cells develop exacerbated disease and present with an increased frequency of Th1/Th17 but a decrease in regulatory T cells. *The Journal of Immunology*. 2011;186(10):5569–5579.

126. Fillatreau S, Sweenie CH, McGeachy MJ, Gray D, Anderton SM. B cells regulate autoimmunity by provision of IL-10. *Nature immunology*. 2002;3(10):944–950.
127. Mauri C, Gray D, Mushtaq N, Londei M. Prevention of arthritis by interleukin 10–producing B cells. *The Journal of experimental medicine*. 2003;197(4):489–501.
128. Rosser EC, Oleinika K, Tonon S, Doyle R, Bosma A, Carter NA, et al. Regulatory B cells are induced by gut microbiota–driven interleukin-1β and interleukin-6 production. *Nature medicine*. 2014;20(11):1334–1339.
129. Yoshizaki A, Miyagaki T, DiLillo DJ, Matsushita T, Horikawa M, Kountikov EI, et al. Regulatory B cells control T-cell autoimmunity through IL-21-dependent cognate interactions. *Nature*. 2012;491(7423):264–268.
130. Wang R-X, Yu C-R, Dambuza IM, Mahdi RM, Dolinska MB, Sergeev YV, et al. Interleukin-35 induces regulatory B cells that suppress autoimmune disease. *Nature medicine*. 2014;20(6):633–641.
131. Blair PA, Noreña LY, Flores-Borja F, Rawlings DJ, Isenberg DA, Ehrenstein MR, et al. CD19+ CD24hiCD38hi B cells exhibit regulatory capacity in healthy individuals but are functionally impaired in systemic lupus erythematosus patients. *immunity*. 2010;32(1):129–140.
132. Bosma A, Abdel-Gadir A, Isenberg DA, Jury EC, Mauri C. Lipid-antigen presentation by CD1d+ B cells is essential for the maintenance of invariant natural killer T cells. *Immunity*. 2012;36(3):477–490.
133. Manjarrez-Orduño N, Quách TD. Sanz I. B cells and immunological tolerance. *Journal of Investigative Dermatology*. 2009;129(2):278–288.
134. Bolland S, Ravetch JV. Spontaneous autoimmune disease in FcγRIIB-deficient mice results from strain-specific epistasis. *Immunity*. 2000;13(2):277–285.
135. Fukuyama H, Nimmerjahn F, Ravetch JV. The inhibitory Fcγ receptor modulates autoimmunity by limiting the accumulation of immunoglobulin G+ anti-DNA plasma cells. *Nature immunology*. 2005;6(1):99–106.
136. Schildberg FA, Klein SR, Freeman GJ, Sharpe AH. Coinhibitory pathways in the B7-CD28 ligand-receptor family. *Immunity*. 2016;44(5):955–972.
137. Khoury SJ, Sayegh MH. The roles of the new negative T cell costimulatory pathways in regulating autoimmunity. *Immunity*. 2004;20(5):529–538.
138. Kostine M, Chiche L, Lazaro E, Halfon P, Charpin C, Arniaud D, et al. Opportunistic autoimmunity secondary to cancer immunotherapy (OASI): an emerging challenge. *La Revue de Médecine Interne*. 2017;38(8):513–525.
139. Chen L. Co-inhibitory molecules of the B7–CD28 family in the control of T-cell immunity. *Nature Reviews Immunology*. 2004;4(5):336–347.
140. Function and regulation of the CD95 (APO-1/Fas) ligand in the immune system. In: Li-Weber M, Krammer PH, eds. Function and regulation of the CD95 (APO-1/Fas) ligand in the immune system. *Seminars in immunology*. 2003.
141. Fas (CD95/Apo-1) ligand regulation in T cell homeostasis, cell-mediated cytotoxicity and immune pathology. In: Brunner T, Wasem C, Torgler R, Cima I, Jakob S, Corazza N, eds. Fas (CD95/Apo-1) ligand regulation in T cell homeostasis, cell-mediated cytotoxicity and immune pathology. *Seminars in immunology*. 2003.
142. Damoiseaux J, Andrade LE, Fritzler MJ, Shoenfeld Y. Autoantibodies 2015: from diagnostic biomarkers toward prediction, prognosis and prevention. *Autoimmunity reviews*. 2015;14(6):555–563.
143. Ohishi K, Kanoh M, Shinomiya H, Hitsumoto Y, Utsumi S. Complement activation by cross-linked B cell-membrane IgM. *The Journal of Immunology*. 1995;154(7):3173–3179.
144. Lleo A, Invernizzi P, Gao B, Podda M, Gershwin ME. Definition of human autoimmunity—Autoantibodies versus autoimmune disease. *Autoimmunity reviews*. 2010;9(5):A259–AA66.
145. Campbell DJ, Kim CH, Butcher EC. Separable effector T cell populations specialized for B cell help or tissue inflammation. *Nature immunology*. 2001;2(9):876–881.
146. Katzman SD, Hoyer KK, Dooms H, Gratz IK, Rosenblum MD, Paw JS, et al. Opposing functions of IL-2 and IL-7 in the regulation of immune responses. *Cytokine*. 2011;56(1):116–121.
147. Gerriets VA, Rathmell JC. Metabolic pathways in T cell fate and function. *Trends in immunology*. 2012;33(4):168–173.
148. Clynes R, Dumitru C, Ravetch JV. Uncoupling of immune complex formation and kidney damage in autoimmune glomerulonephritis. *Science*. 1998;279(5353):1052–1054.

149. Schiffer L, Sinha J, Wang X, Huang W, Von Gonsdorff G, Schiffer M, et al. Short term administration of costimulatory blockade and cyclophosphamide induces remission of systemic lupus erythematosus nephritis in NZB/W F1 mice by a mechanism downstream of renal immune complex deposition. *The Journal of Immunology*. 2003;171(1):489–497.
150. Herrero C, Hu X, Li WP, Samuels S, Sharif MN, Kotenko S, et al. Reprogramming of IL-10 activity and signaling by IFN-γ. *The Journal of Immunology*. 2003;171(10):5034–5041.
151. Mocellin S, Marincola F, Rossi CR, Nitti D, Lise M. The multifaceted relationship between IL-10 and adaptive immunity: putting together the pieces of a puzzle. *Cytokine & growth factor reviews*. 2004;15(1):61–76.
152. Grohmann U, Puccetti P. The Immunosuppressive Activity of Proinflammatory Cytokines in Experimental Models Potential for Therapeutic Intervention in Autoimmunity. *Current Drug Targets-Inflammation & Allergy*. 2002;1(1):77–87.
153. Billiau A. Interferon-γ in autoimmunity. *Cytokine & growth factor reviews*. 1996;7(1):25–34.
154. Rosloniec EF, Latham K, Guedez YB. Paradoxical roles of IFN-γ in models of Th1-mediated autoimmunity. *Arthritis Research & Therapy*. 2002;4(6):333.
155. Valluru M, Staton CA, Reed MWR, Brown NJ. Transforming growth factor-β and endoglin signaling orchestrate wound healing. *Frontiers in physiology*. 2011;2:89.
156. Eming SA, Wynn TA, Martin P. Inflammation and metabolism in tissue repair and regeneration. *Science*. 2017;356(6342):1026–1030.
157. Wynn TA, Ramalingam TR. Mechanisms of fibrosis: therapeutic translation for fibrotic disease. *Nature medicine*. 2012;18(7):1028.
158. Friedman SL, Sheppard D, Duffield JS, Violette S. Therapy for fibrotic diseases: nearing the starting line. *Science translational medicine*. 2013;5(167):167sr1.
159. Hinz B. Tissue stiffness, latent TGF-β1 activation, and mechanical signal transduction: implications for the pathogenesis and treatment of fibrosis. *Current rheumatology reports*. 2009;11(2):120.
160. Huen SC, Cantley LG. Macrophages in renal injury and repair. *Annual review of physiology*. 2017;79:449–469.
161. Stamatiades EG, Tremblay M-E, Bohm M, Crozet L, Bisht K, Kao D, et al. Immune monitoring of trans-endothelial transport by kidney-resident macrophages. *Cell*. 2016;166(4):991–1003.
162. Miller F. Genetics of environmentally-associated rheumatic disease. *Rheumatic diseases and the environment London: Arnold*. 1999:33–45.
163. Miller FW, Alfredsson L, Costenbader KH, Kamen DL, Nelson LM, Norris JM, et al. Epidemiology of environmental exposures and human autoimmune diseases: findings from a National Institute of Environmental Health Sciences Expert Panel Workshop. *Journal of autoimmunity*. 2012;39(4): 259–271.
164. Pollard KM, Hultman P, Kono DH. Toxicology of autoimmune diseases. *Chemical research in toxicology*. 2010;23(3):455–466.
165. Gourley M, Miller FW. Mechanisms of disease: environmental factors in the pathogenesis of rheumatic disease. *Nature clinical practice Rheumatology*. 2007;3(3):172–180.
166. Cooper GS, Miller FW, Pandey JP. The role of genetic factors in autoimmune disease: implications for environmental research. *Environmental Health Perspectives*. 1999;107(suppl 5):693–700.
167. Meng W, Zhu Z, Jiang X, Too CL, Uebe S, Jagodic M, et al. DNA methylation mediates genotype and smoking interaction in the development of anti-citrullinated peptide antibody-positive rheumatoid arthritis. *Arthritis research & therapy*. 2017;19(1):1–10.
168. Javierre BM, Hernando H, Ballestar E. Environmental triggers and epigenetic deregulation in autoimmune disease. *Discovery medicine*. 2011;12(67):535–545.
169. Deane KD. Can rheumatoid arthritis be prevented? *Best practice & research Clinical rheumatology*. 2013;27(4):467–485.
170. Azar M, Rice DB, Kwakkenbos L, Carrier M-E, Shrier I, Bartlett SJ, et al. Exercise habits and factors associated with exercise in systemic sclerosis: a Scleroderma Patient-centered Intervention Network (SPIN) cohort study. *Disability and Rehabilitation*. 2018;40(17):1997–2003.
171. Pinto AJ, Roschel H, de Sá Pinto AL, Lima FR, Pereira RMR, Silva CA, et al. Physical inactivity and sedentary behavior: overlooked risk factors in autoimmune rheumatic diseases? *Autoimmunity reviews*. 2017;16(7):667–674.

172. Aqel SI, Hampton JM, Bruss M, Jones KT, Valiente GR, Wu l-C, et al. Daily moderate exercise is beneficial and social stress is detrimental to disease pathology in murine lupus nephritis. *Frontiers in physiology*. 2017;8:236.
173. Samuel S, Sitrin MD. Vitamin D's role in cell proliferation and differentiation. *Nutrition reviews*. 2008;66(suppl_2):S116–SS24.
174. Antico A, Tampoia M, Tozzoli R, Bizzaro N. Can supplementation with vitamin D reduce the risk or modify the course of autoimmune diseases? A systematic review of the literature. *Autoimmunity reviews*. 2012;12(2):127–136.
175. Agmon-Levin N, Theodor E, Segal RM, Shoenfeld Y. Vitamin D in systemic and organ-specific autoimmune diseases. *Clinical reviews in allergy & immunology*. 2013;45(2):256–266.
176. Watad A, Azrielant S, Bragazzi NL, Sharif K, David P, Katz I, et al. Seasonality and autoimmune diseases: the contribution of the four seasons to the mosaic of autoimmunity. *Journal of Autoimmunity*. 2017;82:13–30.
177. Zhang X, Wang W, Li Y, Wang H, Liu R, Zhu L. Serum 25-hydroxyvitamin D status in chinese children with vitiligo: a case-control study. *Clinical Pediatrics*. 2018;57(7):802–805.
178. Afridi HI, Kazi TG, Talpur FN, Naher S, Brabazon D. Relationship between toxic metals exposure via cigarette smoking and rheumatoid arthritis. *Clinical laboratory*. 2014;60(10):1735–1745.
179. Bang SY, Lee KH, Cho SK, Lee HS, Lee KW, Bae SC. Smoking increases rheumatoid arthritis susceptibility in individuals carrying the HLA–DRB1 shared epitope, regardless of rheumatoid factor or anti–cyclic citrullinated peptide antibody status. *Arthritis & Rheumatism: Official Journal of the American College of Rheumatology*. 2010;62(2):369–377.
180. Perricone C, Versini M, Ben-Ami D, Gertel S, Watad A, Segel MJ, et al. Smoke and autoimmunity: the fire behind the disease. *Autoimmunity reviews*. 2016;15(4):354–374.
181. Ospelt C, Camici GG, Engler A, Kolling C, Vogetseder A, Gay RE, et al. Smoking induces transcription of the heat shock protein system in the joints. *Annals of the rheumatic diseases*. 2014;73(7):1423–1426.
182. Klareskog L, Gregersen PK, Huizinga TW. Prevention of autoimmune rheumatic disease: state of the art and future perspectives. *Annals of the rheumatic diseases*. 2010;69(12):2062–2066.
183. Arnson Y, Shoenfeld Y, Amital H. Effects of tobacco smoke on immunity, inflammation and autoimmunity. *Journal of autoimmunity*. 2010;34(3):J258–JJ65.
184. Chinoy H, Adimulam S, Marriage F, New P, Vincze M, Zilahi E, et al. Interaction of HLA-DRB1* 03 and smoking for the development of anti-Jo-1 antibodies in adult idiopathic inflammatory myopathies: a European-wide case study. *Annals of the rheumatic diseases*. 2012;71(6):961–965.
185. Lilleker JB, Vencovsky J, Wang G, Wedderburn LR, Diederichsen LP, Schmidt J, et al. The EuroMyositis registry: an international collaborative tool to facilitate myositis research. *Annals of the rheumatic diseases*. 2018;77(1):30–39.
186. Mongey A-B, Hess EV. Drug-related lupus. *Current opinion in rheumatology*. 1989;1(3):353–359.
187. Elenkov IJ, Chrousos GP. Stress, cytokine patterns and susceptibility to disease. *Best Practice & Research Clinical Endocrinology & Metabolism*. 1999;13(4):583–595.
188. Winsa B, Adami H-O, Bergstrom R, Gamstedt A, Dahlberg PA, Adamson U, et al. Stressful life events and Graves' disease. *The Lancet*. 1991;338(8781):1475–1479.
189. Wiersinga WM. Clinical relevance of environmental factors in the pathogenesis of autoimmune thyroid disease. *Endocrinology and Metabolism*. 2016;31(2):213–222.
190. Vita R, Lapa D, Trimarchi F, Vita G, Fallahi P, Antonelli A, et al. Certain HLA alleles are associated with stress-triggered Graves' disease and influence its course. *Endocrine*. 2017;55(1):93–100.
191. Faresjo M. The link between psychological stress and autoimmune response in children. *Critical Reviews™ in Immunology*. 2015;35(2).
192. van der Laan JW, Gould S, Tanir JY, Committee ASP. Safety of vaccine adjuvants: focus on autoimmunity. *Vaccine*. 2015;33(13):1507–1514.
193. Robinson CL, Bernstein H, Romero JR, Szilagyi P. Advisory Committee on Immunization Practices recommended immunization schedule for children and adolescents aged 18 years or younger—United States, 2019. *Morbidity and Mortality Weekly Report*. 2019;68(5):112.
194. Atarashi K, Honda K. Microbiota in autoimmunity and tolerance. *Current opinion in immunology*. 2011;23(6):761–768.

195. Fung TC, Olson CA, Hsiao EY. Interactions between the microbiota, immune and nervous systems in health and disease. *Nature neuroscience*. 2017;20(2):145.
196. Paun A, Yau C, Danska JS. The influence of the microbiome on type 1 diabetes. *The Journal of Immunology*. 2017;198(2):590–595.
197. Rosser EC, Mauri C. A clinical update on the significance of the gut microbiota in systemic autoimmunity. *Journal of autoimmunity*. 2016;74:85–93.
198. Kau AL, Ahern PP, Griffin NW, Goodman AL, Gordon JI. Human nutrition, the gut microbiome and the immune system. *Nature*. 2011;474(7351):327–336.
199. Turnbaugh PJ, Ley RE, Mahowald MA, Magrini V, Mardis ER, Gordon JI. An obesity-associated gut microbiome with increased capacity for energy harvest. *nature*. 2006;444(7122):1027.
200. Macia L, Tan J, Vieira AT, Leach K, Stanley D, Luong S, et al. Metabolite-sensing receptors GPR43 and GPR109A facilitate dietary fibre-induced gut homeostasis through regulation of the inflammasome. *Nature communications*. 2015;6:6734.
201. Rook GA, Martinelli R, Brunet LR. Innate immune responses to mycobacteria and the downregulation of atopic responses. *Current opinion in allergy and clinical immunology*. 2003;3(5):337–342.
202. Noverr MC, Huffnagle GB. Does the microbiota regulate immune responses outside the gut? *Trends in microbiology*. 2004;12(12):562–568.
203. Talotta R, Atzeni F, Ditto MC, Gerardi MC, Sarzi-Puttini P. The microbiome in connective tissue diseases and vasculitides: an updated narrative review. *Journal of Immunology Research*. 2017;2017.
204. Shahi SK, Freedman SN, Mangalam AK. Gut microbiome in multiple sclerosis: the players involved and the roles they play. *Gut microbes*. 2017;8(6):607–615.
205. Maeda Y, Takeda K. Role of gut microbiota in rheumatoid arthritis. *Journal of clinical medicine*. 2017;6(6):60.
206. Scher JU, Abramson SB. The microbiome and rheumatoid arthritis. *Nature Reviews Rheumatology*. 2011;7(10):569.
207. Van de Wiele T, Van Praet JT, Marzorati M, Drennan MB. Elewaut D. How the microbiota shapes rheumatic diseases. *Nature Reviews Rheumatology*. 2016;12(7):398.
208. Vatanen T, Kostic AD, d'Hennezel E, Siljander H, Franzosa EA, Yassour M, et al. Variation in microbiome LPS immunogenicity contributes to autoimmunity in humans. *Cell*. 2016;165(4):842–853.
209. Vaarala O, Atkinson MA, Neu J. The "perfect storm" for type 1 diabetes: the complex interplay between intestinal microbiota, gut permeability, and mucosal immunity. *Diabetes*. 2008;57(10):2555–2562.
210. Endesfelder D, zu Castell W, Ardissone A, Davis-Richardson AG, Achenbach P, Hagen M, et al. Compromised gut microbiota networks in children with anti-islet cell autoimmunity. *Diabetes*. 2014;63(6):2006–2014.
211. De Goffau MC, Luopajärvi K, Knip M, Ilonen J, Ruohtula T, Härkönen T, et al. Fecal microbiota composition differs between children with β-cell autoimmunity and those without. *Diabetes*. 2013;62(4):1238–1244.
212. Huttenhower C, Kostic AD, Xavier RJ. Inflammatory bowel disease as a model for translating the microbiome. *Immunity*. 2014;40(6):843–854.
213. Jostins L, Ripke S, Weersma RK, Duerr RH, McGovern DP, Hui KY, et al. Host–microbe interactions have shaped the genetic architecture of inflammatory bowel disease. *Nature*. 2012;491(7422):119–124.
214. Collado MC, Donat E, Ribes-Koninckx C, Calabuig M, Sanz Y. Specific duodenal and faecal bacterial groups associated with paediatric coeliac disease. *Journal of clinical pathology*. 2009;62(3):264–269.
215. Vieira SM, Pagovich OE, Kriegel MA. Diet, microbiota and autoimmune diseases. *Lupus*. 2014;23(6):518–526.
216. Maslowski KM, Mackay CR. Diet, gut microbiota and immune responses. *Nature immunology*. 2011;12(1):5–9.
217. McKenzie C, Tan J, Macia L, Mackay CR. The nutrition-gut microbiome-physiology axis and allergic diseases. *Immunological reviews*. 2017;278(1):277–295.
218. Maslowski KM, Vieira AT, Ng A, Kranich J, Sierro F, Yu D, et al. Regulation of inflammatory responses by gut microbiota and chemoattractant receptor GPR43. *Nature*. 2009;461(7268):1282–1286.
219. Trompette A, Gollwitzer ES, Yadava K, Sichelstiel AK, Sprenger N, Ngom-Bru C, et al. Gut microbiota metabolism of dietary fiber influences allergic airway disease and hematopoiesis. *Nature medicine*. 2014;20(2):159–166.

220. Manzel A, Muller DN, Hafler DA, Erdman SE, Linker RA, Kleinewietfeld M. Role of "Western diet" in inflammatory autoimmune diseases. *Current allergy and asthma reports*. 2014;14(1):404.
221. Alaedini A, Green PH. Narrative review: celiac disease: understanding a complex autoimmune disorder. *Annals of internal medicine*. 2005;142(4):289–298.
222. Mackay IR, Rose NR. *The Autoimmune Diseases*: Elsevier Inc.; 2013.
223. James JA, Robertson JM. Lupus and epstein-barr. *Current opinion in rheumatology*. 2012;24(4):383.
224. Yuki N. Pathogenesis of Guillain-Barre and Miller Fisher syndromes subsequent to Campylobacter jejuni enteritis. *Japanese journal of infectious diseases*. 1999;52(3):99–105.
225. Galvin JE, Hemric ME, Ward K, Cunningham MW. Cytotoxic mAb from rheumatic carditis recognizes heart valves and laminin. *The Journal of clinical investigation*. 2000;106(2):217–224.
226. Guilherme L, Cunha-Neto E, Coelho V, Snitcowsky R, Pomerantzeff P, Assis R, et al. Human heart–infiltrating T-Cell clones from rheumatic heart disease patients recognize both streptococcal and cardiac proteins. *Circulation*. 1995;92(3):415–420.
227. Malkiel S, Liao L, Cunningham MW, Diamond B. T-cell-dependent antibody response to the dominant epitope of streptococcal polysaccharide, N-acetyl-glucosamine, is cross-reactive with cardiac myosin. *Infection and immunity*. 2000;68(10):5803–5808.
228. Guilherme L, Kalil J. Rheumatic fever: from sore throat to autoimmune heart lesions. *International archives of allergy and immunology*. 2004;134(1):56–64.
229. Kuon W, Sieper J. Identification of HLA-B27–restricted peptides in reactive arthritis and other spondyloarthropathies: computer algorithms and fluorescent activated cell sorting analysis as tools for hunting of HLA-B27 restricted chlamydial and autologous crossreactive peptides involved in reactive arthritis and ankylosing spondylitis. *Rheumatic Disease Clinics*. 2003;29(3):595–611.
230. Strassburg CP, Vogel A, Manns MP. Autoimmunity and hepatitis C. *Autoimmunity reviews*. 2003;2(6):322–331.
231. Shlomchik MJ, Craft JE, Mamula MJ. From T to B and back again: positive feedback in systemic autoimmune disease. *Nature Reviews Immunology*. 2001;1(2):147–153.
232. Melki I, Crow YJ. Novel monogenic diseases causing human autoimmunity. *Current opinion in immunology*. 2015;37:1–5.
233. Ulmanen I, Halonen M, Ilmarinen T, Peltonen L. Monogenic autoimmune diseases—Lessons of self-tolerance. *Current opinion in immunology*. 2005;17(6):609–615.
234. Ahonen P, Myllärniemi S, Sipilä I, Perheentupa J. Clinical variation of autoimmune polyendocrinopathy–candidiasis–ectodermal dystrophy (APECED) in a series of 68 patients. *New England Journal of Medicine*. 1990;322(26):1829–1836.
235. Barrera M, Bahamondes V, Sepulveda D, Quest AF, Castro I, Cortés J, et al. Sjögren's syndrome and the epithelial target: a comprehensive review. *Journal of autoimmunity*. 2013;42:7–18.
236. Endo T, Kobayashi T. Immunization of mice with a newly identified thyroid-stimulating hormone receptor splice variant induces Graves'-like disease. *Journal of autoimmunity*. 2013;43:18–25.
237. Nagamine K, Peterson P, Scott HS, Kudoh J, Minoshima S, Heino M, et al. Positional cloning of the APECED gene. *Nature genetics*. 1997;17(4):393–398.
238. Akirav EM, Ruddle NH, Herold KC. The role of AIRE in human autoimmune disease. *Nature Reviews Endocrinology*. 2011;7(1):25–33.
239. Le Deist F, Emile J-F, Rieux-Laucat F, Benkerrou M, Roberts I, Brousse N, et al. Clinical, immunological, and pathological consequences of Fas-deficient conditions. *The Lancet*. 1996;348(9029):719–723.
240. Grodzicky T, Elkon KB. Apoptosis: a case where too much or too little can lead to autoimmunity. The Mount Sinai journal of medicine. *New York*. 2002;69(4):208.
241. Fleisher TA, Straus SE, Bleesing JJ. A genetic disorder of lymphocyte apoptosis involving the fas pathway: the autoimmune lymphoproliferative syndrome. *Current Allergy and Asthma Reports*. 2001;1(6):534–540.
242. Madkaikar M, Mhatre S, Gupta M, Ghosh K. Advances in autoimmune lymphoproliferative syndromes. *European journal of haematology*. 2011;87(1):1–9.
243. Gambineri E, Torgerson TR, Ochs HD. Immune dysregulation, polyendocrinopathy, enteropathy, and X-linked inheritance (IPEX), a syndrome of systemic autoimmunity caused by mutations of FOXP3, a critical regulator of T-cell homeostasis. *Current opinion in rheumatology*. 2003;15(4):430–435.
244. Sakaguchi S. Naturally arising Foxp3-expressing CD25+ CD4+ regulatory T cells in immunological tolerance to self and non-self. *Nature immunology*. 2005;6(4):345–352.

245. Deng Y, Tsao BP. Genetic susceptibility to systemic lupus erythematosus in the genomic era. *Nature Reviews Rheumatology*. 2010;6(12):683.
246. Harley JB, Alarcón-Riquelme ME, Criswell LA, CO Jacob, Kimberly RP, Moser KL, et al. Genome-wide association scan in women with systemic lupus erythematosus identifies susceptibility variants in ITGAM, PXK, KIAA1542 and other loci. *Nature genetics*. 2008;40(2):204–210.
247. Flesher DLT, Sun X, Behrens TW, Graham RR, Criswell LA. Recent advances in the genetics of systemic lupus erythematosus. *Expert review of clinical immunology*. 2010;6(3):461.
248. Sollid LM, Pos W, Wucherpfennig KW. Molecular mechanisms for contribution of MHC molecules to autoimmune diseases. *Current opinion in immunology*. 2014;31:24–30.
249. Wang L, Wang FS, Gershwin ME. Human autoimmune diseases: a comprehensive update. *Journal of internal medicine*. 2015;278(4):369–395.
250. Hu X, Daly M. What have we learned from six years of GWAS in autoimmune diseases, and what is next? *Current opinion in immunology*. 2012;24(5):571–575.
251. Ueda H, Howson JM, Esposito L, Heward J, Chamberlain G, Rainbow DB, et al. Association of the T-cell regulatory gene CTLA4 with susceptibility to autoimmune disease. *Nature*. 2003;423(6939):506–511.
252. Kottyan LC, Zoller EE, Bene J, Lu X, Kelly JA, Rupert AM, et al. The IRF5–TNPO3 association with systemic lupus erythematosus has two components that other autoimmune disorders variably share. *Human molecular genetics*. 2015;24(2):582–596.
253. Zaki MH, Lamkanfi M, Kanneganti T-D. The Nlrp3 inflammasome: contributions to intestinal homeostasis. *Trends in immunology*. 2011;32(4):171–179.
254. Russell RK, Nimmo ER, Satsangi J. Molecular genetics of Crohn's disease. *Current opinion in genetics & development*. 2004;14(3):264–270.
255. Rahman P, Bartlett S, Siannis F, Pellett F, Farewell V, Peddle L, et al. CARD15: a pleiotropic autoimmune gene that confers susceptibility to psoriatic arthritis. *The American Journal of Human Genetics*. 2003;73(3):677–681.
256. Bene L, Falus A, Baffy N, Fulop AK. Cellular and molecular mechanisms in the two major forms of inflammatory bowel disease. *Pathology & Oncology Research*. 2011;17(3):463.
257. Burn GL, Svensson L, Sanchez-Blanco C, Saini M, Cope AP. Why is PTPN22 a good candidate susceptibility gene for autoimmune disease? *FEBS letters*. 2011;585(23):3689–3698.
258. Zhernakova A, Withoff S, Wijmenga C. Clinical implications of shared genetics and pathogenesis in autoimmune diseases. *Nature Reviews Endocrinology*. 2013;9(11):646–659.
259. Achenbach P, Hummel M, Thümer L, Boerschmann H, Höfelmann D, Ziegler A. Characteristics of rapid vs slow progression to type 1 diabetes in multiple islet autoantibody-positive children. *Diabetologia*. 2013;56(7):1615–1622.
260. Lempainen J, Laine A-P, Hammais A, Toppari J, Simell O, Veijola R, et al. Non-HLA gene effects on the disease process of type 1 diabetes: from HLA susceptibility to overt disease. *Journal of autoimmunity*. 2015;61:45–53.
261. Laufer VA, Chen JY, Langefeld CD, Bridges SL. Integrative approaches to understanding the pathogenic role of genetic variation in rheumatic diseases. *Rheumatic Disease Clinics*. 2017;43(3):449–466.
262. Langefeld CD, Ainsworth HC, Graham DSC, Kelly JA, Comeau ME, Marion MC, et al. Transancestral mapping and genetic load in systemic lupus erythematosus. *Nature communications*. 2017;8(1):1–18.
263. Quintero-Ronderos P, Montoya-Ortiz G. Epigenetics and autoimmune diseases. *Autoimmune diseases*. 2012;2012.
264. Zouali M. *The Epigenetics of Autoimmune Diseases*: John Wiley & Sons; 2009.
265. Feil R, Fraga MF. Epigenetics and the environment: emerging patterns and implications. *Nature reviews genetics*. 2012;13(2):97–109.
266. Wang Z, Zheng Y, Hou C, Yang L, Li X, Lin J, et al. DNA methylation impairs TLR9 induced Foxp3 expression by attenuating IRF-7 binding activity in fulminant type 1 diabetes. *Journal of autoimmunity*. 2013;41:50–59.
267. Long H, Yin H, Wang L, Gershwin ME, Lu Q. The critical role of epigenetics in systemic lupus erythematosus and autoimmunity. *Journal of autoimmunity*. 2016;74:118–138.
268. Tost J, Gay S, Firestein G. Epigenetics of the immune system and alterations in inflammation and autoimmunity. *Future Medicine*. 2017.

269. Calabrese R, Zampieri M, Mechelli R, Annibali V, Guastafierro T, Ciccarone F, et al. Methylation-dependent PAD2 upregulation in multiple sclerosis peripheral blood. *Multiple Sclerosis Journal*. 2012;18(3):299–304.
270. Kumagai C, Kalman B, Middleton FA, Vyshkina T, Massa PT. Increased promoter methylation of the immune regulatory gene SHP-1 in leukocytes of multiple sclerosis subjects. *Journal of neuroimmunology*. 2012;246(1–2):51–57.
271. Young DA, Lakey RL, Pennington CJ, Jones D, Kevorkian L, Edwards DR, et al. Histone deacetylase inhibitors modulate metalloproteinase gene expression in chondrocytes and block cartilage resorption. *Arthritis research & therapy*. 2005;7(3):R503.
272. Fradin D, Le Fur S, Mille C, Naoui N, Groves C, Zelenika D, et al. Association of the CpG methylation pattern of the proximal insulin gene promoter with type 1 diabetes. *PloS one*. 2012;7(5):e36278.
273. Yamamura Y, Motegi K, Kani K, Takano H, Momota Y, Aota K, et al. TNF-α inhibits aquaporin 5 expression in human salivary gland acinar cells via suppression of histone H4 acetylation. *Journal of cellular and molecular medicine*. 2012;16(8):1766–1775.
274. Lleo A, Liao J, Invernizzi P, Zhao M, Bernuzzi F, Ma L, et al. Immunoglobulin M levels inversely correlate with CD40 ligand promoter methylation in patients with primary biliary cirrhosis. *Hepatology*. 2012;55(1):153–160.
275. Pauley KM, Cha S, Chan EK. MicroRNA in autoimmunity and autoimmune diseases. *Journal of autoimmunity*. 2009;32(3–4):189–194.
276. Xu W-D, Pan H-F, Li J-H, Ye d-Q. MicroRNA-21 with therapeutic potential in autoimmune diseases. *Expert opinion on therapeutic targets*. 2013;17(6):659–665.
277. Qu Z, Li W, Fu B. MicroRNAs in autoimmune diseases. *BioMed Research International*. 2014;2014.
278. Hu N, Qiu X, Luo Y, Yuan J, Li Y, Lei W, et al. Abnormal histone modification patterns in lupus CD4+ T cells. *The Journal of rheumatology*. 2008;35(5):804–810.
279. Hermansen M-LF, Lindhardsen J, Torp-Pedersen C, Faurschou M, Jacobsen S. Incidence of systemic lupus erythematosus and lupus nephritis in Denmark: a nationwide cohort study. *The Journal of Rheumatology*. 2016;43(7):1335–1339.
280. Chiu Y, Lai C. Nationwide population-based epidemiologic study of systemic lupus erythematosus in Taiwan. *Lupus*. 2010;19(10):1250–1255.
281. Somers EC, Marder W, Cagnoli P, Lewis EE, DeGuire P, Gordon C, et al. Population-based incidence and prevalence of systemic lupus erythematosus: the Michigan Lupus Epidemiology and Surveillance program. *Arthritis & rheumatology*. 2014;66(2):369–378.
282. Rees F, Doherty M, Grainge M, Davenport G, Lanyon P, Zhang W. The incidence and prevalence of systemic lupus erythematosus in the UK, 1999–2012. *Annals of the rheumatic diseases*. 2016;75(1):136–141.
283. Feldman CH, Hiraki LT, Liu J, Fischer MA, Solomon DH, Alarcón GS, et al. Epidemiology and sociodemographics of systemic lupus erythematosus and lupus nephritis among US adults with Medicaid coverage, 2000–2004. *Arthritis & Rheumatism*. 2013;65(3):753–763.
284. Johnson AE, Gordon C, Palmer RG, Bacon PA. The prevalence and incidence of systemic lupus erythematosus in Birmingham, England. *Arthritis & Rheumatism: Official Journal of the American College of Rheumatology*. 1995;38(4):551–558.
285. Rezaei A, Harsini S, Sadr M, Ziaee V, Rezaei N. Interleukin-23 receptor gene polymorphisms in Iranian patients with juvenile systemic lupus erythematosus. *Allergol Immunopathol (Madr)*. 2020;48(1):62–66.
286. Harsini S, Ziaee V, Tahghighi F, Mahmoudi M, Rezaei A, Soltani S, et al. Association of interleukin-2 and interferon-γ single nucleotide polymorphisms with Juvenile systemic lupus erythematosus. *Allergol Immunopathol (Madr)*. 2016;44(5):422–426.
287. Mahmoudi M, Rezaiemanesh A, Salmaninejad A, Harsini S, Poursani S, Bahrami T, et al. PDCD1 single nucleotide genes polymorphisms confer susceptibility to juvenile-onset systemic lupus erythematosus. *Autoimmunity*. 2015;48(7):488–493.
288. Rezaei A, Ziaee V, Sharabian FT, Harsini S, Mahmoudi M, Soltani S, et al. Lack of association between interleukin-10, transforming growth factor-beta gene polymorphisms and juvenile-onset systemic lupus erythematosus. *Clin Rheumatol*. 2015;34(6):1059–1064.
289. Tahghighi F, Ziaee V, Moradinejad MH, Rezaei A, Harsini S, Soltani S, et al. Tumor necrosis factor-alpha single nucleotide polymorphisms in juvenile systemic lupus erythematosus. *Hum Immunol*. 2015;76(8):533–536.

290. Mahmoudi M, Tahghighi F, Ziaee V, Harsini S, Rezaei A, Soltani S, et al. Interleukin-4 single nucleotide polymorphisms in juvenile systemic lupus erythematosus. *Int J Immunogenet*. 2014;41(6):512–517.
291. Ziaee V, Tahghighi F, Moradinejad MH, Harsini S, Mahmoudi M, Rezaei A, et al. Interleukin-6, interleukin-1 gene cluster and interleukin-1 receptor polymorphisms in Iranian patients with juvenile systemic lupus erythematosus. *Eur Cytokine Netw*. 2014;25(2):35–40.
292. Alarcón-Segovia D, Alarcón-Riquelme ME, Cardiel MH, Caeiro F, Massardo L, Villa AR, et al. Familial aggregation of systemic lupus erythematosus, rheumatoid arthritis, and other autoimmune diseases in 1,177 lupus patients from the GLADEL cohort. *Arthritis & Rheumatism*. 2005;52(4):1138–1147.
293. Deafen D, Escalante A, Weinrib L, Horwitz D, Bachman B, Roy-Burman P, et al. A revised estimate of twin concordance in systemic lupus erythematosus. *Arthritis & Rheumatism: Official Journal of the American College of Rheumatology*. 1992;35(3):311–318.
294. Lee-Kirsch MA, Gong M, Chowdhury D, Senenko L, Engel K, Lee Y-A, et al. Mutations in the gene encoding the 3′-5′ DNA exonuclease TREX1 are associated with systemic lupus erythematosus. *Nature genetics*. 2007;39(9):1065–1067.
295. Stetson DB, Ko JS, Heidmann T, Medzhitov R. Trex1 prevents cell-intrinsic initiation of autoimmunity. *Cell*. 2008;134(4):587–598.
296. Lo MS. Monogenic lupus. *Current rheumatology reports*. 2016;18(12):71.
297. Morris DL, Sheng Y, Zhang Y, Wang Y-F, Zhu Z, Tombleson P, et al. Genome-wide association meta-analysis in Chinese and European individuals identifies ten new loci associated with systemic lupus erythematosus. *Nature genetics*. 2016;48(8):940.
298. Hom G, Graham RR, Modrek B, Taylor KE, Ortmann W, Garnier S, et al. Association of systemic lupus erythematosus with C8orf13–BLK and ITGAM–ITGAX. *New England Journal of Medicine*. 2008;358(9):900–909.
299. Kozyrev SV, Abelson A-K, Wojcik J, Zaghlool A, Reddy MPL, Sanchez E, et al. Functional variants in the B-cell gene BANK1 are associated with systemic lupus erythematosus. *Nature genetics*. 2008;40(2):211.
300. Han J-W, Zheng H-F, Cui Y, Sun l-D, Ye d-Q, Hu Z, et al. Genome-wide association study in a Chinese Han population identifies nine new susceptibility loci for systemic lupus erythematosus. *Nature genetics*. 2009;41(11):1234–1237.
301. Yang W, Shen N, Ye d-Q, Liu Q, Zhang Y, Qian X-X, et al. Genome-wide association study in Asian populations identifies variants in ETS1 and WDFY4 associated with systemic lupus erythematosus. *PLoS Genet*. 2010;6(2):e1000841.
302. Autoantibody explosion in systemic lupus erythematosus: more than 100 different antibodies found in SLE patients. In: Sherer Y, Gorstein A, Fritzler MJ, Shoenfeld Y, eds. Autoantibody explosion in systemic lupus erythematosus: more than 100 different antibodies found in SLE patients. *Seminars in arthritis and rheumatism*. 2004.
303. Mariz HA, Sato EI, Barbosa SH, Rodrigues SH, Dellavance A, Andrade LE. Pattern on the antinuclear antibody–HEp-2 test is a critical parameter for discriminating antinuclear antibody–positive healthy individuals and patients with autoimmune rheumatic diseases. *Arthritis & Rheumatism*. 2011;63(1):191–200.
304. Brinkmann V, Reichard U, Goosmann C, Fauler B, Uhlemann Y, Weiss DS, et al. Neutrophil extracellular traps kill bacteria. *science*. 2004;303(5663):1532–1535.
305. Moulton VR, Suarez-Fueyo A, Meidan E, Li H, Mizui M, Tsokos GC. Pathogenesis of human systemic lupus erythematosus: a cellular perspective. *Trends in molecular medicine*. 2017;23(7):615–635.
306. Arbuckle MR, McClain MT, Rubertone MV, Scofield RH, Dennis GJ, James JA, et al. Development of autoantibodies before the clinical onset of systemic lupus erythematosus. *New England Journal of Medicine*. 2003;349(16):1526–1533.
307. Malkiel S, Jeganathan V, Wolfson S, Manjarrez Orduño N, Marasco E, Aranow C, et al. Checkpoints for autoreactive B cells in the peripheral blood of lupus patients assessed by flow cytometry. *Arthritis & rheumatology*. 2016;68(9):2210–2220.
308. Yurasov S, Wardemann H, Hammersen J, Tsuiji M, Meffre E, Pascual V, et al. Defective B cell tolerance checkpoints in systemic lupus erythematosus. *The Journal of experimental medicine*. 2005;201(5):703–711.

309. Zucchi D, Elefante E, Calabresi E, Signorini V, Bortoluzzi A, Tani C. One year in review 2019: systemic lupus erythematosus. *Clin Exp Rheumatol*. 2019;37(5):715–722.
310. Fortuna G, Brennan MT. Systemic lupus erythematosus: epidemiology, pathophysiology, manifestations, and management. *Dental Clinics*. 2013;57(4):631–655.
311. Hahn BH, Mcmahon MA, Wilkinson A, Wallace WD, Daikh DI, Fitzgerald JD, et al. American College of Rheumatology guidelines for screening, treatment, and management of lupus nephritis. *Arthritis care & research*. 2012;64(6):797–808.
312. Bertsias GK, Tektonidou M, Amoura Z, Aringer M, Bajema I, Berden JH, et al. Joint European League Against Rheumatism and European Renal Association–European Dialysis and Transplant Association (EULAR/ERA-EDTA) recommendations for the management of adult and paediatric lupus nephritis. *Annals of the rheumatic diseases*. 2012;71(11):1771–1782.
313. Mackay IR, Rose NR. *The Autoimmune Diseases, 6th*: Elsevier Science & Technology; 2019.
314. Clusters of clinical and immunologic features in systemic lupus erythematosus: analysis of 600 patients from a single center. In: Font J, Cervera R, Ramos-Casals M, García-Carrasco M, Sentís J, Herrero C et al, eds. Clusters of clinical and immunologic features in systemic lupus erythematosus: analysis of 600 patients from a single center. *Seminars in arthritis and rheumatism*. 2004.
315. Ruiz-Irastorza G, Egurbide MV, Pijoan JI, Garmendia M, Villar I, Martinez-Berriotxoa A, et al. Effect of antimalarials on thrombosis and survival in patients with systemic lupus erythematosus. *Lupus*. 2006;15(9):577–583.
316. Alarcón GS, McGwin G, Bertoli AM, Fessler BJ, Calvo-Alén J, Bastian HM, et al. Effect of hydroxychloroquine on the survival of patients with systemic lupus erythematosus: data from LUMINA, a multiethnic US cohort (LUMINA L). *Ann Rheum Dis*. 2007;66(9):1168–1172.
317. Costedoat-Chalumeau N, Galicier L, Aumaître O, Francès C, Le Guern V, Lioté F, et al. Hydroxychloroquine in systemic lupus erythematosus: results of a French multicentre controlled trial (PLUS Study). *Ann Rheum Dis*. 2013;72(11):1786–1792.
318. Marmor MF, Kellner U, Lai TY, Melles RB, Mieler WF. Recommendations on Screening for Chloroquine and Hydroxychloroquine Retinopathy (2016 Revision). *Ophthalmology*. 2016;123(6):1386–1394.
319. Griffiths B, Emery P, Ryan V, Isenberg D, Akil M, Thompson R, et al. The BILAG multi-centre open randomized controlled trial comparing ciclosporin vs azathioprine in patients with severe SLE. *Rheumatology (Oxford)*. 2010;49(4):723–732.
320. Appel GB, Contreras G, Dooley MA, Ginzler EM, Isenberg D, Jayne D, et al. Mycophenolate mofetil versus cyclophosphamide for induction treatment of lupus nephritis. *Journal of the American Society of Nephrology*. 2009;20(5):1103–1112.
321. Ginzler EM, Dooley MA, Aranow C, Kim MY, Buyon J, Merrill JT, et al. Mycophenolate mofetil or intravenous cyclophosphamide for lupus nephritis. *New England Journal of Medicine*. 2005;353(21):2219–2228.
322. Mok CC, Ying KY, Yim CW, Siu YP, Tong KH, To CH, et al. Tacrolimus versus mycophenolate mofetil for induction therapy of lupus nephritis: a randomised controlled trial and long-term follow-up. *Annals of the rheumatic diseases*. 2016;75(1):30–36.
323. Gourley MF, Austin III HA, Scott D, Yarboro CH, Vaughan EM, Muir J, et al. Methylprednisolone and cyclophosphamide, alone or in combination, in patients with lupus nephritis: a randomized, controlled trial. *Annals of internal medicine*. 1996;125(7):549–557.
324. Smith K, Jones R, Burns S, Jayne D. Long-term comparison of rituximab treatment for refractory systemic lupus erythematosus and vasculitis: remission, relapse, and re-treatment. *Arthritis & Rheumatism*. 2006;54(9):2970–2982.
325. Navarra SV, Guzmán RM, Gallacher AE, Hall S, Levy RA, Jimenez RE, et al. Efficacy and safety of belimumab in patients with active systemic lupus erythematosus: a randomised, placebo-controlled, phase 3 trial. *The Lancet*. 2011;377(9767):721–731.
326. Isenberg D, Gordon C, Licu D, Copt S, Rossi CP, Wofsy D. Efficacy and safety of atacicept for prevention of flares in patients with moderate-to-severe systemic lupus erythematosus (SLE): 52-week data (APRIL-SLE randomised trial). *Annals of the rheumatic diseases*. 2015;74(11):2006–2015.
327. Wang D, Zhang H, Liang J, Wang H, Hua B, Feng X, et al. A long-term follow-up study of allogeneic mesenchymal stem/stromal cell transplantation in patients with drug-resistant systemic lupus erythematosus. *Stem Cell Reports*. 2018;10(3):933–941.

328. Kronbichler A, Brezina B, Quintana LF, Jayne DR. Efficacy of plasma exchange and immunoadsorption in systemic lupus erythematosus and antiphospholipid syndrome: a systematic review. *Autoimmunity reviews*. 2016;15(1):38–49.
329. Jayne D, Tyndall A. Autologous stem cell transplantation for systemic lupus erythematosus. *Lupus*. 2004;13(5):359–365.
330. Van Vollenhoven R, Hahn B, Tsokos G, Wagner C, Lipsky P, Hsu B. Efficacy and safety of ustekinumab, an interleukin 12/23 inhibitor, in patients with active systemic lupus erythematosus: results of a phase 2, randomized placebo-controlled study. *Arthritis Rheumatol*. 2017;69(suppl):10.
331. Clowse ME, Wallace DJ, Furie RA, Petri MA, Pike MC, Leszczyński P, et al. Efficacy and safety of epratuzumab in moderately to severely active systemic lupus erythematosus: results from two phase III randomized, double-blind, placebo-controlled trials. *Arthritis & rheumatology*. 2017;69(2):362–375.
332. Khamashta M, Merrill JT, Werth VP, Furie R, Kalunian K, Illei GG, et al. Sifalimumab, an anti-interferon-α monoclonal antibody, in moderate to severe systemic lupus erythematosus: a randomised, double-blind, placebo-controlled study. *Annals of the rheumatic diseases*. 2016;75(11):1909–1916.
333. Kalunian KC, Merrill JT, Maciuca R, McBride JM, Townsend MJ, Wei X, et al. A Phase II study of the efficacy and safety of rontalizumab (rhuMAb interferon-α) in patients with systemic lupus erythematosus (ROSE). *Annals of the rheumatic diseases*. 2016;75(1):196–202.
334. Furie R, Khamashta M, Merrill JT, Werth VP, Kalunian K, Brohawn P, et al. Anifrolumab, an anti–interferon-α receptor monoclonal antibody, in moderate-to-severe systemic lupus erythematosus. *Arthritis & rheumatology*. 2017;69(2):376–386.
335. Alexander T, Sarfert R, Klotsche J, Kühl AA, Rubbert-Roth A, Lorenz H-M, et al. The proteasome inhibitior bortezomib depletes plasma cells and ameliorates clinical manifestations of refractory systemic lupus erythematosus. *Annals of the rheumatic diseases*. 2015;74(7):1474–1478.
336. Silman AJ, Pearson JE. Epidemiology and genetics of rheumatoid arthritis. *Arthritis research & therapy*. 2002;4(S3):S265.
337. Eriksson JK, Neovius M, Ernestam S, Lindblad S, Simard JF, Askling J. Incidence of rheumatoid arthritis in Sweden: a nationwide population-based assessment of incidence, its determinants, and treatment penetration. *Arthritis care & research*. 2013;65(6):870–878.
338. Helmick CG, Felson DT, Lawrence RC, Gabriel S, Hirsch R, Kwoh CK, et al. Estimates of the prevalence of arthritis and other rheumatic conditions in the United States: part I. *Arthritis & Rheumatism*. 2008;58(1):15–25.
339. Uhlig T, Hagen K, Kvien T. Current tobacco smoking, formal education, and the risk of rheumatoid arthritis. *The Journal of rheumatology*. 1999;26(1):47–54.
340. Packard CJ, Bezlyak V, McLean JS, Batty GD, Ford I, Burns H, et al. Early life socioeconomic adversity is associated in adult life with chronic inflammation, carotid atherosclerosis, poorer lung function and decreased cognitive performance: a cross-sectional, population-based study. *BMC public health*. 2011;11(1):42.
341. Callahan LF, Pincus T. Education, self-care, and outcomes of rheumatic diseases: further challenges to the "biomedical model" paradigm. *Arthritis & Rheumatism: Official Journal of the American College of Rheumatology*. 1997;10(5):283–288.
342. Symmons DP, Bankhead CR, Harrison BJ, Brennan P, Silman AJ, Barrett EM, et al. Blood transfusion, smoking, and obesity as risk factors for the development of rheumatoid arthritis. Results from a primary care-based incident case-control study in Norfolk, England. *Arthritis & Rheumatism: Official Journal of the American College of Rheumatology*. 1997;40(11):1955–1961.
343. Mattey DL, Dawes PT, Clarke S, Fisher J, Brownfield A, Thomson W, et al. Relationship among the HLA–DRB1 shared epitope, smoking, and rheumatoid factor production in rheumatoid arthritis. *Arthritis Care & Research*. 2002;47(4):403–407.
344. Glossop J, Dawes P, Mattey D. Association between cigarette smoking and release of tumour necrosis factor α and its soluble receptors by peripheral blood mononuclear cells in patients with rheumatoid arthritis. *Rheumatology*. 2006;45(10):1223–1229.
345. Wu H-J, Ivanov II, Darce J, Hattori K, Shima T, Umesaki Y, et al. Gut-residing segmented filamentous bacteria drive autoimmune arthritis via T helper 17 cells. *Immunity*. 2010;32(6):815–827.
346. Yoshitomi H, Sakaguchi N, Kobayashi K, Brown GD, Tagami T, Sakihama T, et al. A role for fungal β-glucans and their receptor Dectin-1 in the induction of autoimmune arthritis in genetically susceptible mice. *Journal of Experimental medicine*. 2005;201(6):949–960.

347. Abdollahi-Roodsaz S, Joosten LA, Koenders MI, Devesa I, Roelofs MF, Radstake TR, et al. Stimulation of TLR2 and TLR4 differentially skews the balance of T cells in a mouse model of arthritis. *The Journal of clinical investigation*. 2008;118(1):205–216.
348. Viatte S, Plant D, Raychaudhuri S. Genetics and epigenetics of rheumatoid arthritis. *Nature Reviews Rheumatology*. 2013;9(3):141.
349. van der Helm-van Mil AH, Verpoort KN, Breedveld FC, Huizinga TW. Toes RE, de Vries RR. The HLA–DRB1 shared epitope alleles are primarily a risk factor for anti–cyclic citrullinated peptide antibodies and are not an independent risk factor for development of rheumatoid arthritis. *Arthritis & Rheumatism*. 2006;54(4):1117–1121.
350. Deighton C, Walker D, Griffiths I, Roberts D. The contribution of H LA to rheumatoid arthritis. *Clinical genetics*. 1989;36(3):178–182.
351. Begovich AB, Carlton VE, Honigberg LA, Schrodi SJ, Chokkalingam AP, Alexander HC, et al. A missense single-nucleotide polymorphism in a gene encoding a protein tyrosine phosphatase (PTPN22) is associated with rheumatoid arthritis. *The American Journal of Human Genetics*. 2004;75(2):330–337.
352. Plenge RM, Seielstad M, Padyukov L, Lee AT, Remmers EF, Ding B, et al. TRAF1–C5 as a risk locus for rheumatoid arthritis—A genomewide study. *New England Journal of Medicine*. 2007;357(12): 1199–1209.
353. Remmers EF, Plenge RM, Lee AT, Graham RR, Hom G, Behrens TW, et al. STAT4 and the risk of rheumatoid arthritis and systemic lupus erythematosus. *New England Journal of Medicine*. 2007;357(10):977–986.
354. Unraveling the genetics of complex diseases: susceptibility genes for rheumatoid arthritis and psoriasis. In: Li Y, Begovich AB, eds. Unraveling the genetics of complex diseases: susceptibility genes for rheumatoid arthritis and psoriasis. *Seminars in immunology*. 2009.
355. Sigurdsson S, Padyukov L, Kurreeman FA, Liljedahl U, Wiman AC, Alfredsson L, et al. Association of a haplotype in the promoter region of the interferon regulatory factor 5 gene with rheumatoid arthritis. *Arthritis & Rheumatism: Official Journal of the American College of Rheumatology*. 2007;56(7):2202–2210.
356. Lorentzen JC, Flornes L, Eklöw C, Bäckdahl L, Ribbhammar U, Guo JP, et al. Association of arthritis with a gene complex encoding C-type lectin–like receptors. *Arthritis & Rheumatism*. 2007;56(8):2620–2632.
357. Smolen J, Aletaha D. The burden of rheumatoid arthritis and access to treatment: a medical overview. *The European Journal of Health Economics*. 2008;8(2):39–47.
358. Wernick RM, Lipsky PE, Marban-Arcos E, Maliakkal JJ, Edelbaum D, Ziff M. IgG and IgM rheumatoid factor synthesis in rheumatoid synovial membrane cell cultures. *Arthritis & Rheumatism: Official Journal of the American College of Rheumatology*. 1985;28(7):742–752.
359. Kraan M, Haringman J, Post W, Versendaal J, Breedveld F, Tak P. Immunohistological analysis of synovial tissue for differential diagnosis in early arthritis. *Rheumatology*. 1999;38(11):1074–1080.
360. Grabar P. The "globulines-transporteurs" theory and auto-sensitization. *Medical hypotheses*. 1975;1(5):172–175.
361. Van Snick J, Van Roost E, Markowetz B, Cambiaso C, Masson P. Enhancement by IgM rheumatoid factor of in vitro ingestion by macrophages and in vivo clearance of aggregated IgG or antigen-antibody complexes. *European journal of immunology*. 1978;8(4):279–285.
362. Waaler E. On the occurrence of a factor in human serum activating the specific agglutination of sheep blood corpuscles. *Acta Pathologica Microbiologica Scandinavica*. 1940;17(2):172–188.
363. Aletaha D, Alasti F, Smolen JS. Rheumatoid factor determines structural progression of rheumatoid arthritis dependent and independent of disease activity. *Annals of the rheumatic diseases*. 2013;72(6): 875–880.
364. Nielen MM, van Schaardenburg D, Reesink HW, Van de Stadt RJ, van der Horst-Bruinsma IE, de Koning MH, et al. Specific autoantibodies precede the symptoms of rheumatoid arthritis: a study of serial measurements in blood donors. *Arthritis & Rheumatism: Official Journal of the American College of Rheumatology*. 2004;50(2):380–386.
365. The diagnostic and prognostic significance of autoantibodies in patients with very early arthritis. In: Nell V, Machold K, Eberl G, Hiesberger H, Hoefler E, Smolen J et al, eds. The diagnostic and prognostic significance of autoantibodies in patients with very early arthritis. *Annals of the rheumatic diseases*. 2003.

366. Houssien D, Jonsson T, Davies E, Scott D. Clinical significance of IgA rheumatoid factor subclasses in rheumatoid arthritis. *The Journal of rheumatology*. 1997;24(11):2119–2122.
367. Rantapää-Dahlqvist S, De Jong BA, Berglin E, Hallmans G, Wadell G, Stenlund H, et al. Antibodies against cyclic citrullinated peptide and IgA rheumatoid factor predict the development of rheumatoid arthritis. *Arthritis & Rheumatism*. 2003;48(10):2741–2749.
368. Halbert S, Anken M. Auto-antibodies in infectious mononucleosis, as determined by ELISA. *International Archives of Allergy and Immunology*. 1982;69(3):257–261.
369. Elagib K, Børretzen M, Jonsson R, Haga H, Thoen J, Thompson K, et al. Rheumatoid factors in primary Sjögren's syndrome (pSS) use diverse VH region genes, the majority of which show no evidence of somatic hypermutation. *Clinical and experimental immunology*. 1999;117(2):388.
370. Lima I, RCd Oliveira, Atta A, Marchi S, Barbosa L, Reis E, et al. Antibodies to citrullinated peptides in tuberculosis. *Clinical rheumatology*. 2013;32(5):685–687.
371. Bassyouni IH, Ezzat Y, Hamdy S, Talaat RM. Clinical significance of anti-cyclic citrullinated peptide antibodies in Egyptian patients with chronic hepatitis C virus genotype IV infection. *Clinical Chemistry and Laboratory Medicine (CCLM)*. 2009;47(7):842–847.
372. Nielsen SF, Bojesen SE, Schnohr P, Nordestgaard BG. Elevated rheumatoid factor and long term risk of rheumatoid arthritis: a prospective cohort study. *Bmj*. 2012;345:e5244.
373. Winchester R, Agnello V, Kunkel H. Gamma globulin complexes in synovial fluids of patients with rheumatoid arthritis. Partial characterization and relationship to lowered complement levels. *Clinical and experimental immunology*. 1970;6(5):689.
374. Schur P, Britton M, Franco A, Corson J, Sosman J, Ruddy S. Rheumatoid synovitis: complement and immune complexes. *Rheumatology*. 1975;6:34–42.
375. Mallya R, Vergani D, Tee D, Bevis L, De Beer F, Berry H, et al. Correlation in rheumatoid arthritis of concentrations of plasma C3d, serum rheumatoid factor, immune complexes and C-reactive protein with each other and with clinical features of disease activity. *Clinical and experimental immunology*. 1982;48(3):747.
376. Böhler C, Radner H, Smolen JS. Aletaha D. Serological changes in the course of traditional and biological disease modifying therapy of rheumatoid arthritis. *Annals of the rheumatic diseases*. 2013;72(2):241–244.
377. De Rycke L, Verhelst X, Kruithof E, Van den Bosch F, Hoffman IE, Veys EM, et al. Rheumatoid factor, but not anti-cyclic citrullinated peptide antibodies, is modulated by infliximab treatment in rheumatoid arthritis. *Annals of the rheumatic diseases*. 2005;64(2):299–302.
378. Anquetil F, Clavel C, Offer G, Serre G, Sebbag M. IgM and IgA rheumatoid factors purified from rheumatoid arthritis sera boost the Fc receptor–and complement-dependent effector functions of the disease-specific anti–citrullinated protein autoantibodies. *The Journal of Immunology*. 2015;194(8):3664–3674.
379. Hecht C, Schett G, Finzel S. The impact of rheumatoid factor and ACPA on bone erosion in rheumatoid arthritis. *Annals of the Rheumatic Diseases*. 2015;74(1):e4–ee.
380. Steiner G, Hartmuth K, Skriner K, Maurer-Fogy I, Sinski A, Thalmann E, et al. Purification and partial sequencing of the nuclear autoantigen RA33 shows that it is indistinguishable from the A2 protein of the heterogeneous nuclear ribonucleoprotein complex. *The Journal of clinical investigation*. 1992;90(3):1061–1066.
381. Steffen C. Consideration of pathogenesis of rheumatoid arthritis as collagen autoimmunity. *Zeitschrify fur Immunitatsuforschung*. 1970;139:219–220.
382. Trentham DE, Townes AS, Kang AH. Autoimmunity to type II collagen an experimental model of arthritis. *The Journal of experimental medicine*. 1977;146(3):857–868.
383. Trentham DE, Dynesius RA, Rocklin RE, David JR. Cellular sensitivity to collagen in rheumatoid arthritis. *New England Journal of Medicine*. 1978;299(7):327–332.
384. Fritsch R, Eselböck D, Skriner K, Jahn-Schmid B, Scheinecker C, Bohle B, et al. Characterization of autoreactive T cells to the autoantigens heterogeneous nuclear ribonucleoprotein A2 (RA33) and filaggrin in patients with rheumatoid arthritis. *The Journal of Immunology*. 2002;169(2):1068–1076.
385. Albert H, Collin M, Dudziak D, Ravetch JV, Nimmerjahn F. In vivo enzymatic modulation of IgG glycosylation inhibits autoimmune disease in an IgG subclass-dependent manner. *Proceedings of the National Academy of Sciences*. 2008;105(39):15005–15009.

386. Rombouts Y, Ewing E, van de Stadt LA, Selman MH, Trouw LA, Deelder AM, et al. Anti-citrullinated protein antibodies acquire a pro-inflammatory Fc glycosylation phenotype prior to the onset of rheumatoid arthritis. *Annals of the rheumatic diseases*. 2015;74(1):234–241.
387. Pfeifle R, Rothe T, Ipseiz N, Scherer HU, Culemann S, Harre U, et al. Regulation of autoantibody activity by the IL-23–T H 17 axis determines the onset of autoimmune disease. *Nature immunology*. 2017;18(1):104.
388. Aletaha D, Neogi T, Silman AJ, Funovits J, Felson DT, Bingham III CO, et al. 2010 rheumatoid arthritis classification criteria: an American College of Rheumatology/European League Against Rheumatism collaborative initiative. *Arthritis & rheumatism*. 2010;62(9):2569–2581.
389. Smolen JS, Eberl G, Breedveld FC, Jones I, Leeming M, Wylie GL, et al. Validity and reliability of the twenty-eight-joint count for the assessment of rheumatoid arthritis activity. *Arthritis & Rheumatism: Official Journal of the American College of Rheumatology*. 1995;38(1):38–43.
390. Extraarticular manifestations of rheumatoid arthritis. In: Hurd ER, ed. Extraarticular manifestations of rheumatoid arthritis. *Seminars in arthritis and rheumatism*. 1979.
391. Baecklund E, Iliadou A, Askling J, Ekbom A, Backlin C, Granath F, et al. Association of chronic inflammation, not its treatment, with increased lymphoma risk in rheumatoid arthritis. *Arthritis & Rheumatism*. 2006;54(3):692–701.
392. Kitas GD, Gabriel SE. Cardiovascular disease in rheumatoid arthritis: state of the art and future perspectives. *Annals of the rheumatic diseases*. 2011;70(1):8–14.
393. Listing J, Kekow J, Manger B, Burmester G-R, Pattloch D, Zink A, et al. Mortality in rheumatoid arthritis: the impact of disease activity, treatment with glucocorticoids, TNFα inhibitors and rituximab. *Annals of the rheumatic diseases*. 2015;74(2):415–421.
394. Rheumatoid arthritis. *Nat Rev Dis Primers*. 2018;4:18002.
395. Smolen JS, Aletaha D, McInnes IB. Rheumatoid arthritis. *Lancet*. 2016;388(10055):2023–2038.
396. Ravelli A, Martini A. Juvenile idiopathic arthritis. *Lancet*. 2007;369(9563):767–778.
397. Prakken B, Albani S, Martini A. Juvenile idiopathic arthritis. *Lancet*. 2011;377(9783):2138–2149.
398. Petty RE, Southwood TR, Manners P, Baum J, Glass DN, Goldenberg J, et al. International League of Associations for Rheumatology classification of juvenile idiopathic arthritis: second revision, Edmonton, 2001. *The Journal of rheumatology*. 2004;31(2):390.
399. Prahalad S, Ryan MH, Shear ES, Thompson SD, Giannini EH, Glass DN. Juvenile rheumatoid arthritis: linkage to HLA demonstrated by allele sharing in affected sibpairs. *Arthritis & Rheumatism: Official Journal of the American College of Rheumatology*. 2000;43(10):2335–2338.
400. Prahalad S, Glass DN. A comprehensive review of the genetics of juvenile idiopathic arthritis. *Pediatric Rheumatology*. 2008;6(1):11.
401. Prahalad S. Genetics of juvenile idiopathic arthritis: an update. *Current opinion in rheumatology*. 2004;16(5):588–594.
402. Rosen P, Thompson S, Glass D. Pediatric rheumatology review Non-HLA gene polymorphisms in juvenile rheumatoid arthritis. *Clin Exp Rheumatol*. 2003;21:650–656.
403. Harsini S, Saghazadeh A, Nedjat S, Rezaei N. Associations between interleukin-10 polymorphisms and susceptibility to juvenile idiopathic arthritis: a systematic review and meta-analysis. *Eur Cytokine Netw*. 2018;29(1):16–26.
404. Mahmoudi M, Rezaiemanesh A, Harsini S, Salmaninejad A, Poursani S, Bahrami T, et al. PDCD1 Single Nucleotide Polymorphisms in Iranian Patients With Juvenile Idiopathic Arthritis. *Acta Med Iran*. 2017;55(11):676–682.
405. Ziaee V, Maddah M, Harsini S, Rezaei A, Sadr M, Zoghi S, et al. Association of interleukin-1 family gene polymorphisms with juvenile idiopathic arthritis in Iranian population. *Allergol Immunopathol (Madr)*. 2016;44(6):542–546.
406. Ziaee V, Maddah M, Moradinejad MH, Rezaei A, Zoghi S, Sadr M, et al. Association of interleukin-6 single nucleotide polymorphisms with juvenile idiopathic arthritis. *Clin Rheumatol*. 2017;36(1):77–81.
407. Maddah M, Harsini S, Rezaei A, Sadr M, Zoghi S, Moradinejad MH, et al. Association of Interleukin-2, but not Interferon-Gamma, single nucleotide polymorphisms with juvenile idiopathic arthritis. *Allergol Immunopathol (Madr)*. 2016;44(4):303–306.
408. Maddah M, Harsini S, Ziaee V, Moradinejad MH, Rezaei A, Zoghi S, et al. Association of tumour necrosis factor-alpha G/A -238 and G/A -308 single nucleotide polymorphisms with juvenile idiopathic arthritis. *Int J Immunogenet*. 2016;43(6):391–396.

409. Harsini S, Ziaee V, Maddah M, Rezaei A, Sadr M, Zoghi S, et al. Interleukin 10 and transforming growth factor beta 1 gene polymorphisms in juvenile idiopathic arthritis. *Bratisl Lek Listy.* 2016;117(5):258–262.
410. Ziaee V, Rezaei A, Harsini S, Maddah M, Zoghi S, Sadr M, et al. Polymorphisms of genes encoding interleukin-4 and its receptor in Iranian patients with juvenile idiopathic arthritis. *Clin Rheumatol.* 2016;35(8):1943–1948.
411. Gregorio A, Gambini C, Gerloni V, Parafioriti A, Sormani M, Gregorio S, et al. Lymphoid neogenesis in juvenile idiopathic arthritis correlates with ANA positivity and plasma cells infiltration. *Rheumatology.* 2007;46(2):308–313.
412. Wedderburn LR, Patel A, Varsani H, Woo P. Divergence in the degree of clonal expansions in inflammatory T cell subpopulations mirrors HLA-associated risk alleles in genetically and clinically distinct subtypes of childhood arthritis. *International immunology.* 2001;13(12):1541–1550.
413. Wedderburn LR, Robinson N, Patel A, Varsani H, Woo P. Selective recruitment of polarized T cells expressing CCR5 and CXCR3 to the inflamed joints of children with juvenile idiopathic arthritis. *Arthritis & Rheumatism: Official Journal of the American College of Rheumatology.* 2000;43(4):765–774.
414. Jarvis JN, Jiang K, Frank MB, Knowlton N, Aggarwal A, Wallace CA, et al. Gene expression profiling in neutrophils from children with polyarticular juvenile idiopathic arthritis. *Arthritis & Rheumatism.* 2009;60(5):1488–1495.
415. Jarvis J, Diebold M, Chadwell M, Iobidze M, Moore H. Composition and biological behaviour of immune complexes isolated from synovial fluid of patients with juvenile rheumatoid arthritis (JRA). *Clinical & Experimental Immunology.* 1995;100(3):514–518.
416. Foell D, Wittkowski H, Hammerschmidt I, Wulffraat N, Schmeling H, Frosch M, et al. Monitoring neutrophil activation in juvenile rheumatoid arthritis by S100A12 serum concentrations. *Arthritis & Rheumatism: Official Journal of the American College of Rheumatology.* 2004;50(4):1286–1295.
417. De Kleer I, Kamphuis S, Rijkers G, Scholtens L, Gordon G, De Jager W, et al. The spontaneous remission of juvenile idiopathic arthritis is characterized by CD30+ T cells directed to human heat-shock protein 60 capable of producing the regulatory cytokine interleukin-10. *Arthritis & Rheumatism: Official Journal of the American College of Rheumatology.* 2003;48(7):2001–2010.
418. de Kleer I, Vercoulen Y, Klein M, Meerding J, Albani S, van der Zee R, et al. CD30 discriminates heat shock protein 60-induced FOXP3+ CD4+ T cells with a regulatory phenotype. *The Journal of Immunology.* 2010;185(4):2071–2079.
419. Vercoulen Y, van Teijlingen NH, de Kleer IM, Kamphuis S, Albani S, Prakken BJ. Heat shock protein 60 reactive T cells in juvenile idiopathic arthritis: what is new? *Arthritis research & therapy.* 2009;11(3):231.
420. Massa M, Passalia M, Manzoni SM, Campanelli R, Ciardelli L, Yung GP, et al. Differential recognition of heat-shock protein dnaJ–derived epitopes by effector and Treg cells leads to modulation of inflammation in juvenile idiopathic arthritis. *Arthritis & Rheumatism.* 2007;56(5):1648–1657.
421. Kamphuis S, Kuis W, De Jager W, Teklenburg G, Massa M, Gordon G, et al. Tolerogenic immune responses to novel T-cell epitopes from heat-shock protein 60 in juvenile idiopathic arthritis. *The Lancet.* 2005;366(9479):50–56.
422. Nistala K, Moncrieffe H, Newton KR, Varsani H, Hunter P, Wedderburn LR. Interleukin-17–producing T cells are enriched in the joints of children with arthritis, but have a reciprocal relationship to regulatory T cell numbers. *Arthritis & Rheumatism: Official Journal of the American College of Rheumatology.* 2008;58(3):875–887.
423. Nistala K, Adams S, Cambrook H, Ursu S, Olivito B, de Jager W, et al. Th17 plasticity in human autoimmune arthritis is driven by the inflammatory environment. *Proceedings of the National Academy of Sciences.* 2010;107(33):14751–14756.
424. De Benedetti F, Massa M, Pignatti P, Albani S, Novick D, Martini A. Serum soluble interleukin 6 (IL-6) receptor and IL-6/soluble IL-6 receptor complex in systemic juvenile rheumatoid arthritis. *The Journal of clinical investigation.* 1994;93(5):2114–2119.
425. De Benedetti F. Is systemic juvenile rheumatoid arthritis an interleukin 6 mediated disease? *J Rheumatol.* 1998;25(2):203–207.
426. Pascual V, Allantaz F, Arce E, Punaro M, Banchereau J. Role of interleukin-1 (IL-1) in the pathogenesis of systemic onset juvenile idiopathic arthritis and clinical response to IL-1 blockade. *The Journal of experimental medicine.* 2005;201(9):1479–1486.

427. Pascual V, Allantaz F, Patel P, Palucka AK, Chaussabel D, Banchereau J. How the study of children with rheumatic diseases identified interferon-α and interleukin-1 as novel therapeutic targets. *Immunological reviews*. 2008;223(1):39–59.
428. Allantaz F, Chaussabel D, Stichweh D, Bennett L, Allman W, Mejias A, et al. Blood leukocyte microarrays to diagnose systemic onset juvenile idiopathic arthritis and follow the response to IL-1 blockade. *Journal of Experimental Medicine*. 2007;204(9):2131–2144.
429. de Jager W, Vastert SJ, Beekman JM, Wulffraat NM, Kuis W, Coffer PJ, et al. Defective phosphorylation of interleukin-18 receptor β causes impaired natural killer cell function in systemic-onset juvenile idiopathic arthritis. *Arthritis & Rheumatism*. 2009;60(9):2782–2793.
430. de Jager W, Hoppenreijs EP, Wulffraat NM, Wedderburn LR, Kuis W, Prakken BJ. Blood and synovial fluid cytokine signatures in patients with juvenile idiopathic arthritis: a cross-sectional study. *Annals of the rheumatic diseases*. 2007;66(5):589–598.
431. Frosch M, Ahlmann M, Vogl T, Wittkowski H, Wulffraat N, Foell D, et al. The myeloid-related proteins 8 and 14 complex, a novel ligand of toll-like receptor 4, and interleukin-1β form a positive feedback mechanism in systemic-onset juvenile idiopathic arthritis. *Arthritis & Rheumatism: Official Journal of the American College of Rheumatology*. 2009;60(3):883–891.
432. Prakken BJ, Albani S. Using biology of disease to understand and guide therapy of. *JIA. Best Practice & Research Clinical Rheumatology*. 2009;23(5):599–608.
433. Frosch M, Roth J. New insights in systemic juvenile idiopathic arthritis—From pathophysiology to treatment. *Rheumatology*. 2008;47(2):121–125.
434. Foell D, Roth J. Proinflammatory S100 proteins in arthritis and autoimmune disease. *Arthritis & Rheumatism*. 2004;50(12):3762–3771.
435. Foell D, Wulffraat N, Wedderburn LR, Wittkowski H, Frosch M, Gerß J, et al. Methotrexate withdrawal at 6 vs 12 months in juvenile idiopathic arthritis in remission: a randomized clinical trial. *Jama*. 2010;303(13):1266–1273.
436. Foell D, Frosch M, zur Wiesch AS, Vogl T, Sorg C, Roth J. Methotrexate treatment in juvenile idiopathic arthritis: when is the right time to stop? *Annals of the rheumatic diseases*. 2004;63(2):206–208.
437. Ravelli A, Grom A, Behrens E, Cron R. Macrophage activation syndrome as part of systemic juvenile idiopathic arthritis: diagnosis, genetics, pathophysiology and treatment. *Genes & Immunity*. 2012;13(4):289–298.
438. Ravelli A, Minoia F, Davì S, Horne A, Bovis F, Pistorio A, et al. 2016 Classification criteria for macrophage activation syndrome complicating systemic juvenile idiopathic arthritis: a European league against rheumatism/American College of Rheumatology/Paediatric Rheumatology International Trials Organisation Collaborative Initiative. *Annals of the Rheumatic Diseases*. 2016;75(3):481–489.
439. Martini A. It is time to rethink juvenile idiopathic arthritis classification and nomenclature. *Annals of the rheumatic diseases*. 2012;71(9):1437–1439.
440. Martini A. Systemic juvenile idiopathic arthritis. *Autoimmunity reviews*. 2012;12(1):56–59.
441. Gowdie PJ, Tse SM. Juvenile idiopathic arthritis. *Pediatr Clin North Am*. 2012;59(2):301–327.
442. Crayne CB, Beukelman T. Juvenile Idiopathic Arthritis: oligoarthritis and Polyarthritis. *Pediatr Clin North Am*. 2018;65(4):657–674.
443. Martini A. Are the number of joints involved or the presence of psoriasis still useful tools to identify homogeneous disease entities in juvenile idiopathic arthritis? *The Journal of Rheumatology*. 2003;30(9):1900–1903.
444. Ravelli A, Varnier GC, Oliveira S, Castell E, Arguedas O, Magnani A, et al. Antinuclear antibody–positive patients should be grouped as a separate category in the classification of juvenile idiopathic arthritis. *Arthritis & Rheumatism*. 2011;63(1):267–275.
445. Stoll ML, Zurakowski D, Nigrovic LE, Nichols DP, Sundel RP, Nigrovic PA. Patients with juvenile psoriatic arthritis comprise two distinct populations. *Arthritis & Rheumatism: Official Journal of the American College of Rheumatology*. 2006;54(11):3564–3572.
446. Ringold S, Weiss PF, Beukelman T, DeWitt EM, Ilowite NT, Kimura Y, et al. 2013 update of the 2011 American College of Rheumatology recommendations for the treatment of juvenile idiopathic arthritis: recommendations for the medical therapy of children with systemic juvenile idiopathic arthritis and tuberculosis screening among children receiving biologic medications. *Arthritis care & research*. 2013;65(10):1551.

447. Beukelman T, Haynes K, Curtis JR, Xie F, Chen L, Bemrich-Stolz CJ, et al. Rates of malignancy associated with juvenile idiopathic arthritis and its treatment. *Arthritis & Rheumatism*. 2012;64(4):1263–1271.
448. Ruperto N, Murray KJ, Gerloni V, Wulffraat N, Feitosa De Oliveira SK, Falcini F, et al. A randomized trial of parenteral methotrexate comparing an intermediate dose with a higher dose in children with juvenile idiopathic arthritis who failed to respond to standard doses of methotrexate. *Arthritis & Rheumatism: Official Journal of the American College of Rheumatology*. 2004;50(7):2191–2201.
449. Ramanan AV, Dick AD, Jones AP, McKay A, Williamson PR, Compeyrot-Lacassagne S, et al. Adalimumab plus methotrexate for uveitis in juvenile idiopathic arthritis. *New England Journal of Medicine*. 2017;376(17):1637–1646.
450. Brunner HI, Ruperto N, Tzaribachev N, Horneff G, Chasnyk VG, Panaviene V, et al. Subcutaneous golimumab for children with active polyarticular-course juvenile idiopathic arthritis: results of a multicentre, double-blind, randomised-withdrawal trial. *Annals of the rheumatic diseases*. 2018;77(1):21–29.
451. Lovell DJ, Giannini EH, Reiff A, Cawkwell GD, Silverman ED, Nocton JJ, et al. Etanercept in children with polyarticular juvenile rheumatoid arthritis. *New England Journal of Medicine*. 2000;342(11): 763–769.
452. Lovell DJ, Ruperto N, Goodman S, Reiff A, Jung L, Jarosova K, et al. Adalimumab with or without methotrexate in juvenile rheumatoid arthritis. *New England Journal of Medicine*. 2008;359(8):810–820.
453. Ruperto N, Lovell DJ, Quartier P, Paz E, Rubio-Pérez N, Silva CA, et al. Abatacept in children with juvenile idiopathic arthritis: a randomised, double-blind, placebo-controlled withdrawal trial. *The Lancet*. 2008;372(9636):383–391.
454. Brunner HI, Ruperto N, Zuber Z, Keane C, Harari O, Kenwright A, et al. Efficacy and safety of tocilizumab in patients with polyarticular-course juvenile idiopathic arthritis: results from a phase 3, randomised, double-blind withdrawal trial. *Annals of the rheumatic diseases*. 2015;74(6):1110–1117.
455. Elhai M, Meune C, Avouac J, Kahan A, Allanore Y. Trends in mortality in patients with systemic sclerosis over 40 years: a systematic review and meta-analysis of cohort studies. *Rheumatology*. 2012;51(6):1017–1026.
456. Incidence and prevalence of systemic sclerosis: a systematic literature review. In: Chifflot H, Fautrel B, Sordet C, Chatelus E, Sibilia J, eds. Incidence and prevalence of systemic sclerosis: a systematic literature review. *Seminars in arthritis and rheumatism*. 2008.
457. Coral-Alvarado P, Pardo AL, Castaño-Rodriguez N, Rojas-Villarraga A, Anaya J-M. Systemic sclerosis: a world wide global analysis. *Clinical rheumatology*. 2009;28(7):757–765.
458. McCormic ZD, Khuder SS, Aryal BK, Ames AL, Khuder SA. Occupational silica exposure as a risk factor for scleroderma: a meta-analysis. *International archives of occupational and environmental health*. 2010;83(7):763–769.
459. Allanore Y, Simms R, Distler O, Trojanowska M, Pope J, Denton CP, et al. Systemic sclerosis. *Nature reviews Disease primers*. 2015;1(1):1–21.
460. Van Den Hoogen F, Khanna D, Fransen J, Johnson SR, Baron M, Tyndall A, et al. 2013 classification criteria for systemic sclerosis: an American College of Rheumatology/European League against Rheumatism collaborative initiative. *Arthritis & Rheumatism*. 2013;65(11):2737–2747.
461. Masi ATDiagnostic SFSCotARA, Committee T.C. Preliminary criteria for the classification of systemic sclerosis (scleroderma). *Arthritis & Rheumatism*. 1980;23(5):581–590.
462. Feghali-Bostwick C, Medsger Jr TA, Wright TM. Analysis of systemic sclerosis in twins reveals low concordance for disease and high concordance for the presence of antinuclear antibodies. *Arthritis & Rheumatism: Official Journal of the American College of Rheumatology*. 2003;48(7):1956–1963.
463. Allanore Y, Saad M, Dieudé P, Avouac J, Distler JH, Amouyel P, et al. Genome-wide scan identifies TNIP1, PSORS1C1, and RHOB as novel risk loci for systemic sclerosis. *PLoS Genet*. 2011;7(7):e1002091.
464. Radstake TR, Gorlova O, Rueda B, Martin J-E, Alizadeh BZ, Palomino-Morales R, et al. Genome-wide association study of systemic sclerosis identifies CD247 as a new susceptibility locus. *Nature genetics*. 2010;42(5):426–429.
465. Zhou X, Lee JE, Arnett FC, Xiong M, Park MY, Yoo YK, et al. HLA–DPB1 and DPB2 are genetic loci for systemic sclerosis: a genome-wide association study in Koreans with replication in North Americans. *Arthritis & Rheumatism: Official Journal of the American College of Rheumatology*. 2009;60(12):3807–3814.

466. Terao C, Kawaguchi T, Dieude P, Varga J, Kuwana M, Hudson M, et al. Transethnic meta-analysis identifies GSDMA and PRDM1 as susceptibility genes to systemic sclerosis. *Annals of the rheumatic diseases*. 2017;76(6):1150–1158.
467. Mayes MD, Bossini-Castillo L, Gorlova O, Martin JE, Zhou X, Chen WV, et al. Immunochip analysis identifies multiple susceptibility loci for systemic sclerosis. *The American Journal of Human Genetics*. 2014;94(1):47–61.
468. Zochling J, Newell F, Charlesworth JC, Leo P, Stankovich J, Cortes A, et al. An Immunochip-based interrogation of scleroderma susceptibility variants identifies a novel association at DNASE1L3. *Arthritis research & therapy*. 2014;16(5):438.
469. Arora-Singh RK, Assassi S, del Junco DJ, Arnett FC, Perry M, Irfan U, et al. Autoimmune diseases and autoantibodies in the first degree relatives of patients with systemic sclerosis. *Journal of autoimmunity*. 2010;35(1):52–57.
470. Autoantibodies in systemic sclerosis. In: Steen VD, ed. Autoantibodies in systemic sclerosis. *Seminars in arthritis and rheumatism*. 2005.
471. Antinuclear antibody-negative systemic sclerosis. In: Salazar GA, Assassi S, Wigley F, Hummers L, Varga J, Hinchcliff M et al, eds. Antinuclear antibody-negative systemic sclerosis. *Seminars in arthritis and rheumatism;*. 2015.
472. Steen V, Domsic RT, Lucas M, Fertig N, Medsger Jr TA. A clinical and serologic comparison of African American and Caucasian patients with systemic sclerosis. *Arthritis & Rheumatism*. 2012;64(9):2986–2994.
473. Wang J, Assassi S, Guo G, Tu W, Wu W, Yang L, et al. Clinical and serological features of systemic sclerosis in a Chinese cohort. *Clinical rheumatology*. 2013;32(5):617–621.
474. Assassi S, Sharif R, Lasky RE, McNearney TA, Estrada-Y-Martin RM, Draeger H, et al. Predictors of interstitial lung disease in early systemic sclerosis: a prospective longitudinal study of the GENISOS cohort. *Arthritis research & therapy*. 2010;12(5):R166.
475. Nihtyanova SI, Schreiber BE, Ong VH, Rosenberg D, Moinzadeh P, Coghlan JG, et al. Prediction of pulmonary complications and long-term survival in systemic sclerosis. *Arthritis & rheumatology*. 2014;66(6):1625–1635.
476. Assassi S, del Junco D, Sutter K, McNearney TA, Reveille JD, Karnavas A, et al. Clinical and genetic factors predictive of mortality in early systemic sclerosis. *Arthritis Care & Research*. 2009;61(10):1403–1411.
477. Ioannidis JP, Vlachoyiannopoulos PG, Haidich A-B, Medsger Jr TA, Lucas M, Michet CJ, et al. Mortality in systemic sclerosis: an international meta-analysis of individual patient data. *The American journal of medicine*. 2005;118(1):2–10.
478. Aggarwal R, Lucas M, Fertig N, Oddis CV, Medsger Jr TA. Anti–U3 RNP autoantibodies in systemic sclerosis. *Arthritis & Rheumatism: Official Journal of the American College of Rheumatology*. 2009;60(4):1112–1118.
479. Otero CM, Assassi S, Hudson M, Mayes MD, Estrada-Y-Martin R, Pedroza C, et al. Antifibrillarin antibodies are associated with native North American ethnicity and poorer survival in systemic sclerosis. *The Journal of rheumatology*. 2017;44(6):799–805.
480. Ii RK, Fertig N, Lucas M, Domsic R, Medsger Jr T. Anti-PM-Scl antibody in patients with systemic sclerosis. *Clin Exp Rheumatol*. 2012;30(71):S12–S16.
481. D'Aoust J, Hudson M, Tatibouet S, Wick J, Group CSR, Mahler M, et al. Clinical and serologic correlates of anti-PM/Scl antibodies in systemic sclerosis: a multicenter study of 763 patients. *Arthritis & Rheumatology*. 2014;66(6):1608–1615.
482. Nikpour M, Hissaria P, Byron J, Sahhar J, Micallef M, Paspaliaris W, et al. Prevalence, correlates and clinical usefulness of antibodies to RNA polymerase III in systemic sclerosis: a cross-sectional analysis of data from an Australian cohort. *Arthritis research & therapy*. 2011;13(6):R211.
483. Nguyen B, Mayes MD, Arnett FC, Del Junco D, Reveille JD, Gonzalez EB, et al. HLA–DRB1* 0407 and* 1304 are risk factors for scleroderma renal crisis. *Arthritis & Rheumatism*. 2011;63(2):530–534.
484. Ghrénassia E, Avouac J, Khanna D, Derk CT, Distler O, Suliman YA, et al. Prevalence, correlates and outcomes of gastric antral vascular ectasia in systemic sclerosis: a EUSTAR case-control study. *The Journal of Rheumatology*. 2014;41(1):99–105.
485. Shah AA, Rosen A, Hummers L, Wigley F, Casciola-Rosen L. Close temporal relationship between onset of cancer and scleroderma in patients with RNA polymerase I/III antibodies. *Arthritis & Rheumatism*. 2010;62(9):2787–2795.

486. Moinzadeh P, Fonseca C, Hellmich M, Shah AA, Chighizola C, Denton CP, et al. Association of anti-RNA polymerase III autoantibodies and cancer in scleroderma. *Arthritis research & therapy*. 2014;16(1):R53.
487. Lazzaroni M-G, Cavazzana I, Colombo E, Dobrota R, Hernandez J, Hesselstrand R, et al. Malignancies in patients with anti-RNA polymerase III antibodies and systemic sclerosis: analysis of the EULAR scleroderma trials and research cohort and possible recommendations for screening. *The Journal of rheumatology*. 2017;44(5):639–647.
488. Ceribelli A, Cavazzana I, Taraborelli M, Zingarelli S, Franceschini F. Malignancies in Italian patients with systemic sclerosis positive for anti-RNA polymerase III antibodies. *The Journal of rheumatology*. 2011;38(7):1329–1334.
489. Matucci-Cerinic M, Kahaleh B, Wigley FM. Evidence that systemic sclerosis is a vascular disease. *Arthritis & Rheumatism*. 2013;65(8):1953–1962.
490. Tan F, Zhou X, Mayes M, Gourh P, Guo X, Marcum C, et al. Signatures of differentially regulated interferon gene expression and vasculotrophism in the peripheral blood cells of systemic sclerosis patients. *Rheumatology*. 2006;45(6):694–702.
491. Rongioletti F, Ferreli C, Atzori L, Bottoni U, Soda G. Scleroderma with an update about clinico-pathological correlation. *G Ital Dermatol Venereol*. 2018;153(2):208–215.
492. Steen VD, Medsger TA. Changes in causes of death in systemic sclerosis, 1972–2002. *Annals of the rheumatic diseases*. 2007;66(7):940–944.
493. Tyndall AJ, Bannert B, Vonk M, Airò P, Cozzi F, Carreira PE, et al. Causes and risk factors for death in systemic sclerosis: a study from the EULAR Scleroderma Trials and Research (EUSTAR) database. *Annals of the rheumatic diseases*. 2010;69(10):1809–1815.
494. Ferreli C, Gasparini G, Parodi A, Cozzani E, Rongioletti F, Atzori L. Cutaneous manifestations of scleroderma and scleroderma-like disorders: a comprehensive review. *Clinical Reviews in Allergy & Immunology*. 2017;53(3):306–336.
495. Rongioletti F, Ferreli C, Atzori L, Bottoni U, Soda G. Scleroderma with an update about clinico-pathological correlation. *Giornale italiano di dermatologia e venereologia: organo ufficiale, Societa italiana di dermatologia e sifilografia*. 2018;153(2):208–215.
496. Tashkin DP, Roth MD, Clements PJ, Furst DE, Khanna D, Kleerup EC, et al. Mycophenolate mofetil versus oral cyclophosphamide in scleroderma-related interstitial lung disease (SLS II): a randomised controlled, double-blind, parallel group trial. *The Lancet Respiratory Medicine*. 2016;4(9):708–719.
497. Khanna D, Denton CP, Jahreis A, van Laar JM, Frech TM, Anderson ME, et al. Safety and efficacy of subcutaneous tocilizumab in adults with systemic sclerosis (faSScinate): a phase 2, randomised, controlled trial. *The Lancet*. 2016;387(10038):2630–2640.
498. van Laar JM, Farge D, Sont JK, Naraghi K, Marjanovic Z, Larghero J, et al. Autologous hematopoietic stem cell transplantation vs intravenous pulse cyclophosphamide in diffuse cutaneous systemic sclerosis: a randomized clinical trial. *Jama*. 2014;311(24):2490–2498.
499. Distler J, Feghali-Bostwick C, Soare A, Asano Y, Distler O, Abraham D. Review: frontiers of antifibrotic therapy in systemic sclerosis. *Arthritis Rheumatol*. 2017;69(2):257–267.
500. Sieper J, Poddubnyy D. Axial spondyloarthritis. *Lancet*. 2017;390(10089):73–84.
501. Brown M, Wordsworth B, Reveille J. Genetics of ankylosing spondylitis. *Clinical and experimental rheumatology*. 2002;20(6; SUPP/28):S–43.
502. Brewerton D, Hart FD, Nicholls A, Caffrey M, James D, Sturrock R. Ankylosing spondylitis and HL-A 27. *The Lancet*. 1973;301(7809):904–907.
503. Schlosstein L, Terasaki PI, Bluestone R, Pearson CM. High association of an HL-A antigen, W27, with ankylosing spondylitis. *New England Journal of Medicine*. 1973;288(14):704–706.
504. Burton PR, Clayton DG, Cardon LR, Craddock N, Deloukas P, Duncanson A, et al. Association scan of 14,500 nonsynonymous SNPs in four diseases identifies autoimmunity variants. *Nature genetics*. 2007;39(11):1329–1337.
505. Reveille JD, Sims A-M, Danoy P, Evans DM, Leo P, Pointon JJ, et al. Genome-wide association study of ankylosing spondylitis identifies non-MHC susceptibility loci. *Nature genetics*. 2010;42(2):123.
506. Evans DM, Spencer CC, Pointon JJ, Su Z, Harvey D, Kochan G, et al. Interaction between ERAP1 and HLA-B27 in ankylosing spondylitis implicates peptide handling in the mechanism for HLA-B27 in disease susceptibility. *Nature genetics*. 2011;43(8):761–767.

507. Pointon JJ, Harvey D, Karaderi T, Appleton LH, Farrar C, Stone MA, et al. The chromosome 16q region associated with ankylosing spondylitis includes the candidate gene tumour necrosis factor receptor type 1-associated death domain (TRADD). *Annals of the rheumatic diseases*. 2010;69(6): 1243–1246.
508. Zinovieva E, Bourgain C, Kadi A, Letourneur F, Izac B, Said-Nahal R, et al. Comprehensive linkage and association analyses identify haplotype, near to the TNFSF15 gene, significantly associated with spondyloarthritis. *PLoS Genet*. 2009;5(6):e1000528.
509. Danoy P, Pryce K, Hadler J, Ward M, Weisman M, Reveille J. Evidence of genetic overlap between ankylosing spondylitis and Crohn's disease. *Arthritis Rheum*. 2009;60(10).
510. Granfors K, Jalkanen S, von Essen R, Lahesmaa-Rantala R, Isomäki O, Pekkola-Heino K, et al. Yersinia antigens in synovial-fluid cells from patients with reactive arthritis. *New England Journal of Medicine*. 1989;320(4):216–221.
511. Yin Z, Neure L, Grolms M, Eggens U, Radbruch A, Braun J, et al. Th1/Th2 cytokine pattern in the joint of rheumatoid arthritis and reactive arthritis patients: analysis at the single cell level. *Arthritis & Rheumatism*. 1997;40(9).
512. Yin Z, Braun J, Grolms M, Spiller I, Radbruch A, Sieper J. IFNγ, IL-4 and IL-10 positive cells in the CD4+ and CD8+ T cell population of peripheral blood in untreated patients with early rheumatoid arthritis and early reactive arthritis. *Arthritis & Rheumatism*. 1997;40(9).
513. Braun J, Yin Z, Spiller I, Siegert S, Rudwaleit M, Liu L, et al. Low secretion of tumor necrosis factor α, but no other Th1 or Th2 cytokines, by peripheral blood mononuclear cells correlates with chronicity in reactive arthritis. *Arthritis & Rheumatism: Official Journal of the American College of Rheumatology*. 1999;42(10):2039–2044.
514. Stolwijk C, van Tubergen A, Castillo-Ortiz JD, Boonen A. Prevalence of extra-articular manifestations in patients with ankylosing spondylitis: a systematic review and meta-analysis. *Annals of the rheumatic diseases*. 2015;74(1):65–73.
515. Van Praet L, Van den Bosch FE, Jacques P, Carron P, Jans L, Colman R, et al. Microscopic gut inflammation in axial spondyloarthritis: a multiparametric predictive model. *Annals of the rheumatic diseases*. 2013;72(3):414–417.
516. Mielants H, Veys E, Cuvelier C, De Vos M. Ileocolonoscopic findings in seronegative spondylarthropathies. *Rheumatology*. 1988;27(suppl_2):95–105.
517. Appel H, Maier R, Wu P, Scheer R, Hempfing A, Kayser R, et al. Analysis of IL-17+ cells in facet joints of patients with spondyloarthritis suggests that the innate immune pathway might be of greater relevance than the Th17-mediated adaptive immune response. *Arthritis research & therapy*. 2011;13(3):1–9.
518. Moran EM, Heydrich R, Ng CT, Saber TP, McCormick J, Sieper J, et al. IL-17A expression is localised to both mononuclear and polymorphonuclear synovial cell infiltrates. *PloS one*. 2011;6(8): e24048.
519. Appel H, Maier R, Bleil J, Hempfing A, Loddenkemper C, Schlichting U, et al. Situ Analysis of Interleukin–23–and Interleukin-12–Positive Cells in the Spine of Patients With Ankylosing Spondylitis. *Arthritis & Rheumatism*. 2013;65(6):1522–1529.
520. Smith JA, Turner MJ, DeLay ML, Klenk EI, Sowders DP, Colbert RA. Endoplasmic reticulum stress and the unfolded protein response are linked to synergistic IFN-β induction via X-box binding protein 1. *European journal of immunology*. 2008;38(5):1194–1203.
521. Rudwaleit M, Van Der Heijde D, Landewé R, Listing J, Akkoc N, Brandt J, et al. The development of Assessment of SpondyloArthritis international Society classification criteria for axial spondyloarthritis (part II): validation and final selection. *Annals of the rheumatic diseases*. 2009;68(6):777–783.
522. Rudwaleit M, Jurik A-G, Hermann KA, Landewé R, van der Heijde D, Baraliakos X, et al. Defining active sacroiliitis on magnetic resonance imaging (MRI) for classification of axial spondyloarthritis: a consensual approach by the ASAS/OMERACT MRI group. *Annals of the rheumatic diseases*. 2009;68(10):1520–1527.
523. Sieper J, Braun J, Kingsley GH. Report on the Fourth International Workshop on Reactive Arthritis. *Arthritis and rheumatism*. 2000;43(4):720–734.
524. Sieper J, Rudwaleit M, Braun J, van der Heijde D. Diagnosing reactive arthritis: role of clinical setting in the value of serologic and microbiologic assays. *Arthritis & Rheumatism*. 2002;46(2):319–327.

525. Sieper J, Poddubnyy D. New evidence on the management of spondyloarthritis. *Nature Reviews Rheumatology*. 2016;12(5):282–295.
526. Braun J, Sieper J. Biological therapies in the spondyloarthritides—The current state. *Rheumatology*. 2004;43(9):1072–1084.
527. Inman RD, Davis Jr JC, Heijde DVD, Diekman L, Sieper J, Kim SI, et al. Efficacy and safety of golimumab in patients with ankylosing spondylitis: results of a randomized, double-blind, placebo-controlled, phase III trial. *Arthritis & Rheumatism: Official Journal of the American College of Rheumatology*. 2008;58(11):3402–3412.
528. Braun J, Brandt J, Listing J, Rudwaleit M, Sieper J. Biologic therapies in the spondyloarthritis: new opportunities, new challenges. *Current opinion in rheumatology*. 2003;15(4):394–407.
529. Davis Jr JC, Van Der Heijde D, Braun J, Dougados M, Cush J, Clegg DO, et al. Recombinant human tumor necrosis factor receptor (etanercept) for treating ankylosing spondylitis: a randomized, controlled trial. *Arthritis & Rheumatism*. 2003;48(11):3230–3236.
530. Baeten D, Sieper J, Braun J, Baraliakos X, Dougados M, Emery P, et al. Secukinumab, an interleukin-17A inhibitor, in ankylosing spondylitis. *New England journal of medicine*. 2015;373(26):2534–2548.
531. Delaleu N, Jonsson R, Koller MM. Sjögren's syndrome. *European journal of oral sciences*. 2005;113(2): 101–113.
532. Brito-Zeron P, Baldini C, Bootsma H, Bowman SJ, Jonsson R, Mariette X, et al. Sjögren syndrome. *Nature reviews Disease primers*. 2016;2(1):1–20.
533. Fox RI. Sjögren's syndrome. *The Lancet*. 2005;366(9482):321–331.
534. Mitsias D, Tzioufas A, Veiopoulou C, Zintzaras E, Tassios I, Kogopoulou O, et al. The Th1/Th2 cytokine balance changes with the progress of the immunopathological lesion of Sjogren's syndrome. *Clinical & Experimental Immunology*. 2002;128(3):562–568.
535. Ciccia F, Guggino G, Rizzo A, Ferrante A, Raimondo S, Giardina A, et al. Potential involvement of IL-22 and IL-22-producing cells in the inflamed salivary glands of patients with Sjögren's syndrome. *Annals of the rheumatic diseases*. 2012;71(2):295–301.
536. Gliozzi M, Greenwell-Wild T, Jin W, Moutsopoulos NM, Kapsogeorgou E, Moutsopoulos HM, et al. A link between interferon and augmented plasmin generation in exocrine gland damage in Sjögren's syndrome. *Journal of autoimmunity*. 2013;40:122–133.
537. Bikker A, Kruize A, Wenting M, Versnel M, Bijlsma J, Lafeber F, et al. Increased interleukin (IL)-7Rα expression in salivary glands of patients with primary Sjögren's syndrome is restricted to T cells and correlates with IL-7 expression, lymphocyte numbers and activity. *Annals of the rheumatic diseases*. 2012;71(6):1027–1033.
538. Christodoulou MI, Kapsogeorgou EK, Moutsopoulos NM, Moutsopoulos HM. Foxp3+ T-regulatory cells in Sjögren's syndrome: correlation with the grade of the autoimmune lesion and certain adverse prognostic factors. *The American journal of pathology*. 2008;173(5):1389–1396.
539. Katsifis GE, Rekka S, Moutsopoulos NM, Pillemer S, Wahl SM. Systemic and local interleukin-17 and linked cytokines associated with Sjögren's syndrome immunopathogenesis. *The American journal of pathology*. 2009;175(3):1167–1177.
540. Saadoun D, Terrier B, Bannock J, Vazquez T, Massad C, Kang I, et al. Expansion of autoreactive unresponsive CD21−/low B cells in Sjögren's syndrome–associated lymphoproliferation. *Arthritis & Rheumatism*. 2013;65(4):1085–1096.
541. Manoussakis M, Boiu S, Korkolopoulou P, Kapsogeorgou E, Kavantzas N, Ziakas P, et al. Rates of infiltration by macrophages and dendritic cells and expression of interleukin-18 and interleukin-12 in the chronic inflammatory lesions of Sjögren's syndrome: correlation with certain features of immune hyperactivity and factors associated with high risk of lymphoma development. *Arthritis & Rheumatism: Official Journal of the American College of Rheumatology*. 2007;56(12):3977–3988.
542. Christodoulou MI, Kapsogeorgou EK, Moutsopoulos HM. Characteristics of the minor salivary gland infiltrates in Sjögren's syndrome. *Journal of autoimmunity*. 2010;34(4):400–407.
543. Eloranta ML, Alm GV, Rönnblom L. Disease mechanisms in rheumatology—Tools and pathways: plasmacytoid dendritic cells and their role in autoimmune rheumatic diseases. *Arthritis & Rheumatism*. 2013;65(4):853–863.
544. Kawanami T, Sawaki T, Sakai T, Miki M, Iwao H, Nakajima A, et al. Skewed production of IL-6 and TGFβ by cultured salivary gland epithelial cells from patients with Sjögren's syndrome. *PloS one*. 2012;7(10):e45689.

545. Tzioufas AG, Kapsogeorgou EK, Moutsopoulos HM. Pathogenesis of Sjögren's syndrome: what we know and what we should learn. *Journal of autoimmunity*. 2012;39(1–2):4–8.
546. Moutsopoulos H. Sjöc; gren's Syndrome: autoimmune Epithelitis. *Clinical immunology and immunopathology*. 1994;72(2):162–165.
547. Sisto M, Lisi S, Lofrumento DD, Ingravallo G, Maiorano E, D'Amore M. A failure of TNFAIP3 negative regulation maintains sustained NF-κB activation in Sjögren's syndrome. *Histochemistry and cell biology*. 2011;135(6):615.
548. Peng B, Ling J, Lee AJ, Wang Z, Chang Z, Jin W, et al. Defective feedback regulation of NF-κB underlies Sjögren's syndrome in mice with mutated κB enhancers of the IκBα promoter. *Proceedings of the National Academy of Sciences*. 2010;107(34):15193–15198.
549. Napeñas JJ, Rouleau TS. Oral complications of Sjögren's syndrome. *Oral Maxillofac Surg Clin North Am*. 2014;26(1):55–62.
550. Thorne I, Sutcliffe N. Sjögren's syndrome. *British Journal of Hospital Medicine*. 2017;78(8):438–442.
551. Birnbaum J. Peripheral nervous system manifestations of Sjögren syndrome: clinical patterns, diagnostic paradigms, etiopathogenesis, and therapeutic strategies. *The neurologist*. 2010;16(5):287–297.
552. Lynch DA. Lung disease related to collagen vascular disease. *Journal of thoracic imaging*. 2009;24(4): 299–309.
553. Vivino FB, Carsons SE, Foulks G, Daniels TE, Parke A, Brennan MT, et al. New treatment guidelines for Sjögren's disease. *Rheumatic Disease Clinics*. 2016;42(3):531–551.
554. St. Clair EW, Baer AN, Wei C, Noaiseh G, Parke A, Coca A, et al. Clinical Efficacy and Safety of Baminercept, a Lymphotoxin β Receptor Fusion Protein, in Primary Sjögren's Syndrome: results From a Phase II Randomized, Double-Blind, Placebo-Controlled Trial. *Arthritis & Rheumatology*. 2018;70(9):1470–1480.
555. Ginzler EM, Wallace DJ, Merrill JT, Furie RA, Stohl W, Chatham WW, et al. Disease control and safety of belimumab plus standard therapy over 7 years in patients with systemic lupus erythematosus. *The Journal of rheumatology*. 2014;41(2):300–309.
556. Meiners P, Vissink A, Kroese F, Spijkervet F, Smitt-Kamminga NS, Abdulahad W, et al. Abatacept treatment reduces disease activity in early primary Sjögren's syndrome (open-label proof of concept ASAP study). *Annals of the rheumatic diseases*. 2014;73(7):1393–1396.
557. Devauchelle-Pensec V, Mariette X, Jousse-Joulin S, Berthelot J-M, Perdriger A, Puéchal X, et al. Treatment of primary Sjögren syndrome with rituximab: a randomized trial. *Annals of internal medicine*. 2014;160(4):233–242.
558. Pijpe J, Van Imhoff G, Spijkervet F, Roodenburg J, Wolbink G, Mansour K, et al. Rituximab treatment in patients with primary Sjögren's syndrome: an open-label phase II study. *Arthritis & Rheumatism*. 2005;52(9):2740–2750.
559. Carubbi F, Cipriani P, Marrelli A, Di Benedetto P, Ruscitti P, Berardicurti O, et al. Efficacy and safety of rituximab treatment in early primary Sjögren's syndrome: a prospective, multi-center, follow-up study. *Arthritis research & therapy*. 2013;15(5):R172.
560. FBdV Souza, GJM Porfírio, Andriolo BNG, JVd Albuquerque, Trevisani VFM. Rituximab effectiveness and safety for treating primary Sjögren's syndrome (pSS): systematic review and meta-analysis. *PLoS One*. 2016;11(3):e0150749.
561. Mammen AL. Autoimmune myopathies: autoantibodies, phenotypes and pathogenesis. *Nature Reviews Neurology*. 2011;7(6):343.
562. Targoff IN, Reichlin M. The association between Mi-2 antibodies and dermatomyositis. *Arthritis & Rheumatism: Official Journal of the American College of Rheumatology*. 1985;28(7):796–803.
563. Casciola-Rosen LA, Anhalt GJ, Rosen A. DNA-dependent protein kinase is one of a subset of autoantigens specifically cleaved early during apoptosis. *The Journal of experimental medicine*. 1995;182(6):1625–1634.
564. Casciola-Rosen LA, Pluta AF, Plotz PH, Cox AE, Morris S, Wigley FM, et al. The DNA mismatch repair enzyme PMS1 is a myositis-specific autoantigen. *Arthritis & Rheumatism: Official Journal of the American College of Rheumatology*. 2001;44(2):389–396.
565. Suwa A, Hirakata M, Takeda Y, Okano Y, Mimori T, Inada S, et al. Autoantibodies to DNA-dependent protein kinase. Probes for the catalytic subunit. *The Journal of clinical investigation*. 1996;97(6): 1417–1421.

566. Reeves WH, Nigam SK, Blobel G. Human autoantibodies reactive with the signal-recognition particle. *Proceedings of the National Academy of Sciences*. 1986;83(24):9507–9511.
567. Mathews MB, Bernstein RM. Myositis autoantibody inhibits histidyl-tRNA synthetase: a model for autoimmunity. *Nature*. 1983;304(5922):177–179.
568. Okuma T, Honda R, Ichikawa G, Tsumagari N, Yasuda H. In vitroSUMO-1 modification requires two enzymatic steps, E1 and E2. *Biochemical and biophysical research communications*. 1999;254(3):693–698.
569. Mimura Y, Takahashi K, Kawata K, Akazawa T, Inoue N. Two-step colocalization of MORC3 with PML nuclear bodies. *Journal of cell science*. 2010;123(12):2014–2024.
570. Rhodes DA, Ihrke G, Reinicke AT, Malcherek G, Towey M, Isenberg DA, et al. The 52 000 MW Ro/SS-A autoantigen in Sjögren's syndrome/systemic lupus erythematosus (Ro52) is an interferon-γ inducible tripartite motif protein associated with membrane proximal structures. *Immunology*. 2002;106(2):246–256.
571. Sato S, Hoshino K, Satoh T, Fujita T, Kawakami Y, Fujita T, et al. RNA helicase encoded by melanoma differentiation–associated gene 5 is a major autoantigen in patients with clinically amyopathic dermatomyositis: association with rapidly progressive interstitial lung disease. *Arthritis & Rheumatism: Official Journal of the American College of Rheumatology*. 2009;60(7):2193–2200.
572. Interstitial lung disease with autoantibodies againstaminoacyl-tRNA synthetases in the absence of clinically apparent myositis. In: Friedman AW, Targoff IN, Arnett FC, eds. Interstitial lung disease with autoantibodies againstaminoacyl-tRNA synthetases in the absence of clinically apparent myositis. *Seminars in arthritis and rheumatism*. 1996.
573. Fiorentino D, Chung L, Zwerner J, Rosen A, Casciola-Rosen L. The mucocutaneous and systemic phenotype of dermatomyositis patients with antibodies to MDA5 (CADM-140): a retrospective study. *Journal of the American Academy of Dermatology*. 2011;65(1):25–34.
574. Chaisson NF, Paik J, Orbai A-M, Casciola-Rosen L, Fiorentino D, Danoff S, et al. A novel dermato-pulmonary syndrome associated with MDA-5 antibodies: report of 2 cases and review of the literature. *Medicine*. 2012;91(4):220.
575. Fujimoto M, Watanabe R, Ishitsuka Y, Okiyama N. Recent advances in dermatomyositis-specific autoantibodies. *Current opinion in rheumatology*. 2016;28(6):636–644.
576. Satoh M, Tanaka S, Ceribelli A, Calise SJ, Chan EK. A comprehensive overview on myositis-specific antibodies: new and old biomarkers in idiopathic inflammatory myopathy. *Clinical reviews in allergy & immunology*. 2017;52(1):1–19.
577. Betteridge Z, McHugh N. Myositis-specific autoantibodies: an important tool to support diagnosis of myositis. *Journal of internal medicine*. 2016;280(1):8–23.
578. Gunawardena H. The clinical features of myositis-associated autoantibodies: a review. *Clinical reviews in allergy & immunology*. 2017;52(1):45–57.
579. Casciola-Rosen L, Andrade F, Ulanet D, Wong WB, Rosen A. Cleavage by granzyme B is strongly predictive of autoantigen status: implications for initiation of autoimmunity. *The Journal of experimental medicine*. 1999;190(6):815–826.
580. Brouwer R, Hengstman G, Egberts WV, Ehrfeld H, Bozic B, Ghirardello A, et al. Autoantibody profiles in the sera of European patients with myositis. *Annals of the rheumatic diseases*. 2001;60(2):116–123.
581. Rigolet A, Musset L, Dubourg O, Maisonobe T, Grenier P, Charuel J-L, et al. Inflammatory myopathies with anti-Ku antibodies: a prognosis dependent on associated lung disease. *Medicine*. 2012;91(2):95–102.
582. Mahler M, Raijmakers R. Novel aspects of autoantibodies to the PM/Scl complex: clinical, genetic and diagnostic insights. *Autoimmunity reviews*. 2007;6(7):432–437.
583. Pinal-Fernandez I, Fernandez-Codina A, Callejas-Moraga EL, Espinosa J, Marin A, Labrador-Horrillo M, et al. Mixed connective tissue disease and epitope spreading: an historical cohort study. *JCR: Journal of Clinical Rheumatology*. 2017;23(3):155–159.
584. De Padilla CML, Crowson CS, Hein MS, Pendegraft RS, Strausbauch MA, Niewold TB, et al. Gene expression profiling in blood and affected muscle tissues reveals differential activation pathways in patients with new-onset juvenile and adult dermatomyositis. *The Journal of rheumatology*. 2017;44(1):117–124.
585. Miller FW, Chen W, O'Hanlon TP, Cooper RG, Vencovsky J, Rider LG, et al. Genome-wide association study identifies HLA 8.1 ancestral haplotype alleles as major genetic risk factors for myositis phenotypes. *Genes & Immunity*. 2015;16(7):470–480.

586. Greenberg SA, Pinkus JL, Pinkus GS, Burleson T, Sanoudou D, Tawil R, et al. Interferon-α/β–mediated innate immune mechanisms in dermatomyositis. *Annals of Neurology: Official Journal of the American Neurological Association and the Child Neurology Society*. 2005;57(5):664–678.
587. Ohnuki Y, Suzuki S, Shiina T, Uruha A, Watanabe Y, Suzuki S, et al. HLA-DRB1 alleles in immune-mediated necrotizing myopathy. *Neurology*. 2016;87(18):1954–1955.
588. Mammen AL, Gaudet D, Brisson D, Christopher-Stine L, Lloyd TE, Leffell MS, et al. Increased frequency of DRB1* 11: 01 in anti–hydroxymethylglutaryl-coenzyme A reductase–associated autoimmune myopathy. *Arthritis care & research*. 2012;64(8):1233–1237.
589. Christopher-Stine L, Robinson DR, Wu CC, Mark EJ. Case 37-2012: a 21-year-old man with fevers, arthralgias, and pulmonary infiltrates. *New England Journal of Medicine*. 2012;367(22):2134–2146.
590. Miller FW. New approaches to the assessment and treatment of the idiopathic inflammatory myopathies. *Annals of the rheumatic diseases*. 2012;71(Suppl 2):i82–ii5.
591. Robinson AB, Reed AM. Clinical features, pathogenesis and treatment of juvenile and adult dermatomyositis. *Nature Reviews Rheumatology*. 2011;7(11):664.
592. Danoff SK, Casciola-Rosen L. The lung as a possible target for the immune reaction in myositis. *Arthritis research & therapy*. 2011;13(4):230.
593. Labirua A, Lundberg IE. Interstitial lung disease and idiopathic inflammatory myopathies: progress and pitfalls. *Current opinion in rheumatology*. 2010;22(6):633–638.
594. Cervera R, Khamashta MA, Shoenfeld Y, Camps MT, Jacobsen S, Kiss E, et al. Morbidity and mortality in the antiphospholipid syndrome during a 5-year period: a multicentre prospective study of 1000 patients. *Annals of the Rheumatic Diseases*. 2009;68(9):1428–1432.
595. Miyakis S, Lockshin M, Atsumi T, Branch D, Brey R, Cervera R, et al. International consensus statement on an update of the classification criteria for definite antiphospholipid syndrome (APS). *Journal of Thrombosis and Haemostasis*. 2006;4(2):295–306.
596. Biggioggero M, Meroni PL. The geoepidemiology of the antiphospholipid antibody syndrome. *Autoimmunity reviews*. 2010;9(5):A299–A304.
597. Sebastiani GD, Iuliano A, Cantarini L, Galeazzi M. Genetic aspects of the antiphospholipid syndrome: an update. *Autoimmun Rev*. 2016;15(5):433–439.
598. Yin H, Borghi MO, Delgado-Vega AM, Tincani A, Meroni PL. Alarcón-Riquelme ME. Association of STAT4 and BLK, but not BANK1 or IRF5, with primary antiphospholipid syndrome. *Arthritis Rheum*. 2009;60(8):2468–2471.
599. Ochoa E, Iriondo M, Bielsa A, Ruiz-Irastorza G, Estonba A, Zubiaga AM. Thrombotic antiphospholipid syndrome shows strong haplotypic association with SH2B3-ATXN2 locus. *PLoS One*. 2013;8(7):e67897.
600. Bottini N, Vang T, Cucca F, Mustelin T. Role of PTPN22 in type 1 diabetes and other autoimmune diseases. *Semin Immunol*. 2006;18(4):207–213.
601. Lee YH, Choi SJ, Ji JD, Song GG. Association between the valine/leucine247 polymorphism of β2-glycoprotein I and susceptibility to anti-phospholipid syndrome: a meta-analysis. *Lupus*. 2012;21(8):865–871.
602. Bancsi LF, van der Linden IK, Bertina RM. Beta 2-glycoprotein I deficiency and the risk of thrombosis. *Thromb Haemost*. 1992;67(6):649–653.
603. Liestøl S, Sandset PM, Jacobsen EM, Mowinckel MC, Wisløff F. Decreased anticoagulant response to tissue factor pathway inhibitor type 1 in plasmas from patients with lupus anticoagulants. *Br J Haematol*. 2007;136(1):131–137.
604. Breen KA, Seed P, Parmar K, Moore GW, Stuart-Smith SE, Hunt BJ. Complement activation in patients with isolated antiphospholipid antibodies or primary antiphospholipid syndrome. *Thromb Haemost*. 2012;107(3):423–429.
605. Oku K, Amengual O, Hisada R, Ohmura K, Nakagawa I, Watanabe T, et al. Autoantibodies against a complement component 1 q subcomponent contribute to complement activation and recurrent thrombosis/pregnancy morbidity in anti-phospholipid syndrome. *Rheumatology (Oxford)*. 2016;55(8):1403–1411.
606. Arachchillage DR, Efthymiou M, Mackie IJ, Lawrie AS, Machin SJ, Cohen H. Anti-protein C antibodies are associated with resistance to endogenous protein C activation and a severe thrombotic phenotype in antiphospholipid syndrome. *J Thromb Haemost*. 2014;12(11):1801–1809.

607. López-Pedrera C, Buendía P, Cuadrado MJ, Siendones E, Aguirre MA, Barbarroja N, et al. Antiphospholipid antibodies from patients with the antiphospholipid syndrome induce monocyte tissue factor expression through the simultaneous activation of NF-kappaB/Rel proteins via the p38 mitogen-activated protein kinase pathway, and of the MEK-1/ERK pathway. *Arthritis Rheum.* 2006;54(1):301–311.
608. Espinola RG, Pierangeli SS, Gharavi AE, Harris EN. Hydroxychloroquine reverses platelet activation induced by human IgG antiphospholipid antibodies. *Thromb Haemost.* 2002;87(3):518–522.
609. Proulle V, Furie RA, Merrill-Skoloff G, Furie BC, Furie B. Platelets are required for enhanced activation of the endothelium and fibrinogen in a mouse thrombosis model of APS. *Blood.* 2014;124(4):611–622.
610. Romay-Penabad Z, Montiel-Manzano MG, Shilagard T, Papalardo E, Vargas G, Deora AB, et al. Annexin A2 is involved in antiphospholipid antibody-mediated pathogenic effects in vitro and in vivo. *Blood.* 2009;114(14):3074–3083.
611. Pierangeli SS, Chen PP, Raschi E, Scurati S, Grossi C, Borghi MO, et al. Antiphospholipid antibodies and the antiphospholipid syndrome: pathogenic mechanisms. *Semin Thromb Hemost.* 2008;34(3): 236–250.
612. López-Pedrera C, Cuadrado MJ, Herández V, Buendïa P, Aguirre MA, Barbarroja N, et al. Proteomic analysis in monocytes of antiphospholipid syndrome patients: deregulation of proteins related to the development of thrombosis. *Arthritis Rheum.* 2008;58(9):2835–2844.
613. Vega-Ostertag M, Casper K, Swerlick R, Ferrara D, Harris EN, Pierangeli SS. Involvement of p38 MAPK in the up-regulation of tissue factor on endothelial cells by antiphospholipid antibodies. *Arthritis Rheum.* 2005;52(5):1545–1554.
614. Montiel-Manzano G, Romay-Penabad Z, Papalardo de Martínez E, Meillon-García LA, García-Latorre E, Reyes-Maldonado E, et al. In vivo effects of an inhibitor of nuclear factor-kappa B on thrombogenic properties of antiphospholipid antibodies. *Ann NY Acad Sci.* 2007;1108:540–553.
615. Agostinis C, Biffi S, Garrovo C, Durigutto P, Lorenzon A, Bek A, et al. In vivo distribution of β2 glycoprotein I under various pathophysiologic conditions. *Blood.* 2011;118(15):4231–4238.
616. Mulla MJ, Brosens JJ, Chamley LW, Giles I, Pericleous C, Rahman A, et al. Antiphospholipid antibodies induce a pro-inflammatory response in first trimester trophoblast via the TLR4/MyD88 pathway. *Am J Reprod Immunol.* 2009;62(2):96–111.
617. Gladigau G, Haselmayer P, Scharrer I, Munder M, Prinz N, Lackner K, et al. A role for Toll-like receptor mediated signals in neutrophils in the pathogenesis of the anti-phospholipid syndrome. *PLoS One.* 2012;7(7):e42176.
618. Yalavarthi S, Gould TJ, Rao AN, Mazza LF, Morris AE, Núñez-Álvarez C, et al. Release of neutrophil extracellular traps by neutrophils stimulated with antiphospholipid antibodies: a newly identified mechanism of thrombosis in the antiphospholipid syndrome. *Arthritis Rheumatol.* 2015;67(11): 2990–3003.
619. Meng H, Yalavarthi S, Kanthi Y, Mazza LF, Elfline MA, Luke CE, et al. In Vivo Role of Neutrophil Extracellular Traps in Antiphospholipid Antibody-Mediated Venous Thrombosis. *Arthritis Rheumatol.* 2017;69(3):655–667.
620. Shoenfeld Y. APS–more systemic disease than SLE. *Clin Rev Allergy Immunol.* 2007;32(2):129–130.
621. Marai I, Zandman-Goddard G, Shoenfeld Y. The systemic nature of the antiphospholipid syndrome. *Scand J Rheumatol.* 2004;33(6):365–372.
622. Cervera R, Piette JC, Font J, Khamashta MA, Shoenfeld Y, Camps MT, et al. Antiphospholipid syndrome: clinical and immunologic manifestations and patterns of disease expression in a cohort of 1,000 patients. *Arthritis Rheum.* 2002;46(4):1019–1027.
623. Ruiz-Irastorza G, Crowther M, Branch W, Khamashta MA. Antiphospholipid syndrome. *Lancet.* 2010;376(9751):1498–1509.
624. Sciascia S, Radin M, Bazzan M, Roccatello D. Novel diagnostic and therapeutic frontiers in thrombotic anti-phospholipid syndrome. *Intern Emerg Med.* 2017;12(1):1–7.
625. Cohen H, Hunt BJ, Efthymiou M, Arachchillage DR, Mackie IJ, Clawson S, et al. Rivaroxaban versus warfarin to treat patients with thrombotic antiphospholipid syndrome, with or without systemic lupus erythematosus (RAPS): a randomised, controlled, open-label, phase 2/3, non-inferiority trial. *Lancet Haematol.* 2016;3(9):e426–e436.

626. Erkan D, Aguiar CL, Andrade D, Cohen H, Cuadrado MJ, Danowski A, et al. 14th International Congress on Antiphospholipid Antibodies: task force report on antiphospholipid syndrome treatment trends. *Autoimmun Rev*. 2014;13(6):685–696.
627. Levy RA, Dos Santos FC, de Jesús GR, de Jesús NR. Antiphospholipid Antibodies and Antiphospholipid Syndrome during Pregnancy: diagnostic Concepts. *Front Immunol*. 2015;6:205.
628. Tektonidou MG, Laskari K, Panagiotakos DB, Moutsopoulos HM. Risk factors for thrombosis and primary thrombosis prevention in patients with systemic lupus erythematosus with or without antiphospholipid antibodies. *Arthritis Rheum*. 2009;61(1):29–36.
629. Negrini S, Pappalardo F, Murdaca G, Indiveri F, Puppo F. The antiphospholipid syndrome: from pathophysiology to treatment. *Clin Exp Med*. 2017;17(3):257–267.
630. Sciascia S, Branch DW, Levy RA, Middeldorp S, Pavord S, Roccatello D, et al. The efficacy of hydroxychloroquine in altering pregnancy outcome in women with antiphospholipid antibodies. Evidence and clinical judgment. *Thromb Haemost*. 2016;115(2):285–290.
631. Sukara G, Baresic M, Sentic M, Brcic L, Anic B. Catastrophic antiphospholipid syndrome associated with systemic lupus erythematosus treated with rituximab: case report and a review of the literature. *Acta Reumatol Port*. 2015;40(2):169–175.
632. Puente D, Pombo G, Forastiero R. Current management of antiphospholipid syndrome-related thrombosis. *Expert Rev Cardiovasc Ther*. 2009;7(12):1551–1558.
633. Espinosa G, Berman H, Cervera R. Management of refractory cases of catastrophic antiphospholipid syndrome. *Autoimmun Rev*. 2011;10(11):664–668.
634. Stone JH, Zen Y, Deshpande V. IgG4-related disease. *New England Journal of Medicine*. 2012;366(6):539–551.
635. Mahajan VS, Mattoo H, Deshpande V, Pillai SS, Stone JH. IgG4-related disease. *Annual Review of Pathology: Mechanisms of Disease*. 2014;9:315–347.
636. Wallace ZS, Deshpande V, Mattoo H, Mahajan VS, Kulikova M, Pillai S, et al. IgG4-related disease: clinical and laboratory features in one hundred twenty-five patients. *Arthritis & rheumatology*. 2015;67(9):2466–2475.
637. Stone JH. *Immunoglobulin G4-Related Disease. The Autoimmune Diseases*: Elsevier; 2020:715–726.
638. Mattoo H, Mahajan VS, Della-Torre E, Sekigami Y, Carruthers M, Wallace ZS, et al. De novo oligoclonal expansions of circulating plasmablasts in active and relapsing IgG4-related disease. *Journal of allergy and clinical immunology*. 2014;134(3):679–687.
639. Mattoo H, Mahajan VS, Maehara T, Deshpande V, Della-Torre E, Wallace ZS, et al. Clonal expansion of CD4+ cytotoxic T lymphocytes in patients with IgG4-related disease. *Journal of Allergy and Clinical Immunology*. 2016;138(3):825–838.
640. Perugino CA, AlSalem SB, Mattoo H, Della-Torre E, Mahajan V, Ganesh G, et al. Identification of galectin-3 as an autoantigen in patients with IgG4-related disease. *Journal of Allergy and Clinical Immunology*. 2019;143(2):736–745 e6.
641. Perugino CA, Mattoo H, Mahajan VS, Maehara T, Wallace ZS, Pillai S, et al. Emerging treatment models in rheumatology: igG4-related disease: insights into human immunology and targeted therapies. *Arthritis & Rheumatology*. 2017;69(9):1722–1732.
642. Wallace ZS, Mattoo H, Carruthers M, Mahajan VS, Della Torre E, Lee H, et al. Plasmablasts as a biomarker for IgG4-related disease, independent of serum IgG4 concentrations. *Annals of the rheumatic diseases*. 2015;74(1):190–195.
643. Maehara T, Mattoo H, Ohta M, Mahajan VS, Moriyama M, Yamauchi M, et al. Lesional CD4+ IFN-γ+ cytotoxic T lymphocytes in IgG4-related dacryoadenitis and sialoadenitis. *Annals of the Rheumatic Diseases*. 2017;76(2):377–385.
644. Hsi ED, Steinle R, Balasa B, Szmania S, Draksharapu A, Shum BP, et al. CS1, a potential new therapeutic antibody target for the treatment of multiple myeloma. *Clinical Cancer Research*. 2008;14(9): 2775–2784.
645. Pérez-Quintero l-A, Roncagalli R, Guo H, Latour S, Davidson D, Veillette A. EAT-2, a SAP-like adaptor, controls NK cell activation through phospholipase Cγ, Ca++, and Erk, leading to granule polarization. *Journal of Experimental Medicine*. 2014;211(4):727–742.
646. Khosroshahi A, Wallace Z, Crowe J, Akamizu T, Azumi A, Carruthers M, et al. International consensus guidance statement on the management and treatment of IgG4-related disease. *Arthritis and Rheumatology*. 2015;67(7):1688–1699.

647. Khosroshahi A, Bloch DB, Deshpande V, Stone JH. Rituximab therapy leads to rapid decline of serum IgG4 levels and prompt clinical improvement in IgG4-related systemic disease. *Arthritis & Rheumatism.* 2010;62(6):1755–1762.
648. Carruthers MN, Topazian MD, Khosroshahi A, Witzig TE, Wallace ZS, Hart PA, et al. Rituximab for IgG4-related disease: a prospective, open-label trial. *Annals of the rheumatic diseases.* 2015;74(6): 1171–1177.
649. Olek M, Dawson D. *Multiple Sclerosis and Other Inflammatory Demyelinating Diseases of the Central Nervous system. Neurology in Clinical Practice.* New York: Butterworth Heineman; 2002.
650. Schumacher GA, Beebe G, Kibler RF, Kurland LT, Kurtzke JF, McDowell F, et al. Problems of experimental trials of therapy in multiple sclerosis: report by the panel on the evaluation of experimental trials of therapy in multiple sclerosis. *Annals of the New York Academy of Sciences.* 1965;122(1):552–568.
651. Sawcer S, Hellenthal G, Pirinen M, Spencer CC, Patsopoulos NA, Moutsianas L, et al. Genetic risk and a primary role for cell-mediated immune mechanisms in multiple sclerosis. *Nature.* 2011;476(7359):214.
652. Consortium IMSG. Risk alleles for multiple sclerosis identified by a genomewide study. *New England Journal of Medicine.* 2007;357(9):851–862.
653. Ascherio A. Environmental factors in multiple sclerosis. *Expert review of neurotherapeutics.* 2013;13(sup2):3–9.
654. Balashov KE, Rottman JB, Weiner HL, Hancock WW. CCR5+ and CXCR3+ T cells are increased in multiple sclerosis and their ligands MIP-1$\alpha$ and IP-10 are expressed in demyelinating brain lesions. *Proceedings of the National Academy of Sciences.* 1999;96(12):6873–6878.
655. Sørensen TL, Tani M, Jensen J, Pierce V, Lucchinetti C, Folcik VA, et al. Expression of specific chemokines and chemokine receptors in the central nervous system of multiple sclerosis patients. *The Journal of clinical investigation.* 1999;103(6):807–815.
656. Blain M, Nalbantoglu J, Antel JP. Interferon-$\gamma$ mRNA expression in immediately EX vivo CSF T cells. *Journal of Neuroimmunology.* 1994;54(1):149.
657. Hofman F, Hinton D, Johnson K, Merrill J. Tumor necrosis factor identified in multiple sclerosis brain. *The Journal of experimental medicine.* 1989;170(2):607–612.
658. Windhagen A, Schooz C, Höllsberg P, Fukaura H, Sette A, Hafler DA. Modulation of cytokine patterns of human autoreactive T cell clones by a single amino acid substitution of their peptide ligand. *Immunity.* 1995;2(4):373–380.
659. Crawford MP, Yan SX, Ortega SB, Mehta RS, Hewitt RE, Price DA, et al. High prevalence of autoreactive, neuroantigen-specific CD8+ T cells in multiple sclerosis revealed by novel flow cytometric assay. *Blood.* 2004;103(11):4222–4231.
660. Reboldi A, Coisne C, Baumjohann D, Benvenuto F, Bottinelli D, Lira S, et al. CC chemokine receptor 6–regulated entry of TH-17 cells into the CNS through the choroid plexus is required for the initiation of EAE. *Nature immunology.* 2009;10(5):514–523.
661. Steinman L. A brief history of Th 17, the first major revision in the Th 1/Th 2 hypothesis of T cell–mediated tissue damage. *Nature medicine.* 2007;13(2):139–145.
662. El-Behi M, Ciric B, Dai H, Yan Y, Cullimore M, Safavi F, et al. The encephalitogenicity of TH 17 cells is dependent on IL-1-and IL-23-induced production of the cytokine GM-CSF. *Nature immunology.* 2011;12(6):568–575.
663. Codarri L, Gyülvészi G, Tosevski V, Hesske L, Fontana A, Magnenat L, et al. ROR$\gamma$t drives production of the cytokine GM-CSF in helper T cells, which is essential for the effector phase of autoimmune neuroinflammation. *Nature immunology.* 2011;12(6):560–567.
664. Kebir H, Kreymborg K, Ifergan I, Dodelet-Devillers A, Cayrol R, Bernard M, et al. Human TH 17 lymphocytes promote blood-brain barrier disruption and central nervous system inflammation. *Nature medicine.* 2007;13(10):1173–1175.
665. Nylander A. Multiple Sclerosis (Review). *Journal of Clinical Investigations.* 2012;122(4):1180–1188.
666. Haas J, Hug A, Viehöver A, Fritzsching B, Falk CS, Filser A, et al. Reduced suppressive effect of CD4+ CD25high regulatory T cells on the T cell immune response against myelin oligodendrocyte glycoprotein in patients with multiple sclerosis. *European journal of immunology.* 2005;35(11):3343–3352.
667. Lovato L, Willis SN, Rodig SJ, Caron T, Almendinger SE, Howell OW, et al. Related B cell clones populate the meninges and parenchyma of patients with multiple sclerosis. *Brain.* 2011;134(2):534–541.

668. Serafini B, Rosicarelli B, Magliozzi R, Stigliano E, Aloisi F. Detection of ectopic B-cell follicles with germinal centers in the meninges of patients with secondary progressive multiple sclerosis. *Brain pathology*. 2004;14(2):164–174.
669. Barr TA, Shen P, Brown S, Lampropoulou V, Roch T, Lawrie S, et al. B cell depletion therapy ameliorates autoimmune disease through ablation of IL-6–producing B cells. *Journal of Experimental Medicine*. 2012;209(5):1001–1010.
670. Wingerchuk DM, Lucchinetti CF, Noseworthy JH. Multiple sclerosis: current pathophysiological concepts. *Laboratory investigation*. 2001;81(3):263–281.
671. Mattson D, Petrie M, Srivastava DK, McDermott M. Multiple sclerosis: sexual dysfunction and its response to medications. *Archives of Neurology*. 1995;52(9):862–868.
672. Amato M, Bartolozzi M, Zipoli V, Portaccio E, Mortilla M, Guidi L, et al. Neocortical volume decrease in relapsing–remitting MS patients with mild cognitive impairment. *Neurology*. 2004;63(1):89–93.
673. Whitlock F, Siskind M. Depression as a major symptom of multiple sclerosis. *Journal of Neurology, Neurosurgery & Psychiatry*. 1980;43(10):861–865.
674. Hohol MJ, Guttmann CR, Orav J, Mackin GA, Kikinis R, Khoury SJ, et al. Serial neuropsychological assessment and magnetic resonance imaging analysis in multiple sclerosis. *Archives of neurology*. 1997;54(8):1018–1025.
675. Polman CH, Reingold SC, Edan G, Filippi M, Hartung HP, Kappos L, et al. Diagnostic criteria for multiple sclerosis: 2005 revisions to the "McDonald Criteria. *Annals of Neurology: Official Journal of the American Neurological Association and the Child Neurology Society*. 2005;58(6):840–846.
676. Miller DH, Chard DT, Ciccarelli O. Clinically isolated syndromes. *The Lancet Neurology*. 2012;11(2):157–169.
677. Confavreux C, Vukusic S, Moreau T, Adeleine P. Relapses and progression of disability in multiple sclerosis. *New England Journal of Medicine*. 2000;343(20):1430–1438.
678. Weiner HL, Guttmann CR, Khoury SJ, Orav EJ, Hohol MJ, Kikinis R, et al. Serial magnetic resonance imaging in multiple sclerosis: correlation with attacks, disability, and disease stage. *Journal of neuroimmunology*. 2000;104(2):164–173.
679. Filippi M, Paty D, Kappos L, Barkhof F, Compston D, Thompson A, et al. Correlations between changes in disability and T2-weighted brain MRI activity in multiple sclerosis: a follow-up study. *Neurology*. 1995;45(2):255–260.
680. Khoury S, Guttmann C, Orav E, Hohol M, Ahn S, Hsu L, et al. Longitudinal MRI in multiple sclerosis: correlation between disability and lesion burden. *Neurology*. 1994;44(11):2120.
681. Miller DH, Leary SM. Primary-progressive multiple sclerosis. *The Lancet Neurology*. 2007;6(10):903–912.
682. Hutchinson M, Kappos L, Calabresi PA, Confavreux C, Giovannoni G, Galetta SL, et al. The efficacy of natalizumab in patients with relapsing multiple sclerosis: subgroup analyses of AFFIRM and SENTINEL. *Journal of neurology*. 2009;256(3):405–415.
683. Calabresi P, Giovannoni G, Confavreux C, Galetta S, Havrdova E, Hutchinson M, et al. The incidence and significance of anti-natalizumab antibodies: results from AFFIRM and SENTINEL. *Neurology*. 2007;69(14):1391–1403.
684. Cohen JA, Coles AJ, Arnold DL, Confavreux C, Fox EJ, Hartung H-P, et al. Alemtuzumab versus interferon beta 1a as first-line treatment for patients with relapsing-remitting multiple sclerosis: a randomised controlled phase 3 trial. *The Lancet*. 2012;380(9856):1819–1828.
685. Coles AJ, Twyman CL, Arnold DL, Cohen JA, Confavreux C, Fox EJ, et al. Alemtuzumab for patients with relapsing multiple sclerosis after disease-modifying therapy: a randomised controlled phase 3 trial. *The lancet*. 2012;380(9856):1829–1839.
686. Hauser SL, Bar-Or A, Comi G, Giovannoni G, Hartung H-P, Hemmer B, et al. Ocrelizumab versus interferon beta-1a in relapsing multiple sclerosis. *New England Journal of Medicine*. 2017;376(3):221–234.
687. Montalban X, Hauser SL, Kappos L, Arnold DL, Bar-Or A, Comi G, et al. Ocrelizumab versus placebo in primary progressive multiple sclerosis. *New England Journal of Medicine*. 2017;376(3):209–220.
688. Pham TH, Okada T, Matloubian M, Lo CG, Cyster JG. S1P1 receptor signaling overrides retention mediated by Gαi-coupled receptors to promote T cell egress. *Immunity*. 2008;28(1):122–133.
689. Schwab SR, Cyster JG. Finding a way out: lymphocyte egress from lymphoid organs. *Nature immunology*. 2007;8(12):1295–1301.

690. Hartung H-P, Aktas O, Kieseier B, Comi G. Development of oral cladribine for the treatment of multiple sclerosis. *Journal of neurology*. 2010;257(2):163–170.
691. Gold R, Kappos L, Arnold DL, Bar-Or A, Giovannoni G, Selmaj K, et al. Placebo-controlled phase 3 study of oral BG-12 for relapsing multiple sclerosis. *New England Journal of Medicine*. 2012;367(12):1098–1107.
692. Kappos L, Gold R, Miller DH, MacManus DG, Havrdova E, Limmroth V, et al. Efficacy and safety of oral fumarate in patients with relapsing-remitting multiple sclerosis: a multicentre, randomised, double-blind, placebo-controlled phase IIb study. *The Lancet*. 2008;372(9648):1463–1472.
693. Fontoura P, Garren H. *Multiple Sclerosis therapies: Molecular Mechanisms and future. Molecular Basis of Multiple Sclerosis*: Springer; 2010:259–285.
694. Linker RA, Lee d-H, Ryan S, van Dam AM, Conrad R, Bista P, et al. Fumaric acid esters exert neuroprotective effects in neuroinflammation via activation of the Nrf2 antioxidant pathway. *Brain*. 2011;134(3):678–692.
695. PRISMS S. PRISMS-4: long-term efficacy of interferon-beta-1a in relapsing MS. *Neurology*. 2001;56(12):1628.
696. Duda PW, Schmied MC, Cook SL, Krieger JI, Hafler DA. Glatiramer acetate (Copaxone®) induces degenerate, Th2-polarized immune responses in patients with multiple sclerosis. *The Journal of clinical investigation*. 2000;105(7):967–976.
697. Garchon H-J, Djabiri F, Viard J-P, Gajdos P, Bach J-F. Involvement of human muscle acetylcholine receptor alpha-subunit gene (CHRNA) in susceptibility to myasthenia gravis. *Proceedings of the National Academy of Sciences*. 1994;91(11):4668–4672.
698. Dondi E, Gajdos P, Bach J-F, Garchon H-J. Association of Km3 allotype with increased serum levels of autoantibodies against muscle acetylcholine receptor in myasthenia gravis. *Journal of neuroimmunology*. 1994;51(2):221–224.
699. Amdahl C, Alseth EH, Gilhus NE, Nakkestad HL, Skeie GO. Polygenic disease associations in thymomatous myasthenia gravis. *Archives of neurology*. 2007;64(12):1729–1733.
700. Hjelrnström P, Giscombe R, Lefvert A, Pirskanen R, Kockum I, Landin-Olsson M, et al. TAP polymorphisms in Swedish myasthenia gravis patients. *Tissue antigens*. 1997;49(2):176–179.
701. Wang X, Pirskanen R, Giscombe R, Lefvert A. Two SNPs in the promoter region of the CTLA-4 gene affect binding of transcription factors and are associated with human myasthenia gravis. *Journal of internal medicine*. 2008;263(1):61–69.
702. Provenzano C, Ricciardi R, Scuderi F, Maiuri MT, Maestri M, La Carpia F, et al. PTPN22 and myasthenia gravis: replication in an Italian population and meta-analysis of literature data. *Neuromuscular Disorders*. 2012;22(2):131–138.
703. Drosos A, Christou L, Galanopoulou V, Tzioufas A, Tsiakou E. D-penicillamine induced myasthenia gravis: clinical, serological and genetic findings. *Clinical and experimental rheumatology*. 1993;11(4):387–391.
704. Rødgaard A, Nielsen F, Djurup R, Somnier F, Gammeltoft S. Acetylcholine receptor antibody in myasthenia gravis: predominance of IgG subclasses 1 and 3. *Clinical and experimental immunology*. 1987;67(1):82.
705. McConville J, Farrugia ME, Beeson D, Kishore U, Metcalfe R, Newsom-Davis J, et al. Detection and characterization of MuSK antibodies in seronegative myasthenia gravis. *Annals of neurology*. 2004;55(4):580–584.
706. Koneczny I, Stevens JA, De Rosa A, Huda S, Huijbers MG, Saxena A, et al. IgG4 autoantibodies against muscle-specific kinase undergo Fab-arm exchange in myasthenia gravis patients. *Journal of autoimmunity*. 2017;77:104–115.
707. Koneczny I, Cossins J, Waters P, Beeson D, Vincent A. MuSK myasthenia gravis IgG4 disrupts the interaction of LRP4 with MuSK but both IgG4 and IgG1-3 can disperse preformed agrin-independent AChR clusters. *PloS one*. 2013;8(11):e80695.
708. Huijbers MG, Zhang W, Klooster R, Niks EH, Friese MB, Straasheijm KR, et al. MuSK IgG4 autoantibodies cause myasthenia gravis by inhibiting binding between MuSK and Lrp4. *Proceedings of the National Academy of Sciences*. 2013;110(51):20783–20788.
709. Shen C, Lu Y, Zhang B, Figueiredo D, Bean J, Jung J, et al. Antibodies against low-density lipoprotein receptor–related protein 4 induce myasthenia gravis. *The Journal of clinical investigation*. 2013;123(12):5190–5202.

710. Zhang B, Shen C, Bealmear B, Ragheb S, Xiong W-C, Lewis RA, et al. Autoantibodies to agrin in myasthenia gravis patients. *PloS one*. 2014;9(3):e91816.
711. Katarzyna MZ, Belaya K, Leite M, Patrick W, Vincent A, Beeson D. Collagen Q–a potential target for autoantibodies in myasthenia gravis. *Journal of the neurological sciences*. 2015;348(1–2):241–244.
712. Agius MA, Zhu S, Kirvan CA, Schafer AL, Lin MY, Fairclough RH, et al. Rapsyn Antibodies in Myasthenia Gravis a. *Annals of the New York Academy of Sciences*. 1998;841(1):516–521.
713. Cortés-Vicente E, Gallardo E, Martínez MÁ, Díaz-Manera J, Querol L, Rojas-García R, et al. Clinical characteristics of patients with double-seronegative myasthenia gravis and antibodies to cortactin. *JAMA neurology*. 2016;73(9):1099–1104.
714. Gallardo E, Martínez-Hernández E, Titulaer MJ, Huijbers MG, Martínez MA, Ramos A, et al. Cortactin autoantibodies in myasthenia gravis. *Autoimmunity reviews*. 2014;13(10):1003–1007.
715. Åhlberg R, Yi Q, Pirskanen R, Matell G, Swerup C, Rieber E, et al. Treatment of myasthenia gravis with anti-CD4 antibody: improvement correlates to decreased T-cell autoreactivity. *Neurology*. 1994;44(9):1732.
716. Li X, Xiao B-G, Xi J-Y, Lu C-Z, Lu J-H. Decrease of CD4+ CD25highFoxp3+ regulatory T cells and elevation of CD19+ BAFF-R+ B cells and soluble ICAM-1 in myasthenia gravis. *Clinical immunology*. 2008;126(2):180–188.
717. Mu L, Sun B, Kong Q, Wang J, Wang G, Zhang S, et al. Disequilibrium of T helper type 1, 2 and 17 cells and regulatory T cells during the development of experimental autoimmune myasthenia gravis. *Immunology*. 2009;128(1pt2):e826–ee36.
718. Huang YM, Pirskanen R, Giscombe R, Link H, Lefvert AK. Circulating CD4+ CD25+ and CD4+ CD25–T Cells in Myasthenia Gravis and in Relation to Thymectomy. *Scandinavian journal of immunology*. 2004;59(4):408–414.
719. Balandina A, Lécart S, Dartevelle P, Saoudi A. Berrih-Aknin S. Functional defect of regulatory CD4+ CD25+ T cells in the thymus of patients with autoimmune myasthenia gravis. *Blood*. 2005;105(2):735–741.
720. Lee JY, Stathopoulos P, Gupta S, Bannock JM, Barohn RJ, Cotzomi E, et al. Compromised fidelity of B-cell tolerance checkpoints in AChR and MuSK myasthenia gravis. *Annals of clinical and translational neurology*. 2016;3(6):443–454.
721. Yi JS, Russo MA, Massey JM, Juel V, Hobson-Webb LD, Gable K, et al. B10 cell frequencies and suppressive capacity in myasthenia gravis are associated with disease severity. *Frontiers in neurology*. 2017;8:34.
722. Karim MR, Zhang H-Y, Yuan J, Sun Q, Wang Y-F. Regulatory B cells in seropositive myasthenia gravis versus healthy controls. *Frontiers in neurology*. 2017;8:43.
723. Sheng JR, Rezania K, Soliven B. Impaired regulatory B cells in myasthenia gravis. *Journal of neuroimmunology*. 2016;297:38–45.
724. Kohler S, Keil TOP, Hoffmann S, Swierzy M, Ismail M, Rueckert JC, et al. CD4+ FoxP3+ T regulatory cell subsets in myasthenia gravis patients. *Clinical Immunology*. 2017;179:40–46.
725. Wen Y, Yang B, Lu J, Zhang J, Yang H, Li J. Imbalance of circulating CD4+ CXCR5+ FOXP3+ Tfr-like cells and CD4+ CXCR5+ FOXP3− Tfh-like cells in myasthenia gravis. *Neuroscience letters*. 2016;630:176–182.
726. Damato V, Viegas S, Vincent A. *Myasthenia Gravis and Related Disorders. The Autoimmune Diseases*: Elsevier; 2020:1011–1033.
727. Compston D, Vincent A, Newsom-Davis J, Batchelor J. Clinical, pathological, HLA antigen and immunological evidence for disease heterogeneity in myasthenia gravis. *Brain*. 1980;103(3):579–601.
728. Horiki T, Inoko H, Moriuchi J, Ichikawa Y, Arimori S. Combinations of HLA-DPB1 and HLA-DQB1 alleles determine susceptibility to early-onset myasthenia gravis in Japan. *Autoimmunity*. 1994;19(1):49–54.
729. Hill M, Beeson D, Moss P, Jacobson L, Bond A, Corlett L, et al. Early-onset myasthenia gravis: a recurring T-cell epitope in the adult-specific acetylcholine receptor ε subunit presented by the susceptibility allele HLA-DR52a. *Annals of Neurology: Official Journal of the American Neurological Association and the Child Neurology Society*. 1999;45(2):224–231.
730. Janer M, Cowland A, Picard J, Campbell D, Pontarotti P, Newsom-Davis J, et al. A susceptibility region for myasthenia gravis extending into the HLA-class I sector telomeric to HLA-C. *Human immunology*. 1999;60(9):909–917.

731. Carlsson B, Wallin J, Pirskanen R, Matell G, Smith CE. Different HLA DR-DQ associations in subgroups of idiopathic myasthenia gravis. *Immunogenetics*. 1990;31(5–6):285–290.
732. Buckley C, Newsom–Davis J, Willcox N, Vincent A. Do titin and cytokine antibodies in MG patients predict thymoma or thymoma recurrence? *Neurology*. 2001;57(9):1579–1582.
733. Meager A, Wadhwa M, Dilger P, Bird C, Thorpe R, Newsom-Davis J, et al. Anti-cytokine autoantibodies in autoimmunity: preponderance of neutralizing autoantibodies against interferon-alpha, interferon-omega and interleukin-12 in patients with thymoma and/or myasthenia gravis. *Clinical & Experimental Immunology*. 2003;132(1):128–136.
734. Živković SA, Clemens PR. Lacomis D. Characteristics of late-onset myasthenia gravis. *Journal of neurology*. 2012;259(10):2167–2171.
735. Maggi L, Andreetta F, Antozzi C, Confalonieri P, Cornelio F, Scaioli V, et al. Two cases of thymoma-associated myasthenia gravis without antibodies to the acetylcholine receptor. *Neuromuscular Disorders*. 2008;18(8):678–680.
736. Mygland Å, Kuwajima G, Mikoshiba K, Tysnes O-B, Aarli JA, Gilhus NE. Thymomas express epitopes shared by the ryanodine receptor. *Journal of neuroimmunology*. 1995;62(1):79–83.
737. Niks E, Kuks J, Roep B, Haasnoot G, Verduijn W, Ballieux B, et al. Strong association of MuSK antibody–positive myasthenia gravis and HLA-DR14-DQ5. *Neurology*. 2006;66(11):1772–1774.
738. Bartoccioni E, Scuderi F, Augugliaro A, Ranieri SC, Sauchelli D, Alboino P, et al. HLA class II allele analysis in MuSK-positive myasthenia gravis suggests a role for DQ5. *Neurology*. 2009;72(2):195–197.
739. Evoli A, Tonali PA, Padua L, Monaco ML, Scuderi F, Batocchi AP, et al. Clinical correlates with anti-MuSK antibodies in generalized seronegative myasthenia gravis. *Brain*. 2003;126(10):2304–2311.
740. Sanders DB, El-Salem K, Massey J, McConville J, Vincent A. Clinical aspects of MuSK antibody positive seronegative MG. *Neurology*. 2003;60(12):1978–1980.
741. Evoli A, Bianchi MR, Riso R, Minicuci GM, Batocchi AP, Servidei S, et al. Response to therapy in myasthenia gravis with anti-MuSK antibodies. *Annals of the New York Academy of Sciences*. 2008;1132(1):76–83.
742. Leite MI, Jacob S, Viegas S, Cossins J, Clover L, Morgan BP, et al. IgG1 antibodies to acetylcholine receptors in 'seronegative' myasthenia gravis. *Brain*. 2008;131(7):1940–1952.
743. Wolfe GI, Kaminski HJ, Aban IB, Minisman G, Kuo H-C, Marx A, et al. Randomized trial of thymectomy in myasthenia gravis. *New England Journal of Medicine*. 2016;375(6):511–522.
744. Maddison P, McConville J, Farrugia ME, Davies N, Rose M, Norwood F, et al. The use of rituximab in myasthenia gravis and Lambert–Eaton myasthenic syndrome. *Journal of Neurology, Neurosurgery & Psychiatry*. 2011;82(6):671–673.
745. Hadden R, Gregson N. Guillain–Barre syndrome and Campylobacter jejuni infection. *Journal of Applied Microbiology*. 2001;90(S6):145S–154S.
746. Sejvar JJ, Baughman AL, Wise M, Morgan OW. Population incidence of Guillain-Barré syndrome: a systematic review and meta-analysis. *Neuroepidemiology*. 2011;36(2):123–133.
747. Hughes RA, Cornblath DR. Guillain-barre syndrome. *The Lancet*. 2005;366(9497):1653–1666.
748. Rees J, Thompson R, Smeeton N, Hughes R. Epidemiological study of Guillain-Barré syndrome in south east England. *Journal of Neurology, Neurosurgery & Psychiatry*. 1998;64(1):74–77.
749. Geleijns K, Laman JD, van Rijs W, Tio-Gillen AP, Hintzen RQ, van Doorn PA, et al. Fas polymorphisms are associated with the presence of anti-ganglioside antibodies in Guillain–Barré syndrome. *Journal of neuroimmunology*. 2005;161(1–2):183–189.
750. Geleijns K, Schreuder GT, Jacobs B, Sintnicolaas K, Van Koningsveld R, Meulstee J, et al. HLA class II alleles are not a general susceptibility factor in Guillain–Barré syndrome. *Neurology*. 2005;64(1):44–49.
751. Magira EE, Papaioakim M, Nachamkin I, Asbury AK, Li CY, Ho TW, et al. Differential distribution of HLA-DQβ/DRβ epitopes in the two forms of Guillain-Barré syndrome, acute motor axonal neuropathy and acute inflammatory demyelinating polyneuropathy (AIDP): identification of DQβ epitopes associated with susceptibility to and protection from AIDP. *The Journal of Immunology*. 2003;170(6):3074–3080.
752. Hughes RA, Rees JH. Clinical and epidemiologic features of Guillain-Barré syndrome. *Journal of Infectious Diseases*. 1997;176(Supplement_2):S92–SS8.
753. Crawford NW, Cheng A, Andrews N, Charles PG, Clothier HJ, Day B, et al. Guillain-Barré syndrome following pandemic (H1N1) 2009 influenza A immunisation in Victoria: a self-controlled case series. *Medical journal of Australia*. 2012;197(10):574–578.

754. Moran AP, Prendergast MM, Hogan EL. Sialosyl-galactose: a common denominator of Guillain–Barré and related disorders? *Journal of the neurological sciences*. 2002;196(1–2):1–7.
755. Witebsky E, Rose NR, Terplan K, Paine JR, Egan RW. Chronic thyroiditis and autoimmunization. *Journal of the American Medical Association*. 1957;164(13):1439–1447.
756. Chiba A, Kusunoki S, Obata H, Machinami R, Kanazawa I. Ganglioside composition of the human cranial nerves, with special reference to pathophysiology of Miller Fisher syndrome. *Brain research*. 1997;745(1–2):32–36.
757. Chiba A, Kusunoki S, Obata H, Machinami R, Kanazawa I. Serum anti-GQ1b IgG antibody is associated with ophthalmoplegia in Miller Fisher syndrome and Guillain-Barré syndrome: clinical and immunohistochemical studies. *Neurology*. 1993;43(10):1911.
758. Sheikh KA, Zhang G, Gong Y, Schnaar RL, Griffin JW. An anti-ganglioside antibody-secreting hybridoma induces neuropathy in mice. *Annals of Neurology: Official Journal of the American Neurological Association and the Child Neurology Society*. 2004;56(2):228–239.
759. Gong Y, Tagawa Y, Lunn M, Laroy W, Heffer-Lauc M, Li C, et al. Localization of major gangliosides in the PNS: implications for immune neuropathies. *Brain*. 2002;125(11):2491–2506.
760. Willison HJ, Veitch J. Immunoglobulin subclass distribution and binding characteristics of anti-GQ1b antibodies in Miller Fisher syndrome. *Journal of neuroimmunology*. 1994;50(2):159–165.
761. Yuki N, Ichihashi Y, Taki T. Subclass of IgG antibody to GM1 epitope-bearing lipopolysaccharide of Campylobacter jejuni in patients with Guillain-Barré syndrome. *Journal of neuroimmunology*. 1995;60(1–2):161–164.
762. Ho T, Willison H, Nachamkin I, Li C, Veitch J, Ung H, et al. Anti-GD1a antibody is associated with axonal but not demyelinating forms of Guillain-Barré syndrome. *Annals of Neurology: Official Journal of the American Neurological Association and the Child Neurology Society*. 1999;45(2):168–173.
763. Ogino M, Orazio N, Latov N. IgG anti-GM1 antibodies from patients with acute motor neuropathy are predominantly of the IgG1 and IgG3 subclasses. *Journal of neuroimmunology*. 1995;58(1):77–80.
764. Willison HJ, Yuki N. Peripheral neuropathies and anti-glycolipid antibodies. *Brain*. 2002;125(12): 2591–2625.
765. Ogawara K, Kuwabara S, Mori M, Hattori T, Koga M, Yuki N. Axonal Guillain-Barré syndrome: relation to anti-ganglioside antibodies and Campylobacter jejuni infection in Japan. *Annals of Neurology: Official Journal of the American Neurological Association and the Child Neurology Society*. 2000;48(4):624–631.
766. Rees JH, Gregson NA, Hughes RA. Anti-ganglioside GM1 antibodies in Guillain-Barré syndrome and their relationship to Campylobacter jejuni infection. *Annals of Neurology: Official Journal of the American Neurological Association and the Child Neurology Society*. 1995;38(5):809–816.
767. Hadden R, Cornblath D, Hughes R, Zielasek J, Hartung HP, Toyka K, et al. Electrophysiological classification of Guillain-Barré syndrome: clinical associations and outcome. *Annals of neurology*. 1998;44(5):780–788.
768. Ang C, Yuki N, Jacobs B, Koga M, Van Doorn P, Schmitz P, et al. Rapidly progressive, predominantly motor Guillain-Barré syndrome with anti-GalNAc-GD1a antibodies. *Neurology*. 1999;53(9):2122.
769. Yuki N, Sato S, Tsuji S, Ohsawa T, Miyatake T. Frequent presence of anti-GQ1b antibody in Fisher's syndrome. *Neurology*. 1993;43(2):414.
770. Yuki N, Wim Ang C, Koga M, Jacobs BC, Van Doorn PA, Hirata K, et al. Clinical features and response to treatment in Guillain-Barré syndrome associated with antibodies to GM1b ganglioside. *Annals of Neurology: Official Journal of the American Neurological Association and the Child Neurology Society*. 2000;47(3):314–321.
771. Carpo M, Pedotti R, Lolli F, Pitrola A, Allaria S, Scarlato G, et al. Clinical correlate and fine specificity of anti-GQ1b antibodies in peripheral neuropathy. *Journal of the neurological sciences*. 1998;155(2): 186–191.
772. Willison H, Veitch J, Paterson G, Kennedy P. Miller Fisher syndrome is associated with serum antibodies to GQ1b ganglioside. *Journal of Neurology, Neurosurgery & Psychiatry*. 1993;56(2):204–206.
773. Greenshields KN, Halstead SK, Zitman FM, Rinaldi S, Brennan KM, O'Leary C, et al. The neuropathic potential of anti-GM1 autoantibodies is regulated by the local glycolipid environment in mice. *The Journal of clinical investigation*. 2009;119(3):595–610.
774. Kusunoki S, Ki Kaida. Antibodies against ganglioside complexes in Guillain-Barré syndrome and related disorders. *Journal of neurochemistry*. 2011;116(5):828–832.

775. Lopez PH, Zhang G, Zhang J, Lehmann HC, Griffin JW, Schnaar RL, et al. Passive transfer of IgG anti-GM1 antibodies impairs peripheral nerve repair. *Journal of Neuroscience*. 2010;30(28):9533–9541.
776. Lehmann HC, Lopez PH, Zhang G, Ngyuen T, Zhang J, Kieseier BC, et al. Passive immunization with anti-ganglioside antibodies directly inhibits axon regeneration in an animal model. *Journal of Neuroscience*. 2007;27(1):27–34.
777. Sheikh KA, Deerinck TJ, Ellisman MH, Griffin JW. The distribution of ganglioside-like moieties in peripheral nerves. *Brain*. 1999;122(3):449–460.
778. Susuki K, Rasband MN, Tohyama K, Koibuchi K, Okamoto S, Funakoshi K, et al. Anti-GM1 antibodies cause complement-mediated disruption of sodium channel clusters in peripheral motor nerve fibers. *Journal of Neuroscience*. 2007;27(15):3956–3967.
779. Taylor W, Hughes R. T lymphocyte activation antigens in Guillain-Barré syndrome and chronic idiopathic demyelinating polyradiculoneuropathy. *Journal of neuroimmunology*. 1989;24(1–2):33–39.
780. Cornblath DR, Griffin DE, Welch D, Griffin JW, McArthur JC. Quantitative analysis of endoneurial T-cells in human sural nerve biopsies. *Journal of neuroimmunology*. 1990;26(2):113–118.
781. Winer J, Hughes S, Cooper J, Ben-Smith A, Savage C. γδ T cells infiltrating sensory nerve biopsies from patients with inflammatory neuropathy. *Journal of neurology*. 2002;249(5):616–621.
782. Bukowski JF, Morita CT, Band H, Brenner MB. Crucial role of TCRγ chain junctional region in prenyl pyrophosphate antigen recognition by γδ T cells. *The Journal of Immunology*. 1998;161(1):286–293.
783. Exley A, Smith N, Winer J. Tumour necrosis factor-alpha and other cytokines in Guillain-Barre syndrome. *Journal of Neurology, Neurosurgery & Psychiatry*. 1994;57(9):1118–1120.
784. Créange A, Bélec L, Clair B, Degos J-D, Raphaël J-C, Gherardi RK. Circulating transforming growth factor beta 1 (TGF-β1) in Guillain-Barré syndrome: decreased concentrations in the early course and increase with motor function. *Journal of Neurology, Neurosurgery & Psychiatry*. 1998;64(2):162–165.
785. Hartung HP, Reiners K, Schmidt B, Stoll G, Toyka KV. Serum interleukin-2 concentrations in Guillain-Barré syndrome and chronic idiopathic demyelinating polyradiculoneuropathy: comparison with other neurological diseases of presumed immunopathogenesis. *Annals of Neurology: Official Journal of the American Neurological Association and the Child Neurology Society*. 1991;30(1):48–53.
786. Hartung H-P, Willison HJ, Kieseier BC. Acute immunoinflammatory neuropathy: update on Guillain-Barré syndrome. *Current Opinion in Neurology*. 2002;15(5):571–577.
787. Créange A, Chazaud B, Sharshar T, Plonquet A, Poron F, Eliezer M-C, et al. Inhibition of the adhesion step of leukodiapedesis: a critical event in the recovery of Guillain–Barré syndrome associated with accumulation of proteolytically active lymphocytes in blood. *Journal of neuroimmunology*. 2001;114(1–2):188–196.
788. Baggiolini M. Chemokines and leukocyte traffic. *Nature*. 1998;392(6676):565–568.
789. Creange A, Sharshar T, Planchenault T, Christov C, Poron F, Raphael J-C, et al. Matrix metalloproteinase-9 is increased and correlates with severity in Guillain-Barré syndrome. *Neurology*. 1999;53(8):1683.
790. Kieseier BC, Kiefer R, Clements JM, Miller K, Wells G, Schweitzer T, et al. Matrix metalloproteinase-9 and-7 are regulated in experimental autoimmune encephalomyelitis. *Brain: a journal of neurology*. 1998;121(1):159–166.
791. Hughes R, Hadden R, Gregson N, Smith K. Pathogenesis of Guillain–Barré syndrome. *Journal of neuroimmunology*. 1999;100(1–2):74–97.
792. Autoimmune responses in peripheral nerve. In: Hartung H-P, Willison H, Jung S, Pette M, Toyka KV, Giegerich G, eds. Autoimmune responses in peripheral nerve. *Springer seminars in immunopathology;*. 1996.
793. Hafer-Macko C, Hsieh ST, Ho TW, Sheikh K, Cornblath DR, Li CY, et al. Acute motor axonal neuropathy: an antibody-mediated attack on axolemma. *Annals of Neurology: Official Journal of the American Neurological Association and the Child Neurology Society*. 1996;40(4):635–644.
794. Hafer-Macko C, Sheikh K, Li C, Ho T, Cornblath D, McKhann G, et al. Immune attack on the Schwann cell surface in acute inflammatory demyelinating polyneuropathy. *Annals of Neurology: Official Journal of the American Neurological Association and the Child Neurology Society*. 1996;39(5):625–635.
795. Smith KJ, Kapoor R, Felts PA. Demyelination: the role of reactive oxygen and nitrogen species. *Brain pathology*. 1999;9(1):69–92.

796. Redford E, Smith K, Gregson N, Davies M, Hughes P, Gearing A, et al. A combined inhibitor of matrix metalloproteinase activity and tumour necrosis factor-alpha processing attenuates experimental autoimmune neuritis. *Brain: a journal of neurology*. 1997;120(10):1895–1905.
797. Dahle C, Ekerfelt C, Vrethem M, Samuelsson M, Ernerudh J. T helper type 2 like cytokine responses to peptides from P0 and P2 myelin proteins during the recovery phase of Guillain-Barre syndrome. *Journal of the neurological sciences*. 1997;153(1):54–60.
798. Kiefer R, Funa K, Schweitzer T, Jung S, Bourde O, Toyka KV, et al. Transforming growth factor-beta 1 in experimental autoimmune neuritis. Cellular localization and time course. *The American journal of pathology*. 1996;148(1):211.
799. Asbury AK, Cornblath DR. Assessment of current diagnostic criteria for Guillain-Barré syndrome. *Annals of Neurology: Official Journal of the American Neurological Association and the Child Neurology Society*. 1990;27(S1):S21–SS4.
800. Rinaldi S, Brennan KM, Goodyear CS, O'Leary C, Schiavo G, Crocker PR, et al. Analysis of lectin binding to glycolipid complexes using combinatorial glycoarrays. *Glycobiology*. 2009;19(7):789–796.
801. Hall SM, Hughes RA, Atkinson PF, McColl I, Gale A. Motor nerve biopsy in severe Guillain-Barré syndrome. *Annals of Neurology: Official Journal of the American Neurological Association and the Child Neurology Society*. 1992;31(4):441–444.
802. Lunn MP, Lehmann HC, Sheikh KA. *Peripheral Neuropathies. The Autoimmune Diseases*: Elsevier; 2020:987–1009.
803. Kuwabara S, Ogawara K, Mizobuchi K, Koga M, Mori M, Hattori T, et al. Isolated absence of F waves and proximal axonal dysfunction in Guillain-Barre syndrome with antiganglioside antibodies. *Journal of Neurology, Neurosurgery & Psychiatry*. 2000;68(2):191–195.
804. Griffin J, Li C, Ho T, Xue P, Macko C, Gao C, et al. Guillain-Barré syndrome in northern China: the spectrum of neuropathological changes in clinically defined cases. *Brain*. 1995;118(3):577–595.
805. Griffin J, Li C, Ho T, Tian M, Gao C, Xue P, et al. Pathology of the motor-sensory axonal Guillain-Barré syndrome. *Annals of neurology*. 1996;39(1):17–28.
806. Feasby T, Gilbert J, Brown W, Bolton C, Hahn A, Koopman W, et al. An acute axonal form of guillain-barrée polyneuropathy. *Brain*. 1986;109(6):1115–1126.
807. Fisher M. An unusual variant of acute idiopathic polyneuritis (syndrome of ophthalmoplegia, ataxia and areflexia). *New England Journal of Medicine*. 1956;255(2):57–65.
808. Hughes R, Wijdicks E, Barohn R, Benson E, Cornblath D, Hahn AF, et al. Practice parameter: immunotherapy for Guillain–Barré syndrome: report of the Quality Standards Subcommittee of the American Academy of Neurology. *Neurology*. 2003;61(6):736–740.
809. Chevret S, Hughes RA. Annane D. Plasma exchange for Guillain-Barré syndrome. *Cochrane Database of Systematic Reviews*. 2017(2).
810. Swan A, Van Doorn P, Hughes R. Intravenous immunoglobulin for Guillain-Barré syndrome. *Cochrane Database Syst Rev*. 2014;19(9).
811. Willison HJ, Townson K, Veitch J, Boffey J, Isaacs N, Andersen SM, et al. Synthetic disialylgalactose immunoadsorbents deplete anti-GQ1b antibodies from autoimmune neuropathy sera. *Brain*. 2004;127(3):680–691.
812. Okayasu I, Yi-chi MK, Rose NR. Effect of castration and sex hormones on experimental autoimmune thyroiditis. *Clinical immunology and immunopathology*. 1981;20(2):240–245.
813. Ahmed SA, Young P, Penhale W. The effects of female sex steroids on the development of autoimmune thyroiditis in thymectomized and irradiated rats. *Clinical and experimental immunology*. 1983;54(2):351.
814. Eaton WW, Pedersen MG, Atladóttir HÓ, Gregory PE, Rose NR, Mortensen PB. The prevalence of 30 ICD-10 autoimmune diseases in Denmark. *Immunologic research*. 2010;47(1–3):228–231.
815. Tomer Y, Davies TF. Searching for the autoimmune thyroid disease susceptibility genes: from gene mapping to gene function. *Endocrine reviews*. 2003;24(5):694–717.
816. Ji R, Feng Y, Zhan W. Updated analysis of studies on the cytotoxic T-lymphocyte-associated antigen-4 gene A49G polymorphism and Hashimoto's thyroiditis risk. *Genet Mol Res*. 2013;12(2):1421–1430.
817. Cooper JD, Simmonds MJ, Walker NM, Burren O, Brand OJ, Guo H, et al. Seven newly identified loci for autoimmune thyroid disease. *Human molecular genetics*. 2012;21(23):5202–5208.
818. Medici M, Porcu E, Pistis G, Teumer A, Brown SJ, Jensen RA, et al. Identification of novel genetic Loci associated with thyroid peroxidase antibodies and clinical thyroid disease. *PLoS Genet*. 2014;10(2):e1004123.

819. Mortensen KH, Cleemann L, Hjerrild B, Nexo E, Locht H, Jeppesen E, et al. Increased prevalence of autoimmunity in Turner syndrome–influence of age. *Clinical & Experimental Immunology*. 2009;156(2):205–210.
820. Aversa T, Lombardo F, Corrias A, Salerno M, De Luca F, Wasniewska M. In young patients with Turner or Down syndrome, Graves' disease presentation is often preceded by Hashimoto's thyroiditis. *Thyroid*. 2014;24(4):744–747.
821. Pearce EN, Farwell AP, Braverman LE. Thyroiditis. *New England Journal of Medicine*. 2003;348(26):2646–2655.
822. Raber W, Gessl A, Nowotny P, Vierhapper H. Thyroid ultrasound versus antithyroid peroxidase antibody determination: a cohort study of four hundred fifty-one subjects. *Thyroid*. 2002;12(8):725–731.
823. Diana T, Krause J, Olivo P, König J, Kanitz M, Decallonne B, et al. Prevalence and clinical relevance of thyroid stimulating hormone receptor-blocking antibodies in autoimmune thyroid disease. *Clinical & Experimental Immunology*. 2017;189(3):304–309.
824. Brix TH, Hegedüs L, Weetman AP, Kemp HE. Pendrin and NIS antibodies are absent in healthy individuals and are rare in autoimmune thyroid disease: evidence from a Danish twin study. *Clinical endocrinology*. 2014;81(3):440–444.
825. Marazuela M. Lymphocyte traffic and homing in autoimmune thyroid disorders. SCANDINAVIAN UNIVERSITY PRESS PO BOX 2959 TOYEN. *JOURNAL DIVISION CUSTOMER …*. 1999.
826. Liu C, Papewalis C, Domberg J, Scherbaum W, Schott M. Chemokines and autoimmune thyroid diseases. *Hormone and metabolic research*. 2008;40(06):361–368.
827. Aichinger G, Fill H, Wick G. In situ immune complexes, lymphocyte subpopulations, and HLA-DR-positive epithelial cells in Hashimoto thyroiditis. *Laboratory investigation; a journal of technical methods and pathology*. 1985;52(2):132.
828. Iwatani Y, Amino N, Hidaka Y, Kaneda T, Ichihara K, Tamaki H, et al. Decreases in αβ T cell receptor negative T cells and CD8 cells, and an increase in CD4+ CD8+ cells in active Hashimoto's disease and subacute thyroiditis. *Clinical & Experimental Immunology*. 1992;87(3):444–449.
829. Chen C-R, Hamidi S, Braley-Mullen H, Nagayama Y, Bresee C, Aliesky HA, et al. Antibodies to thyroid peroxidase arise spontaneously with age in NOD. H-2h4 mice and appear after thyroglobulin antibodies. *Endocrinology*. 2010;151(9):4583–4593.
830. Menconi F, Huber A, Osman R, Concepcion E, Jacobson EM, Stefan M, et al. Tg. 2098 is a major human thyroglobulin T-cell epitope. *Journal of autoimmunity*. 2010;35(1):45–51.
831. Tandon N, Freeman M, Weetman A. T cell responses to synthetic thyroid peroxidase peptides in autoimmune thyroid disease. *Clinical & Experimental Immunology*. 1991;86(1):56–60.
832. Glick AB, Wodzinski A, Fu P, Levine AD, Wald DN. Impairment of regulatory T-cell function in autoimmune thyroid disease. *Thyroid*. 2013;23(7):871–878.
833. Ajjan R, Watson P, McIntosh R, Weetman A. Intrathyroidal cytokine gene expression in Hashimoto's thyroiditis. *Clinical & Experimental Immunology*. 1996;105(3):523–528.
834. Bottazzo G, Hanafusa T, Pujol-Borrell R, Feldmann M. Role of aberrant HLA-DR expression and antigen presentation in induction of endocrine autoimmunity. *The Lancet*. 1983;322(8359):1115–1119.
835. Marelli-Berg FM, Weetman A, Frasca L, Deacock SJ, Imami N, Lombardi G, et al. Antigen presentation by epithelial cells induces anergic immunoregulatory CD45RO+ T cells and deletion of CD45RA+ T cells. *The Journal of Immunology*. 1997;159(12):5853–5861.
836. Londei M, Bottazzo GF, Feldmann M. Human T-cell clones from autoimmune thyroid glands: specific recognition of autologous thyroid cells. *Science*. 1985;228(4695):85–89.
837. Dayan CM, Chu NR, Londei M, Rapoport B. Feldmann M. T cells involved in human autoimmune disease are resistant to tolerance induction. *The Journal of Immunology*. 1993;151(3):1606–1613.
838. Jonklaas J, Bianco AC, Bauer AJ, Burman KD, Cappola AR, Celi FS, et al. Guidelines for the treatment of hypothyroidism: prepared by the american thyroid association task force on thyroid hormone replacement. *Thyroid*. 2014;24(12):1670–1751.
839. Takasu N, Yamada T, Takasu M, Komiya I, Nagasawa Y, Asawa T, et al. Disappearance of thyrotropin-blocking antibodies and spontaneous recovery from hypothyroidism in autoimmune thyroiditis. *New England Journal of Medicine*. 1992;326(8):513–518.
840. Smith TJ, Hegedüs L. Graves' disease. *New England Journal of Medicine*. 2016;375(16):1552–1565.

841. Brix TH, Kyvik KO, Hegedüs L. What is the evidence of genetic factors in the etiology of Graves' disease? A brief review. *Thyroid*. 1998;8(8):727–734.
842. Yanagawa T, Hidaka Y, Guimaraes V, Soliman M, DeGroot L. CTLA-4 gene polymorphism associated with Graves' disease in a Caucasian population. *The Journal of Clinical Endocrinology & Metabolism*. 1995;80(1):41–45.
843. Tomer Y. Genetic susceptibility to autoimmune thyroid disease: past, present, and future. *Thyroid*. 2010;20(7):715–725.
844. Brand OJ, Barrett JC, Simmonds MJ, Newby PR, McCabe CJ, Bruce CK, et al. Association of the thyroid stimulating hormone receptor gene (TSHR) with Graves' disease. *Human molecular genetics*. 2009;18(9):1704–1713.
845. Chu X, Pan C-M, Zhao S-X, Liang J, Gao G-Q, Zhang X-M, et al. A genome-wide association study identifies two new risk loci for Graves' disease. *Nature genetics*. 2011;43(9):897.
846. Zhao S-X, Xue l-Q, Liu W, Gu Z-H, Pan C-M, Yang S-Y, et al. Robust evidence for five new Graves' disease risk loci from a staged genome-wide association analysis. *Human molecular genetics*. 2013;22(16):3347–3362.
847. Zakarija M. Immunochemical characterization of the thyroid-stimulating antibody (TSAb) of Graves' disease: evidence for restricted heterogeneity. *Journal of clinical & laboratory immunology*. 1983;10(2):77–85.
848. Rapoport B, McLachlan SM. TSH receptor cleavage into subunits and shedding of the A-subunit; a molecular and clinical perspective. *Endocrine reviews*. 2016;37(2):114–134.
849. Morshed SA, Ando T, Latif R, Davies TF. Neutral antibodies to the TSH receptor are present in Graves' disease and regulate selective signaling cascades. *Endocrinology*. 2010;151(11):5537–5549.
850. Weetman A, McGregor A. Autoimmune thyroid disease: further developments in our understanding. *Endocrine reviews*. 1994;15(6):788–830.
851. Okumura M, Hidaka Y, Matsuzuka F, Takeoka K, Tada H, Kuma K, et al. CD30 expression and interleukin-4 and interferon-y production of intrathyroidal lymphocytes in Graves' disease. *Thyroid*. 1999;9(4):333–339.
852. Mao C, Wang S, Xiao Y, Xu J, Jiang Q, Jin M, et al. Impairment of regulatory capacity of CD4+ CD25+ regulatory T cells mediated by dendritic cell polarization and hyperthyroidism in Graves' disease. *The Journal of Immunology*. 2011;186(8):4734–4743.
853. Marazuela M, Garcia-Lopez MA, Figueroa-Vega N, de la Fuente H, Alvarado-Sanchez B, Monsivais-Urenda A, et al. Regulatory T cells in human autoimmune thyroid disease. *The Journal of Clinical Endocrinology & Metabolism*. 2006;91(9):3639–3646.
854. Bahn RS. Graves' ophthalmopathy. *New England Journal of Medicine*. 2010;362(8):726–738.
855. Fatourechi V. Thyroid dermopathy and acropachy. *Best Practice & Research Clinical Endocrinology & Metabolism*. 2012;26(4):553–565.
856. Weetman A, Tandon N, Morgan B. Antithyroid drugs and release of inflammatory mediators by complement-attacked thyroid cells. *The Lancet*. 1992;340(8820):633–636.
857. Ross DS, Burch HB, Cooper DS, Greenlee MC, Laurberg P, Maia AL, et al. 2016 American Thyroid Association guidelines for diagnosis and management of hyperthyroidism and other causes of thyrotoxicosis. *Thyroid*. 2016;26(10):1343–1421.
858. Komiya I, Yamada T, Sato A, Kouki T, Nishimori T, Takasu N. Remission and recurrence of hyperthyroid Graves' disease during and after methimazole treatment when assessed by IgE and interleukin 13. *The Journal of Clinical Endocrinology & Metabolism*. 2001;86(8):3540–3544.
859. Hidaka Y, Amino N, Iwatani Y, Itoh E, Matsunaga M, Tamaki H. Recurrence of thyrotoxicosis after attack of allergic rhinitis in patients with Graves' disease. *The Journal of Clinical Endocrinology & Metabolism*. 1993;77(6):1667–1670.
860. Laurberg P, Wallin G, Tallstedt L, Abraham-Nordling M, Lundell G, Torring O. TSH-receptor autoimmunity in Graves' disease after therapy with anti-thyroid drugs, surgery, or radioiodine: a 5-year prospective randomized study. *European Journal of Endocrinology*. 2008;158(1):69–76.
861. Chiovato L, Latrofa F, Braverman LE, Pacini F, Capezzone M, Masserini L, et al. Disappearance of humoral thyroid autoimmunity after complete removal of thyroid antigens. *Annals of internal medicine*. 2003;139(5_Part_1):346–351.
862. Wiersinga WM. Advances in treatment of active, moderate-to-severe Graves' ophthalmopathy. *The lancet Diabetes & endocrinology*. 2017;5(2):134–142.

863. Atkinson MA, Eisenbarth GS, Michels AW. Type 1 diabetes. *The Lancet*. 2014;383(9911):69–82.
864. Katsarou A, Gudbjörnsdottir S, Rawshani A, Dabelea D, Bonifacio E, Anderson BJ, et al. Type 1 diabetes mellitus. *Nature reviews Disease primers*. 2017;3(1):1–17.
865. Group TS. The environmental determinants of diabetes in the young (TEDDY) study. *Annals of the New York Academy of Sciences*. 2008;1150:1.
866. Rich SS, Concannon P, Erlich H, Julier C, Morahan G, Nerup J, et al. The type 1 diabetes genetics consortium. *Annals of the New York Academy of Sciences*. 2006;1079(1):1–8.
867. Pociot F, Lernmark Å. Genetic risk factors for type 1 diabetes. *The Lancet*. 2016;387(10035):2331–2339.
868. Todd J, Knip M, Mathieu C. Strategies for the prevention of autoimmune type 1 diabetes. *Diabetic medicine*. 2011;28(10):1141–1143.
869. Krischer JP, Lynch KF, Schatz DA, Ilonen J, Lernmark Å, Hagopian WA, et al. The 6 year incidence of diabetes-associated autoantibodies in genetically at-risk children: the TEDDY study. *Diabetologia*. 2015;58(5):980–987.
870. Krischer JP, Lynch KF, Lernmark Å, Hagopian WA, Rewers MJ, She J-X, et al. Genetic and environmental interactions modify the risk of diabetes-related autoimmunity by 6 years of age: the TEDDY study. *Diabetes care*. 2017;40(9):1194–1202.
871. Krischer JP, Liu X, Lernmark Å, Hagopian WA, Rewers MJ, She J-X, et al. The influence of type 1 diabetes genetic susceptibility regions, age, sex, and family history on the progression from multiple autoantibodies to type 1 diabetes: a TEDDY study report. *Diabetes*. 2017;66(12):3122–3129.
872. Lynch KF, Lee H-S, Törn C, Vehik K, Krischer JP, Larsson HE, et al. Gestational respiratory infections interacting with offspring HLA and CTLA-4 modifies incident β-cell autoantibodies. *Journal of autoimmunity*. 2018;86:93–103.
873. Steck AK, Vehik K, Bonifacio E, Lernmark A, Ziegler A-G, Hagopian WA, et al. Predictors of progression from the appearance of islet autoantibodies to early childhood diabetes: the Environmental Determinants of Diabetes in the Young (TEDDY). *Diabetes care*. 2015;38(5):808–813.
874. Association AD. 2. Classification and diagnosis of diabetes: standards of medical care in diabetes—2018. *Diabetes care*. 2018;41(Supplement 1):S13–S27.
875. Xu P, Krischer JP. Prognostic classification factors associated with development of multiple autoantibodies, dysglycemia, and type 1 diabetes—A recursive partitioning analysis. *Diabetes Care*. 2016;39(6):1036–1044.
876. Buysschaert M, Medina J-L, Buysschaert B, Bergman M. Definitions (and Current Controversies) of Diabetes and Prediabetes. *Current diabetes reviews*. 2016;12(1):8.
877. Danne T, Nimri R, Battelino T, Bergenstal RM, Close KL, DeVries JH, et al. International consensus on use of continuous glucose monitoring. *Diabetes care*. 2017;40(12):1631–1640.
878. Vehik K, Cuthbertson D, Boulware D, Beam CA, Rodriguez H, Legault L, et al. Performance of HbA1c as an early diagnostic indicator of type 1 diabetes in children and youth. *Diabetes care*. 2012;35(9):1821–1825.
879. Leslie R, Kolb H, Schloot N, Buzzetti R, Mauricio D, De Leiva A, et al. Diabetes classification: grey zones, sound and smoke: action LADA 1. *Diabetes/metabolism research and reviews*. 2008;24(7):511–519.
880. McLaughlin KA, Richardson CC, Ravishankar A, Brigatti C, Liberati D, Lampasona V, et al. Identification of tetraspanin-7 as a target of autoantibodies in type 1 diabetes. *Diabetes*. 2016;65(6):1690–1698.
881. Insel RA, Dunne JL, Atkinson MA, Chiang JL, Dabelea D, Gottlieb PA, et al. Staging presymptomatic type 1 diabetes: a scientific statement of JDRF, the Endocrine Society, and the American Diabetes Association. *Diabetes care*. 2015;38(10):1964–1974.
882. Dabelea D, Rewers A, Stafford JM, Standiford DA, Lawrence JM, Saydah S, et al. Trends in the prevalence of ketoacidosis at diabetes diagnosis: the SEARCH for diabetes in youth study. *Pediatrics*. 2014;133(4):e938–ee45.
883. Jones A, Hattersley A. The clinical utility of C-peptide measurement in the care of patients with diabetes. *Diabetic medicine*. 2013;30(7):803–817.
884. Grieco FA, Moore F, Vigneron F, Santin I, Villate O, Marselli L, et al. IL-17A increases the expression of proinflammatory chemokines in human pancreatic islets. *Diabetologia*. 2014;57(3):502–511.
885. Cnop M, Welsh N, Jonas J-C, Jörns A, Lenzen S, Eizirik DL. Mechanisms of pancreatic β-cell death in type 1 and type 2 diabetes: many differences, few similarities. *Diabetes*. 2005;54(suppl 2):S97–S107.
886. Eizirik DL, Miani M, Cardozo AK. Signalling danger: endoplasmic reticulum stress and the unfolded protein response in pancreatic islet inflammation. *Diabetologia*. 2013;56(2):234–241.

887. Rojas J, Bermudez V, Palmar J, Martínez MS, Olivar LC, Nava M, et al. Pancreatic beta cell death: novel potential mechanisms in diabetes therapy. *Journal of diabetes research*. 2018:2018.
888. Pociot F, Akolkar B, Concannon P, Erlich HA, Julier C, Morahan G, et al. Genetics of type 1 diabetes: what's next? *Diabetes*. 2010;59(7):1561–1571.
889. Ram R, Mehta M, Nguyen QT, Larma I, Boehm BO, Pociot F, et al. Systematic evaluation of genes and genetic variants associated with type 1 diabetes susceptibility. *The Journal of Immunology*. 2016;196(7):3043–3053.
890. Rich S, Akolkar B, Concannon P, Erlich H, Hilner J, Julier C, et al. Current status and the future for the genetics of type I diabetes. *Genes & Immunity*. 2009;10(1):S128–SS31.
891. Bosi E, Pastore MR, Molteni L, Bazzigaluppi E, Bonifacio E, Piemonti L. Gluten-free diet in subjects at risk for type 1 diabetes: a tool for delaying progression to clinical disease? *Early Nutrition and Its Later Consequences: New Opportunities*: Springer; 2005:157–158.
892. Norris JM, Lee H-S, Frederiksen B, Erlund I, Uusitalo U, Yang J, et al. Plasma 25-hydroxyvitamin D concentration and risk of islet autoimmunity. *Diabetes*. 2018;67(1):146–154.
893. Raab J, Giannopoulou EZ, Schneider S, Warncke K, Krasmann M, Winkler C, et al. Prevalence of vitamin D deficiency in pre-type 1 diabetes and its association with disease progression. *Diabetologia*. 2014;57(5):902–908.
894. Sioofy-Khojine A-B, Lehtonen J, Nurminen N, Laitinen OH, Oikarinen S, Huhtala H, et al. Coxsackievirus B1 infections are associated with the initiation of insulin-driven autoimmunity that progresses to type 1 diabetes. *Diabetologia*. 2018;61(5):1193–1202.
895. Honkanen H, Oikarinen S, Nurminen N, Laitinen OH, Huhtala H, Lehtonen J, et al. Detection of enteroviruses in stools precedes islet autoimmunity by several months: possible evidence for slowly operating mechanisms in virus-induced autoimmunity. *Diabetologia*. 2017;60(3):424–431.
896. Bronson P, Ramsay P, Thomson G, Barcellos L, Consortium DG. Analysis of maternal–offspring HLA compatibility, parent-of-origin and non-inherited maternal effects for the classical HLA loci in type 1 diabetes. *Diabetes, Obesity and Metabolism*. 2009;11:74–83.
897. Bluestone JA, Herold K, Eisenbarth G. Genetics, pathogenesis and clinical interventions in type 1 diabetes. *Nature*. 2010;464(7293):1293–1300.
898. Morran M.P., McInerney M.F., Pietropaolo M. Innate and adaptive autoimmunity in type 1 diabetes. 2008.
899. Woo HJ, Yu C, Reifman J. Collective genetic interaction effects and the role of antigen-presenting cells in autoimmune diseases. *PloS one*. 2017;12(1):e0169918.
900. Hamari S, Kirveskoski T, Glumoff V, Kulmala P, Simell O, Knip M, et al. Analyses of regulatory CD4+ CD25+ FOXP3+ T cells and observations from peripheral T cell subpopulation markers during the development of type 1 diabetes in children. *Scand J Immunol*. 2016;83(4):279–287.
901. Pugliese A, Brown D, Garza D, Murchison D, Zeller M, Redondo M, et al. Self-antigen–presenting cells expressing diabetes-associated autoantigens exist in both thymus and peripheral lymphoid organs. *The Journal of clinical investigation*. 2001;107(5):555–564.
902. Arif S, Tree TI, Astill TP, Tremble JM, Bishop AJ, Dayan CM, et al. Autoreactive T cell responses show proinflammatory polarization in diabetes but a regulatory phenotype in health. *The Journal of clinical investigation*. 2004;113(3):451–463.
903. Karlsen AE, Hagopian WA, Grubin CE, Dube S, Disteche CM, Adler DA, et al. Cloning and primary structure of a human islet isoform of glutamic acid decarboxylase from chromosome 10. *Proceedings of the National Academy of Sciences*. 1991;88(19):8337–8341.
904. Delli AJ, Lindblad B, Carlsson A, Forsander G, Ivarsson SA, Ludvigsson J, et al. Type 1 diabetes patients born to immigrants to Sweden increase their native diabetes risk and differ from Swedish patients in HLA types and islet autoantibodies. *Pediatric diabetes*. 2010;11(8):513–520.
905. Hirai H, Miura J, Hu Y, Larsson H, Larsson K, Lernmark A, et al. Selective screening of secretory vesicle-associated proteins for autoantigens in type 1 diabetes: VAMP2 and NPY are new minor autoantigens. *Clinical immunology*. 2008;127(3):366–374.
906. Wenzlau JM, Hutton JC, Davidson HW. New antigenic targets in type 1 diabetes. Current Opinion in Endocrinology. *Diabetes and Obesity*. 2008;15(4):315–320.
907. Skyler JS. Immune intervention for type 1 diabetes mellitus. *International Journal of Clinical Practice*. 2011;65:61–70.
908. Skyler JS. The year in immune intervention for type 1 diabetes. *Diabetes Technology & Therapeutics*. 2013;15(S1):S-88-S-95.

909. Sherr J, Sosenko J, Skyler JS, Herold KC. Prevention of type 1 diabetes: the time has come. *Nature Clinical Practice Endocrinology & Metabolism*. 2008;4(6):334–343.
910. DiMeglio LA, Evans-Molina C, Oram RA. Type 1 diabetes. *The Lancet*. 2018;391(10138):2449–2462.
911. Björses P, Halonen M, Palvimo JJ, Kolmer M, Aaltonen J, Ellonen P, et al. Mutations in the AIRE gene: effects on subcellular location and transactivation function of the autoimmune polyendocrinopathy-candidiasis–ectodermal dystrophy protein. *The American Journal of Human Genetics*. 2000;66(2): 378–392.
912. Scott HS, Heino M, Peterson P, Mittaz L, Lalioti MD, Betterle C, et al. Common mutations in autoimmune polyendocrinopathy-candidiasis-ectodermal dystrophy patients of different origins. *Molecular Endocrinology*. 1998;12(8):1112–1119.
913. Wang C-Y, Davoodi-Semiromi A, Huang W, Connor E, Shi J-D, She J-X. Characterization of mutations in patients with autoimmune polyglandular syndrome type 1 (APS1). *Human genetics*. 1998;103(6):681–685.
914. Proust-Lemoine E, Saugier-Véber P, Lefranc D, Dubucquoi S, Ryndak A, Buob D, et al. Autoimmune polyendocrine syndrome type 1 in north-western France: AIRE gene mutation specificities and severe forms needing immunosuppressive therapies. *Hormone research in paediatrics*. 2010;74(4):275–284.
915. Heino M, Peterson P, Kudoh J, Nagamine K, Lagerstedt A, Ovod V, et al. Autoimmune regulator is expressed in the cells regulating immune tolerance in thymus medulla. *Biochemical and biophysical research communications*. 1999;257(3):821–825.
916. Pearce SH, Cheetham T, Imrie H, Vaidya B, Barnes ND, Bilous RW, et al. A common and recurrent 13-bp deletion in the autoimmune regulator gene in British kindreds with autoimmune polyendocrinopathy type 1. *The American Journal of Human Genetics*. 1998;63(6):1675–1684.
917. Rosatelli MC, Meloni A, Meloni A, Devoto M, Cao A, Scott HS, et al. A common mutation in Sardinian autoimmune polyendocrinopathy-candidiasis-ectodermal dystrophy patients. *Human genetics*. 1998;103(4):428–434.
918. Giordano C, Modica R, Allotta M, Guarnotta V, Cervato S, Masiero S, et al. Autoimmune Polyendocrinopathy-Candidiasis-Ectodermal-Dystrophy (APECED) in Sicily: confirmation that R203X is the peculiar AIRE gene mutation. *Journal of endocrinological investigation*. 2012;35(4): 384–388.
919. Cetani F, Barbesino G, Borsari S, Pardi E, Cianferotti L, Pinchera A, et al. A novel mutation of the autoimmune regulator gene in an Italian kindred with autoimmune polyendocrinopathy-candidiasis-ectodermal dystrophy, acting in a dominant fashion and strongly cosegregating with hypothyroid autoimmune thyroiditis. *The Journal of Clinical Endocrinology & Metabolism*. 2001;86(10):4747–4752.
920. Oftedal BE, Hellesen A, Erichsen MM, Bratland E, Vardi A, Perheentupa J, et al. Dominant mutations in the autoimmune regulator AIRE are associated with common organ-specific autoimmune diseases. *Immunity*. 2015;42(6):1185–1196.
921. Halonen M, Eskelin P, Myhre A-G, Perheentupa J, Husebye ES, Kämpe O, et al. AIRE mutations and human leukocyte antigen genotypes as determinants of the autoimmune polyendocrinopathy-candidiasis-ectodermal dystrophy phenotype. *The Journal of Clinical Endocrinology & Metabolism*. 2002;87(6):2568–2574.
922. Gylling M, Kääriäinen E, Väisänen R, Kerosuo L, Solin M-L, Halme L, et al. The hypoparathyroidism of autoimmune polyendocrinopathy-candidiasis-ectodermal dystrophy protective effect of male sex. *The Journal of Clinical Endocrinology & Metabolism*. 2003;88(10):4602–4608.
923. Partanen J, Peterson P, Westman P, Aranko S, Krohn K. Major histocompatibility complex class II and III in Addison's disease MHC alleles do not predict autoantibody specificity and 21-hydroxylase gene polymorphism has no independent role in disease susceptibility. *Human immunology*. 1994;41(2):135–140.
924. Maclaren NK, Riley WJ. Inherited Susceptibility to Autoimmune Addison's Disease Is Linked to Juman Leukocyte Antigens-DR3 and/or DR4, except when Associated with Type I Autoimmune Poluglandular Syndrome. *The Journal of Clinical Endocrinology & Metabolism*. 1986;62(3):455–459.
925. Falorni A, Brozzetti A, Torre DL, Tortoioli C, Gambelunghe G. Association of genetic polymorphisms and autoimmune Addison's disease. *Expert review of clinical immunology*. 2008;4(4):441–456.
926. Flesch B, Matheis N, Alt T, Weinstock C, Bux J, Kahaly G. HLA class II haplotypes differentiate between the adult autoimmune polyglandular syndrome types II and III. *The Journal of Clinical Endocrinology & Metabolism*. 2014;99(1):E177–EE82.

927. Erichsen MM, Løvås K, Skinningsrud B, Wolff AB, Undlien DE, Svartberg J, et al. Clinical, immunological, and genetic features of autoimmune primary adrenal insufficiency: observations from a Norwegian registry. *The Journal of Clinical Endocrinology & Metabolism*. 2009;94(12):4882–4890.
928. Baker PR, Baschal EE, Fain PR, Triolo TM, Nanduri P, Siebert JC, et al. Haplotype analysis discriminates genetic risk for DR3-associated endocrine autoimmunity and helps define extreme risk for Addison's disease. *The Journal of Clinical Endocrinology & Metabolism*. 2010;95(10):E263–EE70.
929. Baker PR, Baschal EE, Fain PR, Nanduri P, Triolo TM, Siebert JC, et al. Dominant suppression of Addison's disease associated with HLA-B15. *The Journal of Clinical Endocrinology & Metabolism*. 2011;96(7):2154–2162.
930. Gambelunghe G, Falorni A, Ghaderi M, Laureti S, Tortoioli C, Santeusanio F, et al. Microsatellite polymorphism of the MHC class I chain-related (MIC-A and MIC-B) genes marks the risk for autoimmune Addison's disease. *The Journal of Clinical Endocrinology & Metabolism*. 1999;84(10): 3701–3707.
931. Peterson P, Partanen J, Aavik E, Salmi H, Pelkonen R, Krohn K. Steroid 21-hydroxylase gene polymorphism in Addison's disease patients. *Tissue Antigens*. 1995;46(1):63–67.
932. Brozzetti A, Marzotti S, Tortoioli C, Bini V, Giordano R, Dotta F, et al. Cytotoxic T lymphocyte antigen-4 Ala17 polymorphism is a genetic marker of autoimmune adrenal insufficiency: italian association study and meta-analysis of European studies. *European Journal of Endocrinology*. 2010;162(2):361.
933. Kemp E, Ajjan R, Husebye E, Peterson P, Uibo R, Imrie H, et al. A cytotoxic T lymphocyte antigen-4 (CTLA-4) gene polymorphism is associated with autoimmune Addison's disease in English patients. *Clinical endocrinology*. 1998;49(5):609–613.
934. Wolff ASB, Mitchell AL, Cordell HJ, Short A, Skinningsrud B, Ollier W, et al. CTLA-4 as a genetic determinant in autoimmune Addison's disease. *Genes & Immunity*. 2015;16(6):430–436.
935. Magitta N, Wolff AB, Johansson S, Skinningsrud B, Lie B, Myhr K, et al. A coding polymorphism in NALP1 confers risk for autoimmune Addison's disease and type 1 diabetes. *Genes & Immunity*. 2009;10(2):120–124.
936. Mitchell AL, Cordell HJ, Soemedi R, Owen K, Skinningsrud B, Wolff AB, et al. Programmed death ligand 1 (PD-L1) gene variants contribute to autoimmune Addison's disease and Graves' disease susceptibility. *The Journal of Clinical Endocrinology & Metabolism*. 2009;94(12):5139–5145.
937. Skinningsrud B, Husebye ES, Gervin K, Løvås K, Blomhoff A, Wolff AB, et al. Mutation screening of PTPN22: association of the 1858T-allele with Addison's disease. *European Journal of Human Genetics*. 2008;16(8):977–982.
938. Roycroft M, Fichna M, McDonald D, Owen K, Żurawek M, Gryczyńska M, et al. The tryptophan 620 allele of the lymphoid tyrosine phosphatase (PTPN22) gene predisposes to autoimmune Addison's disease. *Clinical endocrinology*. 2009;70(3):358–362.
939. Owen CJ, Kelly H, Eden JA, Merriman ME, Pearce SH, Merriman TR. Analysis of the Fc receptor-like-3 (FCRL3) locus in Caucasians with autoimmune disorders suggests a complex pattern of disease association. *The Journal of Clinical Endocrinology & Metabolism*. 2007;92(3):1106–1111.
940. Skinningsrud B, Husebye ES, Pearce SH, McDonald DO, Brandal K, Wolff AB, et al. Polymorphisms in CLEC16A and CIITA at 16p13 are associated with primary adrenal insufficiency. *The Journal of Clinical Endocrinology & Metabolism*. 2008;93(9):3310–3317.
941. Ghaderi M, Gambelunghe G, Tortoioli C, Brozzetti A, Jatta K, Gharizadeh B, et al. MHC2TA single nucleotide polymorphism and genetic risk for autoimmune adrenal insufficiency. *The Journal of Clinical Endocrinology & Metabolism*. 2006;91(10):4107–4111.
942. Eriksson D, Bianchi M, Landegren N, Nordin J, Dalin F, Mathioudaki A, et al. Extended exome sequencing identifies BACH2 as a novel major risk locus for Addison's disease. *Journal of Internal Medicine*. 2016;280(6):595–608.
943. Winqvist O, Karlsson FA, Kämpe O. 21-Hydroxylase, a major autoantigen in idiopathic Addison's disease. *The Lancet*. 1992;339(8809):1559–1562.
944. Eriksson D, Dalin F, Eriksson GN, Landegren N, Bianchi M, Hallgren Å, et al. Cytokine autoantibody screening in the Swedish Addison Registry identifies patients with undiagnosed APS1. *The Journal of Clinical Endocrinology & Metabolism*. 2018;103(1):179–186.
945. Bruserud Ø, Oftedal BE, Landegren N, Erichsen MM, Bratland E, Lima K, et al. A longitudinal follow-up of autoimmune polyendocrine syndrome type 1. *The Journal of Clinical Endocrinology & Metabolism*. 2016;101(8):2975–2983.

946. Alimohammadi M, Björklund P, Hallgren Å, Pöntynen N, Szinnai G, Shikama N, et al. Autoimmune polyendocrine syndrome type 1 and NALP5, a parathyroid autoantigen. *New England Journal of Medicine*. 2008;358(10):1018–1028.
947. Winqvist O, Gustafsson J, Rorsman F, Karlsson FA, Kämpe O. Two different cytochrome P450 enzymes are the adrenal antigens in autoimmune polyendocrine syndrome type I and Addison's disease. *The Journal of clinical investigation*. 1993;92(5):2377–2385.
948. Winqvist O, Gebre-Medhin G, Gustafsson J, Ritzén EM, Lundkvist O, Karlsson FA, et al. Identification of the main gonadal autoantigens in patients with adrenal insufficiency and associated ovarian failure. *The Journal of Clinical Endocrinology & Metabolism*. 1995;80(5):1717–1723.
949. Brozzetti A, Marzotti S, La Torre D, Bacosi ML, Morelli S, Bini V, et al. Autoantibody responses in autoimmune ovarian insufficiency and in Addison's disease are IgG1 dominated and suggest a predominant, but not exclusive, Th1 type of response. *European journal of endocrinology*. 2010;163(2):309.
950. Krohn K, Uibo R, Aavik E, Peterson P, Savilahti K. Identification by molecular cloning of an autoantigen associated with Addison's disease as steroid 17α-hydroxylase. *The Lancet*. 1992;339(8796):770–773.
951. Reato G, Morlin L, Chen S, Furmaniak J, Smith BR, Masiero S, et al. Premature ovarian failure in patients with autoimmune Addison's disease: clinical, genetic, and immunological evaluation. *The Journal of Clinical Endocrinology & Metabolism*. 2011;96(8):E1255–E1E61.
952. Gebre-Medhin G, Husebye E, Gustafsson J, Winqvist O, Goksøyr A, Rorsman F, et al. Cytochrome P450IA2 and aromatic L-amino acid decarboxylase are hepatic autoantigens in autoimmune polyendocrine syndrome type I. *FEBS letters*. 1997;412(3):439–445.
953. Husebye ES, Gebre-Medhin G, Tuomi T, Perheentupa J, Landin-Olsson M, Gustafsson J, et al. Autoantibodies against aromatic L-amino acid decarboxylase in autoimmune polyendocrine syndrome type I. *The Journal of Clinical Endocrinology & Metabolism*. 1997;82(1):147–150.
954. Ekwall O, Hedstrand H, Grimelius L, Haavik J, Perheentupa J, Gustafsson J, et al. Identification of tryptophan hydroxylase as an intestinal autoantigen. *The Lancet*. 1998;352(9124):279–283.
955. Hedstrand H, Ekwall O, Haavik J, Landgren E, Betterle C, Perheentupa J, et al. Identification of tyrosine hydroxylase as an autoantigen in autoimmune polyendocrine syndrome type I. *Biochemical and biophysical research communications*. 2000;267(1):456–461.
956. Söderbergh A, Myhre AG, Ekwall O, Gebre-Medhin G, Hk Hedstrand, Landgren E, et al. Prevalence and clinical associations of 10 defined autoantibodies in autoimmune polyendocrine syndrome type I. *The Journal of Clinical Endocrinology & Metabolism*. 2004;89(2):557–562.
957. Sköldberg F, Rorsman F, Perheentupa J, Landin-Olsson M, Husebye ES, Gustafsson J, et al. Analysis of antibody reactivity against cysteine sulfinic acid decarboxylase, a pyridoxal phosphate-dependent enzyme, in endocrine autoimmune disease. *The Journal of Clinical Endocrinology & Metabolism*. 2004;89(4):1636–1640.
958. Tuomi T, Björses P, Falorni A, Partanen J, Perheentupa J, Lernmark A, et al. Antibodies to glutamic acid decarboxylase and insulin-dependent diabetes in patients with autoimmune polyendocrine syndrome type I. *The Journal of Clinical Endocrinology & Metabolism*. 1996;81(4):1488–1494.
959. Landegren N, Sharon D, Shum AK, Khan IS, Fasano KJ, Hallgren Å, et al. Transglutaminase 4 as a prostate autoantigen in male subfertility. *Science translational medicine*. 2015;7(292):292ra101.
960. Landegren N, Sharon D, Freyhult E, Hallgren Å, Eriksson D, Edqvist P-H, et al. Proteome-wide survey of the autoimmune target repertoire in autoimmune polyendocrine syndrome type 1. *Scientific reports*. 2016;6:20104.
961. Fishman D, Kisand K, Hertel C, Rothe M, Remm A, Pihlap M, et al. Autoantibody repertoire in APECED patients targets two distinct subgroups of proteins. *Frontiers in immunology*. 2017;8:976.
962. Meloni A, Furcas M, Cetani F, Marcocci C, Falorni A, Perniola R, et al. Autoantibodies against type I interferons as an additional diagnostic criterion for autoimmune polyendocrine syndrome type I. *The Journal of Clinical Endocrinology & Metabolism*. 2008;93(11):4389–4397.
963. Oftedal BE, Wolff ASB, Bratland E, Kämpe O, Perheentupa J, Myhre AG, et al. Radioimmunoassay for autoantibodies against interferon omega; its use in the diagnosis of autoimmune polyendocrine syndrome type I. *Clinical immunology*. 2008;129(1):163–169.
964. Meager A, Visvalingam K, Peterson P, Möll K, Murumägi A, Krohn K, et al. Anti-interferon autoantibodies in autoimmune polyendocrinopathy syndrome type 1. *PLoS Med*. 2006;3(7):e289.

965. Kisand K, Bøe Wolff AS, Podkrajšek KT, Tserel L, Link M, Kisand KV, et al. Chronic mucocutaneous candidiasis in APECED or thymoma patients correlates with autoimmunity to Th17-associated cytokines. *Journal of Experimental Medicine*. 2010;207(2):299–308.
966. Puel A, Döffinger R, Natividad A, Chrabieh M, Barcenas-Morales G, Picard C, et al. Autoantibodies against IL-17A, IL-17F, and IL-22 in patients with chronic mucocutaneous candidiasis and autoimmune polyendocrine syndrome type IAutoantibodies in patients with APS-I. *The Journal of experimental medicine*. 2010;207(2):291–297.
967. Meyer S, Woodward M, Hertel C, Vlaicu P, Haque Y, Kärner J, et al. AIRE-deficient patients harbor unique high-affinity disease-ameliorating autoantibodies. *Cell*. 2016;166(3):582–595.
968. Kärner J, Pihlap M, Ranki A, Krohn K, Trebusak Podkrajsek K, Bratanic N, et al. IL-6-specific autoantibodies among APECED and thymoma patients. *Immunity, inflammation and disease*. 2016;4(2):235–243.
969. Schoemaker J, Drexhage H, Hoek A. Premature ovarian failure and ovarian autoimmunity. *Endocrine reviews*. 1997.
970. Betterle C, Dal Pra C, Mantero F, Zanchetta R. Autoimmune adrenal insufficiency and autoimmune polyendocrine syndromes: autoantibodies, autoantigens, and their applicability in diagnosis and disease prediction. *Endocrine reviews*. 2002;23(3):327–364.
971. Li D, Streeten EA, Chan A, Lwin W, Tian L, Pellegrino da Silva R, et al. Exome sequencing reveals mutations in AIRE as a cause of isolated hypoparathyroidism. *The Journal of Clinical Endocrinology & Metabolism*. 2017;102(5):1726–1733.
972. Meloni A, Willcox N, Meager A, Atzeni M, Wolff AS, Husebye ES, et al. Autoimmune polyendocrine syndrome type 1: an extensive longitudinal study in Sardinian patients. *The Journal of Clinical Endocrinology & Metabolism*. 2012;97(4):1114–1124.
973. Perheentupa J. Autoimmune polyendocrinopathy-candidiasis-ectodermal dystrophy. *The Journal of Clinical Endocrinology & Metabolism*. 2006;91(8):2843–2850.
974. Wolff AS, Erichsen MM, Meager A, NwF Magitta, Myhre AG, Bollerslev J, et al. Autoimmune polyendocrine syndrome type 1 in Norway: phenotypic variation, autoantibodies, and novel mutations in the autoimmune regulator gene. *The Journal of Clinical Endocrinology & Metabolism*. 2007;92(2):595–603.
975. Ferre EM, Rose SR, Rosenzweig SD, Burbelo PD, Romito KR, Niemela JE, et al. Redefined clinical features and diagnostic criteria in autoimmune polyendocrinopathy-candidiasis-ectodermal dystrophy. *JCI insight*. 2016;1(13).
976. Perheentupa J. APS-I/APECED: the clinical disease and therapy. *Endocrinology and Metabolism Clinics*. 2002;31(2):295–320.
977. Orlova EM, Sozaeva LS, Kareva MA, Oftedal BE, Wolff AS, Breivik L, et al. Expanding the phenotypic and genotypic landscape of autoimmune polyendocrine syndrome type 1. *The Journal of Clinical Endocrinology & Metabolism*. 2017;102(9):3546–3556.
978. Landegren N, Lindberg MP, Skov J, Hallgren Å, Eriksson D, Toft-Bertelsen TL, et al. Autoantibodies Targeting a Collecting Duct–Specific Water Channel in Tubulointerstitial Nephritis. *Journal of the American Society of Nephrology*. 2016;27(10):3220–3228.
979. Alimohammadi M, Dubois N, Sköldberg F, Hallgren Å, Tardivel I, Hedstrand H, et al. Pulmonary autoimmunity as a feature of autoimmune polyendocrine syndrome type 1 and identification of KCNRG as a bronchial autoantigen. *Proceedings of the national academy of Sciences*. 2009;106(11):4396–4401.
980. Orlova EM, Bukina AM, Kuznetsova ES, Kareva MA, Zakharova EU, Peterkova VA, et al. Autoimmune polyglandular syndrome type 1 in Russian patients: clinical variants and autoimmune regulator mutations. *Hormone research in paediatrics*. 2010;73(6):449–457.
981. Sorkina E, Frolova E, Rusinova D, Polyakova S, Roslavtseva E, Vasilyev E, et al. Progressive generalized lipodystrophy as a manifestation of autoimmune polyglandular syndrome type 1. *The Journal of Clinical Endocrinology & Metabolism*. 2016;101(4):1344–1347.
982. Valenzise M, Meloni A, Betterle C, Giometto B, Autunno M, Mazzeo A, et al. Chronic inflammatory demyelinating polyneuropathy as a possible novel component of autoimmune poly-endocrine-candidiasis-ectodermal dystrophy. *European journal of pediatrics*. 2009;168(2):237–240.
983. Harris M, Kecha O, Deal C, Howlett CR, Deiss D, Tobias V, et al. Reversible metaphyseal dysplasia, a novel bone phenotype, in two unrelated children with autoimmunepolyendocrinopathy-candidiasis-ectodermal dystrophy: clinical and molecular studies. *The Journal of Clinical Endocrinology & Metabolism*. 2003;88(10):4576–4585.

984. Gutierrez MJ, Gilson J, Zacharias J, Ishmael F, Bingham C. Childhood polyarthritis as early manifestation of autoimmune polyendocrinopathy with candidiasis and ectodermal dystrophy syndrome. *Frontiers in immunology*. 2017;8:377.
985. Neufeld M, Maclaren NK, Blizzard RM. Two types of autoimmune Addison's disease associated with different polyglandular autoimmune (PGA) syndromes. *Medicine*. 1981;60(5):355–362.
986. Rautemaa R, Richardson M, Pfaller M, Koukila-Kähkölä P, Perheentupa J, Saxén H. Decreased susceptibility of Candida albicans to azole antifungals: a complication of long-term treatment in autoimmune polyendocrinopathy-candidiasis-ectodermal dystrophy (APECED) patients. *Journal of antimicrobial chemotherapy*. 2007;60(4):889–892.
987. Rautemaa R, Richardson M, Pfaller M, Perheentupa J, Saxén H. Reduction of fluconazole susceptibility of Candida albicans in APECED patients due to long-term use of ketoconazole and miconazole. *Scandinavian journal of infectious diseases*. 2008;40(11–12):904–907.
988. Rautemaa R, Richardson M, Pfaller MA, Perheentupa J, Saxén H. Activity of amphotericin B, anidulafungin, caspofungin, micafungin, posaconazole, and voriconazole against Candida albicans with decreased susceptibility to fluconazole from APECED patients on long-term azole treatment of chronic mucocutaneous candidiasis. *Diagnostic microbiology and infectious disease*. 2008;62(2):182–185.
989. Winer KK, Zhang B, Shrader JA, Peterson D, Smith M, Albert PS, et al. Synthetic human parathyroid hormone 1-34 replacement therapy: a randomized crossover trial comparing pump versus injections in the treatment of chronic hypoparathyroidism. *The Journal of clinical endocrinology and metabolism*. 2012;97(2):391.
990. Császár T, Patakfalvi A. Treatment of polyglandular autoimmune syndrome with cyclosporin-A. *Acta Medica Hungarica*. 1992;49(3–4):187.
991. Pearce SH, Mitchell AL, Bennett S, King P, Chandran S, Nag S, et al. Adrenal steroidogenesis after B lymphocyte depletion therapy in new-onset Addison's disease. *The Journal of Clinical Endocrinology & Metabolism*. 2012;97(10):E1927–E1E32.
992. Popler J, Alimohammadi M, Kämpe O, Dalin F, Dishop MK, Barker JM, et al. Autoimmune polyendocrine syndrome type 1: utility of KCNRG autoantibodies as a marker of active pulmonary disease and successful treatment with rituximab. *Pediatric pulmonology*. 2012;47(1):84–87.
993. Ward L, Paquette J, Seidman E, Cl Huot, Alvarez F, Crock P, et al. Severe autoimmune polyendocrinopathy-candidiasis-ectodermal dystrophy in an adolescent girl with a novel AIRE mutation: response to immunosuppressive therapy. *The Journal of Clinical Endocrinology & Metabolism*. 1999;84(3):844–852.
994. Ulinski T, Perrin L, Morris M, Houang M, Cabrol S, Grapin C, et al. Autoimmune polyendocrinopathy-candidiasis-ectodermal dystrophy syndrome with renal failure: impact of posttransplant immunosuppression on disease activity. *The Journal of Clinical Endocrinology & Metabolism*. 2006;91(1):192–195.
995. Carmel R. Prevalence of undiagnosed pernicious anemia in the elderly. *Archives of internal medicine*. 1996;156(10):1097–1100.
996. Ungar B, Mathews J, Tait B, Cowling D. HLA patterns in pernicious anaemia. *Br Med J*. 1977;1(6064):798–800.
997. Faustin B, Lartigue L, Bruey J-M, Luciano F, Sergienko E, Bailly-Maitre B, et al. Reconstituted NALP1 inflammasome reveals two-step mechanism of caspase-1 activation. *Molecular cell*. 2007;25(5):713–724.
998. Silveira PA, Baxter AG, Cain WE, van Driel IR. A major linkage region on distal chromosome 4 confers susceptibility to mouse autoimmune gastritis. *The Journal of Immunology*. 1999;162(9):5106–5111.
999. Silveira PA, Wilson WE, Esteban LM, Jordan MA, van Driel IR, Baxter AG. Identification of the Gasa3 and Gasa4 autoimmune gastritis susceptibility genes using congenic mice and partitioned, segregative and interaction analyses. *Immunogenetics*. 2001;53(9):741–750.
1000. Serafini U, Masala C, Pala A. Studies on gastric autoimmunity. *Folia allergologica*. 1970;17(4):433–434.
1001. Prinz C, Kajimura M, Scott D, Helander H, Shin J, Besancon M, et al. Acid secretion and the H, K ATPase of stomach. *The Yale journal of biology and medicine*. 1992;65(6):577.
1002. Pettitt JM, Humphris DC, Barrett SP, Toh B-H, van Driel IR, Gleeson PA. Fast freeze-fixation/freeze-substitution reveals the secretory membranes of the gastric parietal cell as a network

of helically coiled tubule. A new model for parietal cell transformation. *Journal of Cell Science*. 1995;108(3):1127–1141.
1003. Ma J-Y, Borch K, Mårdh S. Human gastric H, K-adenosine triphosphatase β-subunit is a major autoantigen in atrophic corpus gastritis: expression of the recombinant human glycoprotein in insect cells. *Scandinavian journal of gastroenterology*. 1994;29(9):790–794.
1004. Burman P, Mårdh S, Norberg L, Karlsson FA. Parietal cell antibodies in pernicious anemia inhibit H+, K+-adenosine triphosphatase, the proton pump of the stomach. *Gastroenterology*. 1989;96(6):1434–1438.
1005. Samloff IM, Kleinman MS, Turner MD, Sobel MV, Jeffries GH. Blocking and binding antibodies to intrinsic factor and parietal cell antibody in pernicious anemia. *Gastroenterology*. 1968;55:575–583.
1006. Rothenberg SP, Kantha KK, Ficarra A. Autoantibodies to intrinsic factor: their determination and clinical usefulness. *The Journal of Laboratory and Clinical Medicine*. 1971;77(3):476–484.
1007. Irvine W, Davies S, Teitelbaum S, Delamore I, Williams AW. The clinical and pathological significance of gastric parietal cell antibody. *Annals of the New York Academy of Sciences*. 1965;124(2):657–691.
1008. Kaye MD, Whorwell PJ, Wright R. Gastric mucosal lymphocyte subpopulations in pernicious anemia and in normal stomach. *Clinical immunology and immunopathology*. 1983;28(3):431–440.
1009. Bergman MP, Amedei A, D'Elios MM, Azzurri A, Benagiano M, Tamburini C, et al. Characterization of H+, K+-ATPase T cell epitopes in human autoimmune gastritis. *European journal of immunology*. 2003;33(2):539–545.
1010. MM D'elios, Bergman MP, Azzurri A, Amedei A, Benagiano M, De Pont JJ, et al. H+, K+-ATPase (proton pump) is the target autoantigen of Th1-type cytotoxic T cells in autoimmune gastritis. *Gastroenterology*. 2001;120(2):377–386.
1011. Allen S, Read S, DiPaolo R, McHugh RS, Shevach EM, Gleeson PA, et al. Promiscuous thymic expression of an autoantigen gene does not result in negative selection of pathogenic T cells. *The Journal of Immunology*. 2005;175(9):5759–5764.
1012. Read S, Hogan TV, Zwar TD, Gleeson PA, Van Driel IR. Prevention of autoimmune gastritis in mice requires extra-thymic T-cell deletion and suppression by regulatory T cells. *Gastroenterology*. 2007;133(2):547–558.
1013. Scheinecker C, McHugh R, Shevach EM, Germain RN. Constitutive presentation of a natural tissue autoantigen exclusively by dendritic cells in the draining lymph node. *The Journal of experimental medicine*. 2002;196(8):1079–1090.
1014. Stummvoll GH, DiPaolo RJ, Huter EN, Davidson TS, Glass D, Ward JM, et al. Th1, Th2, and Th17 effector T cell-induced autoimmune gastritis differs in pathological pattern and in susceptibility to suppression by regulatory T cells. *The Journal of Immunology*. 2008;181(3):1908–1916.
1015. Zwar TD, Read S, van Driel IR, Gleeson PA. CD4+ CD25+ regulatory T cells inhibit the antigen-dependent expansion of self-reactive T cells in vivo. *The Journal of Immunology*. 2006;176(3):1609–1617.
1016. Hogan TV, Ang DK, Gleeson PA, van Driel IR. Extrathymic mechanisms of T cell tolerance: lessons from autoimmune gastritis. *Journal of Autoimmunity*. 2008;31(3):268–273.
1017. Toh B-H, van Driel IR, Gleeson PA. Pernicious anemia. *New England Journal of Medicine*. 1997;337(20):1441–1448.
1018. Strickland R, Mackay I. A reappraisal of the nature and significance of chronic atrophic gastritis. *The American journal of digestive diseases*. 1973;18(5):426–440.
1019. Irvine W, Cullen D, Mawhinney H. NATURAL HISTORY OF AUTOIMMUNE ACHLORHYDRIC ATROPHIC GASTRITIS A 1-15-year Follow-up Study. *The Lancet*. 1974;304(7879):482–485.
1020. Glass GBJ. Gastric intrinsic factor and its function in the metabolism of vitamin B12. *Physiological reviews*. 1963;43:529–849.
1021. Donaldson RM, Mackenzie IL, Trier JS. Intrinsic factor-mediated attachment of vitamin B 12 to brush borders and microvillous membranes of hamster intestine. *The Journal of Clinical Investigation*. 1967;46(7):1215–1228.
1022. Lindblom A, Quadt N, Marsh T, Aeschlimann D, Mörgelin M, Mann K, et al. The intrinsic factor-vitamin B12 receptor, cubilin, is assembled into trimers via a coiled-coil α-helix. *Journal of Biological Chemistry*. 1999;274(10):6374–6380.
1023. Carmel R. How I treat cobalamin (vitamin B12) deficiency. *Blood*. 2008;112(6):2214–2221.
1024. Chanarin I. *The Megaloblastic Anaemias*: Blackwell Scientific; 1969.

1025. Varis K, Samloff I, Ihämaki T, Siurala M. An appraisal of tests for severe atrophic gastritis in relatives of patients with pernicious anemia. *Digestive diseases and sciences*. 1979;24(3):187–191.
1026. Carmel R. Pepsinogens and other serum markers in pernicious anemia. *American journal of clinical pathology*. 1988;90(4):442–445.
1027. Samloff IM, Varis K, Ihamaki T, Siurala M, Rotter JI. Relationships among serum pepsinogen I, serum pepsinogen II, and gastric mucosal histology: a study in relatives of patients with pernicious anemia. *Gastroenterology*. 1982;83(1):204–209.
1028. Savage DG, Lindenbaum J. 11 Neurological complications of acquired cobalamin deficiency: clinical aspects. *Bailliere's clinical haematology*. 1995;8(3):657–678.
1029. Hsing AW, Hansson LE, McLaughlin JK, Nyren O, Blot WJ, Ekbom A, et al. Pernicious anemia and subsequent cancer. A population-based cohort study. *Cancer*. 1993;71(3):745–750.
1030. Kokkola A, Sjöblom S-M, Haapiainen R, Sipponen P, Puolakkainen P, Järvinen H. The risk of gastric carcinoma and carcinoid tumours in patients with pernicious anaemia: a prospective follow-up study. *Scandinavian journal of gastroenterology*. 1998;33(1):88–92.
1031. Ardeman S, Chanarin I, Jacobs A, Griffiths L. Family study in Addisonian pernicious anemia. *Blood*. 1966;27(5):599–610.
1032. Whittingham S, Mackay I, Ungar B, Mathews J. The genetic factor in pernicious anaemia: a family study in patients with gastritis. *The Lancet*. 1969;293(7602):951–954.
1033. Wangel A, Callender S, Spray G, Wright R. A Family Study of Pernicious Anaemia: II. Intrinsic Factor Secretion, Vitamin B12 Absorption and Genetic Aspects of Gastric Autoimmunity. *British Journal of Haematology*. 1968;14(2):183–204.
1034. Stabler SP. Vitamin B12 deficiency. *New England Journal of Medicine*. 2013;368(2):149–160.
1035. Murphy K, Biondo M, Toh BH, Alderuccio F. Tolerance established in autoimmune disease by mating or bone marrow transplantation that target autoantigen to thymus. *International immunology*. 2003;15(2):269–277.
1036. Nguyen T-LM, Sullivan NL, Ebel M, Teague RM, DiPaolo RJ. Antigen-Specific TGF-β–Induced Regulatory T Cells Secrete Chemokines, Regulate T Cell Trafficking, and Suppress Ongoing Autoimmunity. *The Journal of Immunology*. 2011;187(4):1745–1753.
1037. Donaldson PT…. Genetics in autoimmune hepatitis. *Seminars in liver disease*. 2002.
1038. Donaldson P. Genetics of liver disease: immunogenetics and disease pathogenesis. *Gut*. 2004;53(4): 599–608.
1039. Furumoto Y, Asano T, Sugita T, Abe H, Chuganji Y, Fujiki K, et al. Evaluation of the role of HLA-DR antigens in Japanese type 1 autoimmune hepatitis. *BMC gastroenterology*. 2015;15(1):144.
1040. van Gerven NM, de Boer YS, Zwiers A, Verwer BJ, Drenth JP, van Hoek B, et al. HLA-DRB1* 03: 01 and HLA-DRB1* 04: 01 modify the presentation and outcome in autoimmune hepatitis type-1. *Genes & Immunity*. 2015;16(4):247–252.
1041. De Boer YS, van Gerven NM, Zwiers A, Verwer BJ, van Hoek B, van Erpecum KJ, et al. Genome-wide association study identifies variants associated with autoimmune hepatitis type 1. *Gastroenterology*. 2014;147(2):443–452 e5.
1042. Djilali-Saiah I, Fakhfakh A, Louafi H, Caillat-Zucman S, Debray D, Alvarez F. HLA class II influences humoral autoimmunity in patients with type 2 autoimmune hepatitis. *Journal of hepatology*. 2006;45(6):844–850.
1043. Agarwal K, Czaja AJ, Jones DE, Donaldson PT. Cytotoxic T lymphocyte antigen-4 (CTLA-4) gene polymorphisms and susceptibility to type 1 autoimmune hepatitis. *Hepatology*. 2000;31(1):49–53.
1044. Cookson S, Constantini PK, Clare M, Underhill JA, Bernal W, Czaja AJ, et al. Frequency and nature of cytokine gene polymorphisms in type 1 autoimmune hepatitis. *Hepatology*. 1999;30(4): 851–856.
1045. Agarwal K, Czaja AJ, Donaldson P. A functional Fas promoter polymorphism is associated with a severe phenotype in type 1 autoimmune hepatitis characterized by early development of cirrhosis. *Tissue Antigens*. 2007;69(3):227–235.
1046. Vergani D, Alvarez F, Bianchi FB, Cançado EL, Mackay IR, Manns MP, et al. Liver autoimmune serology: a consensus statement from the committee for autoimmune serology of the International Autoimmune Hepatitis Group. *Journal of hepatology*. 2004;41(4):677–683.
1047. Hennes EM, Zeniya M, Czaja AJ, Parés A, Dalekos GN, Krawitt EL, et al. Simplified criteria for the diagnosis of autoimmune hepatitis. *Hepatology*. 2008;48(1):169–176.

1048. Liberal R, Mieli-Vergani G, Vergani D. Clinical significance of autoantibodies in autoimmune hepatitis. *Journal of autoimmunity*. 2013;46:17–24.
1049. Autoantibodies and their antigens in autoimmune hepatitis. In: Bogdanos DP, Mieli-Vergani G, Vergani D, eds. Autoantibodies and their antigens in autoimmune hepatitis. *Seminars in liver disease*. 2009.
1050. Longhi MS, Ma Y, Mieli-Vergani G, Vergani D. Aetiopathogenesis of autoimmune hepatitis. *Journal of autoimmunity*. 2010;34(1):7–14.
1051. Heneghan MA, Yeoman AD, Verma S, Smith AD, Longhi MS. Autoimmune hepatitis. *The Lancet*. 2013;382(9902):1433–1444.
1052. Ichiki Y, Aoki CA, Bowlus CL, Shimoda S, Ishibashi H. Gershwin ME. T cell immunity in autoimmune hepatitis. *Autoimmunity reviews*. 2005;4(5):315–321.
1053. Liberal R, Longhi MS, Mieli-Vergani G, Vergani D. Pathogenesis of autoimmune hepatitis. *Best practice & research Clinical gastroenterology*. 2011;25(6):653–664.
1054. Sahebjam F, Vierling JM. Autoimmune hepatitis. *Frontiers of medicine*. 2015;9(2):187–219.
1055. Longhi MS, Ma Y, Grant CR, Samyn M, Gordon P, Mieli-Vergani G, et al. T-regs in autoimmune hepatitis-systemic lupus erythematosus/mixed connective tissue disease overlap syndrome are functionally defective and display a Th1 cytokine profile. *Journal of autoimmunity*. 2013;41:146–151.
1056. Muratori L, Longhi MS. The interplay between regulatory and effector T cells in autoimmune hepatitis: implications for innovative treatment strategies. *Journal of autoimmunity*. 2013;46:74–80.
1057. Grant CR, Liberal R, Holder BS, Cardone J, Ma Y, Robson SC, et al. Dysfunctional CD39POS regulatory T cells and aberrant control of T-helper type 17 cells in autoimmune hepatitis. *Hepatology*. 2014;59(3):1007–1015.
1058. Lohse AW, Chazouilleres O, Dalekos G, Drenth J, Heneghan M, Hofer H, et al. EASL clinical practice guidelines: autoimmune hepatitis. *J Hepatol*. 2015;63(4):971–1004.
1059. Manns MP, Woynarowski M, Kreisel W, Lurie Y, Rust C, Zuckerman E, et al. Budesonide induces remission more effectively than prednisone in a controlled trial of patients with autoimmune hepatitis. *Gastroenterology*. 2010;139(4):1198–1206.
1060. Krawitt EL. Autoimmune hepatitis. *New England Journal of Medicine*. 2006;354(1):54–66.
1061. Al-Chalabi T, Underhill JA, Portmann BC, McFarlane IG, Heneghan MA. Impact of gender on the long-term outcome and survival of patients with autoimmune hepatitis. *Journal of hepatology*. 2008;48(1):140–147.
1062. Oettinger R, Brunnberg A, Gerner P, Wintermeyer P, Jenke A, Wirth S. Clinical features and biochemical data of Caucasian children at diagnosis of autoimmune hepatitis. *Journal of autoimmunity*. 2005;24(1):79–84.
1063. Floreani A, Liberal R, Vergani D, Mieli-Vergani G. Autoimmune hepatitis: contrasts and comparisons in children and adults–a comprehensive review. *Journal of autoimmunity*. 2013;46:7–16.
1064. Crapper R, Bhathal P, Mackay I, Frazer I. 'Acute'autoimmune hepatitis. *Digestion*. 1986;34(3):216–225.
1065. Amontree JS, Stuart TD, Bredfeldt JE. Autoimmune chronic active hepatitis masquerading as acute hepatitis. *Journal of clinical gastroenterology*. 1989;11(3):303–307.
1066. Wong GW, Heneghan MA. Association of extrahepatic manifestations with autoimmune hepatitis. *Digestive Diseases*. 2015;33(Suppl. 2):25–35.
1067. Wong GW, Yeong T, Lawrence D, Yeoman AD, Verma S, Heneghan MA. Concurrent extrahepatic autoimmunity in autoimmune hepatitis: implications for diagnosis, clinical course and long-term outcomes. *Liver International*. 2017;37(3):449–457.
1068. Mieli-Vergani G, Vergani D. Autoimmune hepatitis. *Nature Reviews Gastroenterology & Hepatology*. 2011;8(6):320–329.
1069. Liberal R, Krawitt EL, Vierling JM, Manns MP, Mieli-Vergani G, Vergani D. Cutting edge issues in autoimmune hepatitis. *Journal of autoimmunity*. 2016;75:6–19.
1070. Mackay I. Chronic hepatitis: effect of prolonged suppressive treatment and comparison of azathioprine with prednisolone. *QJM: An International Journal of Medicine*. 1968;37(3):379–392.
1071. Cook G, Mulligan R, Sherlock S. Controlled prospective trial of corticosteroid therapy in active chronic hepatitis. *QJM: An International Journal of Medicine*. 1971;40(2):159–185.

1072. Zizzo AN, Valentino PL, Shah PS, Kamath BM. Second-line agents in pediatric patients with autoimmune hepatitis: a systematic review and meta-analysis. *Journal of pediatric gastroenterology and nutrition*. 2017;65(1):6–15.
1073. Marlaka JR, Papadogiannakis N, Fischler B, Casswall TH, Beijer E, Németh A. Tacrolimus without or with the addition of conventional immunosuppressive treatment in juvenile autoimmune hepatitis. *Acta Paediatrica*. 2012;101(9):993–999.
1074. Cuarterolo M, Ciocca M, Velasco CC, Ramonet M, González T, López S, et al. Follow-up of children with autoimmune hepatitis treated with cyclosporine. *Journal of pediatric gastroenterology and nutrition*. 2006;43(5):635–639.
1075. Peiseler M, Liebscher T, Sebode M, Zenouzi R, Hartl J, Ehlken H, et al. Efficacy and limitations of budesonide as a second-line treatment for patients with autoimmune hepatitis. *Clinical Gastroenterology and Hepatology*. 2018;16(2):260–267 e1.
1076. Hübener S, Oo YH, Than NN, Hübener P, Weiler-Normann C, Lohse AW, et al. Efficacy of 6-mercaptopurine as second-line treatment for patients with autoimmune hepatitis and azathioprine intolerance. *Clinical Gastroenterology and Hepatology*. 2016;14(3):445–453.
1077. Legué C., Legros L., Kammerer-Jacquet S., Jézequel C., Houssel-Debry P., Uguen T., et al. Safety and efficacy of 6-thioguanine as a second-line treatment for autoimmune hepatitis. 2018.
1078. Efe C, Hagström H, Ytting H, Bhanji RA, Müller NF, Wang Q, et al. Efficacy and safety of mycophenolate mofetil and tacrolimus as second-line therapy for patients with autoimmune hepatitis. *Clinical Gastroenterology and Hepatology*. 2017;15(12):1950–1956 e1.
1079. Jothimani D, Cramp ME, Cross TJ. Role of mycophenolate mofetil for the treatment of autoimmune hepatitis—An observational study. *Journal of Clinical and Experimental Hepatology*. 2014;4(3):221–225.
1080. Burak KW, Swain MG, Santodomino-Garzon T, Lee SS, Urbanski SJ, Aspinall AI, et al. Rituximab for the treatment of patients with autoimmune hepatitis who are refractory or intolerant to standard therapy. *Canadian Journal of Gastroenterology*. 2013;27.
1081. D'Agostino D, Costaguta A, Álvarez F. Successful treatment of refractory autoimmune hepatitis with rituximab. *Pediatrics*. 2013;132(2):e526–ee30.
1082. Björnsson ES, Bergmann O, Jonasson JG, Grondal G, Gudbjornsson B, Olafsson S. Drug-induced autoimmune hepatitis: response to corticosteroids and lack of relapse after cessation of steroids. *Clin Gastroenterol Hepatol*. 2017;15(10):1635–1636.
1083. Bovensiepen C, Schakat M, Sebode M, Lohse A, Schramm C, Herkel J, et al. TNFα as therapeutic target in Autoimmune Hepatitis. *Journal of Hepatology*. 2017;66(1):S359.
1084. Rodrigues S, Lopes S, Magro F, Cardoso H, e Vale AMH, Marques M, et al. Autoimmune hepatitis and anti-tumor necrosis factor alpha therapy: a single center report of 8 cases. *World journal of gastroenterology: WJG*. 2015;21(24):7584.
1085. Haridy J, Nicoll A, Sood S. Methotrexate therapy for autoimmune hepatitis. *Clinical Gastroenterology and Hepatology*. 2018;16(2):288–289.
1086. Ytting H, Larsen FS. Everolimus treatment for patients with autoimmune hepatitis and poor response to standard therapy and drug alternatives in use. *Scandinavian Journal of Gastroenterology*. 2015;50(8):1025–1031.
1087. Chatrath H, Allen L, Boyer TD. Use of sirolimus in the treatment of refractory autoimmune hepatitis. *The American journal of medicine*. 2014;127(11):1128–1131.
1088. Kurowski J, Melin-Aldana H, Bass L, Alonso EM, Ekong UD. Sirolimus as rescue therapy in pediatric autoimmune hepatitis. *Journal of pediatric gastroenterology and nutrition*. 2014;58(1):e4–e6.
1089. Petz LD. Cold antibody autoimmune hemolytic anemias. *Blood reviews*. 2008;22(1):1–15.
1090. Packman CH. Hemolytic anemia due to warm autoantibodies. *Blood reviews*. 2008;22(1):17–31.
1091. Sokol R, Booker D, Stamps R. The pathology of autoimmune haemolytic anaemia. *Journal of clinical pathology*. 1992;45(12):1047.
1092. Engelfriet C, ed. *Immune Destruction of Red cells. Seminar On Immune-Mediated Cell Destruction*: American Association of Blood Banks; 1981.
1093. Ruiz-Argüelles A, Llorente L. The role of complement regulatory proteins (CD55 and CD59) in the pathogenesis of autoimmune hemocytopenias. *Autoimmunity reviews*. 2007;6(3):155–161.
1094. Krych-Goldberg M, Atkinson JP. Structure–function relationships of complement receptor type 1. *Immunological reviews*. 2001;180(1):112–122.

1095. Sokol R, Booker D, Stamps R. Paroxysmal cold haemoglobinuria: a clinico-pathological study of patients with a positive Donath-Landsteiner test. *Hematology*. 1999;4(2):137–164.
1096. Kurlander RJ, Rosse WF, Logue GL. Quantitative influence of antibody and complement coating of red cells on monocyte-mediated cell lysis. *The Journal of clinical investigation*. 1978;61(5):1309–1319.
1097. Ross GD, Medof ME. Membrane complement receptors specific for bound fragments of C3. *Advances in immunology*. 1985;37:217–267.
1098. Stott L, Urbaniak S, Barker R. Specific production of regulatory T-cell cytokines, responsiveness to the RhD blood group, and expression of HLA-DRB1* 15. *Immunology-Supplement*. 2002;107.
1099. Pritchard NR, Cutler AJ, Uribe S, Chadban SJ, Morley BJ, Smith KG. Autoimmune-prone mice share a promoter haplotype associated with reduced expression and function of the Fc receptor FcγRII. *Current Biology*. 2000;10(4):227–230.
1100. Kikuchi S, Santiago-Raber M-L, Amano H, Amano E, Fossati-Jimack L, Moll T, et al. Contribution of NZB autoimmunity 2 to Y-linked autoimmune acceleration-induced monocytosis in association with murine systemic lupus. *The Journal of Immunology*. 2006;176(5):3240–3247.
1101. Akbar AN, Fletcher JM. Memory T cell homeostasis and senescence during aging. *Current opinion in immunology*. 2005;17(5):480–485.
1102. Berentsen S, Tjønnfjord GE. Diagnosis and treatment of cold agglutinin mediated autoimmune hemolytic anemia. *Blood reviews*. 2012;26(3):107–115.
1103. Jenkins W, Marsh W, Noades J, Tippett P, Sanger R, Race R. The I antigen and antibody. *Vox sanguinis*. 1960;5(2):97–106.
1104. WL MARSH, Jenkins W. Anti-i: a new cold antibody. *Nature*. 1960;188(4752):753.
1105. Dellagi K., Brouet J.C., Schenmetzler C., Praloran V. Chronic hemolytic anemia due to a monoclonal IgG cold agglutinin with anti-Pr specificity. 1981.
1106. Leddy JP, Falany JL, Kissel GE, Passador ST, Rosenfeld SI. Erythrocyte membrane proteins reactive with human (warm-reacting) anti-red cell autoantibodies. *The Journal of clinical investigation*. 1993;91(4):1672–1680.
1107. Barcellini W, Clerici G, Montesano R, Taioli E, Morelati F, Rebulla P, et al. In vitro quantification of anti-red blood cell antibody production in idiopathic autoimmune haemolytic anaemia: effect of mitogen and cytokine stimulation. *British journal of haematology*. 2000;111(2):452–460.
1108. Ahmad E, Elgohary T, Ibrahim H. 7 Naturally Occurring Regulatory T Cells and Interleukins 10 and 12 in the Pathogenesis of Idiopathic Warm Autoimmune Hemolytic Anemia. *Journal of Investigational Allergology and Clinical Immunology*. 2011;21(4):297.
1109. Kalfa TA. Warm antibody autoimmune hemolytic anemia. *Hematology*. 2016;2016(1):690–697.
1110. Barcellini W. New insights in the pathogenesis of autoimmune hemolytic anemia. *Transfusion medicine and hemotherapy*. 2015;42(5):287–293.
1111. Barros MM, Blajchman MA, Bordin JO. Warm autoimmune hemolytic anemia: recent progress in understanding the immunobiology and the treatment. *Transfusion medicine reviews*. 2010;24(3):195–210.
1112. Liesveld J.L., Rowe J.M., Lichtman M.A. Variability of the erythropoietic response in autoimmune hemolytic anemia: analysis of 109 cases. 1987.
1113. Conley CL, Lippman SM, Ness PM, Petz LD, Branch DR, Gallagher MT. Autoimmune hemolytic anemia with reticulocytopenia and erythroid marrow. *New England Journal of Medicine*. 1982;306(5):281–286.
1114. Lefrère JJ, Courouсé AM, Bertrand Y, Girot R, Soulier JP. Human parvovirus and aplastic crisis in chronic hemolytic anemias: a study of 24 observations. *American journal of hematology*. 1986;23(3):271–275.
1115. Berentsen S, Ulvestad E, Gjertsen BT, Hjorth-Hansen H, Langholm R, Knutsen HV, et al. Rituximab for primary chronic cold agglutinin disease: a prospective study of 37 courses of therapy in 27 patients. *Blood*. 2004;103(8):2925–2928.
1116. Dierickx D, Kentos A, Delannoy A. The role of rituximab in adults with warm antibody autoimmune hemolytic anemia. *Blood, The Journal of the American Society of Hematology*. 2015;125(21):3223–3229.
1117. Crowther M, Chan Y, Garbett IK, Lim W, Vickers MA, Crowther MA. Evidence-based focused review of the treatment of idiopathic warm immune hemolytic anemia in adults. *Blood*. 2011;118(15):4036–4040.

1118. Zanella A, Barcellini W. Treatment of autoimmune hemolytic anemias. *Haematologica*. 2014;99(10):1547–1554.
1119. Fries L, Brickman C, Frank M. Monocyte receptors for the Fc portion of IgG increase in number in autoimmune hemolytic anemia and other hemolytic states and are decreased by glucocorticoid therapy. *The Journal of Immunology*. 1983;131(3):1240–1245.
1120. Sokol R, Hewitt S, Gunson H. Autoimmune hemolysis: a critical review. *Critical reviews in oncology/hematology*. 1985;4(2):125–154.
1121. McMillan R. Chronic idiopathic thrombocytopenic purpura. *New England Journal of Medicine*. 1981;304(19):1135–1147.
1122. Heyns A du P., Badenhorst P.N., Lotter M., Pieters H., Wessels P., Kotze H.F. Platelet turnover and kinetics in immune thrombocytopenic purpura: results with autologous 111In-labeled platelets and homologous 51Cr-labeled platelets differ. 1986.
1123. Moulis G, Palmaro A, Montastruc J-L, Godeau B, Lapeyre-Mestre M, Sailler L. Epidemiology of incident immune thrombocytopenia: a nationwide population-based study in France. *Blood, The Journal of the American Society of Hematology*. 2014;124(22):3308–3315.
1124. Segal JB, Powe N. Prevalence of immune thrombocytopenia: analyses of administrative data. *Journal of Thrombosis and Haemostasis*. 2006;4(11):2377–2383.
1125. Neunert C, Lim W, Crowther M, Cohen A, Solberg L, Crowther MA. The American Society of Hematology 2011 evidence-based practice guideline for immune thrombocytopenia. *Blood*. 2011;117(16):4190–4207.
1126. Cines DB, Bussel JB, Liebman HA, Luning Prak ET. The ITP syndrome: pathogenic and clinical diversity. *Blood*. 2009;113(26):6511–6521.
1127. Rodeghiero F, Stasi R, Gernsheimer T, Michel M, Provan D, Arnold DM, et al. Standardization of terminology, definitions and outcome criteria in immune thrombocytopenic purpura of adults and children: report from an international working group. *Blood*. 2009;113(11):2386–2393.
1128. Shulman NR, Marder VJ, Weinrach RS. Similarities between known antiplatelet antibodies and the factor responsible for thrombocytopenia in idiopathic purpura. Physiologic, serologic and isotopic studies. *Annals of the New York Academy of Sciences*. 1965;124(2):499–542.
1129. Olsson B, Andersson P-O, Jernås M, Jacobsson S, Carlsson B, Carlsson LM, et al. T-cell-mediated cytotoxicity toward platelets in chronic idiopathic thrombocytopenic purpura. *Nature medicine*. 2003;9(9):1123–1124.
1130. Khodadi E, Asnafi AA, Shahrabi S, Shahjahani M, Saki N. Bone marrow niche in immune thrombocytopenia: a focus on megakaryopoiesis. *Annals of hematology*. 2016;95(11):1765–1776.
1131. He R., Reid D.M., Jones C.E., Shulman N.R. Spectrum of Ig classes, specificities, and titers of serum antiglycoproteins in chronic idiopathic thrombocytopenic purpura. 1994.
1132. He R., Reid D., Jones C., Shulman N. Extracellular epitopes of platelet glycoprotein Ib alpha reactive with serum antibodies from patients with chronic idiopathic thrombocytopenic purpura. 1995.
1133. Audia S, Mahévas M, Samson M, Godeau B, Bonnotte B. Pathogenesis of immune thrombocytopenia. *Autoimmunity reviews*. 2017;16(6):620–632.
1134. Kuwana M, Okazaki Y, Ikeda Y. Detection of circulating B cells producing anti-GPIb autoantibodies in patients with immune thrombocytopenia. *PloS one*. 2014;9(1):e86943.
1135. McMillan R, Longmire RL, Yelenosky R, Donnell RL, Armstrong S. Quantitation of platelet-binding IgG produced in vitro by spleens from patients with idiopathic thrombocytopenic purpura. *New England Journal of Medicine*. 1974;291(16):812–817.
1136. Zufferey A, Kapur R, Semple JW. Pathogenesis and therapeutic mechanisms in immune thrombocytopenia (ITP). *Journal of Clinical Medicine*. 2017;6(2):16.
1137. The pathogenesis of chronic immune thrombocytopenic purpura. In: McMillan R, ed. The pathogenesis of chronic immune thrombocytopenic purpura. *Seminars in hematology*. 2007.
1138. Tsubakio T, Tani P, Curd J, McMillan R. Complement activation in vitro by antiplatelet antibodies in chronic immune thrombocytopenic purpura. *British journal of haematology*. 1986;63(2):293–300.
1139. Mahévas M, Patin P, Huetz F, Descatoire M, Cagnard N, Bole-Feysot C, et al. B cell depletion in immune thrombocytopenia reveals splenic long-lived plasma cells. *The Journal of clinical investigation*. 2012;123(1).

1140. Li X, Zhong H, Bao W, Boulad N, Evangelista J, Haider MA, et al. Defective regulatory B-cell compartment in patients with immune thrombocytopenia. *Blood, The Journal of the American Society of Hematology*. 2012;120(16):3318–3325.
1141. Lemoine S, Morva A, Youinou P, Jamin C. Human T cells induce their own regulation through activation of B cells. *Journal of autoimmunity*. 2011;36(3–4):228–238.
1142. Semple JW. Bregging rights in ITP. *Blood, The Journal of the American Society of Hematology*. 2012;120(16):3169.
1143. Wang T, Zhao H, Ren H, Guo J, Xu M, Yang R, et al. Type 1 and type 2 T-cell profiles in idiopathic thrombocytopenic purpura. *Haematologica*. 2005;90(7):914–923.
1144. Zhao C, Li X, Zhang F, Wang L, Peng J, Hou M. Increased cytotoxic T-lymphocyte-mediated cytotoxicity predominant in patients with idiopathic thrombocytopenic purpura without platelet autoantibodies. *Haematologica*. 2008;93(9):1428–1430.
1145. Olsson B, Ridell B, Carlsson L, Jacobsson S, Wadenvik H. Recruitment of T cells into bone marrow of ITP patients possibly due to elevated expression of VLA-4 and CX3CR1. *Blood, The Journal of the American Society of Hematology*. 2008;112(4):1078–1084.
1146. Kuwana M, Kaburaki J, Ikeda Y. Autoreactive T cells to platelet GPIIb-IIIa in immune thrombocytopenic purpura. Role in production of anti-platelet autoantibody. *The Journal of clinical investigation*. 1998;102(7):1393–1402.
1147. Liu B, Zhao H, Poon MC, Han Z, Gu D, Xu M, et al. Abnormality of CD4+ CD25+ regulatory T cells in idiopathic thrombocytopenic purpura. *European journal of haematology*. 2007;78(2):139–143.
1148. Louwes H, Lathori OAZ, Vellenga E, de Wolf JTM. Platelet kinetic studies in patients with idiopathic thrombocytopenic purpura. *The American journal of medicine*. 1999;106(4):430–434.
1149. Nugent D, McMillan R, Nichol JL, Slichter SJ. Pathogenesis of chronic immune thrombocytopenia: increased platelet destruction and/or decreased platelet production. *British journal of haematology*. 2009;146(6):585–596.
1150. Malara A, Abbonante V, Di Buduo CA, Tozzi L, Currao M, Balduini A. The secret life of a megakaryocyte: emerging roles in bone marrow homeostasis control. *Cellular and Molecular Life Sciences*. 2015;72(8):1517–1536.
1151. Makar RS, Zhukov OS, Sahud MA, Kuter DJ. Thrombopoietin levels in patients with disorders of platelet production: diagnostic potential and utility in predicting response to TPO receptor agonists. *American journal of hematology*. 2013;88(12):1041–1044.
1152. Hoffmeister KM. The role of lectins and glycans in platelet clearance. *Journal of thrombosis and haemostasis*. 2011;9:35–43.
1153. Rumjantseva V, Hoffmeister KM. Novel and unexpected clearance mechanisms for cold platelets. *Transfusion and Apheresis Science*. 2010;42(1):63–70.
1154. Hoffmeister KM, Falet H. Platelet clearance by the hepatic Ashwell-Morrell receptor: mechanisms and biological significance. *Thrombosis research*. 2016;141:S68–S72.
1155. Terrell DR, Beebe LA, Vesely SK, Neas BR, Segal JB, George JN. The incidence of immune thrombocytopenic purpura in children and adults: a critical review of published reports. *American journal of hematology*. 2010;85(3):174–180.
1156. Lambert MP, Gernsheimer TB. Clinical updates in adult immune thrombocytopenia. *Blood*. 2017;129(21):2829–2835.
1157. Neunert C, Noroozi N, Norman G, Buchanan G, Goy J, Nazi I, et al. Severe bleeding events in adults and children with primary immune thrombocytopenia: a systematic review. *Journal of Thrombosis and Haemostasis*. 2015;13(3):457–464.
1158. Cortelazzo S., Finazzi G., Buelli M., Molteni A., Viero P., Barbui T. High risk of severe bleeding in aged patients with chronic idiopathic thrombocytopenic purpura. 1991.
1159. Cines DB, Bussel JB. How I treat idiopathic thrombocytopenic purpura (ITP). *Blood*. 2005;106(7):2244–2251.
1160. Doobaree IU, Nandigam R, Bennett D, Newland A, Provan D. Thromboembolism in adults with primary immune thrombocytopenia: a systematic literature review and meta-analysis. *European journal of haematology*. 2016;97(4):321–330.
1161. Sewify EM, Sayed D, RFA AAl, Ahmad HM, Abdou MA. Increased circulating red cell microparticles (RMP) and platelet microparticles (PMP) in immune thrombocytopenic purpura. *Thrombosis Research*. 2013;131(2):e59–e63.

1162. Psaila B, Bussel JB, Frelinger AL, Babula B, Linden MD, Li Y, et al. Differences in platelet function in patients with acute myeloid leukemia and myelodysplasia compared to equally thrombocytopenic patients with immune thrombocytopenia. *Journal of thrombosis and haemostasis*. 2011;9(11):2302–2310.
1163. Cooper N. State of the art–how I manage immune thrombocytopenia. *British journal of haematology*. 2017;177(1):39–54.
1164. Cooper N, Woloski BMR, Fodero EM, Novoa M, Leber M, Beer JH, et al. Does treatment with intermittent infusions of intravenous anti-D allow a proportion of adults with recently diagnosed immune thrombocytopenic purpura to avoid splenectomy? Blood. *The Journal of the American Society of Hematology*. 2002;99(6):1922–1927.
1165. Scaradavou A, Woo B, Woloski B, Cunningham-Rundles S, Ettinger LJ, Aledort LM, et al. Intravenous anti-D treatment of immune thrombocytopenic purpura: experience in 272 patients. *Blood, The Journal of the American Society of Hematology*. 1997;89(8):2689–2700.
1166. Ahmed R, Devasia AJ, Viswabandya A, Lakshmi KM, Abraham A, Karl S, et al. Long-term outcome following splenectomy for chronic and persistent immune thrombocytopenia (ITP) in adults and children. *Annals of hematology*. 2016;95(9):1429–1434.
1167. Kojouri K, Vesely SK, Terrell DR, George JN. Splenectomy for adult patients with idiopathic thrombocytopenic purpura: a systematic review to assess long-term platelet count responses, prediction of response, and surgical complications. *Blood*. 2004;104(9):2623–2634.
1168. Patel VL, Mahévas M, Lee SY, Stasi R, Cunningham-Rundles S, Godeau B, et al. Outcomes 5 years after response to rituximab therapy in children and adults with immune thrombocytopenia. *Blood, The Journal of the American Society of Hematology*. 2012;119(25):5989–5995.
1169. Arnold DM, Dentali F, Crowther MA, Meyer RM, Cook RJ, Sigouin C, et al. Systematic review: efficacy and safety of rituximab for adults with idiopathic thrombocytopenic purpura. *Annals of internal medicine*. 2007;146(1):25–33.
1170. Kuter DJ. New thrombopoietic growth factors. *Blood, The Journal of the American Society of Hematology*. 2007;109(11):4607–4616.
1171. Stirnemann J, Kaddouri N, Khellaf M, Morin AS, Prendki V, Michel M, et al. Vincristine efficacy and safety in treating immune thrombocytopenia: a retrospective study of 35 patients. *European Journal of Haematology*. 2016;96(3):269–275.
1172. Provan D, Moss AJ, Newland AC, Bussel JB. Efficacy of mycophenolate mofetil as single-agent therapy for refractory immune thrombocytopenic purpura. *American journal of hematology*. 2006;81(1):19–25.
1173. Taylor A, Neave L, Solanki S, Westwood JP, Terrinonive I, McGuckin S, et al. Mycophenolate mofetil therapy for severe immune thrombocytopenia. *British journal of haematology*. 2015;171(4):625–630.
1174. Maloisel F, Andrès E, Zimmer J, Noel E, Zamfir A, Koumarianou A, et al. Danazol therapy in patients with chronic idiopathic thrombocytopenic purpura: long-term results. *The American journal of medicine*. 2004;116(9):590–594.
1175. Hou M, Peng J, Shi Y, Zhang C, Qin P, Zhao C, et al. Mycophenolate mofetil (MMF) for the treatment of steroid-resistant idiopathic thrombocytopenic purpura. *European journal of haematology*. 2003;70(6):353–357.
1176. Carapetis JR, Steer AC, Mulholland EK, Weber M. The global burden of group A streptococcal diseases. *The Lancet infectious diseases*. 2005;5(11):685–694.
1177. Settin A, Abdel-Hady H, El-Baz R, Saber I. Gene polymorphisms of TNF-α− 308, IL-10− 1082, IL-6− 174, and IL-1Ra VNTR related to susceptibility and severity of rheumatic heart disease. *Pediatric cardiology*. 2007;28(5):363–371.
1178. Azevedo PM, Bauer R, de Falco Caparbo V, Silva CAA, Bonfá E, Pereira RMR. Interleukin-1 receptor antagonist gene (IL1RN) polymorphism possibly associated to severity of rheumatic carditis in a Brazilian cohort. *Cytokine*. 2010;49(1):109–113.
1179. Beltrame MH, Catarino SJ, Goeldner I, Boldt ABW, de Messias-Reason IJ. The lectin pathway of complement and rheumatic heart disease. *Frontiers in pediatrics*. 2015;2:148.
1180. Sallakci N, Akcurin G, Köksoy S, Kardelen F, Uguz A, Coskun M, et al. TNF-alpha G-308A polymorphism is associated with rheumatic fever and correlates with increased TNF-alpha production. *Journal of autoimmunity*. 2005;25(2):150–154.

1181. Ramasawmy R, Faé KC, Spina G, Victora GD, Tanaka AC, Palácios SA, et al. Association of polymorphisms within the promoter region of the tumor necrosis factor-α with clinical outcomes of rheumatic fever. *Molecular immunology*. 2007;44(8):1873–1878.
1182. Ramasawmy R, Spina GS, Fae KC, Pereira AC, Nisihara R, Reason IJM, et al. Association of mannose-binding lectin gene polymorphism but not of mannose-binding serine protease 2 with chronic severe aortic regurgitation of rheumatic etiology. *Clinical and Vaccine Immunology*. 2008;15(6): 932–936.
1183. Reason IJM, Schafranski MD, Jensenius JC, Steffensen R. The association between mannose-binding lectin gene polymorphism and rheumatic heart disease. *Human immunology*. 2006;67(12):991–998.
1184. Messias-Reason I, Schafranski M, Kremsner P, Ficolin Kun J. 2 (FCN2) functional polymorphisms and the risk of rheumatic fever and rheumatic heart disease. *Clinical & Experimental Immunology*. 2009;157(3):395–399.
1185. Kamal H, Hussein G, Hassoba H, Mosaad N, Gad A, Ismail M. Transforming growth factor-β1 gene C-509T and T869C polymorphisms as possible risk factors in rheumatic heart disease in Egypt. *Acta cardiologica*. 2010;65(2):177–183.
1186. Berdeli A, Celik HA, Özyürek R, Dogrusoz B, Aydin HH. TLR-2 gene Arg753Gln polymorphism is strongly associated with acute rheumatic fever in children. *Journal of molecular medicine*. 2005;83(7):535–541.
1187. Berdeli A, Tabel Y, Celik H, Ozyürek R, Dogrusoz B, Aydin H. Lack of association between TNFα gene polymorphism at position–308 and risk of acute rheumatic fever in Turkish patients. *Scandinavian journal of rheumatology*. 2006;35(1):44–47.
1188. dos Santos Catarino SJ, Boldt ABW, Beltrame MH, Nisihara RM, Schafranski MD, de Messias-Reason IJ. Association of MASP2 polymorphisms and protein levels with rheumatic fever and rheumatic heart disease. *Human Immunology*. 2014;75(12):1197–1202.
1189. Col-Araz N, Pehlivan S, Baspinar O, Sever T, Oguzkan-Balci S, Balat A. Association of macrophage migration inhibitory factor and mannose-binding lectin-2 gene polymorphisms in acute rheumatic fever. *Cardiology in the Young*. 2013;23(4):486–490.
1190. Chou H-T, Chen C-H, Tsai C-H, Tsai F-J. Association between transforming growth factor-β1 gene C-509T and T869C polymorphisms and rheumatic heart disease. *American heart journal*. 2004;148(1):181–186.
1191. Hernández-Pacheco G, Flores-Domínguez C, Rodríguez-Pérez JM, Pérez-Hernández N, Fragoso JM, Saul A, et al. Tumor necrosis factor-alpha promoter polymorphisms in Mexican patients with rheumatic heart disease. *Journal of autoimmunity*. 2003;21(1):59–63.
1192. Hirsch E, Irikura VM, Paul SM, Hirsh D. Functions of interleukin 1 receptor antagonist in gene knockout and overproducing mice. *Proceedings of the National Academy of Sciences*. 1996;93(20): 11008–11013.
1193. Düzgün N, Duman T, Haydardedeoğlu F, Tutkak H. Cytotoxic T lymphocyte-associated antigen-4 polymorphism in patients with rheumatic heart disease. *Tissue Antigens*. 2009;74(6):539–542.
1194. Guilherme L, Kalil J. Rheumatic fever and rheumatic heart disease: cellular mechanisms leading autoimmune reactivity and disease. *Journal of clinical immunology*. 2010;30(1):17–23.
1195. Guilherme L, Köhler K, Kalil J. Rheumatic heart disease: mediation by complex immune events. *Advances in clinical chemistry*. 2011;53(2):31–50.
1196. Guilherme L, Alba MP, Ferreira FM, Oshiro SE, Higa F, Patarroyo ME, et al. Anti-Group A streptococcal vaccine epitope structure, stability, and its ability to interact with HLA Class II molecules. *Journal of Biological Chemistry*. 2011;286(9):6989–6998.
1197. Cunningham MW. Pathogenesis of group A streptococcal infections. *Clinical microbiology reviews*. 2000;13(3):470–511.
1198. Yeğin O, Coşkun M, Ertuğ H. Cytokines in acute rheumatic fever. *European journal of pediatrics*. 1996;156(1):25–29.
1199. Kemeny E, Grieve T, Marcus R, Sareli P, Zabriskie J. Identification of mononuclear cells and T cell subsets in rheumatic valvulitis. *Clinical immunology and immunopathology*. 1989;52(2):225–237.
1200. Fraser W, Haffejee Z, Jankelow D, Wadee A, Cooper K. Rheumatic Aschoff nodules revisited. II: cytokine expression corroborates recently proposed sequential stages. *Histopathology*. 1997;31(5):460–464.

1201. Mota CCC, Aiello VD, Anderson RH. Chronic rheumatic heart disease*Paediatric Cardiology*: Elsevier; 2010:1115–1134.

1202. Dajani AS, Ayoub E, Bierman FZ, Bisno AL, Denny FW, Durack DT, et al. Guidelines for the diagnosis of rheumatic fever: jones criteria, 1992 update. *Jama*. 1992;268(15):2069–2073.

1203. Liu M, Lu L, Sun R, Zheng Y, Zhang P. Rheumatic heart disease: causes, symptoms, and treatments. *Cell biochemistry and biophysics*. 2015;72(3):861–863.

# CHAPTER 4

# Tumor immunology

**Pouya Mahdavi Sharif[a,b], Amin Pastaki Khoshbin[a,b], Elaheh Nasrollahzadeh[b,c], Mahsa Keshavarz-Fathi[a,b,d], Nima Rezaei[d,e,f]**
[a]School of Medicine, Tehran University of Medical Sciences, Tehran, Iran
[b]Cancer Immunology Project (CIP), Universal Scientific Education and Research Network (USERN), Tehran, Iran
[c]School of Medicine, Guilan University of Medical Sciences, Rasht, Iran
[d]Research Center for Immunodeficiencies, Children's Medical Center, Tehran University of Medical Sciences, Tehran, Iran
[e]Department of Immunology, School of Medicine, Tehran University of Medical Sciences, Tehran, Iran
[f]Network of Immunity in Infection, Malignancy and Autoimmunity (NIIMA), Universal Scientific Education and Research Network (USERN), Tehran, Iran

## Introduction

Cancer is a burdensome disease globally. It leads to a tremendous impact on human health, with an estimated 18.1 million new incident cases and 9.6 million deaths worldwide in 2018.[1,2] Cancer has been a well-liked focus of research in the past decade, and much effort has been undertaken to identify the underlying etiologies, elucidate pathophysiological mechanisms and develop efficacious treatments for this condition.[3] This growing body of research has been granting better survival for cancer patients.[4]

Cancer is a complex disorder caused by unopposed dysregulated cell proliferation.[5] During neoplastic transformation, a normal cell acquires new characteristics that enable cell survival, replication, invasiveness, and dissemination.[5] Despite the fact that cancer cells demonstrate substantial heterogeneity in phenotype and function,[6] they share some salient features that allow malignant behavior. These common traits were subsumed by Hanahan and Weinberg under eight "hallmarks of cancer".[5] The hallmarks of cancer constitute sustaining proliferating signaling, defective proliferation suppression, recalcitrance to programmed cell death, overcoming telomere shortening, inducing angiogenesis, capability to invade the surrounding tissue and disseminate to distant organs, altered cellular metabolism, and evading immune responses against cancer.[5] Collectively, cancer cells are autonomous proliferators that have circumvented intrinsic checkpoints of cellular dysfunction and conquered the surrounding environment to foster their growth and progression.

The immune system is a key player in the biology of cancer. Beyond intrinsic cellular regulatory mechanisms and other defenses at the level of tissue organization, the immune system significantly contributes to preventing the outgrowth of transformed cells and their progression.[7] The idea that the immune system may be involved in eliminating cancer cells traces back to Paul Ehrlich. Thereupon, accumulating evidence culminated in the formulation of the cancer immune surveillance theory by Burnet in 1957. Burnet hypothesized that abnormal cells with malignant potential possess

*Clinical Immunology*
DOI: https://doi.org/10.1016/B978-0-12-818006-8.00003-7

specific antigens that are recognized by the host immune system and are destroyed by immunological reactions.[8] Considering the ability of the immune system to demolish transformed cells, it was postulated that the evasion of immune responses was a distinctive and essential tenet for malignant cells to grow and progress.[9] Intriguingly, it was subsequently revealed that the immune system may contribute to cancer progression by affecting cancer cell survival, proliferation, angiogenesis, invasion, and metastasis.[10] Thus, the immune system plays important and multifaceted roles in cancer pathogenesis.

Harnessing the immune system for cancer therapy was a revolutionary step to fight against cancer. Cancer immunotherapy exploits the components of the immune system to directly kill malignant cells or enhance host immune responses against cancer. Several cancer immunotherapeutic approaches such as passive antibody therapy, immune checkpoint inhibition, and adoptive immune cell therapy are currently being used for the treatment of cancer patients.[11] Cancer immunotherapy has come of age, and ongoing research on cancer immunology and immunotherapy is a hope for better cancer treatment options in the future. In this chapter, we have reviewed the status of cancer immunology while discussing various components of the immune system, either inhibiting or supporting tumor outgrowth and invasion. Immunotherapeutic methods for a variety of established tumors have been detailed, and phenotypes of tumor immune microenvironment after cancer treatment have been provided as well.

## Cancer immunoediting

Although a growing number of experiments had been continually confirmed the role of the immune system in eradicating cancer cells, the fact that cancer occurs in immunocompetent hosts led to the proposal of cancer immunoediting theory. Cancer immunoediting theory conceptualizes the states of immunological reactions in relation to tumor development. In this theory, the contribution of the immune system in tumor growth control is divided into three phases: elimination, equilibrium, and escape.[12]

Elimination: in the elimination phase, the immune system detects cancerous cells and eliminates them.[12] The presence of anti-cancer immune responses in the elimination phase is supported by multiple lines of evidence that reports increased incidence of malignancies in transgenic mouse models that lack particular elements of the innate or adaptive immune system and human patients with primary and secondary immunodeficiency.[12–16]

Equilibrium: it is postulated that in the equilibrium phase, the immune system is not capable of complete eradication of cancerous cells, but still, the immune system may prevent overt growth of the tumor by immunological reactions. The equilibrium state may be explained by cancer cell heterogeneity. Cancer cells in a tumor may harbor different genetic and epigenetic alterations, and each cancer cell clone may express its specific set of antigens. Thus, only part of them can be recognized and eradicated by the adaptive immune system.[12] There are some clinical conditions that might be explained by the equilibrium phase of cancer immunoediting theory. The metastasized cancer cells may remain in quiescence in a distant site, a state called metastatic cancer cell dormancy.[17] The state of the interplay between the immune system and dormant cancer cells may be put into the equilibrium phase. Monoclonal gammopathy of undetermined significance (MGUS) is the precursor state of multiple myeloma (MM). In contrast to patients with MM, the bone marrow of patients with MGUS contains effective cluster of differentiation (CD)4+ and CD8+ T cells. These T cells are specifically reactive to MGUS cell antigens.[18]

Escape: in this phase, anti-cancer immune responses are not effective, and consequently, cancer grows and progresses.[12] A Darwinian natural selection model is proposed for the transition from equilibrium to escape phase. In the early equilibrium phase, the immune system destroys cancer cell clones that are susceptible to anti-cancer immune responses, and other clones that are either unrecognizable by the immune system or can employ mechanisms to suppress anti-tumor immune responses survive and repopulate the tumor mass.[19]

Therefore, cancer immunoediting theory is a framework for understanding the many aspects of interactions between the immune system and cancer.

## Immune profiles in malignancy

Given that the immune system takes part significantly in cancer pathogenesis, it is not surprising that characteristics of tumor-infiltrating and circulating immune cells may prognosticate survival or predict response to cancer therapies, especially immunotherapies.[20–22] Immune cell density, spatial distribution, phenotype, function, cytokine production, transcriptomics, and proteomics may be used for immune profiling of cancer.[23–25] Many models for cancer immune landscape have been developed,[26] but one of the earliest models is still in use for anti-cancer immune response conceptualization and has been proved to be clinically reliable in solid tumors.[27] This model is based on the density and spatial distribution of tumor infiltration by lymphocytes. Drew on this model, solid tumors are categorized into three immune profile subtypes (Fig. 4.1). Inflamed (hot) tumors contain an abundance of T cells all over the tumor, including in the proximity of cancer cells. In immune-excluded tumors, the inflammatory cells are only present at the stroma of the tumor, not in the cancer cell nests. Immune-desert (cold) tumors are devoid of T cells in the whole tumor.[27] Inflamed (hot) immune phenotype has been associated with better prognosis in several cancer types, including microsatellite instability (MSI)-high colon cancer, pancreatic cancer, and melanoma.[28–31]

The regulation of T cell infiltration into tumor tissue seems to be dependent on host factors and the genetic and epigenetic composition of cancer cells.[27,32] Chen et al.[33]

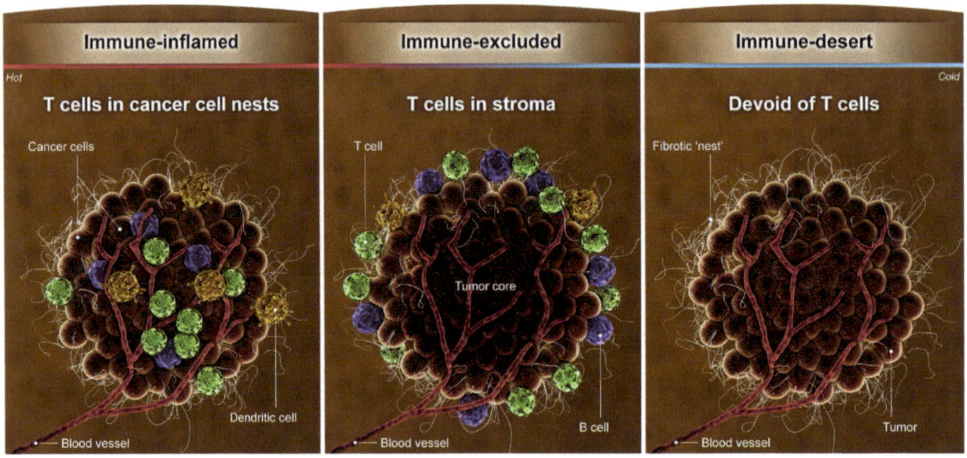


**Fig. 4.1** ***Immune profiles in malignancies.*** This illustration recapitulates three immune phenotypes of solid tumors. Inflamed tumors show infiltration of lymphocytes all over the tumor tissue, including tumor nests. In immune-excluded tumors, tumor-infiltrating lymphocytes (TIL) are not present in the cancer cell nests and are only found in the tumor stroma, sometimes forming tertiary lymphoid structures. Immune-desert tumors are devoid of TIL in the whole tumor.

adroitly summarized the mechanisms underpinning each immune phenotype. Immune-desert phenotype may be the result of the absence of immunogenic antigens, down-regulation or modulation of antigen-presenting machinery in cancer cells, the presence of immunosuppressive cells and cytokines in the tumor microenvironment (TME), or impaired antigen presentation by antigen-presenting cells (APC). Immune-excluded phenotype may arise out of high extracellular density in some parts of the tumor, chemokine alteration that incapacitates their ability to recruit T cells, and defective vascular networks. Many factors contribute to the regulation of the above immunopathological mechanisms, such as the genetic and epigenetic composition of cancer cells, host germline genetic and epigenetic state, and microbiota.[33] Consistent among several studies, a higher somatic tumor mutational burden (TMB) is associated with improved survival across many cancer types. This has shown to be related to more neoantigen generation in tumors with a higher mutational burden.[34] To summarize, tumor-host-environment interaction regulates immune system response to cancer.

## Cancer antigens and cancer antigen presentation

Cancer cells are derived from host cells. As the adaptive immune system is tolerant to self-antigens, it is expected that no adaptive immune response could be mounted against cancer cells. However, tumor antigen-specific lymphocytes are present in cancer patients and can exert potent anti-cancer immune responses in vitro and in vivo.[35] Therefore, cancer cells should display antigens that central and peripheral tolerance has not been developed toward them. In this section, antigen presentation machinery function, mechanisms of cancer cell antigenicity, and types of cancer antigens will be discussed.

## Antigen presentation machinery

Major histocompatibility complex (MHC) molecules are membrane molecules committed to antigen presentation to T cells. T cells recognize their target cells through interaction ofT cell receptor (TCR)-MHC/peptide complex. Fig. 4.2 illustrates cellular antigen processing and presentation machinery. Briefly, MHC class I molecules present intracellular protein fragments to CD8+ T cells, and MHC class II molecules present extracellular protein fragments to CD4+ T cells. MHC class I molecule is expressed by almost all nucleated cells, while MHC class II molecule is expressed almost exclusively by professional APCs, namely dendritic cells (DCs), macrophages, and B lymphocytes. MHC class I heavy chain is encoded by three genes: *human leukocyte antigen (HLA)-A*,

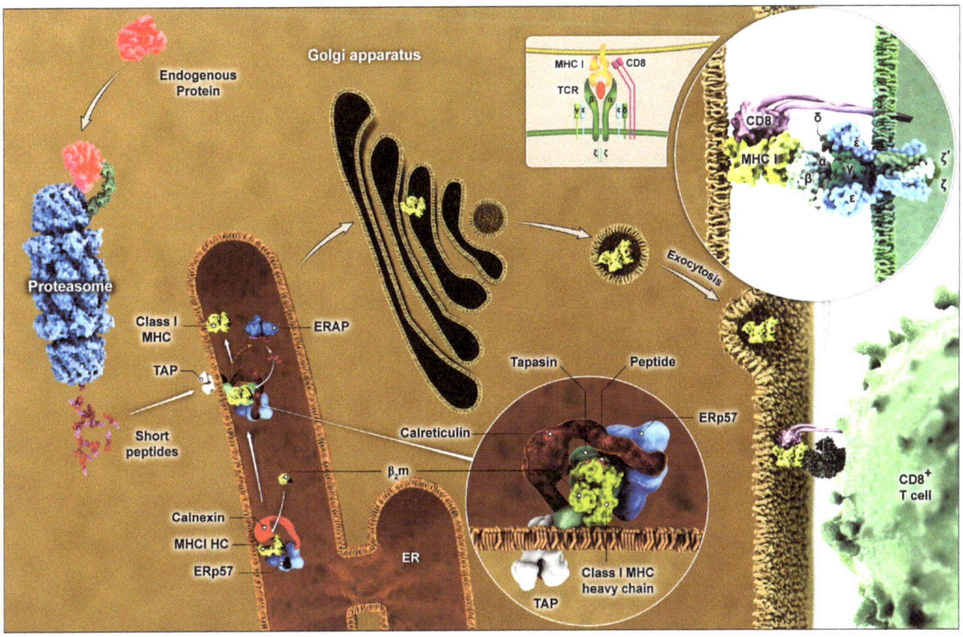


**Fig. 4.2** ***Antigen presentation machinery of cancer cells.*** The cytoplasmic or nuclear proteins are degraded by proteasome complex, and the resulting peptide fragments give entrance to endoplasmic reticulum (ER) through transporter associated with antigen processing (TAP). In the ER, peptide-loading complex composed of major histocompatibility complex (MHC) class I heavy chain, β2-microglobulin, Tap, Tapsin, Calreticulin, and ERp57 acts to load antigenic peptide fragment on MHC class I molecule. The MHC class I/antigen complex then leaves ER and resides in the cytoplasmic membrane.

B2M, Beta2-microglobulin; CD, Cluster of differentiation; ERAP, Endoplasmic reticulum amino peptidase, MHCI HC, Major histocompatibility complex class I heavy chain; TAP, Transporter associated with antigen processing; TCR, T cell receptor.

*HLA-B*, and *HLA-C*. MHC class II monomer is encoded by three distinct genes: *HLA-DR*, *HLA-DQ*, and *HLA-DP*.[36]

Cytosolic and nuclear proteins are degraded by the proteasome complex, and the resultant peptides are transported into the endoplasmic reticulum (ER) by a transmembrane protein of ER membrane called transporter associated with antigen processing (TAP). In ER, the peptides may be further affected to N-terminal cleavage by ER aminopeptidase ½ (ERAP1/2).[37] MHC class I complex is composed of a heavy chain, a light chain called β2-microglobulin, and a peptide fragment of 8–9 amino acid chain length. The assembly of this complex requires the activity of many proteins such as TAP, Tapsin, ERp57, and Calreticulin.[36] Then, the peptide-MHC class I complex is transported to the cell membrane.[37] Of note, MHC class I antigen presentation may occur in cancer cells in proteasome-independent or TAP-independent manners.[37–40]

An intricate antigen-presenting system is involved in CD8+ T cell priming. T cell priming requires antigen presentation and providing co-stimulatory signals to T cells by APC. The main entrance pathway of exogenous antigens such as cancer cell antigen to APC is the endocytosis of dead cell remnants. CD8+ T cell priming is dependent on MHC class I-TCR interaction. Notwithstanding, the conventional pathway for exogenous antigen presentation is through MHC class II molecules. Conventional DC can present exogenous antigens by MHC class I molecules, a process known as "antigen cross-presentation".[41] Two main pathways for antigen cross-presentation exist: the endosome-to-cytosol and vacuolar pathways. In the endosome-to-cytosol pathway, proteins are transported from the endosome to DC cytosol and get degraded by the proteasome and follow the same route for MHC class I antigen presentation. In the vacuolar pathway, exogenous proteins undergo cleavage by lysosomal Cathepsin enzymes and subsequently get loaded on MHC class I molecule in the endosome organelle environment. The exact mechanisms of antigen cross-presentation are still waiting to be unraveled.[41,42] While most exogenous antigens are conveyed to APC by endocytosis, there are other routes for exogenous antigen capture by APC as well. Proteins can be directly transported from cancer cells to DC by gap junctions. The transferred proteins then utilize MHC class I machinery to be presented.[43]

## Cancer cell antigenicity

In normal conditions, a protein-encoding gene is transcribed in the nucleus. The produced messenger RNA exits the nucleus and enters cytosol. Ribosome decodes the messenger RNA and synthesizes a peptide chain. The resultant protein may be affected by post-translational modification. The protein then may be degraded by the proteasome complex. Some but not all of the peptide fragments generated by the proteasome complex can be loaded on MHC class I molecules and be presented by them if the cell contains MHC class I machinery. MHC class I/peptide complexes that can be recognized by TCR in normal conditions would not result in T cell responses as these antigens had been subjected to central or peripheral tolerance.

The above course of action may be altered in cancer cells so that immunogenic antigens ensue. A number of mechanisms may explain cancer antigen generation on most occasions. A cancer cell may express a protein that is normally expressed by cells that have no antigen presentation machinery. As these proteins are not presented in normal conditions, the adaptive immune system is not tolerant to them. This is the case for cancer germline antigens. These proteins are normally present in male germline cells and trophoblasts that do not have antigen-presenting machinery. The expression of these genes is repressed in most other normal cells causing promoter hypermethylation. Demethylation of cancer germline antigen genes in cancer cells as the result of global hypomethylation in cancer cells leads to their expression.[35,44–47] Viral gene expression, gene mutation, or alternative post-transcriptional or post-translational modifications may result in the production of proteins, that upon degradation by the proteasome complex, generates peptide fragments that are not present in normal cells and can be presented by MHC class I molecules. Apparently, these peptides are immunogenic if the MHC class I/peptide complex can match TCR. The protein that is presented in this way may never be presented on normal occasions or may be presented by a different antigenic fragment.[35,48] The proteasome content of cancer cells may be different from normal cells. The proteasome content may affect the resulting peptide generated and the peptide presented by MHC class I accordingly.[35,49–51] Cancer cells may possess mutations in MHC class I genes. The resultant MHC protein may present antigens that are not normally presented by the non-mutated MHC molecule of the host. Therefore, the presented peptide fragment may be immunogenic.[48,52]

## Cancer antigen categories

Although no uniform classification system for cancer antigens currently exists, some families of cancer antigens have been arbitrarily described in the literature. The separation of these groups of antigens is mostly reliant on the mechanism and origin of cancer antigens.

Neoantigen: neoantigen is a totally new antigenic peptide, which is originated from the host genome and is generated through gene mutation or altered gene expression.[35,53,54] Neoantigen may be derived from single nucleotide substitution, frameshift mutation, gene fusion, expression of retrotransposons, messenger RNA alternative splicing, alternative translation, and post-translational modifications.[48]

Neoantigen can be the result of a driver or passenger mutation. Driver mutation is crucial to the oncogenic transformation, such as proto-oncogene and tumor suppressor gene mutations. One notable example of cancer antigen derived from a driver mutation is the antigenic peptide from BCR-ABL fusion protein generated by *bcr-abl* translocation during chronic myelogenous leukemia oncogenesis. Passenger mutations are haphazard mutations as a result of genomic instability of cancer.[35,55,56] Neoantigen can make a highly tumor-specific anti-cancer immune response.

**Table 4.1** Viral-encoded cancer antigens.

| Virus | Virus family/genome | Associated cancer type(s) | Antigen(s) |
|---|---|---|---|
| HPV | Papillomaviridae/DNA | Cervical SCC, oropharyngeal SCC, vulvar SCC, anal and rectal SCC, penile SCC, vaginal SCC | E6, E7 |
| HBV | Hepadnaviridae/DNA | Hepatocellular Carcinoma | HBx |
| HCV | Flaviviridae/RNA | Hepatocellular Carcinoma, NHL | |
| EBV | Herpesviridae/DNA | Nasopharyngeal carcinoma, Hodgkin disease, NHL, gastric carcinoma | EBNA1, EBNA3, LMP1, LMP3, gp350 |
| HHV-8 | Herpesviridae/DNA | Kaposi sarcoma, primary effusion lymphoma | K12, ORF-gB, ORF-6, ORF-61, ORF-65 |
| HTLV-½ | Retroviridae/RNA | Adult T-cell leukemia/lymphoma | Tax, HBz |

HPV, Human Papilloma Virus; DNA, Deoxyribonucleic Acid; SCC, Squamous Cell Carcinoma; HBV, Hepatitis B Virus; HCV, Hepatitis C Virus; RNA, Ribonucleic Acid; EBV, Epstein Bar Virus; NHL, Non-Hodgkin Lymphoma; EBNA, Epstein Bar Virus Nuclear Antigen; LMP, Latent membrane Protein; HHV, Human Herpes Virus; ORF, Open Reading Frame; HTLV, Human T Cell Lymphotropic Virus.

Viral-encoded cancer antigens: some viral infections are capable of triggering oncogenesis in humans (Table 4.1). They can cause cancer either by governing host cell proliferation, enhancing genomic instability, propagating chronic inflammation, or suppressing the host immune system.[57] *Human Papillomavirus (HPV), Hepatitis B Virus (HBV), Hepatitis C Virus (HCV), Epstein Bar Virus (EBV), Human Herpes Virus (HHV)−8, Human T-Lymphotropic Virus (HTLV)−½* collectively attribute to around 1,400,000 cancer cases each year.[58] Virus-encoded proteins in the host cell can be presented by MHC class I molecules using the host cell machinery for self-antigen presentation. Transformed cells infected by viruses present virus-encoded antigens that can be recognized by the host's adaptive immune system. As these antigens are not self-antigens, the immune responses against them are highly specific.[57,59,60]

Cancer germline antigens: several cancer germline antigens have been discovered so far. Some of the most studied cancer germline antigens are MAGE antigens, GAGE antigens, SSX, BAGE, Cyclin A, KMHN1 and SPA17.[35,61-63] Immune response against cancer germline antigens is highly specific.[35]

Differentiation antigens: differentiation antigens are so-called since the tissue of origin also expresses the antigen. Some remarkable examples are Tyrosinase and Melan-A in melanoma, prostatic-specific antigen (PSA) in prostate cancer, carcinoembryonic antigen (CEA) in colorectal, pancreatic, ovarian and breast cancers, and alpha-fetoprotein in hepatocellular carcinoma.[35,37] Immune response against these antigens is of low tumor specificity.[35]

Overexpressed antigens: some of the immune responses against cancer cells are toward proteins whose genes are overexpressed in cancer cells. One noteworthy example is WT1 in acute myelogenous leukemia (AML).[35,64,65]

## Immunity to cancer

The immune system is the preeminent obstacle for transformed cells to survive and progress. Both adaptive and innate arms of the immune system are able to mount effective immune responses against cancer cells. T cells were historically recognized as the main effectors of immunity against cancer. However, B cells and antibody production are integral to cancer immunity. Components of innate immunity encompassing natural killer (NK) cells, macrophages, neutrophils, and innate lymphoid cells take part in the fight of the immune system against cancer as well. In this section, we review the role of immune cells in cancer immunity.

## T cells

### Basic immunobiology of T cells

T cells are lymphoid progenitor-derived cells that undergo thymic maturation and selection. Unique to the T cell population is the expression of TCR. TCR is composed of either α and β or γ and δ heterodimers. TCRαβ-T cells constitute the major proportion of T cells in the peripheral blood. Each TCR chain contains a constant and a variable region. TCR gene recombination generates a diverse repertoire of TCR variable regions and the ability to bind to different antigens. As a member of the adaptive immune system, TCRαβ-T cells act in an antigen-specific manner. Cardinal to this antigen specificity is MHC-restricted antigen recognition and the presence of a vast array of T cell clones that express their unique TCR.[66,67] On the T cell surface, TCRαβ makes a complex with three CD3 molecules.[68,69] Upon binding to its complementary antigen, a signal is relayed to the T cell interior by the TCR-CD3 complex.[70] TCR-αβ-T cells are divided into some subpopulations with distinct phenotype, function, cytokine profile, and relation to cancer progression (Table 4.2).

The fate of T cell activation status upon antigen recognition and TCR-CD3 signaling is dependent on co-stimulatory and co-inhibitory signals. T cells express a wide array of co-stimulatory or co-inhibitory receptors that upon interaction with their ligands regulate T cell activation. The particular set of receptors present on the T cell surface and their ligands in the surrounding environment determines the ultimate destiny of TCR-CD3 signaling.[71]

**Table 4.2** T cell subpopulations.

| Subpopulation | Chemokine receptors | Transcription factor(s) | Cytokine production | Function(s) | Role in cancer |
|---|---|---|---|---|---|
| CTL | CXCR3, CCR5 | T-bet | IFN-γ | Perforin/Granzymes cell killing<br>Death receptor cell killing | Anti-tumor |
| Th1 | CXCR3, CCR5 | T-bet, STAT1, STAT4 | IFN-γ, TNF-α | CTL↑<br>Th1↑<br>B cell: IgG production<br>NK cell↑<br>M1-macrophage↑ | Anti-tumor |
| Th2 | CCR3, CCR4, CCR8 | GATA3, STAT6 | IL-4, IL-5, IL-13 | Th2↑<br>B cell: IgE production<br>NK cell↓<br>M2-macrophage↑<br>Eosinophil↑ | Pro-tumor |
| Th9 | CXCR3, CCR3, CCR6 | IRF4, PU.1, STAT6 | IL-3, IL-9, IL-21 | Diverse | Both pro/anti-tumor |
| Th17 | CCR6 | RORγt, STAT3 | IL-8, IL-17, IL-21, IL-22 | Th17↑<br>Neutrophil↑ | Both pro/anti-tumor |
| Th22 | CCR10 | AhR, FOXO4 | IL-22 | Epithelial cells: Defensins↑ | Both pro/anti-tumor |
| Treg | CXCR3, CCR4, CCR5, CCR8 | FOXP3 | IL-10, TGF-β | CTL↓<br>Th17↑<br>B cell: IgA production<br>NK cell↓<br>M2-macrophage↑ | Pro-tumor |

CTL, Cytotoxic T Lymphocytes; CXCR, CXC Chemokine Receptor; CCR, CC Chemokine Receptor; T-bet, T-Box Transcription Factor; IFN, Interferon; Th, T helper; STAT, Signal Transducer and Activator of Transcription; TNF, Tumor-Necrosis Factor; Ig Immunoglobulin; NK, Natural Killer; IL, Interleukin; IRF, Interferon-Regulating Factor; PU, Purine Rich; RORγt; Retinoic Acid Receptor-Related Orphan Receptor Gamma t; AhR, Aryl Hydrocarbon Receptor; FOXO, Forkhead Box O; Treg, Regulatory T cell; FOXP, Forkhead Box P; TGF, Tumor Growth Factor.

Many co-stimulatory and co-inhibitory receptors have been identified to be implicated in T cell biology. CD28 is a costimulatory molecule that may be expressed on the T cell surface. It binds to B7-1 (CD80) and B7-2 (CD86) on APC and directs T cells toward an active state.[71,72] Some clinically relevant co-inhibitory molecules are cytotoxic

T lymphocyte-associated protein (CTLA)−4, programmed cell death protein (PD)−1, lymphocyte activation gene (LAG)−3, T cell immunoglobulin and mucin domain (TIM) 3, and T cell immunoglobulin and ITIM domain (TIGIT).[33,71] CTLA-4 is structurally similar to CD28. Like CD28, CTLA-4 binds to B7-1 and B7-2 on APC. This interaction impairs T cell activation and proliferation through dysregulating many T cell intracellular pathways such as activator protein (AP) 1, nuclear factor kappa B (NF-κB), and nuclear factor of activated T cells (NFAT). The affinity of CTLA-4 to B7-1 and B7-2 is higher than CD28 to B7-1 and B7-2 and consequently, CTLA-4 competes with CD28 to bind their ligands. Interestingly, CTLA-4 binding to B7-1 and B7-2 on DC results in ligand internalization. Furthermore, DC may acquire immunosuppressive functions through B7-1 and B7-2 interaction with CTLA-4.[71,73,74] Activated T cells may express PD-1. PD-1 interacts with programmed death ligand (PD-L)1 and PD1L2, which are expressed in TME by B cells, regulatory T cells (Treg), myeloid-derived suppressor cells (MDSCs), tumor-associated macrophages (TAMs), cancer-associated fibroblasts (CAFs), and cancer cells. This ligand binding inhibits T cell function, which is mainly mediated by directly stagnating TCR-CD3 complex signaling.[33,71,73-76]

### *Activation, recruitment and the effector functions of T cells in tumor setting*

The first encounter of naïve T cells with tumor antigen generally occurs in tumor-draining lymph nodes or tertiary lymphoid structures in the tumor. CD103+ DCs are recognized as the principal APCs in the context of tumor immunity. After that, naïve T cells are primed by DCs in the draining lymph nodes, T cells upregulate C—C chemokine receptor (CCR)5 and C-X-C chemokine receptor (CXCR)3. Tumor microenvironmental cells secret C—C chemokine ligand (CCL)2, CCL3, CCL4, CCL5, C-X-C chemokine ligand (CXCL)9, and CXCL10 that recruit CCR5 and CXCR3 expressing T cells. Primed T cells leave the lymph nodes into circulation and infiltrate the tumor tissue.[27,77,78] Tumor-infiltrating T cells proliferate in TME, a process that is orchestrated by CD103+ DCs.[32]

The role of cytotoxic T lymphocytes (CTL) in cancer immunity is central. After infiltration into TME, CTLs recognize cancer cells by MHC class I/TCR interaction. This interaction activates its effector functions. CTLs elicit anti-cancer immune response via granule exocytosis, using cell death ligand/receptor system, and cytokine and chemokine production.[79,80]

Two main components of CTL granules are Perforin and Granzymes, which are crucial for CTL-mediated cytolysis. Upon release from CTL into the synaptic cleft, Perforin undergoes calcium-dependent oligomerization on the target cancer cell membrane and makes transmembrane pores on it (Fig. 4.3). Granzymes are a group of serine proteases that are delivered into target cancer cells in a Perforin-dependent manner. They orchestrate many intracellular pathways to the eventual regulated cell death.[79-81]

Granule exocytosis happens through a four-step process. Once CTLs are activated, an immunological synapse is formed between CTLs and target cancer cells. After synapse

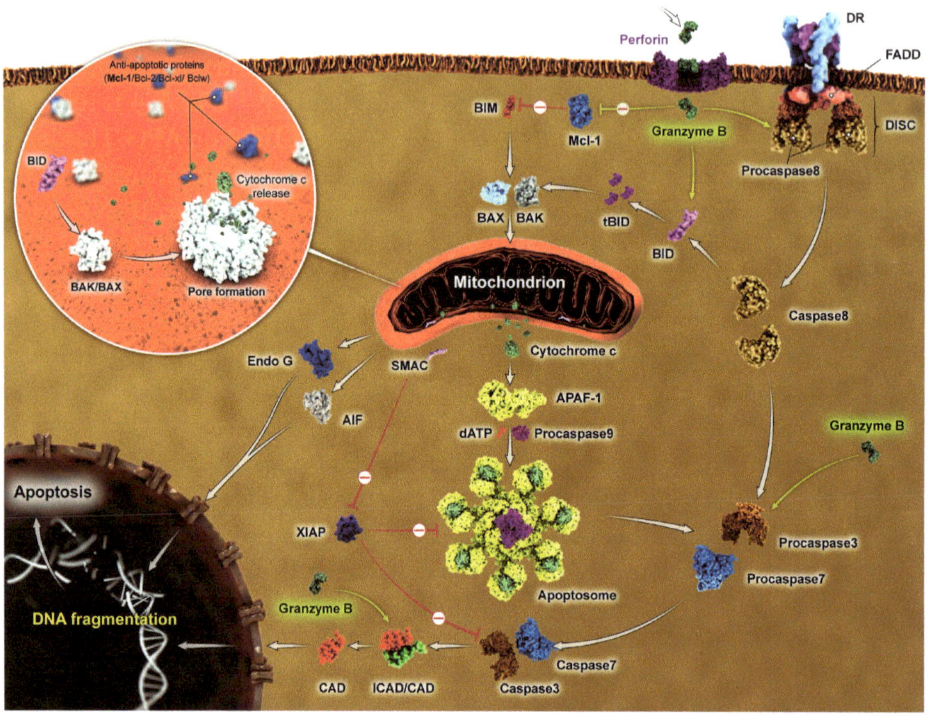


**Fig. 4.3** ***Cancer cell killing by cytotoxic lymphocytes.*** Cytotoxic lymphocytes, i.e., cytotoxic T lymphocytes (CTL) and natural killer (NK) cells destroy cancer cells using either Perforin/Granzymes pathway or the death-ligand/death receptor pathway. Perforin polymerizes on the cancer cell surface and produces transmembrane routes through it. This may result in osmotic cell lysis. Granzymes get into cancer cells either through perforin-produced membrane pores or endocytosis of the perforin/Granzyme complex. Granzymes B, A, M, K, and other Granzymes have been shown to have the ability to induce cell death. However, only Granzyme B-mediated apoptosis mechanism is better understood. Granzyme B can induce apoptosis through mitochondrion-dependent and mitochondrion-independent pathways. Granzyme B cleaves BH3-interacting domain death agonist (Bid), which produces truncated Bid. Truncated Bid activates proapoptotic proteins BCL-2-antagonist/killer (Bak) and BCL-2-associated X (Bax). Activated Bak and Bax disrupt the mitochondrial membrane, which allows proapoptotic factors, notably Cytochrome c, release into the cytoplasm. In addition, Granzyme B can inhibit myeloid leukemia cell differentiation protein (MLC)–1. MLC-1 stabilizes the BCL-2-interacting mediator of cell death (Bim), while Bim itself activates Bak and Bax. MLC-1 inhibition consequently results in Bim-mediated Bak and Bax activation. Cytochrome c, nucleotides, apoptotic protease activating factor (APAF) 1, and procaspase-9 form apoptosome complex, which activates procaspase-3 and procaspase-7. Granzyme B can directly cleave procaspase-3 or procaspase-7, or it can first activate procaspase-8, which subsequently renders procaspase-3/7 active. Death receptors such as Fas and tumor necrosis factor-related apoptosis-inducing ligand receptor (TRAILR) bind to their corresponding ligands FasL and TRAIL, respectively. Upon ligand binding and conformational change, the death receptor interacts with Fas-associated protein with death domain (FADD) and procaspase-8, which collectively form death-inducing signaling complex (DISC). Activated caspase-8 then mediates proteolytic activation of procaspase-3/7. Caspase-3/7 catalyzes the inhibitor of caspase-activated DNase (ICAD). CAD then translocates to the nucleus and fragments DNA, and apoptosis ensues. In an independent pathway, death receptors can also stimulate another type of regulated cell death called necroptosis, which is not shown in this Fig.
APAF, Apoptotic protease activating factor; Bak, BCL2-antagonist/killer; Bax, BCL2-associated X; Bid, BH3-interacting domain death agonist; Bim, BCL2-interacting mediator of cell death; CAD, Caspase-activated DNase; dATP, Deoxyadenosine triphosphate; DR, Death receptor; FADD, Fas-associated protein with death domain; ICAD, Inhibitor of caspase-activated DNase; MLC, Myeloid leukemia cell differentiation protein.

is formed, cytoskeletal rearrangement leads to polarization of microtubule-organizing center (MTOC) toward immunological synapse. Along with MTOC, lysosomal-related lytic granules are brought to the site of the immunological synapse. Lytic granules get attached to the synaptic cell membrane, a process called "docking". Finally, the secretory granules get fused with the plasma membrane and secreted.[79,82]

CTLs may express tumor necrosis factor (TNF) superfamily members, TNF-α, Fas ligand (FasL), and TNF-related apoptosis-inducing ligand (TRAIL), on their cell membrane or release exosomes containing these molecules. FasL and TRAIL induce apoptosis or necroptosis in target cancer cells by binding to their cognate receptors.[79,82,83]

T helper (Th) cells are coordinators of immune response in TME. They influence several immune cells in TME, including DCs, CTLs, B cells, and macrophages. In response to interleukin (IL)−12 produced by DCs, Th cells confer Th1 phenotype. Th1 reciprocally activates DCs through CD40 ligand (CD40L)-CD40 interaction. Th1 augments CTLs' anti-cancer function by cytokine production, especially interferon (IFN)-γ, IL-2, and IL-21. Pivotal for B cell activation, differentiation to plasma cell and acquisition of antigen-presenting capabilities is priming B cell through upregulation of CD40L in surrounding microenvironment, primarily Th cells.[84,85]

IFN-γ is a critical cytokine in anti-cancer immunity. The major sources of IFN-γ production in the cancerous microenvironment are CD8+ T cells, Th1, and NK cells. Upon binding to the IFN-γ receptor, they alter target cell function mainly through Janus kinase (JAK) ½-signal transducer and activator of transcription (STAT) 1/3 pathways. IFN-γ inhibits cancer cell proliferation through suppressing β-Catenin as well as CDK4/6 pathways and activation of p21 and p27 tumor suppressors. Moreover, IFN-γ induces regulated cell death that is mediated by cleaving Caspases and activating the Ras pathway.[86-92] IFN-γ upregulates MHC class I expression of cancer cells, hence potentiating immune responses against cancer cells through increased antigen presentation.[93] Additionally, IFN-γ induces the expression of Class II MHC trans-activator (CIITA) in cancer cells. CIITA is a prime regulator of MHC class II and IFN-γ-mediated CIITA induction upregulates MHC class II expression in cancer cells. MHC class II expression by cancer cells provides activating signals for Th cells in TME.[88,94-97] IFN-γ lines up immune cells in TME to propagate anti-tumor immunity. IFN-γ activates CD8+ T cells, Th1 cells, NK cells, and M1-like macrophages.[86]

## B cell and immunoglobulin

B cells infiltrate the cancerous microenvironment. They may exert anti-cancer immune responses in antibody-independent or antibody-dependent ways. Activated B cells act as intra-tumoral APCs and prime antigen-specific CD4+ and CD8+ T cells. Cancer antigen-specific B cells expand and differentiate into plasma cells that produce high-affinity antibodies against cancer antigens. These antibodies may contribute to anti-tumor immunity. Antibody-dependent immune responses may be mediated by antibody-dependent cellular cytotoxicity (ADCC) by NK cells, fostering phagocytosis by macrophages and neutrophils and probably activating the classical complement pathway. Furthermore, the binding of the immunoglobulin to cancer antigen may augment antigen recognition by APCs. It seems that immunoglobulin G (IgG)1 among all classes of immunoglobulins contributes to anti-tumor immunity.[98-101]

## NK cells

NK cells are innate effector cells. They descend from common lymphoid progenitor and attack stressed cells such as virus-infected or transformed cells.[102,103] Even though NK cells and CTLs are unalike in immunophenotype, antigen specificity and the mode of activation, their effector functions are closely the same.[104]

NK cells do not express TCR-CD3 complex, and their target cell recognition relies on detecting the change in cellular stress marker expression. Those NK cell receptors that are essential for NK cell function and their corresponding ligands that are increased during cellular stress are celled stimulatory receptors. On the contrary, some NK cell receptors transmit inhibitory intracellular signals, and their ligands are reduced in stressed cells. These receptors are called inhibitory receptors. The interaction of NK cell stimulatory and inhibitory receptors and their ligands in TME and the effect of inflammatory and immunosuppressive cytokines in the surrounding milieu regulate the functional status of NK cells.[105]

Many cancerous cells downregulate MHC class I expression.[106] NK cells harbor killer immunoglobulin-like receptor (KIR) 2DL1, KIR2DL2, and KIR2DL3 on their cell surface membrane. They are immunoglobulin-like receptor molecules with the conserved cytoplasmic tail of immunoreceptor tyrosine-based inhibition motif (ITIM).[107] Upon binding to HLA-C, a member of the MHC class I molecule, these receptors transmit inhibitory signals that eventually suppress NK cell cytotoxic functions.[105,107] Natural killer group (NKG) 2A/CD94 complex recognizes HLA-E molecule on cancer cells and inhibits NK cell activation.[105,108] Cancer cells may diminish MHC class I expression, which removes the inhibitory effect of MHC class I expression on NK cell function and leads to cancer cell destruction by NK cells.[105] NK cell inhibitory receptors may also recognize non-MHC ligands. TIGIT inhibits NK cell function through binding to CD155 and CD112 on tumor cells.[105,109]

The most widely known stimulatory NK cell receptor is natural killer group 2D (NKG2D) that binds to MHC class I polypeptide-related sequence A (MICA), MICB, and some other ligands.[105,110] Although MICA and MICB are expressed in normal cells constitutively, localization in the cytoplasmic membrane is limited mostly to cells that suffer from a viral infection, DNA damage, or malignant transformation.[111] Two B7 family proteins, B7-H6 and B7-H7, interact with their cognate stimulatory NK cell receptors, NKp30 and CD28H, respectively.[105,112-114] The interaction of well-known costimulatory T cell protein CD2 on NK cells with CD58/48 on cancer cells is essential for nanotube formation and NK cell cytotoxic function.[115] NKp46 is a stimulatory receptor with a yet unknown ligand that plays an important part in triggering the polarization of NK cell granules into the immunological synapse between NK cells and target cells.[116] The binding of NK cell receptor NKp44 to platelet-derived growth factor (PDGF) DD on tumor cells enhances NK cell function.[117,118]

Inflammatory and immunosuppressive cytokine milieu in TME can modulate the set point of NK cell activation. IL-2, IL-12, Il-15, IL-18, and IL-21 lower the threshold for NK cell activation.[105] Type I Interferon cytokines are potent stimulators of NK cell function. DNA damage during oncogenic transformation causes fragments of double-stranded DNA release into the cancer cell cytoplasm. Interaction of cytosolic DNA with cyclic Guanosine monophosphate (GMP) Adenosine monophosphate (AMP) synthase (CGAS) produces 2′, 3′-cGAMP, which induces type I Interferon production through STING-mediated signaling.[119,120] Transforming growth factor (TGF)-β and adenosine act directly on NK cells and inhibit their anti-cancer functions.[105]

There are four main categories of anti-cancer immune functions exerted by NK cells. First, NK cells release cytolytic granules and directly kill cancer cells, a process mainly mediated by Perforin and Granzymes. The process of granule exocytosis and Perforin and Granzymes functions are similar to what was explained for T cells to a great extent.[81,82,121] Second, NK cells can induce regulated cell death by FasL and TRAIL.[121] Third, NK cells produce inflammatory cytokines and chemokines in TME and promote tumor immunity. Among these cytokines and chemokines are IFN-γ, TNF-α, CCL3, CCL4, CCL5, XCL1, and granulocyte-macrophage colony-stimulating factor (GM-CSF).[82,121,122] These cytokines are particularly involved in enhancing T cell recruitment and anti-tumor function.[122] Fourth, NK cell CD16 binding to the Fc portion of antibodies that target cancer cells results in ADCC.[121,123]

## Macrophages

Macrophages contribute to a huge pool of tumor microenvironmental cells with a vast diversity of phenotypes and functions. Based on phenotype and functional status, macrophages were classified into M1 (classically-activated or pro-inflammatory) and M2 (alternatively-activated or anti-inflammatory) macrophages. In the context of tumor immunology, M1 macrophages were considered to exert anti-tumor immune responses and control tumor growth, whereas M2 macrophages promoted an immunosuppressive milieu and contributed to cancer progression. However, further evidence elucidated the great plasticity and wide functional capabilities of cancer macrophages and found the concept of M1/M2 macrophage polarization too simplistic in order to fully explain the macrophage's versatility of function.[124]

Tumor macrophages either may have been present in the primary tissue before cancer initiation or may be derived from the circulating monocyte pool after tumor formation. Prior to tumor initiation, macrophages emanated from embryonic/feta hematopoietic precursor cells with self-maintaining properties constitute the predominant portion of tissue-resident macrophages besides the macrophages that belonged to post-partum circulating monocyte pool and migrated to tissues. It seems that macrophages with embryonic/fetal or post-partum hematopoietic precursor origins may behave differently in TME.[124-126]

The microenvironmental factors regulate macrophage function. While IFN-γ, TNF-α, IL-12, and CD40L can stimulate macrophages to confer anti-tumor properties, IL-4, IL-13, IL-10, IL-33, TGF-β, and hypoxia induce immunosuppressive macrophages that propagate tumorigenesis.[124,127,128] Macrophage may express PD-1 on its surface, which upon interaction with microenvironmental PD-L1 leads to the anti-inflammatory phenotype of macrophage.[129]

M1-like macrophages promote anti-cancer immune responses by antigen-presentation to T cells, inflammatory cytokine production, and phagocytosis of opsonized cancer cells. M1-like macrophages express high levels of MHC class II and co-stimulatory protein B7-2 (CD86), which is required for antigen presentation. They overexpress IL-12, IL-23, and TNF-α that fuel Th1 and Th17 and activate cytotoxicity by CD8+ T cells and NK cells.[124,128,130-132]

A discussion on the immunosuppressive potentials of macrophages in cancer will be provided in the next section of this chapter.

## The interaction of immune system with other components of TME

Apart from cancerous and immune cells, various non-immune cells and extracellular matrix components constitute TME. The interaction between these elements is one of the determinants of the fate of tumorigenesis and cancer progression. Non-immune cells of TME include, but are not limited to, CAF, vascular and lymphatic endothelial cells, pericytes, adipocytes, mesenchymal stem cells, and neural cells.[133]

CAF is a non-immune cellular constituent of TME with typical elongated fibroblast morphology. They lack endothelial, epithelial, and leukocyte lineage markers and are often identified by the expression of a mesenchymal marker such as Vimentin, fibroblast activation protein (FAP), or PDGF receptor (PDGFR)α.[134] In TME, CAFs are largely derived from the expansion and reprogramming of tissue-resident fibroblasts, but they may also originate from endothelial cells, pericytes, adipocytes, smooth muscle cells, myoepithelial cells, and bone marrow-derived mesenchymal stem cells.[133,134] The main function of CAFs is the production and remodeling of ECM. CAF improves survival, proliferation, and migration of cancer cells through extracellular matrix (ECM) remodeling, contact-mediated signal transduction, and the secretion of growth factors and cytokines.[134] CAFs also drive tumor-associated angiogenesis,[135,136] and they may contribute to cancer immune escape. CAFs produce CCL2, CXCL1, CXCL2, CXCL5, and CXCL12, which recruit MDSCs and TAMs to TME. CXCL12 increases the infiltration of Tregs into TME.[137] CAFs can cross-present cancer cell-derived antigens to CTLs and induce antigen-specific T cell death and exhaustion by expressing FasL and PD-L2.[138] CAFs produce TGF-β and IL-6, which inhibit DCs' antigen-presenting functions.[137] Immunosuppressive cytokine production by CAFs fosters Treg differentiation.[139]

Endothelial cells have historically been recognized as crucial players in tumor biology. Their principal roles were considered to be supplying oxygen and nutrients and the removal of metabolic waste products. They are a doorway that lets cancer cells egress from their primary site and enter circulation.[5] They are also capable of adding to the migratory potential of cancer cells, thus contributing to cancer progression and metastasis.[140]

Besides the increased density of blood and lymphatic vessels in the tumor bed, tumor vasculature differs from normal vessels in cellular and architectural levels.[141] Tumor endothelial cells contrast with their normal counterparts by the increased incidence of chromosomal abnormalities, divergent transcriptome and methylome, enhanced and alternative expression of proangiogenic factors, better responsiveness to angiogenic stimuli from the environment, amplified proliferative capacity, larger size, and more fenestrae. The tumor vasculature shows weakened adhesion to pericytes, fewer pericytes, non-uniformed vessel wall thickness, and increased leakiness.[141-143]

Tumor endothelium regulates T cell trafficking to the tumor bed. Despite the inflammatory nature of the tumor microenvironment that is expected to activate endothelial cells to upregulate the expression of molecules involved in T cell extravasation, cancer and other microenvironmental cells may produce factors that inhibit endothelial cell activation.[144] The overexpression of Endothelin B receptor on ovarian tumor endothelium impedes T cell adhesion to tumor endothelial cell surface.[145] Further, endothelial cells may exclude T cells either by anergy induction or direct killing. Tumor endothelial cells stimulate apoptosis of CD8+ T cells in the FasL-dependent manner. Vascular endothelial growth factor (VEGF)A, IL-10, and prostaglandin (PG)E2 induce expression of FasL on tumor endothelial cells.[146] Endothelial cells may hamper T cell responses through the expression of inhibitory checkpoint molecules such as PD-L1.[143,147]

ECM is the non-cellular constituent of TME, which provides a scaffold for the settlement of the cellular components. ECM is composed of water, proteins, proteoglycans, glycoproteins, and polysaccharides. In addition to creating a physical platform and anchorage, ECM regulates associated cell functions, and its derangement during tumorigenesis is particularly instrumental.[148,149]

ECM is dynamic and it may be remodeled quantitatively or qualitatively in the cancerous microenvironment. ECM remodeling in TME may be caused by increased construction of ECM components by tumor microenvironmental cells, especially CAFs and cancer cells, post-translational modifications of ECM molecules, and ECM degradation by matrix-degrading enzymes produced by cellular components of TME.[150] ECM remodeling may alter tissue biomechanical properties and ECM-tumor microenvironmental cells interaction and significantly affect malignant behavior. Collagen cross-linking in TME provides survival and proliferation advantages for cancer cells through integrin signaling.[149] ECM remodeling is also essential for the development of a sustaining cancer stem cell (CSC) niche, regulating epithelial-to-mesenchymal transition (EMT) and angiogenesis.[149] As previously stated, ECM remodeling is a critical coordinator of cancer cell invasion. Collagen fibers may be reorganized in a linear alignment, which facilitates the invasion of cancer cell clusters.[149,151]

ECM shapes tumor immune microenvironment by affecting immune cell recruitment, extravasation, migration in TME, and their activation and differentiation states. T cell migration is greatly impaired in dense, Collagen- and Fibronectin-rich areas of tumor stroma compared to loose areas.[152] ECM degradation generates cleaved fragments of ECM components, which can recruit or regulate the activation and differentiation of immune cells. Biglycan induces macrophage inflammatory cytokine production through interaction with toll-like receptor (TLR)-2 and −4.[150] The proteoglycan Versican can be cleaved and liberate a new protein fragment called Versikine. Versikine was shown to promote CD103+ DCs, which were able to activate CD8+ T cells.[153] ECM remodeling has an important role to play in the accumulation of immune cells in the premetastatic niche. In response to primary tumor-derived factors, the glycoprotein Fibronectin becomes more abundant in premetastatic lung. Fibronectin may enhance the infiltration of bone marrow-derived hematopoietic cells to the lung through interaction with its cognate receptor, very late antigen (VLA)-4, on bone marrow-derived hematopoietic cells.[154] Monocytic-MDSCs (M-MDSCs) in metastatic lung produce Versican. Versican could support metastatic colonization through induction of mesenchymal-to-epithelial transition (MET) in metastatic cancer cells.[155]

## Evading immune destruction and immune escape mechanisms

As already reviewed, the immune system is a body defender against malignant growth. However, this armament may become defective, and cancer growth and progression may eventuate. Malignant cells themselves govern immune evasion. They may become intrinsically resistant to immune responses, gain control of the local immune microenvironment of the tumor, or systemically alter hematopoiesis. Mechanisms underlying cancer immune evasion are complex, interconnected, pleiotropic, and redundant. In this section, we will describe the principle immune evasion strategies involved in cancer progression. The following classification of immune evasion strategies is arbitrary, and some mechanisms can be put in more than one category.

To activate adaptive immunity, cancer cells must contain immunogenic antigens. Only a small fraction (nearly 10 percent) of tumor-specific point mutations in the exome of cancer cells are predicted to result in the generation of neoepitopes that can be presented by MHC class I molecules, and only a small portion of these neoepitopes is immunogenic.[27,156] Immune escape is partly related to the heterogeneity of cancer cells and the pressure exerted by the immune system. The immune system may eradicate cancer cells that express recognizable antigens, and the remaining cancer cells do not express those immunogenic antigens expressed by the ancestor cells. The tumor cells that do not express immunogenic antigens are naturally selected. Hyper methylation of neoantigen genes has been discovered as the contributor to this type of immune evasion.[157] Genetic mutation or the regulation of genes implicated in cancer cell antigen presentation such as MHC class I, TAP, Tapsin, the proteasome complex, and β2-microglobulin may lead to defective cancer cell antigen presentation. The cancer cells with abnormal MHC class I machinery are consequently poor activators of adaptive immunity.[158-162]

Another prerequisite for effective adaptive immune response is that functional APCs should be present and be recruited to tumor-draining lymph nodes. In a tumor-bearing host, DCs may lose their capability to prime T cells. Frequently in the cancer context, DCs downregulate co-stimulatory molecules such as B7-1 (CD80), B7-2 (CD86), and CD40 for T cell and B cell priming while enhancing the production of immunosuppressive molecules, including PD-L1, IL-10, and indoleamine 2, 3-dioxygenase (IDO).[27,163,164]

The primed T cells in the tumor-draining lymph nodes must be recruited to the tumor tissue. Cancer cells may downregulate the production of T cell-recruiting chemokines through DNA methylation.[165] Reactive oxygen species (ROS) and reactive nitrogen species (RNS) generation is elevated in many cancerous tissues. RNS can post-translationally regulate protein function by adding nitro-complexes to them. Nitrosylated CCL2 is incapable of recruiting T cells, but it can still recruit immunosuppressive monocytes to tumor beds.[166] As a further matter, endothelial cells may be affected by RNS and downregulate E-Selectin expression. E-Selectin is required for T cell trafficking. Impaired E-Selectin expression hampers T cell infiltration.[167]

Perforin/Granzymes and death ligand/death receptor pathways rely for the most part on cellular apoptotic pathways for cancer cell killing. Dysregulation in apoptosis machinery is a frequent finding in cancer, and aside from providing intrinsic survival advantages for cancer cells, inhibition of cancer cell apoptosis also hinders CTL and NK cell cytolysis by Perforin/Granzymes and death ligand/death receptor pathways.[168] Downregulation of components of death receptor-mediated apoptosis pathway or upregulation of inhibitors of this pathway such as cellular FLICE inhibitory protein (cFLIP) causes resistance of cancer cells to apoptosis induction by CTL and NK cells.[169]

When T cells are chronically activated, they overexpress exhaustion markers PD-1, LAG-3, T-cell immunoglobulin mucin (TIM)−3, and TIGIT. Cancer cells and other microenvironmental cells express their corresponding ligands and inhibit T cell function.[162]

The overexpression of MHC class I molecules by cancer cells may prevent the anti-cancer immune reaction of NK cells.[105] Cancer cells downregulate the expression of NKG2D ligands to escape from NK cell-mediated cytotoxicity. The regulation of

NKG2D ligands may be reduced by hypermethylation or histone-deacetylation of their genes. MicroRNA-93 and microRNA-10b regulate MICA and MICB expression.[170] ADAM family metalloproteinases cleave membrane-bound MICA from the cancer cell surface. Shed MICA binds to the NKG2D receptor and down modulate the NKG2D receptor on NK cells through receptor endocytosis and lysosomal degradation.[171-173] Similarly, ADAM10 and ADAM17 cleave the extracellular domain of B7-H6. B7-H6 sheds from the tumor cell surface, thereby preventing NK cell-mediated cytotoxicity through B7-H6-NKp30 reaction.[174] Autophagy promotes NK cell immune evasion by disrupting gap junction Connexin43 accumulation in cancer cell-NK cell immune synapse.[175] NK cells are the main eliminators of circulating cancer cells. Platelets wrap malignant cells in the circulation and protect them from immune killing by NK cells through the production of immunosuppressive cytokines and making a physical barrier against NK cell cytotoxicity.[176]

Tumor cells upregulate the surface glycoprotein CD47 that upon interaction with signal receptor protein alpha (SIRPα) on phagocytic cells, suppress the phagocytosis of cancer cells.[177,178] Cancer cell β2-microglobulin binds to leukocyte immunoglobulin-like receptor (LILR) B1 present on TAM and inhibits TAM phagocytic activity.[179]

TME is rich in extracellular adenosine triphosphate (ATP). Ectonuleotidases CD39 and CD73 hydrolyze ATP to adenosine. Many tumor microenvironmental cells, including cancer cells, Tregs, TAMs, MDSCs, CAFs, and exhausted T cells, express CD39 and CD73. Adenosine binds to adenosine receptors on T cells, NK cells, DCs, MDSCs, and macrophages. In this way, it inhibits T cell proliferation, differentiation, and anti-tumor function, impairs NK cell cytotoxicity and promotes immunosuppressive macrophage phenotype.[180]

Amino acid deprivation in TME is a metabolic strategy for suppressing anti-tumor immune responses. This may contribute to cancer progression either by the reduction in the availability of amino acids that are vital for T cell function or the production of byproducts with detrimental effects. Amino acids that have been recognized to be related to this mode of cancer immune evasion are L-arginine, Tryptophan, and Cysteine. A common mechanism that underlies the interference posed by amino acid starvation on cellular function is the global downregulation of the protein translation process through the GCN2-eIF2D pathway.[181]

T cells cannot synthesize L-arginine and are dependent on the surrounding environment arginine for their cellular functions. L-arginine depletion in TME is mediated by arginase activity, inducible nitric oxide synthase (iNOS) production, and active transport of L-arginine to the interior of immune cells.[182] Arginase hydrolyzes L-arginine to Urea and L-Ornithine. Two isoforms of arginase exist. Arginase1 locates in the cell cytosol, and arginase2 is a mitochondrial enzyme. Malignant cells, TAMs, MDSCs, and CAFs express arginase in TME.[182] L-arginine is essential for T cell's CD3ζ chain expression. In the absence of L-arginine, T cell anergy or apoptosis may occur.[183] L-Ornithine, which is the byproduct of arginase activity, can be converted to polyamines such as Putrescine by Ornithine decarboxylase. Polyamines reinforce cancer cell proliferation.[184]

IDO in TME is expressed by TAMs as well as MDSCs, DCs, and cancer cells. It depletes Tryptophan in TME, which is essential for T cell function. IDO inhibits CD8+ T cells, CD4+ T cells, and NK cells proliferation and function and enhances the differentiation and immunosuppressive functions of Tregs. The anti-proliferative capacity is mediated by the depletion of Tryptophan together with the production of Tryptophan catabolism byproducts such L-Kynurenine and Picolinic acid.[185-187] L-Kynurenine induces T cells to exhibit exhausted phenotype and upregulate PD-1 expression.[188] NK cells decrease NKG2D expression following the exposure to L-Kynurenine.[172,189] Furthermore, L-Kynurenine is a potent stimulus for T cell and NK cell apoptosis.[190,191]

TME is characterized by the accumulation of immune cell populations that specialize in actively suppressing immune responses. In the following paragraphs, we will review the immunosuppressive functions of Tregs, regulatory B cells (Bregs), TAMs, and MDSCs in relation to cancer immunology.

Tregs are the main contributors to maintaining peripheral self-tolerance and curbing inflammatory reactions to prevent pathologic overresponse. FOXP3 is a crucial transcription factor for Treg development. They are immunosuppressive cells that interfere with anti-tumor immune responses.[192,193] Tregs in TME can originate from circulating regulatory Tregs or be differentiated from naïve T cells in TME under the influence of microenvironmental factors such as TGF-β.[194]

Tregs produce TGF-β, IL-10, and IL-35 that inhibit T cell proliferation and function. Tregs express high-affinity IL-2 receptors that deprive IL-2 availability for naïve T cells. IL-2 is crucial for naïve T cell proliferation and the acquisition of anti-tumor functions.[193]

Unlike other TCRαβ-T cells that express CTLA-4 after antigen activation, Tregs constitutively express CTLA-4. Tregs inhibit the priming function of DCs by CTLA-4 by interfering with the B7-1/B7-2-CD28 pathway.[195]

Tregs express CD39 and CD73 that generate adenosine. Adenosine's contribution to immunosuppression has been already discussed. Adenosine also acts in an autocrine manner and further enhances the immunosuppressive abilities of Tregs.[196,197]

Tregs strongly adhere to DCs. This attachment seems to be dependent on lymphocyte function-associated antigen (LFA)−1 and intercellular adhesion molecule (ICAM)−1 presence on Tregs and DCs, respectively. The Treg-DC adherence interferes with T cell activation by DCs.[198]

Bregs are B lymphocytes with immunosuppressive functions. Bregs secrete IL-10, TGF-β, and IL-35 and express PD-L1 and through them inhibit T cell proliferation, skew Th cell polarization toward Th2 and promote Tregs. IL-10 produced by Bregs inhibits NK cell anti-tumor function.[100,199]

M2-like macrophages overexpress IL-10, TGF-β, IL-1 receptor antagonist, arginase1, and PGE2. Macrophages with M2-like features promote Th2 and Treg responses, suppress CTL, and inhibit APCs' functions.[124,127,128] TAMs express PD-L1, which inhibits T cell responses through interaction with PD-1.[200] ROS enhances the expression of PD-L1 by TAMs, thus increasing their immunosuppressive potential.[201]

MDSCs are immature cells of hematopoietic origin that have immunosuppressive potential. They are raised in a variety of pathological conditions such as cancer.[202] Chronic inflammatory conditions associated with malignancy alter physiological differentiation of polymorphonuclear and myeloid cell lineages. The generated cells have a relatively immature phenotype and are rather suppressors of innate and adaptive immunity than be capable of exerting anti-tumor immune responses. Cancer cells and the associated stromal cells produce exosomes and cytokines such as granulocyte colony-stimulating factor (G-CSF), macrophage colony-stimulating factor (M-CSF), GM-CSF, and VEGF, which trigger the accumulation of immature granulocytic and myelomonocytic cells in the body through STAT3, STAT5, retinoic acid receptor-related orphan receptor C (RORC)1, C/EBPB, Notch, and NF-κB pathways. The accumulated immature cells then acquire immunosuppressive functions in response to IL-1β, IL-6, IL-4, IL-13, TNF-α, and PGE2 through STAT3, STAT1, STAT6, and NF-κB pathways.[203-206]

MDSCs are categorized into two main subsets based on morphological and phenotypic resemblance to their normal counterparts: polymorphonuclear (PMN)-MDSC and M-MDSC with phenotypic characteristics similar to polymorphonuclear cells and monocytes, respectively.[202] Proper characterization of MDSCs requires both demonstration of morphological and phenotypic features and confirmation of immunosuppressive function.[207] Murine PMN-MDSC and M-MDSC are phenotypically identified by CD11b+Ly6G+Ly6C low and CD11b+Ly6G-Ly6C high combination of markers, respectively. Human PMN-MDSC and M-MDSC are identified as CD11b+CD14-CD15+ and CD11b+CD14+CD15-HLA-DR-/low cells, respectively.[203,207] Lectin-type oxidized LDL receptor (LOX)1 is a particularly specific marker for PMN-MDSC to discriminate from neutrophils.[208] Downregulation of HLA-DR distinguishes M-MDSC from monocytes.[202]

MDSCs deploy a variety of mechanisms to suppress innate and adaptive anti-cancer immune responses. They impair CTL survival, activation, cytotoxicity, and trafficking. MDSCs deplete amino acids required for T cell proliferation and function by expressing arginase1, internalizing L-arginine by cationic amino acid transporter 2B, iNOS and IDO expression, and sequestering Cysteine.[181,209] MDSCs express NADPH oxidase (NOX)2, which reduces oxygen and generates superoxide. Superoxide reacts with nitric oxide (NO), and peroxynitrite is the result of the reaction. Concertedly, NO is produced by the activity of iNOS in M-MDSC.[209,210] Peroxynitrite impedes TCR replenishment in CTL and simultaneously down-modulates the MHC class I repertoire of tumor cells. Therefore, Peroxynitrite significantly impairs cancer antigen presentation.[211] PMN-MDSCs inhibit antigen cross-presentation by DCs and, in consequence, hinder antigen presentation.[212] iNOS catabolizes L-arginine and generates NO. NO inhibits T cell function as well as antigen presentation by DCs through altering many intracellular signaling molecules.[181,213,214] MDSCs downregulate endothelial cell E-selectin expression, a process which is at least partly dependents on NO.[215] MDSCs express plasma membrane-bound ADAM17, which shed L-selectin from the T cell surface, thereby compromising T cell recruitment to tumor-draining lymph nodes.[216] Some MDSCs express PD-L1, which upon interaction with PD-1 on T cells impairs their function.[181] MDSCs also induce cancer cells and B cells to upregulate PD-L1 expression. MDSCs produce TGF-β, which renders CD8+ T cells express PD-1.[217] MDSCs can induce CD4+ T cells to confer Tregs' phenotype by secretion of IL-10 and TGF-β.[181,218] The interaction of CD40 on MDSCs and CD40L on T cells is required for MDSC-induced Treg expansion.[219] MDSCs fuel the accumulation and immunosuppressive functions of TAMs. In TME, M-MDSCs may directly convert to TAMs.[202,209,211]

## Immune regulation of cancer progression and metastasis

Metastasis is defined as the outgrowth of neoplastic cells in tissues that are not in direct contiguity to the primary tumor. Metastasis is a dreadful upshot in cancer progression and poses a serious pathophysiologic crisis in the host. A multi-step cascade is theorized for the cancer metastasis process. Cancer cells must detach from the surrounding cells, and ECM components in the primary site then migrate to the primary tissue site to give entrance to blood and lymphatic vessels, disseminate to distant sites via circulation, extravasate, establish dormant clones in the metastatic site and finally make metastatic outgrowths.[217,220]

The metastasis formation process is in the tight regulation of genetic and epigenetic properties of malignant cells and the interaction with host microenvironmental elements that are adjusted by the germline genetic composition of the host, epigenetic imprints, environmental exposures, and microbiota.[217,220-229] The immune system is involved in determining the fate of the metastatic process. The immune system can either prevent or control metastasis or contribute to fostering it. The immune system may promote metastasis by providing an immunosuppressed environment, augmenting cancer cell proliferation and survival, inducing EMT or MET, CSC formation, enhancing angiogenesis and lymphangiogenesis, ECM remodeling, and increasing local invasion.[217,230,231]

The primary tumor may influence the distant site characteristics before the arrival of disseminated cells to prepare an environment capable of maintaining metastasized cells, a process called "premetastatic niche formation".[232-235] A prominent feature of the premetastatic niche is the accumulation of immunosuppressive cell populations. The primary tumor may produce cytokines and exosomes that mobilize hematopoietic cells to accumulate in premetastatic and metastatic sites. Moreover, in response to factors released by the primary tumor, distant organs may change so that they will become receptive to immune cell recruitment.[236,237] The myeloid-lineage cells in the premetastatic niche create a permissive environment for upcoming cancer cells by suppressing effector immune cells in the premetastatic niche, upregulating E-selectin expression on premetastatic tissue endothelium to arrest cancer cells in target organ vasculature, promoting aberrant vessel permeability to facilitate cancer cell extravasation, and the secretion of factors for chemoattraction of cancer cells.[217,230]

CTLs and NK cells that are the main immune system players in the elimination of malignant cells in the primary tumor are also present in metastatic sites and eradicate cancer cells. Immune suppression may enhance cancer metastasis. Accumulation of Tregs, Bregs, TAMs, and MDSCs occurs both in primary and metastatic tumor sites and provides an immunosuppressive microenvironment. In metastatic sites, these immunosuppressive cell populations inhibit anti-cancer immune responses and let cancer cells survive in metastatic sites.[230,238]

EMT is an elaborate phenomenon characterized by the loss of epithelial cell features and gaining mesenchymal traits. EMT accompanies the attainment of many properties that are required for carcinoma cell invasiveness and metastasis.[176] TGF-β has an established role in EMT induction in TME. Treg and Breg cells produce TGF-β, which mediates EMT.[100,239] TGF-β, TNF-α, IL-8, and IL-6 are the main culprits of TAM-induced EMT.[240] MDSCs may prompt EMT by upregulating the β-Catenin/TCF-4 pathway in cancer cells. The induction of EMT was dependent on nitric oxide synthase (NOS) activity in MDSCs.[241,242] Additionally, MDSCs produce IL-28, which activates the STAT3 signaling pathway in cancer cells and promotes EMT.[243]

A minority of transformed cells in a tumor are known to possess characteristics of a stem cell, including asymmetric replication and self-renewal capacity. These cells are called CSCs, and their presence in the primary tumor and metastatic sites are speculated to be essential for enabling repopulating and heterogeneity of a tumor.[244] CSCs may result from neoplastic transformation of tissue-resident stem cells or the reprogramming of cells without stemness features to obtain those traits.[244] TAMs activate the EGFR/STAT3/SOX2 pathway in breast cancer cells, which contributes to CSC formation.[245] TAMs promote the generation of lymphoma and glioblastoma CSCs by producing Pleiotrophin (PTN), which upregulates the β-Catenin pathway upon binding to its receptor on cancer cells.[246,247] MDSC-mediated upregulation of microRNA-101 decreases C-terminal-binding protein (CtBP)2 in ovarian cancer cells and results in CSC formation.[248] MDSCs produce IL-6 and NO, which induce the formation of breast CSCs through STAT3 and Notch signaling pathways in cancer cells.[249]

Immune cells may potentiate the migration of cancer cells. Cancer cell ability to invade the surrounding tissue is essential for reaching tumor vasculature and intravasation. Immune cells contribute to ECM remodeling and propagate cancer cell invasiveness. TAMs, MDSCs, and mast cells produce matrix metalloproteinases (MMPs) that their inhibition ameliorates the migratory potential of cancer cells.[217,250,251] TAM-derived Cathepsin proteases are involved in ECM remodeling and promotion of cancer cell invasiveness.[252] TAMs produce epidermal growth factor (EGF), which increases proliferation and invasion of multiple carcinoma cell lines. Intriguingly, cancer cells secret colony-stimulating factor (CSF)1, which stimulates TAMs to approach cancer cells and produce EGF.[253-257] TAMs release microRNA-223-containing microvesicles, which enhance breast cancer cell invasiveness through β-Catenin activation.[258]

Angiogenesis and lymphangiogenesis are indispensable for cancer growth and dissemination. Blood vessel network provides essential oxygen, and nutrient elements for cancer cell survival in primary tumor and metastatic sites, and the affluence and structural aberrancy of tumor blood and lymphatic vasculature provide an escape gate for cancer cell dissemination.[259] Immune cells can contribute to tumor angiogenesis and lymphangiogenesis through the production of inducers of angiogenesis, stimulating cancer cells to produce proangiogenic factors, ECM degradation, and direct conversion to endothelial cells. TAMs produce angiogenesis-promoting cytokines such as VEGFA, Semaphorin 4D, and Adrenomedullin.[260-262] MDSCs secrete proangiogenic molecules VEGFA, fibroblast growth factor (FGF)2, and Bv8.[217] TAM-derived IL-1β and TGF-β induce cancer cells to produce VEGFA, FGF2, and IL-8, which increase tumor neovasculogenesis.[260] A pool of VEGF is retained within ECM and MMPs cleave ECM-bound VEGFA to release a bioavailable form of VEGFA.[263] TAMs and MDSCs produce MMP2 and MMP9 in TME of several tumor types and enhance angiogenesis in this manner.[217,260] Myeloid cells have been found to be contributing to tumor angiogenesis by directly converting to endothelial-like cells.[264]

## Immunolopathology and immunotherapy of hematologic malignancies

Perhaps hematological malignancies are the best-known targets for cancer immunotherapies. In 1997, the Food and Drug Administration (FDA) announced rituximab as the first approved monoclonal antibody (mAb) for the treatment of B cell non-Hodgkin lymphoma (NHL)[265] and later, in 2009 for chronic lymphocytic leukemia (CLL), discussed later. Since then, incredible discoveries about the different aspects of immune cell functions and tumoral escape mechanisms have led to the innovation of novel agents with different approaches to enforcing the immune system to defeat cancer cells. Of these, immune checkpoint inhibitors (ICIs), chimeric antigen receptor T-cells (CART-cells), bispecific T cell engagers (BiTEs), and to a lesser extent, vaccines have shown promising results. As the molecular mechanisms of action of these therapies are discussed earlier, clinical aspects of such interventions will be reviewed here.

### Immunopathology

#### *Lymphoma*

Lymphomas are subdivided into NHL and Hodgkin lymphoma (HL), with 10 percent of all lymphoma cases present with HL.[266] HL further has two pathologic subtypes[1]:

classic HL and[2] nodular lymphocyte predominant (NLPHL), the latter is present in less than 10 percent of HL patients.[267] The NHL has numerous subtypes, according to the morphologic and pathologic features.[267]

Pathologic findings of HL include the distribution of sparse malignant cells in a dense but suppressed background of a wide variety of immune cells. These characteristic neoplastic cells are known as Reed-Sternberg cells (RS cells). These cells have a CD15+, CD30+, and CD45- immunophenotype.[267] Copy number gain of chromosome 9p24.1 is another feature usually seen in RS cells, which is imperative from the immunological point of view (discussed later). The underlying etiologies of HL are not fully understood. However, there is evidence that infection with *EBV*, immunosuppressive states (*Human immunodeficiency virus* (*HIV*) infection, transplantation), and autoimmunity might increase the incidence of HL. Despite its highly malignant nature, most cases of HL respond well to conventional chemotherapeutic regimens.[266] However, a fraction of cases has a refractory disease (i.e., do not respond to the therapy), and some with an early response will be afflicted by the disease again (defined as relapse). Treatment options for such groups are limited to high-dose salvage chemotherapy, radiation therapy, targeted therapy (including brentuximab vedotin), autologous hematopoietic stem cell transplantation (HSCT), and immunotherapies, which will be discussed in this part.

NHLs are derived from either B cells, T cells, NK cells, or their precursors. Based on the morphologic, genetic, and clinical features, NHLs are subdivided into a huge number of entities.[267] However, about 65 percent of NHL cases are either diffuse large B cell lymphoma (DLBCL) or follicular lymphoma.[268] Risk factors underpinning the development of NHL are generally similar to HL, as *EBV*, *HCV*, and helicobacter pylori infections, autoimmune disorders, and immunosuppression are identified as the possible culprits.[269] Genetic alterations also play a role in both the initial development and further evolution of the NHL. Some chromosomal translocations are quite characteristic for certain subtypes of NHL. For example, t(11;14)(q13;q32) and t(14;18)(q32;q21) translocation in the mantle cell lymphoma, and t(8;14)(q24;q32) translocation in Burkitt lymphoma frequently occur, leading to the overexpression of *cyclin D1*, *MYC*, and *B-cell lymphoma protein* (*BCL*)−*2*, respectively.[270] Double-hit lymphomas are those harboring mutations related to *MYC* and either *BCL2* or *BCL6*. The prognosis and the response to therapy are substantially decreased in such lymphomas.[271] Of note, like classic HL, amplification of 9p24.1 is also identified in primary mediastinal large B cell lymphoma (PMBCL).[272] The addition of rituximab to the traditional CHOP regimen (cyclophosphamide, doxorubicin, vincristine, and prednisone) improves the scope of patients with DLBCL.[273] However, depending on the stage and risk factors, between 20 percent to 50 percent of them will have refractory disease or relapse after demonstrating a response.[274] Follicular lymphoma has an indolent course in the early stages, with a watch and wait strategy accepted as an effective approach for such cases. However, it is estimated that up to 40 percent of follicular lymphoma cases finally transform into a more aggressive NHL (usually DLBCL).[275] The management of relapsed or refractory (R/R) DLBCL and follicular lymphoma is generally consisting of salvage chemotherapy, followed by autologous HSCT. Some studies have shown the benefit of the administration of ibrutinib for both and idelalisib (a phosphoinositide 3-kinase inhibitor) and venetoclax (BCL-2 inhibitor) for follicular lymphoma.[270] Immunotherapies come into action when the aforementioned interventions fail, too.

### Leukemia

Acute and chronic myeloid leukemia (AML and CML, respectively) are the result of the increased proliferation of multipotent hematopoietic stem cells. Single progenitor B cell or T cell multiplications will manifest as either acute lymphocytic leukemia (ALL) or CLL.[267] Each of the mentioned disorders has specific subtypes, etiologic factors, and target populations, which are not discussed here. Blast cells of AML stem from one of these two populations: granulocyte-monocyte progenitors (CD34+CD38+CD45RA+CD110+) or myeloid progenitors (CD34+CD45RA+CD38–CD90–).[276] Two of them, CD13 and CD33, are present in most subtypes of AML. Common genetic alterations of AML include t(8;21)(q22;q22), t(9;11)(p22;q23), t(9;22)(q34;q22), t(15;17)(q31;q22), t(16;16)(p13.1;q22), Inv(16)(p13.1;q22), Inv(3)(q21q26.2), del(7) and del(5).[267] Regarding ALL, genetic abnormalities are quite specific and complex for each subtype,[277] but immunophenotype is similar to those of B and T cell lineage (CD19+CD22+cytoplasmic CD79+; and cytoplasmic CD3+CD10+, respectively).[278] Compared with lymphomas, the therapeutic approaches for AML and ALL are more consistent. However, despite the early response in the majority, relapse will occur in 50 percent of AML[279] and 80 percent of adults with ALL.[280] Regarding immunotherapies, patients with R/R AML and ALL have been studied for the effectiveness of such agents, which will be reviewed in detail throughout this part.

CLL is mainly originated from inhibited apoptosis of mature B cells that results in their accumulation in lymphoid organs.[267] This disease is largely limited to the elderly and is probably the most common type of leukemias in developed countries.[266] Patients usually have genetic aberrations exhibited as del(13q14), trisomy 12, del(11q22.3), del(17p13.1), and del(6q21), in order of frequency.[281] Since the *TP53* gene is located on chromosome 17, its mutation along with del(17) are considered poor prognostic factors.[281] Neoplastic B cells usually express CD5, CD23, CD27, CD43, and CD200, and lower levels of CD19, CD20, and CD79b compared with normal B cells.[282] Elevated levels of CD23, CD38, and CD49d are associated with poor prognosis.[283] The initiation of treatment for CLL patients usually is confined to those with symptomatic disease (according to IWCLL-2008 guidelines).[284] Chlorambucil and cyclophosphamide are the traditional agents being used for the treatment of CLL and have had acceptable outcomes. In recent years, the introduction of anti CD20 antibodies (rituximab), Bruton tyrosine kinase, and phosphatidylinositol 3 kinase inhibitors (ibrutinib and idelalisib, respectively), and BCL-2 antagonist venetoclax has elongated the survival of high risk and relapsed patients.[282]

### Multiple myeloma (MM)

MM is another lymphoid malignancy with neoplastic cells that are originated from the post-germinal center plasma cells located in the bone marrow.[267] Almost all cases of MM are evolved from an asymptomatic disorder named MGUS that progresses to MM with a rate of 1 percent each year.[285] Early genetic derangements usually include translocations and number gains (trisomy) of the immunoglobulin heavy chain locus (IGH). More complex cytogenetic abnormalities occur during the progression, with some implicated as prognostic factors, with t(4;14), t(14;16), t(14;20), del(17p), gain 1q and *TP53* mutations as indicators of a dismal prognosis.[285] Malignant plasma cells have a CD38+, CD44+, CD138+, CD319 (SLAMF7)+, CD19-, and CD45- immunophenotype.[286] The presence of CD19 and high levels of CD138 are indicators of poor prognosis. B cell maturation antigen (BCMA) is a transmembrane glycoprotein that belongs to the TNF receptor superfamily member 17 (TNFRSF17) and is expressed on both normal and neoplastic plasma cells.[287] B cell maturation antigen, along with B cell-activating factor (BAFF), a proliferation-inducing ligand (APRIL), and IL-6 enhance proliferation and survival of plasma cells.[287] Immunosuppression is one of the most striking clinical and pathologic hallmarks of MM. It seems that a complex network of immunosuppressive cells (MDSCs and Tregs) and cytokines (IL-10 and TGF-β) are conducive. In recent years, with the development of novel drugs, the treatment of patients with MM has improved drastically. Such agents include immunomodulators (IMiDS, such as thalidomide, lenalidomide, and pomalidomide), proteasome inhibitors (bortezomib, ixazomib, and carfilzomib), anti-SLAMF7 (elotuzumab), and anti-CD38 (daratumumab and isatuximab) antibodies. Nevertheless, relapse is still the final destiny of almost all patients with MM.[285] Options for the treatment of R/R disease are limited. However, novel immunotherapeutic approaches (particularly against BCMA) have shown robust results for such patients, as discussed later.

## Immunotherapies

### Immune checkpoint inhibitors (ICIs)

ICIs are among the most guarded candidates for the treatment of hematological malignancies. Nivolumab, a mAb against PD-1, is one of the most studied ICIs. A phase I study of nivolumab for previously treated patients with R/R classic HL showed quite promising results. 87 percent of patients had an objective response rate (ORR), 86 percent had progression-free survival (PFS) at 24 weeks, and the incidence of grade three or more adverse events (AEs) was 21 percent.[288] The extended follow-up of these patients showed that seven had a durable response for more than 1.5 years.[289] In a phase II trial (CheckMate 205) of 243 R/R classic HL patients with failure of autologous HSCT, 69 percent achieved overall response after a median of 2.1 months, and 37 percent experienced grade 3 and 4 AEs, with no related deaths.[290] The median duration of response (DOR) was 16.6 months.[290] Another phase II study recruited 80 R/R classic HL patients after failure of autologous HSCT and brentuximab vedotin (BV) administration. Of these, 66.3 percent achieved an overall response after a median of 2.1 months after the initiation of therapy. Patients received a median of 16 doses of nivolumab, and the median DOR was 7.8 months. Of 53 patients with overall response, 11 had progressive disease. One patient suffered from multi-organ failure during the therapy (a grade 5 AE).[291] A recent phase I/II trial of nivolumab for pediatric and young adult patients with different types of cancers has shown that among 10 patients with classic HL, one achieved CR, two showed partial remission (PR), and five showed stable disease, after a median of 4.5 courses of therapy.[292] One patient with mediastinal large B cell lymphoma (MLBL) exhibited a PR, but no overall response was observed in other NHL cases, along with all solid tumors. Grade three and more AEs were reported in 27 of 75 available patients for the evaluation of toxicity.[292] In another cohort of 99 patients with R/R classic HL, nivolumab led to ORR and median PFS of 68 percent and 19.4 months, respectively. After 21 months, 48.5 percent of patients have been still alive. However, this study has used a new index for reporting the outcomes (lymphoma response to immunomodulatory therapy criteria).[293] Of note, 18 percent of patients had grade three, four, and five (bacterial pneumonia) AEs.[293]

As it is obvious, most clinical trials of nivolumab are carried out on patients with classic HL. This is mostly because those early preclinical studies showed that the RS cells usually express relatively high amounts of PD-L due to amplification of chromosome 9p24.1, which contains the genes encoding the PD-L, *PDL1* and *PDL2* (also known as *CD274* and *PDCD1LG2*, respectively), and *JAK2* that can further induce the expression of PD-L.[272,288] Younes and colleagues showed a significant difference in 9p24.1 alterations between patients with complete remission (CR) and progressive disease,[291] and in another trial, all 10 available tumor samples showed amplification, copy gain, or polysomy of the chromosome 9p.[288] Furthermore, this amplification can also be seen in malignant cells of PMBCL, another amenable target for PD-1 blockade therapy.[272]

Nivolumab has also been investigated for patients with other types of hematological neoplasms. For patients with R/RDLBCL, ORR has been only 10 percent and 3 percent for autologous HSCT-failed and autologous HSCT-naïve patients, respectively, which is quite disappointing.[294] Fortunately, among 30 patients with R/R PMBCL who had been included in a phase II study of the combination of nivolumab and BV (CheckMate 436), 73 percent achieved an ORR after a median of 1.3 months.[295] The safety profile of this combination therapy was also acceptable, with 53 percent of patients experiencing grade three and more treatment-related AEs.[295] There are also two phase 2 trials for the combination therapy of nivolumab and conventional chemotherapies[296,297] for patients with AML, which have shown relatively auspicious outcomes (Table 4.3). There are also studies

**Table 4.3** Selected clinical studies for the usage of immune checkpoint inhibitors (ICIs) for patients with hematological malignancies.

| References | Study decide/ phase | Agent (s) | Patients | Type of neoplasm | Previous treat-ment (S) | Dosage | Objective response rate (ORR) (percent percent) | Progression-free survival (PFS) | Overall survival (OS) | Grade 3 or more adverse events (AEs) (percent percent) | Response assessment tool |
|---|---|---|---|---|---|---|---|---|---|---|---|
| Ansell et al. 2015[288] | I | Nivolumab | 23 | R/R classic HL, 22 NS 1 MC | 18 BV 18 autologous HSCT 19 radiotherapy | 3 mg/kg, weeks 1 and 4, then every 2 weeks until disease pro-gression or CR for a maximum of 2 years | 17 percent CR 70 percent PR | 86 percent at 24 weeks | | 21 percent | Revised response criteria for malignant lymphoma |
| Armand et al. 2018[290] | II | Nivolumab | 243 | R/R classic HL | 243 AHSCT 63 BV naïve 80 BV received after autologous HSCT 100 BV received before and/or after autologous HSCT | 3 mg/kg every 2 weeks until disease pro-gression/ unaccept-able toxicity | 16 percent CR 53 percent PR | Median of 14.7 months | 92 percent at 1 year | 37 percent | IRRC |
| Younes et al. 2016[291] | II | Nivolumab | 81 | | autologous HSCT and BV | 3 mg/kg every 2 weeks until progression, unaccept-able toxicity, and death | 8.8 percent CR 57.5 percent PR | 76.9 percent at 6 months Median of 10 months | 98.7 percent at 6 months | 41 percent | IRRC |

| References | Study decide/ phase | Agent (s) | Patients | Type of neoplasm | Previous treatment (S) | Dosage | Objective response rate (ORR) (percent percent) | Progression-free survival (PFS) | Overall survival (OS) | Grade 3 or more adverse events (AEs) (percent percent) | Response assessment tool |
|---|---|---|---|---|---|---|---|---|---|---|---|
| Davis et al. 2020[292] | I-II | Nivolumab | 85 (aged between 1 and 30) | 22 neuroblastomas<br>13 osteosarcomas<br>12 rhabdomyosarcomas<br>12 classic HL (6 NS)<br>10 NHL<br>16 others | 71 chemotherapy<br>46 radiotherapy | 3 mg/kg on days 1 and 15 of a 28-day cycle | 1 CR and 2 PR among classic HL patients | NR | NR | 36 percent | RECIST |
| Lepik et al. 2019[293] | Cohort | Nivolumab | 99 | Classic HL | 65 radiotherapy<br>40 autologous HSCT<br>49 BV<br>39 Chemotherapy only | 3 mg/kg every 2 weeks until unacceptable toxicity or disease progression | 31 percent CR<br>33 percent PR | 48.5 percent at 21 months<br>Median of 19 months | Not reached | 18 percent | LYRIC |
| Ansell et al. 2019[294] | II | Nivolumab | 121 | DLBCL | Cohort 1: 87 autologous HSCT<br>Cohort 2: 34 without autologous HSCT | Nivolumab 3 mg/kg every 2 weeks until disease progression, unacceptable toxicity, or withdrawal | Cohort 1: 10 percent<br>Cohort 2: 3 percent | Cohort 1: median of 1.9 months<br>Cohort 2: median of 1.4 months | Cohort 1: median of 12.2 months<br>Cohort 2: median of 5.8 months | 24 percent | IRC |

(Continued)

**Table 4.3** Cont'd

| References | Study decide/ phase | Agent (s) | Patients | Type of neoplasm | Previous treatment (S) | Dosage | Objective response rate (ORR) (percent percent) | Progression-free survival (PFS) | Overall survival (OS) | Grade 3 or more adverse events (AEs) (percent percent) | Response assessment tool |
|---|---|---|---|---|---|---|---|---|---|---|---|
| Zinzani et al.[295] | II | Nivolumab and BV | 30 | PMBCL | NR | Nivolumab 240 mg every 3 weeks until disease progression or unacceptable toxicity | 37 percent CR<br>37 percent PR | NR | NR | 53 percent | LYRIC |
| Ravandi et al. 2019[296] | II | Nivolumab + idarubicin + cytarabine | 44 | 42 Newly diagnosed AML, 2 High-risk MDS | 6 Hypomethylating agents for MDS | Nivolumab 3 mg/kg on day 24 (range 22–26) and every 2 weeks for up to a year in responders | 78 percent CR | | Median of 18.54 months | 13.6 percent | Revised International Working Group criteria for acute myeloid leukemia |
| Dacer et al. 2019[297] | II | Nivolumab + azacitidine | 70 | R/R AML | 45 Hypomethylating agents | 3 mg/kg on Day 1 and 14, every 4 to 6 weeks | 22 percent CR<br>1 percent PR | NR | Median of 6.3 months | 11 percent | Revised International Working Group criteria for acute myeloid leukemia |

| References | Study decide/ phase | Agent (s) | Patients | Type of neoplasm | Previous treatment (S) | Dosage | Objective response rate (ORR) (percent percent) | Progression-free survival (PFS) | Overall survival (OS) | Grade 3 or more adverse events (AEs) (percent percent) | Response assessment tool |
|---|---|---|---|---|---|---|---|---|---|---|---|
| Armand et al. 2019[299] | Ib-II | Pembrolizumab | 21 in KEYNOTE -13<br>53 in KEYNOTE -170 | R/R PMBCL | Multiple different therapies | 10 mg/kg every 2 weeks or 200 mg every 3 weeks | KEYNOTE-13: 33 percent CR, 14 percent PR<br>KEYNOTE-170: 13 percent CR, 32 percent PR | Median of 10.4 months in KEYNOTE-13 and 5.5 months in KEYNOTE-170 | Median of 31.4 months in KEYNOTE-13 and not reached in KEYNOTE-170 | 24 percent in KEYNOTE-13 and 23 percent in kEY-NOTE-170 | International working group cheson 2007 |
| Armand et al. 2016[300] | II | Pembrolizumab | 31 | R/R classic HL | BV and other different agents | 10 mg/kg every 2 weeks | 16 percent CR<br>48 percent PR | 46 percent at 52 weeks | 100 percent at 24 weeks | 16 percent | International harmonization project on lymphoma |
| Chen et al. 2019[301] | II | Pembrolizumab | 210 | R/R classic HL | Cohort 1: after autologous HSCT/BV<br>Cohort 2: after BV<br>Cohort 3: no BV after autologous HSCT | 200 mg every 3 weeks | Cohort 1: 26 percent CR, 51 percent PR<br>Cohort 2: 26 percent CR, 41 percent PR<br>Cohort 3: 28 percent CR, 44 percent PR | Cohort 1: median of 16.4 months<br>Cohort 2: median of 11.1 months<br>Cohort 3: median of 19.4 months | Not reported separately | 12 percent | International harmonization project on Lymphoma |

ORR, objective response rate; PFS, progression-free survival; OS, overall survival; AE, adverse effect; R/R, relapsed or refractory; HL, Hodgkin lymphoma; NS, nodular sclerosing; MC, mixed cellularity; BV, brentuximab vedotin; HSCT, hematopoietic stem cell transplantation; CR, complete remission; PR, partial remission; IRRC, independent radiologic review committee; NR, not reported; NHL, non-Hodgkin lymphoma; RECIST, Response Evaluation criteria in solid tumors; LYRIC, lymphoma response to immunomodulatory therapy criteria; DLBCL; diffuse large B cell lymphoma; IRC, International working group response criteria for malignant lymphoma; PMBCL, Primary mediastinal large B cell lymphoma; AML, acute myeloid leukemia; MDS, myelodysplastic syndrome.

about combination strategies of nivolumab and other immunotherapies, which will be discussed later. To date, the FDA has approved nivolumab for the treatment of R/R classic HL patients who have received autologous HSCT and BV, or more than 2 lines of systemic therapies (including autologous HSCT).[298]

Pembrolizumab is another anti-PD-1 antibody and like nivolumab, has been studied mainly for R/R classic HL and PMBCL. Among 21 enrolled patients in KEYNOTE-13 and 53 patients in KEYNOTE-170 trials who had R/RPMBCL, 48 percent and 45 percent showed an OR, respectively, with only 17 patients experiencing treatment-related grade three and more AEs.[299] Administration of pembrolizumab for patients with R/R classic HL has shown robust results and acceptable safety profile, similar to those of nivolumab[300,301] (Table 4.3).

As discussed earlier, MM induces generalized immunosuppression along with an increased expression of PD-1. Therefore, some trials aimed to investigate the effectiveness of pembrolizumab in combination with other conventional agents for patients with R/R or treatment-naïve MM.[302-304] However, all of them culminated in unfavorable outcomes, which made the FDA put an alert regarding the stoppage of these trials.[305] Of note, the long-term results of these trials are not published yet.

Atezolizumab and durvalumab are anti-PD-L1 antibodies and, until now, have been studied in young patients with different types of malignancies[306] and in combination with ibrutinib for R/R follicular lymphoma or DLBL,[307] respectively, with no encouraging outcomes. Ipilimumab, another ICI against CTLA-4, is also used for patients with hematological malignancies in relatively small trials with overall modest results[291,308,309] (not shown in Table 4.3).

### Chimeric antigen receptor T-cell therapies

CART-cells are mostly studied for patients with ALL and NHL and have shown remarkable results, but at the expense of severe toxicities, difficult manufacturing due to lymphopenia and highly personalized technique, extensive financial costs, and somehow unpredictable in vivo expansion rates of manipulated T cells. Patients who are candidates for CART-cell therapy routinely receive lymphodepleting regimens before receiving the therapy and generally have complications of severe cytokine release syndrome (CRS) and neurotoxicity. Neurologic side effects are generally mild and manageable and include delirium, confusion, lethargy, tremor, seizure, encephalopathy, and rarely cerebral edema.[310] The American Society for Blood and Marrow Transplantation has defined CRS as an immunologic event with the presence of fever and hypotension, hypoxia, and multi-organ failure.[310]

In 2011, 19–28z+ second-generation CART-cells infused for 8 patients with relapsed CLL following lymphodepletion with cyclophosphamide in 5 cases.[311] One case died after the therapy, probably due to underlying infections. 3 subjects achieved stable disease lasting between two to six months.[311] This study also reported that the longer persistence of CART-cells was associated with cyclophosphamide lymphodepletion and lower tumoral burden.[311] Later in 2013, 19–28z+ CART-cells were infused for 5 patients with relapsed B cell ALL following lymphodepletion with cyclophosphamide.[312] All patients showed negative minimal residual disease (MRD) after therapy, examined by deep sequencing polymerase chain reaction (PCR). 4 cases then undergo allogeneic HSCT, and the ineligible patient had a relapse 90 days after the infusion of CART-cell, probably because of the administered corticosteroid for CRS.[312] It was also shown that there is an association between the level of inflammatory cytokines and the bulk of the neoplasm at the time of CART-cell therapy.[312] Maude and colleagues administered CTL019 (now known as tisagenlecleucel) for 25 pediatric and 5 adult patients with R/R ALL.[313] 27 of them demonstrated CR, and among them, 22 had negative MRD (assessed using multiparametric flow cytometry). After a median follow-up of seven months (range, one to 24 months), 19 cases were still in CR.[313] Regarding side effects, 8 patients showed severe CRS, requiring the administration of tocilizumab. Patients with a higher tumor burden had a greater probability of having severe CRS. Neurologic toxicities were all self-limited.[313] All patients had prolonged B cell aplasia and, therefore, had to receive immunoglobulin replacements.[313] A phase 2 trial of tisagenlecleucel for young patients (age < 21) with R/R B cell ALL showed an overall remission rate of 81 percent, with negative MRD (determined by flow cytometry) in all of such cases.[314] After one year, the response was still present in 59 percent of cases. Tisagenlecleucel could be detected in responsive cases between 20 and 617 days after the administration (median, 168 days), regardless of dosage or response status. As of previous studies, the safety profile of the therapy has not been encouraging, as all patients had B cell aplasia, 77 percent developed CRS (including 47 percent that required intensive care unit admission), and 40 percent showed neurologic abnormalities. 37 percent of patients with CRS received tocilizumab. Only 9 percent of cases undergo allogeneic HSCT after CART-cell therapy.[314]

Long-term follow-up of 53 B cell ALL patients treated with 19–28z+ CART-cells showed that among 44 cases who went into CR, 25 relapsed later, including all 9 cases who had positive MRD.[315] Of the responsive group, 17 underwent transplantation. Interestingly, there was no association between CR and the dosage or lymphodepleting regiment (i.e., cyclophosphamide alone or cyclophosphamide and fludarabine). Treatment-related toxicities were similar to that of other studies. Also, the authors found a relation between the higher disease burden and increased probability of CRS and neurotoxicity.[315] Somehow surprisingly, this study found no correlation between the persistence of CART-cells and survival.[315]

Another area of interest for CART-cell therapy has been NHL. As an example of this, among 101 adult patients with R/R NHL who were enrolled in the ZUMA-1 trial and received axicabtagene ciloleucel, 82 percent showed an OR after a median of 15.4 months, with a median duration of 8.1 months.[316] Long-term analysis of 108 patients with a minimum of one-year follow-up revealed an ORR of 82 percent, with

42 percent still in the response at the time of data cutoff. Outcomes were similar for patients with DLBCL and PMBCL/transformed follicular lymphoma (TFL).[316] Despite the reports of preliminary studies,[317] this trial did not find any relation between the CD4+ to CD8+ ratio of CART-cells and the response rate (RR). Another report of these patients showed that after a median of 27.1 months, 83 percent of patients still have had an overall response, with CR in 58 percent, which is quite paramount.[318]

JULIET was a phase II study for evaluating the effectiveness of tisagenlecleucel for adult patients with R/R NHL.[319] Among 93 patients, 52 percent achieved a response, which was persistent in 65 percent of them after 12 months. Like the ZUMA-1 study, there was no association between the level of CD19 expression and the RR.[319] These findings were consistent with the results of a previous study of tisagenlecleucel for 28 cases with DLBCL and follicular lymphoma[320] (not shown in Table 4.4). Table 4.5 represents the FDA-approved immunotherapies for the treatment of hematologic malignancies.

The outcome of CART-cell therapy in patients with MM is also guarded. Beginning in 2018, CART-cells against BCMA (named as CAR-BCMA, LCAR-B38M, and bb2121) have been administered for patients with R/R MM in phase I studies, with ORRs of 81 percent, 88 percent, and 85 percent.[321-323] It seems that the neurologic side effects are less common for anti-BCMACART-cells (Table 4.4). Despite robust early responses, the relatively high relapse rates, even in the short-term follow-ups, are disappointing. Nevertheless, now there are more than 30 phase II and III active trials aiming to evaluate the efficacy and safety of CART-cells (mostly against BCMA) for patients with MM.

### *Bispecific T cell engagers*

Until now, Blinatumomab is the only FDA-approved BiTE, which is being administered for the B cell ALL patients who have R/R disease or have achieved first or second CR but with MRD ≥0.1 percent.[326] Early studies for the evaluation of blinatumomab in patients with hematological malignancies began before 2010, and their observations were consistent with profound toxicities and almost no overall response. As a result, administration protocols changed, and acceptable overall responses were observed in patients with B cell NHLs, in addition to B cell ALL.[326] The safety profile of blinatumomab is favorable, with CRS and neurologic toxicities generally present in less than 10 percent of cases.[326] In 2017, the TOWER trial enrolled heavily pretreated Philadelphia negative B cell ALL patients to either receive conventional chemotherapies (109 cases) or blinatumomab (267 cases). The median overall survival (OS) was significantly higher in the blinatumomab group (7.7 compared to 4 months), with a similar rate of adverse effects in both groups.[327] AMG 330 (binds to CD3 and CD33) and AMG 420 (binds to CD3 and BCMA) are BiTEs that have been studied in patients with R/R AML[328] and R/R MM,[329] respectively, and have shown modest results after early analyses. Now ongoing trials are investigating different features of therapies with BiTEs (specific for CD3 and either CD16, CD20, CD33, or BCMA) for different types of hematologic malignancies.

**Table 4.4** Selected clinical studies for chimeric antigen receptor T-cells (CAR T-cells) therapy in patients with hematological malignancies.

| Study | Design/ phase | Agent | No of treated Patients | Previous treatment(s) | Dosage | Median follow-up | Response rate | The relapse rate in CAR responses | Overall survival (OS) | Toxicity(s) |
|---|---|---|---|---|---|---|---|---|---|---|
| Maude et al. 2014[313] | I-II | CTL019 | 30 R/R ALL | 18 allogeneic HSCT<br>3 Blinatumomab | $0.76 \times 10^6$ to $20.6 \times 106$ CTL019 cells/kg | 7 months | 90 percent CR | 26 percent of those with CR | 78 percent at 6 months | 100 percent CRS, severe in 27 percent<br>100 percent B cell aplasia<br>43 percent neurologic toxicities |
| Maude et al. 2018[314] | II | Tisagenlecleucel | 75 R/R B cell ALL | 46 allogeneic HSCT<br>All received 1 to 8 therapies | $0.2 \times 10^6$ to $5.4 \times 10^6$ cells/kg | 13.1 months | 60 percent CR<br>21 percent CR with incomplete hematological recovery | 20 percent at 6 months<br>41 percent at 12 months | 90 percent at 6 months<br>76 percent at 12 months | 100 percent B cell aplasia<br>77 percent CRS<br>40 percent neurologic toxicities |
| Park et al. 2018[315] | I | 19–28z$^+$ | 53 R/R B cell ALL | 19 allogeneic HSCT<br>13 Blinatumomab<br>All received at least 2 treatments | $1 \times 10^7$, $3 \times 10^7$, or $1 \times 10^8$ 19–28z$^+$ T cells/kg | 29 months | 83 percent CR | 56.8 percent | Median of 12.9 months | 85 percent CRS, severe in 26 percent<br>44 percent neurologic toxicities |

*(Continued)*

**Table 4.4** Cont'd

| Study | Design/ phase | Agent | No of treated Patients | Previous treatment(s) | Dosage | Median follow-up | Response rate | The relapse rate in CAR responses | Overall survival (OS) | Toxicity(s) |
|---|---|---|---|---|---|---|---|---|---|---|
| Neelapu et al. 2017[316] | II | Axicabtagene ciloleucel | 77 DLBCL<br>16 TFL<br>8 PMBCL | 21 autologous HSCT | $2 \times 10^6$ cells/kg | 15.4 months | 82 percent OR, including 54 percent with CR | NR | 52 percent at 18 months | 93 percent CRS<br>64 percent neurologic toxicities |
| Schuster et al. 2019[319] | IIa | Tisagenlecleucel | 93 DLBCL or TFL | 93 rituximab<br>93 an anthracycline<br>41 autologous HSCT | $0.1 \times 10^8$ to $6 \times 10^8$ | 14 months | 40 percent CR<br>12 percent PR | NR | Median of 12 months | 58 percent CRS<br>21 percent neurologic toxicities |
| Brudno et al. 2018[321] | I | CAR-BCMA | 16 R/R MM | Multiple agents | $9 \times 10^6$ anti-BCMA CAR T-cells/kg | NR | 81 percent ORR | 54 percent | NR | 100 percent CRS |
| Zhao et al. 2018[323] | I | LCAR-B38M | 57 R/R MM | 39 bortezomib<br>39 thalidomide<br>25 lenalidomide<br>10 autologous HSCT | 0.07 to $2.1 \times 10^6$ anti BCMA CAR T-cells | 8 months | 68 percent CR<br>5 percent very good PR<br>14 percent PR | 20 percent | Not reached | 90 percent CRS<br>2 percent neurologic toxicity |

| Study | Design/ phase | Agent | No of treated Patients | Previous treatment(s) | Dosage | Median follow-up | Response rate | The relapse rate in CAR responses | Overall survival (OS) | Toxicity(s) |
|---|---|---|---|---|---|---|---|---|---|---|
| Raje et al. 2019[322] | I | bb2121 | 33 R/R MM | 33 bortezomib<br>33 lenalidomide<br>32 autologous HSCT<br>31 pomalidomide<br>30 carfilzomib<br>27 daratumumab | 5 to $45 \times 10^7$ anti BCMA CAR T-cells | 11.3 months | 45 percent CR | 43 percent | NR | 76 percent CRS<br>42 percent neurologic toxicity |

CAR, chimeric antigen receptor; OS, overall survival; R/R, relapsed or refractory; ALL, acute lymphocytic leukemia; HSCT, hematopoietic stem cell transplantation; CR, complete remission; CRS, cytokine release syndrome; DLBCL, diffuse large B cell lymphoma; TFL, transformed follicular lymphoma; PMBCL, primary mediastinal B cell lymphoma; NR, not reported; PR, partial remission; MM, multiple myeloma; BCMA, B cell maturation antigen; ORR, overall response rate.

**Table 4.5** List of the FDA-approved immune checkpoint inhibitors (ICIs) and CAR T-cells for hematologic malignancies.

| Agent | Indications | Trial identifier |
|---|---|---|
| Nivolumab | Classic HL in adult patients that have relapsed or progressed after autologous HSCT and brentuximab vedotin, or<br>3 or more lines of systemic therapy that includes autologous HSCT. | CheckMate 205[290] and CheckMate 039 |
| Pembrolizumab | R/R (after 3 or more prior lines of therapy) classic HL in adults and pediatrics | KEYNOTE-087[324] |
| Pembrolizumab | R/R (after 2 or more prior lines of therapy) PMBCL in adults and pediatrics | KEYNOTE-170[299] |
| Axicabtagene ciloleucel | R/R large B cell lymphoma after 2 or more lines of systemic therapy in adult patients (including DLBCL not otherwise specified, PMBCL, high-grade B cell lymphoma, and DLBCL arising from follicular lymphoma) | Different trials |
| Tisagenlecleucel | Patientsup to 25 years of age with B cell precursor ALL that is refractory or in second or later relapse.<br>Adult patients with R/R large B cell lymphoma after two or more lines of systemic therapy (including DLBCL not otherwise specified, high-grade B cell lymphoma, and DLBCL arising from follicular lymphoma) | ELIANA (NCT02228096)<br>JULIET[325] |

HL, Hodgkin lymphoma; HSCT, hematopoietic stem-cell transplantation; R/R, relapsed or refractory; DLBCL, diffuse large B cell lymphoma; PMBCL, primary mediastinal large B cell lymphoma; ALL, acute lymphocytic leukemia.

### *Cancer vaccines*

Attempts to develop vaccines for the treatment of hematological malignancies have long been studied for the management of hematological and other neoplasms. However, except for certain limited cancers (e.g., melanoma, as discussed later), vaccines have not had prominent activities and have not received administration approvals. Among hematological malignancies, follicular lymphoma and AML have been interesting targets for cancer vaccines. MyVax was an idiotype vaccine that exhibited promising activities in phase I and II trials of follicular lymphoma cases.[330] However, in a randomized phase III trial, the addition of MyVax to control immunotherapy (keyhole limpet hemocyanin [KLH] and GM-CSF) did not enhance the PFS and the interval to subsequent therapies.[331] Likewise, other similar vaccines have not achieved any success in follicular lymphoma.[332]

Regarding leukemia, administration of a peptide-based vaccine (PR1) for HLA-A2-positive patients with AML ($n$ = 42), CML ($n$ = 13), and myelodysplastic syndrome (MDS) ($n$ = 11) resulted in a promising immune RR (defined as at least a two-fold increase in PR1-specific CTLs) and ORR of 53 percent and 24 percent, respectively.[333] In another attempt, Wilms' tumor 1 mRNA expressing DCs could induce molecular remission in 30 percent of pretreated AML patients with a very high probability of relapse.[334] Besides, after a median follow-up of 109 months, 55 percent of responses were sustained.[334]

## Antibodies against clusters of differentiation

mAbs against CDs are well-accepted immunotherapies and constitute the mainstay of treatments for some malignancies. Rituximab, an anti-CD20 mAb, is indicated for patients with B cell NHL and CLL.[335] Obinutuzumab is another anti-CD20 mAb that was designed to overcome the resistance to rituximab and now is approved for the treatment of follicular lymphoma and CLL as a combination therapy with chemotherapeutic agents.[335] Other approved anti-CD20 mAbs include ofatumumab (combined with chemotherapy for CLL),[336] ibritumomab tiuxetan (a radiotherapeutic agent linked to rituximab, as second-line therapy for NHLs),[337] and Iodine I 131 tositumomab (another radiotherapeutic agent for rituximab-refractory NHL).[338]

Inotuzumab ozogamicin is an antibody-drug conjugate against CD22, which has been used for R/R B cell ALL.[339] Brentuximab vedotin is an anti-CD30 antibody drug-conjugate that is indicated for treatment-naïve stage III or IV classic HL (as combination therapy with chemotherapy), following failure or high probability of the relapse of classic HL after autologous HSCT and other rare hematological malignancies.[340] Another antibody-drug conjugate is gemtuzumab ozogamicin, which is directed against CD33 and is approved for the treatment of newly-diagnosed (only for adults) and R/R CD33-positive AML.[341] Two mAbs against CD38, daratumumab[342-344] and isatuximab,[345] have shown acceptable clinical activities against MM and recently have received the FDA approval as the fourth-line monotherapy (daratumumab)[346] or combined with other agents as first-line (daratumumab for autologous HSCT ineligible subjects)[346] or later (daratumumab and isatuximab)[346,347] therapies.

## Future perspective

Almost all the cutting-edge immunotherapies have been studied for hematological malignancies. Despite the astonishing outcome, the duration of response and the fraction of responding patients are not striking yet. In addition, severe toxicities and difficulties in manufacturing (mostly for CART-cells) are substantial issues that should be resolved by prospective trials. Although the old approach, mAbs against surface molecules, is being extensively studied[348] for hematological and other malignancies and has yielded significant outcomes in recent years (in case of MM). What is apparent is that cellular and checkpoint immunotherapies will shape the future of the therapeutic armamentarium for hematological malignancies.

## Immunolopathology and immunotherapy of central nervous system tumors

Central nervous system (CNS) malignancies have an incidence of about 30 and 5.9 per 100 000 adults and pediatric (less than 19 years) population, respectively.[349] Although nervous system tumors are estimated to comprise less than 1.4 percent of all newly diagnosed cancers in the United States, disproportionately cause 3 percent of cancer-related deaths.[266] In adults, less than one-third of CNS tumors are malignant. However, this is two-thirds for pediatrics, whom which about 20 percent of their cancers are originated from CNS.[349] CNS tumors have unique pathologic and clinical features as no premalignant lesions have been identified for them yet, their surrounding microenvironment is highly immunosuppressed, despite local invasion (even in low-grade tumors) virtually never metastasize, and their management is highly dependent on the anatomic site of the tumor. The presence of the blood-brain barrier (BBB) further complicates the delivery of chemotherapeutic agents. The 2016 revised World Health Organization (WHO) classification of CNS tumors has combined molecular (e.g., *IDH* and *H3K27M* mutations, 1p/19q codeletion, etc.) and pathologic features and, therefore, has fundamentally evolved and involuted in some parts.[350] For example, due to genetic similarities between diffuse astrocytomas and oligodendrogliomas, the term diffuse glioma is now being used instead of both.[350]

Gliomas are the most common primary malignant neoplasms of the CNS.[349] It is presumed that gliomas arise from the neuroectodermal glial cells that provide structural and metabolic support for neurons and construct BBB. Traditionally, gliomas were disaggregated to astrocytoma, oligodendroglioma, and ependymoma according to their morphologic features. However, in the 2016 CNS WHO classification, this has been replaced with terms low-grade glioma, high-grade glioma, and ependymoma, with different subtypes in each category.[350]

### Immunopathology

Gliomas evade the immune system harnessing different paths. Malignant glioma cells and their surrounding Tregs and MDSCs can produce IDO[351] and arginase1,[352] catalytic enzymes for tryptophan and arginine, respectively. Tryptophan depletion will enhance the recruitment of Tregs and hinder normal T cell functions. Interestingly, the level of IDO expression has a direct relation to the grade of the tumor.[351,353] Similarly, arginine deficiency will result in impaired T cell function and proliferation.[352] Roles for NO and

ROS are also implicated in inducing the immunosuppressive state in gliomas.[352] TGF-β and IL-10 are well-known anti-inflammatory cytokines that are produced by MDSCs in considerable amounts.[354] TGF-β is conducive to the carcinogenesis of gliomas not only by suppression of DCs and T cells but also via enhanced angiogenesis and local invasion.[354]

It had long been shown that despite the absence of a structured lymphatic system, the brain extracellular fluid could be drained via the arachnoid sheaths of the olfactory nerve to the nasal submucosa.[355] In recent years, the discovery of the glymphatic system has made a paradigm shift in our understanding of CNS physiology, as it facilitates the connection of CNS immune cells and antigens to the peripheral lymphatic system.[356]

One of the most prominent features of gliomas is the scarcity of immune cells within their microenvironment.[357] Tumor-infiltrating lymphocytes (TILs) are almost absent, and only Tregs and tumor-associated myeloid cells (TAMCs, including MDSCs, microglia, and TAMs) can be found.[354] This theoretically serves as a solid barrier against immunotherapies. Besides, the very low number of the recruited T cells exhibits an extremely exhausted phenotype. This is largely due to the high expression of PD-1, TIM-3, and LAG-3.[358] Glioma cells and TAMCs can express PD-L1 on their surface.[354] However, blockade of PD-L1 might not result in the regression of the tumor, as the PD-L1 expression on tumor-adjacent brain tissues can surprisingly induce the death of glioma cells.[359]

CNS tumors exhibit different genetic alterations. More prominent examples are *IDH* mutations in grade 2 and 3 astrocytoma and oligodendroglioma, 1p/19q codeletion in oligodendroglioma, H3K27M mutation in diffuse midline glioma, $O^6$-methylguanine-DNA methyltransferase (MGMT) promoter methylation in IDH-wildtype glioblastoma and oligodendrogliomas, and *epidermal growth factor receptor variant III* (*EGFRvIII*) mutation in glioblastoma.[360] More importantly, CNS tumors have a low mutational burden, and there is a median of 1.5 mutations per megabase.[357] Regarding the therapy with ICIs, it is postulated that more robust outcomes generally will be seen in tumors that have more than 10 mutations per megabase.[361] The putative reason behind this observation is that lower mutations will result in lower tumor neoantigens and, therefore, immune cells cannot recognize and invade cancer cells. The recognition of TMB as a predictor of the response to ICIs seems applicable in the context of CNS tumors (discussed later). However, this must be interpreted together with other factors (e.g., intra-tumoral heterogeneity of antigens).

The management of CNS tumors is generally based on surgical resection, if feasible, followed by chemotherapy and radiation therapy for high-grade tumors. The addition of temozolomide (an alkylating agent) to the radiation therapy for glioblastoma added 2.5 months and 8 percent to the median OS and five-year OS, resulting in values of 14.6 months and 10 percent, respectively.[362,363] Until now, no immunotherapeutic approach is approved for the management of CNS tumors. Nevertheless, some trials have described modest outcomes, which bolsters the ongoing attempts. As mentioned earlier, more than 66 percent of adult primary brain tumors are benign and usually are manageable with surgery. Hence most efforts in unriddling immunologic aspects are dedicated to glioblastomas. As a result, the following discussion will primarily focus on glioblastoma and some malignant pediatric neoplasms. Metastatic brain cancers are discussed separately, based on their tumor of origin.

## Immunotherapies

### *Immune checkpoint inhibitors (ICIs)*

According to the 2016 CNS WHO classification, the term diffuse gliomas refers to diffuse astrocytoma and oligodendrogliomas (WHO grade II), anaplastic astrocytoma and oligodendrogliomas (WHO grade III), glioblastoma (GBM), and diffuse midline glioma (WHO grade IV).[350] Five-year survival rates of diffuse astrocytoma, anaplastic oligodendroglioma, and anaplastic astrocytoma are 50 percent, 57 percent, and 30 percent, respectively, while it is only 5.5 percent for glioblastoma.[364] Almost all high-grade gliomas will eventually recur, and until now, there is no widely accepted and effective therapeutic approach for them.[364]

Among multiple different immunotherapies, ICIs are studied most for the treatment of glioblastomas. Until now, no promising result is reported after the ICI therapy for glioblastomas. Compared with anti-VEGF agent bevacizumab, nivolumab showed no prior benefit in enhancing the OS of patients with recurrent GBM.[365] The median OS was 9.8 months for nivolumab and 10 months for bevacizumab, and the one-year OS rate was 42 percent for both arms. Conversely, the median PFS of the nivolumab arm was two months less than that of bevacizumab (1.5 months versus 3.5 months). Similarly, ORRs were 8 percent and 32 percent for nivolumab and bevacizumab arms, respectively. In fact, the only priority of nivolumab was its longer duration of response (median of 11.1 months versus 5.3 months).[365] In summary, this cohort 2 of the CheckMate 143 trial could not meet its primary endpoint (OS).[365] In addition, in the CheckMate 143 trial (of 40 patients with grade IV GBM or gliosarcoma), no difference was found between the outcome of nivolumab with or without ipilimumab therapy and conventional regimens.[366] Similar discouraging results are seen for atezolizumab (one PR among 16 patients and a median OS of 4.2 months).[367]

Regarding the neoadjuvant setting, a trial[368] aimed to explore the added benefit of neoadjuvant pembrolizumab compared to only adjuvant therapy. Among 35 patients with recurrent surgically resectable glioblastoma, neoadjuvant therapy significantly enhanced OS and PFS (13.7 months versus 7.5 months; hazard ratio (HR), 0.39; 95 percent confidence interval (CI), 0.17 – 0.94; $p$ = 0.04, and 3.3 months versus 2.4 months; HR, 0.43; 95 percent CI, 0.20–0.90; $p$ = 0.03) over adjuvant-only group. Intriguingly, overexpression of T cell-related and IFN-γ and under-expression of cell cycle genes, focal increase in tumoral CTL densities, and enhanced PD-L1 expression were observed in the neoadjuvant arm.[368] Similar findings to the above are also reported after neoadjuvant therapy with nivolumab.[369]

Despite these findings, ongoing trials are still evaluating the efficacy of ICIs combined with chemotherapies (mostly temozolomide) or radiation therapy (NCT02667587 and NCT02617589). Interestingly, there are studies aiming to describe the outcome of anti-LAG-3 (NCT02658981) or anti-TIM-3 (NCT03961971) therapies with or without nivolumab.

### *Cancer vaccines*

Unlike many other cancers, oncolytic viruses have shown modest efficacy in the field of glioblastoma. PVSRIPO is a recombinant nonpathogenic polio-rhinovirus chimera (poliovirus Sabin type 1). The internal ribosome entry site of polio is replaced by human rhinovirus type 2 to prevent its neuropathogenic effects.[370] Based on the observation of high expression amounts of CD155 (poliovirus receptor) on neoplastic cells and its direct cytotoxic activity and stimulation of APCs and subsequently T cells, PVSRIPO was elicited as novel immunotherapy against gliomas.[370] A phase I study enrolled 61 patients with single supratentorial recurrent grade IV glioma to administrate intra-tumoral PVSRIPO.[370] Compared with a historical control cohort, PVSRIPO added 1.3 months to the median OS of patients (11.3 months versus 12.5 months). Interestingly, despite the descriptions of historical control, the OS rate of PVSRIPO did not decline and remained stable (21 percent) after 24 and 36 months, regardless of *IDH1 (R132)* mutation status.[370] Besides, the vaccine had a manageable safety profile[370] and, owing to its considerable activities, is now under investigation in a phase II trial (NCT01491893). G207 is an oncolytic vaccine based on modified herpes simplex virus (HSV)−1.[371] G207 direct delivery to tumoral margins in combination with radiotherapy could induce stable disease in of 9 patients with recurrent GBM, without any serious AEs.[371] Another oncolytic vaccine, DNX-2401 (tasadenoturev, *Adenovirus*-based vaccine), has been able to exert some anti-tumoral activities against recurrent malignant gliomas.[372] Another sound approach for cancer immunotherapies is neoantigen vaccines. In a phase Ib trial, the administration of the neoantigen-targeting vaccine for patients with newly diagnosed MGMT-unmethylated glioblastoma has been able to increase the density of TILs and primer peripheral CD8+ and CD4+ T cells against the neoantigens.[373]

The mentioned outcomes of cancer vaccines seem very encouraging. However, they should be interpreted with great caution, as all of them are stemmed from phase I trials. Lastly, despite early favorable results, larger studies of peptide vaccines against EGFRvIII (PEPvIII and rindopepimut),[374,375] Wilms tumor 1 (WT1),[376] IDH1-R132H,[377] and a DC-based vaccine for six antigens (ICT-107)[378] have not shown significant clinical benefits.

### *Other immunotherapies*

CART-cells therapies are another approach studied for the treatment of gliomas. In 2017, a small study administered EGFRvIII specific CART-cells for patients with recurrent GBM.[379] Despite the documented infiltration of CART-cells in the tumoral tissue and acceptable safety profile, the authors found that compared with pretreatment samples, there was a more extreme immunosuppressive environment (including recruitment of Tregs and overexpression of IDO, PD-L1, and IL-10) after the infusion of CART-cells. In addition, heterogeneity in the expression of EGFRvIII, its decreased expression after therapy, and possible antigen escape mechanism were other challenges facing this therapy.[379] CART-cells specific for human epidermal growth factor receptor (HER)2 (in 17 cases),[380] and IL-13Rα2 positive GBM (in three cases)[381] have shown modest results.

Preclinical studies of CART-cells specific for HER2 and PRAME have shown considerable activity against pediatric medulloblastoma cell lines.[382,383] Until now, there is only one phase I trial for the usage of HER2-specific CART-cells in pediatric patients with recurrent or refractory CNS tumors (NCT03500991). At last, it also should be noted that targeting TGF-β (using galunisertib, a TGF-β receptor 1 kinase inhibitor) has not gained success in defeating recurrent glioblastoma.[384]

## Future perspective

Despite astonishing outcomes after the therapy with novel immunotherapies in a variety of malignancies (e.g., melanoma, non-small cell lung cancer (NSCLC), AML, NHL, and renal cancer), none of them have concurred the grim course of GBM. The main reasons for this formidable behavior of GBM are discussed earlier. Besides, there are ongoing efforts to elucidate specific challenges encountering each modality. For instance, treatment with temozolomide and radiation can lead to the suppression of PD-L1 expression, which in turn might make the subsequent ICI therapy futile.[385] For the reduction of vasogenic edema, corticosteroids are administered in almost all cases of brain tumors early after the diagnosis. This can hamper the response to cancer vaccines.[386] The direction of novel immunotherapies for brain tumors is now shifted toward more personalized methods. Examples are personalized multiple neoantigen vaccines,[386,387] engineered T cells with specific receptors for tumor-associated antigens (TAAs) (TCR instead of the CAR),[357] and targeting multiple immune checkpoints simultaneously, as discussed earlier. It is now clear that future attempts should focus on the resolution of the extensive immunosuppressive state seen in high-grade brain tumors.

# Immunolopathology and immunotherapy of head and neck cancers

Head and neck cancers are referred to as malignancies that originate from the mucosa lining the upper aerodigestive tract, including the oral cavity (lips, gingiva, tongue, buccal surface, the floor of the mouth, retromolar triangle, and hard palate), pharynx (nasopharynx, oropharynx, and hypopharynx), larynx (supraglottic, glottic, and subglottic larynx), nasal cavity and the paranasal sinuses, and major and minor salivary glands.[388] More than 90 percent of head and neck cancers are squamous cell carcinoma (SCC).[389] It was estimated that in 2019, more than 3.7 percent of newly diagnosed cancers in the United States might be head and neck related (including laryngeal cancer).[266] The global incidence of head and neck cancers is about 4.9 percent.[390] However, in southeast Asia, it can be the most common malignancy[391] due to exclusive risk factors (discussed later). Unlike most other neoplasms, several strong risk factors have been identified for the development of head and neck squamous cell carcinoma (HNSCC). Cigarette smoking and alcohol consumption are the strongest risk factors. They can increase the probability of developing head and neck cancer by three and two times, respectively.[392,393] Furthermore, the synergy between alcohol and cigarette will increase the chance of up to 35 times.[394] *HPV*, especially subtypes 16 and 18, has a significant role in the development of oropharyngeal SCC, especially in young non-smoker individuals, with somehow exclusive molecular signatures compared with those of other etiologies (discussed later).[395] *EBV* has an established role in the pathogenesis of nasopharyngeal carcinoma.[396] Betel nut chewing is somehow common in the Southeast Asia regions and is ascribed as the etiology of high incidence rates of HNSCC in such regions.[397] Other contributing risk factors include radiation exposure, marijuana usage, immunosuppressive state, Plummer-Vinson syndrome, Bloom's syndrome, Fanconi anemia, and dyskeratosis congenita.[389]

## Immunopathology

HNSCCs exhibit a severe immunosuppressive TMEPD-L1 is detected in more than 50 percent of HNSCC samples, and some studies have reported significantly higher expression levels in *HPV+* cases compared with negative ones.[398] It is reported that the higher expression of TIM-3 is associated with lymph node metastasis and a higher TME population of MDSCs.[399] Another study has found that the expression of LAG-3 on TILs is higher in malignant samples and is associated with advanced-stage disease.[400] On the other hand, another article has reported that PD-1, TIM-3, LAG-3, and TIGIT expression is significantly higher in *HPV+* cases and implicate a better prognosis.[401] Overexpression of epidermal growth factor receptor (EGFR) is seen in almost all head and neck cancer cells and has shown to be imperative for the establishment of the neoplasm, as it is involved in cell proliferation, survival, angiogenesis, and invasion.[388] Higher expression of EGFR is also associated with poor prognosis.[388] Aberrations in amounts of suppressive cytokines and immune cells are also common in HNSCC. The accumulation and suppressive potential of Tregs inside the tumor are higher than that of the circulating Tregs.[402] Besides, the authors have concluded that CTLA-4, TGF-β1, and CD39 are the key elements of Treg suppressive activities, and their inhibition might enhance the anti-tumor effects of the immune system.[402] However, it should be mentioned that the preclinical models have shown early in the course of malignant transformation, TGF-β might paradoxically act as an anti-neoplastic cytokine, as the deletion of *Tgfbr1* and *Pten* genes are conducive to the carcinogenesis.[403] Compared with normal controls, HNSCC patients show higher levels of IL-10, a potent anti-inflammatory cytokine.[404] In addition, an increased amount of IL-6, a pro-inflammatory cytokine, is a predictor of recurrence[405] and is associated with enhanced expression of PD-L1 and recruitment of MDSCs.[406] Another feature of these neoplastic cells is the reduced MHC-dependent presentation of their antigens. As discussed earlier, this is a major immune-escape mechanism and largely is caused by derangements in *HLA-A* and *HLA-B* genes[407] and different constitutes of antigen processing machinery (APM) due to increased signaling of STAT1.[408]

In 2015, The Cancer Genome Atlas (TCGA) project tried to identify frequent genetic aberrations in 279 HNSCC cases based on *HPV* status.[409] It turned out that all samples harbored frequent amplifications of *TP63*, *SOX2*, and *PIK3CA* genes, all located on the 3q26/28 region. Such genes are mostly involved in the differentiation and survival of epithelial cells. *HPV*+ samples showed recurrent deletions and mutations of *TRAF3* and amplification of *E2F1*. *TRAF3* encoded protein is a part of CD40, which is known for its integral role in response to viral infections (e.g., *HPV*, *HIV*, and *EBV*), inhibition of NF-κB activation, and production of interferons. E2F1 is a transcription factor that regulates cell cycle apoptosis mainly via binding to RB1.[409]

Samples with the negative status of *HPV* were distinguished with deletion of *CDKN2A*, *SMAD4*, and *NOTCH1*, amplification of *FADD*, and inactivating mutations of *TP53*, *CASP8*, and *FAT1*. The first three genes are well-recognized tumor suppressors. FADD encoded protein is an activator of the caspase-8, a key modulator of apoptosis. It is well characterized that *HPV* E6 and E7 proteins interfere with the functions of p53 and Rb proteins.[410] However, *TP53* mutation is one of the most common genetic signatures of HNSCC in heavy-smoker cases but is relatively rare in *HPV*+ patients.[409] *FAT1* is involved in the Wnt/β-catenin signaling pathway.[409] Interestingly, the authors observed no difference between the mutation rates of *HPV*+ and *HPV*- cases.[409] Finally, the mean mutational burden of HNSCCs is five mutations per megabase, which is around the average.[361]

## Immunotherapies

Around 30 percent to 40 percent of patients with HNSCC are diagnosed while their disease is confined to stage I or II. The mainstay of treatment for such groups is surgery alone or definitive radiotherapy alone, and their five-year OS is between 70 percent to 90 percent after such therapies.[388] Advances in robotic surgery and laser microsurgery in recent years have culminated in better performance and quality of life and limited morbidity for such patients. The remaining have the advanced-stage disease (stage III and IV). The approach to the treatment of these groups is complex and tailored to the anatomical site, pathological characteristics, and performance status.[411] Nevertheless, more than 65 percent of HNSCC cases will have recurrent disease, metastasis, or both.[388] The median OS for such cases is less than 10 months after the administration of the more accepted regimens based on cetuximab, platinum, and fluorouracil.[412]

### *Immune checkpoint inhibitors (ICIs)*

ICIs have shown unprecedented outcomes for certain subpopulations of subjects with HNSCC. In 2016, the Phase IKEYNOTE-012 trial enrolled pretreated patients with recurrent or metastatic (R/M) HNSCC who were at least 1 percent positive for PD-L1 immunohistochemistry (IHC) staining for the administration of pembrolizumab.[413] The overall RR was 18 percent, which endured for 12.2 months. The median PFS and median OS were reported as 2 and 13 months, respectively.[413]

A phase III randomized trial (KEYNOTE-040) evaluated the long-term efficacy of pembrolizumab compared with the investigator's choice of drugs (IC, consisting of methotrexate, docetaxel, or cetuximab) for patients with R/M HNSCC.[414] After a median follow-up of 7.5 and 7.1 months in the treatment groups, the median OS was 8.4 and 6.9 months for pembrolizumab and IC groups, respectively (HR for death: 0.8; 95 percent CI: 0.65 - 0.98), which was acceptable, although less robust than previous trials.[413,415] The safety profile was also more favorable for pembrolizumab.[414]

Another phase III randomized trial (KEYNOTE-048) aimed to investigate the efficacy of three different regimens for treatment-naïve R/M HNSCC patients: pembrolizumab alone, pembrolizumab with chemotherapy, and cetuximab with chemotherapy (the regimen of EXTREME trial).[416] After a median follow-up duration of at least 10.7 months, pembrolizumab monotherapy did not significantly improve OS in the total population. However, it was superior to cetuximab with chemotherapy in patients with PD-L1 combined positive score (CPS) of 20 and more (median of 14.9 versus 10.7 months; HR, 0.61; 95 percent CI, 0.45–0.83), and in those with CPS of 1 and more (12.3 versus 10.3 months; HR, 0.78; 95 percent CI, 0.64–0.96). Pembrolizumab with chemotherapy was superior to cetuximab with chemotherapy in improving OS, regardless of CPS.[416] However, PFS was not prolonged in those who received the pembrolizumab-based regimen. Based on these findings, the authors have proposed pembrolizumab combined with platinum and 5-fluorouracil as a suitable upfront treatment for R/M HNSCC and pembrolizumab monotherapy as the first-line therapy for R/M HNSCCs with PD-L1 positivity in IHC.[416]

CheckMate 141 was a phase III trial of patients with recurrent HNSCC who were randomized to receive nivolumab or investigator's choice single agent (methotrexate, docetaxel, or cetuximab).[417] Compared with the investigator group, patients who received nivolumab had a significantly greater OS (7.5 versus 5.1 months) and RR (13.3 versus 5.8 percent). Interestingly, the rate of severe AEs was lower in the nivolumab group (13.1 versus 35.1 percent)(417). The encouraging outcomes of nivolumab therapy have been continuing even after a minimum follow-up of 24 months (OS rate of 16.9 vs 6 percent), regardless of PD-L1 expression.[418] Based on the findings of the CeckMate-141 trial, the FDA approved nivolumab for patients with R/M HNSCC who have disease progression on or after platinum-based therapy.[419] FDA approval of pembrolizumab was first for patients with R/M HNSCC who had disease progression on or after a platinum-based therapy, which was due to reports of the KEYNOTE-012 trial. However, in 2019 and after the publication of results of the KEYNOTE-048 trial, pembrolizumab combined with platinum and fluorouracil was also announced as upfront therapy for patients with metastatic or with unresectable, recurrent HNSCC, and as a single agent for the first-line treatment of patients with metastatic or with unresectable, recurrent HNSCC who have a CPS of one or higher.[420] One caveat is that the laboratory kit used in the KEYNOTE-048 trial for the measurement of PD-L1 expression is not approved by the FDA.[420]

It should be mentioned that other ICIs are being investigated in patients with HNSCC. For example, in 2018, the administration of durvalumab for high expressing PD-L1 (defined as more than 25 percent) R/M HNSCC patients who were enrolled in a phase II trial resulted in a median OS and PFS of 7.1 and 2.1 months, respectively, with 18 of 111 cases had an overall response.[421] CONDOR was a phase II randomized trial of durvalumab or tremelimumab (an anti-CTLA-4 mAb) therapy, either alone or in combination for R/M HNSCC patients with low or negative PD-L1 expression.[422] The ORR and median OS in durvalumab, tremelimumab, and the combination arm were 9.2 percent and six months, 1.6 percent and 5.5 months, and 7.8 percent and 7.6 months, respectively. The median duration of response was 9.4 months in the combination arm and was not reached in two other groups. Although this study lacks enough power to compare treatment arms, the authors suggest there is more benefit in combination therapy over durvalumab monotherapy.[422]

### Other immunotherapies

In 2019, a phase II study tried to investigate the usage of ISA 101, a synthetic long-peptide *HPV*-16 vaccine with *HPV*-specific T cells, combined with nivolumab for the treatment of HPV-16 related cancers.[423] Among 24 patients who received the therapy, 22 had incurable R/M oropharyngeal cancer. After a median follow-up of 12.2 months, the ORR was 33 percent (all in patients with oropharyngeal cancer), which was ongoing in 63 percent of them.[423] Despite a considerable median OS (17.5 months), the efficacy of this combination therapy must be evaluated in larger trials.

Other approaches, such as adoptive T cell therapies, BiTEs, and vaccines are being investigated in ongoing trials for HNSCC patients.[416] Furthermore, several novel approaches are under active evaluation, such as photo-immunotherapy (NCT02422979), combination therapy with multikinase inhibitors (MKIS) (NCT02501096), oncolytic immunotherapies (NCT02626000), and anti-OX40-mAbs (NCT02274155).

## Future perspective

Before the integration of pembrolizumab and nivolumab with the standard of care guidelines for pretreated R/MHNSCC, the ORR was as low as 4 percent.[422] The impact of ICIs on the survival of this group of patients is guarded. However, there are still some issues, as the duration of responses is not long, and many will have progressive disease after the therapy. Now, many authors are attempting to determine the feasibility and efficacy of combination strategies (either two ICIs or ICI with conventional regimens) and the administration of ICIs as neoadjuvant or definite agents.[416] It seems that the identification of biomarkers of response, prognostic factors, and delicate immunosuppressive mechanisms will shape the future care of HNSCC

## Immunolopathology and immunotherapy of respiratory system cancer

Lung cancer is the leading cause of death due to malignancies in both sexes combined. Worldwide, it is estimated that more than 18.6 percent of cancer-related deaths (near 1.8 million) are due to lung cancers and mesothelioma.[424] In 2019, it was anticipated that about 13.2 percent of newly diagnosed cancers and 23.6 percent of malignancy-related deaths might be attributed to lung and respiratory system neoplasms.[266] Based on histopathologic findings, lung cancers traditionally are subdivided into small cell lung cancer (SCLC) and NSCLC. NSCLC itself has different subtypes, including lung adenocarcinoma (LUAD), lung squamous cell carcinoma (LUSC), large cell carcinoma, and large cell neuroendocrine carcinoma. In 2015, WHO changed some parts of the nosology and integrated genetic and molecular signatures to the diagnostic categories.[425] For example, SCLC is now a subtype of neuroendocrine carcinomas, LUAD, LUSC, and large cell carcinoma are distinct entities, and the latter one is now a diagnosis of exclusion.[425] After the approval of novel targeted therapies, the distinction between LUAD and LUSC has become more critical, as some therapeutic approaches for one of them might be catastrophic for the other one (discussed later).

Approximately 85 percent of lung cancers are NSCLC.[426] Cigarette smoking has long been recognized as an imperative risk factor for the development of lung cancers and is implicated as a causative agent in more than 80 percent of lung cancers. Later, with trends toward decreased smoking among males, an increased proportion of LUAD, and the fact that LUAD is the most common type of lung cancer in females and never-smokers culminated in the identification of other risk factors, like exposure to radon, uranium, vinyl chloride, arsenic, asbestos, chromium, and cadmium.[426,427] The risk of developing lung cancer is also higher in those with chronic obstructive pulmonary disease (COPD), emphysema, and other chronic inflammatory conditions of the lungs.[428]

## Immunopathology

Like other neoplasms, immunosuppression is a prerequisite for the establishment and further invasion of lung cancers. It long has been shown that PD-L1 can be detected in NSCLC,[429] but its impact on the accumulation of TILs and the overall prognosis is not similar throughout different studies.[429,430] Of note, a recent study has revealed an association between the PD-L1 expression status and advanced-stage disease and also reported that patients with positive PD-L1 expression have had a greater probability of having LUAD.[431] A role for other immune checkpoints is also implicated in NSCLC. For instance, a small study has shown that TIM-3 expression on CD4+ TILs is associated with nodal metastasis and advanced-stage disease.[432] Another small survey has found that 27 percent of NSCLC cases express LAG-3 on their TILs, which positively correlates with PD-1 and PD-L1 expression and recurrence rate.[433] IL-35 is expressed by Tregs and TAMs of the NSCLC microenvironment and might serve as another potential target for therapeutic interventions.[434]

Similar to GBM, lung cancers are generally recognized as cold tumors (i.e., lack the inflammatory TME and T cell infiltrations).[435] However, unprecedented outcomes after the administration of ICIs made researchers reconsider the old belief. Subsequent observations of the relatively high amounts of migratory effector T cells and the detection of "pre-exhausted" T cells in TME provided an explanatory theory about the underpinning triggers of this response.[436] In fact, there are large studies that have shown that the increased accumulation of TME CD8+ T cells is an indicator of a favorable clinical course, although there are exceptions.[437]

As with other cancers, cytokines play an important role in the enhanced immunosuppression and metastasis of NSCLC. Increased levels of circulating IL-6 are associated with decreased survival and enhanced capability to metastasize,[438,439] and the opposite is reported for IL-10 and IL-12.[438] A decreased level of blood IL-8 soon after the ICI therapy might be associated with prolonged survival in melanoma and NSCLC patients.[440] IL-17 might contribute to the metastasis of NSCLC, probably via induction of lymphangiogenesis, and is considered a poor prognostic factor.[441] TNF-$\alpha$ is a well-known conducive cytokine for the metastasis of lung cancers.[439]

The process of obtaining tissue biopsies is quite cumbersome for SCLC, and as a result, the number of studies dedicated to unraveling its immunologic features is quite scarce. A study tried to identify the PD-L1 expression status and CD8+ T cell infiltration of 159 cases of pulmonary neuroendocrine tumors.[442] About 45 percent showed a PD-L1 expression of more than 1 percent, which was associated with advanced pathologic grade and histologic type, but not with PFS or OS.[442] In contrast, CD8+ T cell infiltration was correlated to a lower stage, absence of lymph node metastases, and prolonged OS.[442] Unexpectedly, the presence of FOXP3+ T cells was shown to be associated with a better prognosis for non-metastatic stage I to III SCLC.[443]

Lung cancers harbor a wide variety of genetic alterations. For instance, between 18 percent to 30 percent of SCLCs have amplification of the MYC family of oncogenes (*MYC*, *MYCN*, and *MYCL*), which are linked to the refractory disease.[444] For LUAD, a group of driver mutations with pivotal roles in its development are identified, including RTK/RAS/RAF activation (76 percent of cases), *MET* and *ERBB2/HER2* amplification, and *NF1* and *RIT1* mutations.[445] Other prevalent genetic aberrations in LUAD include *EGFR*, *TP53*, *NF1*, and *STK11* mutations. Interestingly, approximately all LUSCs have *TP53* mutation, and *CDKN2A* and *RB1* are mutated in more than 70 percent. Of note, *EGFR* mutation is almost rare in LUSC.[446] Translocations involving *ALK*, *ROS1*, and *RET* are identified in a few cases with LUAD, although they have clinical importance.[445] Regrading SCLC, its genomic profile is similar to that of LUSC, with roughly all cases having detectable *TP53* and *RB1* mutations.[447] The mean of mutations per megabase is 8.9 and 8.1 for LUAC and LUSC, respectively,[445,446] which makes them good targets for ICI therapies.[361] Cytogenetic analysis of premalignant lesions has shown that almost all types of lung cancers exhibit loss of heterozygosity and deletions of chromosome 3p. Hence, it seems that several tumor suppressor genes might be located in this region.[448]

Since the therapeutic approaches for SCLC and different subtypes of NSCLC have evolved exquisitely during the last decade, it is important to distinguish them from each other. Several cell-surface and cytoplasmic markers are elicited for this purpose. CD56, neural cell adhesion molecule (NCAM), synaptophysin, and chromogranin are positive in neuroendocrine tumors, thyroid transcription factor-1 (TTF-1) and Napsin-A are positive in LUAD, and p40, p63, and CK5/6 are expressed by LUSC cells.[425] The progress in delineating the genetic and immunologic features of lung cancers has led to the development of potent, targeted therapies, and some of them (those against EGFR, ALK, and ROS1) are approved by the FDA for the treatment of certain subpopulations with lung cancers, especially LUAD.[449]

Mesotheliomas are aggressive neoplasms that emanate from serous membranes lining the pleura, peritoneum, pericardium, and tunica vaginalis.[450] Although rare, almost all of them are lethal. In recent years, molecular and genetic analyses have shed light on the pathophysiology and the development process of this cancer (e.g., identification of mutations in tumor suppressor genes *CDKN2A*, BRCA1 associated protein 1, and *NF2*), which are discussed elsewhere in detail.[450] At the end of this part, novel immunotherapies for mesothelioma will be discussed in brief.

## Immunotherapies for non-small cell lung cancer

Treatment of stage I and II NSCLC is based on surgical resection, with five-year survival rates falling between 53 percent to 92 percent.[449] However, less than 20 percent of patients are diagnosed with localized disease.[266] Therapy of advanced-stage NSCLC is quite personalized, but the cornerstones are platinum-based chemotherapies, with or without radiation therapy.[449] The introduction of targeted therapies against certain driver oncogene-derived molecules made a breakthrough in the management of lung cancer. However, the promising outcomes of these agents do not last long, and only a small subset of patients harbor such genetic alterations.[449] Hence, the five-year survival for all patients with lung cancer is still less than 20 percent.[266]

The prognosis of SCLC is even more dismal. Although about one-third of cases have the limited-stage disease (LS-SCLC), their five-year survival rate is as low as 10 percent.[451] This is less than 5 percent for those with extensive-stage disease (ES-SCLC), which has not improved substantially during the last three decades.[452]

There is no widely accepted approach for the management of malignant mesothelioma, and all modalities (surgery, chemotherapy, and radiotherapy) are being used.[453] Although targeted therapies (such as anti-angiogenic and anti-EGFR agents) hold some promise, none of them have received FDA approval yet.[453]

### *Immune checkpoint inhibitors (ICIs)*

The efficacy of anti-PD-1 and anti-PD-L1 antibodies in overcoming NSCLC were first reported by two landmark trials in 2012.[454,455] Later in 2015, the results of pembrolizumab administration for 495 patients in the NSCLC cohort of the KEYNOTE-001 trial showed an ORR of 19.4 percent and a median OS of 12 months[456] (Table 4.6). The authors found that the outcome is more significant in those with a history of smoking (probably due to higher TMB). However, this was not true for those with a PD-L1 proportion score of at least 50 percent (of the neoplastic cells). Responses were not affected by the dosage of therapy. Most importantly, this trial reported improved RR and prolonged OS and PFS in those with at least 50 percent PD-L1 expression, and it took as a cutoff value by the succeeding trials.[456] Reports of the long-term follow-up (51.8 to 77.9 months) of patients in the expanded cohort revealed an estimated five-year OS of 23.2 percent, 15.5 percent, 29.6 percent, and 25.0 percent for untreated, previously treated, PD-L1 ≥50 percent untreated, and PD-L1 ≥50 percent previously treated groups, respectively.[457]

One year later, the KEYNOTE-010 trial (comparing pembrolizumab and docetaxel) provided accreditation for the robustness of this agent for those with advanced NSCLC.[458] The considerable outcomes of this study have remained consistent after a median follow-up of 42.6 months (range, 35.2 to 53.2), as the three-year OS is 35 percent and 13 percent for patients with tumor proportion score (TPS) ≥50 percent in pembrolizumab and docetaxel arms, respectively.[459]

Since chemotherapeutic regimens presumably can reinforce the immune system against neoplastic cells (via epitope spreading, increasing CTL accumulation, and impeding MDSC functions),[460] Phase IIKEYNOTE-021 trial aimed to assess the efficacy of adding pembrolizumab to the conventional chemotherapeutic regiment (carboplatin plus pemetrexed) for advanced-stage treatment-naïve NSCLC.[461] Although ORR and

**Table 4.6** Selected trials of immune checkpoint inhibitors (ICIs) for patients with non-small cell lung cancer (NSCLC).

| Study ID | Phase | Treatment arms (n) | Patients & type of cancer | Previous treatment | dosage | Median duration of follow-up | Objective response rate (ORR) (percent percent) | Median duration of response | Progression-free survival (PFS) | Median survival | Biomarker | Grade 3 or more adverse events (AEs) (percent percent) |
|---|---|---|---|---|---|---|---|---|---|---|---|---|
| KEYNOTE-001[456] | I | Pembrolizumab | 495 locally advanced or metastatic NSCLC | 495 in total | 2 mg or 10 mg per kilogram of body weight every 3 weeks or 10 mg per kilogram every 2 weeks | 10.9 months | 19.4 percent | 12.5 months | 3.7 months | 12 months | Significantly improved RR, PFS, and OS in those with PD-L1 expression ≥ 50 percent, compared with 1–49 percent and <1 percent, for both treated and untreated patients | 14 percent (including 19 with dyspnea and 9 with pneumonitis) |
| | | | | 101 previously untreated | | | 24.8 percent | 23.3 months | 6 months | 16.2 months | | |
| | | | | 394 previously treated | | | 18 percent | 10.4 months | 3 months | 9.3 months | | |
| KEYNOTE-010[458] | III | Pembrolizumab[344] | 1034 Advanced NSCLC with at least 1 percent PD-L1 expression | 2 or more cycles of platinum-doublet Chemotherapy | pembrolizumab 2 mg/kg, every 3 weeks | 13.1 months | 18 percent | Not reached | 3.9 months | 10.4 months | Due to the exclusion of those with negative PD-L1, effects of PD-L1 expression on outcome could not be evaluated | 13 percent (including 7 pneumonitis) |
| | | Pembrolizumab[346] | | | Pembrolizumab10 mg/kg, every 3 weeks | | 18 percent | Not reached | 4 months | 12.7 months | | 16 percent (including 7 pneumonitides and 6 severe skin reaction) |
| | | Docetaxel[343] | | | Docetaxel 75 mg/m² every 3 weeks | | 9 percent | 6 months | 4 months | 8.5 months | | 35 percent (including 38 neutropenia) |

*(Continued)*

**Table 4.6** Cont'd

| Study ID | Phase | Treatment arms (n) | Patients & type of cancer | Previous treatment | dosage | Median duration of follow-up | Objective response rate (ORR) (percent percent) | Median duration of response | Progression-free survival (PFS) | Median survival | Biomarker | Grade 3 or more adverse events (AEs) (percent percent) |
|---|---|---|---|---|---|---|---|---|---|---|---|---|
| KEYNOTE-021[461] | II | Carboplatin and pemetrexed and pembrolizumab[60] | 123 Stage IIIb or IV non-squamous NSCLC and absence of ALK or EGFR gene aberrations | Chemotherapy naïve | 4 cycles of pembrolizumab 200 mg, pemetrexed 500 mg/ $m^2$, and carboplatin AUC 5 mg/mL per min administered over 15–60 min, every 3 weeks followed by pembrolizumab for 24 months | 10.6 months | 55 percent | NR | 13 months | NR | No significant difference between groups with PD-L1 expression of <1 percent and >1 percent | 29 percent (including 1 death |
| | | Carboplatin and pemetrexed[63] | | | 4 cycles of pemetrexed 500 mg/$m^2$ and carboplatin AUC 5 mg/mL per min | | 29 percent | NR | 8.9 months | NR | | 26 percent (including 2 deaths) |
| KEYNOTE-024[463] | III | Pembrolizumab[154] | 305 untreated stage IV NSCLC with at least 50 percent PD-L1 expression and absence of *ALK* or *EGFR* gene aberrations | None for metastatic disease | 200 mg every 3 weeks | 11.2 months | 44.8 percent | Not reached | 10.3 months | Not reached | None | 26.6 percent (including 6 diarrhea, 6 skin reaction, 4 pneumonitides, and 1 death) |
| | | One of five IC regimens[151] | | | Different | | 27.8 percent | 6.3 months | 6 months | Not reached | | 53.3 percent (including 49 anemia or neutropenia, and 3 deaths) |

| Study ID | Phase | Treatment arms (n) | Patients & type of cancer | Previous treatment | dosage | Median duration of follow-up | Objective response rate (ORR) (percent percent) | Median duration of response | Progression-free survival (PFS) | Median survival | Biomarker | Grade 3 or more adverse events (AEs) (percent percent) |
|---|---|---|---|---|---|---|---|---|---|---|---|---|
| KEYNOTE-189[460] | III | Pembrolizumab combination[410] | 616 metastatic non-squamous NSCLC and absence of ALK or EGFR gene aberrations | None for metastatic disease | Pembrolizumab 200 mg or saline placebo, every 3 weeks for up to 35 cycles; and for all patients, four cycles cisplatin (75 mg/m$^2$ or carboplatin 5 mg/mL/min plus pemetrexed 500 mg/m$^2$ every 3 weeks, followed by pemetrexed 500 mg/m$^2$ every 3 weeks | 10.5 months | 47.6 percent | 11.2 months | 8.8 months | Not reached | No significant difference between outcome parameters in different TPS groups | 67.2 percent (including 27 deaths) |
| | | Placebo combination[206] | | | | | 18.9 percent | 7.8 months | 4.9 months | 11.3 months | | 65.8 percent (including 12 deaths) |
| KEYNOTE-407[462] | III | Pembrolizumab combination[278] | 559 stage IV squamous NSCLC without evidence of CNS metastasis | No systemic therapy for metastatic disease | Pembrolizumab 200 mg or saline placebo on day 1 for up to 35 cycles; For the first 4 cycles, all patients received carboplatin 6 mg/mL/min on day 1 and either paclitaxel 200 mg/m$^2$ on day 1 or nab-paclitaxel 100 mg/m$^2$ on days 1, 8, and 15, every 3 weeks | 7.8 months | 57.9 percent | 7.7 months | 6.4 months | 15.9 months | No significant difference between outcome parameters in different TPS groups | 69.8 percent (including 23 deaths) |
| | | Placebo combination[281] | | | | | 38.4 percent | 4.8 months | 4.8 months | 11.3 months | | 68.2 percent (including 18 deaths) |

*(Continued)*

**Table 4.6** Cont'd

| Study ID | Phase | Treatment arms (n) | Patients & type of cancer | Previous treatment | dosage | Median duration of follow-up | Objective response rate (ORR) (percent percent) | Median duration of response | Progression-free survival (PFS) | Median survival | Biomarker | Grade 3 or more adverse events (AEs) (percent percent) |
|---|---|---|---|---|---|---|---|---|---|---|---|---|
| KEYNOTE-042[464] | III | Pembrolizumab[637] | 1274 locally advanced or metastatic NSCLC with PD-L1 TPS≥1 percent and absence of ALK or EGFR gene aberrations | No previous therapy for locally advanced or metastatic disease | Pembrolizumab 200 mg | 12.8 months | 27 percent | 20.2 months | 5.4 months | 16.7 months | In the pembrolizumab arm, the lowest HR for survival belonged to those with PD-L1 TPS ≥50 percent but was acceptable in those with ≥1 percent | 18 percent (including 13 deaths) |
| | | Chemotherapy[637] | | | Carboplatin with AUC of 5–6 mg/mL/min plus paclitaxel 200 mg/m² or pemetrexed 500 mg/m² | | 27 percent | 8.3 months | 6.5 months | 12.1 months | | 41 percent (including 14 deaths) |
| OAK*,[469] | III | Atezolizumab[425] | 850 stage IIIb and IV NSCLC | All had received 1–2 previous cytotoxic chemotherapy Regimens (≥1 platinum-based combination therapy) | Atezolizumab 1200 mg every 3 weeks | 21 months | 14 percent | 16.3 months | 2.8 months | 13.8 months | OS enhanced regardless of PD-L1 expression. However, those with the highest TC or IC PD-L1 score achieved the most benefit from atezolizumab therapy | 37 percent |
| | | Docetaxel[425] | | | Docetaxel 75 mg/m² every 3 weeks | | 13 percent | 6.2 months | 4 months | 9.6 months | | 54 percent (including 1 death) |

| Study ID | Phase | Treatment arms (n) | Patients & type of cancer | Previous treatment | dosage | Median duration of follow-up | Objective response rate (ORR) (percent percent) | Median duration of response | Progression-free survival (PFS) | Median survival | Biomarker | Grade 3 or more adverse events (AEs) (percent percent) |
|---|---|---|---|---|---|---|---|---|---|---|---|---|
| IMpower130[†,471] | III | Atezolizumab plus carboplatin and nab-paclitaxel[451] | 679 stage IV non-squamous NSCLC | No previous chemotherapy for stage IV disease | Atezolizumab 1200 mg every 3 weeks and carboplatin AUC 6 mg/mL/min every 3 and nab-paclitaxel 100 $mg/m^2$ every week, 4 or 6 21-day cycles followed by maintenance therapy | 18.5 months | 49.2 percent | 8.4 months | 7 months | 18.6 months | TC or IC PD-L1 score did not affect the outcome | 75 percent (including 152 neutropenia, 138 anemia) |
| | | Carboplatin and nab-paclitaxel[228] | | | As above | 19.2 months | 31.9 percent | 6.1 months | 5.5 months | 13.9 months | | 61 percent (including 65 neutropenia, 47 anemia) |
| PACIFIC[473] | III | Durvalumab[473] | 709 stage III, unresectable NSCLC who did not have a disease progression after concurrent chemoradiotherapy | at least two cycles of platinum-based chemotherapy ( etoposide, vinblastine, vinorelbine, a taxane, or pemetrexed) concurrently with definitive radiation therapy | Durvalumab 10 m/kg every 2 weeks | 25.2 months | 30 percent | Not reached | 17.2 months | NR | PD-L1 expression was not measured for all patients (details provided in the appendix of the article) | 30.5 percent (of any cause) |
| | | Placebo[236] | | | Placebo matched with durvalumab | | 17.8 percent | 18.4 months | 5.6 months | NR | | 26.1 percent (of any cause) |

*(Continued)*

**Table 4.6** Cont'd

| Study ID | Phase | Treatment arms (n) | Patients & type of cancer | Previous treatment | dosage | Median duration of follow-up | Objective response rate (ORR) (percent percent) | Median duration of response | Progression-free survival (PFS) | Median survival | Biomarker | Grade 3 or more adverse events (AEs) (percent percent) |
|---|---|---|---|---|---|---|---|---|---|---|---|---|
| IMpower110[472] | III | Atezolizumab[277] | 554 chemotherapy naïve with stage IV NSCLC and PD-L1 expression ≥1 percent on TC or IC | NR | 1200 mg every 3 weeks | 15.7 months | NR | NR | NR | 17.5 months | OS for TC3 or IC3: HR, 0.595; 95 percent CI, 0.398–0.89 OS for TC2/3 or IC 2/3: HR, 0.717; 95 percent CI 0.52–0.989 | 12.9 percent |
| | | Chemotherapy[277] | | | Different based on histologic type | | NR | NR | NR | 14.1 months | | 44.1 percent |

*Except for AEs, other clinical outcomes are based on intention-to-treat groups.

†Based on the intention-to-treat wild-type population values, except for AEs.NSCLC, non-small cell lung cancer; RR, response rate; PFS, progression-free survival; OS, overall survival; PD-L1, programmed death ligand 1; EGFR, epidermal growth factor receptor; NR, not reported; TPS, tumor proportion score; CNS, Central nervous system; HR, hazard ratio; TC, tumor cells; IC, immune cells.

PFS improved significantly, no difference in OS was observed between the two arms.[461] Besides, similar to the results of the phase IKEYNOTE-021,[461] the PD-L1 expression score did not significantly alter the response to therapy, but this must be interpreted cautiously due to the relatively small number of cases. Following the results of this trial, two phase III studies reported significant benefits (enhanced OS, PFS, and RR) in adding pembrolizumab to conventional chemotherapies for metastatic nonsquamous[460] and squamous[462] NSCLC, regardless of TPS

In KEYNOTE-024 randomized trial, the impact of pembrolizumab on enhancing OS (HR for death, 0.60; 95 percent CI, 0.41–0.89; $P = 0.005$) and PFS (HR for disease progression or death, 0.50; 95 percent CI, 0.37–0.68; $P < 0.001$) of untreated patients with advanced NSCLC was so encouraging that 43.7 percent of patients in the chemotherapy arm went on pembrolizumab.[463] In addition, these promising results were also seen in those with LUSC, and for PFS, it was independent of brain metastasis status.[463] A similar phase III trial, but for those with PD-L1 TPS ≥1 percent, confirmed the achievements of the KEYNOTE-024 trial, although the differences between the two arms were less significant.[464]

The efficacy of nivolumab monotherapy for patients with advanced NSCLC is a matter of debate. Although two phase III trials of nivolumab for pretreated stage IIIB or IV or recurrent squamous[465] and nonsquamous[465] NSCLC, unveiled its superior activity over chemotherapy (in both early and two-year follow-up assessments),[466] but compared with chemotherapy, except for a more favorable safety profile, nivolumab showed no clinical advantage for untreated stage IV or recurrent NSCLC[467] (not shown in Table 4.6).

Based on the promising results of a phase II trial[468] of atezolizumab versus docetaxel (not shown in Table 4.6), the phase III OAK trial was designed for the advanced-stage pretreated NSCLC patients.[469] These two trials grouped patients according to PD-L1 expression score on tumor cells (TCs) or tumor-infiltrating immune cells (ICs). Achieved improvements in OS were independent of PD-L1 expression level or histologic types (squamous versus nonsquamous).[469] Notably, as also reported for nivolumab, PFS was shorter for atezolizumab, although not significantly. Proposed etiologies for this phenomenon include delayed immune responses to the neoplastic cells and early increment in the infiltrated immune cells inside the tumor. ORR was also close in two groups.[469] The findings of the IMpower150 randomized phase III trial revealed a meaningful benefit in adding atezolizumab to the chemotherapeutic regimen consisting of bevacizumab plus carboplatin plus paclitaxel, as the first-line treatment for metastatic nonsquamous NSCLC (not shown in Table 4.6).[470] The added benefit was achieved regardless of PD-L1 expression level or effector T cell gene signature status (*PD-L1*, *CXCL9*, and *IFN-γ* mRNA expression).[470] Later, the IMpower130 trial showed meaningful improvements in the OS, ORR, and also PFS in stage IV nonsquamous NSCLC cases who had received atezolizumab in combination with carboplatin and nab-paclitaxel as the front-line therapy.[471] Such benefits were derived regardless of PD-L1 expression status, but interestingly, on the contrary to IMpower150 conclusions, patients with liver metastases and those with *ALK* or *EGFR* gene aberrations achieved no superior outcome of the combination therapy, which bears putative effectiveness of bevacizumab for such groups into the mind.[471] The interim analysis of the IMpower110 trial is consistent with a considerable increment in the OS after administration of atezolizumab as first-line therapy for stage IV NSCLC with PD-L1 TC ≥50 percent or IC ≥10 percent.[472]

Compared with placebo, durvalumab exhibited superiority in enhancing the OS and PFS of pretreated patients with unresectable stage III NSCLC.[473] The updated report of this trial showed a three-year OS rate of 66.3 percent versus 43.5 percent for durvalumab and placebo, respectively.[474] As a third-line agent, durvalumab also showed modest clinical activity (enhancing RR) in *EGFR+/ALK+* heavily pretreated advanced NSCLC patients with TCPD-L1 ≥25 percent, as well as in those without these genetic aberrations,[475] necessitating the conduction of phase III trials.

For progressive stage IIIB, IV, or recurrent platinum-doublet-treated NSCLC, avelumab was not superior to docetaxel in meeting the primary endpoint of the phase III trial (JAVELIN Lung 200), as median OS did not differ significantly between the two arms (HR, 0.90; 96 percent CI, 0.72–1.12; one-sided $p = 0.16$).[476]

Efforts are also made to evaluate whether the combination therapy with two ICIs will culminate in improved clinical response and manageable side effects or not. Phase III trial Checkmate 227 concluded that first-line ipilimumab and nivolumab combination regiment is superior to nivolumab monotherapy and conventional chemotherapy in prolonging PFS among stage IV or recurrent NSCLCs who have a TMB of at least 10 per megabase, irrespective of histologic type or PD-L1 expression values.[477] This trial later showed improved OS with this combination therapy. However, the role of TMB as a biomarker became less evident.[478] Modest results of this combination therapy are also observed in phase I[479] and II[480] trials for the treatment-naïve patients with recurrent stage IIIb or IVNSCLC, with a TMB cutoff of 10 per megabase as an indicator of favorable RR and PFS.[480]

Recently, the results of the MYSTIC phase III randomized trial were published, which showed no added clinical value of the combined tremelimumab and durvalumab therapy, compared with conventional chemotherapy, in prolonging OS and PFS, and for durvalumab monotherapy, in improving OS of stage IV NSCLC cases with TCPD-L1 ≥25 percent.[481] However, in those with blood-derived TMB ≥20 per megabase, combination therapy exhibited significantly enhanced OS (unadjusted HR, 0.49; 95 percent CI, 0.32–0.74) and also increased PFS and RR.[481]

The remarkable outcomes of ICI therapy for advanced NSCLC have made them potential agents for the treatment of the early-stage or driver-oncogene mutated NSCLCs (combined with targeted therapies). For example, a small phase I trial showed that despite serious toxicities, a combination therapy consisting of ipilimumab and either erlotinib or crizotinib (for *EGFR* and *ALK* gene aberrations, respectively) might have the potentials for improving PFS and OS.[482] Recently, in a phase II trial of NSCLC patients who have been amenable to surgical resection (stage IB to III), neoadjuvant combination therapy with atezolizumab, carboplatin, and nab-paclitaxel has shown robust outcomes. 57 percent achieved a major pathological response, including 33 percent with CR (which is less than 10 percent for neoadjuvant conventional chemotherapies), 68 percent of those with N2 stage showed nodal downstaging, and 87 percent underwent successful surgery.[483] Obviously, due to the small sample size and limitations in assessing responses, larger phase III trials are needed to validate these descriptions.

### *Other immunotherapies*

Because of the high prevalence and extensive mortality rates, a wide variety of immunotherapies have been explored in patients with lung cancer. As was expected, most of them have resulted in severe toxicities and/or minimal clinical benefits. Here, only some of the more prominent interventions will be reviewed.

Co-administration of nivolumab and ALT-803 (an IL-15 superagonist that acts on the IL-2Rβγ pathway) for 21 previously treated stage IIIB or IV NSCLC patients provided evidence for its manageable adverse effects and possible roles in restoring response to anti-PD-1 therapy in the case of resistance.[484]

Cancer vaccines have been evaluated in patients with NSCLC. However, the outcomes have been discouraging. Immunotherapies with recMAGE-A3 (combined with AS15 immunostimulant) and tecemotide (MUC1 antigen-specific immunotherapy) were similar to placebo in improving OS of NSCLC patients.[485,486] Of note, TG4010 (an IL-2 contained MUC1 immunotherapy) in combination with chemotherapy as first-line therapy could increase PFS of stage IV NSCLC.[487]

Until now, to our knowledge, there are no published results of a large trial for the investigation of CART-cell therapies. Hopefully, ongoing trials are evaluating this modality for NSCLC (e.g., NCT03638206 and NCT04153799). The list of FDA-approved immunotherapies for NSCLC is provided in Table 4.7.

## Immunotherapies for small cell lung cancer

### *Immune checkpoint inhibitors (ICIs)*

Although modest, but ICIs have also altered the care of patients with SCLC. Based on the investigations of the landmark IMpower133 trial, the FDA approved combination therapy with atezolizumab, carboplatin, and etoposide as upfront therapy for ED-SCLC.[501] Recently, the FDA also approved a regiment composed of durvalumab combined with etoposide and either carboplatin or cisplatin for the same indication as to the previous one.[502] Nivolumab and pembrolizumab are also approved for metastatic SCLC with progression after (and for pembrolizumab during) platinum-based chemotherapy and at least one other line of therapy. The key features of other trials of ICI for SCLC are provided in Table 4.8.

**Table 4.7** List of currently FDA-approved immune checkpoint inhibitors (ICIs) for the treatment of non-small cell lung cancer.

| Agent (s) | Indication | Trial identifier |
|---|---|---|
| Ipilimumab plus nivolumab | As the first-line treatment for metastatic NSCLC expressing PD-L1 ≥1 percent with no *EGFR* or *ALK* genomic aberrations, in combination with nivolumab | CheckMate 227[488] |
| Ipilimumab plus nivolumab | As the first-line treatment for adult patients with metastatic or recurrent NSCLC with no *EGFR* or *ALK* genomic aberrations, in combination with nivolumab and 2 cycles of platinum-doublet chemotherapy | CheckMate 9LA[489] |
| Nivolumab | Metastatic NSCLC and progression on or after platinum-based chemotherapy. Patients with EGFR or ALK genomic tumor aberrations should have disease progression on FDA-approved therapy for these aberrations prior to receiving nivolumab. | CheckMate 017[490] and CheckMate 057[491] |
| Pembrolizumab | As the first-line treatment for metastatic non-squamous NSCLC with no EGFR or ALK genomic aberrations, in combination with pemetrexed and platinum chemotherapy | KEYNOTE-189[492] |
| Pembrolizumab | As the first-line treatment for metastatic squamous NSCLC, in combination with carboplatin and either paclitaxel or paclitaxel protein-bound | KEYNOTE-407[493] |
| Pembrolizumab | As the first-line treatment of patients with NSCLC expressing PD-L1 (tumor proportion score)<br>≥1 percent, with no EGFR or ALK genomic aberrations, and stage III where patients are not candidates for surgical resection or definitive chemoradiation, or metastatic disease | KEYNOTE-042[494] |
| Pembrolizumab | NSCLC expressing PD-L1 (tumor proportion score) ≥1 percent with disease progression on or after platinum-containing chemotherapy. Patients with EGFR or ALK genomic aberrations should have disease progression on FDA-approved therapy for these aberrations prior to receiving pembrolizumab. | KEYNOTE-010[495] |
| Atezolizumab | As first-line treatment of adult patients with metastatic NSCLC TC PD-L1 ≥50 percent or IC PD-L1 ≥10 percent and without EGFR or ALK genomic aberrations | IMpower110[496] |
| Atezolizumab | In combination with bevacizumab, paclitaxel, and carboplatin, for the first-line treatment of adult patients with metastatic nonsquamous NSCLC without EGFR or ALK genomic aberrations | IMpower150[497] |

| Agent (s) | Indication | Trial identifier |
|---|---|---|
| Atezolizumab | In combination with paclitaxel protein-bound and carboplatin for the first-line treatment of adult patients with metastatic nonsquamous NSCLC without EGFR or ALK genomic aberrations | IMpower130[498] |
| Atezolizumab | Metastatic NSCLC and progression on or after platinum-based chemotherapy. Patients with EGFR or ALK genomic tumor aberrations should have disease progression on FDA-approved therapy for these aberrations prior to receiving nivolumab | OAK[499] |
| Durvalumab | Inadult patients with unresectable, stage III NSCLC that has not progressed after concurrent platinum-based chemotherapy and radiation therapy | PACIFIC[500] |

NSCLC, non-small cell lung cancer; EGFR, epidermal growth factor receptor; FDA, Food and Drug Administration; PD-L1, programmed death ligand 1; TC, tumor cells; IC, immune cells.

### *Other therapies*

Now there are active trials investigating other novel immunotherapies (such as CAR T-cells or BiTEs) and the combination of ICIs (e.g., NCT03708328) for SCLC. Delta-like protein 3 (DDL3) is exclusively expressed on SCLC cells and interacts with Notch and Snail signaling pathways to further promote neoplastic development.[503] Although rovalpituzumab tesirine (an antibody-drug conjugate against DDL3) administration was associated with serious toxicities and only modest outcomes,[504] a CAR T-cell (AMG 119) and a BiTE (AMG 757) specific for DDL3 are currently under evaluation for patients with R/R SCLC (NCT03392064 and NCT03319940, respectively).

## Immunotherapies for mesothelioma

### *Immune checkpoint inhibitors (ICIs)*

The proportion of malignant mesotheliomas that express PD-L1 or have high TMB is not large.[517,518] However, the outcome of ICI therapy for such patients has been acceptable in some (but not all) phase II trials (Table 4.9). The results of the post-hoc analysis for investigation of associations between PD-L1 expression level and OS are not consistent among different studies (significant association in[519] and[520] but not in[521]). Interestingly, preliminary analysis of a phase III trial (CheckMate 743) has shown the superiority of nivolumab and ipilimumab combination to chemotherapy in enhancing OS as first-line therapy.[522]

**Table 4.8** Selected trials of immune checkpoint inhibitors (ICIs) for small cell lung cancer.

| Trial | Treatment arms (*n*) | Objective response rate (ORR) (percent percent) | Progression-free survival (PFS) | Overall survival (OS) | Grade 3 or more adverse events (AEs) (percent percent) |
|---|---|---|---|---|---|
| **Fist-line setting** | | | | | |
| IMPower133[505] | Chemotherapy plus atezolizumab[201] vs chemotherapy[202] | 60 vs 64 | Median PFS 5.2 months vs 4.3 months; 1-year PFS 12.6 percent vs 5.4 percent | Median OS 12.3 months vs 10.3 months (HR 0.70, 95 percent CI 0.54–0.91, $P = 0.007$); 1-year OS 51.7 percent vs 38.2 percent | 56.6 vs 56.1 |
| CASPIAN[506] | Chemotherapyplus durvalumab[268] vs chemotherapy[269] | 79.5 vs 70.3 | Median PFS 5.1 months vs 5.4 months (HR 0.78, 95 percent CI 0.65–0.94); 1-year PFS 17.5 percent vs 4.7 percent | Median OS 13 months vs 10.3 months (HR 0.73, 95 percent CI 0.59–0.91, $P = 0.0047$); 1-year OS 53.7 percent vs 39.8 percent | 62 vs 62 |
| Reck et al.[507] | Chemotherapyplus ipilimumab[478] vs chemotherapy[476] | 62 vs 62 | Median PFS 4.6 months vs 4.4 months (HR 0.85, 95 percent CI 0.75–0.97, $P = 0.016$) | Median OS 11 months versus 10.9 months (HR 0.94, 95 percent CI 0.81–1.09, $P = 0.38$); 1-year OS 40 percent vs 40 percent | 48 vs 45 |
| **First-line maintenance** | | | | | |
| Gadgeel et al.[508] | Chemotherapy followed by pembrolizumab[45] | 14.7 | Median PFS 1.4 months; 1-year PFS 13 percent | Median OS 9.6 months; 1-year OS 37 percent | Grade ≥3 NR; grade 5: 4 percent |
| CheckMate 451[509] | Chemotherapyfollowed by nivolumab plus ipilimumab[279] vs nivolumab[280] vs placebo[275] | NR | Median PFS 1.7 months (HR 0.72, 95 percent CI 0.60–0.87) vs 1.9 months (HR 0.67, 95 percent CI 0.56–0.81) vs 1.4 months | Median OS 9.2 months (HR 0.92, 95 percent CI 0.75–1.12, $P = 0.37$) vs 10.4 months (HR 0.84, 95 percent CI 0.69–1.02) vs 9.6 months; 1-year OS 41 percent vs 44 percent vs 40 percent | 52 vs 12 vs 8 |

| Trial | Treatment arms (*n*) | Objective response rate (ORR) (percent percent) | Progression-free survival (PFS) | Overall survival (OS) | Grade 3 or more adverse events (AEs) (percent percent) |
|---|---|---|---|---|---|
| ***Second-line or later*** | | | | | |
| CheckMate 032[510] | Nivolumab[98] | 10 | 1.4 months; 1-year PFS 11 percent | 4.4 months; 1-year OS 33 percent | 13 |
| | Nivolumab 1 mg/kg plus ipilimumab 3 mg/kg[61] | 23 | 2.6 months; 1-year PFS 19 percent | 7.7 months; 1-year OS 43 percent | 30 |
| | Nivolumab 3 mg/kg plus ipilimumab 1 mg/kg[54] | 19 | 1.4 months; 1-year PFS NR | 6 months; 1-year OS 35 percent | 19 |
| CheckMate 032[511] | Nivolumab[109] | 11.9 | 1.4 months; 1-year PFS NR | 5.6 months; 1-year OS 28.3 percent | 11.9 |
| CheckMate 032[512] | Nivolumab 3 mg/kg[147] | 11.6 | 1.4 months; 1-year PFS 9.5 percent | 5.7 months; 2-year OS 17.9 percent | 12.9 |
| | Nivolumab 1 mg/kg plus ipilimumab 3 mg/kg[96] | 21.9 | 1.5 months; 1-year PFS 11.9 percent | 4.7 months; 2-year OS 16.9 percent | 37.5 |
| CheckMate 331[513] | Nivolumab[284] vs chemo-therapy[285] | NR | 1.5 months vs 3.8 months (HR 1.41, 95 percent CI 1.18–1.69); 1-year PFS 11 percent vs 10 percent | 7.5 months vs 8.4 months (HR 0.86, 95 percent CI 0.72–1.04, $P = 0.11$); 1-year OS 37 percent vs 34 percent | 14 vs 73 |

*(Continued)*

**Table 4.8** Cont'd

| Trial | Treatment arms (*n*) | Objective response rate (ORR) (percent percent) | Progression-free survival (PFS) | Overall survival (OS) | Grade 3 or more adverse events (AEs) (percent percent) |
|---|---|---|---|---|---|
| KEYNOTE-028[514] | Pembrolizumab(24, with PD-L1 ≥1 percent) | 33 | 1.9 months; 1-year PFS 23.8 percent | 9.7 months; 1-year OS 37.7 percent | 4.2 |
| KEYNOTE-158[515] | Pembrolizumab$^{107}$ | 18.7 | 2 months | 9.1 months | Grade ≥3 NR; grade 5: 0.9 percent |
| IFCT-1603[516] | Atezolizumab$^{49}$ vs chemotherapy$^{24}$ | 2 vs 10 | 1.4 months vs 4.3 months | 9.5 months vs 8.7 months (HR 0.84, 95 percent CI 0.45–1.58, *P* = 0.60); 1-year OS 42.5 percent vs NR | 4.2 vs NR (at least 33.3) |

PFS, progression-free survival; OS, overall survival; HR, hazard ratio; CI, confidence-interval; NR, not reported.

**Table 4.9** Selected trials of immune checkpoint inhibitors (ICIs) for mesotheliomas.

| Trial and phase | Treatment arms (*n*) | Disease control rate (DCR) (percent percent) | Objective response rate (ORR) (percent percent) | Progression-free survival (PFS) | Overall survival (OS) | Grade 3 or more adverse events (AEs) (percent percent) |
|---|---|---|---|---|---|---|
| **Second line and later** | | | | | | |
| IFCT-1501 MAPS2[519] | Nivolumab | 40 | 19 (primary analysis) | Median: 4 months; 1-year PFS: 15.9 percent | Median: 11.9 months; 1-year OS: 49.2 percent | 14 |
| | Nivolumab plus ipilimumab | 52 | 28 (primary analysis) | Median: 5.6 months; 1-year PFS: 22.6 percent | Median: 15.9 months; 1-year OS: 58.1 percent | 26 |
| INITIATE[520] | Nivolumab plus ipilimumab | 68 | 38 | Median: 6.2 months; 6-months PFS: 50 percent | Median: not reached; 1-year OS: 64 percent | 38 |
| MERIT[524] | Nivolumab | 68 | 29 | Median: 6.1 months; 1-year PFS: 32 percent | Median: 17.3 months; 1-year OS: 59 percent | 47 |
| DETERMINE*[525] | Tremelimumab vs placebo | 27 vs 22 | 4.5 vs 11 | Did not differ significantly between 2 arms | Median of 7.7 months vs 7.3 months (HR, 0.92; 95 percent CI, 0.76–1.12; $p = 0.41$) | 65 vs 48 |
| **First or second line** | | | | | | |
| NIBIT-MESO-1[521] | Tremelimumab plus durvalumab | 63 | 25 | Median: 5.7 months; 1-year PFS: 32 percent | Median: 16.6 months; 1-year OS: 62 percent | 18 |

*Including patients with peritoneal malignant mesothelioma.
PFS, progression-free survival; OS, overall survival; HR, hazard ratio; CI, confidence-interval.

### *Other immunotherapies*

There are other modalities of interest for the treatment of this grim malignancy. Mesothelin and WT1 are potential candidates for different immunotherapies, including CAR T-cells (NCT02414269) and vaccines.[523] However, to date, no immunotherapy has been approved by the FDA for malignant mesothelioma.

## Immunolopathology and immunotherapy of breast cancer

Breast cancer is the most common female malignancy and is also the leading cause of death among women.[424] It is estimated that in the United States, about 30 percent of newly diagnosed cancers and around 14 percent of cancer-related deaths will be related to breast cancer.[266] Owing to impressive advances in developing screening protocols, conservative surgical techniques, and targeted and endocrine therapies, and also due to deciphering underpinning molecular and genetic features carcinogenesis, the five-year survival rate of breast cancer is now more than 90 percent, with curability of roughly all stage 0 and I tumors.[266,526] However, the tide turns for those with stage IV metastatic disease, as only 27 percent will be alive after five years.[266] Increased expression of estrogen receptor (ER), progesterone receptor (PgR), or both are seen in more than 80 percent of patients with breast cancer.[527] Likewise, HER2 is overexpressed in about 16 percent of cases.[527] Endocrine therapies (including ER blockers, aromatase inhibitors, and oophorectomy) and targeted therapies against HER2 (namely, trastuzumab) have improved the short-term prognosis of patients. However, as the drug resistance develops, most patients will eventually have progressive disease after long-term periods.[528]

## Immunopathology

An investigation of 410 breast cancer samples demonstrated that the proportion of tumors with at least 1 percent PD-L1 expression is about 53 percent, 73 percent, and 84 percent for ER+HER2-, HER2+, and triple-negative breast cancer (TNBC), respectively.[529] Naturally, disparities remain, as proportions as low as 40 percent to more than 85 percent are reported.[530-532] Besides, a relation between IC PD-L1 ≥50 percent and a favorable outcome is implicated for TNBC.[529] Memory T cells express high amounts of PD-1 and CTLA-4, and their accumulation within TME of TNBC has been associated with a better prognosis.[533] Recently, the prognostic value of PD-L1 expression is also validated for early breast cancers.[534] In addition to PD-L1, TIM-3 and LAG-3 are expressed in about 11 percent of breast cancers, and the latter one is associated with increased survival.[535,536]

Well-established documents reported the association of TNF-α, IFN-γ, and IL-6 with cancer cell dissemination within the bone marrow,[537] IL-6, IL-8, and IL-10 with metastasis,[538] and IL-17 with reduced disease-free survival.[539]

TILs are present in the TME of breast cancers and probably have imperative roles in determining the prognosis of patients. Several studies have shown a link between the higher TIL population and a more desirable outcome in different clinical scenarios of breast cancer.[441,540,541] Of note, evaluation of 897 TNBC samples revealed 22 percent had TIL ≥50 percent (so-called lymphocyte-predominant breast cancer), with a median of 20 percent across all samples.[542] The prognostic values of TILs were like previous reports.[542] On the other hand, a meta-analysis has shown that higher densities of Tregs are indicators of a poor OS.[543] In fact, there seem to be considerable populations of TILs, especially in TNBC and luminal B subtypes of breast cancer (but not in luminal A and HER2).[544] Further, single-cell transcriptome analysis has disaggregated three different populations of immune cells within TME: B-lymphocytes, T-lymphocytes (generally with Treg or exhausted phenotype), and TAMs (mainly M2 subtype).[544] Like other neoplasms, TAMs promote the CTL suppression and invasion, angiogenesis, and metastasis of breast cancer.[545] Their accumulation within stroma is related to HR- status and worse survival.[546] Along with these populations, NK cells can also be detected in the TME and are predictors of a better pathological complete response (pCR) after anti-HER2 therapy.[547]

Near 10 percent of breast cancers are hereditary and mainly result from mutations in *BRCA1*, *BRCA2*, *TP53*, *PTEN*, *PALB1*, and *STK11*.[548] The first two genes are involved in the genomic stabilizing system and almost always give rise to TNBC and ER+/PgR+ breast cancer, respectively.[548] Common somatic mutations in different subtypes of breast cancer include *PIK3CA* in luminal A, *PIK3CA* and *TP53* in luminal B, *TP53* in basal-like, and *TP53* along with *HER2* amplification in HER2-enriched (HER2E).[549]

Current treatment options for metastatic breast cancer (MBT) are limited to endocrine or targeted therapies, with or without chemotherapy (depending on molecular characteristics and previous therapies).[526] Similarly, therapeutic options for TNBC are limited to chemotherapy and surgery.[526] There are countless ongoing trials intending to investigate the impact of novel immunotherapies on certain groups of patients with breast cancers. The findings of a few have been published and will be discussed here.

## Immunotherapies

### *Immune checkpoint inhibitors (ICIs)*

The yield of standard chemotherapy for metastatic TNBC is an OS less than 17 months.[550] Hence, trials have first begun to assess the effectiveness of ICIs for such patients. KEYNOTE-012[551] was a landmark study that paved the way for using ICIs against TNBC and subsequently other subtypes (Table 4.10).

In 2019, the KEYNOTE-086 phase II trial reported a median OS of 18 and 9 months for treatment-naïve[552] and pretreated[550] patients with metastatic TMBC who had received single-agent pembrolizumab. However, the RRs were not high. Therefore, ICI monotherapies generally gave their place to the combination therapy strategies. Particularly, neoadjuvant combination therapy with pembrolizumab and platinum-based chemotherapies for early-stage TNBC has been associated with acceptable rates

**Table 4.10** Selected trials of immune checkpoint inhibitors (ICIs) for the treatment of breast cancers.

| Trial | Condition | Treatment arms (*n*) | Median follow-up | Response rate (RR) (percent percent) | Median duration of response (m) | Progression-free survival (PFS) | Overall survival (OS) | Biomarker | Grade 3 or more adverse events (AEs) (percent percent) |
|---|---|---|---|---|---|---|---|---|---|
| **First-line** | | | | | | | | | |
| Impassion130/ III/2018[530], 2020[559] | Unresectable locally advanced or metastatic TNBC | Atezolizumab plus nab-paclitaxel[445] | 18.5 | 56 | 7.4 | Median of 7.2 months vs 5.5 months (HR, 0.8; 95 percent CI 0.69–0.92; $P = 0.0021$); 2-year PFS of 10 percent vs 6 percent | Median of 21 months vs 18.7 months (stratified HR, 0.86; 95 percent CI 0.72–1.02; $P = 0.078$) 2-year OS of 42.4 percent vs 38.7 percent | In those with IC PD-L1 ≥1 percent, median OS of 25 vs 18 months (Stratified HR, 0.71; 95 percent CI, 0.54–0.94); 2-year OS of 50.7 percent vs 36.9 percent Median PFS of 7.5 vs 5.3 months (stratified HR, 0.63; 95 percent CI, 0.5–0.8; $P < 0.0001$); 2-year PFS of 12.4 percent vs 7.4 percent | 49 |
| | | Placebo plus nab-paclitaxel[445] | 17.5 | 45.9 | 5.6 | | | | 43 |

| Trial | Condition | Treatment arms (*n*) | Median follow-up | Response rate (RR) (percent percent) | Median duration of response (m) | Progression-free survival (PFS) | Overall survival (OS) | Biomarker | Grade 3 or more adverse events (AEs) (percent percent) |
|---|---|---|---|---|---|---|---|---|---|
| KEYNOTE-522/III/2020[553] | Previously untreated stage II or stage III TNBC | Pembrolizumabplus paclitaxel and carboplatin[784]<br>Placebo plus paclitaxel and carboplatin[390] | 15.5 | The primary analysis of pCR[1]: 64.8 vs 51.2, estimated treatment difference, 13.6 percentage points; 95 percent CI, 5.4–21.8; $P < 0.001$ | NR | HR for disease progression (precluding definitive surgery), local or distant recurrence or a second primary tumor, or death from any cause: 0.63; 95 percent CI, 0.43–0.93 (favored pembrolizumab) | Not reached<br>Not reached | PD-L1 expression status did not affect the acquisition of pCR | 77<br>72 |
| KEYNOTE-086/II/2019[552] | Metastatic TNBC with positive PD-L1 | Cohort B: Pembrolizumab[84] | 12.3 | 21.4 | 10.4 | Median of 2.1 months; 6-months PFS of 27 percent | Median of 18 months, 1-year OS of 61.7 percent | None | 9.5 |

*(Continued)*

**Table 4.10** Cont'd

| Trial | Condition | Treatment arms (*n*) | Median follow-up | Response rate (RR) (percent percent) | Median duration of response (m) | Progression-free survival (PFS) | Overall survival (OS) | Biomarker | Grade 3 or more adverse events (AEs) (percent percent) |
|---|---|---|---|---|---|---|---|---|---|
| KEYNOTE-173/ Ib/2020[554] | High risk early-stage TNBC | Pembrolizumab plus different chemotherapeutic regimens[60] | 19.6 | 60 pCR[1] | NR | NR | OS rate of 98 percent for platinum-containing regimens vs 80 percent for other regimens | Higher PD-L1 CPS and pre-treatment and on-treatment sTILs were significantly associated with pCR rate | 90 |
| **First-line or later** | | | | | | | | | |
| KEYNOTE-012/ Ib/2016[551] | Advanced TNBC with TC PD-L1 ≥1 percent | Pembrolizumab[32] | 10 | 18.5 | Not reached | Median of 1.9 months; 6-month PFS of 24.4 percent | Median of 11.2 months, 1-year OS of 43.1 percent | PD-L1 expression increased the chance of response | 15.6 |

| Trial | Condition | Treatment arms (*n*) | Median follow-up | Response rate (RR) (percent percent) | Median duration of response (m) | Progression-free survival (PFS) | Overall survival (OS) | Biomarker | Grade 3 or more adverse events (AEs) (percent percent) |
|---|---|---|---|---|---|---|---|---|---|
| Vinayak et al./ II/2019[560] | Advanced or metastatic TNBC | Niraparib plus pembrolizumab[55] | 14.8 | 18 | Not reached | Median of 2.3 months; 1-year PFS of 14 percent | NR | Numerically higher response in those with *BRCA* mutation or PD-L1+ status | 58 |
| Ho et al. / II/2020[561] | Metastatic TNBC | Pembrolizumab plus radiation therapy[17] | 34.5 weeks | 17.6 | 4.5 | Median of 2.6 months; 6-months PFS of 18 percent | Median of 7.6 months, 1-year OS of 41 percent | PD-L1 expression status did not correlate to RR or PFS | 24 |
| **Second-line or later** | | | | | | | | | |
| KEYNOTE-086/ II/2019[550] | Metastatic TNBC | Cohort A: pembrolizumab[170] | 9.6 | 5.3 | Not reached | Median of 2 months; 6-months PFS of 14.9 percent | Median of 9 months, 1-year OS of 69.1 percent | None | 12.9 |

*(Continued)*

**Table 4.10** Cont'd

| Trial | Condition | Treatment arms (*n*) | Median follow-up | Response rate (RR) (percent percent) | Median duration of response (m) | Progression-free survival (PFS) | Overall survival (OS) | Biomarker | Grade 3 or more adverse events (AEs) (percent percent) |
|---|---|---|---|---|---|---|---|---|---|
| PANACEA/IB-II/2019[557] | Advanced HER2+ breast cancer with progression on previous trastuzumab-based therapy | PD-L1+[40] vs PD-L1-[12] patients received Pembrolizumab plus standard trastuzumab[52] | 13.6 vs 12.2 | 15 vs 0 | 3.5 | Median of 2.7 months; 1-year PFS of 12 percent VS median of 2.5 months; 1-year PFS of 0 percent | Median OS not reached, 1-year OS of 65 percent VS Median of 7 months, 1-year OS of 12 percent | PD-L1 expression status and density of TILs in metastatic lesions conferred benefit from this combination therapy | 29 |

1. defined as ypT0/Tis ypN0.
TNBC, triple-negative breast cancer; PFS, progression-free survival; HR, hazard ratio; OS, overall survival; PD-L1, programmed death ligand 1; IC PD-L1, immune cell PD-L1 expression; pCR, pathological complete response; NR, not reported; CI, confidence-interval; CPS, combine positive score; sTIL, stromal tumor-infiltrating lymphocyte; RR, response rate.

of pCR[553,554] (Table 4.10). It is also estimated that neoadjuvant chemotherapy plus pembrolizumab for early-stage high-risk TNBC and HR+ HER2- breast cancer will increase the chance of achieving a pCR more than two times.[555]

Despite the limited number of trials with published results, major advances have been made in understanding the immunologic and molecular mechanisms of breast cancer's response to therapy with ICIs. One of the best examples of such efforts is the phase II TONIC trial.[531] The authors designed 5 cohorts to receive doxorubicin, cisplatin, cyclophosphamide, radiation therapy, or nothing as induction therapy, followed by administration of nivolumab. Among 67 cases with metastatic TNBC, the highest ORRs were observed for doxorubicin and cisplatin cohorts (35 percent and 23 percent, respectively), whereas only 8 percent of patients in the radiation therapy and cyclophosphamide showed a response.[531] It was then demonstrated that higher stromal tumor-infiltrating lymphocyte (sTIL), CD8+, and PD-L1+ immune cells, upregulation of inflammatory-related genes (e.g., those involved in the TNF-α and JAK-STAT signaling pathways), and lower levels of cancer antigen 15–3 (CA 15–3) all correlate with the response to therapy. In fact, the increased TIL infiltration and inflammatory-genes upregulation were observed after induction therapy with doxorubicin and cisplatin.[531] Noteworthy, this study did not find any relationship between the TMB or *BRCA1/2* mutations (but not *BRCA1*-like amplification) and response to therapy.[531] The role of TILs in enhancing anti-tumor activities of ICIs is also proven by at least two other trials of ICI for TNBC[554,556] and HER2+ breast cancer.[557]

Trastuzumab induces tumor suppression mainly via inhibition of HER2 tyrosine kinase. However, it is proposed that its performance is also based on an immunologic-related fashion.[558] Interestingly, a study of pembrolizumab for HER2+ trastuzumab-resistant breast cancer has suggested that resistance to trastuzumab might be mediated via immunologic derangements.[557]

To date, the FDA has given accelerated approval to atezolizumab usage in combination with nab-paclitaxel for patients with unresectable, locally advanced, or metastatic TNBC with IC PD-L1 expression of ≥1 percent (based on improved PFS described in Impassion 130 trial[530]).

### *Other immunotherapies*

A type of CAR T-cells against c-Met-has been explored for a small number of patients with metastatic disease and has resulted in considerable tissue necrosis and induction of inflammation, evident under microscopic tissue examinations.[562] There are ongoing trials investigating CAR T-cells against MUC1 (NCT04020575 and NCT04025216) and mesothelin (NCT02792114) for patients with breast cancer. Reparixin, an anti CXCR1/2 (IL-8 receptors) antagonist (NCT02370238), M7824, a bifunctional agent that acts via inhibition of PD-L1 and sequestration of TGF-β (NCT03524170, NCT03524170, and NCT03620201), and NKTR-214 (an IL-2 agonist) in combination with nivolumab (NCT02983045) is under investigation for the treatment of breast cancer.

XmAb22841 is a novel bispecific antibody against LAG-3 and CTLA-4 that is planned to be administered alone or in combination with pembrolizumab for various cancers, including TNBC (NCT03849469). Likewise, MGD013 is another bispecific antibody targeting PD-1 and LAG-3 and is going to be studied in a phase I trial in patients with different neoplasms (NCT03219268). There are other trials underway to test different regimens of antibodies against LAG-3 (e.g., NCT03499899, NCT03742349, and NCT03250832) and TIM-3 (NCT03652077) for breast cancer.

## Future prospective

The stimulator of interferon genes (STING) is a DNA sensing regulatory molecule for the transcription of several immune-related genes.[435] Activation of STING will trigger CTL and DC activation and facilitate their infiltration inside the TME.[435] In preclinical studies, the administration of STING agonists has induced significant regression of different neoplastic cell lines, including breast carcinoma.[563] Together with the evidence of putative ICI resistance mechanisms (T cell exhaustion as an example),[564] at least theoretically, it seems reasonable that co-administration of ICIs and STING agonists will culminate in enhanced immune system performance and forbiddance of the development of resistance to ICIs. Nevertheless, the limitations of ICI for breast cancer are identical to those of other neoplasms. Only a fraction of patients respond well to ICIs, and even the responses do not last long enough. Perhaps the most required next steps in the field of immunotherapies are to construct validated inclusion criteria, establish robust strategies of combination therapies, and increase the immunogenicity of neoplastic cells.

## Immunolopathology and immunotherapy of gastrointestinal system cancers

Gastrointestinal system malignancies (including esophageal, gastric, colorectal, anal, hepatobiliary, and pancreatic cancers) together are estimated to comprise more than 27 percent of new cancer cases and about 37 percent of cancer-related deaths worldwide.[424] These statistics are less prominent in western countries (18.6 percent and 27.1 percent in the United States, respectively), mainly due to lower incidence rates of esophageal and gastric cancers.[266] Neoplasms of the pancreas, liver, and esophagus are the first three deadliest cancers, and their five-year survival rates are around 9 percent, 18 percent, and 19 percent, respectively.[266] Fortunately, because of the early detection of colorectal cancer by screening programs and the declined prevalence of Helicobacter pylori infection, the burden of colorectal and gastric cancers has reduced in recent years.[424] Putative risk factors for gastrointestinal cancers are diverse and encompass genetic alterations, dietary habits, infections, metabolic derangements, and environmental exposures.[424] The cornerstone of the treatment of gastrointestinal cancers is surgical resection, with the aid of chemotherapy and/or radiation therapy for advanced-stage diseases. Particularly, because of increasing trends in the incidence of pancreatic and esophageal cancers in western countries[266] and virtually no effective therapy for pancreatic and advanced-stage esophageal cancers, there is an urgent need for developing novel therapeutic modalities.

## Immunopathology

### *Esophageal cancers*

The vast majority of esophageal cancers are either squamous cell carcinoma (ESCC) or adenocarcinoma (EAS).[565] Although these two subtypes have different etiologic factors overall, their clinical feature and therapeutic approaches are similar. Historically, ESCC outnumbered EAS and still comprises more than 90 percent of esophageal cancers in eastern Asia, but the trend in western countries is now towards EAS.[566]

Like other neoplasms, immune checkpoints can be detected in esophageal cancers and probably have prognostic values. In one study, it has shown that PD-L2 is expressed on the neoplastic cells of about 50 percent of EASs and even can be detected in samples of Barrett's esophagus (precursor lesions of EAS), and their expression is probably induced by cytokines secreted from Th2 cells.[567] PD-L1 has been detectable on the tumor cells and the infiltrating immune cells of about 30 percent and 40 percent of 347 samples of ESCC, respectively, and has been linked to a dismal prognosis.[568] These findings are in concordance with a previously published meta-analysis, which concluded that PD-L1 is detectable in 43.7 percent of ESCCs and is significantly associated with an unfavorable OS and distant metastasis.[569] Pro-inflammatory cytokines IL-6[570,571] and IL-8,[572] and circulating MDSCs[573] are suggested to be an indicator of the poor prognosis of esophageal cancers. As it is expected, two meta-analyses have found that the bulk of TILs and CD8+ TILs are positively correlated to the OS of patients with esophageal cancers[574] and specifically ESCC.[575]

Devastating genetic mutations (i.e., in *TP53* and *CDKN2A* genes) are present even in Barrett's esophagus and ESCC samples. Other notable genetic alterations include *ERBB2* and *VEGFA* amplification in 32 percent and 28 percent of EASs, respectively, and EGFR amplification and *PIK3CA/PTEN* mutations in 19 percent and 24 percent of ESCCs, respectively.[565]

### *Gastric cancer*

More than 85 percent of gastric cancers are adenocarcinomas, which are further subclassified into intestinal and diffuse types (Lauren classification) according to histologic features,[576] with each type conferring different risk factors and prognostic implications. Unlike what has been reported for some other neoplasms (e.g., breast cancer), a meta-analysis has shown that PD-L1 expression in gastric cancers is associated with lymph node metastasis, larger tumor size, and poor OS.[577] Likewise, a small study of 52 gastric cancer samples found a significant association between TIM-3 expression and the three mentioned parameters for PD-L1 expression.[578] A recent study has found higher LAG-3 and also OX40 expression on the circulating T cells in patients with advanced gastric cancers who achieve longer PFS after therapy with nivolumab.[579] The prognostic values for different cytokines and immune cells are generally identical to what was discussed for esophageal cancer and other neoplasms.[580]

One of the most paramount breakthroughs in understanding the molecular biology of gastric adenocarcinomas is its classification to four groups based on the genetic features: chromosomal instability (CIN), genomically stable (GS), MSI-associated, and *EBV* positive, that constitutes about 50 percent, 20 percent, 22 percent and 9 percent of cases, respectively.[576] Each of these subtypes harbors its unique set of genetic aberrations. For example, the *EBV* subtype has frequent *PIK3CA* mutations, a high rate of DNA hypermethylation, and most importantly, 9p amplifications in about 15 percent of cases.[576] *JAK2*, *CD274* (encoding PD-L1), and *PDCD1LG2* (encoding PD-L2) are located on chromosome 9p and can turn the *EBV* subtype into a suitable target for ICIs.[576] Gastrointestinal stromal tumors (GIST) represent a minority of gastric cancers. There is solid evidence consisting of the presence of immune checkpoint molecules and other immunosuppressive components inside their TME, and hence, makes them potentially suitable targets for immunotherapies.[581] However, because of their rarity and lack of enough space, GISTs will not be discussed anymore.

### Colorectal and anal cancer

PD-L1 expression in colorectal cancer is generally confined to the relatively uncommon types that have harbored unique genomic alterations (discussed later). However, like other gastrointestinal cancers, PD-L1 expression in colorectal cancer is associated with grim OS and shorter disease-free survival, as suggested by a meta-analysis.[582] The role of the immune system in modifying the behavior of colorectal cancers and affecting their prognosis has been long documented. For instance, the presence of CTLs and effector memory T cells inside the tumor inversely correlates with the probability of metastasis and is an indicator of favorable survival.[583,584] The accumulation of immune cells inside TME has further shown to be correlated with higher neoantigen loads.[585]

Based on the mutational burden, TCGA classified colorectal cancers into two groups: those with low TMB (defined as less than 8.24 mutations per megabase) and those with high TMB (≥12 mutations per megabase), which represent about 16 percent of cases.[586] Further, 77 percent, 25 percent, and 25 percent of those with high TMB harbored *MSI*, *polymerase epsilon* (*POLE*), and *MMR* gene mutations, respectively, and *ERBB* gene family mutations or amplifications were present in 53 percent of cases.[586] Intriguingly, DNA mismatch repair-deficient/MSI-high (dMMR/MSI-H) colorectal cancers have higher densities of CTL and Th1 cells and enhanced expression of CTLA-4, PD-1, PD-L1, and IDO.[587] Likewise, another study aimed to delineate effective factors on PD-L1 expression in colorectal cancers found significant associations with B-Raf proto-oncogene (*BRAF*) mutations, MSI, less differentiation, and also higher CD8+ T cell infiltration.[588]

### *Hepatobiliary and pancreatic cancers*

Approximately 85 percent to 90 percent of all liver malignancies are hepatocellular carcinoma.[589] The majority of liver cancers are originated from highly inflamed precursor lesions. Thus, immune system suppression is of the greatest importance for the development of hepatocellular carcinoma.[589] The expression of PD-L1 in hepatocellular carcinoma is associated with post-surgical recurrence,[590,591] Tregs infiltration, and poorer OS.[590] Such prognostic values for PD-L1 are also confirmed by a recent meta-analysis.[592] In addition, the inflammatory gene signature (including signaling pathways of TNF-α, NF-κB, and interferons) is associated with a dismal prognosis of hepatocellular carcinoma.[593]

Pancreatic ductal adenocarcinoma (PDAC) comprises around 90 percent of all pancreatic cancers.[594] One of the pathologic hallmarks of PDAC is the scarcity of neoplastic cells, as they constitute less than 20 percent of the cellularity.[595] Therefore, most of the tumoral volume is made of a dense desmoplastic stroma that surprisingly plays an important role in the development of the neoplasm.[596] Myofibroblasts and fibrous stroma establish a hypoxic environment, produce growth cytokines for neoplastic and immunosuppressive cells,[596] and like other neoplasms, can also disturb T cell activities by producing high amounts of NO,[597] IL-10, TGF-β, and arginase.[598] FAP positive fibroblasts of the stroma can produce CXCL12, that when localizing on the cancer cells, will prevent the recruitment of CD8+ T cells into the TME.[599] Therefore, unlike hepatocellular carcinoma, pancreatic cancers are not recognized as immunogenic tumors.[600] Although functional T cells are almost entirely absent in the TME of PDAC but is prevailed by Tregs, MDSCs, TAMs, and other immunosuppressive cells.[601] Recruitment and maturations of MDSCs probably depend on the GM-CSF. On the other hand, CD40 and its agonists might trigger a shifting in macrophages towards an anti-neoplastic phenotype.[601,602] Of note, PDAC has one of the lowest TMBs among cancers.[361] Preclinical studies in mice have demonstrated that the co-administration of chemotherapy and an αCD40-agonist mAb can overcome the hard-bitten resistance of PDAC to ICIs, and enhance survival.[603] Similarly, the addition of CSF1 receptor (CSF1R, one of myeloid growth factor receptors) blockers to ICIs has instigated tumor regression in a mouse model of PDAC.[604] As with other gastrointestinal malignancies, PD-L1 expression of PDAC is associated with reduced OS, lower differentiation, positive lymph node status, and advanced T stage.[605]

## Immunotherapies for esophageal and gastric cancers

### *Immune checkpoint inhibitors (ICIs)*

ICIs have shown unprecedented outcomes for patients with advanced-stage gastric and esophageal cancers. The phase III ATTRACTION-2 trial enrolled 493 pretreated patients with gastric or gastro-esophageal junction (GEJ) tumors to receive either placebo or nivolumab.[606] After a median follow-up of about 8 months, nivolumab significantly reduced the risk of death (HR for death, 0.63; 95 percent CI, 0.51–0.78; $p < 0.0001$), irrespective of PD-L1 expression status or different Lauren subtypes.[606] Nivolumab also has shown superior benefit over chemotherapy in prolonging the OS of patients with advanced ESCC, as second-line therapy (HR for death, 0.77; 95 percent CI, 0.62–0.96; $p = 0.019$).[607]

Regarding pembrolizumab, added value in increasing OS over the second-line chemotherapy was only observed in those with PD-L1 CPS of ≥10 (for both EAS and ESCC).[608] Similarly, among GEJ and gastric cancer subjects, only those with CPS ≥10 or high MSI would achieve a response after receiving pembrolizumab as the second-line therapy.[609] Camrelizumab (an anti-PD-1 mAb) has enhanced the OS of patients with advanced or metastatic ESCC in a phase III trial, as compared with second-line chemotherapy.[610] To date, the FDA has only approved pembrolizumab for the treatment of gastric and esophageal cancers (Table 4.11).

### *Other immunotherapies*

The addition of relatlimab (an anti-LAG-3 agent) to nivolumab plus chemotherapy is now being tested in a large phase II trial for patients with locally advanced, unresectable, or metastatic gastric or GEJ cancers as first-line therapy (NCT03662659). Some studies have developed vaccines against different cancer antigens expressed in esophageal cancer cells, but minor activities have been observed.[611] According to the outcomes of the mentioned trials, ICIs are suitable modalities for gastric and esophageal cancers, and future attempts should focus on improving their duration of responses.

## Immunotherapies for colorectal cancers

### *Immune checkpoint inhibitors (ICIs)*

Early trials of different ICIs for metastatic colorectal cancer did not report any response to the therapy.[454,455,612,613] Due to Compelling immunologic and genetic features of dMMR/MSI-H colorectal cancer, and the restricted robust outcomes after the therapy with pembrolizumab to those with mismatch-repair deficient colorectal cancer,[614] and also the emergence of new evidence demonstrating the effectiveness of anti-PD-1 therapy for other mismatch-repair deficient tumors,[615] succeeding trials focused on this specific type and reached to convincing outcomes. In a phase II trial of nivolumab for pretreated dMMR/MSI-H metastatic colorectal cancer patients, 31 percent of cases achieved a PR, and the one-year OS and PFS were found to be 73 percent and 50 percent, respectively.[616]

**Table 4.11** The list of the FDA-approved immune checkpoint inhibitors (ICIs) for the treatment of gastrointestinal malignancies.

| Agent | Indication | Trial |
|---|---|---|
| Pembrolizumab | Recurrent locally advanced or metastatic gastric or GEJ adenocarcinoma with PD-L1 CPS ≥1 with disease progression on or after 2 or more prior lines of therapy, including fluoropyrimidine- and platinum-containing chemotherapy and if appropriate, HER2 targeted therapy. | KEYNOTE-059[642] |
| Pembrolizumab | Recurrent locally advanced or metastatic ESCC with PD-L1 CPS ≥10 with disease progression after one or more prior lines of systemic therapy. | KEYNOTE-181[608] |
| Nivolumab | dMMR/MSI-H metastatic colorectal cancer in patients aged ≥12 who have progressed disease following treatment with fluoropyrimidine, oxaliplatin, and irinotecan (single therapy or in combination with ipilimumab). | CheckMate 142[643] |
| Ipilimumab plus nivolumab | dMMR/MSI-H metastatic colorectal cancer in patients aged ≥12 who have progressed disease following treatment with fluoropyrimidine, oxaliplatin, and irinotecan (only in combination with nivolumab). | CheckMate 142[644] |
| Pembrolizumab | dMMR/MSI-H unresectable or metastatic colorectal cancer that has progressed following treatment with fluoropyrimidine, oxaliplatin, and irinotecan. | Several trials |
| Ipilimumab plus nivolumab | previously treated with sorafenib hepatocellular carcinoma (only in combination with nivolumab). | CheckMate 040[645] |
| Nivolumab | previously treated with sorafenib hepatocellular carcinoma (single therapy or in combination with ipilimumab). | CheckMate 040[645] |
| Pembrolizumab | previously treated with sorafenib hepatocellular carcinoma | KEYNOTE-224[646] |

GEJ, gastro-esophageal junction; PD-L1, programmed death ligand 1; CPS, combined positive score; ESCC, Esophageal squamous cell carcinoma; dMMR/MSI-H, DNA mismatch repair-deficient/ microsatellite instability-high.

Of note, exhibiting a response was independent of PD-L1 expression status and *BRAF* or *KRAS* mutations. In fact, the RR of patients with *BRAF* mutation to nivolumab was higher than that of other regimens.[616]

Administration of nivolumab plus ipilimumab for another cohort of the previously mentioned trial (CheckMate-142) showed tremendous activities. 54.6 percent achieved a response (including CR in 3.4 percent), with a one-year OS of 85 percent.[616] Similar to the nivolumab monotherapy cohort, PD-L1 expression and *BRAF* or *KRAS* mutations did not affect the acquisition of response.[616] Furthermore, nivolumab plus low-dose ipilimumab therapy has shown to be effective even as the first-line therapy in such patients, with an ORR of 60 percent.[617] Avelumab monotherapy also exhibited a modest clinical activity in patients with dMMR/MSI-H metastatic colorectal cancer but not in those with *POLE* mutation. Albeit, the small size of the trial permits reaching definitive conclusions.[618]

A phase III trial tried to overcome the cold immune environment of colorectal cancer by adding cobimetinib (a MAP kinase pathway inhibitor, which is postulated to be involved in the immunosuppressive mechanisms of neoplasms) to atezolizumab and compared this combination against regorafenib monotherapy. Unfortunately, this trial did not meet its primary endpoint (increasing OS).[619] However, this is probably because the trial tried to close the proportion of patients with MSI-H status to that of the general population (5 percent).[619] The same disappointing findings have been reported for combination therapy with durvalumab and trametinib (another MAP kinase pathway inhibitor) for microsatellite-stable (MSS) patients.[620] Recently, a phase II trial composed mainly of MSS metastatic colorectal cancer patients has described only mild superior benefit in adding durvalumab and tremelimumab to best supportive care (BSC) (HR for death, 0.72; 90 percent CI, 0.54–0.97; $p$ = 0.07), but notably, those with a plasma TMB ≥28 per megabase have had significantly elongated OS after the ICI therapy, compared with only BSC (median OS, 5.5 versus 3.0 months; $p$ = 0.004).[621]

Interestingly, preliminary analysis of a trial combining pembrolizumab, tremelimumab, and modified FOLFOX6 (oxaliplatin, 5-fluorouracil, and leucovorin) as the first-line therapy for MSS metastatic colorectal cancer with *RAS* mutation has been intriguing, as 5 of 16 patients have shown a CR.[622] In addition, a combination therapy consisting of avelumab, cetuximab, and modified FOLFOX6 as first-line therapy for *BRAF/RAS* wild-type MSS metastatic colorectal cancer has shown unprecedented results.[623] The List of the FDA-approved ICIs for colorectal cancers is mentioned in Table 4.11.

### *Other immunotherapies*

The CEA-CD3 TCB is a BiTE specific for CD3 and CEA, which has been used for metastatic colorectal cancer and demonstrated modest clinical activities.[624] Likewise, a CAR T-cell specific for CEA has been studied in colorectal cancer, and the preliminary outcomes have been promising.[625,626] Now there are various trials underway to evaluate different agents (e.g., antibodies against LAG-3, TIM-3, TIGIT, and glucocorticoid-induced tumor necrosis factor receptor (GITR)), alone or combined with each other for the treatment of colorectal cancers (e.g., NCT01968109, NCT03219268, NCT03119428, NCT02740270, and NCT02318394).

## Immunotherapies for hepatocellular carcinoma

### *Immune checkpoint inhibitors (ICIs)*

Early attempts for integrating ICIs in the therapeutic approach of patients with hepatocellular carcinoma were done using anti-CTLA-4 antibodies. Administration of tremelimumab for a small number of advanced hepatocellular carcinoma cases with concurrent *HCV* infection resulted in an ORR of 17.6 percent.[627] Of note, the RR of the FDA-approved agent, sorafenib (an inhibitor of Raf-1, B-Raf, VEGF receptor (VEGFR), and PDGFR-β) is only 2 percent for patients with advanced hepatocellular carcinoma.[628] In the CheckMate 040 trial, nivolumab demonstrated encouraging clinical activity in advanced hepatocellular carcinoma patients, as 20 percent achieved an overall response, and nine-month PFS and OS were 28 percent and 74 percent, respectively.[629] Of note, the responses were seen regardless of PD-L1 positivity, the setting of the therapy (first-line or after sorafenib), and the presence of viral infections.[629] In addition, combination therapy with nivolumab and ipilimumab as the second-line therapy for advanced hepatocellular carcinoma has resulted in even higher clinical benefit, with an ORR and two-year OS of 31 percent and 40 percent, respectively.[630]

Despite promising anti-tumor activities of nivolumab as second-line therapy for hepatocellular carcinoma, its administration as the frontline agent for advanced hepatocellular carcinoma did not meet the significance level in prolonging OS over sorafenib in the CheckMate 459 trial.[631] However, both OS and ORR were numerically higher in the nivolumab arm (median OS of 16.4 versus 14.7 months, the two-year OS of 36.8 percent versus 33.1 percent, and ORR of 15 percent versus 7 percent).[631]

Pembrolizumab has shown similar efficacy as second-line therapy for advanced hepatocellular carcinoma, with ORR, one-year PFS, and one-year OS of 17 percent, 28 percent, and 54 percent, respectively, as described by a phase II trial (KEYNOTE-224).[632] Unfortunately, in a large phase III trial aimed to compare pembrolizumab versus placebo as the second-line therapy, despite the superior risk-to-benefit ratio of pembrolizumab, the OS and PFS did not differ significantly (due to prespecified p values) between the pembrolizumab and placebo arms.[592]

The results of the IMbrave150 phase III trial, which enrolled patients with locally advanced metastatic and/or unresectable hepatocellular carcinoma to receive either atezolizumab plus bevacizumab or sorafenib as the first-line therapy are published recently.[633] After a median follow-up duration of 8.6 months, the combination therapy culminated in both superior OS (one-year OS of 67.2 percent versus 54.6 percent; HR for death 0.58; 95 percent CI, 0.42–0.79; $p < 0.001$) and PFS (median of 6.8 versus 4.3 months; HR for disease progression or death, 0.59; 95 percent CI, 0.47–0.76; $p < 0.001$)[633] and, hence, makes this combination therapy a potential candidate for such groups of patients.

Finally, camrelizumab has shown modest anti-tumor activities in the context of advanced hepatocellular carcinoma as a second-line or later therapy (with an ORR of 14.7 percent and six-month OS probability of 74.4 percent).[634] To date, three ICIs have received accelerated FDA approval for the usage in patients with hepatocellular carcinoma (Table 4.11).

### *Other immunotherapies*

A trial conducted late in the 1990s demonstrated lower rates of post-surgical recurrence and longer time to the first recurrence in those who had received adoptive T cell therapy.[635] In recent years, this kind of modality has come to the interest once more, and modest outcomes have described.[636-638] Glypican3 (GPC3) is a glycoprotein, which is exclusively expressed on hepatocellular carcinoma cancer cells, but not normal liver tissue.[639] While the vaccine therapies against GPC3 generally did not alter the course of hepatocellular carcinoma,[640,641] several ongoing trials are aiming to evaluate the applicability and efficacy of CAR T-cells specific for GPC3 (e.g., NCT02905188, NCT03884751, and NCT03980288). Combination therapies of checkpoint inhibitors with each other (NCT03298451 and NCT03680508) or with targeted therapies (NCT03713593, NCT03847428, and NCT03794440) seem reasonable strategies and are being pursued by the mentioned trials.

## Immunotherapies for pancreatic cancers

### *Immune checkpoint inhibitors (ICIs)*

Until now, all ICI-based therapies, including BMS-936,559 (anti-PD-L1 mAb),[455] ipilimumab,[647,648] tremelimumab,[649,650] tremelimumab plus durvalumab,[650] and pembrolizumab[651] have failed to alter the clinical course of PDAC. Beyond the well-established role of the extreme immunosuppressive environment, fairly low TMB probably is another major barrier that ICIs are faced with.[652] A comprehensive investigation of the different aspects of tumoral immune evasion has shed new light on identifying novel putative mechanisms leading to resistance to ICIs. For instance, reduced MHC class I expression (by an autophagy-dependent fashion) is an important mechanism of resistance and has been reported in other neoplasms as well as PDAC.[653] TGF-β is also implicated in response to ICIs, as its blockade can result in increased PD-L1 expression.[654] CXCL12, mainly produced by FAP+ fibroblasts, is another culprit since the inhibition of one of its receptors named CXCR4 has resulted in the accumulation of T cells and response to anti-PD-L1 therapy.[599] Similarly, preventing the activation of CCR2 will facilitate CD8+ T cell and ICI activation by reducing the recruitment of monocytes.[655] One of the well-studied molecules involved in the induction of extremely fibrotic and T cell-depleted TME of PDAC is focal adhesion kinases (FAK).[656] Like the previously mentioned studies, FAK inhibition has resulted in the restoration of the response to anti-PD-1 therapy in a preclinical model.[656]

Nevertheless, as with other gastrointestinal neoplasms, a subset of pancreatic cancers demonstrates high rates of MSI.[657] Among 22 patients with dMMR/MSI-H pancreatic cancer who participated in the KEYNOTE-158 trial, 4 achieved a response (one CR and three PR) after receiving pembrolizumab.[658] Regarding the similar observations seen in colorectal cancer (discussed earlier), and also high RR reported by another very small trial,[659] now there are several active trials underway to test the activity of ICIs for this subset of patients with PDAC.[660]

### Vaccine therapies

GVAX is an irradiated allogeneic vaccine composed of tumor cells genetically modified to express GM-SCF. The mild activity of this vaccine as adjuvant therapy after surgical resection showed by two phase I and II trials.[661,662] It is also reported that the addition of cyclophosphamide can enhance GVAX anti-tumor activities.[663]

CRS-207 is another cancer vaccine that contains live attenuated *Listeria monocytogenes* expressing mesothelin.[664] Despite early encouraging outcomes,[664,665] compared with chemotherapy, combined GVAX and CRS-207 could not elongate the OS of patients with metastatic PDAC.[666] Other vaccine therapies (for instance, those against CEA, MUC1, Kirsten rat sarcoma virus (KRAS), gastrin, and telomerase) generally have not exhibited robust activities in PDAC.[667-669]

### Other immunotherapies

Failure of ICIs in defeating PDAC has forced clinicians to focus on delineating other constructors of the desmoplastic immunosuppressed TME of pancreatic cancers. As a result, trials now are headed toward targeting metabolic pathways, structural molecules, novel immune checkpoints, and tumor-specific antigens.[660] Moreover, depicting genetic underpinnings of each of these factors might help properly categorize candidates for different immunotherapies.

## Immunolopathology and immunotherapy of endocrine system cancers

It was expected that in 2019, more than 54,000 new cases of endocrine system cancers (including thyroid, parathyroid, adrenal, and endocrine pancreas) might be detected in the United States, accounting for about 3.1 percent of all cancers.[266] More than 95 percent of these patients were expected to have thyroid cancers.[266] Based on pathological findings, thyroid cancers are generally categorized as papillary (85 percent), follicular (2 to 5 percent), anaplastic-poorly differentiated (6 percent), or medullary (3 to 5 percent).[670] The cornerstones of therapy for thyroid cancers are surgery, radioiodine ablation (RAI), and systemic chemotherapy for advanced-stage cases.[670] Fortunately, the five-year survival for these patients is 98 percent. However, about 10 percent of differentiated and most medullary and anaplastic cancers exhibit resistance to therapies, and the survival rate of metastatic disease is around 56 percent.[671] The development of several targeted therapies (e.g., MKIs) has modestly enhanced the survival of such patients,[670] but there is a need for novel therapies against less-differentiated as well as advanced-stage papillary and follicular cancers. Malignancies of other endocrine organs are quite rare, and due to the lack of enough space, are not discussed here.

## Immunopathology

Regarding PD-L1, Tregs extracted from tumoral-involved lymph nodes of patients with papillary thyroid cancer were expressing high amounts of PD-L1 on their surface.[672] It was reported by a study that about 52 percent of patients with papillary thyroid cancer have detectable PD-L1, and it is associated with poorer prognosis,[673] which was also concluded by another study.[674] Another study has linked PD-L1 expression status in papillary thyroid cancer to lymphocytic thyroiditis because 39 percent of such patients were positive for PD-L1, compared with 6.9 percent of those without thyroiditis.[675] However, in contrast to previous reports, this study found no association between PD-L1 expression status and overall prognosis, which might be justified by its relatively small sample size.[675] Like other neoplasms, various immune cells and cytokines can contribute to the tumoral invasion or regression. However, the exact mechanism and prognostic roles of such factors are less studied in thyroid cancers.

## Immunotherapies for thyroid cancers

To our knowledge, to date, there is only one trial of ICIs for thyroid cancer that has published its results.[676] In this phase Ib trial, 22 patients with PD-L1 positive, locally advanced, or metastatic follicular or papillary thyroid cancers enrolled to receive pembrolizumab.[676] After a median follow-up duration of 31 months, two patients (both with papillary thyroid cancer) achieved a response, with a median PFS of 7 months.[676] Although disappointing, definite conclusions should be made after larger phase II and III trials. There are also a relatively small number of trials assessing the efficacy of ICIs, either alone or in combination with other regimens, mainly MKIs (Table 4.12).

## Future perspective

Fortunately, most thyroid cancers are treatment-responsive papillary and follicular carcinoma, but the therapeutic options for metastatic disease and less-differentiated cancers are limited. In addition to assessing the effectiveness of immunotherapies, ongoing trials should focus on defining validated predictive biomarkers for such therapies. Furthermore, as it was shown for lung cancers, immunotherapy as a neoadjuvant modality can potentially synergize with the current standard-of-cares for advanced-stage carcinomas, but the effectiveness of such approaches is yet to be determined.

Table 4.12 Selected ongoing trials evaluating novel immunotherapies for thyroid cancers.

| Agent | Trial identifier | Phase | Indication | Notes |
|---|---|---|---|---|
| Pembrolizumab | NCT02628067 | II | Advanced (non-resectable and/or metastatic) solid tumors | Second-line or later therapy |
| Pembrolizumab | NCT02688608 | II | Anaplastic/undifferentiated thyroid cancer | |
| Pembrolizumab plus lenvatinib | NCT04171622 | II | Advanced-stage anaplastic thyroid cancer | |
| Pembrolizumab plus docetaxel | NCT03360890 | II | Poorly chemo-responsive thyroid and salivary gland tumors | Radiation therapy-refractory and after failure, intolerance to or refusal of anti-antiangiogenic therapy, or with evidence of dedifferentiated or anaplastic histology |
| Nivolumab plus ipilimumab | NCT03246958 | II | Metastatic RAI refractory differentiated thyroid cancer | Exploratory Cohorts in Medullary and Anaplastic Thyroid Cancer |
| Nivolumab, ipilimumab, and cabozantinib | NCT03914300 | II | Advanced differentiated thyroid cancer | Anaplastic thyroid cancer or medullary thyroid cancer are not eligible |
| Atezolizumab plus chemotherapy | NCT03181100 | II | Anaplastic or poorly differentiated thyroid cancer | |
| Atezolizumab plus cabozantinib | NCT04400474 | II | Advanced and progressive neoplasms of the endocrine system, including anaplastic thyroid cancer | |
| Avelumab plus regorafenib | NCT03475953 | II | Radioiodine-refractory differentiated thyroid cancer | |
| Durvalumab plus tremelimumab | NCT03753919 | II | Progressive, refractory advanced thyroid carcinoma | |

*(Continued)*

**Table 4.12** Cont'd

| Agent | Trial identifier | Phase | Indication | Notes |
|---|---|---|---|---|
| AIC100 CAR T-cell | NCT04420754 | II | R/R thyroid cancer | CAR T-cells containing the I domain of LFA-1and targeting its overexpressed physiological ligand, ICAM-1 on thyroid cancer. |
| GI-6207 cancer vaccine | NCT01856920 | II | Recurrent medullary thyroid cancer | Recombinant yeast-based vaccine engineered to express the full-length human carcinoembryonic antigen. |

RAI, radioiodine ablation; R/R, relapsed or refractory; CAR T-cells, chimeric antigen receptor T-cells; LFA-1, lymphocyte function-associated antigen-1; ICAM-1, intercellular adhesion molecule-1.

## Immunolopathology and immunotherapy of urinary system cancers

With more than 158 000 estimated new cases of urinary system cancers in 2019, these neoplasms constitute about 9 percent of all cancers in the United States.[266] The great preponderance of urinary system neoplasms is originated from the kidney and its pelvis (50 percent) and bladder (46 percent).[266] Generally, the prognosis of these two neoplasms is relatively good, and their five-year survival rates are around 75 percent. However, this comes to rates as low as 12 percent and 5 percent for metastatic renal and bladder cancers, respectively.[266]

About 90 percent of all kidney cancers are renal cell carcinoma (RCC), and the remaining are mostly urothelial carcinoma of the renal pelvis.[677] Based on pathological and genetic features, RCCs are further subdivided into various subtypes, with clear-cell RCC (ccRCC, 70 to 90 percent of cases), papillary RCC (pRCC, 10 to 15 percent), and chromophobe RCC (chRCC, 3 to 5 percent) as the most common ones.[678] Well-known risk factors of RCC are obesity, cigarette smoking, and hypertension, but a role for chronic kidney disease, diabetes, and red meat consumption is implicated by some reports.[679] Historically, kidney cancers are recognized as silent tumors, as exhibit no clinical signs and symptoms until the advanced-stage disease, but owing to the growing trends in the acquisition of abdominal imaging (mainly by computed tomography), more renal masses are incidentally detected.[680] This along with advances in developing novel therapeutic techniques has culminated in increased OS of RCC during the past decades.[680] Notwithstanding, still 16 percent of RCCs are detected when have metastasized to distant sites.[266] Surgery is the cornerstone of the treatment of localized and regional RCC.[680] Interestingly, the approach to early-stage disease is now experiencing a shift toward active surveillance for selected cases, which mainly results from observations showing slow growth rates and a low probability of metastasis in such tumors.[680] Metastatic RCC is one of the oldest targets for cancer immunotherapies. In the 1980s, IL-2 and IFN-α started to be administered to those with such tumors.[680] Although these agents did not significantly improve the OS of patients, remained the main therapeutic options for metastatic RCC for many years, and high-dose IL-2 even received FDA approval in 1992.[680] The characterization of the underpinning signaling pathways involved in tumorigenesis of renal neoplasms paved the way for developing novel targeted therapies against PDGFR, VEGFR, receptor tyrosine kinase (c-Kit), and mammalian target of rapamycin (mTOR) that are now approved as the first-line agents against metastatic RCC.[680] However, the short duration of responses is still one of the major drawbacks of these drugs.[680]

Between 90 to 95 percent of bladder cancers are originated from the urothelium lining the inner surface of the bladder.[681] Cigarette smoking is an established risk factor for bladder cancer.[680] Besides, schistosomiasis (associated with squamous cell cancer, which constitutes 10–40 percent of bladder cancers in endemic areas, such as Egypt),[682] diets low in vegetables and high in alcohol,[683,684] occupational exposure to dyes, arsenic, and petroleum,[685,686] and ambient air pollution[685] are all linked to increased risk of developing bladder cancers, although controversies remain.[687] Tumoral invasion of the detrusor muscle is one of the most important determinants of subsequent therapeutic strategies. At diagnosis, about 75 percent of patients have non-muscle-invasive bladder cancer (NMIBC), 20 percent present with muscle-invasive bladder cancer (MIBC), and the remaining 5 percent have the metastatic disease.[681] It is believed that the precursor lesions of NMIBC and MIBC have different genetic and pathological features and are recognized as papillary and non-papillary (solid) tumors, respectively.[688] Papillary tumors harbor del[9] and activating mutations in *FGFR3*, *telomerase reverse transcriptase* (*TERT*), and *PIK3CA*. In contrast, solid tumors show mutations in *TP53*, *RB1*, and *PTEN*, features that are also seen in flat dysplasia and carcinoma in situ of the bladder.[688] Another categorization of bladder cancer is based on the patterns of gene expression and consists of basal and luminal types.[681] The first one usually expresses markers of EMT, upon which metastasis is a usual phenomenon in this type. The basal type is indolent and usually is found in NMIBC. Another important aspect of this classification is the differences seen in their immune cell infiltrations, as discussed later.[681] The common approach to NMIBC is to first classify the disease into three groups according to the various factors, including number, size, grade, and stage of the tumor, the risk of recurrence, and the presence of carcinoma in situ.[688] After the resection of the tumor using transurethral resection of bladder tumor (TURBT), bacillus Calmette-Guérin (BCG) for high and intermediate-risk groups and immediate intravesical chemotherapy (most commonly, mitomycin or doxorubicin) for the low-risk group will be administered.[689] Along with IL-2 for RCC, BCG is one of the earliest immunotherapies approved by the FDA in 1990 for the treatment of bladder cancers and has significantly reduced the risk of tumoral recurrence and progression.[688] Certain high-risk patients and those who fail after adjuvant immunotherapy usually undergo cystectomy. MIBC is managed by radical cystectomy and concurrent pelvic lymphadenectomy.[688] However, about 50 percent of MIBCs will relapse after radical cystectomy, usually in the form of metastatic disease.[690] The five-year survival rate of patients with metastatic disease is less than 15 percent after systemic chemotherapy, which depicts the need for novel, more efficient therapies.[681]

## Immunopathology

### Kidney cancer

A study of 738 resected localized RCC samples has demonstrated that 8.2 percent and 7.6 percent of tumors are positive (defined as tumoral and immune cell PD-1 expression of ≥5 percent) for PD-L1 and PD-1, respectively.[691] For PD-L1 expression, proportions as high as 29 percent are also reported in those with metastatic RCC.[692] In these studies, PD-L1 expression status has been linked to a worse outcome[693] after surgical resection[691] and targeted therapies.[692,694] A recent meta-analysis of 3389 RCC patients has reported the pooled prevalence of PD-L1 positivity as 27 percent that again has been strongly and negatively correlated to the OS, PFS, and cancer-specific survival.[695]

Although ccRCC is recognized as one of the most extensively CD8+ T cell infiltrated neoplasms,[696] but T cells often exhibit an exhausted phenotype, which is thought to result due to alterations in metabolic pathways and expression of immunosuppressive molecules and cytokines, such as VEGF.[697,698] The prognostic value of infiltrating CTLs for ccRCC is interpreted in the presence of other immune cells: high CD8+ T cell/Treg ratio[696] and high CD8+ T cell and mature DC infiltration along with low immune checkpoint expression[699] are associated with a more favorable prognosis. The importance of cytokines in the clinical course of RCC is mainly studied in the milieu of targeted therapies, where high levels of IL-6 and IL-8 have been associated with a shorter PFS.[700] Although the TMB of RCC is not high, it has the highest rate of indel mutations among tumors.[701] Somehow paradoxical, a study has observed high TMB RCCs are less infiltrated with CD8+ T cells and DCs, which has further correlated with a poor prognosis.[702]

### Bladder cancer

The PD-L1 positivity of urothelial bladder cancers is associated with a higher-grade tumor, reduced survival,[703-706] BCG-therapy resistance, and mononuclear cell infiltration.[704] In contrast to these findings, *PD-L1* mRNA expression is reported to be positively correlated to a better outcome for patients with T1 NMIBC.[707] Likewise, the presence of PD-L1 positive infiltrating mononuclear cells (but not cancer cells) can be an indicator of longer survival in patients with metastatic disease.[708] Discouragingly, urothelial bladder cancers are not hot, as about 36 percent of MIBCs are non-T cell inflamed (i.e., lacking expression of PD-L1, TIM-3, LAG-3, IDO, and FOXP3).[709] The impact of CTLs, Tregs, and MDSCs is similar to those of other types of neoplasms, as discussed throughout this chapter.[710-713] The genetic landscape of bladder cancers is quite complicated, and different studies have proposed several models for both NMIBC and MIBC, discussed elsewhere in detail.[688] The prognostic value of such classifications is not fully elucidated yet. However, the identification of certain candidate gene alterations for targeted therapies (e.g., *FGFR3*, *PARPG*, *HER2*, and *EGFR*) have shaped the efforts toward engineering novel therapies.[688] Regarding TMB, urothelial bladder cancer is amongst neoplasms with substantial loads,[361] which can partly explain its relatively high response to ICIs.[714] Also, a study has reported that higher TMB is associated with increased CTL infiltrations and improved survival of affected individuals.[715]

## Immunotherapies for renal cell carcinoma

### *Immune checkpoint inhibitors (ICIs)*

Like most of the advanced-stage neoplasms discussed throughout this chapter, ICIs have yielded most among immunotherapies for RCC. A phase III trial from 2015 (CheckMate 025) showed that compared with everolimus (an mTOR inhibitor), nivolumab administration for patients with advanced ccRCC (previously treated with anti-angiogenic agents) could significantly increase median OS and ORR (irrespective of PD-L1 expression status) with a favorably lower rate of side effects.[693] Intriguingly, the PFS was not different across the total population, but the difference was significantly favored nivolumab arm among those who had no disease progression or death at 6 months,[693] which is in concordance with the delayed responses to immunotherapies seen in other cancers (discussed earlier) and ccRCC.[716] Recently, the results of the extended follow-up (minimum of 64 months) of this trial were published and are in concordance with the previous reports.[717] Importantly, five-year OS probabilities have been 26 percent and 18 percent, respectively, and nivolumab has inferred an increment in the median survival by 6.1 months. In addition, PFS has remained in favor of nivolumab (HR, 0.84; 95 percent CI, 0.72–0.99; $P$ = 0.0331).[717]

Subsequently, first-line combination therapy with nivolumab and ipilimumab resulted in higher OS and overall response among patients with advanced ccRCC with intermediate- and poor-risk diseases (based on International etastatic Renal Cell Carcinoma Database Consortium (IMDC)), as compared with sunitinib.[716] Such benefits were observed across all PD-L1 expression groups but were higher among those with at least 1 percent expression level. Notably, a benefit from sunitinib in improving overall response and PFS was observed among patients with the favorable-risk disease, although it was not significant and definitive interpretations were limited by the low sample size of such patients.[716] The findings of the extended follow-up of these patients were consistent with previous results, with the addition of significantly prolonged PFS observed for the combination therapy group.[694] Furthermore, the outperformance of sunitinib for favorable-risk patients became less prominent than the preliminary analysis. Finally, a worrisome caveat revealed by this study was greater death rates among the combination therapy group (8 versus 4 deaths).[694]

Regarding combination therapies, another phase III trial demonstrated the superiority of first-line avelumab and axitinib combination therapy over sunitinib in improving ORR and PFS of advanced ccRCC patients.[718] Similar prominent outcomes, in addition to enhanced OS, were also described for pembrolizumab plus axitinib frontline therapy, compared with sunitinib.[719] Notably, the efficacy of these combined immunotherapies has been observed across all groups of PD-L1 expression status and prognostic risk groups (according to Memorial Sloan Kettering Cancer Center (MSKCC) and IMDC criteria).[718,719]

Despite these encouraging results, ICI-based combination therapies have not always ended up in robust outcomes. For instance, the added benefit of frontline atezolizumab and bevacizumab combination therapy over sunitinib was limited to enhanced PFS of patients with a PD-L1 expression of at least 1 percent.[720] Interestingly, this study found that tumors harboring a sarcomatoid histology component show a substantial response to dual therapy, which was observed across all PD-L1 expression groups.[720] Better responses of RCCs with sarcomatoid features to ICIs are also described in the CheckMate 214 trial.[694,721] Besides, this post-hoc analysis found a higher prevalence of tumors with PD-L1 expression ≥1 percent among those with sarcomatoid features, compared with the total pool of samples.[721]

Most clinical trials of ICIs are conducted for patients with ccRCC, and little is known about their efficacy in non-clear cell renal cell carcinoma (nccRCC). As an example, the first-line pembrolizumab for advanced nccRCC culminated in ORRs of 25.4 percent for papillary, 9.5 percent for chromophobe, and 34.6 percent for unclassified subtypes.[722] Notably, 33.3 percent of patients with CPS ≥1 percent achieved a response, compared with only 10.3 percent of cases with CPS <1.[722] A small retrospective study on metastatic nccRCC cases who received nivolumab revealed that 20 percent showed a PR and 29 percent achieved stable disease, mostly seen for unclassified, papillary, and collecting duct subtypes.[723] These data suggest the effectiveness of ICIs for nccRCC too, which is now being tested by some ongoing trials (Table 4.14).

Taking the PD-L1 expression status as a biomarker for response to ICIs has shown to be inconclusive by different trials. Generally, problems such as different measurement methods, heterogeneity in the expression across tumoral tissue,[724] and variable expression in the primary and metastatic sites leading to sampling bias,[724] temporal alterations in the level of expression,[725] and more importantly, its potential effects on the overall prognosis of RCC patients (discussed earlier) prevent establishing PD-L1 expression status as a predictive biomarker. The importance of other commonly recognized biomarkers is not fully delineated in the field of RCC. The IMmotion 150 was a Phase II trial for the evaluation of atezolizumab alone or in combination with bevacizumab versus sunitinib for advanced treatment-naïve RCC.[726] At the end of the study, it was revealed that TMB and neoantigen burden do not alter the PFS, whereas angiogenic, effector T cells and myeloid inflammatory gene expression signatures are significantly associated with enhanced PFS in response to anti-VEGF, anti-PD-L1, and combination therapy, respectively.[726] However, the subsequent phase III IMmotion 151 trial only reported a positive association between effector T cell gene signature and improved OS after combined atezolizumab and bevacizumab therapy.[720] Analysis of patients enrolled in JAVELIN Renal 101 trial[718] demonstrated the positive impact of an immunologic gene expression signature (consisted of genes involved in effector and inflamed T cells, angiogenesis, and pathways related to T- and NK-cell activation and IFN-γ signaling) on PFS after administration of avelumab combined with axitinib.[727] In addition, no impact was found for TMB as a predictor of PFS.[727]

It also should be noted that, like other trials of ICIs, the pre-specified amendments for enrollment in ICI trials for RCC include a good performance status and the absence of active CNS metastases. Together, the robust performance of ICI-based combination therapies has led to a striking transformation in the therapeutic armamentarium of advanced RCC. The list of current FDA-approved ICIs for the treatment of RCC is provided in Table 4.13.

### *Future perspective*

Now several phase III trials are testing the efficacy of combination ICIs with targeted therapies as adjuvant or even neoadjuvant regimens for localized or advanced ccRCC and nccRCC (Table 4.14). IMA901 is a cancer vaccine containing nine HLA class

**Table 4.13** List of FDA-approved immune checkpoint inhibitors (ICIs) for the treatment of renal cell carcinoma (RCC).

| Agent | Indication | Trial |
|---|---|---|
| Avelumab | In combination with axitinib, as the frontline therapy for advanced RCC | JAVELIN Renal 101[694] |
| Pembrolizumab | In combination with axitinib, as the frontline therapy for advanced RCC | KEYNOTE-426[728] |
| Ipilimumab plus nivolumab | As first-line combination therapy for intermediate- or poor-risk, advanced RCC | CheckMate 214[716] |
| Nivolumab | Asthe second-line therapy for advanced RCC, after the disease progression on at least one anti-angiogenic agent | CheckMate 025[729] |

RCC, renal cell carcinoma.

**Table 4.14** List of selected ongoing trials of novel immunotherapies for renal cell carcinoma (RCC).

| Agent (s) | Trial identifier | Phase | Indications | Notes |
|---|---|---|---|---|
| **Advanced or metastatic ccRCC** | | | | |
| Nivolumab plus cabozantinib vs sunitinib | NCT03141177 | III | As the first-line therapy for advanced/metastatic RCC | ccRCC,including those with sarcomatoid features, are eligible. Based on interim analyses, the trial has met its primary and secondary endpoints in improving ORR, PFS, and OS[732]. |
| Nivolumab plus ipilimumab and cabozantinib vs nivolumab plus ipilimumab | NCT03937219 | III | As the first-line therapy for advanced/metastatic ccRCC with intermediate- or poor-risk disease | |
| **Adjuvant setting** | | | | |
| Nivolumab vs nivolumab plus ipilimumab vs placebo | NCT03138512 | III | As adjuvant therapy for localized RCC after radical or partial nephrectomy and high risk of relapse | patients with RCC with predominantly clear cell histology, including sarcomatoid features, are included. |
| Atezolizumab vs placebo | NCT03024996 | III | As adjuvant therapy for non-metastatic RCC after radical or partial nephrectomy and high risk of recurrence/metastasis | Patients with RCC with a component of either clear cell histology or sarcomatoid histology that has not been previously treated in the adjuvant or neoadjuvant setting are included |
| Pembrolizumab vs placebo | NCT03142334 | III | As adjuvant therapy after radical or partial nephrectomy and presence of intermediate-high risk, high risk, or "M1 with NED" RCC | RCC with clear cell components with or without sarcomatoid features is included. |

| Agent (s) | Trial identifier | Phase | Indications | Notes |
|---|---|---|---|---|
| Durvalumab plus tremelimumab vs durvalumab vs placebo | NCT03288532 | III | As adjuvant therapy for localized RCC after radical or partial nephrectomy and intermediate or high risk of relapse | All cell types of RCC are eligible, except for pure oncocytoma, collecting duct, medullary and transitional cell cancer. |
| **Neoadjuvant setting** | | | | |
| Nivolumab | NCT03055013 | III | Nivolumab administration and then partial or radical nephrectomy of RCC, 7 to 28 days after the final round | |
| **Non-clear-cell RCC** | | | | |
| Nivolumab plus Ipilimumab | NCT02982954 | IIIb/IV | Previously untreated, advanced, or metastatic RCC | patients with nccRCC with KPS ≥70 percent and RCC regardless of any histology or existing non-active brain metastasis, with KPS 50 percent–60 percent, are also included. |
| Nivolumab plus ipilimumab vs sunitinib | NCT03075423 | II | Previously untreated, advanced (unresectable or metastatic) nccRCC | At least 50 percent non-clear cell component according to actual WHO classification is needed. Patients with active brain metastases requiring corticosteroids are excluded. |
| **Combination therapy of ICI with other novel immunotherapies** | | | | |
| Nivolumab plus NKTR-214 (bempegaldesleukin) and other agents | NCT02983045 | I | Advanced RCC and other solid tumors | |
| Nivolumab plus NKTR-214 (bempegaldesleukin) vs sunitinib or cabozantinib | NCT03729245 | III | Previously untreated advanced RCC | RCCs with a clear-cell component, with or without sarcomatoid features are included. |

*(Continued)*

**Table 4.14** Cont'd

| Agent (s) | Trial identifier | Phase | Indications | Notes |
|---|---|---|---|---|
| Durvalumab plus tremelimumab and personalized neoantigen DNA vaccine | NCT03598816 | II | As the second or third-line therapy for advanced metastatic RCC | |
| Neovax (personalized neoantigen cancer vaccine combined with poly-ICLC) plus ipilimumab | NCT02950766 | I | High-risk RCC | |
| GEN-009 (personalized cancer vaccine combined with poly-ICLC) in combination with nivolumab or pembrolizumab | NCT03633110 | I/Ia | Advanced RCC who with prior anti-angiogenic therapy, or treatment-naïve intermediate or poor-risk RCC based on the IMDC | |

RCC, renal cell carcinoma; ccRCC, clear-cell renal cell carcinoma; ORR, objective response rate; PFS, progression-free survival; OS, overall survival; NED, no evidence of disease; nccRCC, non-clear cell renal cell carcinoma; KPS, Karnofsky Performance Status Scale; WHO, world health organization; ICI, immune checkpoint inhibitor; IMDC, International metastatic renal-cell carcinoma database consortium.

I and one HLA class II binding tumor-associated peptides.[730] Although the results of a phase II trial of IMA901 were promising, the phase III trial (IMPRINT) did not show any added value of its combination therapy with sunitinib versus sunitinib monotherapy in the first-line setting for advanced RCC.[730] Another trial examining the combination therapy of autologous tumor lysate DC vaccine with IL-2, IFN-α, and bevacizumab for advanced RCC was terminated due to low efficacy (NCT00913913). Generally, cancer vaccines, including DC-based (NCT00050323) and anti-von Hippel-Lindau (VHL) (NCT00001703) ones have not been successful in treating RCC. Hence, trials of novel personalized vaccines are now underway to evaluate their effectiveness for this malignancy. NKTR-214 (also known as bempegaldesleukin) is a novel CD122 agonist that acts via stimulation of IL-2 related pathways, leading to enhanced proliferation and activation of CTLs and NK cells.[731] NKTR-214 combined with nivolumab is being tested for patients with advanced RCC (Table 4.14).

## Immunotherapies for bladder cancer

### *Immune checkpoint inhibitors (ICIs)*

Unlike RCC, to date, there are only three phase III randomized trials that have explored the efficacy of ICIs for bladder cancers.[733-735] It is also important to consider that these trials have been conducted on patients with locally advanced or metastatic urothelial carcinoma that mostly but not exclusively originates from the bladder (other sites of origin include ureter, urethra, and renal pelvis).

The first phase III trial in 2017 (KEYNOTE-045) met one of its primary endpoints. Compared with the investigator's choice of chemotherapy (vinflunine, paclitaxel, or docetaxel), pembrolizumab significantly increased OS (and also ORR) of patients who had progressive disease after receiving platinum-based chemotherapy. This was achieved regardless of the PD-L1 expression level. However, PFS did not differ significantly between the two arms.[733] Later in 2018, phase III IMvigor211, with similar inclusion criteria and chemotherapeutic regimens to the KEYNOTE-045 trial, failed to prove the superiority of atezolizumab in increasing OS and ORR of patients with PD-L1 IC ≥5 percent.[734] This was in contrast to the descriptions of cohort 2 of the phase II IMvigor210 trial[736] and made the FDA put new restrictions on the indications for atezolizumab administration against advanced urothelial carcinoma.[737] Notwithstanding, atezolizumab is still considered eligible by the FDA for certain subgroups of these patients (Table 4.15).[738] The results of the IMvigor130 trial published recently, revealing the effectiveness of frontline combination therapy with atezolizumab and platinum-based chemotherapy over their monotherapies in prolonging PFS of patients with locally advanced or metastatic urothelial carcinoma.[735]

Putting phase III trials aside, there are several phase I and II trials with promising outcomes out of ICI therapy for advanced urothelial cancers (discussed elsewhere in detail[739]). Of note, the FDA approval of some ICIs is based on these phase II trials (Table 4.15). Hence, it is not unexpected that the current approvals might change substantially as more mature outcomes will be published by phase III trials.

### *Future perspective*

There are now several large phase III trials aiming to determine the performance of ICIs, either alone or in combination with each other or chemotherapeutic regimens, in patients with advanced urothelial carcinomas (NCT02603432, NCT03036098, and NCT02516241). Among numerous novel immunotherapies, anti-B7-H3 (enoblituzumab, also known as MGA271, in NCT01391143 and NCT02475213), anti-CD3 bispecific antibody (MGD009, NCT02628535), and combination therapy of atezolizumab plus recombinant human IL-7 (CYT107, NCT03513952) are remarkable ones being under investigation for urothelial carcinoma and other tumors in phase I trials. As briefly mentioned, the immunogenetic of urothelial cancers are quite intricate, and numerous dark sides are yet to be elucidated. What is currently apparent is that ICIs solely will

**Table 4.15** List of the FDA-approved immune checkpoint inhibitors (ICIs) for the treatment of urothelial carcinomas.

| Agent | Indications | Trial |
|---|---|---|
| Avelumab | As a maintenance therapy for patients with locally advanced or metastatic urothelial carcinoma that has not progressed with frontline platinum-based chemotherapy. | JAVELIN Bladder 100 (NCT02603432, official results are not published yet) |
| Avelumab | For patients with locally advanced or metastatic urothelial carcinoma who have disease progression during or following platinum-containing chemotherapy or within 12 months of treatment with a platinum-containing neoadjuvant or adjuvant chemotherapy. | JAVELIN Solid Tumor[740] |
| Nivolumab | Same as above | CheckMate 275[741] |
| Durvalumab | Same as above | NCT01693562[742] |
| Atezolizumab | Patients with locally advanced or metastatic who:<br>Are ineligible for cisplatin-containing therapy, and have IC PD-L1 ≥5 percent; or<br>Are not eligible for any platinum-containing therapy, regardless of PD-L1 expression status. | Cohort 1 of IMvigor210[738] |
| Pembrolizumab | Patients with locally advanced or metastatic who:<br>Are ineligible for cisplatin-containing therapy and have CPS PD-L1 ≥10 percent; or<br>Are ineligible for any platinum-containing chemotherapy regardless of PD-L1 expression status; or<br>Have disease progression during or following treatment with platinum-containing chemotherapy, or within 12 months of neoadjuvant or adjuvant therapy with platinum-containing chemotherapy. | KEYNOTE-052[743]<br>KEYNOTE-045[733] |
| Pembrolizumab | Highrisk, NMIBC with carcinoma in situ, with or without papillary tumors, which is unresponsive to Bacillus Calmette-Guérin and is not eligible for cystectomy. | KEYNOTE-057[744] |

IC, immune cell; PD-L1, programmed death ligand 1; CPS, combined Positive Score; NMIBC, non-muscle-invasive bladder cancer.

not substantially change the treatment armamentarium of urothelial cancers. The best example is enfortumab vedotin, an antibody-drug conjugate against Nectin-4, which received FDA approval for being used by patients with advanced/metastatic urothelial carcinoma who have received platinum-containing chemotherapy and an anti-PD-1 or anti-PD-L1 antibody.[745] Therefore, developing strategies devoted to clarifying eligibility criteria (including predictive biomarkers) and illustrating protocols of combination therapies are desired for future efforts.

## Immunolopathology and immunotherapy of skin cancers

It was expected that in 2019, melanomas of the skin (cutaneous melanoma) might be detected in 5.4 percent of American patients who are newly diagnosed with cancer.[266] Data from the 2008–14 time period demonstrate that about 84 percent of melanomas are first detected in the localized form, while regional and distant diseases constitute 9 percent and 4 percent of all cases, respectively.[266] These statistics translate into favorable survival rates. In the same period, the five-year survival rate of all stages of cutaneous melanomas has been 92 percent. The five-year survival rates are disaggregated to 98 percent for localized, 64 percent for regional, and 23 percent for distant forms.[266] Uncommonly, melanomas can arise from sites other than the skin, including mucosal melanomas of the oral and nasal cavity, upper esophagus, anogenital area, and also meningeal and uveal melanomas which can be found in a small subset of patients.[746]

Exposure to the ultraviolet radiation emitted from the sun (and also tanning beds), the existence of melanocytic, dysplastic, or giant congenital nevi, light pigmentation of the skin, and fair skin phenotype are known risk factors contributing to the development of melanoma.[747] The first phase of the malignant proliferation of melanocytes gives rise to the radial growth, from which different traditional clinicopathological subtypes can be derived, including superficial spreading, the most common subtype (50–70 percent) that usually is seen in sun-exposed areas stemming from a precursor melanocytic nevus, the indolent lentigo maligna (10 percent), nodular that is an aggressive subtype with minimal radial growth (10–30 percent), acral lentiginous (30 percent) that is considered as a subtype unrelated to the sun exposure, and desmoplastic melanoma, with characteristic neuronal invasion and fibrotic reactions.[748]

Melanomas are the first among all cancers that have achieved FDA approval for the administration of ICIs. Based on the results of a landmark trial conducted by Hodi and colleagues,[749] in 2011 FDA approved ipilimumab for stage III and IV unresectable melanoma. Since then, numerous large-scale trials have evaluated the effectiveness of a variety of combination therapies and even different ICIs against each other, upon which solid predictive biomarkers and inclusion criteria have been generated.

Basal cell carcinoma (BCC) and cutaneous squamous cell carcinoma (CSCC) are the most diagnosed malignancies worldwide and comprise almost all cases of non-melanoma skin cancer (NMSC). Most cases of these neoplasms are facilely managed by wide excision and, therefore, are not documented in cancer registries, which estimates their incidence inconvenient.[266] According to the latest predictions, more than 4.3 million cases of BCC and one million cases of CSCC are diagnosed in the United States each year.[750] BCCs very rarely metastasize, their five-year cure rate is near 100 percent,[751] and therefore, are not discussed here anymore. CSCCs generally proffer a good prognosis, and their five-year cure rate can reach 98 percent with the Mohs micrographic surgical technique.[752] However, there is a small but considerable chance of metastasis. For instance, a prospective study found that 4 percent of CSCCs with a thickness between 2.1 to 6 mm, and 16 percent of those with more than 6 mm in thickness metastasized.[753] Other features related to the increased probability of metastasis are immunosuppressive state, radiation exposure, an origin from burn scars, greater horizontal size, localization of the lesions at ear, invasive Bowen's disease, and de novo lesions.[753,754] In recent years, metastatic CSCC has been studied by some trials as a potential candidate for immunotherapies.

Merkel cell carcinoma (MCC) is an uncommon neuroendocrine tumor of the skin (in the United States, 2000 new cases are diagnosed each year),[755] which infers a less favored prognosis compared with other skin cancers.[756] ICIs have earned triumphs in hampering the aggressive behavior of this cancer and are almost the only effective therapeutic options for metastatic MCC. However, due to the lack of enough space, immunotherapies for MCC[756,757] and CSCC[758-760] will not be discussed here.

## Immunopathology

Based on various reports, between 30 percent to 40 percent of metastatic cutaneous melanomas have a PD-L1 expression level of ≥5 percent.[761,762] When the cutoff is 1 percent, proportions as high as 72 percent are reported.[763] Like other tumors, there are discrepancies in PD-L1 expression levels across tumoral tissue and between primary and metastatic sites.[763,764] The role of PD-L1 expression status in predicting response to ICI therapy is extensively studied by different trials and retrospective studies, and as expected, the conclusions are in absolute discordance. Although it is stated as a valid predictor of overall response, OS, and PFS,[747] until the development of sound criteria, the patient selection for ICI therapy should not be based on the sole PD-L1 expression status. What is clear now is that the expression of immune checkpoints is strongly correlated to the infiltration densities of immune cells, important determinants of the response to ICIs.[763,764]

Efforts are now toward unraveling the different determinants of PD-L1 expression and the mechanisms behind resistance to ICI therapy. For example, in a preclinical melanoma model, continuous activation of the WNT/β-catenin pathway could result in the depletion of infiltrating DCs and CTLs, upon which resistance to ICIs would appear.[765] Further, the administration of a small-molecule tankyrase inhibitor (G007-LK) for a mouse melanoma model has resulted in the reversal of anti-PD-1 resistance and enhanced IFN-γ and CTL mediated anti-tumor responses.[766]

PD-L1 can also be expressed on the surface of exosomes (exoPD-L1). In a cohort of metastatic melanoma patients, responders to anti-PD-1 therapy had significantly higher levels of exoPD-L1 early after the initiation of therapy,[767] making it an attractive candidate for further investigations for identifying predictive biomarkers for ICIs. It is also reported that metastatic melanoma cases who receive anti-PD-1 antibody and have higher baseline levels of serum PD-1 and PD-L1 achieve significantly higher PFS and OS, respectively.[768] LAG-3, another immune checkpoint, can be found on the surface of T cells[769] and plasmacytoid DCs[770] infiltrating melanomas and are being tested as other targets for immunotherapies (discussed later). Likewise, TIM-3 can be detected on the melanoma TILs and seems to be co-expressed with PD-1.[771]

The role of immune cell infiltrates in bridling the behavior of malignant melanocytes is well established. Higher accumulation of B cells, CTLs, and other T cells is linked to enhanced survival of patients with metastatic melanoma.[772,773] Similarly, the presence of PD-1 or PD-L1 expressing CTLs with a more clonal receptor repertoire within and on the invasive brink of tumors can predict the response to ICIs.[774]

Historically, the genetic alterations of melanomas related to ultraviolet were separated into two different signatures, and each was associated with an exclusive pattern of ultraviolet exposure.[747] Early, intermittent ultraviolet exposure in those with a tendency to develop nevi would result in *BRAF* mutations, while chronic sun exposure would induce mutations in *N-RAS*.[747] Besides, ultraviolet-related melanomas usually harbor characteristic C > T transitions.[775] More recently, TCGA has divided melanomas into 4 genetic subgroups: *BRAF* mutated (52 percent), *RAS* (including *H-*, *K-*, and *N-RAS*) mutated (28 percent), NF1 mutated (14 percent), and the triple wild-type subtype (6 percent).[773] In addition, three transcriptomic subgroups (immune, keratin, and melanocyte lineage-specific oncogene (MITF)-low) were defined, and as expected, the presence of the immune subgroups was a predictor of a favorable survival. Furthermore, this analysis found that higher expression of lymphocyte-specific protein tyrosine kinase (LCK), a protein involved in T cell signaling pathways, is another predictor of enhanced survival.[773] Of note, Melanomas have one of the highest mutational loads among all cancers,[361,775] which partially accounts for their robust response to ICIs. In recent years, the attempts have deviated toward altering the genetic regulators of the expression of cancer-related immunologic molecules. Such strategies have gained success in down-regulating PD-L1 expression.[776,777]

The therapeutic landscape of advanced-stage melanoma has changed substantially in recent years, owing to the delineation of their exquisite genetic, molecular, and immunologic features upon which multiple targeted therapies (e.g., BRAF, mitogen-activated protein kinase (MEK), and KIT inhibitors) and immunotherapies have gained approval for the treatment of such tumors (Fig. 4.4).

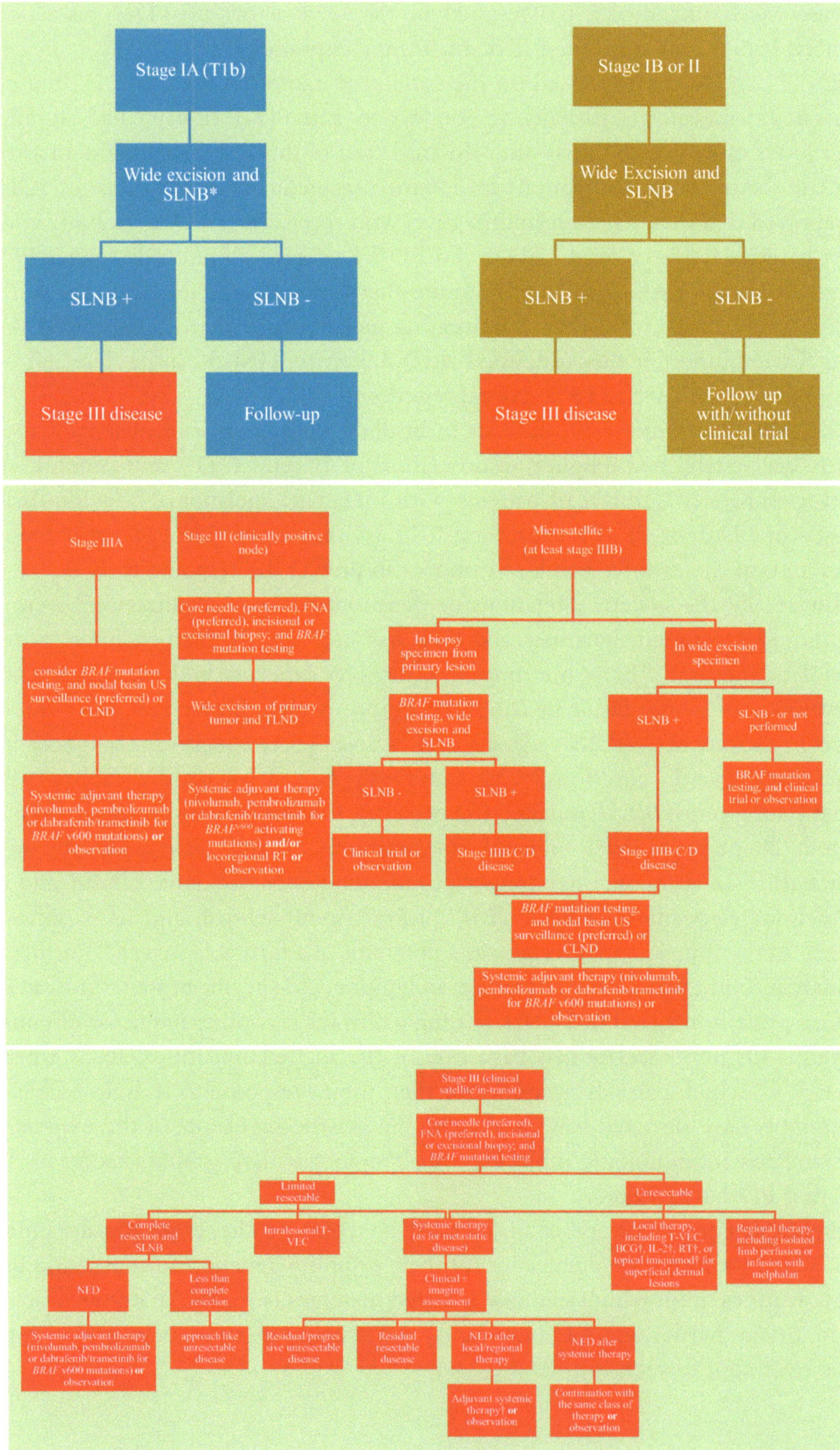
Stage IA (T1b)
Wide excision and SLNB*
SLNB +
SLNB -
Stage III disease
Follow-up
Stage IB or II
Wide Excision and SLNB
SLNB +
SLNB -
Stage III disease
Follow up with/without clinical trial
Stage IIIA
consider BRAF mutation testing, and nodal basin US surveillance (preferred) or CLND
Systemic adjuvant therapy (nivolumab, pembrolizumab or dabrafenib/trametinib for BRAF v600 mutations) or observation
Stage III (clinically positive node)
Core needle (preferred), FNA (preferred), incisional or excisional biopsy; and BRAF mutation testing
Wide excision of primary tumor and TLND
Systemic adjuvant therapy (nivolumab, pembrolizumab or dabrafenib/trametinib for BRAF v600 activating mutations) and/or locoregional RT or observation
Microsatellite + (at least stage IIIB)
In biopsy specimen from primary lesion
BRAF mutation testing, wide excision and SLNB
SLNB -
SLNB +
Clinical trial or observation
Stage IIIB/C/D disease
In wide excision specimen
SLNB +
SLNB - or not performed
BRAF mutation testing, and clinical trial or observation
Stage IIIB/C/D disease
BRAF mutation testing, and nodal basin US surveillance (preferred) or CLND
Systemic adjuvant therapy (nivolumab, pembrolizumab or dabrafenib/trametinib for BRAF v600 mutations) or observation
Stage III (clinical satellite/in-transit)
Core needle (preferred), FNA (preferred), incisional or excisional biopsy; and BRAF mutation testing
Limited resectable
Unresectable
Complete resection and SLNB
Intralesional T-VEC
Systemic therapy (as for metastatic disease)
Local therapy, including T-VEC, BCG†, IL-2†, RT†, or topical imiquimod† for superficial dermal lesions
Regional therapy, including isolated limb perfusion or infusion with melphalan
NED
Less than complete resection
Clinical + imaging assessment
Systemic adjuvant therapy (nivolumab, pembrolizumab or dabrafenib/trametinib for BRAF v600 mutations) or observation
approach like unresectable disease
Residual/progressive unresectable disease
Residual resectable dusease
NED after local/regional therapy
NED after systemic therapy
Adjuvant systemic therapy† or observation
Continuation with the same class of therapy or observation

*(Continued)*

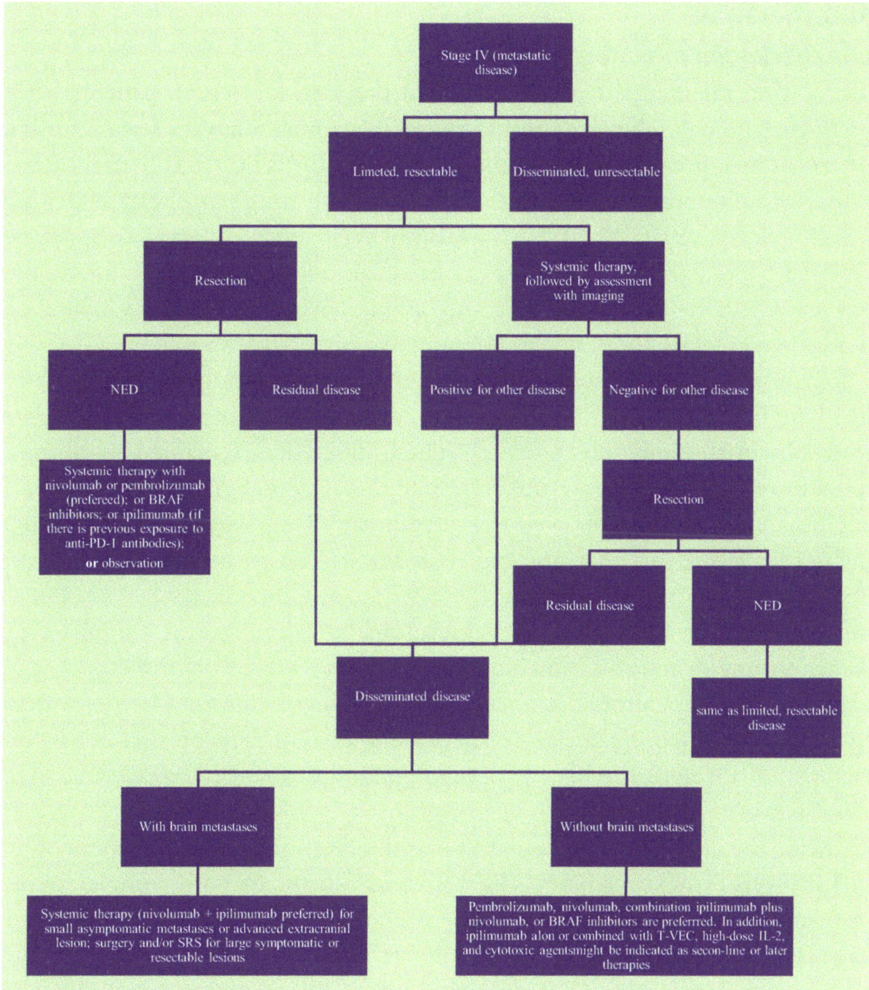


**Fig. 4.4** ***Simplified algorithm for the treatment of stage II, III, and IV melanomas.*** Designed based on the guidelines.[747,826-828] Note that the algorithms are based on the eighth Edition of the American Joint Committee on Cancer (AJCC) staging system. However, protocols of most trials have been based on the seventh Edition.

**Sentinel lymph node biopsy is recommended for lesions >1 mm thick and lesions 0.75–1 mm thick with high-risk features (e.g., ulceration or lymphovascular invasion).*

*†Not recommended as the first-line option.*

SLNB, sentinel lymph node biopsy; US, ultrasound; CLND, completion lymph node dissection; FNA, fine needle aspiration; TLND, therapeutic lymph node dissection; SRS, stereotactic radiosurgery; T-VEC, Talimogene laherparepvec; NED, no evidence of disease; RT, radiation therapy.

## Immunotherapies

### *Immune checkpoint inhibitors (ICIs)*

ICIs are now an integral part of the treatment program for certain patients with stage III and IV melanoma (Table 4.17 and Fig. 4.4). Regarding adjuvant setting for stage III and IV melanoma, five-year follow-up of patients in EORTC 18,071 trial showed the superiority of ipilimumab (10 mg/kg) over placebo in improving relapse-free survival (RFS, 40.8 percent versus 30.3 percent; HR for recurrence or death, 0.76; 95 percent CI, 0.64–0.89; $p < 0.001$), OS (65.4 percent versus 54.4 percent; HR for death, 0.72; 95.1 percent CI, 0.58–0.88; $p = 0.001$), and distant metastasis-free survival (48.3 percent versus 38.9 percent; HR for death or distant metastasis, 0.76; 95.8 percent CI, 0.64–0.92; $p = 0.002$) of patients with surgically resected stage III melanoma with metastasis to regional lymph nodes.[778] However, these outcomes came at the cost of five immune-related deaths in the ipilimumab arm.[778] These differences remained significant even after a median of 6.9 years follow-up.[779] Despite these encouraging outcomes, the results of the CheckMate 238 trial showed that nivolumab (3 mg/kg) could outperform ipilimumab (10 mg/kg) in enhancing one-year RFS (70.5 percent versus 60.8 percent; HR for disease recurrence or death, 0.65; 97.56 percent CI, 0.51–0.83; $p < 0.001$) of patients with stage IIIB, IIIC, or IV melanoma who underwent complete regional lymphadenectomy or resection (including those with resected brain metastases), with a remarkably better safety profile (rate of grade three or more AEs, 14.4 percent vs 45.9 percent, treatment discontinuation in 9.7 percent vs 42.6 percent, two deaths in ipilimumab arm).[780] Of note, the benefit of nivolumab was observed irrespective of *BRAF* mutation status.[780]

Following the effectiveness of anti-PD-1 antibodies, long-term follow-up of patients enrolled in EORTC 1325/KEYNOTE-057 trial[781] (patients with completely resected stage IIIA melanoma with a high risk of recurrence, i.e., sentinel node diameter >1 mm, and stage IIIB or IIIC (without in-transit metastasis)) showed that after a median follow-up of 3 years, pembrolizumab (200 mg) could still significantly elongate RFS among the overall population (64 percent for pembrolizumab versus 44 percent for placebo; HR, 0.56; 95 percent CI, 0.47–0.68) and those with PD-L1 positive status (65 percent versus 46 percent; HR, 0.57; 95 percent CI, 0.43–0.74).[782]

For the neoadjuvant setting, the data are generally limited to small phase I and II trials. In 2018, findings of a randomized, noncomparative phase II trial of neoadjuvant combination therapy with ipilimumab and nivolumab or nivolumab alone were published.[783] The combination therapy resulted in an ORR of 73 percent and a pCR of 45 percent, but as expected, caused grade three or more AEs in 73 percent of patients. Also, nivolumab monotherapy led to ORRs and pCRs of 25 percent, with only 8 percent grade three or more AEs.[783] As expected, responders exhibited higher immune cell infiltrations after neoadjuvant therapy.[783] A phase I study reported that single-dose pembrolizumab as neoadjuvant therapy for patients with resectable stage III/IV melanoma

**Table 4.16** Randomized trials on the effect of immune checkpoint inhibitors (ICIs) in the palliative therapy of melanoma. Reprinted with permission from[747].

| Trial identifier | Design | Treatment groups and regimen | Overall response rate (percent percent) | Duration of response (median, months) | Progression-free survival (PFS) (median, months) | Overall survival (OS) (median, months) |
|---|---|---|---|---|---|---|
| Hodiet al. (2010)[749] | Pretreated patients; double-blind, phase 3 trial | Ipilimumab 3 mg per kg + gp100 ($n = 403$) vs ipilimumab 3 mg per kg ($n = 137$) vs gp100 ($n = 136$) | 5.7 percent vs 11.0 percent vs 1.5 percent, $p = 0.04$ | 11.5 months vs not reached vs not reached | Ipilimumab + gp100 2.76 months (HR vs gp100 0.81, $p < 0.05$); ipilimumab 2.86 months (HR vs gp100 0.64, $p < 0.001$); gp100 2.76 months | Ipilimumab + gp100 10.0 months (HR vs gp100 0.68, $p < 0.001$); ipilimumab 10.1 months (HR vs gp100 0.66, $p = 0.003$); gp100 6.4 months |
| Robertet al. (2011)[785] | Untreated patients; double-blind, phase 3 trial | Ipilimumab 10 mg per kg + dacarbazine ($n = 250$) vs placebo + dacarbazine ($n = 252$) | 15.2 percent vs 10.3 percent, $p = 0.09$ | 19.3 months vs 8.1 months, $p = 0.03$ | Median survival in both groups similar, HR 0.76, $p < 0.006$ in favor of ipilimumab + dacarbazine | 11.2 months vs 9.1 months, HR 0.72, $p < 0.001$ |
| Asciertoet al. (2017)[786] | Pretreated and untreated patients; double-blind, phase 3 trial (CA184-169) | Ipilimumab 10 mg per kg ($n = 364$) vs ipilimumab 3 mg per kg ($n = 362$) | 15 percent vs 12 percent | •• | 2.8 months vs 2.8 months, HR 0.89, $p = 0.16$ | 15.7 months vs 11.5 months, HR 0.84, $p = 0.04$ |
| Ribaset al. (2013)[787] | Untreated patients; open-label, phase 3 trial | Tremelimumab ($n = 328$) vs chemotherapy ($n = 327$) | 10.7 percent vs 9.8 percent | 35.8 months vs 13.7 months, $p = 0.0011$ | •• | 12.6 months vs 10.7 months, HR 0.88, $p = 0.127$ |

(Continued)

**Table 4.16** Cont'd

| Trial identifier | Design | Treatment groups and regimen | Overall response rate (percent percent) | Duration of response (median, months) | Progression-free survival (PFS) (median, months) | Overall survival (OS) (median, months) |
|---|---|---|---|---|---|---|
| Robertet al. (2015)[788] | Untreated patients (with melanoma without *BRAF* mutation); double-blind, phase 3 trial (Checkmate 66) | Nivolumab ($n = 210$) vs dacarbazine ($n = 208$) | 40.0 percent vs 13.9 percent, $p < 0.001$ | Not reached vs 6.0 months | 5.1 months vs 2.2 months, HR 0.43, $p < 0.001$ | Not reached vs 10.8 months, HR 0.42, $p < 0.001$ |
| Weberet al. (2015)[789] and Larkin et al. (2018)[790] | Patients pretreated with ipilimumab and *BRAF* inhibitor; open-label, phase 3 trial (Checkmate 37) | Nivolumab ($n = 272$) vs chemotherapy ($n = 133$) | 27 percent vs 10 percent | 31.9 months vs 12.8 months | 3.1 months vs 3.7 months, HR 1.0 | 15.7 months vs 14.4 months, HR 0.95 |
| Weberet al. (2016)[791] | Untreated and pretreated patients; open-label, phase 2 trial (Checkmate 64) | Nivolumab followed by ipilimumab ($n = 68$) vs ipilimumab followed by nivolumab ($n = 70$) | 56 percent vs 31 percent | not reached vs not reached | •• | Not reached vs 16.9 months, HR 0.48 |
| Larkinet al. (2015)[792] and Wolchok et al. (2017)[793] | Untreated patients; double-blind, phase 3 trial (Checkmate 67) | Nivolumab + ipilimumab ($n = 314$) vs nivolumab ($n = 316$) vs ipilimumab ($n = 315$) | 58 percent vs 44 percent vs 19 percent | not reached vs not reached vs 19.3 months | Nivolumab + ipilimumab 11.5 months (HR vs ipilimumab 0.43, $p < 0.001$; HR vs nivolumab 0.78, 95 percent CI 0.64–0.96); nivolumab 6.9 months (HR vs ipilimumab 0.55, $p < 0.001$); ipilimumab 2.9 months | Nivolumab + ipilimumab not reached (HR vs ipilimumab 0.55, $p < 0.001$; HR vs nivolumab 0.85, 95 percent CI 0.68–1.07); nivolumab 37.6 months (HR vs ipilimumab 0.65, $p < 0.001$); ipilimumab 19.9 months |

| Trial identifier | Design | Treatment groups and regimen | Overall response rate (percent percent) | Duration of response (median, months) | Progression-free survival (PFS) (median, months) | Overall survival (OS) (median, months) |
|---|---|---|---|---|---|---|
| Postowet al. (2015)[794] and Hodi et al. (2016)[795] | Untreated patients; double-blind, phase 2 trial (Checkmate 69) | Nivolumab + ipilimumab ($n = 95$) vs ipilimumab ($n = 47$) | 59 percent vs 11 percent, $p < 0.0001$ | not reached vs not reached | not reached vs 3.0 months, HR 0.36, $p < 0.0001$ | Crossover from ipilimumab to nivolumab allowed; median overall survival not reached in both groups, HR 0.74, $p = 0.26$ |
| Ribaset al. (2015)[796] and Hamid et al. (2017)[797] | Patients pretreated with ipilimumab and *BRAF* inhibitor; open-label, phase 2 trial (Keynote 2) | Pembrolizumab 2 mg per kg ($n = 180$) vs pembrolizumab 10 mg per kg ($n = 181$) vs chemotherapy ($n = 179$) | 22 percent vs 28 percent vs 4 percent, $p < 0.0001$ | 22.8 months vs not reached vs 6.8 months | Pembrolizumab (2 mg per kg) 2.9 months (HR vs chemotherapy 0.57, $p < 0.0001$); pembrolizumab (10 mg per kg) 2.9 months (HR vs chemotherapy 0.50, $p < 0.0001$); chemotherapy 2.7 months | Crossover allowed; pembrolizumab (2 mg per kg) 13.4 months (HR vs chemotherapy 0.86, $p = 0.117$); pembrolizumab (10 mg per kg) 14.7 months (HR 0.74, $p = 0.011$); chemotherapy 11.0 months |
| Schachteret al. (2017)[798] and Robert et al. (2015)[799] | Untreated and pretreated patients; double-blind, phase 3 trial (Keynote 6) | Pembrolizumab once every 2 weeks ($n = 279$) vs pembrolizumab once every 3 weeks ($n = 277$) vs ipilimumab ($n = 278$) | 37 percent vs 36 percent vs 13 percent | not reached vs not reached vs not reached | 5.6 months vs 4.1 months vs 2.8 months; pooled pembrolizumab groups vs ipilimumab HR 0.61, $p < 0.0001$ | Pembrolizumab once every 2 weeks not reached (HR vs ipilimumab 0.68, $p = 0.0009$); pembrolizumab once every 3 weeks not reached (HR vs ipilimumab 0.68, $p = 0.0008$); ipilimumab 16.0 months |

HR, hazard ratio.

**Table 4.17** List of novel FDA-approved immunotherapies for melanoma.

| Agent | Indication | Trial |
|---|---|---|
| Ipilimumab | For unresectable or metastatic melanoma in previously treated patients older than 12. | MDX010-20[749] |
| Ipilimumab | As adjuvant therapy for cutaneous melanoma with pathologic involvement of regional lymph nodes of more than 1 mm, after the complete resection (including total lymphadenectomy). | EORTC 18,071[808] |
| Pembrolizumab | For unresectable or metastatic melanoma | KEYNOTE-006[798]<br>KEYNOTE-002[796] |
| Pembrolizumab | As adjuvant treatment for melanoma with involvement of lymph node(s) following complete resection. | KEYNOTE-054[781] |
| Nivolumab (alone or in combination with nivolumab) | For unresectable or metastatic melanoma | CheckMate 037[789]<br>CheckMate 066[788]<br>CheckMate 067[793] |
| Nivolumab | As adjuvant treatment for melanoma with involvement of lymph node(s) or metastasis following complete resection. | CheckMate 238[780] |
| Talimogenelaherparepvec | For the local treatment of unresectable cutaneous, subcutaneous, and nodal lesions in patients with recurrent disease after the initial surgery. | OPTiM[809] |

can induce a complete or major (defined as less than 10 percent viable tumor cells) pathological response in 29.6 percent of subjects.[784] In concordance with the previous study, this trial also observed an increment in TILs after therapy.[784]

In line with advanced-stage/metastatic melanomas, several trials have been conducted before 2018, and their advantages and disadvantages are discussed elsewhere in detail (Table 4.16). Here, the results of newer trials will be discussed.

The efficacy of nivolumab (either as a single agent or combined with ipilimumab) for patients with resected or radiation-treated stage IV melanoma with no evidence of disease (NED) was evaluated in a randomized phase II trial.[800] After a median follow-up of 28.4 months, both nivolumab monotherapy and combination therapy groups had significantly lower HR of recurrence, as compared with placebo (0.23; 97.5 percent CI, 0.12–0.45; $p < 0.0001$ for combination therapy; and 0.56; 0.33 – 0.94; $p = 0.011$ for nivolumab monotherapy). In line with these findings, the two-year RFS was 70 percent, 42 percent, and 14 percent for combination therapy, nivolumab, and placebo, respectively.[800] However, combination therapy culminated in treatment-related grade three and more AEs in 71 percent of cases, upon which 53 percent discontinued the therapy (62 percent due to any grade AEs). Of note, the prevalence of grade three or higher AEs in the placebo group has been 26 percent, which is attributed, at least partly, to the advanced-stage of the enrolled patients.[800] Another highlight of this trial is the enhanced benefit of patients with *BRAF* mutations from the combination therapy, as also reported by other trials, but with unknown reasons.[800]

Recently, a randomized trial found that the addition of atezolizumab to vemurafenib and cobimetinib (BRAF and MEK inhibitors, respectively) as frontline therapy for stage IIIC/IV melanoma can significantly elongate PFS from 10.6 to 15.1 months (HR, 0.78; 95 percent CI, 0.63–0.97; $p = 0.025$), regardless of PD-L1 expression status, and with comparable side effects.[801] Although the RR did not differ between the two arms but based on the immature survival data, the two-year event-free survival rate has been estimated as 60 percent for atezolizumab and 53 percent for control arms.[801] Similarly, in a phase I study of trametinib, dabrafenib, and pembrolizumab for metastatic melanoma with *BRAF*[600] mutations,[802] 11 of 15 patients exhibited a response, and 11 experienced grade three or more AEs (including three grade four). Another finding of this study was an observed increment in the number and function of CTLs and the expression of PD-L1 and several MHC class I and class II molecules.[802]

Regarding brain metastases, a fascinating trial[803] aimed to test the performance of combined nivolumab and ipilimumab therapy in controlling the brain metastases of melanoma. Among 94 enrolled patients with no neurologic symptoms and at least one measurable nonirradiated metastasis to the brain, 24 achieved CR, 28 achieved PR, and 2 showed stable disease.[803] Another trial[804] found that among patients with asymptomatic untreated melanoma brain metastases, 57 percent of those who received combined nivolumab and ipilimumab and 20 percent of those who received nivolumab showed an intracranial response (either CR, PR, or stable disease). In addition, estimated intracranial six-months PFS was 53 percent and 20 percent for these groups, respectively.[804] Altogether, these data propose a novel approach in managing melanoma brain metastases, meaning that immunotherapies can precede surgery and stereotactic radiotherapies, which in turn can lead to less cognitive-related side effects and radionecrosis.[803,804]

Predictors of the response to ICI therapy are extensively studied in melanoma patients, and as expected, the conclusions are quite heterogeneous in some instances. Molecular analysis of patients with metastatic melanoma revealed that MHC class II expression, *TAP2* (a component of MHC class I) and MHC-I amplification, higher tumor ploidy, and immune gene signature expression are associated with response to anti-PD-1 therapy, while tumor heterogeneity (proportion of sub-clonal mutations) and loss of heterozygosity of *JAK1* are linked to progressive disease after such therapies.[805] Notably, this study found no significant association between the number of immune infiltrated cells and loss of heterozygosity of *HLA-A*, *HLA-B*, or *HLA-C* with the response to therapy.[805] As other examples, analysis of enrolled patients in the CheckMate 064 trial showed that suppressed transcriptions of *HLA-A*, *HLA-B*, *HLA-C*, and *B2M* and subsequent under-expression of MHC class I are linked to the resistance to anti-CTLA-4 therapy.[806] Besides, higher MHC class II expression has been shown to be a predictor of response to anti-PD-1 antibodies.[806] Another retrospective analysis of patients with advanced melanoma who were treated with combined nivolumab and ipilimumab (CheckMate 067 trial) revealed that higher levels of baseline IL-8 (≥23 pg/ml) are associated with shortened survival (HR, 3.06; 95 percent CI, 2.13–4.41).[807] Further, higher tumoral expression of IL-8 could increase the infiltration of tolerogenic monocytes and neutrophils inside the tumoral tissues.[807]

### Oncolytic viruses

Talimogene laherparepvec (T-VEC) is a genetically modified HSV-1 based oncolytic immunotherapy that has shown clinical activity for both injected and uninjected melanoma lesions. This vaccine can eliminate lesions by replicating inside and lysing neoplastic cells and also by producing GM-CSF that can enhance the local and systemic immune responses against tumoral tissues.[809]

The effectiveness of T-VEC for melanoma has been proved by a phase III randomized trial of patients with unresected stages IIIB and IV melanoma.[809] Compared with GM-CSF, T-VEC exhibited significantly higher rates of durable responses (defined as overall response lasting continuously for at least 6 months, 16.3 percent versus 2.1 percent; odds ratio (OR), 8.9; $p < 0.001$). Similar trend also observed for ORR (26.4 percent; 95 percent CI, 21.4 percent−31.5 percent vs 5.7 percent; 95 percent CI, 1.9 percent−9.5 percent).[809] Further investigation of the patients enrolled in the T-VEC arm showed that injected administration of T-VEC could decrease the size by ≥50 percent in 64 percent of lesions, whereas systemic effects of T-VEC induced the same shrinkage in 34 percent of non-visceral lesions.[810] In addition, 47 percent of injected and 22 percent of uninjected non-visceral lesions were completely resolved. Furthermore, 10.8 percent of patients in the T-VEC arm achieved a CR, and 15.6 percent achieved a PR.[810] Common AEs reported after T-VEC therapy were fatigue (50 percent), chills (49 percent), pyrexia (43 percent), nausea (36 percent), influenza-like illness (30 percent), and injection-site pain (28 percent).[809] Besides, 36 percent of T-VEC arm patients experienced grade three or more AEs, compared with 21 percent of those in the GM-CSF arm ($p = 0.003$).[809] An intriguing observation in this trial was the pseudo-progression of lesions, as more than 50 percent of patients who achieved a response initially showed *a* ≥ 25 percent increase in the size of their lesion or appearance of new lesions.[809]

Owing to the considerable efficacy of T-VEC, a phase II trial[811] planned to compare the combination therapy with ipilimumab and T-VEC with ipilimumab monotherapy. Of 198 patients with unresectable stages IIIB to IV melanoma, 39 percent in the combination arm and 18 percent in ipilimumab arm exhibited an OR (2.9; 95 percent CI, 1.5–5.5; $p = 0.002$). The rate of grade three or more AEs was 45 percent and 35 percent for combination and ipilimumab arms, respectively.[811] Interestingly, 18.4 percent of responders in combination arm initially experienced a pseudo-progression pattern of lesions, emphasizing the continuation of therapy irrespective of early progression of the lesion (unless occurrence life-threatening events).[809,812]

### *Interferon-α*

In the era before the introduction of immunotherapies and targeted therapies, the only available systemic therapies for high-risk resectable melanomas were usually confined to IFN-α.[747] A meta-analysis showed that compared with observation or vaccination (GMK and GM2-KLH/QS-21), IFN-α significantly increase the event-free survival (HR, 0.86; CI, 0.81–0.91; $p < 0.00001$) and OS (HR, 0.90; CI, 0.85–0.97; $p = 0.003$), with absolute differences of 3.5 percent and 3 percent at five-year, respectively.[813] More importantly, this meta-analysis found that higher doses of IFN-α confer no added benefit.[813] The clinical activity of IFN-α seems trivial and with considerable side effects.[814] As a matter of fact, the results of an ongoing phase III trial (ECOG 1609) confirmed that ipilimumab (3 mg/kg, but not 10 mg/kg) could modestly but significantly increase the OS of patients with resected stage IIIB, IIIC, M1a, and M1b melanoma over high-dose IFN-α−2β (HR, 0.78, 95.6 percent repeated confidence interval (RCI), 0.61–1.00; $p = 0.044$).[814] In conclusion, ICIs and targeted therapies have supplanted IFN-α, and it is not recommended anymore as first-choice adjuvant therapy for high-risk melanomas.[815]

### *Interleukins*

Discussions about the fate of IFN-α can be imputed for IL-2. In the past, it was the first-choice option for systemic therapy of metastatic melanomas and even gained FDA approval in 1998. A meta-analysis of 34 studies about the application of IL-2 (alone or combined with different modalities) found that CR rate is 4 percent (range, 0 percent−23 percent; 95 percent CI, 2.8 percent−5.3 percent), PR rate is 12.5 percent (95 percent CI, 10.1 percent−15 percent), and ORR is 19.7 percent (95 percent CI, 15.9 percent−23.5 percent).[816] In addition, low-dose IL-2 was found superior to both intermediate- and high-dose IL-2 in inducing CR.[816] Despite these modest results, side-effects of systemic IL-2 injection are serious and, therefore, systemic IL-2 should be administered only in advanced medical centers with experienced staff.[815]

Another advantage of IL-2 is its intralesional injection for cutaneous and subcutaneous metastases seen in locoregional disease (in-transit melanoma).[817] A meta-analysis about this therapeutic modality concluded that 50 percent of patients and 78 percent of lesions completely responded to intralesional IL-2, and it was associated with only three grade three AEs.[817] Commonly reported grade one and two AEs were pain and swelling restricted to the injection site and flu-like symptoms.[817]

Other ILs are also studied for patients with melanoma. For instance, Pegilodecakin, a pegylated IL-10 receptor agonist, in combination with pembrolizumab administered for 31 patients with stage IV melanoma, of whom 20 were anti-PD-1 refractory.[818] Unfortunately, only 3 patients achieved an overall response, all belonging to the "not PD-1 refractory" group, a finding that hampered the advancement of trial for melanoma patients.[818] As another example, an IL-15 analog has shown promising activities in a mouse melanoma model.[819]

### Other immunotherapies

One of the oldest immunotherapies for melanoma was the topical injection of BCG for metastatic lesions.[820] Although the responses were considerable[821] due to its serious regional AEs, today, its administration is not generally recommended.

Imiquimod is a TLR-7 agonist and an immune response modifier that acts via the induced production of various pro-inflammatory cytokines (e.g., IFN-α and IL-1).[822] This will result in enhanced activation of Langerhans cells and CTLs.[822] Indications for the application of imiquimod for melanoma (Fig. 4.4) are usually confined to lesions with positive margins after resection and lesions of patients who are ineligible for surgery or radiation therapy.[815]

Before the major advancements in the characterization of immune checkpoints, adoptive cell therapy with TILs was an area of interest for cutting-edge research. Using this approach, a phase II trial of patients with metastatic melanoma refractory to IL-2 and chemotherapy reported a promising ORR of 50 percent.[823] However, due to technical complexities[823] and unprecedented results of ICIs, adoptive cell therapy lost much of its popularity, although is still under limited investigation. For example, results of a more recent trial of adoptive cell therapy and low dose IL-2 for treatment-refractory metastatic melanoma are consistent with an ORR of 42 percent and a median OS of 21.8 months.[824] Administration of such regiment for 12 metastatic melanoma patients with progression after therapy with ICI (except one patient) has been able to induce PR in 3 patients (one unconfirmed) and stabilize the disease in another 6 ones.[825]

## Future perspective

Adaptive cell therapies are now under investigation as a part of combination therapies (NCT03374839, NCT03475134, and NCT03158935). Regarding CAR T-cells, active trials are generally limited to melanomas that express disialoganglioside (GD)2 (NCT03635632) or CD70 (NCT02830724).

RO7247669 (NCT04140500) and RO7121661 (NCT03708328) are bispecific antibodies (anti-PD-1/LAG-3, and anti-PD-1/TIM-3, respectively), which are now being evaluated for patients with metastatic melanoma and other solid tumors. XmAb20717 (anti-CTLA-4/PD-1), XmAb23104 (anti-PD-1/T cell co-stimulator inducible co-stimulatory (ICOS)), and XmAb22841 (anti-CTLA-4/LAG-3) are other bispecific antibodies that are being evaluated in phase I trials for a variety of solid tumors, including melanoma (NCT03517488, NCT03752398, and NCT03849469).

Despite unprecedented results of ICI therapies in melanoma, only a subset of patients will gain a clinical benefit, and the duration of response are not universally high. Some of the mechanisms behind resistance to ICIs are characterized (discussed earlier). However, until now, no clinical benefit can be extracted from them. Hence, there is an urgent need in classifying best candidates for ICIs, adjusting the dosing and combination therapy strategies (e.g., integrating radiation therapy with immunotherapies, such as NCT04042506 and NCT02318771),[829] and developing novel and personalized[830] immunotherapies for those who do not benefit from ICIs.

## Immunolopathology and immunology of soft tissue and bone cancers

Sarcomas are rare mesenchymal malignancies and generally are divided into soft tissue sarcomas (STS, including sarcomas of nerves, vessels, muscles, tendons, and synovial tissue) and bone sarcomas. Soft tissue sarcomas constitute about 80 percent of all sarcomas.[266] Based on estimates, in 2019, approximately 0.9 percent of all newly diagnosed cancers in the United States were sarcomas.[266] Albeit, sarcomas are among common pediatric cancers and even represent about 20 percent of pediatric solid tumors.[831] Besides, bone sarcomas and STSs are the third and fourth most common causes of cancer deaths in patients less than 20 years old.[266]

Histologically, more than 50 subtypes of sarcomas are identified. However, therapeutic approaches are not as heterogeneous as subtypes.[832] The underpinnings of sarcoma development are diverse and somehow exclusive to certain types. Surgical resection, chemotherapy, and for some subtypes, targeted therapy are the only available therapeutic options.[832] The five-year survival rate of sarcomas generally falls between 60 percent to 70 percent. Unfortunately, this rate is 16 percent for distant STS.[833]

### Immunopathology

The proportion of PD-L1 positive STSs (defined as an expression on at least 1 percent of tumor cells) ranges from 0 percent in malignant peripheral nerve sheath tumor to 50 percent in angiosarcoma.[834] About 3 percent of Synovial sarcomas, 12 percent of leiomyosarcomas (LMS), and dedifferentiated liposarcoma, and 23 percent of undifferentiated pleomorphic sarcomas (UPS) have had detectable PD-L1.[834] Furthermore, PD-L1 expression is found to be associated with PD-1 positivity, a higher grade of the tumor, and a more dismal five-year survival.[834] These descriptions corroborate the findings of previous studies.[835] Such correlations between PD-1/PD-L1 positivity and grim prognosis of STS are also suggested by other studies.[836-838]

In line with the suggestions of TCGA about the importance of immune cells in STS,[839] an astonishing study[840] analyzed the immune gene expression profiles of patients with sarcoma, and after validating the results with immunohistochemical evaluations, proposed a classification system according to the features of TME. Sarcoma immune class (SIC) A is characterized by a negligible immune gene signature (immune desert). SIC C is featured with high endothelial cell-related gene expression (vascularized type). SIC E has the highest expression of immune-related genes (e.g., those related to CTLs, NK cells, chemotaxis of T cells and myeloid cells, MHC class I and B cell lineage, and the tertiary lymphoid structure-related chemokine CXCL13). Eventually, SIC B and SIC

D are considered immune-low and immune-high subclasses.[840] In line with immune checkpoints, PD-1, PD-L2, CTLA-4, and TIM-3 are highly expressed in SIC E and SIC D, while LAG-3 expression is generally limited to SIC E.[840] An association between SIC and survival was also implicated. In multivariate analysis, SIC E appeared to be associated with more favorable survival. Albeit unexpectedly, no association between CTL density and survival was inferred. Instead, the B cell lineage signature was found to be significantly associated with prolonged OS ($p = 0.0004$).[840] Other noteworthy findings of this study are homogeneously low TMB across different SICs and the significant association between SIC E and response to anti-PD-1 therapy ($p = 0.026$).[840] The latter finding is also reported by another study[841] of the same patients enrolled in a trial (SARC028, discussed later). Of note, PD-L1 positivity has been reported in all five subclasses, and it might be deducted that the prognostic role of PD-L1 should only be interpreted with the constellation of other immunologic components. To make the maze of PD-L1 more complex, a study has shown that higher levels of soluble PD-L1 (sPD-L1), but not tumoral PD-L1, are associated with shortened metastasis-free survival and OS of STS patients.[842]

The proportion of PD-L1 positive osteosarcomas varies widely among different studies and ranges between 5.9 percent to 75 percent.[843] Regarding Ewing's sarcoma, the prevalence of PD-L1 positive tumors is reported to be 19 percent, which is also unrelated to the prognosis of patients.[844] Albeit, higher proportions (33 percent and 39 percent) are also reported[838,845] and is linked to a worse prognosis.[838] Like other sarcomas, Ewing's sarcoma is generally considered a "cold" tumor. They have low HLA class I expression,[846] are depleted of CD8+ T cells,[844] and instead have measurable clusters of CD68+ macrophages.[847]

Different subtypes of chondrosarcoma exhibit considerable discrepancies in expressing PD-L1. A study found that none of the conventional, mesenchymal, and clear-cell, but 41 percent (and 52 percent in the validation cohort) of dedifferentiated subtypes are positively stained for PD-L1.[848] In this study, PD-L1 expression has been associated with a higher accumulation of TILs, but not with the OS.[848] Further characterization of the immune cells of dedifferentiated chondrosarcomas has revealed that 85 percent of them are heavily infiltrated with CD14+ CD163+ immunosuppressive macrophages, and 45 percent harbor high populations of T cells (predominantly CTLs).

In summary, based on the results of a meta-analysis, PD-L1 expression in osteosarcoma and chondrosarcoma is negatively associated with OS (HR, 1.987; 95 percent CI, 1.22–3.22; $p = 0.005$) and event-free survival (HR, 3.868; 95 percent CI, 2.298–6.511; $p = 0.000$), but positively with accumulation of PD-1-positive T cells (OR, 4.012; 95 percent CI, 2.391–6.733; $p = 0.000$).[843]

As previously discussed, the neutrophil-to-lymphocyte ratio is known as a prognostic factor and a predictor of response to immunotherapies for some cancers. A large retrospective survey of patients with STS has provided information about the negative associations between higher neutrophil-to-lymphocyte ratio (>2.5) and OS, irrespective of the stage or histologic type of tumors.[849] Besides, neutrophil-to-lymphocyte ratio has been higher in tumors with a larger size, higher grade, and metastases.[849] Still, the therapeutic advantage of these findings is yet to be determined. Likewise, higher values of neutrophil-to-lymphocyte ratio, c-reactive protein, platelet-lymphocyte ratio, and lower values of the lymphocyte-monocyte ratio are described as predictors of a worse prognosis for patients with osteosarcoma.[850]

Immunohistochemical analysis of 1242 sarcoma specimens has shown that the density of CD163+ macrophages (M2-like) is higher than that of CD68+ macrophages (M1-like) and TILs. Also, this study found that non-translocation associated sarcomas (especially undifferentiated pleomorphic sarcoma and dedifferentiated liposarcoma) have higher densities of macrophages compared with translocation-associated tumors (discussed later).

Following in the path of immunology, the influence of cytokines on different aspects of sarcomas behavior has also been explored. In osteosarcoma, significantly higher levels of IL-8 are seen in patients with metastatic disease.[851] This probably results from its secretion by circulating tumor cells, which in turn enhances cancer cell proliferation and invasiveness.[851] A similar role in promoting capability to metastasize is also implicated for IL-6 in osteosarcoma[852] and Ewing's sarcoma,[853] and IL-1 and TNF-α in osteosarcoma.[854]

The genetic landscape of STSs is[855] quite intricate. However, by and large, can be classified into simple (20 percent, euploid with chromosomal translocations, including Ewing's sarcoma and synovial sarcoma) and complex (80 percent, aneuploid or polyploid, including UPS and LMS) karyotypes. Of note, the TMB of STSs is quite low (about 1 mutation per megabase)(839).

## Immunotherapies

### *Immune checkpoint inhibitors (ICIs)*

As expected, most of the scarce trials of novel immunotherapies for sarcomas are dedicated to ICIs.

SARC028 phase II landmark trial[832] aimed to evaluate the response of different types of unresectable/metastatic sarcomas to pembrolizumab. Unfortunately, after a median follow-up of 17.8 months, only 18 percent of all STS patients showed an overall response, including 40 percent of UPS, 20 percent of dedifferentiated liposarcoma, and 10 percent of synovial sarcoma patients. Among 40 patients with bone sarcoma, only two (one with osteosarcoma and another with chondrosarcoma) showed an overall response. None of the patients with Ewing's sarcoma and LMS achieved a response. Therefore, patients with UPS and LPS enrolled in two expansion cohorts. Unfortunately, the ORR for UPS and LPS in the expansion cohort is reported as 16.6 percent and 6.6 percent, respectively.[856] The pre-determined cutoff for ORR to be meaningful has been 25 percent, and rates less than 10 percent have been considered ineffective. Hence, despite encouraging outcomes of the original trial, pembrolizumab is not effective for at least LPS.[856] In concordance with these observations, no response was observed after the administration of nivolumab for patients with advanced uterine LMS,[857] and also ipilimumab in patients with synovial sarcoma.[858]

Another trial of nivolumab has culminated in PRs only in 3 of 24 sarcoma patients (one dedifferentiated chondrosarcoma, one epithelioid sarcoma, and one maxillary osteosarcoma).[859] Likewise, despite the modest clinical activity, camrelizumab plus apatinib combination therapy for advanced osteosarcoma has not met its pre-specified cutoff for six-month PFS to be considered effective.[860]

Transforming the preclinical data to clinical benefits, a phase II trial of combined pembrolizumab and cyclophosphamide for STS has proposed that the extremely low activity of ICIs (only one PR among 50 patients and a six-month non-progression rate of 0 percent for LMS and UPS) is attributed to the high accumulation of CD163+ IDO1 producing macrophages, low expression of PD-L1, and low densities of CD8+ T cells.[859] As confirmation, the only patients with PR have had an IC PD-L1 >10 percent and high accumulation of CD8+ T cells.[859]

The futility of nivolumab monotherapy is also documented by another trial. Alliance A091401,[861] a phase II non-comparative trial, administered single nivolumab or combined with ipilimumab for patients with advanced, unresectable, or metastatic sarcoma. Despite nivolumab monotherapy, the combination therapy met its primary endpoint in inducing acceptable ORR (5 percent versus 16 percent, including one uterine LMS, one non-uterine LMS, one myxofibrosarcoma, two UPS or malignant fibrous histiocytoma, and one angiosarcoma). However, this activity is offset by serious yet manageable toxicities.[861] Although the benefits seem modest, the authors have claimed the ORR and median OS (14.3 months; 95 percent CI, 9.6-not reached) of treated patients with combination therapy is comparable to those who are being treated with standard chemotherapies.[861]

Alveolar soft part sarcoma (ASPS) is a rare sarcoma characterized by uninhibited transcription of *hypoxia-inducible factor* (*HIF*)$-1\alpha$ that results in overexpression of VEGF.[862] The immunosuppressive essence of VEGF has been discussed earlier (part 13). Therefore, the combination of VEGFR inhibitors and ICIs seems rationale. A phase II study[862] was designed to test the performance of such combination therapy (plus pembrolizumab) on the PFS of STS patients. After a median follow-up of 14.7 months, three-month, six-month, and 12-month, PFS was revealed to be 65.5 percent, 46.9 percent, and 27.5 percent, respectively. Strikingly, 54.5 percent of ASPS patients, but 9.5 percent of all other patients achieved a PR. Albeit, the difference in PFS of the two groups was not as such.[862] The added benefits of this combination therapy were achieved regardless of PD-L1 expression status or TIL. However, neutrophil-to-lymphocyte ratio >5 was found to be associated with progressive disease.[862] For non-ASPS patients, the added benefit of pembrolizumab over axitinib monotherapy has been negligible. However, at a six-month cutoff, the added benefit has become considerable. For ASPS patients, compared with axitinib monotherapy, the combination therapy has resulted in substantially higher rates of overall response, but PFS has been comparable.[862]

### Cancer vaccines

In a phase II trial,[863] 7 of 20 patients with locally advanced/metastatic sarcoma exhibited a PR after receiving pembrolizumab and T-VEC (part 14) combination therapy (two angiosarcomas of head and neck, two UPS, one myxofibrosarcoma, one epithelioid sarcoma, and one unclassified sarcoma). The 24-week PFS rate was 39.4 percent. Thus, the trial met its primary endpoint.[863] Histologic analysis of tumor samples showed that responding patients had more clusters of CD8+ T cells in the infiltrating border of their tumors.[863]

Treatment of pediatric patients with metastatic or recurrent sarcoma with a tumor-lysate primed DC vaccine (and with autologous lymphocytes, with or without IL-17) resulted in a five-year OS of 63 percent for patients with Ewing's sarcoma and rhabdomyosarcoma.[864] Vigil is a personalized vaccine that contains DNA-transfected tumor cells by GMCSF/bi-shRNA$^{furin}$ (which induces expression of GM-CSF and prevents the production of functional TGF-$\beta_1$ and TGF-$\beta_2$).[865] A three-year follow-up of patients with advanced-stage Ewing's sarcoma showed that those who received Vigil had an increase in OS by 17.2 months.[865] In addition, the one-year OS of patients who received and those who did not receive Vigil was 73 percent and 23 percent, respectively.[865] Given these promising outcomes, Vigil is now being tested in a phase IIb trial for patients with Ewing's sarcoma (NCT02511132). The outreaching outcomes of these two trials and virtually no response to ICIs will shape the future direction of immunotherapies against Ewing's sarcoma. As a matter of proof, another study has examined neoadjuvant injection of DCs in combination with radiotherapy for large high-grade resectable STS and has reached a one-year PFS of 70.6 percent.[866]

Sarcoma cells can express different types of TAAs on their surface. Several cancer vaccines and adoptive immunotherapies have been developed based on these antigens. Administration of an SYT-SSX-derived peptide vaccine with and without IFN-$\alpha$ led to radiologically stable disease in 6 of 12 and 1 of 9 patients with synovial sarcoma, respectively.[867]

### Adoptive cell therapy

For patients with refractory metastatic synovial sarcoma, administration of autologous T cells transduced with TCR against NY-ESO-1 demonstrated an extraordinary activity, as 4 of 6 treated patients achieved a response.[868] The outcome of the expansion cohort of this trial corroborates the mentioned outcome, which was 11 of 18 enrolled patients with synovial sarcoma demonstrated objective clinical response.[869]

### Other immunotherapies

In addition to these novel modalities, older methods of immunotherapies have also been tested for sarcomas. For instance, mifamurtide (liposomal muramyl tripeptide phosphatidylethanolamine or MTP-PE) is an immunomodulator that is supposed to act by activating the nucleotide-binding oligomerization domain (NOD)2 receptor that eventually leads to NF-κB activation and promotion of the innate immune system.[870] The clinical activity of mifamurtide was examined in a large phase III trial of patients with newly diagnosed resectable osteosarcoma.[871] The addition of mifamurtide to the conventional chemotherapeutic regimens increased the six-year event-free survival by 8 percent ($p = 0.03$) and also demonstrated a minor but significant benefit in enhancing OS (HR, 0.71; 95 percent CI, 0.52–0.96).[872] However, the trial was not originally designed to compare combination therapy and chemotherapy. Thereby, mifamurtide is not approved by the FDA for administration in osteosarcoma.

## Future perspective

The immune and genomic landscape of sarcomas and CNS tumors share several common features, including both having low TMB, being "immune desert", and having diverse mutations that are potential candidates for targeted therapies.[873] ICIs have not exerted clinical activity in sarcomas and ideally will be candidates just for a minority of tumors with high immune cell infiltrates. Also, vaccine and adoptive immunotherapies have demonstrated unprecedented results in some instances and are potential immunotherapies of the future for sarcomas. Indeed, most active trials of sarcomas belong to these modalities (NCT02992743, NCT01169584, NCT02239861, and NCT04052334).

## Immunolopathology and immunotherapy of cancers of men reproductive system

It was expected that in 2019, more than 174 000 prostate cancer patients might be diagnosed in the United States, making it the most common malignancy of men.[266] Fortunately, the wide availability of PSA-based screening programs have prevented delays in the diagnosis, and now, only 10 percent of cancer-related death among men are attributed to prostate cancer.[266] More than 90 percent of prostate cancers are detected in localized or regional forms, and their five-year survival rates are more than 99 percent. Adversely, just 30 percent of patients with a distant form of the disease will be alive after five years.[266] The principles of therapy for localized high-risk prostate cancer are radical prostatectomy, radiation therapy (using external-beam radiotherapy and brachytherapy), and adjuvant androgen deprivation. Active surveillance can be appropriate for certain patients with the localized low-risk disease.[874] Castration (via surgical or medical interventions) is the initial step for the management of the advanced disease.[874] Unfortunately, recurrence after treatment of both localized and metastatic disease is common, which eventually leads to metastatic castration-resistant prostate cancer (mCRPC). There are several therapeutic options for such subjects, but there are ongoing debates about the best choices for them.[874] Conventional immunotherapies for prostate cancer constitute different types of vaccines.[874] ICIs have come to the interest in recent years. Hence until now, there are not many robust trials of those, and their role in treating prostate cancer is still evolving (discussed later).

The vast majority of testicular cancers are germ cell tumors that are further categorized as seminomas and nonseminomas.[875] Testicular cancers are rare, as less than 10,000 new cases were estimated to be diagnosed in 2019.[266] Fortunately, more than 95 percent of all stages and 80 percent of metastatic testicular cancers are curable, an achievement that has not been accomplished for any other cancer yet.[875] The therapeutic options for refractory cases are limited and ineffective, prompting the need for more novel effective therapies.

## Immunopathology

Like what was mentioned in the previous parts, there are profound debates about the percentage of PD-L1 positive prostate cancers. However, a large survey on 508 prostate acinar adenocarcinomas and 57 mCRPC has detected PD-L1 in 7.7 percent and 31.6 percent of samples, respectively.[876] Another immune regulator TIM-3 is reported to be expressed by 25.2 percent of metastatic prostate cancers and surprisingly can be used as a predictor of hormone sensitivity of disease and a better OS of patients with mCRPC.[877]

Prostate cancers have long been considered immunologically "cold" tumors. This fact can create challenges in the way of developing effective immunotherapeutic strategies against the disease. Hence, a better understanding of its microenvironment and classifying it with regard to the immunological aspects is guarded. A recent study has introduced a classification for prostate adenocarcinoma with eight clusters according to the different mechanisms of tumoral immune evasion.[878] Of note, 89 percent of included samples showed an immunological ignorance phenotype, corroborating older reports. Some of these clusters are characterized by more than one immune ignorance and immune tolerance mechanisms.[878] Thereby, at least theoretically, single-agent immunotherapies will not demonstrate considerable activities in such tumors.[878] Another sound strategy is to turn these immune desert tumors into "hot" ones. As an example, high dose-rate brachytherapy has been shown to do such in localized prostate cancer.[879]

Like other neoplasms, different roles of cytokines and ILs in contributing to or prohibiting tumorigenesis of prostate cancers have been described. Examples are IL-17 and IL-7 that can enhance invasiveness by increasing the expression of MMP7[880] and other EMT markers,[881] respectively. Several different models have been proposed for the genetic aberrations in prostate cancer. In brief, about 19 percent of primary prostate carcinomas[882] and 23 percent of mCRPCs[883] exhibit mutations in DNA repair genes (e.g., *BRCA2*, *CDK12*, and *ATM*). The discrepancy between primary prostate carcinoma and mCRPC also comes to mean mutational burden, whereas it is only 0.94 per megabase for the first one[882] but is as high as 2,[884] 2.7,[885] or 4.4 per megabase[883] for mCRPC. Of note, almost all tumors with MSI have higher TMB (defined as more than 10 mutations per megabase).[883,885]

## Immunotherapies for prostate cancer

### *Immune checkpoint inhibitors (ICIs)*

A randomized phase III trial (CA184-043) enrolled patients with mCRPC with at least one bone metastasis that had progressed after docetaxel to explore the efficacy of ipilimumab plus radiation therapy versus radiation therapy alone in improving OS.[886] Despite some activity, the resulted p-value was greater than the prespecified cutoff (HR, 0.85, 95 percent CI, 0.72–1.00; $p = 0.053$). Also, the benefit of ipilimumab came at the cost of four treatment-related deaths.[886] Following the lead of the previous trial, another large randomized phase III trial of ipilimumab for asymptomatic/minimally symptomatic patients with chemotherapy-naïve mCRPC without any visceral metastases could not meet its primary endpoint in lengthening OS.[887] Indeed, median OS was one month longer in the placebo arm (probably attributed to therapies after study discontinuation). Besides, nine treatment-related deaths occurred in the ipilimumab arm. However, ipilimumab could significantly improve PFS (HR, 0.67; 95.87 percent CI, 0.55–0.81) and PSA response (23 percent versus 8 percent).[887] Of note, one of the hypotheses of the CA184-043 trial, the superior activity of ipilimumab among patients without visceral metastases,[886] was rejected by the disappointing results of this trial. Overexpression of V-domain Ig suppressor of T cell activation (VISTA, an inhibitory immune checkpoint) and PD-L1 on T cells and CD68+ macrophages was documented after treatment with ipilimumab and was considered as a putative mechanism of resistance to this agent.[888]

Regarding pembrolizumab, three cohorts of patients with mCRPC (PD-L1 positive (CPS ≥1), PD-L1 negative, and bone predominant disease) enrolled in phase II KEYNOTE-199 trial[889] to receive the agent as at least third-line therapy (after docetaxel and targeted endocrine therapies). Median OS and disease control rates (DCRs) for these cohorts were 9.5 months and 10 percent, 7.9 months and 9 percent, and 14.1 months and 22 percent, respectively.[889] Although seems trivial, the median duration of responses has been acceptable (not reached; range, 1.9 to ≥21.8 months; and 10.6 months; range, 4.4 to 16.8 months; respectively), making further exploration of pembrolizumab for such patients reasonable. Of note, this study has not reported any apparent association between DNA damage repair gene mutation or PD-L1 expression status and response to therapy.[889] Pembrolizumab is collectively approved by the FDA for dMMR/MSI-H solid tumors.[890] Only a small fraction (3.1 percent) of prostate cancers is dMMR/MSI-H.[891] However, it might proffer predicting roles. For example, among 11 patients with dMMR/MSI-H mCRPC, 6 (54.5 percent) had a PSA reduction of ≥50 percent after treatment with anti–PD-1/PD-L1 agents.[891] Similarly, a retrospective study on dMMR and/or MSI-H metastatic PC showed that 53 percent of patients had a PSA reduction of ≥50 percent in response to pembrolizumab.[892] These promising outcomes heralded the importance of MSI in determining response to pembrolizumab. Pembrolizumab is being evaluated along with other therapies (olaparib, abiraterone, enzalutamide, and prednisone) for patients with mCRPC in phase Ib/II KEYNOTE-365 trial

(NCT02861573). The interim analysis of cohort A (pembrolizumab plus olaparib for docetaxel pretreated subjects) has shown modest efficacy (PSA decline ≥50 percent in 9 percent).[893]

Nivolumab has been explored in combination with ipilimumab in patients with asymptomatic/minimally symptomatic mCRPC who have received second-generation hormone therapy alone (cohort 1) or with taxane-based chemotherapies (cohort 2).[894] After a minimum follow-up of six months, ORRs have been 26 percent for cohort 1 and 10 percent for cohort 2. Intriguingly, the RR has been higher in patients with DNA-repair defects, PD-L1 expression ≥1 percent, and above-median TMB.[894] Likewise, significant differences have been observed in PSA responses, ORR, PSA-PFS, and PFS after nivolumab plus ipilimumab administration between those with DNA-repair deficiencies (*BRCA2*, *ATM*, and *ERCC4* mutations) and those without.[895]

Based on the observations of increased PD-L1 expression on APCs after the development of resistance to enzalutamide (an androgen receptor inhibitor),[896] a trial was designed to investigate the effects of combined pembrolizumab and enzalutamide on decreasing PSA of mCRPC.[897] Among 28 participants, 5 (18 percent) experienced a reduction in PSA ≥50 percent that appeared to be independent of PD-L1 expression status or DNA-repair defects.[897]

### *Vaccines*

*Poxvirus*-based PSA-targeting vaccines are more conventional immunotherapies for prostate cancer. One of them (PROSTVAC-VF, encoding PSA, B7-1, ICAM-1, and LFA-3, and in combination with GM-CSF) was investigated in a phase II trial for patients with mCRPC, and although could not meet its primary endpoint (PFS), it showed significantly prolonged OS of treated patients (median of 25.1 months versus 16.6 months for placebo arm) and reduced rate of death by 44 percent.[898] Unfortunately, the phase III trial of PROSTVAC-VF did not reach its effectiveness criteria and, therefore, stopped prematurely.[899] Another therapeutic approach included GVAX in combination with ipilimumab, and despite demonstrating modest outcomes in a phase I trial,[900] further evaluations were halted by the manufacturer (NCT01510288).

A novel vaccine is now being explored in patients with early-stage prostate cancer. VANCE is a virus-based vaccine targeting oncofetal self-antigen 5T4 and has been able to induce immune responses.[901] It is now being investigated in combination with nivolumab for mCRPC in the ADVANCE trial.

The most known vaccine therapy for mCRPC is sipuleucel-T.[902] It is an active autologous mononuclear cell-derived immunotherapy. Derived cells are activated *ex vivo* by a recombinant fusion protein named PA2024 (contained a prostate antigen, prostatic acid phosphatase, and GM-CSF).[902] Being tested by a phase III trial, sipuleucel overperformed placebo in reducing the risk of death by 22 percent (HR, 0.78; 95 percent CI; 0.61–0.98; $p = 0.03$) and increasing median OS by 4.1 months[902] among patients with asymptomatic mCRPC. The vaccine was well-tolerated, and its major side effect was flu-like symptoms.[902] However, there were several drawbacks. The vaccine could not increase time to objective disease progression (although this might be due to pseudo-progression), the manufacturing process was personalized and costly,[902] and there were some interfering differences in harvesting cells of two arms.[903] Nevertheless, sipuleucel-T is still approved by the FDA for the treatment of patients with asymptomatic or minimally symptomatic mCRPC.[904]

## Immunotherapies for testicular cancer

Studies with published results of immunotherapies for testicular cancers are limited to case series[905,906] and two phase II trials. The first one administered pembrolizumab for 12 refractory nonseminomas (including one in mediastinum), and only two achieved radiologically stable disease, which made the trial close prematurely.[907] In the second trial, durvalumab monotherapy led to catastrophic hyperprogressive disease, but the combination with tremelimumab resulted in one PR, one stable disease, and also four hyperprogressive.[908]

## Future perspective

Putting cancer vaccines aside, cancer immunotherapies had not been studied for prostate and testicular cancers until very recent years. Just like some of the other previously reviewed neoplasms (CNS tumors and sarcomas), these cancers harbor a cold immunophenotype. Hence, future strategies should focus on evading this phenotype or targeting more than one immunosuppressive pathway (Table 4.18) and controlling its subsequent side effects. As an example, a double checkpoint blockade has demonstrated promising clinical activities, but the high rate of grade three or more AEs makes its widespread usage troublesome.

# Immunolopathology and immunotherapy of cancers of women reproductive system

Ovarian and uterine cervical cancers constitute a large proportion of gynecological malignancies.[266] Worldwide, uterine cervical cancer is the fourth commonly diagnosed and fourth lethal cancer among women.[424] However, their incidence varies widely around the world, as cervical cancer is the most common cancer in 28 countries and the leading cause of cancer-related deaths in 42 countries.[424] In contrast, it was predicted that in 2019, 22,000 new cases of ovarian cancer and 13,000 new cases of cervical cancer might be detected among the United States population.[266] In the United States, ovarian cancer ranks fourth for cancer-related mortalities among females, while cervical cancer is not even among the 10 most common cancers for both incidence and mortality, owing to the widespread screening programs and vaccination against *HPV*.[266] When diagnosed, more than 80 percent of uterine cervical cancers are localized or regional. Conversely, about 60 percent of ovarian cancers have metastasized at the time of detection.[266] Thereby, five-year survival rates for all stages of cervical and ovarian cancers are 66 percent and 47 percent, respectively.[266]

Table 4.18 Selected ongoing trials of novel immunotherapies for male cancers.

| Agent | Trial identifier | Phase | Indication | Notes |
|---|---|---|---|---|
| **Prostate cancer** | | | | |
| DCVAC (autologous immunotherapy) with chemotherapy | NCT02111577 | III | Chemotherapy eligible mCRPC | |
| Nivolumab and ipilimumab | NCT03570619 | II | CDK12 mutated mCRPC | |
| MVA-BN-Brachyury plus PROSTVAC-V plus atezolizumab | NCT04020094 | II | Unfavorable intermediate, high-risk, or very high-risk localized prostate adenocarcinoma | In the neoadjuvant (pre-operative) setting |
| Pembrolizumab | NCT04009967 | II | Non-metastatic localized Gleason ≥8 prostate cancer with positive tumor by 18FDG-PET Scanning (PICT-01) | In the neoadjuvant (pre-operative) setting |
| Pembrolizumab pTVG-HP plus pTVG-AR plus rhGM-CSF plus | NCT04090528 | II | mCRPC | pTVG-HP contains plasmid DNA encoding human prostatic acid phosphatase<br>pTVG-AR contains plasmid DNA encoding the human androgen receptor ligand-binding domain |
| Sipuleucel-T plus ipilimumab | NCT01804465 | II | mCRPC | Immediate versus delayed administration of ipilimumab after the final dose of sipuleucel-R |
| Sipuleucel-T plus CYT107 | NCT01881867 | II | Asymptomatic or minimally symptomatic mCRPC | CYT107 is a glycosylated recombinant human IL-7. |
| Durvalumab plus Tremelimumab | NCT03204812 | II | Asymptomatic or minimally symptomatic chemotherapy-naïve mCRPC | |

*(Continued)*

**Table 4.18** Cont'd

| Agent | Trial identifier | Phase | Indication | Notes |
|---|---|---|---|---|
| Nivolumab plus degarelix plus BMS-986,253 (HuMax IL8) | NCT03689699 | Ib/II | Hormone-sensitive prostate cancer with rising PSA | BMS-986,253 is a fully human-sequence IgG1κ mAb directed against human IL-8 |
| Utolimumab, PF-04,518,600, avelumab, and radiation therapy | NCT03217747 | I/II | mCRPC and other advanced malignancies | Utolimumab is a fully human IgG2 agonist mAb that binds to human 4–1BB/CD137 PF-04,518,600 is a fully human, mAb that targets the OX40 protein (CD134) Various combination regimens are designed in the trial |
| Adenoviral PSA, MUC1, and brachyury vaccine | NCT03481816 | I | mCRPC | |
| **Testicular cancer** | | | | |
| Nivolumab plus ipilimumab | NCT02834013 | II | Testicular cancer and other rare tumors | |
| Durvalumab plus tremelimumab | NCT03158064 | II | R/R germ cell tumors | |

mCRPC, metastatic castration-resistant prostate cancer; IL, interleukin; PSA, prostate-specific antigen; mAb, monoclonal antibody, Ig, immunoglobulin; R/R, relapsed/refractory.

## Immunopathology

There is wide variability of the percentage of PD-L1 expressing ovarian tumors and their prognostic values. Analysis of high-grade serous carcinomas revealed that about 54 percent of the samples are positive for PD-L1 staining, and its expression is an indicator of better prognosis.[909] However, the results of a recent meta-analysis showed that except for a negative correlation between PD-L1 mRNA expression and PFS, there is no association between PD-L1 protein expression and clinical variables (OS, PFS, grade, stage, histologic type, and lymph node involvement).[910]

The positive prognostic role of CD3+ tumor-infiltrating T cells has long been shown for ovarian cancer.[911] Also, it has been reported that only 54.8 percent of the samples are positive for such cells.[911] Further characterization of immune cell infiltrates shows that a higher CD8+ T cell density and higher CD8+ T cell to Treg ratio are associated with elongated survival.[912] On the other hand, IL-4, IL-6, IL-10, and TGF-β are implicated as conducive cytokines in the tumorigenesis of ovarian cancers.[913]

Unlike ovarian cancer, high PD-L1 expression in cervical cancer is a marker of adverse OS.[914] Of note, the mean TMB for cervical and ovarian cancer is less than the average number.[361,915]

## Immunotherapies for ovarian cancer

### *Immune checkpoint inhibitors (ICIs)*

One of the earliest trials of ICIs was designed to evaluate the effectiveness of an anti-PD-L1 antibody (MDX1105-01) for several advanced cancers, including ovarian cancer.[916] Unfortunately, among 17 cases of ovarian cancer, only 1 achieved a PR.[916]

The response of recurrent ovarian carcinoma to pembrolizumab monotherapy has been correlated to PD-L1 positivity, as 4.1 percent of cases with CPS <1 and 10 percent of those with CPS ≥10 have achieved a response.[917] However, in this trial, the performance of pembrolizumab has not been promising, with only 7.4 percent of patients in cohort A (one to three prior therapies) and 9.9 percent of patients in cohort B (four to six prior therapies) showing a response.[917] Of note, PFS (2.1 months) and DCR (37.2 percent and 37.4 percent) was similar between the two cohorts.[917] In addition, pembrolizumab has demonstrated remarkable activity in patients with dMMR/MSI-H ovarian cancer. In the CheckMate 158 trial, two CRs and three PRs recorded for such patients after receiving pembrolizumab, which comes to a promising ORR of 33.3 percent.[918]

Following in the path of ICI monotherapy, avelumab has shown modest activity among patients with recurrent/refractory ovarian cancer (ORR of 9.6 percent, an overall DCR of 52 percent, a one-year PFS rate of 10.2 percent, and median OS of 11.2 months).[919] The response to therapy has been independent of PD-L1 expression status or *BRCA* mutations, but a positive correlation was found for the lower number of prior treatments.[919]

Regarding combination therapies, administration of durvalumab plus olaparib (a poly adenosine diphosphate-ribose polymerase (PARP) inhibitor) for germline *BRCA* mutated platinum-sensitive relapsed ovarian cancer has resulted in very encouraging outcomes. Among 32 enrolled patients, 26 achieved disease control at 12 weeks, including 6 with a CR (all with one or two prior chemotherapies) and 14 with a PR.[920] Likewise, combination therapy with pembrolizumab and niraparib (another PARP inhibitor) for recurrent ovarian carcinoma have resulted in promising durable ORR and DCR of 18 percent and 65 percent, regardless of PD-L1 positivity, platinum sensitivity, and *BRCA* mutations.[921] Another trial of combined nivolumab and bevacizumab for subjects with relapsed epithelial ovarian cancer culminated in an ORR of 28.9 percent with an acceptable safety profile (23.7 percent grade three or higher treatment-related

AEs).[922] Notably, the RR was 40 percent for platinum-sensitive and 16.7 percent for platinum-resistant patients. Also, PD-L1 expression status has not been an indicator of response to therapy.[922]

More recently, the superiority of dual checkpoint blockade over monotherapy has been confirmed by a phase II study, in which nivolumab and ipilimumab combination therapy for recurrent/persistent ovarian cancer led to significantly higher ORR and PFS compared with nivolumab monotherapy (RR of 12.2 percent versus 31.4 percent; overall response, 3.28; 85 percent CI, 1.54-infinity; $p = 0.034$; and median PFS of 2 versus 3.9 months; HR, 0.53; 95 percent CI, 0.34–0.82).[923] Similar to some other trials, there was not a possible correlation between PD-L1 positivity and response to therapy.[923]

### *Other immunotherapies*

Regarding cancer vaccines, combination therapy with durvalumab and TPIV200 (a cancer vaccine against folate receptor-α) against advanced platinum-resistant ovarian cancer was not successful, as only 1 unconfirmed PR and 9 stable disease have been recorded among 27 participated patients.[924]

The application of CAR T-cells against ovarian cancers has been an area of interest during recent years. A phase I study of mesothelin-directed CAR T-cells reported that there was evidence of infiltrated CAR T-cells in three of four available samples.[925] Besides, all 6 patients were in stable disease one month after receiving the therapy.[925] Other types of CAR T-cells have shown promising activities in preclinical models of ovarian cancer.[913,926]

## Immunotherapies for cervical cancer

### *Immune checkpoint inhibitors (ICIs)*

There are few trials with published results about the outcome of therapy with ICIs in patients with cervical cancers. A phase I/II trial of pretreated patients with metastatic *HPV*-related cervical carcinoma showed that ipilimumab has little efficacy for such patients.[927] Among 42 subjects, only 1 achieved a PR, and 10 showed stable disease, with a median PFS and OS of 2.5 months and 8.5 months, respectively.[927] Administration of pembrolizumab for a similar cohort of patients resulted in an overall response in 12 subjects (including three CRs)(928). Although ORR and median OS were like those of conventional regimens, the duration of responses was higher for pembrolizumab (median duration of response was not reached; range, ≥3.7 to ≥18.6 months). Of note, all responses were seen in patients with CPS ≥. However, the small size of PD-L1 negative patients (16 cases) prevents reaching definite conclusions.[928] Based on the results of this trial (KEYNOTE-158), the FDA approved pembrolizumab for patients with R/M cervical cancer with disease progression on or after chemotherapy and a CPS ≥1.[929]

Regarding nivolumab, its effectiveness has been very promising in the CheckMate 358 trial.[930] In this phase I/II trial, 19 pretreated patients with recurrent/metastatic SCC of cervix enrolled. After a median follow-up of 19.2 months, 5 cases (26.2 percent) achieved an overall response, which was persistent in 3 of them at the time of data cutoff. The DCR was 68.4 percent, and median OS and PFS were 21.9 months and 5.1 months, respectively.[930]

### Cancer vaccines

Several *Listeria monocytogenes*-based vaccines have been investigated for cervical cancers. One of them is Lm-LLO-E7, a live-attenuated vaccine that secretes a fusion protein composed of HPV-16 E7 antigen and a non-hemolytic fragment of listeriolysin O.[931] Being evaluated by a phase I trial of 15 advanced cervical cancers, Lm-LLO-E7 was able to induce PR in 1 case and stable disease in another 7 cases.[931]

Following these results, axalimogene filolisbac (ADXS11-001, a cancer vaccine similar to Lm-LLO-E7) was explored in combination with cisplatin for recurrent/refractory cervical cancer in phase II randomized trial.[932] Compared with cisplatin monotherapy, the combination therapy showed similar median OS, median PFS, and ORR. However, the one-year survival rate was 8 percent higher for the combination arm (38.9 percent versus 30.9 percent).[932]

### Adaptive cell therapies

Administration of cultured TILs against HPV-16 or HPV-18 E6 and E7 for patients with metastatic cervical cancer culminated in an ORR of 28 percent (5 of 18 subjects, including two CRs with durations of 53 and 67 months).[933] This outcome is quite prominent. However, in addition to technical difficulties (discussed in previous parts), no definite biomarker of response was detected in this study.[933]

## Future perspective

The results of novel immunotherapies for gynecological cancers are still immature. Nevertheless, considering modest activities of single-agent immunotherapies and the extreme immune desert phenotype of ovarian cancers, the only putative triumphant strategies are combination therapies. For cervical cancer, the administration of single-agent ICI has been promising and is now being explored by some phase III trials (Table 4.19). This finding is reminiscent of the tumor control described in patients with unresectable stage IV melanoma treated with nivolumab plus ipilimumab, who discontinued because of treatment-related AEs.

## Immunotherapy in combination with other therapeutic approaches

Considering tumor sub-clones and TME heterogeneity in addition to host systemic reaction as the major determinants of final therapeutic response, apparently, none of the

**Table 4.19** Selected ongoing trials of novel immunotherapies for ovarian and cervical cancers.

| Agents | Trial identifier | Phase | Indication | Notes |
|---|---|---|---|---|
| Ovarian cancer | | | | |
| Atezolizumab, bevacizumab, and acetylsalicylic acid | NCT02659384 | II | Recurrent, histologically proven, platinum-resistant, epithelial ovarian, fallopian tube, and primary peritoneal cancer in advanced or metastatic stage | |
| Atezolizumab versus placebo, plus bevacizumab plus platinum-based chemotherapy | NCT02891824 | III | Progressive non-mucinous epithelial ovarian cancer, primary peritoneal adenocarcinoma, and/or fallopian tube adenocarcinoma | |
| Nivolumab and/or rucaparib | NCT03522246 | III | Newly diagnosed advanced (stage III or IV) epithelial ovarian, fallopian tube, or primary peritoneal cancer, with complete cytoreductive surgery, including at least a bilateral salpingo-oophorectomy and partial omentectomy, either prior to chemotherapy (primary surgery) or following neoadjuvant chemotherapy (interval debulking) and completed first-line platinum-based chemotherapy and surgery with a response. | As for maintenance therapy |
| Atezolizumab versus Placebo plus paclitaxel, carboplatin, and bevacizumab | NCT03038100 | III | Newly diagnosed stage III or IV ovarian, fallopian tube, or primary peritoneal carcinoma | As frontline therapy |
| Chemotherapy plus pembrolizumab or placebo followed by olaparib or placebo | NCT03740165 | III | *BRCA* non-mutated advanced (stage III or IV) epithelial ovarian cancer with completed primary debulking surgery or eligibility for primary or interval debulking surgery | As frontline therapy |
| Durvalumab, olaparib, bevacizumab, and chemotherapy | NCT03737643 | III | Advanced (stage III or IV) high grade epithelial ovarian (including serous, endometrioid, and clear cell) cancer or carcinosarcoma, primary peritoneal cancer, and/or fallopian tube cancer | As frontline and maintenance therapy |

| Agents | Trial identifier | Phase | Indication | Notes |
|---|---|---|---|---|
| REGN4018 with or without cemiplimab | NCT03564340 | I/II | Relapsed/progressive advanced, epithelial ovarian cancer (except carcinosarcoma), primary peritoneal, or fallopian tube cancer which has received a platinum-containing therapy | REGN4018 is a bispecific antibody against CD3 and MUC16 |
| MGD013 with or without margetuximab | NCT03219268 | I | Unresectable or metastatic ovarian cancer | MGD013 is a bispecific antibody against PD-1 and LAG-3 |
| CDX-527 | NCT04440943 | I | Recurrent, locally advanced, or metastatic ovarian cancer | CDX-527 is a bispecific antibody against PD-L1 and CD27 |
| **Cervical cancer** | | | | |
| Cemiplimab | NCT03257267 | III | Recurrent, persistent, and/or metastatic cervical cancer with squamous cell histology and resistance to platinum-based chemotherapy | |
| Chemotherapy plus pembrolizumab or placebo | NCT03635567 | III | As frontline therapy for persistent, recurrent, or metastatic squamous cell carcinoma, adenosquamous carcinoma, or adenocarcinoma of the cervix which has not been treated with systemic chemotherapy and is not amenable to curative treatment (surgery and/or radiation) | |
| Chemotherapy (cisplatin and paclitaxel) plus bevacizumab with or without atezolizumab | NCT03556839 | III | As frontline therapy for metastatic (stage IVB), persistent, or recurrent squamous cell, adenocarcinoma, or adenosquamous cervical cancer which is not amenable for curative treatment with surgery and/or radiation therapy | |
| ALT-803, pembrolizumab, nivolumab, avelumab and atezolizumab | NCT03228667 | II | R/M cervical cancer with progression on or after pembrolizumab, with combine positive score ≥1, and other solid tumors | ALT-803 is an IL-15 superagonist |

*(Continued)*

**Table 4.19** Cont'd

| Agents | Trial identifier | Phase | Indication | Notes |
|---|---|---|---|---|
| Ipilimumab | NCT01693783 | II | R/M HPV-related cervical cancer of squamous, adeno-carcinoma, or mixed histology type not suited to definitive localized therapy | |
| Nivolumab | NCT02257528 | II | R/M squamous cell carcinoma, adenosquamous carcinoma, or adenocarcinoma of the cervix with documented disease progression and at least one target lesion | |
| Brachytherapy plus chemotherapy and concurrent or adjuvant pembrolizumab | NCT02635360 | II | Advanced cervical cancer | |
| Radiotherapy plus chemotherapy with or without atezolizumab | NCT03612791 | II | Squamous cell carcinoma, adenosquamous carcinoma, or adenocarcinoma of the cervix with at least one evaluable lesion | |
| AGEN2034 (anti-PD-1) with or without AGEN1884 (anti-CTLA-4) | NCT03894215 | II | Metastatic, locally advanced, and/or unresectable squamous-cell carcinoma, adenosquamous carcinoma, or adenocarcinoma of the cervix and measurable disease on imaging | |
| AK104 | NCT04380805 | II | R/M squamous carcinoma or adenosquamous carcinoma of the cervix, measurable disease on imaging, and no more than two prior therapies for R/M disease | AK104 is a bispecific antibody against CTLA-4 and PD-1 |
| ADXS11-001 | NCT02853604 | III | As adjuvant therapy (after chemoradiation) for locally advanced squamous cell, adenocarcinoma, or adenosquamous carcinoma of the cervix | |

| Agents | Trial identifier | Phase | Indication | Notes |
|---|---|---|---|---|
| **Ovarian and cervical cancer** | | | | |
| XmAb22841 with or without pembrolizumab | NCT03849469 | I | Advanced or metastatic epithelial ovarian cancer, fallopian tube cancer, or primary peritoneal cancer<br>Advanced or metastatic cervical carcinoma<br>Oher advanced solid tumors | XmAb22841 is a bispecific antibody against CTLA-4 and LAG-3 |
| XmAb20717 | NCT03517488 | I | Advanced ovarian or fallopian tube carcinoma<br>Advanced cervical carcinoma<br>Other advanced solid tumors | XmAb20717 is a bispecific antibody against CTLA-4 and PD-1 |
| SNK01, trastuzumab, and cetuximab | NCT04464967 | I/II | Advanced HER2 or EGFR cancers, including ovarian and cervical carcinoma | SNK01 is a natural-killer cell-based therapy |

R/M, recurrent or metastatic; PD-1, programmed cell death protein-1; LAG-3, lymphocyte activation gene-3; PD-L1, programmed death ligand 1; R/M, recurrent or metastatic; IL, interleukin; HPV, Human Papillomavirus; CTLA-4, cytotoxic T lymphocyte-associated protein-4; EGFR, epidermal growth factor receptor.

cytotoxic or surgical therapeutic modalities are alone efficient enough to overcome these pre-existing barriers or their tumor-promoting side effects.[934-936] Interestingly, cytotoxic therapies can go beyond expectations through inducing an intramural pool of TAA and danger signal (damage-associated molecular patterns (DAMPs)), overexpressing antigen-presenting MHC I that stimulates APCs, activate tumor-resident CD8+ T cells, and attract more CTLs toward tumor to prime a fatal anti-tumor response.[937] Paradoxically chemotherapy, radiotherapy, and surgery have an undeniable dark side. Post-therapy tumor immune microenvironment (TIME) and systemic inflammatory response create a potent cellular and molecular immunosuppressive collection that harshly compete with CTL-mediated anti-tumor response. Indeed the winning force drives tumors fate and patients prognosis.[938] Knowing these complex post-therapeutic interactions brings to mind that adding immune-modulating modalities for either augmenting the induced anti-tumor response or eliminating the local and systemic immunosuppressive condition might significantly increase the chance of positive clinical response.[934,935,939] Although choosing the appropriate time window and optional immunotherapy plan for combination therapy is still challenging.

Desirable immunotherapeutic approaches for combination are those that directly or indirectly enhance CTLs infiltration and functions.[940,941] For instance, using viral vaccines or using potent cytokines such as IFN-I that is the key mediator of the adaptive immune response, would sensitize and stimulate APCs and adaptive T cells.[942-944] Transferring adaptive T cells immediately after chemotherapy or stimulating their intra-tumoral infiltration can augment anti-tumor response and break the post-chemotherapy peri-tumoral ring of Tregs.[945] Also, DC-based therapies or systemic administration of TLR agonists might improve CTLs activation.[946,947] Although chemotherapy and radiotherapy increase expression and presentation of MHC type I molecules on tumor cells and target them to synapse with T cells, in parallel, tumor cells or therapy-induced immunosuppressive tumor-infiltrating myeloid cells (TIMs) express T cells inhibitory molecules such as PD-L1 and CTLA-4 that results in T cells exhaustion and dysfunction following binding to associated receptors. Therefore, combining ICIs such as systemic anti-PD-1/PD-L1 therapy and CTLA-4 antagonists with cytotoxic therapies might prevent further local T cells dysfunction and overcome therapeutic resistance.[948-955] Further, in the case of radiotherapy, CTLA-4 blockade enhances CTLs anti-tumor performance in distant sites and consequently increase the efficacy of the abscopal effect.[956] In addition, immune modulation of solid tumors can sensitize therapy-resistant variant tumor cells or modify tumor immune phenotype.[936,957] As it was discussed, conventional cancer therapies are often followed by systemic host inflammatory response and mobilization of bone marrow-derived progenitor cells (BMDCs), leading to an increased crowding of TIMs or Tregs with pro-tumor features. Thus, targeting this inflammatory burst and immunosuppressive infiltrating cells seems to be a rationale option for combination therapies. This purpose can be yielded through either using systemic anti-inflammatory agents, antagonizing chemo-attractants such as CCL2, and CSF-1, blocking recruiting pathways, eliminating Tregs and TIMs, and skewing TAMs toward an anti-tumor phenotype.[938,945,958-964]

## Tumor immune microenvironment (TIME) after other therapeutic approaches

### TIME Post-Chemotherapy

As unwelcome strangers in the TME, chemotherapeutic agents do not merely kill tumor cells. Not only does chemotherapy induces DNA damage and upcoming cell death in a number of cancer cells, but also visualizes them to the host immune system and provokes a local inflammatory status that re-builds the cellular and molecular composition of the TME.[937,965] The latter occurred mainly through reprogramming the pre-existing stromal and non-stromal cells along with recruiting innate and adaptive immune cells toward the tumor site. However, the recruited cells might behave unexpectedly in the post-chemotherapy microenvironment.[966-968] Since altered TIME at early hours of therapy later brings both immunogenic and immune-suppressive responses, the unpredictable balance of these forces drives the tumor's final destiny.[969]

Cellular death frequently happens in tumors as a natural consequence of tumor growth. By focusing on the morphology of dying cells, cell death could be broadly categorized into two types of apoptosis and necrosis.[970,971] While remains of apoptotic cells are silently engulfed by resident phagocytes, during necrosis, the DAMPs released from smudged tumor cells signal the adjacent cells and macrophages via pattern recognition receptors (PRRs), namely TLRs, priming an extensive inflammatory immune response followed by migration of more macrophages and aiding adaptive immune cells seeking released TAAs.[967] Along with this, by considering the reaction of the immune system to dead cells, it is assumed that while necrosis is a noisy immunogenic death, apoptosis is silent and tolerogenic.[971,972] Although cytotoxic drug-induced death is mainly apoptotic, a number of chemotherapy agents such as anthracyclines, cyclophosphamide, and oxaliplatin are capable of inducing DNA damage, ER stress, and ROS production in exposed tumor cells and drive them toward an apparently apoptotic death, but in nature similar to necrosis with the upcoming immunogenicity named as immunogenic cell death (ICD).[973-977]

The chemotherapy-induced ICD is tightly engaged with a collection of DAMPs and stress-associated molecules and their tandem translocation to the extracellular milieu.[972] Instantly after the cytotoxic exposure, tumor cells accept and declare their obligatory pre-apoptotic state via translocating a chaperon named Calreticulin from ER to the cell surface.[978] Appearing Calreticulin on the outer surface of injured tumor cells is translated as an "eat me" signal to immature DCs or other APCs in the neighbor and prompts ICD.[978] Synchronously, tumor cells reduce the presentation of regular "don't eat me" signals on their outer surface that make them more visible to APCs. Small interfering (si)RNA-mediated knocking down of Calreticulin in a mice model of anthracycline-induced ICD was associated with abolished APCs' phagocytic and antigen processing functions.[979] Hours later, other chaperons, namely heat shock protein (HSP)70 and 90, are translocated from ER to the cell surface as another waving white flag for DCs, similar to Calreticulin.[971] These signals attract immature DCs and pro-apoptotic tumor cells to each other and induce a multi-step process leading to activation and maturation of DCs and eventually uptake of blebbing tumor cells.[978,980] In addition, high mobility group protein B1 (HMGB1), another DAMP that leaks from the nucleus of dying tumor cells attaches, and signals the activated DCs in a TLR-2/4-dependent manner to optimize the antigen processing of released TAAs from engulfed tumor cells. ATP, IFN, and IL-1β are among the last released molecules from the dying tumor cells that induce local inflammation and regulate the final steps of DC maturation.[978] Actually, ATP secretion from dying tumor cells is an inseparable characteristic of ICD.[968] Before chemotherapy, the tumor-infiltrating CD11b+ DCs are low in density and immature in phenotype.[968,981] Indeed, chemotherapy-induced ICD promotes the maturation of pre-existing DCs. ICD also causes an influx of myeloid precursors toward the tumor nest to become fully matured DCs in an ATP-dependent manner.[968,981] Maturity shifts DCs' immune-suppressive secretory profile to an immune-stimulating one. Specifically, released ATP provokes the activation of pyrin-containing NOD-like receptor (NLRP)3 inflammasome and secretion of IL-1β consequently. This is essential for recruiting and skewing the recruited T cells to polarize into cytotoxic INF-γ producing CD8+ T cells and CD4+ T cells.[981]

Following ICD, DCs receive the "eat me" signals and in tandem catch TAAs and particles released from dying tumor cells. TAA processing-DCs migrate to the tumor-draining lymph nodes, where they present the processed antigens to cytotoxic T cells and conduct a T cell-mediated anti-tumor response.[969] However, a report indicates that removing the tumor-draining lymph node could not suppress the efficacy of anthracycline-induced T cell responses.[968] Concluding that, probably TAA presenting DCs might not have to travel to lymph nodes and instead recruit T cells to DCs rich sites of tumor nests.[968,982] Tumor antigens are processed via APCs and presented to naïve cytotoxic T cells. This process is called cross-presentation.[981] In the pre-chemotherapy settings, DCs are not capable of priming the cross-presentation of TAAs. Although it is a consequence of local immune suppression rather than a persistent innate disability.[981] In the regular state, tumor cells downregulate the expression and presentation of MHC type I that is a strictly essential marker to notice naïve cytotoxic T cells to attack tumor cells and remove them.[983] This deceptive strategy keeps tumors safe from immune attacks and turns them into neglected enemies of immunosurveillance right inside the body. Surprisingly, chemotherapy can visualize tumor cells to the immune system via increasing the expression of MHC class I via an NF-kB pathway in survived tumor cells and guide the seeking T cells to hunt them.[983-987] In summary, chemotherapy can induce immunogenicity, broaden the load of TAAs, and increase the visibility of tumor cells.[978,988] Chemotherapy agents inducing ICD indirectly vaccinate the host as they kill tumor cells and spread their corpses, and overloaded specific antigens in the tumor bed following by adaptive immune responses.[937,971]

The post-chemotherapy microenvironment of tumors is hardly predictable due to the paradoxical effects of drugs on different cell types. The favorable anti-tumor response of adaptive immune cells following chemotherapy is explained here in a step-by-step approach. Even so, chemotherapy itself can hinder this response and paradoxically induce a supportive condition for tumor cells to escape. It has been reported that chemotherapy can temporarily alter the expression of immune inhibitory molecules, such as increasing the expression of PD-L1 in tumor cells.[984,989-991] Since activated cytotoxic T cells express PD-1 checkpoint, their connection with PD-L1 positive tumor cells could bring anergy or exhaustion.[984,992] Interestingly, in a mouse model of prostate cancer treated with oxaliplatin, which is an ICD-induced agent, Shalapour et al. indicated that oxaliplatin can induce the expression of PD-L1 and IL-10 not in tumor cells but in IgA+ CD20+ plasma cells, instead.[992] The yielded PD-L1+ IL-10+ plasmocytes harnessed the proper function of CTLs and inconsistently neutralized the immune-stimulating effect of ICD.[992]

Furthermore, in some studies, a number of chemotherapy agents such as gemcitabine, 5-fluorouracil, doxorubicin, and cyclophosphamide in some tumors were associated with the expansion of a population of myeloid cells functionally identical to MDSCs.[966,970,993-995] Mechanistically, chemotherapy causes cell stress and turns on the inflammatory pathways in tumor cells, specifically the NF-kB pathway, which leads to the expression of various inflammatory mediators.[970] GM-CSF is one of these mediators and is known as a critical factor in generating MDSCs following chemotherapy.[970,993] It has been shown that MDSCs exert at least one of their immunosuppressive tricks through the PD-1/PD-L1 axis to impede CD4+ T cells.[966] Surprisingly, these or some other drugs are reported as MDSCS eliminating agents in some other experiments.[996-1000] In addition to MDSCs, tumor-infiltrating macrophages are another myeloid population that are involved in post-chemotherapy immune escape.[1001,1002] Mechanistically, released DAMPs following chemotherapy attach to macrophages and stimulate them to hyper product IL-10.[1001] It has been reported that IL-10 does not silent CTLs directly but hinders the production of IL-12 in inflammatory DCs. IL-12 subunit B positively regulates the expression of granzyme B, IFN-γ, and CD8A in CTLs, which are required for a proper immune response.[1001]

## TIME post-radiation therapy

Radiation therapy is a conventional modality for local ablation of tumors. Ionizing radiation is cytotoxic due to inducing destructive DNA damages in exposed cells. Albeit, genetic material does rarely exposed to high energy photons directly.[1003] Actually, radiotherapy promotes intracellular water molecules' breakdown that produces high concentrations of ROS and NOS.[1003] The radiotherapy-induced oxidative burst is associated with oxidation of various cellular macromolecules, and single and double-strand DNA breaks, and consequently cell death.[1003] Indeed, tumor cells are not selectively exposed to ionizing rays, but as they lack proper DNA repair machinery, they are more prone to radiotherapy-induced DNA damage and upcoming cell death rather than normal cells around.[1004] Although it seems that basically low dose radiation is associated with a clean apoptotic cell death that is followed by a silent dead body clearance, high doses of radiotherapy, as they are utilized in clinical settings, induce noisy immunologic cell death, identical to chemotherapy-induced ICD.[1005,1006] Tumor debris, DAMPs (danger signals), and damaged genetic material promote "eat me" signals that attract and activate DCs or other APCs and prime an IFN-1-mediated CD8+ T cell-dependent anti-tumor response.[1007–1010] Radiotherapy upregulates the expression of lymphocyte chemoattractants such as CXCL9 and CXCL16 that attract helper and cytotoxic T cells.[1011] Interestingly, radiotherapy puts a "come and catch me" sign on tumor cells via increasing MHC class I expression that sensitizes cytotoxic T cells.[1012–1014] Surprisingly, radiotherapy-induced CTL-mediated response can go beyond the area of radiation in primary tumors and kill disseminated tumor cells in distant sites, a not common but considerable event known as the abscopal effect.[1015–1018] Radiotherapy turns on inflammatory signaling pathways in the irradiated tumor, stromal and endothelial cells such as NF-kB pathway that promote the production of a collection of pro-inflammatory cytokines (such as TNF-α, IL-1, and IL-6), chemokines (such as CXCL4, CCL2, and CSF-1) and growth factors such as TGF-β that attract bone marrow-derived cells, especially suppressive myeloid cells such as MDSCs and macrophages toward irrigation site.[1003,1019–1024] In addition to CTLs activation, the abscopal effect can be also a result of radiotherapy-induced MDSCs reduction in peripheral blood and distant sites. Hence, they are attracted to the primary tumor site.[1025] Radiotherapy also increases the accumulation and cytotoxic activity of NK cells and activates associated pathways via overexpressing the NKG2D ligand.[1005,1026]

Tumor vasculature network and precisely endothelial cells are harshly impressed by high-dose radiotherapy. Radiotherapy-induced oxidative burst induces apoptosis in endothelial cells that results in hyper-permeable and dysfunctional micro-vessels and consequently hypoxia.[1003,1005] Since oxygen is the major mediator of radiotherapy-induced DNA damage, hypoxia can impede tumor radiosensitivity.[1027] However, radiotherapy mainly shrinkages the tumor size via destroying clusters of oxygenated tumor cells at first, leaving behind hypoxic and pre-necrotic areas.[1011] These remaining hypoxic areas later find a chance to re-oxygenate as the tumor volume is reduced.[1003] Inflamed and damaged vessels also reduce the accumulation of cytotoxic T cells, and in turn, attract immunosuppressive populations such as MDSCs and Tregs.[1005,1011] Immune-suppressive crowding, in turn, enhances vascular damage and following hypoxia that consequently induce a defective loop and limit tumor radiosensitivity.[1011] In lower doses, endothelial cells are activated and express integrins and adhesion molecules such as ICAM-1, vascular cell adhesion protein (VCAM)−1, and E-selectin that in turn facilitates rolling and arrest of leukocytes in the irritated areas.[1005] The attracted leukocytes, precisely macrophages, and neutrophils show different faces depending on the local polarization cues. Indeed, radiotherapy confusingly can induce both tumor-suppressive and tumor-progenic TAMs and tumor-associated neutrophils (TANs).[1007,1022,1028–1031]

Collectively, radiotherapy-induced ICD, released chemokines, inflammatory mediators, vascular damage, and endothelial activation conduct an intra-tumoral vaccine through activating innate and adaptive immune responses.[1011,1032] Albeit, radiation contradictory reduces this vaccine-like effect via attracting tumor-supportive stromal and inflammatory cells and upregulation of immune inhibitory molecules such as PD-L1 or reducing expression of co-stimulatory molecules on APCs that impede adaptive immune response.[1011,1026,1033]

## Immune regulation of therapeutic-resistance

### Chemo-resistance

During their development, tumors continuously undergo selective environmental pressures such as early immune attacks, hypoxia, and acidosis. Indeed, each of them can be life challenging as they select which tumor cells are strong enough to survive. Similarly, chemotherapy also seems to be another selection pressure for tumor cells.[972,1034]

In most cases, chemotherapy insult is not tolerated by tumors. Resisting against chemotherapy is broadly divided into an instantly de novo program and a lately acquired one. De novo resistance is in part due to stochastic pre-existing variants of tumor cells that were assumed ordinary before chemotherapy exposure, unaware that they silently carry death-resisting mutations. The winning mutations might code changes in cellular transporters or metabolic pathways that cause drug efflux or reduced drug uptake and metabolism.[1034] In addition, tumor cells containing dysfunctional variants of ICD mediators and danger signals, which might not be considered as an advantage before, now turn to extraordinary resisting cells.[972,1035] Besides, this intrinsic side of the de novo resistance program that is more randomly in nature, the extrinsic side known as environment-mediated drug resistance (EMDR) that actively interferes in inducing chemo-resistance.[1034,1036] Briefly, EMDR is defined by two mechanisms, soluble factor mediated-drug resistance (SFM-DR) and cell adhesion-mediated drug resistance (CAM-DR). The first occurs when passing inflammatory cells and neighboring stromal cells in TME that are insulted by chemotherapy themselves, contact with tumor cells through soluble factors and paracrine loops as a damage response, and the second occurs while the tumor cells adhere to the surrounding ECM or a distinct stromal component such as collagen, fibronectin or laminin. SFM-DR or CAM-DR both eventually support tumor cells similarly through inducing them to turn on survival signals, inactivating apoptotic complexes, and beginning to express anti-apoptotic proteins. While chemotherapy rapidly kills sensitive phenotypes, EMDR buys time for tumors via generating a transiently-resistant population of tumor cells that survive as minimal residual of disease. As time passes, further pressures of therapy result in more acquired mutations and transcriptional advantages to permanently rescue chemotherapy and cause local/distant relapse.[1034]

### *Role of macrophages in environment-mediated drug resistance*

Sensitive tumor cells cannot overcome the cyclophosphamide-induced damage or ICD, but not all tumor cells are as sensitive to being killed. Therefore, the entire tumor is more like a wound rather than a corpse, and wounds tend to be healed.[973] Several studies on different tumor types and under different chemotherapeutic settings have shown that chemotherapy-induced damage causes tumor cells to produce monocytes' chemotactic factors. CSF1/CSF1-R and CCL2/CCR2 pathways are the best-known macrophages recruitment pathways so far.[959,991,1037–1039] IL-34, a second ligand for CSF1-R is produced as a result of the activated NF-kB pathway in damaged tumor cells and promotes macrophages recruitment.[1040] In a study on pancreatic tumor cells treated with gemcitabine, IL-8 is introduced as the chemotactic factor involved in macrophage infiltration.[1002] Monocytes' migration toward the wounded tumor is accompanied by an M2 phenotype polarization.[1040–1043] Gene signatures and expression profiles show the predominantly upregulation of M2 genes and markers such as arginase1 and TGF-β.[1002,1037] In a study on cervical and ovarian cell lines, cisplatin and carboplatin-induced DNA damage caused tumor cells to produce IL-6 and PGE2 in an NF-kB and STAT3 dependent manner, that in turn, skew recruited macrophages toward an M2 phenotype.[1042] In another study on NSCLC cell lines, cisplatin induced a similar polarization program via promoting tumor cells to secrete macrophage inhibitory factor (MIF).[1044]

Tumor-infiltrating macrophages are one of the predominant populations of TME and the key member of the tumor immune microenvironment. Thus, it is not surprising that they actively participate in EMDR.[1045] Evidence regards TAMs activation in drug resistance indicates that they exert their functions mainly by releasing cytokines, chemokines, exosomes, and other soluble factors or in a cell-contact basis that starts a paracrine or juxtacrine signaling pathway in tumor cells. The activated pathways support tumor cells against drug-induced cell death or induce survival signals.

M2 TAMs infiltrated following chemotherapy, suppress drug-induced apoptosis as the first plan to transiently rescue tumor cells. Caspase-dependent ICD could be stopped by reduced cleavage of caspases or triggered expression of anti-apoptotic genes like *BCL-2*. In a model of pancreatic tumor treaded with gemcitabine, M2 TAMs induce tumor cells to overexpress cytidine deaminase, the enzyme that metabolizes the drug after its transport into the cells, in order to reduce the activation of caspase-3 and upcoming apoptosis.[1046] In other settings, 5-fluorouracil-induced JNK/caspase-3 activation in colorectal tumors has been suppressed by TAMs.[1047] A different mechanism with a similar consequence has been reported in MM treated with melphalan. Protective macrophages physically contact MM cells and impede caspase-dependent apoptosis in a juxtacrine manner through P-selectin glycoprotein ligand-1 (PSGL-1)/selectin and ICAM-1/CD18 interactions.[1048,1049] In a study on tissues derived from a colorectal tumor, it has been showed that TAMs-derived IL-6 induces overexpression of *IL-6R*, *multiple drug resistance* (*MDR*) *1*, and *BCL-2* genes and thus, protect tumor cells against chemotherapy-induced apoptosis. This study also recognized that the IL-6/pSTAT3 signaling pathway inhibits mir-204–5p, a tumor suppressor.[1045] Paclitaxel-treated breast cancer cells also showed the same mechanism to escape paclitaxel-induced programmed cell death but in response to IL-10 instead. Following chemotherapy, TAMs-derived IL-10 activates the STAT3/BCL-2 pathway.[1043] Probably, there might be other mechanisms and pathways for macrophage-derived apoptosis protection that are not fully understood yet. As an example, in a model of hepatocellular carcinoma, macrophages induce autophagy in tumor cells to protect them from oxaliplatin-mediated apoptosis.[1050]

TAMs transfer regulatory miRNAs via exosomes as another route of connection with in-danger tumor cells. In two different reports, macrophages-derived exosomes, mir-21 in gastric cancer cells and mir-233 in ovarian cancer cell lines activate PTEN/PI3K/AKT pathway and induce survival signals.[1051,1052] Interestingly, another report investigating seven different tumor cell lines describes a macrophage-tumor cell dialogue mediated by exosomes, leading to regulation of transferrin receptor protein (TFR)1, a telomerase inhibitor, and consequently cellular survival against chemotherapy.[1053]

## Radio-resistance

Similar to chemotherapy, tumor response to radiotherapy is in part dependent on inherent cellular radiosensitivity, existing mutations, and DNA repair machine integrity that determines whether the injured tumor cell can survive upcoming cell death or not.[1054] However, radio-resistance is a complicated program beyond merely intrinsic cellular mutations. In fact, as irradiation insult is sensed by different molecules and pathways, conducts a DNA-damage response program that modifies tumor cells transcriptional profile and eventually might yield acquired radio-resistance.[1055] A major part of radiotherapy response is due to CTL-dependent anti-tumor response at the primary tumor and magic abscopal effect. Thereafter, acquired radiation resistance is in part based on restricting anti-tumor response that indeed is mediated through different mechanisms. For instance, DNA-damage response program induces expression and release of a collection of inflammatory cytokines and mediators, including but not limited to CCL2, CSF-1, CXCL12, and IL-6 that in turn attract and recruit myeloid bone marrow-derived myeloid cells such as macrophages, MDSCs, and neutrophils toward the irritated area, where they often exert immune suppressive functions and impede radiotherapy-induced anti-tumor immune response.[390,940,958,1056–1058] HMGB1, another molecule released as a result of DNA damage, not only directs tumor cells toward autophagy to escape radiotherapy-induced apoptosis but also further promotes infiltration of TAMs and MDSCs to restrict tumor radiosensitivity.[1059] Interestingly, attracted TANs are able to induce proliferation in tumor cells via stimulating mitogen-activated protein kinase (MAPK), a pro-survival pathway.[1060] In addition to attracted TAMs and TANs, it has been reported that in brain tumor microglias, CNS resident macrophages rescue tumor cells from radiotherapy-induced cell death and cause radiation resistance.[1061,1062] Interestingly, it seems that the transcriptional profile of radio-resistant tumor cells is altered and can limit CD8+ T cells infiltration.[1063] Furthermore, tumor-derived TGF-β under radiotherapy settings hijack resident T cells and alter their cytotoxic programs.[1064] Surprisingly, CTLs might point the pistol toward themselves via augmenting expression of PD-L1 on tumor cells in an IFN-γ dependent manner.[1065] Radiotherapy is often assumed to harshly destroy tumor vascular architecture and induce tumor hypoxia. As oxygen is the major mediator of radiotherapy-induced DNA damage, hypoxia can directly restrict radiation cytotoxic capacity. Hypoxia also causes the production of HIF-1 that attracts and mobilizes BMDCs with pro-angiogenic properties to promote angiogenesis, which maybe initially increases radiosensitivity but in the long-term is a hallmark of therapeutic relapse.[1005,1066,1067]

## Immune regulation of therapeutic-induced relapse

Almost all available cancer therapies, including chemo- and radiation therapy, surgery, and targeted therapies (especially anti-angiogenic drugs) are paradoxically linked to tumor relapse, local re-growth, or outgrowth in distant sites, despite their proven beneficial effects.[1054,1068,1069] It is worth mentioning that relapse in this context is not a consequence of therapy failure but a result of therapy-induced reactions. Drugs, radiotherapy, and surgical manipulations like biopsies, incisions, and partial resections all shrink the tumor or harshly disrupt its structure.[1069] In the previous section, it was discussed that how these therapeutic-induced alternations are twisted to tumor-resistance. It is hard to distinguish the invisible border between tumor-resistance and relapse-bearing events from each other.

## Therapy induces a dual tumor-host inflammatory response

Apparently, a dual tumor-host response to therapy mediates both resistance, and consequently, local and distant tumor relapse.[1070] Briefly, therapy stress causes DNA damage response and associated inflammatory and secretory programs in both tumor and stromal cells in TME. Besides, induced hypoxia, tumor-derived debris, and microparticles all lead to a chemokine /cytokine burst with local (tumor) and systemic (host) effec ts.[1069,1071,1072] As we explained before, the local effects, as a part of de novo resistance, lead to early survival of minor tumor populations that later may earn more aggressive phenotypes (future metastatic seeds). The cytokine burst systemically affects normal tissues and reactive host stress-sensing cells in different sites, especially bone marrow that consequently causes an acute mobilization of myeloid BMDCs with pro-angiogenic features and huge production of inflammatory mediators and growth factors. Mobilized BMDCs infiltrate tumor sites and hostile distant sites to create promising niches for angiogenesis and re-growth of survived tumor cells at the primary site and successful colonization of disseminated seeds in the distant sites (the soil). Thus, it seems that the host response can be the missing link between therapy-induced resistance and upcoming relapse.

## Loco-Regional relapse

### *Angiogenesis*

Several studies on preclinical and clinical models of cancer have introduced neoangiogenesis as a potent mechanism of tumor local re-growth following different therapeutic modalities.[1073–1079] In addition to epithelial progenitor cells (EPCs), bone marrow-derived myelomonocytic cells (CD11b+) are also a critical source for chemotherapy-induced angiogenesis, mobilizing toward tumor as a consequence of host response.[1074,1080] Chemotherapy increases the quantity and pro-cancer properties of tumor cell-derived microparticles (TMPs). Treating EMT/6 murine breast cancer cells with paclitaxel increased TMPs and their osteopontin expression, a factor associated with recruitment of myeloid progenitor cells from BMDCs.[1071] It has also been shown that paclitaxel can imitate the LPS-mediated activation of the TLR-4 pathway in breast cancer cells that induces a systemic inflammatory response and produces IL-1β, IL-6, and IL-10 that results in the migration of CD11b+ Ly6C+ myeloid BMDCs toward the primary tumor site to increase angiogenesis.[1081] Furthermore, chemotherapy derives a specific population of M2 TAMs with CD206+ TIE2+ CXCR4 high VEGFA+ phenotype.[1082] Apparently, infiltration of CD206+ TAMs is an initial bad omen, predicting upcoming relapse.[1083] TIE2+, which is a receptor tyrosine kinase protects macrophages from chemotherapy-induced apoptosis via activating the AKT pathway, and it is a hallmark of pro-angiogenic features.[1073] Interestingly, cyclophosphamide-derived hypoxia can induce the expression of TIE2 in previously TIE2- CD11b+ myeloid cells in TME.[1073] Chemotherapy, in part by inducing oxidative stress causes upregulation of CXCL12, a ligand of CXCR4, in specific spaces nearby the vessels that are known as perivascular niches (PVNs), and thereby, guide TIE2+ CXCR4 high angiogenic TAMs.[1066,1082] A similar interaction between perivascular expressed CXCL12 and CXCR4hi recruited bone marrow-derived myeloid cells also was shown following tumor local radiation and vascular-disruptive drugs.[1075,1084]

Anti-angiogenic targeted therapies and irradiation both destruct the tumor vascular network and cause hypoxia.[1078,1085–1087] This promotes release of chemo-attractants such as G-CSF and host inflammatory response that acutely attract MMP-9 expressing CD11b+ VEGF+ myeloid cells as regulators of vasculogenesis to recover the damaged vessels.[1077,1087–1090]

Surgery stress caused either by direct trauma, induced hypoxia, or vascular damage is associated with increased levels of pro-angiogenic factors such as VEGF and Angiopoietin-2 (Ang-2) and bone marrow-derived endothelial- and myeloid progenitor cells in the circulation.[1072,1079,1091,1092]

### *Immune escape and proliferation*

Refractory relapses following therapy are not merely due to acquired aggressive behaviors in tumor cells, but it is also a result of immune evasion and breaking immune-mediated limited proliferation.[1093,1094] It seems that surgical stress is a well-established cue for inducing local and systemic responses. For example, in needle biopsy or partial resections, the injured residual tumor mimics a wound and promotes a systemic wound-healing response that is initiated by attracting neutrophils, macrophages, and fibroblasts, releasing inflammatory and regenerative factors such as PGs and TGF-β in TME and circulation that eventually continuous with ECM remodeling, angiogenesis, and down-regulation of the adaptive immune response.[1094–1097] Apparently, under the wound-healing condition, the inflammatory environment recruits and alternatively activates macrophages and Tregs that can promptly hinder Th1 and consequently Th2 responses.[1098–1100] TGF-β acts as a critical chemotactic molecule for M2-TAMs and Tregs.[1100] Interestingly, a report on investigating the effect of surgical stress on a mouse model of breast cancer showed that surgery induces mobilization of MDSCs toward the wounded site, and MDSCs, in turn, produce high amounts of IL-10 and TGF-β that can attract more

Tregs.[1092] As it was mentioned earlier, surgery stress increases the serum level of Ang-2, a pro-angiogenic factor that binds to the TIE2 receptor on TIE2+ TAMs. Surprisingly, the Ang-2/TIE2 connection activates TIE2+ TAMs to express and release more IL-10, which harshly impede CD8+ T cells proliferation and function, and also CCL17, a potent chemo-attractant that expands the Treg population in tumors.[1101] In addition to breaking immune-limited growth, it seems that M2 TAMs can also directly increase the proliferation of residual tumor cells.[1100,1102]

## Distant relapse

### *At the primary site*

The tumor heterogeneity, at least in part, is due to the existence of special subpopulations of tumor-initiating cells with stem-like features commonly known as CSCs.[1103] Although classical cytotoxic therapies such as chemotherapy and radiotherapy eliminate a massive number of non-CSC, they merely can affect CSCs, remaining a crowd of survivors leading to further relapse.[1104] It has been reported that treatment-induced inflammatory state or post-surgery wound condition can directly induce CSCs proliferation via stimulating their stemness-related signaling pathways such as NF-kB and Wnt/β-catenin.[1105–1107] Furthermore, mobilization of bone marrow-derived myeloid-lineage cells, precisely monocytes/macrophages as prompt host response, is linked to therapy-dependent self-renewal of CSCs.[1108] Attracted TAMs are able to release stemness-inducing cytokines/chemokines such as IL-1β, IL-6, and TNF-α to enhance the quantity of CSCs and their stem-like features.[1039,1109,1110] CSCs express mesenchymal-related genes, exert more invasive properties, and have less sensitivity to drugs cytotoxicity. Thus, their niches can potentially turn into undeniable pockets of pro-metastatic seeds.[1110] Surprisingly, the therapy-induced tumor-host response is able to provoke partial EMT, a phenotype-determining program that can finely tune the expression of stemness-related genes in cancer cells and promote a reversible conversion of non-CSCs to CSCs that yield more seeds.[1054,1110–1113] Indeed, EMT turns on a collection of genes, morphological and functional properties that physically enhances the chance of cancer cells (seeds) to overcome the obstacles of distant dissemination.[1114] Cyclophosphamide-caused inflammatory burst generally stimulates TAMs, probably both M1 and M2 phenotypes, to induce EMT in non-CSCs, and therefore, increases the number of motile chemo-resistance cells with metastatic abilities.[1115,1116] Few reports indicate that PVNs restore CSCs in mouse models of brain tumors.[1117–1119] Considering this and the accumulation of TAMs in PVNs following chemotherapy, another possible CSCs-protective function of macrophages might be attributed to pro-vascular TAMs (PV-TAMs), though it is still not defined.[1120] In addition to macrophages, it seems that other types of bone marrow-derived myeloid cells such as MDSCs and neutrophils also can drive the EMT program in cancer cells.[1121,1122] For instance, post-surgical stress in a mouse model of breast cancer was associated with the accumulation of CD11b+ Gr1+ MDSCs in the primary tumor, where they stimulate expression of EMT-related genes in cancer cells and promote metastasis.[1092]

It has been shown that there must be a correlation between the number of viable disseminated tumor cells and a higher chance for successful colonization in distant sites. The number of disseminated tumor cells is dependent on the number of tumor cells that can enter the bloodstream and survive from the shear stress and intravascular immune recognition.[1054] Intravasation seems to occur both in passive and active routs.[1123] Different conventional therapies can increase the number of circulating tumor cells.[1124–1126] Chemotherapy, radiotherapy, and especially surgical procedures are accompanied by damage or at least increased permeability of vascular bed and structural disruption of tumor nests.[1112,1127–1129] Thus, probably shedding viable or apoptotic tumor cells and debris can passively enter the fragile and broken blood vessels.[1086,1123,1130,1131] However, as these populations of circulating tumor cells have been accidentally entered the vasculature while they have not the opportunity to acquire invasive traits, they might not find the chance to survive and home at distant sites. Therefore, there must be another reason to link the increased number of circulating tumor cells and the increased rate of successful seeding following therapy. For instance, the increased number of circulating tumor cells might be also attributed to the expansion of stem-like and resistant cancer cells following therapy-induced host response, as was discussed earlier. Surprisingly, there is evidence that cyclophosphamide plus paclitaxel also push survived cancer cells actively inside the blood vessels not by inducing a novel mechanism but via enhancing the classical routes of active intravasation like through the tumor microenvironment of metastasis (TMEM).[1132] TMEMs are micro-anatomical gateways through blood vessels, predominantly in points with less pericyte coverage, assembled from joining streaming Mena-invasive tumor cells to a TIE2+ perivascular TAMs and the neighbor endothelial cells.[1133,1134] At TMEM, TIE2+ TAMs release VEGFA to transiently loosen tight junctions between endothelial cells and create a tiny tunnel for cancer cells to cross (trans-endothelial migration).[1134] For doing so, tumor cells must be able to form degrading feet or invadopodium that is associated with overexpressing Mena-invasive, the invasive isoform of an actin-regulatory protein.[1135,1136] Apparently, Mena-invasive expression in cancer cells is induced through the Notch1 pathway in physical contact with macrophages.[1136] Two different reports on breast cancer mouse models and patients showed that chemotherapy-induced BMDMs mobilization enhances active intravasation via increasing TMEM assembly and function and decreasing pericyte coating.[1036,1137,1138] Indeed, chemotherapy-induced host response mobilizes TIE2+ CXCR4 high monocytes from bone marrow to find CXCL12 rich PVNs and reside there, expecting an invasive tumor cell to assembly another TMEM.[1082,1138,1139] Interestingly, chemotherapy-induced inflammation provokes EMT program that in turn increases motile tumor cells.[1140] Also, it recruits more bone marrow-derived monocytes that enhance the possibility of tumor cells-macrophages physical contacts, and hence, Notch1-dependent

Mena-invasive expression, an additional road to resistance.[1138,1141] It has not been clearly understood whether the stimulation of angiogenesis as a part of tissue-repair response after therapy is associated with more intravasation or not, but apparently, it is correlated with distant relapse.[1108,1142] Even so, it seems that chemotherapy-induced lymphangiogenesis is correlated with higher rates of intravasation and distant metastasis.[1143] Interestingly, the chemotherapeutic agent, paclitaxel, induces infiltration of VEGFR3+ cathepsin producer TAMs in TME that further promotes lymphangiogenesis-mediated distant metastasis.[1144] Actually, M2 TAMs are associated with lymphangiogenesis, lymphovascular invasion, and lymph node metastasis that eventually lead to distant metastasis both in pre- and post-chemotherapy settings.[1083,1143–1147]

### At distant sites

Cytotoxic therapies and surgical stress both induce a systemic inflammatory state that impedes circulating tumor cells clearance machinery driven by intraluminal innate immune cells, precisely NK cells, and in parallel, provokes their arrest and adhesion via modulating the endothelial barrier at pre-metastatic sites. Thus, therapy-induced inflammation facilitates circulating tumor cells intraluminal struggle for survival and eventually increases the number of survived circulating tumor cells.[1069,1100,1137,1148–1150]

Interestingly, surgery-induced stress can induce neutrophilia and hijack circulating neutrophils to join circulating tumor cells during the last events of the metastatic cascade. Briefly, neutrophils increase retention of tumor cells in the pre-metastatic sites mainly through three steps. First, they suppress circulatory NK cells, saving circulating tumor cells from following clearance.[1151] Second, neutrophils capture circulating tumor cells, promote their adhesion to endothelial cells, and extravasation.[1151–1153] Mechanistically, the systemic inflammation following surgery-induced hypoxia or infection triggers neutrophils to spread a net made of protruded chromatin fibers known as neutrophil extracellular trap (NET) that physically entraps tumor cells.[1150,1154,1155] However, NET is not only a physical web to capture circulating tumor cells, as these DNA fibers are decorated with various inflammatory molecules that aid arrested tumor cells adhesion to endothelial wall and extravasation, at least in part with a TLR-9 dependent manner.[1150,1154] Neutrophils also express integrins that bind to adhesion molecules expressed on circulating tumor cells, make a steady complex to promote their anchorage to endothelial cells or release pro-metastatic molecules such as IL-1$\beta$, MMP-9, and cathepsins that promote extravasation and following colonization in pre-metastatic sites like liver and lung.[1151–1153,1156] Third, neutrophils' secretions such as leukotrienes and NETosis promote colonization through inducing survival signals and proliferation in metastatic seeds.[1150,1156,1157]

The normal microenvironment in tissues far from the primary tumor site seems to be a hostile soil for foreign metastatic seeds. This normal microenvironment may reject the foreign metastatic seeds. Therefore, tumors intelligently release soluble factors, microparticles, and extracellular vesicles into the circulation to affect distant sites and prepare a proper niche for circulating tumor cells to arrest and reside, which consequently prevent their early rejection.[1158] Pre-metastatic niches are inflamed and immune-suppressed niches, with re-programmed resident cells, precisely macrophages and fibroblasts, remodeled ECM, and leaky vessels prone to arrest and adhesion of circulating tumor cells.[1159] The question is how conventional cancer therapies might induce/amplify these hallmarks in normal tissues far from the disrupted tumor? Evidently, therapy-induced local stress, inflammation, and hypoxia ease the production of tumor-derived soluble factors and debris such as extracellular vehicles (EVs) and microparticles.[1071,1160–1163] For instance, surgery-induced local hypoxia stimulates the production and systemic release of lysyl oxidase (LOX) from residual tumor cells. At the lungs, released LOX crosslinks type IV collagen fibers and induces adhesion signaling.[1161] Besides surgery, chemotherapy induces tumor cells to send away exosomes, covered with ECM remodeling enzymes.[1164] Thus, therapy might promote matrix remodeling as the first hallmark of pre-metastatic niche formation.[1158,1161,1164] Inflammation and immunosuppression, as the second hallmark of pre-metastatic niche formation, is due to the accumulation of BMDCs, especially the myelomonocytic lineage.[1159,1165] As it was mentioned earlier, chemotherapy-induced repair response can both directly or indirectly, via increasing tumor-derived secretion and debris, rapidly stimulate the mobilization of BMDCs toward primary tumor and pre-metastatic sites.[1112,1160,1166] Furthermore, it seems that tumor-derived microparticles that are over-released under chemotherapy settings also independently accumulate in distant sites like lungs and reprogram resident macrophages to produce CCL2, a potent chemo-attractant for CD11b+ Ly6c+ CCR2+ monocytes.[1071,1167] In addition to microparticles, chemotherapy-induced EVs from breast cancer cells that contain annexin-A6 induce the NF-kB pathway in endothelial cells of lung and liver vessels to produce CCL2.[1162] Local radiotherapy also generates a similar host response and induces BMDCS-dependent pre-metastatic niche formation.[1160,1168,1169] Attracted monocytes turn to metastasis-associated macrophages, adhere to the remodeled matrix, and promote further matrix remodeling via releasing MMPs, express inflammatory cytokines and growth factors, and increase vascular permeability by producing VEGFA to assist circulating tumor cells extravasation and seeding.[1167,1170] MDSCs are another predominant population of BMDCs that induce the infiltration of the PMNs, precisely following surgical stress. MDSCs exert their immune-suppressive functions via suppressing NK cells' expansion and cytotoxicity and consequently reduce the chance of circulating tumor cells elimination after extravasation.[1092,1171,1172]

Interestingly, in parallel with attracting inflammatory macrophages and MDSCs to pre-metastatic niches, chemotherapy can also activate specific resident macrophages in the pre-metastatic tissues or induce differentiation of their progenitor cells to expand their population. In the case of bone as the pre-metastatic site, osteoclasts and bone-specific resident macrophages are "giant bone eaters" that degrade bone via secreting

MMPs and consequently create a growth factor-rich lodge for arrived circulating tumor cells, resulting in osteolytic bone metastasis. Osteoclasts also turn off the "dormancy switch" and awaken quiescent cancer cells. Chemotherapeutic agents such as doxorubicin, melphalan, and methotrexate induce a stress response or release inflammatory cytokines such as TNF-α in bone and increase osteoclast progenitor cells and their differentiation, which subsequently create a trophic pre-metastatic niche.[1173–1176] Chemotherapy also induces the expression of jagged-1, a ligand that activates the Notch pathway, in osteoblast and augments osteoclastogenesis and associated bone reabsorption.[1177,1178] Interestingly, chemotherapy-induced CCL2 overproduction might also have a pro-metastatic effect on the bone marrow niche since CCL2 is a key regulator of osteoclast formation.[1179–1181] Specific resident macrophages in the liver microenvironment, namely Kupffer cells, are activated in response to colorectal surgery and produce ROS that damage endothelial cell lining, leading to matrix exposure, which is a selective adhesion site for shedding colon tumor cells.[1182,1183]

Metastatic seeds find themselves in completely foreign soil after extravasation in distant sites. Disseminated tumor cells' innate capacities and interactions with the new microenvironment determine whether they will survive or not. However, it seems that their fate is not harshly limited to these two ends, but alternatively, they might find a chance to remain in a "dormant state" somewhere between apoptosis and mitosis, waiting for a second chance to overcome environmental obstacles and escape dormancy.[1184–1186] Tumor dormancy in metastatic sites is mainly limited to three types. Cellular dormancy, angiogenic dormancy, and immunologic dormancy.[1186,1187] The two latter are related to the foreign microenvironment and can be altered by therapy-induced host responses.[1184] Indeed, permissive niches such as stem cell niche, PVNs, and immune niche support disseminated tumor cells dormancy state while existing pre-metastatic niches augment their chance of proliferation and outgrowth initially after arrival at distant sites.[17,1185,1188–1191] Thus, therapy-induced pre-metastatic niche formation provides newcomers supportive signals from their new microenvironment that bypass dormancy program and accelerate clinical overt metastatic outgrowth.[1069,1098,1184]

In addition, some tumor cells might detach at earlier stages of tumor progression precisely before therapeutic interventions and lodge in named permissive niches in a dormant state.[1185,1192,1193] Surprisingly chemotherapy might hijack dormancy permissive niches. For instance, inducing osteoclast formation that reabsorbs endosteal surface awakens pre-existing dormant cells in bone marrow stem cell niche and facilities their growth.[1173,1194] It seems that primary tumor prime innate and adaptive mediated anti-tumor responses in secondary sites eliminate early disseminated tumor cells or derive them toward immunologic dormancy, and thus, limit metastatic lesion formation.[1170,1193,1195] Interestingly, surgical systemic stress and upcoming inflammation impede CD8+ T cell-mediated response and set free immune-restricted dormant disseminated tumor cells.[1094,1193,1196] Furthermore, therapy-induced inflammation promotes neutrophils and NETosis that in turn remodel extracellular matrix in dormant niches and enhance matrix adhesion molecules, and awakening proliferation signals in dormant disseminated tumor cells.[1150,1197]

Even so, disseminated tumor cells, whether as solitary cells or clusters, would not proliferate further to form macro-metastatic lesions until they lack adequate vasculature.[1186] Cytotoxic therapies and surgery both induce a systemic inflammatory state, increase pro-angiogenic factors and mobilize BMDCs that altogether turn on angiogenesis switch in metastatic sites, in addition to the primary tumor and assist new micro-metastatic foci to break angiogenic dormancy. Surprisingly, angiogenic dormancy is closely related to primary tumor existence since, in different preclinical models and patients, complete resection of the primary tumor is followed by higher and earlier metastatic attacks. It is hypothesized that primary tumor paradoxically produces and releases both pro- and anti-angiogenic factors such as angiostatin in circulation, while anti-angiogenic factors would drive disseminated tumor cells toward angiogenic dormancy. Resection of primary tumor means eliminating a source of angiogenesis inhibitory factors.[1198,1199] Thus, surgical removal of primary tumor induces a somehow ghost effect since the removed tumor can continuously grow in distant sites. Overall, therapy-induced inflammation and wound-healing responses following surgery directly or indirectly promote dormancy escape and reactivate dormant disseminated tumor cells and pre-existing silent micro-metastases.[964,1102,1184,1200,1201]

## References


1. Siegel RL, Miller KD, Jemal A. Cancer statistics, 2020. *CA Cancer J. Clin.* 2020;70(1):7–30.
2. Bray F, Ferlay J, Soerjomataram I, Siegel RL, Torre LA, Jemal A. Global cancer statistics 2018: GLOBOCAN estimates of incidence and mortality worldwide for 36 cancers in 185 countries. *CA Cancer J. Clin.* 2018;68(6):394–424.
3. Shao H, Yu Q, Bo X, Duan Z. Analysis of oncology research from 2001 to 2010: a scientometric perspective. *Oncol. Rep.* 2013;29(4):1441–1452.
4. Allemani C, Matsuda T, Di Carlo V, Harewood R, Matz M, Nikšić M, et al. Global surveillance of trends in cancer survival 2000-14 (CONCORD-3): analysis of individual records for 37 513 025 patients diagnosed with one of 18 cancers from 322 population-based registries in 71 countries. *Lancet.* 2018;391(10125):1023–1075.
5. Hanahan D, Weinberg RA. Hallmarks of cancer: the next generation. *Cell.* 2011;144(5):646–674.
6. Meacham CE, Morrison SJ. Tumour heterogeneity and cancer cell plasticity. *Nature.* 2013;501(7467):328–337.
7. Weinberg RA. *The Biology of Cancer.* W.W. Norton; 2013.
8. Dunn GP, Bruce AT, Ikeda H, Old LJ, Schreiber RD. Cancer immunoediting: from immunosurveillance to tumor escape. *Nat. Immunol.* 2002;3(11):991–998.
9. Kim R, Emi M, Tanabe K. Cancer immunoediting from immune surveillance to immune escape. *Immunology.* 2007;121(1):1–14.
10. Zamarron BF, Chen W. Dual roles of immune cells and their factors in cancer development and progression. *Int J Biol Sci.* 2011;7(5):651–658.
11. Zhang Y, Zhang Z. The history and advances in cancer immunotherapy: understanding the characteristics of tumor-infiltrating immune cells and their therapeutic implications. *Cell. Mol. Immunol.* 2020;17(8):807–821.

12. Swann JB, Smyth MJ. Immune surveillance of tumors. *J. Clin. Invest.* 2007;117(5):1137–1146.
13. Heydari K, Shamshirian A, Lotfi-Foroushani P, Aref A, Hedayatizadeh-Omran A, Ahmadi M, et al. The risk of malignancies in patients receiving hematopoietic stem cell transplantation: a systematic review and meta-analysis. *Clinical and Translational Oncology.* 2020;22(10):1825–1837.
14. Kiaee F, Azizi G, Rafiemanesh H, Zainaldain H, Sadaat Rizvi F, Alizadeh M, et al. Malignancy in common variable immunodeficiency: a systematic review and meta-analysis. *Expert Rev Clin Immunol.* 2019;15(10):1105–1113.
15. Shiels MS, SR C, Kirk GD, Poole C. A meta-analysis of the incidence of non-AIDS cancers in HIV-infected individuals. *J. Acquir. Immune Defic. Syndr.* 2009;52(5):611–622.
16. Haas OA. Primary Immunodeficiency and Cancer Predisposition Revisited: embedding Two Closely Related Concepts Into an Integrative Conceptual Framework. *Front. Immunol.* 2019;9:3136.
17. Goddard ET, Bozic I, Riddell SR, Ghajar CM. Dormant tumour cells, their niches and the influence of immunity. *Nat. Cell Biol.* 2018;20(11):1240–1249.
18. Dhodapkar MV, Krasovsky J, Osman K, Geller MD. Vigorous premalignancy-specific effector T cell response in the bone marrow of patients with monoclonal gammopathy. *J. Exp. Med.* 2003;198(11):1753–1757.
19. Wilkie KP, Hahnfeldt P. Mathematical models of immune-induced cancer dormancy and the emergence of immune evasion. *Interface Focus.* 2013;3(4):20130010.
20. Hsu DS, Kim MK, Balakumaran BS, Acharya CR, Anders CK, Clay T, et al. Immune signatures predict prognosis in localized cancer. *Cancer Invest.* 2010;28(7):765–773.
21. Quigley DA, Kristensen V. Predicting prognosis and therapeutic response from interactions between lymphocytes and tumor cells. *Mol Oncol.* 2015;9(10):2054–2062.
22. Miao Y-R, Zhang Q, Lei Q, Luo M, Xie G-Y, Wang H, et al. ImmuCellAI: a Unique Method for Comprehensive T-Cell Subsets Abundance Prediction and its Application in Cancer Immunotherapy. *Advanced Science.* 2020;7(7):1902880.
23. Lyons YA, Wu SY, Overwijk WW, Baggerly KA, Sood AK. Immune cell profiling in cancer: molecular approaches to cell-specific identification. *npj Precision Oncology.* 2017;1(1):26.
24. Chuah S, Chew V. High-dimensional immune-profiling in cancer: implications for immunotherapy. *J. Immunother. Cancer.* 2020;8(1):e000363.
25. Thorsson V, Gibbs DL, Brown SD, Wolf D, Bortone DS, Ou Yang T-H, et al. The immune landscape of cancer. *Immunity.* 2018;48(4):812–830 e14.
26. Bruni D, Angell HK, Galon J. The immune contexture and Immunoscore in cancer prognosis and therapeutic efficacy. *Nat. Rev. Cancer.* 2020.
27. Lanitis E, Dangaj D, Irving M, Coukos G. Mechanisms regulating T-cell infiltration and activity in solid tumors. *Ann. Oncol.* 2017;28:xii18–xii32.
28. Guidoboni M, Gafà R, Viel A, Doglioni C, Russo A, Santini A, et al. Microsatellite instability and high content of activated cytotoxic lymphocytes identify colon cancer patients with a favorable prognosis. *Am. J. Pathol.* 2001;159(1):297–304.
29. Dolcetti R, Viel A, Doglioni C, Russo A, Guidoboni M, Capozzi E, et al. High prevalence of activated intraepithelial cytotoxic T lymphocytes and increased neoplastic cell apoptosis in colorectal carcinomas with microsatellite instability. *Am. J. Pathol.* 1999;154(6):1805–1813.
30. Nakata B, Qing Wang Y, Yashiro M, Nishioka N, Tanaka H, Ohira M, et al. Prognostic Value of Microsatellite Instability in Resectable Pancreatic Cancer. *Clin. Cancer Res.* 2002;8(8):2536.
31. Fu Q, Chen N, Ge C, Li R, Li Z, Zeng B, et al. Prognostic value of tumor-infiltrating lymphocytes in melanoma: a systematic review and meta-analysis. *Oncoimmunology.* 2019;8(7):1593806.
32. Joyce JA, Fearon DT. T cell exclusion, immune privilege, and the tumor microenvironment. *Science.* 2015;348(6230):74.
33. Chen DS, Mellman I. Elements of cancer immunity and the cancer–immune set point. *Nature.* 2017;541(7637):321–330.
34. Samstein RM, Lee C-H, Shoushtari AN, Hellmann MD, Shen R, Janjigian YY, et al. Tumor mutational load predicts survival after immunotherapy across multiple cancer types. *Nat. Genet.* 2019;51(2):202–206.
35. Coulie PG, Van den Eynde BJ, van der Bruggen P, Boon T. Tumour antigens recognized by T lymphocytes: at the core of cancer immunotherapy. *Nat. Rev. Cancer.* 2014;14(2):135–146.

36. Neefjes J, Jongsma MLM, Paul P, Bakke O. Towards a systems understanding of MHC class I and MHC class II antigen presentation. *Nat. Rev. Immunol.* 2011;11(12):823–836.
37. Vigneron N. Human Tumor Antigens and Cancer Immunotherapy. *Biomed. Res. Int.* 2015;2015:948501.
38. Merzougui N, Kratzer R, Saveanu L, van Endert P. A proteasome-dependent, TAP-independent pathway for cross-presentation of phagocytosed antigen. *EMBO Rep.* 2011;12(12):1257–1264.
39. Oliveira CC, van Hall T. Alternative Antigen Processing for MHC Class I: multiple Roads Lead to Rome. *Front. Immunol.* 2015;6(298).
40. Leclerc D, Beauseigle D, Denis J, Morin H, Paré C, Lamarre A, et al. Proteasome-Independent Major Histocompatibility Complex Class I Cross-Presentation Mediated by Papaya Mosaic Virus-Like Particles Leads to Expansion of Specific Human T Cells. *J. Virol.* 2007;81(3):1319.
41. Embgenbroich M, Burgdorf S. Current Concepts of Antigen Cross-Presentation. *Front. Immunol.* 2018;9(1643).
42. Gros M, Amigorena S. Regulation of Antigen Export to the Cytosol During Cross-Presentation. *Front. Immunol.* 2019;10(41).
43. Gleisner MA, Navarrete M, Hofmann F, Salazar-Onfray F, Tittarelli A. Mind the Gaps in Tumor Immunity: impact of Connexin-Mediated Intercellular Connections. *Front. Immunol.* 2017;8(1067).
44. Akers SN, Odunsi K, Karpf AR. Regulation of cancer germline antigen gene expression: implications for cancer immunotherapy. *Future Oncol.* 2010;6(5):717–732.
45. James SR, Link PA, Karpf AR. Epigenetic regulation of X-linked cancer/germline antigen genes by DNMT1 and DNMT3b. *Oncogene.* 2006;25(52):6975–6985.
46. Kim R, Kulkarni P, Hannenhalli S. Derepression of Cancer/Testis Antigens in cancer is associated with distinct patterns of DNA Hypomethylation. *BMC Cancer.* 2013;13(1):144.
47. Fratta E, Coral S, Covre A, Parisi G, Colizzi F, Danielli R, et al. The biology of cancer testis antigens: putative function, regulation and therapeutic potential. *Mol Oncol.* 2011;5(2):164–182.
48. Smith CC, Selitsky SR, Chai S, Armistead PM, Vincent BG, Serody JS. Alternative tumour-specific antigens. *Nat. Rev. Cancer.* 2019;19(8):465–478.
49. Kalaora S, Lee JS, Barnea E, Levy R, Greenberg P, Alon M, et al. Immunoproteasome expression is associated with better prognosis and response to checkpoint therapies in melanoma. *Nat. Commun.* 2020;11(1):896.
50. Morozov AV, Karpov VL. Proteasomes and Several Aspects of Their Heterogeneity Relevant to Cancer. *Front. Oncol.* 2019;9:761.
51. Vigneron N, Van den Eynde BJ. Proteasome subtypes and the processing of tumor antigens: increasing antigenic diversity. *Curr. Opin. Immunol.* 2012;24(1):84–91.
52. Huang J, El-Gamil M, Dudley ME, Li YF, Rosenberg SA, Robbins PF. T cells associated with tumor regression recognize frameshifted products of the CDKN2A tumor suppressor gene locus and a mutated HLA class I gene product. *J. Immunol.* 2004;172(10):6057–6064.
53. Jiang T, Shi T, Zhang H, Hu J, Song Y, Wei J, et al. Tumor neoantigens: from basic research to clinical applications. *J. Hematol. Oncol.* 2019;12(1):93.
54. Schumacher TN, Scheper W, Kvistborg P. Cancer Neoantigens. *Annual Review of Immunology.* 2019;37(1):173–200.
55. Ueda N, Zhang R, Tatsumi M, Liu T-Y, Kitayama S, Yasui Y, et al. BCR–ABL-specific CD4+ T-helper cells promote the priming of antigen-specific cytotoxic T cells via dendritic cells. *Cell. Mol. Immunol.* 2018;15(1):15–26.
56. van Denderen J, Hermans A, Meeuwsen T, Troelstra C, Zegers N, Boersma W, et al. Antibody recognition of the tumor-specific bcr-abl joining region in chronic myeloid leukemia. *J. Exp. Med.* 1989;169(1):87–98.
57. Tashiro H, Brenner MK. Immunotherapy against cancer-related viruses. *Cell Res.* 2017;27(1):59–73.
58. de Martel C, Georges D, Bray F, Ferlay J, Clifford GM. Global burden of cancer attributable to infections in 2018: a worldwide incidence analysis. *The Lancet Global Health.* 2020;8(2):e180–e190.
59. Habel K. Virus Tumor Antigens: specific Fingerprints? *Cancer Res.* 1966;26(9 Part 1):2018.
60. Gilden RV, Beddow TG, Huebner RJ. Production of high-titer antibody in serum and ascitic fluid of hamsters for a variety of virus-induced tumor antigens. *Appl. Microbiol.* 1967;15(3):657–660.
61. Weon JL, Potts PR. The MAGE protein family and cancer. *Curr. Opin. Cell Biol.* 2015;37:1–8.
62. Smith HA, McNeel DG. The SSX family of cancer-testis antigens as target proteins for tumor therapy. *Clin. Dev. Immunol.* 2010;2010:150591.

63. Arsenic R, Braicu EI, Letsch A, Dietel M, Sehouli J, Keilholz U, et al. Cancer-testis antigen cyclin A1 is broadly expressed in ovarian cancer and is associated with prolonged time to tumor progression after platinum-based therapy. *BMC Cancer*. 2015;15(1):784.
64. Dao T, Korontsvit T, Zakhaleva V, Jarvis C, Mondello P, Oh C, et al. An immunogenic WT1-derived peptide that induces T cell response in the context of HLA-A*02:01 and HLA-A*24:02 molecules. *Oncoimmunology*. 2016;6(2):e1252895.
65. Anguille S, Van Tendeloo VF, Berneman ZN. Leukemia-associated antigens and their relevance to the immunotherapy of acute myeloid leukemia. *Leukemia*. 2012;26(10):2186–2196.
66. Kumar BV, Connors TJ, Farber DL. Human T Cell Development, Localization, and Function throughout Life. *Immunity*. 2018;48(2):202–213.
67. Krangel MS. Mechanics of T cell receptor gene rearrangement. *Curr. Opin. Immunol*. 2009;21(2):133–139.
68. Wucherpfennig KW, Gagnon E, Call MJ, Huseby ES, Call ME. Structural biology of the T-cell receptor: insights into receptor assembly, ligand recognition, and initiation of signaling. *Cold Spring Harb. Perspect. Biol*. 2010;2(4):a005140.
69. Dong D, Zheng L, Lin J, Zhang B, Zhu Y, Li N, et al. Structural basis of assembly of the human T cell receptor–CD3 complex. *Nature*. 2019;573(7775):546–552.
70. Minguet S, Swamy M, Alarcón B, Luescher IF, Schamel WWA. Full Activation of the T Cell Receptor Requires Both Clustering and Conformational Changes at CD3. *Immunity*. 2007;26(1):43–54.
71. Chen L, Flies DB. Molecular mechanisms of T cell co-stimulation and co-inhibition. *Nat. Rev. Immunol*. 2013;13(4):227–242.
72. Esensten JH, Helou YA, Chopra G, Weiss A, Bluestone JA. CD28 Costimulation: from Mechanism to Therapy. *Immunity*. 2016;44(5):973–988.
73. Brunner-Weinzierl MC, Rudd CE. CTLA-4 and PD-1 Control of T-Cell Motility and Migration: implications for Tumor Immunotherapy. *Front. Immunol*. 2018;9(2737).
74. Waldman AD, Fritz JM, Lenardo MJ. A guide to cancer immunotherapy: from T cell basic science to clinical practice. *Nat. Rev. Immunol*. 2020.
75. Mizuno R, Sugiura D, Shimizu K, Maruhashi T, Watada M, Okazaki I-m, et al. PD-1 Primarily Targets TCR Signal in the Inhibition of Functional T. *Cell Activation. Front Immunol*. 2019;10(630).
76. Zuazo M, Gato-Cañas M, Llorente N, Ibañez-Vea M, Arasanz H, Kochan G, et al. Molecular mechanisms of programmed cell death-1 dependent T cell suppression: relevance for immunotherapy. *Ann. Transl. Med*. 2017;5(19):385.
77. Aires DJ, Yoshida M, Richardson SK, Bai M, Liu L, Moreno R, et al. T-cell trafficking plays an essential role in tumor immunity. *Lab. Invest*. 2019;99(1):85–92.
78. Slaney CY, Kershaw MH, Darcy PK. Trafficking of T Cells into Tumors. *Cancer Res*. 2014;74(24):7168.
79. Martínez-Lostao L, Anel A, Pardo J. How Do Cytotoxic Lymphocytes Kill Cancer Cells? *Clin. Cancer Res*. 2015;21(22):5047.
80. Durgeau A, Virk Y, Corgnac S, Mami-Chouaib F. Recent Advances in Targeting CD8 T-Cell Immunity for More Effective Cancer Immunotherapy. *Front. Immunol*. 2018;9(14).
81. Voskoboinik I, Whisstock JC, Trapani JA. Perforin and granzymes: function, dysfunction and human pathology. *Nat. Rev. Immunol*. 2015;15(6):388–400.
82. Paul S, Lal G. The Molecular Mechanism of Natural Killer Cells Function and Its Importance in Cancer Immunotherapy. *Front. Immunol*. 2017;8(1124).
83. Tang D, Kang R, Berghe TV, Vandenabeele P, Kroemer G. The molecular machinery of regulated cell death. *Cell Res*. 2019;29(5):347–364.
84. Tay RE, Richardson EK, Toh HC. Revisiting the role of CD4+ T cells in cancer immunotherapy—New insights into old paradigms. *Cancer Gene Ther*. 2020.
85. Borst J, Ahrends T, Bąbała N, Melief CJM, Kastenmüller W. CD4+ T cell help in cancer immunology and immunotherapy. *Nat. Rev. Immunol*. 2018;18(10):635–647.
86. Mojic M, Takeda K, Hayakawa Y. The Dark Side of IFN-γ: its Role in Promoting Cancer Immunoevasion. *Int. J. Mol. Sci*. 2017;19(1):89.
87. Ni L, Lu J. Interferon gamma in cancer immunotherapy. *Cancer Med*. 2018;7(9):4509–4516.
88. Castro F, Cardoso AP, Gonçalves RM, Serre K, Oliveira MJ. Interferon-Gamma at the Crossroads of Tumor Immune Surveillance or Evasion. *Front. Immunol*. 2018;9:847.

89. Li W, Huang X, Tong H, Wang Y, Zhang T, Wang W, et al. Comparison of the regulation of β-catenin signaling by type I, type II and type III interferons in hepatocellular carcinoma cells. *PLoS ONE.* 2012;7(10):e47040.
90. Kochupurakkal BS, Wang ZC, Hua T, Culhane AC, Rodig SJ, Rajkovic-Molek K, et al. RelA-Induced Interferon Response Negatively Regulates Proliferation. *PLoS ONE.* 2015;10(10):e0140243.
91. Schmitt MJ, Philippidou D, Reinsbach SE, Margue C, Wienecke-Baldacchino A, Nashan D, et al. Interferon-γ-induced activation of Signal Transducer and Activator of Transcription 1 (STAT1) up-regulates the tumor suppressing microRNA-29 family in melanoma cells. *Cell Commun Signal.* 2012;10(1):41.
92. Wang Q-S, Shen S-Q, Sun H-W, Xing Z-X, Yang H-L. Interferon-gamma induces autophagy-associated apoptosis through induction of cPLA2-dependent mitochondrial ROS generation in colorectal cancer cells. *Biochem. Biophys. Res. Commun.* 2018;498(4):1058–1065.
93. Martini M, Testi MG, Pasetto M, Picchio MC, Innamorati G, Mazzocco M, et al. IFN-γ-mediated upmodulation of MHC class I expression activates tumor-specific immune response in a mouse model of prostate cancer. *Vaccine.* 2010;28(20):3548–3557.
94. Axelrod ML, Cook RS, Johnson DB, Balko JM. Biological Consequences of MHC-II Expression by Tumor Cells in Cancer. *Clin. Cancer Res.* 2019;25(8):2392.
95. Kamma H, Yazawa T, Ogata T, Horiguchi H, Iijima T. Expression of MHC class II antigens in human lung cancer cells. *Virchows Archiv B.* 1991;60(1):407.
96. Steimle V, Siegrist CA, Mottet A, Lisowska-Grospierre B, Mach B. Regulation of MHC class II expression by interferon-gamma mediated by the transactivator gene CIITA. *Science.* 1994;265(5168):106.
97. Park IA, Hwang S-H, Song IH, Heo S-H, Kim Y-A, Bang WS, et al. Expression of the MHC class II in triple-negative breast cancer is associated with tumor-infiltrating lymphocytes and interferon signaling. *PLoS ONE.* 2017;12(8):e0182786.
98. Yuen GJ, Demissie E, Pillai S. B lymphocytes and cancer: a love-hate relationship. *Trends Cancer.* 2016;2(12):747–757.
99. Tsou P, Katayama H, Ostrin EJ, Hanash SM. The Emerging Role of B Cells in Tumor Immunity. *Cancer Res.* 2016;76(19):5597.
100. Guo FF, Cui JW. The Role of Tumor-Infiltrating B Cells in Tumor Immunity. *J. Oncol.* 2019;2019:2592419.
101. Sharonov GV, Serebrovskaya EO, Yuzhakova DV, Britanova OV, Chudakov DM. B cells, plasma cells and antibody repertoires in the tumour microenvironment. *Nat. Rev. Immunol.* 2020;20(5):294–307.
102. Abel AM, Yang C, Thakar MS, Malarkannan S. Natural Killer Cells: development, Maturation, and Clinical Utilization. *Front. Immunol.* 2018;9(1869).
103. Tarazona R, Lopez-Sejas N, Guerrero B, Hassouneh F, Valhondo I, Pera A, et al. Current progress in NK cell biology and NK cell-based cancer immunotherapy. *Cancer Immunology, Immunotherapy.* 2020;69(5):879–899.
104. Chiang SCC, Theorell J, Entesarian M, Meeths M, Mastafa M, Al-Herz W, et al. Comparison of primary human cytotoxic T-cell and natural killer cell responses reveal similar molecular requirements for lytic granule exocytosis but differences in cytokine production. *Blood.* 2013;121(8):1345–1356.
105. Huntington ND, Cursons J, Rautela J. The cancer–natural killer cell immunity cycle. *Nat. Rev. Cancer.* 2020;20(8):437–454.
106. Morrison BJ, Steel JC, Morris JC. Reduction of MHC-I expression limits T-lymphocyte-mediated killing of Cancer-initiating cells. *BMC Cancer.* 2018;18(1):469.
107. Pende D, Falco M, Vitale M, Cantoni C, Vitale C, Munari E, et al. Killer Ig-Like Receptors (KIRs): their Role in NK Cell Modulation and Developments Leading to Their Clinical Exploitation. *Front. Immunol.* 2019;10(1179).
108. Braud VM, Allan DSJ, O'Callaghan CA, Söderström K, D'Andrea A, Ogg GS, et al. HLA-E binds to natural killer cell receptors CD94/NKG2A, B and C. *Nature.* 1998;391(6669):795–799.
109. Zhang Q, Bi J, Zheng X, Chen Y, Wang H, Wu W, et al. Blockade of the checkpoint receptor TIGIT prevents NK cell exhaustion and elicits potent anti-tumor immunity. *Nat. Immunol.* 2018;19(7):723–732.
110. Frazao A, Rethacker L, Messaoudene M, Avril M-F, Toubert A, Dulphy N, et al. NKG2D/NKG2-Ligand Pathway Offers New Opportunities in Cancer Treatment. *Front. Immunol.* 2019;10:661.

111. Ghadially H, Brown L, Lloyd C, Lewis L, Lewis A, Dillon J, et al. MHC class I chain-related protein A and B (MICA and MICB) are predominantly expressed intracellularly in tumour and normal tissue. *Br. J. Cancer.* 2017;116(9):1208–1217.
112. Matta J, Baratin M, Chiche L, Forel J-M, Cognet C, Thomas G, et al. Induction of B7-H6, a ligand for the natural killer cell–activating receptor NKp30, in inflammatory conditions. *Blood.* 2013;122(3):394–404.
113. Bjørnsen EG, Thiruchelvam-Kyle L, Hoelsbrekken SE, Henden C, Saether PC, Boysen P, et al. B7H6 is a functional ligand for NKp30 in rat and cattle and determines NKp30 reactivity toward human cancer cell lines. *Eur. J. Immunol.* 2019;49(1):54–65.
114. Zhuang X, Long EO. CD28 Homolog Is a Strong Activator of Natural Killer Cells for Lysis of B7H7(+) Tumor Cells. *Cancer Immunol. Res.* 2019;7(6):939–951.
115. Comerci CJ, Mace EM, Banerjee PP, Orange JS. CD2 Promotes Human Natural Killer Cell Membrane Nanotube Formation. *PLoS ONE.* 2012;7(10):e47664.
116. Hadad U, Thauland TJ, Martinez OM, Butte MJ, Porgador A, Krams SM. NKp46 Clusters at the Immune Synapse and Regulates NK Cell Polarization. *Front. Immunol.* 2015;6(495).
117. Parodi M, Favoreel H, Candiano G, Gaggero S, Sivori S, Mingari MC, et al. NKp44-NKp44 Ligand Interactions in the Regulation of Natural Killer Cells and Other Innate Lymphoid Cells in Humans. *Front. Immunol.* 2019;10(719).
118. Barrow AD, Edeling MA, Trifonov V, Luo J, Goyal P, Bohl B, et al. Natural Killer Cells Control Tumor Growth by Sensing a Growth Factor. *Cell.* 2018;172(3):534–548 e19.
119. Müller L, Aigner P. Stoiber D. Type I Interferons and Natural Killer Cell Regulation in Cancer. *Front. Immunol.* 2017;8:304.
120. Marcus A, Mao AJ, Lensink-Vasan M, Wang L, Vance RE, Raulet DH. Tumor-Derived cGAMP Triggers a STING-Mediated Interferon Response in Non-tumor Cells to Activate the NK Cell Response. *Immunity.* 2018;49(4):754–763 e4.
121. Shimasaki N, Jain A, Campana D. NK cells for cancer immunotherapy. *Nat. Rev. Drug Discovery.* 2020;19(3):200–218.
122. Schmidt L, Eskiocak B, Kohn R, Dang C, Joshi NS, DuPage M, et al. Enhanced adaptive immune responses in lung adenocarcinoma through natural killer cell stimulation. *Proc Natl Acad Sci U S A.* 2019;116(35):17460–17469.
123. Wang W, Erbe AK, Hank JA, Morris ZS, Sondel PM. NK Cell-Mediated Antibody-Dependent Cellular Cytotoxicity in Cancer Immunotherapy. *Front Immunol.* 2015;6(368).
124. DeNardo DG, Ruffell B. Macrophages as regulators of tumour immunity and immunotherapy. *Nat. Rev. Immunol.* 2019;19(6):369–382.
125. Laviron M, Boissonnas A. Ontogeny of Tumor-Associated Macrophages. *Front Immunol.* 2019;10(1799).
126. Kielbassa K, Vegna S, Ramirez C, Akkari L. Understanding the Origin and Diversity of Macrophages to Tailor Their Targeting in Solid Cancers. *Front. Immunol.* 2019;10:2215.
127. Hao N-B, Lü M-H, Fan Y-H, Cao Y-L, Zhang Z-R, Yang S-M. Macrophages in Tumor Microenvironments and the Progression of Tumors. *Clinical and Developmental Immunology.* 2012;2012:948098.
128. Biswas SK, Mantovani A. Macrophage plasticity and interaction with lymphocyte subsets: cancer as a paradigm. *Nat. Immunol.* 2010;11(10):889–896.
129. Gordon SR, Maute RL, Dulken BW, Hutter G, George BM, McCracken MN, et al. PD-1 expression by tumour-associated macrophages inhibits phagocytosis and tumour immunity. *Nature.* 2017;545(7655):495–499.
130. Weiskopf K, Weissman IL. Macrophages are critical effectors of antibody therapies for cancer. *MAbs.* 2015;7(2):303–310.
131. Huls G, Heijnen IAFM, Cuomo E, van der Linden J, Boel E, van de Winkel JGJ, et al. Antitumor Immune Effector Mechanisms Recruited by Phage Display-derived Fully Human IgG1 and IgA1 Monoclonal Antibodies. *Cancer Res.* 1999;59(22):5778.
132. Gül N, van Egmond M. Antibody-Dependent Phagocytosis of Tumor Cells by Macrophages: a Potent Effector Mechanism of Monoclonal Antibody Therapy of Cancer. *Cancer Res.* 2015;75(23):5008.
133. Balkwill FR, Capasso M, Hagemann T. The tumor microenvironment at a glance. *J. Cell Sci.* 2012;125(23):5591.

134. Sahai E, Astsaturov I, Cukierman E, DeNardo DG, Egeblad M, Evans RM, et al. A framework for advancing our understanding of cancer-associated fibroblasts. *Nat. Rev. Cancer*. 2020;20(3):174–186.
135. Unterleuthner D, Neuhold P, Schwarz K, Janker L, Neuditschko B, Nivarthi H, et al. Cancer-associated fibroblast-derived WNT2 increases tumor angiogenesis in colon cancer. *Angiogenesis*. 2020;23(2):159–177.
136. Huang B, Huang M, Li Q. Cancer-Associated Fibroblasts Promote Angiogenesis of Hepatocellular Carcinoma by VEGF-Mediated EZH2/VASH1 Pathway. *Technol. Cancer Res. Treat*. 2019;18:1533033819879905.
137. Monteran L, Erez N. The Dark Side of Fibroblasts: cancer-Associated Fibroblasts as Mediators of Immunosuppression in the Tumor Microenvironment. *Front. Immunol*. 2019;10(1835).
138. Lakins MA, Ghorani E, Munir H, Martins CP, Shields JD. Cancer-associated fibroblasts induce antigen-specific deletion of CD8+T Cells to protect tumour cells. *Nat. Commun*. 2018;9(1):948.
139. Kato T, Noma K, Ohara T, Kashima H, Katsura Y, Sato H, et al. Cancer-Associated Fibroblasts Affect Intratumoral CD8<sup>+</sup> and FoxP3<sup>+</sup>T Cells Via IL6 in the Tumor Microenvironment. *Clinical Cancer Research*. 2018;24(19):4820.
140. Hida K, Maishi N, Annan DA, Hida Y. Contribution of Tumor Endothelial Cells in Cancer Progression. *Int. J. Mol. Sci*. 2018;19(5):1272.
141. Hida K, Maishi N. Abnormalities of tumor endothelial cells and cancer progression. *Oral Science International*. 2018;15(1):1–6.
142. Jin H, Cheng X, Pei Y, Fu J, Lyu Z, Peng H, et al. Data from a comparative proteomic analysis of tumor-derived lung-cancer CD105+ endothelial cells. *Data Brief*. 2016;7:927–939.
143. Nagl L, Horvath L, Pircher A, Wolf D. Tumor Endothelial Cells (TECs) as Potential Immune Directors of the Tumor Microenvironment – New Findings and Future Perspectives. *Front. Cell Dev. Biol*. 2020;8(766).
144. McDowell SAC, Quail DF. Immunological Regulation of Vascular Inflammation During Cancer Metastasis. *Front. Immunol*. 2019;10:1984 -.
145. Buckanovich RJ, Facciabene A, Kim S, Benencia F, Sasaroli D, Balint K, et al. Endothelin B receptor mediates the endothelial barrier to T cell homing to tumors and disables immune therapy. *Nat. Med*. 2008;14(1):28–36.
146. Motz GT, Santoro SP, Wang l, Garrabrant T, Lastra RR, Hagemann IS, et al. Tumor endothelium FasL establishes a selective immune barrier promoting tolerance in tumors. *Nat. Med*. 2014;20(6):607–615.
147. Liu S, Qin T, Liu Z, Wang J, Jia Y, Feng Y, et al. anlotinib alters tumor immune microenvironment by downregulating PD-L1 expression on vascular endothelial cells. *Cell Death. Dis*. 2020;11(5):309.
148. Frantz C, Stewart KM, Weaver VM. The extracellular matrix at a glance. *J. Cell Sci*. 2010;123(24):4195.
149. Lu P, Weaver VM, Werb Z. The extracellular matrix: a dynamic niche in cancer progression. *J. Cell Biol*. 2012;196(4):395–406.
150. Winkler J, Abisoye-Ogunniyan A, Metcalf KJ, Werb Z. Concepts of extracellular matrix remodelling in tumour progression and metastasis. *Nat. Commun*. 2020;11(1):5120.
151. Eble JA, Niland S. The extracellular matrix in tumor progression and metastasis. *Clin. Exp. Metastasis*. 2019;36(3):171–198.
152. Salmon H, Franciszkiewicz K, Damotte D, Dieu-Nosjean M-C, Validire P, Trautmann A, et al. Matrix architecture defines the preferential localization and migration of T cells into the stroma of human lung tumors. *J. Clin. Invest*. 2012;122(3):899–910.
153. Hope C, Emmerich PB, Papadas A, Pagenkopf A, Matkowskyj KA, Van De Hey DR, et al. Versican-Derived Matrikines Regulate Batf3-Dendritic Cell Differentiation and Promote T Cell Infiltration in Colorectal Cancer. *J. Immunol*. 2017;199(5):1933–1941.
154. Kaplan RN, Riba RD, Zacharoulis S, Bramley AH, Vincent L, Costa C, et al. VEGFR1-positive haematopoietic bone marrow progenitors initiate the pre-metastatic niche. *Nature*. 2005;438(7069):820–827.
155. Gao D, Joshi N, Choi H, Ryu S, Hahn M, Catena R, et al. Myeloid Progenitor Cells in the Premetastatic Lung Promote Metastases by Inducing Mesenchymal to Epithelial Transition. *Cancer Res*. 2012;72(6):1384.
156. Yadav M, Jhunjhunwala S, Phung QT, Lupardus P, Tanguay J, Bumbaca S, et al. Predicting immunogenic tumour mutations by combining mass spectrometry and exome sequencing. *Nature*. 2014;515(7528):572–576.

157. Yi M, Dong B, Chu Q, Wu K. Immune pressures drive the promoter hypermethylation of neoantigen genes. *Exp Hematol Oncol*. 2019;8(1):32.
158. Angell TE, Lechner MG, Jang JK, LoPresti JS, Epstein AL. MHC class I loss is a frequent mechanism of immune escape in papillary thyroid cancer that is reversed by interferon and selumetinib treatment in vitro. *Clin. Cancer Res*. 2014;20(23):6034–6044.
159. Ritz U, Seliger B. The Transporter Associated With Antigen Processing (TAP): structural Integrity, Expression, Function, and Its Clinical Relevance. *Mol. Med*. 2001;7(3):149–158.
160. Töpfer K, Kempe S, Müller N, Schmitz M, Bachmann M, Cartellieri M, et al. Tumor Evasion from T Cell Surveillance. *J. Biomed. Biotechnol*. 2011(2011):918471.
161. Restifo NP, Marincola FM, Kawakami Y, Taubenberger J, Yannelli JR, Rosenberg SA. Loss of functional beta 2-microglobulin in metastatic melanomas from five patients receiving immunotherapy. *J. Natl. Cancer Inst*. 1996;88(2):100–108.
162. Vinay DS, Ryan EP, Pawelec G, Talib WH, Stagg J, Elkord E, et al. Immune evasion in cancer: mechanistic basis and therapeutic strategies. *Semin. Cancer Biol*. 2015;35:S185–SS98.
163. Veglia F, Gabrilovich DI. Dendritic cells in cancer: the role revisited. *Curr. Opin. Immunol*. 2017;45:43–51.
164. Berglund A, Mills M, Putney RM, Hamaidi I, Mulé J, Kim S. Methylation of immune synapse genes modulates tumor immunogenicity. *J. Clin. Invest*. 2020;130(2):974–980.
165. Peng D, Kryczek I, Nagarsheth N, Zhao L, Wei S, Wang W, et al. Epigenetic silencing of TH1-type chemokines shapes tumour immunity and immunotherapy. *Nature*. 2015;527(7577):249–253.
166. Molon B, Ugel S, Del Pozzo F, Soldani C, Zilio S, Avella D, et al. Chemokine nitration prevents intratumoral infiltration of antigen-specific T cells. *J. Exp. Med*. 2011;208(10):1949–1962.
167. Afanasiev OK, Nagase K, Simonson W, Vandeven N, Blom A, Koelle DM, et al. Vascular E-Selectin Expression Correlates with CD8 Lymphocyte Infiltration and Improved Outcome in Merkel Cell Carcinoma. *J. Invest. Dermatol*. 2013;133(8):2065–2073.
168. Sordo-Bahamonde C, Lorenzo-Herrero S, Payer ÁR, Gonzalez S. López-Soto A. Mechanisms of Apoptosis Resistance to NK Cell-Mediated Cytotoxicity in Cancer. *Int. J. Mol. Sci*. 2020;21(10):3726.
169. French LE, Tschopp J. Defective death receptor signaling as a cause of tumor immune escape. *Semin. Cancer Biol*. 2002;12(1):51–55.
170. Schmiedel D, Mandelboim O. NKG2D Ligands-Critical Targets for Cancer Immune Escape and Therapy. *Front. Immunol*. 2018;9:2040.
171. Groh V, Wu J, Yee C, Spies T. Tumour-derived soluble MIC ligands impair expression of NKG2D and T-cell activation. *Nature*. 2002;419(6908):734–738.
172. Duan S, Guo W, Xu Z, He Y, Liang C, Mo Y, et al. Natural killer group 2D receptor and its ligands in cancer immune escape. *Mol. Cancer*. 2019;18(1):29.
173. Ferrari de Andrade L, Tay RE, Pan D, Luoma AM, Ito Y, Badrinath S, et al. Antibody-mediated inhibition of MICA and MICB shedding promotes NK cell–driven tumor immunity. *Science*. 2018;359(6383):1537.
174. Schlecker E, Fiegler N, Arnold A, Altevogt P, Rose-John S, Moldenhauer G, et al. Metalloprotease-mediated tumor cell shedding of B7-H6, the ligand of the natural killer cell-activating receptor NKp30. *Cancer Res*. 2014;74(13):3429–3440.
175. Tittarelli A, Janji B, Van Moer K, Noman MZ, Chouaib S. The Selective Degradation of Synaptic Connexin 43 Protein by Hypoxia-induced Autophagy Impairs Natural Killer Cell-mediated Tumor Cell Killing. *J. Biol. Chem*. 2015;290(39):23670–23679.
176. Lambert AW, Pattabiraman DR, Weinberg RA. Emerging Biological Principles of Metastasis. *Cell*. 2017;168(4):670–691.
177. Weiskopf K. Cancer immunotherapy targeting the CD47/SIRPα axis. *Eur. J. Cancer*. 2017;76:100–109.
178. Gu S, Ni T, Wang J, Liu Y, Fan Q, Wang Y, et al. CD47 Blockade Inhibits Tumor Progression through Promoting Phagocytosis of Tumor Cells by M2 Polarized Macrophages in Endometrial Cancer. *J Immunol Res*. 2018;2018:6156757.
179. Feng M, Jiang W, Kim BYS, Zhang CC, Fu Y-X, Weissman IL. Phagocytosis checkpoints as new targets for cancer immunotherapy. *Nat. Rev. Cancer*. 2019;19(10):568–586.
180. Vigano S, Alatzoglou D, Irving M, Ménétrier-Caux C, Caux C, Romero P, et al. Targeting Adenosine in Cancer Immunotherapy to Enhance T-Cell Function. *Front. Immunol*. 2019;10:925.

181. Parker KH, Beury DW, Ostrand-Rosenberg S. Chapter Three - Myeloid-Derived Suppressor Cells: critical Cells Driving Immune Suppression in the Tumor Microenvironment. In: Wang X-Y, Fisher PB, eds. *Advances in Cancer Research*: Academic Press; 2015:95–139 128.
182. Timosenko E, Hadjinicolaou AV, Cerundolo V. Modulation of cancer-specific immune responses by amino acid degrading enzymes. *Immunotherapy*. 2016;9(1):83–97.
183. Rodriguez PC, Quiceno DG, Zabaleta J, Ortiz B, Zea AH, Piazuelo MB, et al. Arginase I Production in the Tumor Microenvironment by Mature Myeloid Cells Inhibits T-Cell Receptor Expression and Antigen-Specific T-Cell Responses. *Cancer Res*. 2004;64(16):5839.
184. Chang C-I, Liao JC, Kuo L. Macrophage Arginase Promotes Tumor Cell Growth and Suppresses Nitric Oxide-mediated Tumor Cytotoxicity. *Cancer Res*. 2001;61(3):1100.
185. Munn DH, Mellor AL. IDO in the Tumor Microenvironment: inflammation, Counter-Regulation, and Tolerance. *Trends Immunol*. 2016;37(3):193–207.
186. Zhao Q, Kuang DM, Wu Y, Xiao X, Li XF, Li TJ, et al. Activated CD69+ T cells foster immune privilege by regulating IDO expression in tumor-associated macrophages. *J. Immunol*. 2012;188(3):1117–1124.
187. Frumento G, Rotondo R, Tonetti M, Damonte G, Benatti U, Ferrara GB. Tryptophan-derived catabolites are responsible for inhibition of T and natural killer cell proliferation induced by indoleamine 2,3-dioxygenase. *J. Exp. Med*. 2002;196(4):459–468.
188. Liu Y, Liang X, Dong W, Fang Y, Lv J, Zhang T, et al. Tumor-Repopulating Cells Induce PD-1 Expression in CD8+ T Cells by Transferring Kynurenine and AhR Activation. *Cancer Cell*. 2018;33(3):480–494 e7.
189. Chiesa MD, Carlomagno S, Frumento G, Balsamo M, Cantoni C, Conte R, et al. The tryptophan catabolite L-kynurenine inhibits the surface expression of NKp46- and NKG2D-activating receptors and regulates NK-cell function. *Blood*. 2006;108(13):4118–4125.
190. Song H, Park H, Kim Y-S, Kim KD, Lee H-K, Cho d, et al. L-Kynurenine-induced apoptosis in human NK cells is mediated by reactive oxygen species. *Int. Immunopharmacol*. 2011;11(8):932–938.
191. Fallarino F, Grohmann U, Vacca C, Bianchi R, Orabona C, Spreca A, et al. T cell apoptosis by tryptophan catabolism. *Cell Death & Differentiation*. 2002;9(10):1069–1077.
192. Yano H, Andrews LP, Workman CJ, Vignali DAA. Intratumoral regulatory T cells: markers, subsets and their impact on anti-tumor immunity. *Immunology*. 2019;157(3):232–247.
193. Han S, Toker A, Liu ZQ, Ohashi PS. Turning the Tide Against Regulatory T Cells. *Front. Oncol*. 2019;9(279).
194. Li C, Jiang P, Wei S, Xu X, Wang J. Regulatory T cells in tumor microenvironment: new mechanisms, potential therapeutic strategies and future prospects. *Mol. Cancer*. 2020;19(1):116.
195. Tanaka A, Sakaguchi S. Regulatory T cells in cancer immunotherapy. *Cell Res*. 2017;27(1):109–118.
196. Deaglio S, Dwyer KM, Gao W, Friedman D, Usheva A, Erat A, et al. Adenosine generation catalyzed by CD39 and CD73 expressed on regulatory T cells mediates immune suppression. *J. Exp. Med*. 2007;204(6):1257–1265.
197. Ohta A, Kini R, Ohta A, Subramanian M, Madasu M, Sitkovsky M. The development and immunosuppressive functions of CD4(+) CD25(+) FoxP3(+) regulatory T cells are under influence of the adenosine-A2A adenosine receptor pathway. *Front. Immunol*. 2012;3:190.
198. Chen J, Ganguly A, Mucsi AD, Meng J, Yan J, Detampel P, et al. Strong adhesion by regulatory T cells induces dendritic cell cytoskeletal polarization and contact-dependent lethargy. *J. Exp. Med*. 2017;214(2):327–338.
199. Zhao Y, Shen M, Feng Y, He R, Xu X, Xie Y, et al. Regulatory B cells induced by pancreatic cancer cell-derived interleukin-18 promote immune tolerance via the PD-1/PD-L1 pathway. *Oncotarget*. 2017;9(19):14803–14814.
200. Kuang d, Zhao Q, Peng C, Xu J, Zhang J-P, Wu C, et al. Activated monocytes in peritumoral stroma of hepatocellular carcinoma foster immune privilege and disease progression through PD-L1. *J. Exp. Med*. 2009;206(6):1327–1337.
201. Roux C, Jafari SM, Shinde R, Duncan G, Cescon DW, Silvester J, et al. Reactive oxygen species modulate macrophage immunosuppressive phenotype through the up-regulation of PD-L1. *Proc Natl Acad Sci U S A*. 2019;116(10):4326–4335.
202. Tcyganov E, Mastio J, Chen E, Gabrilovich DI. Plasticity of myeloid-derived suppressor cells in cancer. *Curr. Opin. Immunol*. 2018;51:76–82.

203. Veglia F, Perego M, Gabrilovich D. Myeloid-derived suppressor cells coming of age. *Nat. Immunol.* 2018;19(2):108–119.
204. Katoh H, Watanabe M. Myeloid-Derived Suppressor Cells and Therapeutic Strategies in Cancer. *Mediators Inflamm.* 2015;2015:159269.
205. Zhao Y, Wu T, Shao S, Shi B, Zhao Y. Phenotype, development, and biological function of myeloid-derived suppressor cells. *Oncoimmunology*. 2016;5(2):e1004983.
206. Vetsika E-K, Koukos A, Kotsakis A. Myeloid-Derived Suppressor Cells: major Figs. that Shape the Immunosuppressive and Angiogenic Network in. *Cancer. Cells*. 2019;8(12):1647.
207. Bronte V, Brandau S, Chen S-H, Colombo MP, Frey AB, Greten TF, et al. Recommendations for myeloid-derived suppressor cell nomenclature and characterization standards. *Nat. Commun.* 2016;7(1):12150.
208. Condamine T, Dominguez GA, Youn J-I, Kossenkov AV, Mony S, Alicea-Torres K, et al. Lectin-type oxidized LDL receptor-1 distinguishes population of human polymorphonuclear myeloid-derived suppressor cells in cancer patients. *Science Immunology*. 2016;1(2):aaf8943.
209. Ostrand-Rosenberg S, Fenselau C. Myeloid-Derived Suppressor Cells: immune-Suppressive Cells That Impair Antitumor Immunity and Are Sculpted by Their Environment. *J. Immunol.* 2018;200(2):422–431.
210. Ohl K, Tenbrock K. Reactive Oxygen Species as Regulators of MDSC-Mediated Immune Suppression. *Front. Immunol.* 2018;9(2499).
211. Gabrilovich DI. Myeloid-Derived Suppressor Cells. *Cancer Immunol. Res.* 2017;5(1):3–8.
212. Ugolini A, Tyurin VA, Tyurina YY, Tcyganov EN, Donthireddy L, Kagan VE, et al. Polymorphonuclear myeloid-derived suppressor cells limit antigen cross-presentation by dendritic cells in cancer. *JCI Insight*. 2020;5(15).
213. Raber PL, Thevenot P, Sierra R, Wyczechowska D, Halle D, Ramirez ME, et al. Subpopulations of myeloid-derived suppressor cells impair T cell responses through independent nitric oxide-related pathways. *Int. J. Cancer*. 2014;134(12):2853–2864.
214. Markowitz J, Wang J, Vangundy Z, You J, Yildiz V, Yu L, et al. Nitric oxide mediated inhibition of antigen presentation from DCs to CD4+ T cells in cancer and measurement of STAT1 nitration. *Sci. Rep.* 2017;7(1):15424.
215. Gehad AE, Lichtman MK, Schmults CD, Teague JE, Calarese AW, Jiang Y, et al. Nitric Oxide–Producing Myeloid-Derived Suppressor Cells Inhibit Vascular E-Selectin Expression in Human Squamous Cell Carcinomas. *J. Invest. Dermatol.* 2012;132(11):2642–2651.
216. Ku AW, Muhitch JB, Powers CA, Diehl M, Kim M, Fisher DT, et al. Tumor-induced MDSC act via remote control to inhibit L-selectin-dependent adaptive immunity in lymph nodes. *Elife*. 2016;5:e17375.
217. Pastaki Khoshbin A, Eskian M, Keshavarz-Fathi M, Rezaei N. Roles of Myeloid-Derived Suppressor Cells in Cancer Metastasis: immunosuppression and Beyond. *Arch. Immunol. Ther. Exp. (Warsz.).* 2019;67(2):89–102.
218. Hoechst B, Ormandy LA, Ballmaier M, Lehner F, Krüger C, Manns MP, et al. A New Population of Myeloid-Derived Suppressor Cells in Hepatocellular Carcinoma Patients Induces CD4+CD25+Foxp3+ T Cells. *Gastroenterology*. 2008;135(1):234–243.
219. Pan P-Y, Ma G, Weber KJ, Ozao-Choy J, Wang G, Yin B, et al. Immune stimulatory receptor CD40 is required for T-cell suppression and T regulatory cell activation mediated by myeloid-derived suppressor cells in cancer. *Cancer Res.* 2010;70(1):99–108.
220. Sahai E. Illuminating the metastatic process. *Nat. Rev. Cancer*. 2007;7(10):737–749.
221. Jinesh GG, Brohl AS. The genetic script of metastasis. *Biological Reviews*. 2020;95(1):244–266.
222. Nakayama J, Ito E, Fujimoto J, Watanabe S, Semba K. Comparative analysis of gene regulatory networks of highly metastatic breast cancer cells established by orthotopic transplantation and intra-circulation injection. *Int. J. Oncol.* 2017;50(2):497–504.
223. Chan S-H, Wang l. Regulation of cancer metastasis by microRNAs. *J. Biomed. Sci.* 2015;22(1):9.
224. Chatterjee A, Rodger EJ, Eccles MR. Epigenetic drivers of tumourigenesis and cancer metastasis. *Semin. Cancer Biol.* 2018;51:149–159.
225. Alderton GK. Epigenetic and genetic heterogeneity in metastasis. *Nat. Rev. Cancer*. 2017;17(3):141.
226. Fares J, Fares MY, Khachfe HH, Salhab HA, Fares Y. Molecular principles of metastasis: a hallmark of cancer revisited. *Signal Transduction and Targeted Therapy*. 2020;5(1):28.

227. Koual M, Cano-Sancho G, Bats A-S, Tomkiewicz C, Kaddouch-Amar Y, Douay-Hauser N, et al. Associations between persistent organic pollutants and risk of breast cancer metastasis. *Environ. Int.* 2019;132:105028.
228. Whisner CM, Athena Aktipis C. The Role of the Microbiome in Cancer Initiation and Progression: how Microbes and Cancer Cells Utilize Excess Energy and Promote One Another's Growth. *Curr Nutr Rep*. 2019;8(1):42–51.
229. Zhu Z, Huang J, Li X, Xing J, Chen Q, Liu R, et al. Gut microbiota regulate tumor metastasis via circRNA/miRNA networks. *Gut Microbes*. 2020;12(1):1788891.
230. Kitamura T, Qian B-Z, Pollard JW. Immune cell promotion of metastasis. *Nat. Rev. Immunol.* 2015;15(2):73–86.
231. Janssen LME, Ramsay EE, Logsdon CD, Overwijk WW. The immune system in cancer metastasis: friend or foe? *J. Immunother. Cancer*. 2017;5(1):79.
232. Peinado H, Zhang H, Matei IR, Costa-Silva B, Hoshino A, Rodrigues G, et al. Pre-metastatic niches: organ-specific homes for metastases. *Nat. Rev. Cancer*. 2017;17(5):302–317.
233. Kaplan RN, Rafii S, Lyden D. Preparing the "soil": the premetastatic niche. *Cancer Res.* 2006;66(23):11089–11093.
234. Doglioni G, Parik S, Fendt S-M. Interactions in the (Pre)metastatic Niche Support Metastasis Formation. *Front. Oncol.* 2019;9:219.
235. Doglioni G, Parik S, Fendt S-M. Interactions in the (Pre)metastatic Niche Support Metastasis Formation. *Front. Oncol.* 2019;9(219).
236. Guo Y, Ji X, Liu J, Fan D, Zhou Q, Chen C, et al. Effects of exosomes on pre-metastatic niche formation in tumors. *Mol. Cancer*. 2019;18(1):39.
237. Peinado H, Lavotshkin S, Lyden D. The secreted factors responsible for pre-metastatic niche formation: old sayings and new thoughts. *Semin. Cancer Biol.* 2011;21(2):139–146.
238. Li P, Lu M, Shi J, Hua L, Gong Z, Li Q, et al. Dual roles of neutrophils in metastatic colonization are governed by the host NK cell status. *Nat. Commun.* 2020;11(1):4387.
239. Shi C, Chen Y, Chen Y, Yang Y, Bing W, Qi J. CD4(+) CD25(+) regulatory T cells promote hepatocellular carcinoma invasion via TGF-β1-induced epithelial-mesenchymal transition. *Onco Targets Ther.* 2018;12:279–289.
240. Song W, Mazzieri R, Yang T, Gobe GC. Translational Significance for Tumor Metastasis of Tumor-Associated Macrophages and Epithelial–Mesenchymal Transition. *Front. Immunol.* 2017;8(1106).
241. Ouzounova M, Lee E, Piranlioglu R, El Andaloussi A, Kolhe R, Demirci MF, et al. Monocytic and granulocytic myeloid derived suppressor cells differentially regulate spatiotemporal tumour plasticity during metastatic cascade. *Nat. Commun.* 2017;8(1):14979.
242. Li Z-L, Ye S-B, OuYang l, Zhang H, Chen Y-S, He J, et al. COX-2 promotes metastasis in nasopharyngeal carcinoma by mediating interactions between cancer cells and myeloid-derived suppressor cells. *Oncoimmunology*. 2015;4(11):e1044712.
243. Mucha J, Majchrzak K, Taciak B, Hellmén E, Król M. MDSCs Mediate Angiogenesis and Predispose Canine Mammary Tumor Cells for Metastasis via IL-28/IL-28RA (IFN-λ) Signaling. *PLoS ONE*. 2014;9(7):e103249.
244. Saygin C, Matei D, Majeti R, Reizes O, Lathia JD. Targeting Cancer Stemness in the Clinic: from Hype to Hope. *Cell Stem Cell*. 2019;24(1):25–40.
245. Yang J, Liao D, Chen C, Liu Y, Chuang T-H, Xiang R, et al. Tumor-Associated Macrophages Regulate Murine Breast Cancer Stem Cells Through a Novel Paracrine EGFR/Stat3/Sox-2 Signaling Pathway. *Stem Cells*. 2013;31(2):248–258.
246. Wei X, Yang S, Pu X, He S, Yang Z, Sheng X, et al. Tumor-associated macrophages increase the proportion of cancer stem cells in lymphoma by secreting pleiotrophin. *Am. J. Transl. Res.* 2019;11(10):6393–6402.
247. Shi Y, Ping Y-F, Zhou W, He Z-C, Chen C, Bian B-S-J, et al. Tumour-associated macrophages secrete pleiotrophin to promote PTPRZ1 signalling in glioblastoma stem cells for tumour growth. *Nat. Commun.* 2017;8(1):15080.
248. Cui TX, Kryczek I, Zhao L, Zhao E, Kuick R, Roh MH, et al. Myeloid-derived suppressor cells enhance stemness of cancer cells by inducing microRNA101 and suppressing the corepressor CtBP2. *Immunity*. 2013;39(3):611–621.

249. Peng D, Tanikawa T, Li W, Zhao L, Vatan L, Szeliga W, et al. Myeloid-Derived Suppressor Cells Endow Stem-like Qualities to Breast Cancer Cells through IL6/STAT3 and NO/NOTCH Cross-talk Signaling. *Cancer Res.* 2016;76(11):3156–3165.
250. Fu l, Du W-L, Cai M-H, Yao J-Y, Zhao Y-Y, Mou X-Z. The roles of tumor-associated macrophages in tumor angiogenesis and metastasis. *Cell. Immunol.* 2020;353:104119.
251. Rigoni A, Colombo MP, Pucillo C. The Role of Mast Cells in Molding the Tumor Microenvironment. *Cancer Microenviron.* 2015;8(3):167–176.
252. Gocheva V, Wang H-W, Gadea BB, Shree T, Hunter KE, Garfall AL, et al. IL-4 induces cathepsin protease activity in tumor-associated macrophages to promote cancer growth and invasion. *Genes Dev.* 2010;24(3):241–255.
253. Haque ASMR, Moriyama M, Kubota K, Ishiguro N, Sakamoto M, Chinju A, et al. CD206+ tumor-associated macrophages promote proliferation and invasion in oral squamous cell carcinoma via EGF production. *Sci. Rep.* 2019;9(1):14611.
254. Rigo A, Gottardi M, Zamò A, Mauri P, Bonifacio M, Krampera M, et al. Macrophages may promote cancer growth via a GM-CSF/HB-EGF paracrine loop that is enhanced by CXCL12. *Mol. Cancer.* 2010;9:273.
255. Carroll MJ, Kapur A, Felder M, Patankar MS, Kreeger PK. M2 macrophages induce ovarian cancer cell proliferation via a heparin binding epidermal growth factor/matrix metalloproteinase 9 intercellular feedback loop. *Oncotarget.* 2016;7(52):86608–86620.
256. Zeng X-Y, Xie H, Yuan J, Jiang X-Y, Yong J-H, Zeng D, et al. M2-like tumor-associated macrophages-secreted EGF promotes epithelial ovarian cancer metastasis via activating EGFR-ERK signaling and suppressing lncRNA LIMT expression. *Cancer Biol. Ther.* 2019;20(7):956–966.
257. Goswami S, Sahai E, Wyckoff JB, Cammer M, Cox D, Pixley FJ, et al. Macrophages Promote the Invasion of Breast Carcinoma Cells via a Colony-Stimulating Factor-1/Epidermal Growth Factor Paracrine Loop. *Cancer Res.* 2005;65(12):5278.
258. Yang M, Chen J, Su F, Yu B, Su F, Lin L, et al. Microvesicles secreted by macrophages shuttle invasion-potentiating microRNAs into breast cancer cells. *Mol. Cancer.* 2011;10(1):117.
259. Bielenberg DR, Zetter BR. The Contribution of Angiogenesis to the Process of Metastasis. *Cancer J.* 2015;21(4):267–273.
260. Riabov V, Gudima A, Wang N, Mickley A, Orekhov A, Kzhyshkowska J. Role of tumor associated macrophages in tumor angiogenesis and lymphangiogenesis. *Front Physiol.* 2014;5:75.
261. Albini A, Bruno A, Noonan DM, Mortara L. Contribution to Tumor Angiogenesis From Innate Immune Cells Within the Tumor Microenvironment: implications for Immunotherapy. *Front. Immunol.* 2018;9:527.
262. Sierra JR, Corso S, Caione L, Cepero V, Conrotto P, Cignetti A, et al. Tumor angiogenesis and progression are enhanced by Sema4D produced by tumor-associated macrophages. *J. Exp. Med.* 2008;205(7):1673–1685.
263. Lee S, Jilani SM, Nikolova GV, Carpizo D, Iruela-Arispe ML. Processing of VEGF-A by matrix metalloproteinases regulates bioavailability and vascular patterning in tumors. *J. Cell Biol.* 2005;169(4):681–691.
264. Yang L, DeBusk LM, Fukuda K, Fingleton B, Green-Jarvis B, Shyr Y, et al. Expansion of myeloid immune suppressor Gr+CD11b+ cells in tumor-bearing host directly promotes tumor angiogenesis. *Cancer Cell.* 2004;6(4):409–421.
265. Maloney DG, Grillo-Lopez AJ, Bodkin DJ, White CA, Liles TM, Royston I, et al. IDEC-C2B8: results of a phase I multiple-dose trial in patients with relapsed non-Hodgkin's lymphoma. *J. Clin. Oncol.* 1997;15(10):3266–3274.
266. Siegel RL, Miller KD, Jemal A. Cancer statistics, 2019. *CA Cancer J. Clin.* 2019;69(1):7–34.
267. Swerdlow SH C E, Harris NL, Jaffe ES, Pileri SA, Stein H, Thiele J. WHO Classification of Tumours of Haematopoietic and Lymphoid Tissues. Revised Fourth Edition; 2017.
268. Smith A, Crouch S, Lax S, Li J, Painter D, Howell D, et al. Lymphoma incidence, survival and prevalence 2004-2014: sub-type analyses from the UK's Haematological Malignancy Research Network. *Br. J. Cancer.* 2015;112(9):1575–1584.
269. Morton LM, Slager SL, Cerhan JR, Wang SS, Vajdic CM, Skibola CF, et al. Etiologic heterogeneity among non-Hodgkin lymphoma subtypes: the InterLymph Non-Hodgkin Lymphoma Subtypes Project. *J. Natl. Cancer Inst. Monogr.* 2014;2014(48):130–144.

270. Armitage JO, Gascoyne RD, Lunning MA, Cavalli F. Non-Hodgkin lymphoma. *Lancet*. 2017;390(10091):298–310.
271. Landsburg DJ, Petrich AM, Abramson JS, Sohani AR, Press O, Cassaday R, et al. Impact of oncogene rearrangement patterns on outcomes in patients with double-hit non-Hodgkin lymphoma. *Cancer*. 2016;122(4):559–564.
272. Green MR, Monti S, Rodig SJ, Juszczynski P, Currie T, O'Donnell E, et al. Integrative analysis reveals selective 9p24.1 amplification, increased PD-1 ligand expression, and further induction via JAK2 in nodular sclerosing Hodgkin lymphoma and primary mediastinal large B-cell lymphoma. *Blood*. 2010;116(17):3268–3277.
273. Sehn LH, Donaldson J, Chhanabhai M, Fitzgerald C, Gill K, Klasa R, et al. Introduction of combined CHOP plus rituximab therapy dramatically improved outcome of diffuse large B-cell lymphoma in British Columbia. *J. Clin. Oncol*. 2005;23(22):5027–5033.
274. Crump M, Neelapu SS, Farooq U, Van Den Neste E, Kuruvilla J, Westin J, et al. Outcomes in refractory diffuse large B-cell lymphoma: results from the international SCHOLAR-1 study. *Blood*. 2017;130(16):1800–1808.
275. Al-Tourah AJ, Gill KK, Chhanabhai M, Hoskins PJ, Klasa RJ, Savage KJ, et al. Population-based analysis of incidence and outcome of transformed non-Hodgkin's lymphoma. *J. Clin. Oncol*. 2008;26(32):5165–5169.
276. Majeti R, Weissman IL. Human acute myelogenous leukemia stem cells revisited: there's more than meets the eye. *Cancer Cell*. 2011;19(1):9–10.
277. Inaba H, Greaves M, Mullighan CG. Acute lymphoblastic leukaemia. *Lancet*. 2013;381(9881):1943–1955.
278. Bene MC, Nebe T, Bettelheim P, Buldini B, Bumbea H, Kern W, et al. Immunophenotyping of acute leukemia and lymphoproliferative disorders: a consensus proposal of the European LeukemiaNet Work Package 10. *Leukemia*. 2011;25(4):567–574.
279. Dohner H, Estey E, Grimwade D, Amadori S, Appelbaum FR, Buchner T, et al. Diagnosis and management of AML in adults: 2017 ELN recommendations from an international expert panel. *Blood*. 2017;129(4):424–447.
280. Oriol A, Vives S, Hernandez-Rivas JM, Tormo M, Heras I, Rivas C, et al. Outcome after relapse of acute lymphoblastic leukemia in adult patients included in four consecutive risk-adapted trials by the PETHEMA Study Group. *Haematologica*. 2010;95(4):589–596.
281. Stilgenbauer S, Bullinger L, Lichter P, Dohner H, Cllsgcll G. Genetics of chronic lymphocytic leukemia: genomic aberrations and V(H) gene mutation status in pathogenesis and clinical course. *Leukemia*. 2002;16(6):993–1007.
282. Hallek M, Shanafelt TD, Eichhorst B. Chronic lymphocytic leukaemia. *Lancet*. 2018;391(10129):1524–1537.
283. Chen C, Puvvada S. Prognostic Factors for Chronic Lymphocytic Leukemia. *Curr Hematol Malig Rep*. 2016;11(1):37–42.
284. Hallek M, Cheson BD, Catovsky D, Caligaris-Cappio F, Dighiero G, Dohner H, et al. Guidelines for the diagnosis and treatment of chronic lymphocytic leukemia: a report from the International Workshop on Chronic Lymphocytic Leukemia updating the National Cancer Institute-Working Group 1996 guidelines. *Blood*. 2008;111(12):5446–5456.
285. Rajkumar SV. Multiple myeloma: 2020 update on diagnosis, risk-stratification and management. *Am. J. Hematol*. 2020;95(5):548–567.
286. Rawstron AC, Orfao A, Beksac M, Bezdickova L, Brooimans RA, Bumbea H, et al. Report of the European Myeloma Network on multiparametric flow cytometry in multiple myeloma and related disorders. *Haematologica*. 2008;93(3):431–438.
287. Cho SF, Anderson KC, Tai YT. Targeting B Cell Maturation Antigen (BCMA) in Multiple Myeloma: potential Uses of BCMA-Based Immunotherapy. *Front. Immunol*. 2018;9:1821.
288. Ansell SM, Lesokhin AM, Borrello I, Halwani A, Scott EC, Gutierrez M, et al. PD-1 blockade with nivolumab in relapsed or refractory Hodgkin's lymphoma. *N. Engl. J. Med*. 2015;372(4):311–319.
289. Ansell S, Armand P, Timmerman JM, Shipp MA, Bradley Garelik MB, Zhu L, et al. Nivolumab in Patients (Pts) with Relapsed or Refractory Classical Hodgkin Lymphoma (R/R cHL): clinical Outcomes from Extended Follow-up of a Phase 1 Study (CA209-039). *Blood*. 2015;126(23):583.
290. Armand P, Engert A, Younes A, Fanale M, Santoro A, Zinzani PL, et al. Nivolumab for Relapsed/Refractory Classic Hodgkin Lymphoma After Failure of Autologous Hematopoietic Cell

Transplantation: extended Follow-Up of the Multicohort Single-Arm Phase II CheckMate 205 Trial. *J. Clin. Oncol.* 2018;36(14):1428–1439.
291. Younes A, Santoro A, Shipp M, Zinzani PL, Timmerman JM, Ansell S, et al. Nivolumab for classical Hodgkin's lymphoma after failure of both autologous stem-cell transplantation and brentuximab vedotin: a multicentre, multicohort, single-arm phase 2 trial. *Lancet Oncol.* 2016;17(9):1283–1294.
292. Davis KL, Fox E, Merchant MS, Reid JM, Kudgus RA, Liu X, et al. Nivolumab in children and young adults with relapsed or refractory solid tumours or lymphoma (ADVL1412): a multicentre, open-label, single-arm, phase 1-2 trial. *Lancet Oncol.* 2020;21(4):541–550.
293. Lepik KV, Mikhailova NB, Moiseev IS, Kondakova EV, Tsvetkova LA, Zalyalov YR, et al. Nivolumab for the treatment of relapsed and refractory classical Hodgkin lymphoma after ASCT and in ASCT-naive patients. *Leuk. Lymphoma.* 2019;60(9):2316–2319.
294. Ansell SM, Minnema MC, Johnson P, Timmerman JM, Armand P, Shipp MA, et al. Nivolumab for Relapsed/Refractory Diffuse Large B-Cell Lymphoma in Patients Ineligible for or Having Failed Autologous Transplantation: a Single-Arm, Phase II Study. *J. Clin. Oncol.* 2019;37(6):481–489.
295. Zinzani PL, Santoro A, Gritti G, Brice P, Barr PM, Kuruvilla J, et al. Nivolumab Combined With Brentuximab Vedotin for Relapsed/Refractory Primary Mediastinal Large B-Cell Lymphoma: efficacy and Safety From the Phase II CheckMate 436 Study. *J. Clin. Oncol.* 2019;37(33):3081–3089.
296. Ravandi F, Assi R, Daver N, Benton CB, Kadia T, Thompson PA, et al. Idarubicin, cytarabine, and nivolumab in patients with newly diagnosed acute myeloid leukaemia or high-risk myelodysplastic syndrome: a single-arm, phase 2 study. *Lancet Haematol.* 2019;6(9):e480–e488.
297. Daver N, Garcia-Manero G, Basu S, Boddu PC, Alfayez M, Cortes JE, et al. Efficacy, Safety, and Biomarkers of Response to Azacitidine and Nivolumab in Relapsed/Refractory Acute Myeloid Leukemia: a Nonrandomized, Open-Label. *Phase II Study. Cancer Discov.* 2019;9(3):370–383.
298. Kasamon YL, de Claro RA, Wang Y, Shen YL, Farrell AT, Pazdur R. FDA Approval Summary: nivolumab for the Treatment of Relapsed or Progressive Classical Hodgkin Lymphoma. *Oncologist.* 2017;22(5):585–591.
299. Armand P, Rodig S, Melnichenko V, Thieblemont C, Bouabdallah K, Tumyan G, et al. Pembrolizumab in Relapsed or Refractory Primary Mediastinal Large B-Cell Lymphoma. *J. Clin. Oncol.* 2019;37(34):3291–3299.
300. Armand P, Shipp MA, Ribrag V, Michot JM, Zinzani PL, Kuruvilla J, et al. Programmed Death-1 Blockade With Pembrolizumab in Patients With Classical Hodgkin Lymphoma After Brentuximab Vedotin Failure. *J. Clin. Oncol.* 2016;34(31):3733–3739.
301. Chen R, Zinzani PL, Lee HJ, Armand P, Johnson NA, Brice P, et al. Pembrolizumab in relapsed or refractory Hodgkin lymphoma: 2-year follow-up of KEYNOTE-087. *Blood.* 2019;134(14):1144–1153.
302. Mateos MV, Blacklock H, Schjesvold F, Oriol A, Simpson D, George A, et al. Pembrolizumab plus pomalidomide and dexamethasone for patients with relapsed or refractory multiple myeloma (KEYNOTE-183): a randomised, open-label, phase 3 trial. *Lancet Haematol.* 2019;6(9):e459–ee69.
303. Mateos MV, Orlowski RZ, Ocio EM, Rodriguez-Otero P, Reece D, Moreau P, et al. Pembrolizumab combined with lenalidomide and low-dose dexamethasone for relapsed or refractory multiple myeloma: phase I KEYNOTE-023 study. *Br. J. Haematol.* 2019;186(5):e117–ee21.
304. Usmani SZ, Schjesvold F, Oriol A, Karlin L, Cavo M, Rifkin RM, et al. Pembrolizumab plus lenalidomide and dexamethasone for patients with treatment-naive multiple myeloma (KEYNOTE-185): a randomised, open-label, phase 3 trial. *Lancet Haematol.* 2019;6(9):e448–ee58.
305. United States Food and Drug Administration. FDA Alerts Healthcare Professionals and Oncology Clinical Investigators about Two Clinical Trials on Hold Evaluating KEYTRUDA® (pembrolizumab) in Patients with Multiple Myeloma. September 2017, [Available from: www.fda.gov/drugs/drug-safety-and-availability/fda-alerts-healthcare-professionals-and-oncology-clinical-investigators-about-two-clinical-trials].
306. Geoerger B, Zwaan CM, Marshall LV, Michon J, Bourdeaut F, Casanova M, et al. Atezolizumab for children and young adults with previously treated solid tumours, non-Hodgkin lymphoma, and Hodgkin lymphoma (iMATRIX): a multicentre phase 1-2 study. *Lancet Oncol.* 2020;21(1):134–144.

307. Herrera AF, Goy A, Mehta A, Ramchandren R, Pagel JM, Svoboda J, et al. Safety and activity of ibrutinib in combination with durvalumab in patients with relapsed or refractory follicular lymphoma or diffuse large B-cell lymphoma. *Am. J. Hematol.* 2020;95(1):18–27.
308. Ansell SM, Hurvitz SA, Koenig PA, LaPlant BR, Kabat BF, Fernando D, et al. Phase I study of ipilimumab, an anti-CTLA-4 monoclonal antibody, in patients with relapsed and refractory B-cell non-Hodgkin lymphoma. *Clin. Cancer Res.* 2009;15(20):6446–6453.
309. Tuscano JM, Maverakis E, Groshen S, Tsao-Wei D, Luxardi G, Merleev AA, et al. A Phase I Study of the Combination of Rituximab and Ipilimumab in Patients with Relapsed/Refractory B-Cell Lymphoma. *Clin. Cancer Res.* 2019;25(23):7004–7013.
310. Lee DW, Santomasso BD, Locke FL, Ghobadi A, Turtle CJ, Brudno JN, et al. ASTCT Consensus Grading for Cytokine Release Syndrome and Neurologic Toxicity Associated with Immune Effector Cells. *Biol. Blood Marrow Transplant.* 2019;25(4):625–638.
311. Brentjens RJ, Riviere I, Park JH, Davila ML, Wang X, Stefanski J, et al. Safety and persistence of adoptively transferred autologous CD19-targeted T cells in patients with relapsed or chemotherapy refractory B-cell leukemias. *Blood.* 2011;118(18):4817–4828.
312. Brentjens RJ, Davila ML, Riviere I, Park J, Wang X, Cowell LG, et al. CD19-targeted T cells rapidly induce molecular remissions in adults with chemotherapy-refractory acute lymphoblastic leukemia. *Sci. Transl. Med.* 2013;5(177):177ra38.
313. Maude SL, Frey N, Shaw PA, Aplenc R, Barrett DM, Bunin NJ, et al. Chimeric antigen receptor T cells for sustained remissions in leukemia. *N. Engl. J. Med.* 2014;371(16):1507–1517.
314. Maude SL, Laetsch TW, Buechner J, Rives S, Boyer M, Bittencourt H, et al. Tisagenlecleucel in Children and Young Adults with B-Cell Lymphoblastic Leukemia. *N. Engl. J. Med.* 2018;378(5):439–448.
315. Park JH, Riviere I, Gonen M, Wang X, Senechal B, Curran KJ, et al. Long-Term Follow-up of CD19 CAR Therapy in Acute Lymphoblastic Leukemia. *N. Engl. J. Med.* 2018;378(5):449–459.
316. Neelapu SS, Locke FL, Bartlett NL, Lekakis LJ, Miklos DB, Jacobson CA, et al. Axicabtagene Ciloleucel CAR T-Cell Therapy in Refractory Large B-Cell Lymphoma. *N. Engl. J. Med.* 2017;377(26):2531–2544.
317. Gardner RA, Finney O, Annesley C, Brakke H, Summers C, Leger K, et al. Intent-to-treat leukemia remission by CD19 CAR T cells of defined formulation and dose in children and young adults. *Blood.* 2017;129(25):3322–3331.
318. Locke FL, Ghobadi A, Jacobson CA, Miklos DB, Lekakis LJ, Oluwole OO, et al. Long-term safety and activity of axicabtagene ciloleucel in refractory large B-cell lymphoma (ZUMA-1): a single-arm, multicentre, phase 1-2 trial. *Lancet Oncol.* 2019;20(1):31–42.
319. Schuster SJ, Bishop MR, Tam CS, Waller EK, Borchmann P, McGuirk JP, et al. Tisagenlecleucel in Adult Relapsed or Refractory Diffuse Large B-Cell Lymphoma. *N. Engl. J. Med.* 2019;380(1):45–56.
320. Schuster SJ, Svoboda J, Chong EA, Nasta SD, Mato AR, Anak O, et al. Chimeric Antigen Receptor T Cells in Refractory B-Cell Lymphomas. *N. Engl. J. Med.* 2017;377(26):2545–2554.
321. Brudno JN, Maric I, Hartman SD, Rose JJ, Wang M, Lam N, et al. T Cells Genetically Modified to Express an Anti-B-Cell Maturation Antigen Chimeric Antigen Receptor Cause Remissions of Poor-Prognosis Relapsed Multiple Myeloma. *J. Clin. Oncol.* 2018;36(22):2267–2280.
322. Raje N, Berdeja J, Lin Y, Siegel D, Jagannath S, Madduri D, et al. Anti-BCMA CAR T-Cell Therapy bb2121 in Relapsed or Refractory Multiple Myeloma. *N. Engl. J. Med.* 2019;380(18):1726–1737.
323. Zhao WH, Liu J, Wang BY, Chen YX, Cao XM, Yang Y, et al. A phase 1, open-label study of LCAR-B38M, a chimeric antigen receptor T cell therapy directed against B cell maturation antigen, in patients with relapsed or refractory multiple myeloma. *J. Hematol. Oncol.* 2018;11(1):141.
324. Chen R, Zinzani PL, Fanale MA, Armand P, Johnson NA, Brice P, et al. Phase II Study of the Efficacy and Safety of Pembrolizumab for Relapsed/Refractory Classic Hodgkin Lymphoma. *J. Clin. Oncol.* 2017;35(19):2125–2132.
325. Schuster SJ, Bishop MR, Tam CS, Waller EK, Borchmann P, McGuirk JP, et al. Tisagenlecleucel in Adult Relapsed or Refractory Diffuse Large B-Cell Lymphoma. *N. Engl. J. Med.* 2018;380(1):45–56.
326. Goebeler ME, Bargou RC. T cell-engaging therapies - BiTEs and beyond. *Nat. Rev. Clin. Oncol.* 2020.
327. Kantarjian H, Stein A, Gokbuget N, Fielding AK, Schuh AC, Ribera JM, et al. Blinatumomab versus Chemotherapy for Advanced Acute Lymphoblastic Leukemia. *N. Engl. J. Med.* 2017;376(9):836–847.
328. Ravandi F, Stein AS, Kantarjian HM, Walter RB, Paschka P, Jongen-Lavrencic M, et al. A Phase 1

First-in-Human Study of AMG 330, an Anti-CD33 Bispecific T-Cell Engager (BiTE (R)) Antibody Construct, in Relapsed/Refractory Acute Myeloid Leukemia (R/R AML). *Blood*. 2018;132:4.
329. Topp MS, Duell J, Zugmaier G, Attal M, Moreau P, Langer C, et al. Anti-B-Cell Maturation Antigen BiTE Molecule AMG 420 Induces Responses in Multiple Myeloma. *J. Clin. Oncol.* 2020;38(8):775–783.
330. Schuster SJ, Neelapu SS, Gause BL, Janik JE, Muggia FM, Gockerman JP, et al. Vaccination With Patient-Specific Tumor-Derived Antigen in First Remission Improves Disease-Free Survival in Follicular Lymphoma. *J. Clin. Oncol.* 2011;29(20):2787–2794.
331. Levy R, Ganjoo KN, Leonard JP, Vose JM, Flinn IW, Ambinder RF, et al. Active Idiotypic Vaccination Versus Control Immunotherapy for Follicular Lymphoma. *J. Clin. Oncol.* 2014;32(17):1797–1803.
332. Freedman A, Neelapu SS, Nichols C, Robertson MJ, Djulbegovic B, Winter JN, et al. Placebo-Controlled Phase III Trial of Patient-Specific Immunotherapy With Mitumprotimut-T and Granulocyte-Macrophage Colony-Stimulating Factor After Rituximab in Patients With Follicular Lymphoma. *J. Clin. Oncol.* 2009;27(18):3036–3043.
333. Qazilbash MH, Wieder E, Thall PF, Wang X, Rios R, Lu S, et al. PR1 peptide vaccine induces specific immunity with clinical responses in myeloid malignancies. *Leukemia*. 2017;31(3):697–704.
334. Anguille S, Van de Velde AL, Smits EL, Van Tendeloo VF, Juliusson G, Cools N, et al. Dendritic cell vaccination as postremission treatment to prevent or delay relapse in acute myeloid leukemia. *Blood*. 2017;130(15):1713–1721.
335. Freeman CL, Sehn LH. A tale of two antibodies: obinutuzumab versus rituximab. *Br. J. Haematol.* 2018;182(1):29–45.
336. AlDallal SM. Ofatumumab - a valid treatment option for chronic lymphocytic leukemia patients. *Ther Clin Risk Manag*. 2017;13:905–907.
337. Rizzieri D. Zevalin(®) (ibritumomab tiuxetan): after more than a decade of treatment experience, what have we learned? *Crit. Rev. Oncol. Hematol.* 2016;105:5–17.
338. Srinivasan A, Mukherji SK. Tositumomab and Iodine I 131 Tositumomab (Bexaar). *Am. J. Neuroradiol.* 2011;32(4):637.
339. ZT A-S. Inotuzumab Ozogamicin: a Review in Relapsed/Refractory B-Cell Acute Lymphoblastic Leukaemia. *Target Oncol*. 2018;13(4):525–532.
340. Milunović V, Mišura Jakobac K, Kursar M, Mandac Rogulj I, Ostojić Kolonić S. FDA's and EMA's approval of brentuximab vedotin for advanced Hodgkin lymphoma: another player in the town? *Eur. J. Haematol.* 2019;103(3):145–151.
341. Norsworthy KJ, Ko CW, Lee JE, Liu J, John CS, Przepiorka D, et al. FDA Approval Summary: mylotarg for Treatment of Patients with Relapsed or Refractory CD33-Positive Acute Myeloid Leukemia. *Oncologist*. 2018;23(9):1103–1108.
342. Lokhorst HM, Plesner T, Laubach JP, Nahi H, Gimsing P, Hansson M, et al. Targeting CD38 with Daratumumab Monotherapy in Multiple Myeloma. *N. Engl. J. Med.* 2015;373(13):1207–1219.
343. Facon T, Kumar S, Plesner T, Orlowski RZ, Moreau P, Bahlis N, et al. Daratumumab plus Lenalidomide and Dexamethasone for Untreated Myeloma. *N. Engl. J. Med.* 2019;380(22):2104–2115.
344. Mateos M-V, Nahi H, Legiec W, Grosicki S, Vorobyev V, Spicka I, et al. Subcutaneous versus intravenous daratumumab in patients with relapsed or refractory multiple myeloma (COLUMBA): a multicentre, open-label, non-inferiority, randomised, phase 3 trial. *Lancet Haematol.* 2020;7(5):e370–ee80.
345. Attal M, Richardson PG, Rajkumar SV, San-Miguel J, Beksac M, Spicka I, et al. Isatuximab plus pomalidomide and low-dose dexamethasone versus pomalidomide and low-dose dexamethasone in patients with relapsed and refractory multiple myeloma (ICARIA-MM): a randomised, multicentre, open-label, phase 3 study. *Lancet North Am. Ed.* 2019;394(10214):2096–2107.
346. United States Food and Drug Administration. FDA approves daratumumab and hyaluronidase-fihj for multiple myeloma. 2020 [Available from: https://www.fda.gov/drugs/drug-approvals-and-databases/fda-approves-daratumumab-and-hyaluronidase-fihj-multiple-myeloma.
347. United States Food and Drug Administration. FDA approves isatuximab-irfc for multiple myeloma. 2020 [Available from: https://www.fda.gov/drugs/development-approval-process-drugs/fda-approves-isatuximab-irfc-multiple-myeloma.
348. Cuesta-Mateos C, Alcaraz-Serna A, Somovilla-Crespo B, Muñoz-Calleja C. Monoclonal Antibody

Therapies for Hematological Malignancies: not Just Lineage-Specific Targets. *Front Immunol.* 2018;8:1936.
349. Ostrom QT, Gittleman H, Truitt G, Boscia A, Kruchko C, Barnholtz-Sloan JS. CBTRUS Statistical Report: primary Brain and Other Central Nervous System Tumors Diagnosed in the United States in 2011-2015. *Neuro. Oncol.* 2018;20(suppl_4):iv1–iv86.
350. Louis DN, Perry A, Reifenberger G, von Deimling A, Figarella-Branger D, Cavenee WK, et al. The 2016 World Health Organization Classification of Tumors of the Central Nervous System: a summary. *Acta Neuropathol.* 2016;131(6):803–820.
351. Wainwright DA, Balyasnikova IV, Chang AL, Ahmed AU, Moon KS, Auffinger B, et al. IDO expression in brain tumors increases the recruitment of regulatory T cells and negatively impacts survival. *Clin. Cancer Res.* 2012;18(22):6110–6121.
352. Zhang I, Alizadeh D, Liang J, Zhang L, Gao H, Song Y, et al. Characterization of Arginase Expression in Glioma-Associated Microglia and Macrophages. *PLoS ONE.* 2016;11(12):e0165118.
353. Mitsuka K, Kawataki T, Satoh E, Asahara T, Horikoshi T, Kinouchi H. Expression of indoleamine 2,3-dioxygenase and correlation with pathological malignancy in gliomas. *Neurosurgery.* 2013;72(6):1031–1038 discussion 8-9.
354. Perng P, Lim M. Immunosuppressive Mechanisms of Malignant Gliomas: parallels at Non-CNS Sites. *Front. Oncol.* 2015;5:153.
355. Cserr HF, Knopf PM. Cervical lymphatics, the blood-brain barrier and the immunoreactivity of the brain: a new view. *Immunol. Today.* 1992;13(12):507–512.
356. Iliff JJ, Wang M, Liao Y, Plogg BA, Peng W, Gundersen GA, et al. A paravascular pathway facilitates CSF flow through the brain parenchyma and the clearance of interstitial solutes, including amyloid beta. *Sci. Transl. Med.* 2012;4(147):147ra11.
357. Sampson JH, Gunn MD, Fecci PE, Ashley DM. Brain immunology and immunotherapy in brain tumours. *Nat. Rev. Cancer.* 2020;20(1):12–25.
358. Woroniecka K, Chongsathidkiet P, Rhodin K, Kemeny H, Dechant C, Farber SH, et al. T-Cell Exhaustion Signatures Vary with Tumor Type and Are Severe in Glioblastoma. *Clin. Cancer Res.* 2018;24(17):4175–4186.
359. Liu Y, Carlsson R, Ambjorn M, Hasan M, Badn W, Darabi A, et al. PD-L1 expression by neurons nearby tumors indicates better prognosis in glioblastoma patients. *J. Neurosci.* 2013;33(35):14231–14245.
360. Park SH, Won J, Kim SI, Lee Y, Park CK, Kim SK, et al. Molecular Testing of Brain Tumor. *J Pathol Transl Med.* 2017;51(3):205–223.
361. Chalmers ZR, Connelly CF, Fabrizio D, Gay L, Ali SM, Ennis R, et al. Analysis of 100,000 human cancer genomes reveals the landscape of tumor mutational burden. *Genome Med.* 2017;9(1):34.
362. Stupp R, Mason WP, van den Bent MJ, Weller M, Fisher B, Taphoorn MJ, et al. Radiotherapy plus concomitant and adjuvant temozolomide for glioblastoma. *N. Engl. J. Med.* 2005;352(10):987–996.
363. Stupp R, Hegi ME, Mason WP, van den Bent MJ, Taphoorn MJ, Janzer RC, et al. Effects of radiotherapy with concomitant and adjuvant temozolomide versus radiotherapy alone on survival in glioblastoma in a randomised phase III study: 5-year analysis of the EORTC-NCIC trial. *Lancet Oncol.* 2009;10(5):459–466.
364. Lapointe S, Perry A, Butowski NA. Primary brain tumours in adults. *Lancet.* 2018;392(10145):432–446.
365. Reardon DA, Brandes AA, Omuro A, Mulholland P, Lim M, Wick A, et al. Effect of Nivolumab vs Bevacizumab in Patients With Recurrent Glioblastoma: the CheckMate 143 Phase 3 Randomized Clinical Trial. *JAMA Oncol.* 2020;6(7):1–8.
366. Omuro A, Vlahovic G, Lim M, Sahebjam S, Baehring J, Cloughesy T, et al. Nivolumab with or without ipilimumab in patients with recurrent glioblastoma: results from exploratory phase I cohorts of CheckMate 143. *Neuro. Oncol.* 2018;20(5):674–686.
367. Lukas RV, Rodon J, Becker K, Wong ET, Shih K, Touat M, et al. Clinical activity and safety of atezolizumab in patients with recurrent glioblastoma. *J. Neurooncol.* 2018;140(2):317–328.
368. Cloughesy TF, Mochizuki AY, Orpilla JR, Hugo W, Lee AH, Davidson TB, et al. Neoadjuvant anti-PD-1 immunotherapy promotes a survival benefit with intratumoral and systemic immune responses in recurrent glioblastoma. *Nat. Med.* 2019;25(3):477–486.
369. Schalper KA, Rodriguez-Ruiz ME, Diez-Valle R, López-Janeiro A, Porciuncula A, Idoate MA, et al.

Neoadjuvant nivolumab modifies the tumor immune microenvironment in resectable glioblastoma. *Nat. Med.* 2019;25(3):470–476.
370. Desjardins A, Gromeier M, Herndon 2nd JE, Beaubier N, Bolognesi DP, Friedman AH, et al. Recurrent Glioblastoma Treated with Recombinant Poliovirus. *N. Engl. J. Med.* 2018;379(2):150–161.
371. Markert JM, Razdan SN, Kuo HC, Cantor A, Knoll A, Karrasch M, et al. A phase 1 trial of oncolytic HSV-1, G207, given in combination with radiation for recurrent GBM demonstrates safety and radiographic responses. *Mol. Ther.* 2014;22(5):1048–1055.
372. Lang FF, Conrad C, Gomez-Manzano C, Yung WKA, Sawaya R, Weinberg JS, et al. Phase I Study of DNX-2401 (Delta-24-RGD) Oncolytic Adenovirus: replication and Immunotherapeutic Effects in Recurrent Malignant Glioma. *J. Clin. Oncol.* 2018;36(14):1419–1427.
373. Keskin DB, Anandappa AJ, Sun J, Tirosh I, Mathewson ND, Li S, et al. Neoantigen vaccine generates intratumoral T cell responses in phase Ib glioblastoma trial. *Nature.* 2019;565(7738):234–239.
374. Sampson JH, Heimberger AB, Archer GE, Aldape KD, Friedman AH, Friedman HS, et al. Immunologic escape after prolonged progression-free survival with epidermal growth factor receptor variant III peptide vaccination in patients with newly diagnosed glioblastoma. *J. Clin. Oncol.* 2010;28(31):4722–4729.
375. Weller M, Butowski N, Tran DD, Recht LD, Lim M, Hirte H, et al. Rindopepimut with temozolomide for patients with newly diagnosed, EGFRvIII-expressing glioblastoma (ACT IV): a randomised, double-blind, international phase 3 trial. *Lancet Oncol.* 2017;18(10):1373–1385.
376. Izumoto S, Tsuboi A, Oka Y, Suzuki T, Hashiba T, Kagawa N, et al. Phase II clinical trial of Wilms tumor 1 peptide vaccination for patients with recurrent glioblastoma multiforme. *J. Neurosurg.* 2008;108(5):963–971.
377. Schumacher T, Bunse L, Pusch S, Sahm F, Wiestler B, Quandt J, et al. A vaccine targeting mutant IDH1 induces antitumour immunity. *Nature.* 2014;512(7514):324–327.
378. Wen PY, Reardon DA, Armstrong TS, Phuphanich S, Aiken RD, Landolfi JC, et al. A Randomized Double-Blind Placebo-Controlled Phase II Trial of Dendritic Cell Vaccine ICT-107 in Newly Diagnosed Patients with Glioblastoma. *Clin. Cancer Res.* 2019;25(19):5799–5807.
379. O'Rourke DM, Nasrallah MP, Desai A, Melenhorst JJ, Mansfield K, Morrissette JJD, et al. A single dose of peripherally infused EGFRvIII-directed CAR T cells mediates antigen loss and induces adaptive resistance in patients with recurrent glioblastoma. *Sci. Transl. Med.* 2017;9(399).
380. Ahmed N, Brawley V, Hegde M, Bielamowicz K, Kalra M, Landi D, et al. HER2-Specific Chimeric Antigen Receptor-Modified Virus-Specific T Cells for Progressive Glioblastoma: a Phase 1 Dose-Escalation Trial. *JAMA Oncol.* 2017;3(8):1094–1101.
381. Brown CE, Badie B, Barish ME, Weng L, Ostberg JR, Chang WC, et al. Bioactivity and Safety of IL13Ralpha2-Redirected Chimeric Antigen Receptor CD8+ T Cells in Patients with Recurrent Glioblastoma. *Clin. Cancer Res.* 2015;21(18):4062–4072.
382. Nellan A, Rota C, Majzner R, Lester-McCully CM, Griesinger AM, Mulcahy Levy JM, et al. Durable regression of Medulloblastoma after regional and intravenous delivery of anti-HER2 chimeric antigen receptor T cells. *J. Immunother. Cancer.* 2018;6(1):30.
383. Orlando D, Miele E, De Angelis B, Guercio M, Boffa I, Sinibaldi M, et al. Adoptive Immunotherapy Using PRAME-Specific T Cells in Medulloblastoma. *Cancer Res.* 2018;78(12):3337–3349.
384. Brandes AA, Carpentier AF, Kesari S, Sepulveda-Sanchez JM, Wheeler HR, Chinot O, et al. A Phase II randomized study of galunisertib monotherapy or galunisertib plus lomustine compared with lomustine monotherapy in patients with recurrent glioblastoma. *Neuro. Oncol.* 2016;18(8):1146–1156.
385. Heynckes S, Daka K, Franco P, Gaebelein A, Frenking JH, Doria-Medina R, et al. Crosslink between Temozolomide and PD-L1 immune-checkpoint inhibition in glioblastoma multiforme. *BMC Cancer.* 2019;19(1):117.
386. Keskin DB, Anandappa AJ, Sun J, Tirosh I, Mathewson ND, Li S, et al. Neoantigen vaccine generates intratumoral T cell responses in phase Ib glioblastoma trial. *Nature.* 2019;565(7738):234–239.
387. Hilf N, Kuttruff-Coqui S, Frenzel K, Bukur V, Stevanovic S, Gouttefangeas C, et al. Actively personalized vaccination trial for newly diagnosed glioblastoma. *Nature.* 2019;565(7738):240–245.
388. Argiris A, Karamouzis MV, Raben D, Ferris RL. Head and neck cancer. *Lancet.* 2008;371(9625):1695–1709.
389. Vigneswaran N, Williams MD. Epidemiologic trends in head and neck cancer and aids in diagnosis. *Oral Maxillofac Surg Clin North Am.* 2014;26(2):123–141.

390. Wu C-T, Chen W-C, Chen M-F. The Response of Prostate Cancer to Androgen Deprivation and Irradiation Due to Immune Modulation. *Cancers (Basel)*. 2019;11(1):20.
391. Joshi P, Dutta S, Chaturvedi P, Nair S. Head and neck cancers in developing countries. *Rambam Maimonides Med J*. 2014;5(2):e0009.
392. Wyss A, Hashibe M, Chuang SC, Lee YC, Zhang ZF, Yu GP, et al. Cigarette, cigar, and pipe smoking and the risk of head and neck cancers: pooled analysis in the International Head and Neck Cancer Epidemiology Consortium. *Am. J. Epidemiol.* 2013;178(5):679–690.
393. Hashibe M, Brennan P, Benhamou S, Castellsague X, Chen C, Curado MP, et al. Alcohol drinking in never users of tobacco, cigarette smoking in never drinkers, and the risk of head and neck cancer: pooled analysis in the International Head and Neck Cancer Epidemiology Consortium. *J. Natl. Cancer Inst.* 2007;99(10):777–789.
394. Hashibe M, Brennan P, Chuang SC, Boccia S, Castellsague X, Chen C, et al. Interaction between tobacco and alcohol use and the risk of head and neck cancer: pooled analysis in the International Head and Neck Cancer Epidemiology Consortium. *Cancer Epidemiol. Biomarkers Prev.* 2009;18(2):541–550.
395. Bosch FX, Lorincz A, Munoz N, Meijer CJ, Shah KV. The causal relation between human papillomavirus and cervical cancer. *J. Clin. Pathol.* 2002;55(4):244–265.
396. Young LS, Dawson CW. Epstein-Barr virus and nasopharyngeal carcinoma. *Chin. J. Cancer.* 2014;33(12):581–590.
397. Chourasia NR, Borle RM, Vastani A. Concomitant Association of Oral Submucous Fibrosis and Oral Squamous Cell Carcinoma and Incidence of Malignant Transformation of Oral Submucous Fibrosis in a Population of Central India: a Retrospective Study. *J Maxillofac Oral Surg*. 2015;14(4):902–906.
398. Zandberg DP, Strome SE. The role of the PD-L1:PD-1 pathway in squamous cell carcinoma of the head and neck. *Oral Oncol.* 2014;50(7):627–632.
399. Liu JF, Ma SR, Mao L, Bu LL, Yu GT, Li YC, et al. T-cell immunoglobulin mucin 3 blockade drives an antitumor immune response in head and neck cancer. *Mol Oncol.* 2017;11(2):235–247.
400. Deng WW, Mao L, Yu GT, Bu LL, Ma SR, Liu B, et al. LAG-3 confers poor prognosis and its blockade reshapes antitumor response in head and neck squamous cell carcinoma. *Oncoimmunology*. 2016;5(11):e1239005.
401. Gameiro SF, Ghasemi F, Barrett JW, Koropatnick J, Nichols AC, Mymryk JS, et al. Treatment-naïve HPV+ head and neck cancers display a T-cell-inflamed phenotype distinct from their HPV- counterparts that has implications for immunotherapy. *Oncoimmunology*. 2018;7(10):e1498439.
402. Jie HB, Gildener-Leapman N, Li J, Srivastava RM, Gibson SP, Whiteside TL, et al. Intratumoral regulatory T cells upregulate immunosuppressive molecules in head and neck cancer patients. *Br. J. Cancer.* 2013;109(10):2629–2635.
403. Bian Y, Hall B, Sun ZJ, Molinolo A, Chen W, Gutkind JS, et al. Loss of TGF-beta signaling and PTEN promotes head and neck squamous cell carcinoma through cellular senescence evasion and cancer-related inflammation. *Oncogene*. 2012;31(28):3322–3332.
404. Jebreel A, Mistry D, Loke D, Dunn G, Hough V, Oliver K, et al. Investigation of interleukin 10, 12 and 18 levels in patients with head and neck cancer. *J. Laryngol. Otol.* 2007;121(3):246–252.
405. Duffy SA, Taylor JM, Terrell JE, Islam M, Li Y, Fowler KE, et al. Interleukin-6 predicts recurrence and survival among head and neck cancer patients. *Cancer*. 2008;113(4):750–757.
406. Tsai MS, Chen WC, Lu CH, Chen MF. The prognosis of head and neck squamous cell carcinoma related to immunosuppressive tumor microenvironment regulated by IL-6 signaling. *Oral Oncol.* 2019;91:47–55.
407. Seiwert TY, Zuo Z, Keck MK, Khattri A, Pedamallu CS, Stricker T, et al. Integrative and comparative genomic analysis of HPV-positive and HPV-negative head and neck squamous cell carcinomas. *Clin. Cancer Res.* 2015;21(3):632–641.
408. Leibowitz MS, Andrade Filho PA, Ferrone S, Ferris RL. Deficiency of activated STAT1 in head and neck cancer cells mediates TAP1-dependent escape from cytotoxic T lymphocytes. *Cancer Immunol. Immunother.* 2011;60(4):525–535.
409. Lawrence MS, Sougnez C, Lichtenstein L, Cibulskis K, Lander E, Gabriel SB, et al. Comprehensive genomic characterization of head and neck squamous cell carcinomas. *Nature*. 2015;517(7536):576–582.
410. Moody CA, Laimins LA. Human papillomavirus oncoproteins: pathways to transformation. *Nat. Rev. Cancer*. 2010;10(8):550–560.

411. Wuthrick EJ, Zhang Q, Machtay M, Rosenthal DI, Nguyen-Tan PF, Fortin A, et al. Institutional clinical trial accrual volume and survival of patients with head and neck cancer. *J. Clin. Oncol.* 2015;33(2):156–164.
412. Vermorken JB, Mesia R, Rivera F, Remenar E, Kawecki A, Rottey S, et al. Platinum-based chemotherapy plus cetuximab in head and neck cancer. *N. Engl. J. Med.* 2008;359(11):1116–1127.
413. Seiwert TY, Burtness B, Mehra R, Weiss J, Berger R, Eder JP, et al. Safety and clinical activity of pembrolizumab for treatment of recurrent or metastatic squamous cell carcinoma of the head and neck (KEYNOTE-012): an open-label, multicentre, phase 1b trial. *Lancet Oncol.* 2016;17(7):956–965.
414. Cohen EEW, Soulieres D, Le Tourneau C, Dinis J, Licitra L, Ahn MJ, et al. Pembrolizumab versus methotrexate, docetaxel, or cetuximab for recurrent or metastatic head-and-neck squamous cell carcinoma (KEYNOTE-040): a randomised, open-label, phase 3 study. *Lancet.* 2019;393(10167):156–167.
415. Bauml J, Seiwert TY, Pfister DG, Worden F, Liu SV, Gilbert J, et al. Pembrolizumab for Platinum- and Cetuximab-Refractory Head and Neck Cancer: results From a Single-Arm, Phase II Study. *J. Clin. Oncol.* 2017;35(14):1542–1549.
416. Cohen EEW, Bell RB, Bifulco CB, Burtness B, Gillison ML, Harrington KJ, et al. The Society for Immunotherapy of Cancer consensus statement on immunotherapy for the treatment of squamous cell carcinoma of the head and neck (HNSCC). *J. Immunother. Cancer.* 2019;7(1):184.
417. Ferris RL, Blumenschein Jr G, Fayette J, Guigay J, Colevas AD, Licitra L, et al. Nivolumab for Recurrent Squamous-Cell Carcinoma of the Head and Neck. *N. Engl. J. Med.* 2016;375(19):1856–1867.
418. Ferris RL, Blumenschein Jr G, Fayette J, Guigay J, Colevas AD, Licitra L, et al. Nivolumab vs investigator's choice in recurrent or metastatic squamous cell carcinoma of the head and neck: 2-year long-term survival update of CheckMate 141 with analyses by tumor PD-L1 expression. *Oral Oncol.* 2018;81:45–51.
419. United States Food and Drug Administration. Nivolumab for SCCHN. November 2016. [Available from: https://www.fda.gov/drugs/resources-information-approved-drugs/nivolumab-scchn.
420. United States Food and Drug Administration. FDA approves pembrolizumab for first-line treatment of head and neck squamous cell carcinoma. November 2019. [Available from: https://www.fda.gov/drugs/resources-information-approved-drugs/fda-approves-pembrolizumab-first-line-treatment-head-and-neck-squamous-cell-carcinoma.
421. Zandberg DP, Algazi AP, Jimeno A, Good JS, Fayette J, Bouganim N, et al. Durvalumab for recurrent or metastatic head and neck squamous cell carcinoma: results from a single-arm, phase II study in patients with >/=25% tumour cell PD-L1 expression who have progressed on platinum-based chemotherapy. *Eur. J. Cancer.* 2019;107:142–152.
422. Siu LL, Even C, Mesia R, Remenar E, Daste A, Delord JP, et al. Safety and Efficacy of Durvalumab With or Without Tremelimumab in Patients With PD-L1-Low/Negative Recurrent or Metastatic HNSCC: the Phase 2 CONDOR Randomized Clinical Trial. *JAMA Oncol.* 2019;5(2):195–203.
423. Massarelli E, William W, Johnson F, Kies M, Ferrarotto R, Guo M, et al. Combining Immune Checkpoint Blockade and Tumor-Specific Vaccine for Patients With Incurable Human Papillomavirus 16-Related Cancer: a Phase 2 Clinical Trial. *JAMA Oncol.* 2019;5(1):67–73.
424. Bray F, Ferlay J, Soerjomataram I, Siegel RL, Torre LA, Jemal A. Global cancer statistics 2018: GLOBOCAN estimates of incidence and mortality worldwide for 36 cancers in 185 countries. *CA Cancer J. Clin.* 2018;68(6):394–424.
425. Travis WD, Brambilla E, Nicholson AG, Yatabe Y, Austin JHM, Beasley MB, et al. The 2015 World Health Organization Classification of Lung Tumors: impact of Genetic, Clinical and Radiologic Advances Since the 2004 Classification. *J. Thorac. Oncol.* 2015;10(9):1243–1260.
426. Inamura K. Lung Cancer: understanding Its Molecular Pathology and the 2015 WHO Classification. *Front. Oncol.* 2017;7:193.
427. Malhotra J, Malvezzi M, Negri E, La Vecchia C, Boffetta P. Risk factors for lung cancer worldwide. *Eur. Respir. J.* 2016;48(3):889–902.
428. Seijo LM, Zulueta JJ. Understanding the Links Between Lung Cancer, COPD, and Emphysema: a Key to More Effective Treatment and Screening. *Oncology (Williston Park).* 2017;31(2):93–102.
429. Konishi J, Yamazaki K, Azuma M, Kinoshita I, Dosaka-Akita H, Nishimura M. B7-H1 expression on non-small cell lung cancer cells and its relationship with tumor-infiltrating lymphocytes and their PD-1 expression. *Clin. Cancer Res.* 2004;10(15):5094–5100.

430. Kim MY, Koh J, Kim S, Go H, Jeon YK, Chung DH. Clinicopathological analysis of PD-L1 and PD-L2 expression in pulmonary squamous cell carcinoma: comparison with tumor-infiltrating T cells and the status of oncogenic drivers. *Lung Cancer.* 2015;88(1):24–33.
431. Skov BG, Rorvig SB, Jensen THL, Skov T. The prevalence of programmed death ligand-1 (PD-L1) expression in non-small cell lung cancer in an unselected, consecutive population. *Mod. Pathol.* 2020;33(1):109–117.
432. Gao X, Zhu Y, Li G, Huang H, Zhang G, Wang F, et al. TIM-3 expression characterizes regulatory T cells in tumor tissues and is associated with lung cancer progression. *PLoS ONE.* 2012;7(2):e30676.
433. He Y, Yu H, Rozeboom L, Rivard CJ, Ellison K, Dziadziuszko R, et al. LAG-3 Protein Expression in Non-Small Cell Lung Cancer and Its Relationship with PD-1/PD-L1 and Tumor-Infiltrating Lymphocytes. *J. Thorac. Oncol.* 2017;12(5):814–823.
434. Heim L, Kachler K, Siegmund R, Trufa DI, Mittler S, Geppert CI, et al. Increased expression of the immunosuppressive interleukin-35 in patients with non-small cell lung cancer. *Br. J. Cancer.* 2019;120(9):903–912.
435. Duan Q, Zhang H, Zheng J, Zhang L. Turning Cold into Hot: firing up the Tumor Microenvironment. *Trends Cancer.* 2020.
436. Guo X, Zhang Y, Zheng L, Zheng C, Song J, Zhang Q, et al. Global characterization of T cells in non-small-cell lung cancer by single-cell sequencing. *Nat. Med.* 2018;24(7):978–985.
437. Bremnes RM, Busund LT, Kilvaer TL, Andersen S, Richardsen E, Paulsen EE, et al. The Role of Tumor-Infiltrating Lymphocytes in Development, Progression, and Prognosis of Non-Small Cell Lung Cancer. *J. Thorac. Oncol.* 2016;11(6):789–800.
438. Enewold L, Mechanic LE, Bowman ED, Zheng YL, Yu Z, Trivers G, et al. Serum concentrations of cytokines and lung cancer survival in African Americans and Caucasians. *Cancer Epidemiol. Biomarkers Prev.* 2009;18(1):215–222.
439. Landskron G, De la Fuente M, Thuwajit P, Thuwajit C, Hermoso MA. Chronic inflammation and cytokines in the tumor microenvironment. *J Immunol Res.* 2014;2014:149185.
440. Sanmamed MF, Perez-Gracia JL, Schalper KA, Fusco JP, Gonzalez A, Rodriguez-Ruiz ME, et al. Changes in serum interleukin-8 (IL-8) levels reflect and predict response to anti-PD-1 treatment in melanoma and non-small-cell lung cancer patients. *Ann. Oncol.* 2017;28(8):1988–1995.
441. Denkert C, Loibl S, Noske A, Roller M, Muller BM, Komor M, et al. Tumor-associated lymphocytes as an independent predictor of response to neoadjuvant chemotherapy in breast cancer. *J. Clin. Oncol.* 2010;28(1):105–113.
442. Wang H, Li Z, Dong B, Sun W, Yang X, Liu R, et al. Prognostic significance of PD-L1 expression and CD8+ T cell infiltration in pulmonary neuroendocrine tumors. *Diagn Pathol.* 2018;13(1):30.
443. Bonanno L, Pavan A, Dieci MV, Di Liso E, Schiavon M, Comacchio G, et al. The role of immune microenvironment in small-cell lung cancer: distribution of PD-L1 expression and prognostic role of FOXP3-positive tumour infiltrating lymphocytes. *Eur. J. Cancer.* 2018;101:191–200.
444. Wistuba II, Gazdar AF, Minna JD. Molecular genetics of small cell lung carcinoma. *Semin. Oncol.* 2001;28(2 Suppl 4):3–13.
445. Cancer Genome Atlas Research N. Comprehensive molecular profiling of lung adenocarcinoma. *Nature.* 2014;511(7511):543–550.
446. Cancer Genome Atlas Research N. Comprehensive genomic characterization of squamous cell lung cancers. *Nature.* 2012;489(7417):519–525.
447. George J, Lim JS, Jang SJ, Cun Y, Ozretic L, Kong G, et al. Comprehensive genomic profiles of small cell lung cancer. *Nature.* 2015;524(7563):47–53.
448. Zabarovsky ER, Lerman MI, Minna JD. Tumor suppressor genes on chromosome 3p involved in the pathogenesis of lung and other cancers. *Oncogene.* 2002;21(45):6915–6935.
449. Hirsch FR, Scagliotti GV, Mulshine JL, Kwon R, Curran Jr WJ, Wu YL, et al. Lung cancer: current therapies and new targeted treatments. *Lancet.* 2017;389(10066):299–311.
450. Yap TA, Aerts JG, Popat S, Fennell DA. Novel insights into mesothelioma biology and implications for therapy. *Nat. Rev. Cancer.* 2017;17(8):475–488.
451. National Cancer Institute. *Small Cell Lung Cancer Treatment (PDQ®)–Health Professional Version*; 2020. [Available from: https://www.cancer.gov/types/lung/hp/small-cell-lung-treatment-pdq#section/all.
452. Wang S, Tang J, Sun T, Zheng X, Li J, Sun H, et al. Survival changes in patients with small cell lung cancer and disparities between different sexes, socioeconomic statuses and ages. *Sci. Rep.* 2017;7(1):1339.

453. Tsao AS, Lindwasser OW, Adjei AA, Adusumilli PS, Beyers ML, Blumenthal GM, et al. Current and Future Management of Malignant Mesothelioma: a Consensus Report from the National Cancer Institute Thoracic Malignancy Steering Committee, International Association for the Study of Lung Cancer, and Mesothelioma Applied Research Foundation. *J. Thorac. Oncol.* 2018;13(11):1655–1667.
454. Topalian SL, Hodi FS, Brahmer JR, Gettinger SN, Smith DC, McDermott DF, et al. Safety, activity, and immune correlates of anti-PD-1 antibody in cancer. *N. Engl. J. Med.* 2012;366(26):2443–2454.
455. Brahmer JR, Tykodi SS, Chow LQ, Hwu WJ, Topalian SL, Hwu P, et al. Safety and activity of anti-PD-L1 antibody in patients with advanced cancer. *N. Engl. J. Med.* 2012;366(26):2455–2465.
456. Garon EB, Rizvi NA, Hui R, Leighl N, Balmanoukian AS, Eder JP, et al. Pembrolizumab for the treatment of non-small-cell lung cancer. *N. Engl. J. Med.* 2015;372(21):2018–2028.
457. Garon EB, Hellmann MD, Rizvi NA, Carcereny E, Leighl NB, Ahn MJ, et al. Five-Year Overall Survival for Patients With Advanced NonSmall-Cell Lung Cancer Treated With Pembrolizumab: results From the Phase I KEYNOTE-001 Study. *J. Clin. Oncol.* 2019;37(28):2518–2527.
458. Herbst RS, Baas P, Kim DW, Felip E, Perez-Gracia JL, Han JY, et al. Pembrolizumab versus docetaxel for previously treated, PD-L1-positive, advanced non-small-cell lung cancer (KEYNOTE-010): a randomised controlled trial. *Lancet.* 2016;387(10027):1540–1550.
459. Herbst RS, Garon EB, Kim DW, Chul Cho B, Pérez Gracia JL, Han JY, et al. Long-term follow-up in the KEYNOTE-010 study of pembrolizumab (pembro) for advanced NSCLC, including in patients (pts) who completed 2 years of pembro and pts who received a second course of pembro. *Ann. Oncol.* 2018;29:x42–xx3.
460. Gandhi L, Rodriguez-Abreu D, Gadgeel S, Esteban E, Felip E, De Angelis F, et al. Pembrolizumab plus Chemotherapy in Metastatic Non-Small-Cell Lung Cancer. *N. Engl. J. Med.* 2018;378(22):2078–2092.
461. Langer CJ, Gadgeel SM, Borghaei H, Papadimitrakopoulou VA, Patnaik A, Powell SF, et al. Carboplatin and pemetrexed with or without pembrolizumab for advanced, non-squamous non-small-cell lung cancer: a randomised, phase 2 cohort of the open-label KEYNOTE-021 study. *Lancet Oncol.* 2016;17(11):1497–1508.
462. Paz-Ares L, Luft A, Vicente D, Tafreshi A, Gumus M, Mazieres J, et al. Pembrolizumab plus Chemotherapy for Squamous Non-Small-Cell Lung Cancer. *N. Engl. J. Med.* 2018;379(21):2040–2051.
463. Reck M, Rodriguez-Abreu D, Robinson AG, Hui R, Csoszi T, Fulop A, et al. Pembrolizumab versus Chemotherapy for PD-L1-Positive Non-Small-Cell Lung Cancer. *N. Engl. J. Med.* 2016;375(19):1823–1833.
464. Mok TSK, Wu YL, Kudaba I, Kowalski DM, Cho BC, Turna HZ, et al. Pembrolizumab versus chemotherapy for previously untreated, PD-L1-expressing, locally advanced or metastatic non-small-cell lung cancer (KEYNOTE-042): a randomised, open-label, controlled, phase 3 trial. *Lancet.* 2019;393(10183):1819–1830.
465. Borghaei H, Paz-Ares L, Horn L, Spigel DR, Steins M, Ready NE, et al. Nivolumab versus Docetaxel in Advanced Nonsquamous Non-Small-Cell Lung Cancer. *N. Engl. J. Med.* 2015;373(17):1627–1639.
466. Horn L, Spigel DR, Vokes EE, Holgado E, Ready N, Steins M, et al. Nivolumab Versus Docetaxel in Previously Treated Patients With Advanced Non-Small-Cell Lung Cancer: two-Year Outcomes From Two Randomized, Open-Label, Phase III Trials (CheckMate 017 and CheckMate 057). *J. Clin. Oncol.* 2017;35(35):3924–3933.
467. Carbone DP, Reck M, Paz-Ares L, Creelan B, Horn L, Steins M, et al. First-Line Nivolumab in Stage IV or Recurrent Non-Small-Cell Lung Cancer. *N. Engl. J. Med.* 2017;376(25):2415–2426.
468. Fehrenbacher L, Spira A, Ballinger M, Kowanetz M, Vansteenkiste J, Mazieres J, et al. Atezolizumab versus docetaxel for patients with previously treated non-small-cell lung cancer (POPLAR): a multicentre, open-label, phase 2 randomised controlled trial. *Lancet.* 2016;387(10030):1837–1846.
469. Rittmeyer A, Barlesi F, Waterkamp D, Park K, Ciardiello F, von Pawel J, et al. Atezolizumab versus docetaxel in patients with previously treated non-small-cell lung cancer (OAK): a phase 3, open-label, multicentre randomised controlled trial. *Lancet.* 2017;389(10066):255–265.
470. Socinski MA, Jotte RM, Cappuzzo F, Orlandi F, Stroyakovskiy D, Nogami N, et al. Atezolizumab for First-Line Treatment of Metastatic Nonsquamous NSCLC. *N. Engl. J. Med.* 2018;378(24):2288–2301.
471. West H, McCleod M, Hussein M, Morabito A, Rittmeyer A, Conter HJ, et al. Atezolizumab in combination with carboplatin plus nab-paclitaxel chemotherapy compared with chemotherapy alone as first-line treatment for metastatic non-squamous non-small-cell lung cancer (IMpower130): a multicentre, randomised, open-label, phase 3 trial. *Lancet Oncol.* 2019;20(7):924–937.

472. Spigel D, de Marinis F, Giaccone G, Reinmuth N, Vergnenegre A, Barrios CH, et al. IMpower110: interim overall survival (OS) analysis of a phase III study of atezolizumab (atezo) vs platinum-based chemotherapy (chemo) as first-line (1L) treatment (tx) in PD-L1-selected NSCLC. *Ann. Oncol.* 2019;30:915.
473. Antonia SJ, Villegas A, Daniel D, Vicente D, Murakami S, Hui R, et al. Overall Survival with Durvalumab after Chemoradiotherapy in Stage III NSCLC. *N. Engl. J. Med.* 2018;379(24):2342–2350.
474. Gray JE, Villegas A, Daniel D, Vicente D, Murakami S, Hui R, et al. Three-Year Overall Survival with Durvalumab after Chemoradiotherapy in Stage III NSCLC-Update from PACIFIC. *J. Thorac. Oncol.* 2020;15(2):288–293.
475. Garassino MC, Cho BC, Kim JH, Mazieres J, Vansteenkiste J, Lena H, et al. Durvalumab as third-line or later treatment for advanced non-small-cell lung cancer (ATLANTIC): an open-label, single-arm, phase 2 study. *Lancet Oncol.* 2018;19(4):521–536.
476. Barlesi F, Vansteenkiste J, Spigel D, Ishii H, Garassino M, de Marinis F, et al. Avelumab versus docetaxel in patients with platinum-treated advanced non-small-cell lung cancer (JAVELIN Lung 200): an open-label, randomised, phase 3 study. *Lancet Oncol.* 2018;19(11):1468–1479.
477. Hellmann MD, Ciuleanu TE, Pluzanski A, Lee JS, Otterson GA, Audigier-Valette C, et al. Nivolumab plus Ipilimumab in Lung Cancer with a High Tumor Mutational Burden. *N. Engl. J. Med.* 2018;378(22):2093–2104.
478. Hellmann MD, Paz-Ares L, Bernabe Caro R, Zurawski B, Kim SW, Carcereny Costa E, et al. Nivolumab plus Ipilimumab in Advanced Non-Small-Cell Lung Cancer. *N. Engl. J. Med.* 2019;381(21):2020–2031.
479. Hellmann MD, Rizvi NA, Goldman JW, Gettinger SN, Borghaei H, Brahmer JR, et al. Nivolumab plus ipilimumab as first-line treatment for advanced non-small-cell lung cancer (CheckMate 012): results of an open-label, phase 1, multicohort study. *Lancet Oncol.* 2017;18(1):31–41.
480. Ready N, Hellmann MD, Awad MM, Otterson GA, Gutierrez M, Gainor JF, et al. First-Line Nivolumab Plus Ipilimumab in Advanced Non-Small-Cell Lung Cancer (CheckMate 568): outcomes by Programmed Death Ligand 1 and Tumor Mutational Burden as Biomarkers. *J. Clin. Oncol.* 2019;37(12):992–1000.
481. Rizvi NA, Cho BC, Reinmuth N, Lee KH, Luft A, Ahn MJ, et al. Durvalumab With or Without Tremelimumab vs Standard Chemotherapy in First-line Treatment of Metastatic Non-Small Cell Lung Cancer: the MYSTIC Phase 3 Randomized Clinical Trial. *JAMA Oncol.* 2020.
482. Chalmers AW, Patel S, Boucher K, Cannon L, Esplin M, Luckart J, et al. Phase I Trial of Targeted EGFR or ALK Therapy with Ipilimumab in Metastatic NSCLC with Long-Term Follow-Up. *Target Oncol.* 2019;14(4):417–421.
483. Shu CA, Gainor JF, Awad MM, Chiuzan C, Grigg CM, Pabani A, et al. Neoadjuvant atezolizumab and chemotherapy in patients with resectable non-small-cell lung cancer: an open-label, multicentre, single-arm, phase 2 trial. *Lancet Oncol.* 2020.
484. Wrangle JM, Velcheti V, Patel MR, Garrett-Mayer E, Hill EG, Ravenel JG, et al. ALT-803, an IL-15 superagonist, in combination with nivolumab in patients with metastatic non-small cell lung cancer: a non-randomised, open-label, phase 1b trial. *Lancet Oncol.* 2018;19(5):694–704.
485. Vansteenkiste JF, Cho BC, Vanakesa T, De Pas T, Zielinski M, Kim MS, et al. Efficacy of the MAGE-A3 cancer immunotherapeutic as adjuvant therapy in patients with resected MAGE-A3-positive non-small-cell lung cancer (MAGRIT): a randomised, double-blind, placebo-controlled, phase 3 trial. *Lancet Oncol.* 2016;17(6):822–835.
486. Butts C, Socinski MA, Mitchell PL, Thatcher N, Havel L, Krzakowski M, et al. Tecemotide (L-BLP25) versus placebo after chemoradiotherapy for stage III non-small-cell lung cancer (START): a randomised, double-blind, phase 3 trial. *Lancet Oncol.* 2014;15(1):59–68.
487. Quoix E, Lena H, Losonczy G, Forget F, Chouaid C, Papai Z, et al. TG4010 immunotherapy and first-line chemotherapy for advanced non-small-cell lung cancer (TIME): results from the phase 2b part of a randomised, double-blind, placebo-controlled, phase 2b/3 trial. *Lancet Oncol.* 2016;17(2):212–223.
488. Hellmann MD, Paz-Ares L, Bernabe Caro R, Zurawski B, Kim S-W, Carcereny Costa E, et al. Nivolumab plus Ipilimumab in Advanced Non–Small-Cell Lung Cancer. *N. Engl. J. Med.* 2019;381(21):2020–2031.

489. Reck M, Ciuleanu T-E, Dols MC, Schenker M, Zurawski B, Menezes J, et al. Nivolumab (NIVO) + ipilimumab (IPI) + 2 cycles of platinum-doublet chemotherapy (chemo) vs 4 cycles chemo as first-line (1L) treatment (tx) for stage IV/recurrent non-small cell lung cancer (NSCLC): checkMate 9LA. *J. Clin. Oncol.* 2020;38(15_suppl):9501.
490. Brahmer J, Reckamp KL, Baas P, Crinò L, Eberhardt WEE, Poddubskaya E, et al. Nivolumab versus Docetaxel in Advanced Squamous-Cell Non–Small-Cell Lung Cancer. *N. Engl. J. Med.* 2015;373(2):123–135.
491. Borghaei H, Paz-Ares L, Horn L, Spigel DR, Steins M, Ready NE, et al. Nivolumab versus Docetaxel in Advanced Nonsquamous Non–Small-Cell Lung Cancer. *N. Engl. J. Med.* 2015;373(17):1627–1639.
492. Gandhi L, Rodríguez-Abreu D, Gadgeel S, Esteban E, Felip E, De Angelis F, et al. Pembrolizumab plus Chemotherapy in Metastatic Non–Small-Cell Lung Cancer. *N. Engl. J. Med.* 2018;378(22):2078–2092.
493. Paz-Ares L, Luft A, Vicente D, Tafreshi A, Gümüş M, Mazières J, et al. Pembrolizumab plus Chemotherapy for Squamous Non–Small-Cell Lung Cancer. *N. Engl. J. Med.* 2018;379(21):2040–2051.
494. Mok TSK, Wu Y-L, Kudaba I, Kowalski DM, Cho BC, Turna HZ, et al. Pembrolizumab versus chemotherapy for previously untreated, PD-L1-expressing, locally advanced or metastatic non-small-cell lung cancer (KEYNOTE-042): a randomised, open-label, controlled, phase 3 trial. *Lancet North Am. Ed.* 2019;393(10183):1819–1830.
495. Herbst RS, Baas P, Kim d, Felip E, Pérez-Gracia JL, Han J-Y, et al. Pembrolizumab versus docetaxel for previously treated, PD-L1-positive, advanced non-small-cell lung cancer (KEYNOTE-010): a randomised controlled trial. *Lancet North Am. Ed.* 2016;387(10027):1540–1550.
496. Jassem J, Herbst RS, de Marinis F, Cadranel J, Csőszi T, Isla D, et al. IMpower110: clinical safety in a phase III study of atezolizumab (atezo) monotherapy (mono) vs platinum-based chemotherapy (chemo) in first-line non-small cell lung cancer (NSCLC). *J. Clin. Oncol.* 2020;38(15_suppl):e21623.
497. Socinski MA, Jotte RM, Cappuzzo F, Orlandi F, Stroyakovskiy D, Nogami N, et al. Atezolizumab for First-Line Treatment of Metastatic Nonsquamous NSCLC. *N. Engl. J. Med.* 2018;378(24):2288–2301.
498. West H, McCleod M, Hussein M, Morabito A, Rittmeyer A, Conter HJ, et al. Atezolizumab in combination with carboplatin plus nab-paclitaxel chemotherapy compared with chemotherapy alone as first-line treatment for metastatic non-squamous non-small-cell lung cancer (IMpower130): a multicentre, randomised, open-label, phase 3 trial. *Lancet Oncol.* 2019;20(7):924–937.
499. Rittmeyer A, Barlesi F, Waterkamp D, Park K, Ciardiello F, von Pawel J, et al. Atezolizumab versus docetaxel in patients with previously treated non-small-cell lung cancer (OAK): a phase 3, open-label, multicentre randomised controlled trial. *Lancet North Am. Ed.* 2017;389(10066):255–265.
500. Gray JE, Villegas AE, Daniel DB, Vicente D, Murakami S, Hui R, et al. Three-year overall survival update from the PACIFIC trial. *J. Clin. Oncol.* 2019;37(15_suppl):8526.
501. united States Food and Drug Administration. FDA approves atezolizumab for extensive-stage small cell lung cancer. 2019 [Available from: https://www.fda.gov/drugs/drug-approvals-and-databases/fda-approves-atezolizumab-extensive-stage-small-cell-lung-cancer.
502. united States Food and Drug Administration. FDA approves durvalumab for extensive-stage small cell lung cancer 2020 [Available from: https://www.fda.gov/drugs/resources-information-approved-drugs/fda-approves-durvalumab-extensive-stage-small-cell-lung-cancer.
503. Furuta M, Kikuchi H, Shoji T, Takashima Y, Kikuchi E, Kikuchi J, et al. DLL3 regulates the migration and invasion of small cell lung cancer by modulating Snail. *Cancer Sci.* 2019;110(5):1599–1608.
504. Morgensztern D, Besse B, Greillier L, Santana-Davila R, Ready N, Hann CL, et al. Efficacy and Safety of Rovalpituzumab Tesirine in Third-Line and Beyond Patients with DLL3-Expressing, Relapsed/Refractory Small-Cell Lung Cancer: results From the Phase II TRINITY Study. *Clin. Cancer Res.* 2019;25(23):6958–6966.
505. Horn L, Mansfield AS, Szczesna A, Havel L, Krzakowski M, Hochmair MJ, et al. First-Line Atezolizumab plus Chemotherapy in Extensive-Stage Small-Cell Lung Cancer. *N. Engl. J. Med.* 2018;379(23):2220–2229.
506. Paz-Ares L, Chen Y, Reinmuth N, Hotta K, Trukhin D, Statsenko G, et al. PL02.11 Overall Survival with Durvalumab Plus Etoposide-Platinum in First-Line Extensive-Stage SCLC: results from the CASPIAN Study. *J. Thorac. Oncol.* 2019;14(10):S7–S8.

507. Reck M, Luft A, Szczesna A, Havel L, Kim SW, Akerley W, et al. Phase III Randomized Trial of Ipilimumab Plus Etoposide and Platinum Versus Placebo Plus Etoposide and Platinum in Extensive-Stage Small-Cell Lung Cancer. *J. Clin. Oncol.* 2016;34(31):3740–3748.
508. Gadgeel SM, Pennell NA, Fidler MJ, Halmos B, Bonomi P, Stevenson J, et al. Phase II Study of Maintenance Pembrolizumab in Patients with Extensive-Stage Small Cell Lung Cancer (SCLC). *J. Thorac. Oncol.* 2018;13(9):1393–1399.
509. Owonikoko TK, Kim HR, Govindan R, Ready N, Reck M, Peters S, et al. Nivolumab (nivo) plus ipilimumab (ipi), nivo, or placebo (pbo) as maintenance therapy in patients (pts) with extensive disease small cell lung cancer (ED-SCLC) after first-line (1L) platinum-based chemotherapy (chemo): results from the double-blind, randomized phase III CheckMate 451 study. *Ann. Oncol.* 2019;30:ii77.
510. Antonia SJ, Lopez-Martin JA, Bendell J, Ott PA, Taylor M, Eder JP, et al. Nivolumab alone and nivolumab plus ipilimumab in recurrent small-cell lung cancer (CheckMate 032): a multicentre, open-label, phase 1/2 trial. *Lancet Oncol.* 2016;17(7):883–895.
511. Ready N, Farago AF, de Braud F, Atmaca A, Hellmann MD, Schneider JG, et al. Third-Line Nivolumab Monotherapy in Recurrent SCLC: checkMate 032. *J. Thorac. Oncol.* 2019;14(2):237–244.
512. Ready NE, Ott PA, Hellmann MD, Zugazagoitia J, Hann CL, de Braud F, et al. Nivolumab Monotherapy and Nivolumab Plus Ipilimumab in Recurrent Small Cell Lung Cancer: results From the CheckMate 032 Randomized Cohort. *J. Thorac. Oncol.* 2020;15(3):426–435.
513. Reck M, Vicente D, Ciuleanu T, Gettinger S, Peters S, Horn L, et al. Efficacy and safety of nivolumab (nivo) monotherapy versus chemotherapy (chemo) in recurrent small cell lung cancer (SCLC): results from CheckMate 331. *Ann. Oncol.* 2018;29:43.
514. Ott PA, Elez E, Hiret S, Kim DW, Morosky A, Saraf S, et al. Pembrolizumab in Patients With Extensive-Stage Small-Cell Lung Cancer: results From the Phase Ib KEYNOTE-028 Study. *J. Clin. Oncol.* 2017;35(34):3823–3829.
515. Chung HC, Lopez-Martin JA, Kao SC-H, Miller WH, Ros W, Gao B, et al. Phase 2 study of pembrolizumab in advanced small-cell lung cancer (SCLC): KEYNOTE-158. *J. Clin. Oncol.* 2018;36(15_suppl):8506.
516. Pujol JL, Greillier L, Audigier-Valette C, Moro-Sibilot D, Uwer L, Hureaux J, et al. A Randomized Non-Comparative Phase II Study of Anti-Programmed Cell Death-Ligand 1 Atezolizumab or Chemotherapy as Second-Line Therapy in Patients With Small Cell Lung Cancer: results From the IFCT-1603 Trial. *J. Thorac. Oncol.* 2019;14(5):903–913.
517. Cedres S, Ponce-Aix S, Zugazagoitia J, Sansano I, Enguita A, Navarro-Mendivil A, et al. Analysis of expression of programmed cell death 1 ligand 1 (PD-L1) in malignant pleural mesothelioma (MPM). *PLoS ONE.* 2015;10(3):e0121071.
518. Bueno R, Stawiski EW, Goldstein LD, Durinck S, De Rienzo A, Modrusan Z, et al. Comprehensive genomic analysis of malignant pleural mesothelioma identifies recurrent mutations, gene fusions and splicing alterations. *Nat. Genet.* 2016;48(4):407–416.
519. Scherpereel A, Mazieres J, Greillier L, Lantuejoul S, Do P, Bylicki O, et al. Nivolumab or nivolumab plus ipilimumab in patients with relapsed malignant pleural mesothelioma (IFCT-1501 MAPS2): a multicentre, open-label, randomised, non-comparative, phase 2 trial. *Lancet Oncol.* 2019;20(2):239–253.
520. Disselhorst MJ, Quispel-Janssen J, Lalezari F, Monkhorst K, de Vries JF, van der Noort V, et al. Ipilimumab and nivolumab in the treatment of recurrent malignant pleural mesothelioma (INITIATE): results of a prospective, single-arm, phase 2 trial. *Lancet Respir Med.* 2019;7(3):260–270.
521. Calabrò L, Morra A, Giannarelli D, Amato G, D'Incecco A, Covre A, et al. Tremelimumab combined with durvalumab in patients with mesothelioma (NIBIT-MESO-1): an open-label, non-randomised, phase 2 study. *The Lancet Respiratory Medicine.* 2018;6(6):451–460.
522. Bristol Myers Squibb. Bristol Myers Squibb Announces Positive Topline Result from Pivotal Phase 3 Trial Evaluating Opdivo® (nivolumab) plus Yervoy® (ipilimumab) vs. Chemotherapy in Previously Untreated Malignant Pleural Mesothelioma. 2020 [Available from: https://news.bms.com/press-release/corporatefinancial-news/bristol-myers-squibb-announces-positive-topline-result-pivotal.
523. Hassan R, Alley E, Kindler H, Antonia S, Jahan T, Honarmand S, et al. Clinical Response of Live-Attenuated, Listeria monocytogenes Expressing Mesothelin (CRS-207) with Chemotherapy in Patients with Malignant Pleural Mesothelioma. *Clin. Cancer Res.* 2019;25(19):5787–5798.

524. Okada M, Kijima T, Aoe K, Kato T, Fujimoto N, Nakagawa K, et al. Clinical Efficacy and Safety of Nivolumab: results of a Multicenter, Open-label, Single-arm, Japanese Phase II study in Malignant Pleural Mesothelioma (MERIT). *Clin. Cancer Res.* 2019;25(18):5485–5492.
525. Maio M, Scherpereel A, Calabro L, Aerts J, Perez SC, Bearz A, et al. Tremelimumab as second-line or third-line treatment in relapsed malignant mesothelioma (DETERMINE): a multicentre, international, randomised, double-blind, placebo-controlled phase 2b trial. *Lancet Oncol.* 2017;18(9):1261–1273.
526. Harbeck N, Gnant M. Breast cancer. *Lancet North Am. Ed.* 2017;389(10074):1134–1150.
527. Howlader N, Altekruse SF, Li CI, Chen VW, Clarke CA, Ries LA, et al. US incidence of breast cancer subtypes defined by joint hormone receptor and HER2 status. *J. Natl. Cancer Inst.* 2014;106(5).
528. Osborne CK, Schiff R. Mechanisms of endocrine resistance in breast cancer. *Annu. Rev. Med.* 2011;62:233–247.
529. Sobral-Leite M, Van de Vijver K, Michaut M, van der Linden R, Hooijer GKJ, Horlings HM, et al. Assessment of PD-L1 expression across breast cancer molecular subtypes, in relation to mutation rate, BRCA1-like status, tumor-infiltrating immune cells and survival. *Oncoimmunology.* 2018;7(12):e1509820.
530. Schmid P, Adams S, Rugo HS, Schneeweiss A, Barrios CH, Iwata H, et al. Atezolizumab and Nab-Paclitaxel in Advanced Triple-Negative Breast Cancer. *N. Engl. J. Med.* 2018;379(22):2108–2121.
531. Voorwerk L, Slagter M, Horlings HM, Sikorska K, van de Vijver KK, de Maaker M, et al. Immune induction strategies in metastatic triple-negative breast cancer to enhance the sensitivity to PD-1 blockade: the TONIC trial. *Nat. Med.* 2019;25(6):920–928.
532. Emens LA, Cruz C, Eder JP, Braiteh F, Chung C, Tolaney SM, et al. Long-term Clinical Outcomes and Biomarker Analyses of Atezolizumab Therapy for Patients With Metastatic Triple-Negative Breast Cancer: a Phase 1 Study. *JAMA Oncol.* 2019;5(1):74–82.
533. Savas P, Virassamy B, Ye C, Salim A, Mintoff CP, Caramia F, et al. Single-cell profiling of breast cancer T cells reveals a tissue-resident memory subset associated with improved prognosis. *Nat. Med.* 2018;24(7):986–993.
534. Zerdes I, Sifakis EG, Matikas A, Chretien S, Tobin NP, Hartman J, et al. Programmed death-ligand 1 gene expression is a prognostic marker in early breast cancer and provides additional prognostic value to 21-gene and 70-gene signatures in estrogen receptor-positive disease. *Mol Oncol.* 2020;14(5):951–963.
535. Burugu S, Gao D, Leung S, Chia SK, Nielsen TO. TIM-3 expression in breast cancer. *Oncoimmunology.* 2018;7(11):e1502128.
536. Burugu S, Gao D, Leung S, Chia SK, Nielsen TO. LAG-3+ tumor infiltrating lymphocytes in breast cancer: clinical correlates and association with PD-1/PD-L1+ tumors. *Ann. Oncol.* 2017;28(12):2977–2984.
537. Semesiuk NI, Zhylchuk A, Bezdenezhnykh N, Lykhova A, Vorontsova AL, Zhylchuk VE, et al. Disseminated tumor cells and enhanced level of some cytokines in bone marrow and peripheral blood of breast cancer patients as predictive factors of tumor progression. *Exp. Oncol.* 2013;35(4):295–302.
538. Wang H, Yang X. Association between serum cytokines and progression of breast cancer in Chinese population. *Medicine (Baltimore).* 2017;96(49):e8840.
539. Kawaguchi K, Sakurai M, Yamamoto Y, Suzuki E, Tsuda M, Kataoka TR, et al. Alteration of specific cytokine expression patterns in patients with breast cancer. *Sci. Rep.* 2019;9(1):2924.
540. Loi S, Michiels S, Salgado R, Sirtaine N, Jose V, Fumagalli D, et al. Tumor infiltrating lymphocytes are prognostic in triple negative breast cancer and predictive for trastuzumab benefit in early breast cancer: results from the FinHER trial. *Ann. Oncol.* 2014;25(8):1544–1550.
541. Adams S, Gray RJ, Demaria S, Goldstein L, Perez EA, Shulman LN, et al. Prognostic value of tumor-infiltrating lymphocytes in triple-negative breast cancers from two phase III randomized adjuvant breast cancer trials: ECOG 2197 and ECOG 1199. *J. Clin. Oncol.* 2014;32(27):2959–2966.
542. Pruneri G, Vingiani A, Bagnardi V, Rotmensz N, De Rose A, Palazzo A, et al. Clinical validity of tumor-infiltrating lymphocytes analysis in patients with triple-negative breast cancer. *Ann. Oncol.* 2016;27(2):249–256.
543. Shou J, Zhang Z, Lai Y, Chen Z, Huang J. Worse outcome in breast cancer with higher tumor-infiltrating FOXP3+ Tregs : a systematic review and meta-analysis. *BMC Cancer.* 2016;16:687.

544. Chung W, Eum HH, Lee HO, Lee KM, Lee HB, Kim KT, et al. Single-cell RNA-seq enables comprehensive tumour and immune cell profiling in primary breast cancer. *Nat. Commun.* 2017;8:15081.
545. Qiu SQ, Waaijer SJH, Zwager MC, de Vries EGE, van der Vegt B, Schroder CP. Tumor-associated macrophages in breast cancer: innocent bystander or important player? *Cancer Treat. Rev.* 2018;70:178–189.
546. Zhao X, Qu J, Sun Y, Wang J, Liu X, Wang F, et al. Prognostic significance of tumor-associated macrophages in breast cancer: a meta-analysis of the literature. *Oncotarget.* 2017;8(18):30576–30586.
547. Muntasell A, Rojo F, Servitja S, Rubio-Perez C, Cabo M, Tamborero D, et al. NK Cell Infiltrates and HLA Class I Expression in Primary HER2(+) Breast Cancer Predict and Uncouple Pathological Response and Disease-free Survival. *Clin. Cancer Res.* 2019;25(5):1535–1545.
548. Apostolou P, Fostira F. Hereditary breast cancer: the era of new susceptibility genes. *Biomed. Res. Int.* 2013;2013:747318.
549. Cancer Genome Atlas N. Comprehensive molecular portraits of human breast tumours. *Nature.* 2012;490(7418):61–70.
550. Adams S, Schmid P, Rugo HS, Winer EP, Loirat D, Awada A, et al. Pembrolizumab monotherapy for previously treated metastatic triple-negative breast cancer: cohort A of the phase II KEYNOTE-086 study. *Ann. Oncol.* 2019;30(3):397–404.
551. Nanda R, Chow LQ, Dees EC, Berger R, Gupta S, Geva R, et al. Pembrolizumab in Patients With Advanced Triple-Negative Breast Cancer: phase Ib KEYNOTE-012 Study. *J. Clin. Oncol.* 2016;34(21):2460–2467.
552. Adams S, Loi S, Toppmeyer D, Cescon DW, De Laurentiis M, Nanda R, et al. Pembrolizumab monotherapy for previously untreated, PD-L1-positive, metastatic triple-negative breast cancer: cohort B of the phase II KEYNOTE-086 study. *Ann. Oncol.* 2019;30(3):405–411.
553. Schmid P, Cortes J, Pusztai L, McArthur H, Kummel S, Bergh J, et al. Pembrolizumab for Early Triple-Negative Breast Cancer. *N. Engl. J. Med.* 2020;382(9):810–821.
554. Schmid P, Salgado R, Park YH, Munoz-Couselo E, Kim SB, Sohn J, et al. Pembrolizumab plus chemotherapy as neoadjuvant treatment of high-risk, early-stage triple-negative breast cancer: results from the phase 1b open-label, multicohort KEYNOTE-173 study. *Ann. Oncol.* 2020;31(5):569–581.
555. Nanda R, Liu MC, Yau C, Shatsky R, Pusztai L, Wallace A, et al. Effect of Pembrolizumab Plus Neoadjuvant Chemotherapy on Pathologic Complete Response in Women With Early-Stage Breast Cancer: an Analysis of the Ongoing Phase 2 Adaptively Randomized I-SPY2 Trial. *JAMA Oncol.* 2020.
556. Loibl S, Untch M, Burchardi N, Huober J, Sinn BV, Blohmer JU, et al. A randomised phase II study investigating durvalumab in addition to an anthracycline taxane-based neoadjuvant therapy in early triple-negative breast cancer: clinical results and biomarker analysis of GeparNuevo study. *Ann. Oncol.* 2019;30(8):1279–1288.
557. Loi S, Giobbie-Hurder A, Gombos A, Bachelot T, Hui R, Curigliano G, et al. Pembrolizumab plus trastuzumab in trastuzumab-resistant, advanced, HER2-positive breast cancer (PANACEA): a single-arm, multicentre, phase 1b-2 trial. *Lancet Oncol.* 2019;20(3):371–382.
558. Luque-Cabal M, Garcia-Teijido P, Fernandez-Perez Y, Sanchez-Lorenzo L, Palacio-Vazquez I. Mechanisms Behind the Resistance to Trastuzumab in HER2-Amplified Breast Cancer and Strategies to Overcome It. *Clin Med Insights Oncol.* 2016;10(Suppl 1):21–30.
559. Schmid P, Rugo HS, Adams S, Schneeweiss A, Barrios CH, Iwata H, et al. Atezolizumab plus nab-paclitaxel as first-line treatment for unresectable, locally advanced or metastatic triple-negative breast cancer (IMpassion130): updated efficacy results from a randomised, double-blind, placebo-controlled, phase 3 trial. *Lancet Oncol.* 2020;21(1):44–59.
560. Vinayak S, Tolaney SM, Schwartzberg L, Mita M, McCann G, Tan AR, et al. Open-Label Clinical Trial of Niraparib Combined With Pembrolizumab for Treatment of Advanced or Metastatic Triple-Negative Breast Cancer. *JAMA Oncol.* 2019.
561. Ho AY, Barker CA, Arnold BB, Powell SN, Hu ZI, Gucalp A, et al. A phase 2 clinical trialassessing theefficacy and safety of pembrolizumab and radiotherapy in patients with metastatic triple-negative breast cancer. *Cancer.* 2020;126(4):850–860.
562. Tchou J, Zhao Y, Levine BL, Zhang PJ, Davis MM, Melenhorst JJ, et al. Safety and Efficacy of Intratumoral Injections of Chimeric Antigen Receptor (CAR) T Cells in Metastatic Breast Cancer. *Cancer Immunol. Res.* 2017;5(12):1152–1161.

563. Corrales L, Glickman LH, McWhirter SM, Kanne DB, Sivick KE, Katibah GE, et al. Direct Activation of STING in the Tumor Microenvironment Leads to Potent and Systemic Tumor Regression and Immunity. *Cell Rep.* 2015;11(7):1018–1030.
564. Nowicki TS, Hu-Lieskovan S, Ribas A. Mechanisms of Resistance to PD-1 and PD-L1 Blockade. *Cancer J.* 2018;24(1):47–53.
565. Cancer Genome Atlas Research N, Analysis Working Group: Asan U, Agency BCC, Brigham, Women's HBroad I, et al. Integrated genomic characterization of oesophageal carcinoma. *Nature.* 2017;541(7636):169–175.
566. Zhang HZ, Jin GF, Shen HB. Epidemiologic differences in esophageal cancer between Asian and Western populations. *Chin. J. Cancer.* 2012;31(6):281–286.
567. Derks S, Nason KS, Liao X, Stachler MD, Liu KX, Liu JB, et al. Epithelial PD-L2 Expression Marks Barrett's Esophagus and Esophageal Adenocarcinoma. *Cancer Immunol. Res.* 2015;3(10):1123–1129.
568. Rong L, Liu Y, Hui Z, Zhao Z, Zhang Y, Wang B, et al. PD-L1 expression and its clinicopathological correlation in advanced esophageal squamous cell carcinoma in a Chinese population. *Diagn Pathol.* 2019;14(1):6.
569. Guo W, Wang P, Li N, Shao F, Zhang H, Yang Z, et al. Prognostic value of PD-L1 in esophageal squamous cell carcinoma: a meta-analysis. *Oncotarget.* 2018;9(17):13920–13933.
570. Chen MF, Kuan FC, Yen TC, Lu MS, Lin PY, Chung YH, et al. IL-6-stimulated CD11b+ CD14+ HLA-DR- myeloid-derived suppressor cells, are associated with progression and poor prognosis in squamous cell carcinoma of the esophagus. *Oncotarget.* 2014;5(18):8716–8728.
571. Chen MF, Chen PT, Lu MS, Lin PY, Chen WC, Lee KD. IL-6 expression predicts treatment response and outcome in squamous cell carcinoma of the esophagus. *Mol. Cancer.* 2013;12:26.
572. Ogura M, Takeuchi H, Kawakubo H, Nishi T, Fukuda K, Nakamura R, et al. Clinical significance of CXCL-8/CXCR-2 network in esophageal squamous cell carcinoma. *Surgery.* 2013;154(3):512–520.
573. Gabitass RF, Annels NE, Stocken DD, Pandha HA, Middleton GW. Elevated myeloid-derived suppressor cells in pancreatic, esophageal and gastric cancer are an independent prognostic factor and are associated with significant elevation of the Th2 cytokine interleukin-13. *Cancer Immunol. Immunother.* 2011;60(10):1419–1430.
574. Zheng X, Song X, Shao Y, Xu B, Hu W, Zhou Q, et al. Prognostic Role of Tumor-Infiltrating Lymphocytes in Esophagus Cancer: a Meta-Analysis. *Cell. Physiol. Biochem.* 2018;45(2):720–732.
575. Hao J, Li M, Zhang T, Yu H, Liu Y, Xue Y, et al. Prognostic Value of Tumor-Infiltrating Lymphocytes Differs Depending on Lymphocyte Subsets in Esophageal Squamous Cell Carcinoma: an Updated Meta-Analysis. *Front. Oncol.* 2020;10:614.
576. Cancer Genome Atlas Research N. Comprehensive molecular characterization of gastric adenocarcinoma. *Nature.* 2014;513(7517):202–209.
577. Zhang M, Dong Y, Liu H, Wang Y, Zhao S, Xuan Q, et al. The clinicopathological and prognostic significance of PD-L1 expression in gastric cancer: a meta-analysis of 10 studies with 1,901 patients. *Sci. Rep.* 2016;6:37933.
578. Cheng G, Li M, Wu J, Ji M, Fang C, Shi H, et al. Expression of Tim-3 in gastric cancer tissue and its relationship with prognosis. *Int J Clin Exp Pathol.* 2015;8(8):9452–9457.
579. Ohmura H, Yamaguchi K, Hanamura F, Ito M, Makiyama A, Uchino K, et al. OX40 and LAG3 are associated with better prognosis in advanced gastric cancer patients treated with anti-programmed death-1 antibody. *Br. J. Cancer.* 2020;122(10):1507–1517.
580. Chang WJ, Du Y, Zhao X, Ma LY, Cao GW. Inflammation-related factors predicting prognosis of gastric cancer. *World J. Gastroenterol.* 2014;20(16):4586–4596.
581. Indio V, Astolfi A, Urbini M, Nannini M, Pantaleo MA. Genetics and treatment of gastrointestinal stromal tumors with immune checkpoint inhibitors: what do we know? *Pharmacogenomics.* 2020;21(4):231–234.
582. Li Y, He M, Zhou Y, Yang C, Wei S, Bian X, et al. The Prognostic and Clinicopathological Roles of PD-L1 Expression in Colorectal Cancer: a Systematic Review and Meta-Analysis. *Front Pharmacol.* 2019;10:139.
583. Pages F, Berger A, Camus M, Sanchez-Cabo F, Costes A, Molidor R, et al. Effector memory T cells, early metastasis, and survival in colorectal cancer. *N. Engl. J. Med.* 2005;353(25):2654–2666.

584. Galon J, Costes A, Sanchez-Cabo F, Kirilovsky A, Mlecnik B, Lagorce-Pages C, et al. Type, density, and location of immune cells within human colorectal tumors predict clinical outcome. *Science.* 2006;313(5795):1960–1964.
585. Giannakis M, Mu XJ, Shukla SA, Qian ZR, Cohen O, Nishihara R, et al. Genomic Correlates of Immune-Cell Infiltrates in Colorectal Carcinoma. *Cell Rep.* 2016;15(4):857–865.
586. Cancer Genome Atlas N. Comprehensive molecular characterization of human colon and rectal cancer. *Nature.* 2012;487(7407):330–337.
587. Llosa NJ, Cruise M, Tam A, Wicks EC, Hechenbleikner EM, Taube JM, et al. The vigorous immune microenvironment of microsatellite instable colon cancer is balanced by multiple counter-inhibitory checkpoints. *Cancer Discov.* 2015;5(1):43–51.
588. Rosenbaum MW, Bledsoe JR, Morales-Oyarvide V, Huynh TG, Mino-Kenudson M. PD-L1 expression in colorectal cancer is associated with microsatellite instability, BRAF mutation, medullary morphology and cytotoxic tumor-infiltrating lymphocytes. *Mod. Pathol.* 2016;29(9):1104–1112.
589. Ringelhan M, Pfister D, O'Connor T, Pikarsky E, Heikenwalder M. The immunology of hepatocellular carcinoma. *Nat. Immunol.* 2018;19(3):222–232.
590. Gao Q, Wang XY, Qiu SJ, Yamato I, Sho M, Nakajima Y, et al. Overexpression of PD-L1 significantly associates with tumor aggressiveness and postoperative recurrence in human hepatocellular carcinoma. *Clin. Cancer Res.* 2009;15(3):971–979.
591. Shi F, Shi M, Zeng Z, Qi RZ, Liu ZW, Zhang JY, et al. PD-1 and PD-L1 upregulation promotes CD8(+) T-cell apoptosis and postoperative recurrence in hepatocellular carcinoma patients. *Int. J. Cancer.* 2011;128(4):887–896.
592. Finn RS, Ryoo BY, Merle P, Kudo M, Bouattour M, Lim HY, et al. Pembrolizumab As Second-Line Therapy in Patients With Advanced Hepatocellular Carcinoma in KEYNOTE-240: a Randomized, Double-Blind, Phase III Trial. *J. Clin. Oncol.* 2020;38(3):193–202.
593. Hoshida Y, Villanueva A, Kobayashi M, Peix J, Chiang DY, Camargo A, et al. Gene expression in fixed tissues and outcome in hepatocellular carcinoma. *N. Engl. J. Med.* 2008;359(19):1995–2004.
594. Cascinu S, Falconi M, Valentini V, Jelic SGroup EGW. Pancreatic cancer: ESMO Clinical Practice Guidelines for diagnosis, treatment and follow-up. *Ann. Oncol.* 2010;21(Suppl 5):v55–v58.
595. Cancer Genome Atlas Research Network. Electronic address aadhe, Cancer Genome Atlas Research N. Integrated Genomic Characterization of Pancreatic Ductal Adenocarcinoma. *Cancer Cell.* 2017;32(2):185–203 e13.
596. Ryan DP, Hong TS, Bardeesy N. Pancreatic adenocarcinoma. *N. Engl. J. Med.* 2014;371(11):1039–1049.
597. Lunardi S, Muschel RJ, Brunner TB. The stromal compartments in pancreatic cancer: are there any therapeutic targets? *Cancer Lett.* 2014;343(2):147–155.
598. Gabrilovich DI. Myeloid-Derived Suppressor Cells. *Cancer Immunol. Res.* 2017;5(1):3–8.
599. Feig C, Jones JO, Kraman M, Wells RJ, Deonarine A, Chan DS, et al. Targeting CXCL12 from FAP-expressing carcinoma-associated fibroblasts synergizes with anti-PD-L1 immunotherapy in pancreatic cancer. *Proc Natl Acad Sci U S A.* 2013;110(50):20212–20217.
600. Karamitopoulou E. Tumour microenvironment of pancreatic cancer: immune landscape is dictated by molecular and histopathological features. *Br. J. Cancer.* 2019;121(1):5–14.
601. Vonderheide RH, Bayne LJ. Inflammatory networks and immune surveillance of pancreatic carcinoma. *Curr. Opin. Immunol.* 2013;25(2):200–205.
602. Beatty GL, Chiorean EG, Fishman MP, Saboury B, Teitelbaum UR, Sun W, et al. CD40 agonists alter tumor stroma and show efficacy against pancreatic carcinoma in mice and humans. *Science.* 2011;331(6024):1612–1616.
603. Winograd R, Byrne KT, Evans RA, Odorizzi PM, Meyer AR, Bajor DL, et al. Induction of T-cell Immunity Overcomes Complete Resistance to PD-1 and CTLA-4 Blockade and Improves Survival in Pancreatic Carcinoma. *Cancer Immunol. Res.* 2015;3(4):399–411.
604. Zhu Y, Knolhoff BL, Meyer MA, Nywening TM, West BL, Luo J, et al. CSF1/CSF1R blockade reprograms tumor-infiltrating macrophages and improves response to T-cell checkpoint immunotherapy in pancreatic cancer models. *Cancer Res.* 2014;74(18):5057–5069.
605. Hu Y, Chen W, Yan Z, Ma J, Zhu F, Huo J. Prognostic value of PD-L1 expression in patients with pancreatic cancer: a PRISMA-compliant meta-analysis. *Medicine (Baltimore).* 2019;98(3):e14006.

606. Kang YK, Boku N, Satoh T, Ryu MH, Chao Y, Kato K, et al. Nivolumab in patients with advanced gastric or gastro-oesophageal junction cancer refractory to, or intolerant of, at least two previous chemotherapy regimens (ONO-4538-12, ATTRACTION-2): a randomised, double-blind, placebo-controlled, phase 3 trial. *Lancet.* 2017;390(10111):2461–2471.
607. Kato K, Cho BC, Takahashi M, Okada M, Lin CY, Chin K, et al. Nivolumab versus chemotherapy in patients with advanced oesophageal squamous cell carcinoma refractory or intolerant to previous chemotherapy (ATTRACTION-3): a multicentre, randomised, open-label, phase 3 trial. *Lancet Oncol.* 2019;20(11):1506–1517.
608. Kojima T, Muro K, Francois E, Hsu C-H, Moriwaki T, Kim S-B, et al. Pembrolizumab versus chemotherapy as second-line therapy for advanced esophageal cancer: phase III KEYNOTE-181 study. *J. Clin. Oncol.* 2019;37(4_suppl):2.
609. Shitara K, Ozguroglu M, Bang YJ, Di Bartolomeo M, Mandala M, Ryu MH, et al. Pembrolizumab versus paclitaxel for previously treated, advanced gastric or gastro-oesophageal junction cancer (KEYNOTE-061): a randomised, open-label, controlled, phase 3 trial. *Lancet.* 2018;392(10142):123–133.
610. Huang J, Xu J, Chen Y, Zhuang W, Zhang Y, Chen Z, et al. Camrelizumab versus investigator's choice of chemotherapy as second-line therapy for advanced or metastatic oesophageal squamous cell carcinoma (ESCORT): a multicentre, randomised, open-label, phase 3 study. *Lancet Oncol.* 2020;21(6):832–842.
611. Kono K, Iinuma H, Akutsu Y, Tanaka H, Hayashi N, Uchikado Y, et al. Multicenter, phase II clinical trial of cancer vaccination for advanced esophageal cancer with three peptides derived from novel cancer-testis antigens. *J. Transl. Med.* 2012;10:141.
612. Chung KY, Gore I, Fong L, Venook A, Beck SB, Dorazio P, et al. Phase II study of the anti-cytotoxic T-lymphocyte-associated antigen 4 monoclonal antibody, tremelimumab, in patients with refractory metastatic colorectal cancer. *J. Clin. Oncol.* 2010;28(21):3485–3490.
613. O'Neil BH, Wallmark JM, Lorente D, Elez E, Raimbourg J, Gomez-Roca C, et al. Safety and antitumor activity of the anti-PD-1 antibody pembrolizumab in patients with advanced colorectal carcinoma. *PLoS ONE.* 2017;12(12):e0189848.
614. Le DT, Uram JN, Wang H, Bartlett BR, Kemberling H, Eyring AD, et al. PD-1 Blockade in Tumors with Mismatch-Repair Deficiency. *N. Engl. J. Med.* 2015;372(26):2509–2520.
615. Le DT, Durham JN, Smith KN, Wang H, Bartlett BR, Aulakh LK, et al. Mismatch repair deficiency predicts response of solid tumors to PD-1 blockade. *Science.* 2017;357(6349):409–413.
616. Overman MJ, McDermott R, Leach JL, Lonardi S, Lenz HJ, Morse MA, et al. Nivolumab in patients with metastatic DNA mismatch repair-deficient or microsatellite instability-high colorectal cancer (CheckMate 142): an open-label, multicentre, phase 2 study. *Lancet Oncol.* 2017;18(9):1182–1191.
617. Lenz H-J, Lonardi S, Zagonel V, Cutsem EV, Limon ML, Wong KYM, et al. Nivolumab plus low-dose ipilimumab as first-line therapy in microsatellite instability-high/DNA mismatch repair deficient metastatic colorectal cancer: clinical update. *J. Clin. Oncol.* 2020;38(4_suppl):11.
618. Kim JH, Kim SY, Baek JY, Cha YJ, Ahn JB, Kim HS, et al. A Phase II Study of Avelumab Monotherapy in Patients with Mismatch Repair-Deficient/Microsatellite Instability-High or POLE-Mutated Metastatic or Unresectable Colorectal Cancer. *Cancer Res. Treat.* 2020.
619. Eng C, Kim TW, Bendell J, Argiles G, Tebbutt NC, Di Bartolomeo M, et al. Atezolizumab with or without cobimetinib versus regorafenib in previously treated metastatic colorectal cancer (IMblaze370): a multicentre, open-label, phase 3, randomised, controlled trial. *Lancet Oncol.* 2019;20(6):849–861.
620. Johnson B, Thomas JV, Dasari A, Raghav KPS, Sanchez EV, Kee BK, et al. A phase II study of durvalumab (MEDI4736) (anti-PD-L1) and trametinib (MEKi) in microsatellite stable (MSS) metastatic colorectal cancer (mCRC). *J. Clin. Oncol.* 2020;38(4_suppl):152.
621. Chen EX, Jonker DJ, Loree JM, Kennecke HF, Berry SR, Couture F, et al. Effect of Combined Immune Checkpoint Inhibition vs Best Supportive Care Alone in Patients With Advanced Colorectal Cancer: the Canadian Cancer Trials Group CO.26 Study. *JAMA Oncol.* 2020.
622. Ghiringhelli F, Chibaudel B, Taieb J, Bennouna J, Martin-Babau J, Fonck M, et al. Durvalumab and tremelimumab in combination with FOLFOX in patients with RAS-mutated, microsatellite-stable, previously untreated metastatic colorectal cancer (MCRC): results of the first intermediate analysis of the phase Ib/II MEDETREME trial. *J. Clin. Oncol.* 2020;38(15_suppl):3006.

623. Stein A, Binder M, Goekkurt E, Lorenzen S, Riera-Knorrenschild J, Depenbusch R, et al. Avelumab and cetuximab in combination with FOLFOX in patients with previously untreated metastatic colorectal cancer (MCRC): final results of the phase II AVETUX trial (AIO-KRK-0216). *J. Clin. Oncol.* 2020;38(4_suppl):96.
624. Segal NH, Saro J, Melero I, Ros W, Argiles G, Marabelle A, et al. Phase I studies of the novel carcinoembryonic antigen T-cell bispecific (CEA-CD3 TCB) antibody as a single agent and in combination with atezolizumab: preliminary efficacy and safety in patients (pts) with metastatic colorectal cancer (mCRC). *Ann. Oncol.* 2017;28:v134.
625. Zhang C, Wang Z, Yang Z, Wang M, Li S, Li Y, et al. Phase I Escalating-Dose Trial of CAR-T Therapy Targeting CEA(+) Metastatic Colorectal Cancers. *Mol. Ther.* 2017;25(5):1248–1258.
626. Parkhurst MR, Yang JC, Langan RC, Dudley ME, Nathan DA, Feldman SA, et al. T cells targeting carcinoembryonic antigen can mediate regression of metastatic colorectal cancer but induce severe transient colitis. *Mol. Ther.* 2011;19(3):620–626.
627. Sangro B, Gomez-Martin C, de la Mata M, Inarrairaegui M, Garralda E, Barrera P, et al. A clinical trial of CTLA-4 blockade with tremelimumab in patients with hepatocellular carcinoma and chronic hepatitis C. *J. Hepatol.* 2013;59(1):81–88.
628. Llovet JM, Ricci S, Mazzaferro V, Hilgard P, Gane E, Blanc JF, et al. Sorafenib in advanced hepatocellular carcinoma. *N. Engl. J. Med.* 2008;359(4):378–390.
629. El-Khoueiry AB, Sangro B, Yau T, Crocenzi TS, Kudo M, Hsu C, et al. Nivolumab in patients with advanced hepatocellular carcinoma (CheckMate 040): an open-label, non-comparative, phase 1/2 dose escalation and expansion trial. *Lancet.* 2017;389(10088):2492–2502.
630. Yau T, Kang Y-K, Kim T-Y, El-Khoueiry AB, Santoro A, Sangro B, et al. Nivolumab (NIVO) + ipilimumab (IPI) combination therapy in patients (pts) with advanced hepatocellular carcinoma (aHCC): results from CheckMate 040. *J. Clin. Oncol.* 2019;37(15_suppl):4012.
631. Yau T, Park JW, Finn RS, Cheng AL, Mathurin P, Edeline J, et al. CheckMate 459: a randomized, multi-center phase III study of nivolumab (NIVO) vs sorafenib (SOR) as first-line (1L) treatment in patients (pts) with advanced hepatocellular carcinoma (aHCC). *Ann. Oncol.* 2019;30:v874–v8v5.
632. Zhu AX, Finn RS, Edeline J, Cattan S, Ogasawara S, Palmer D, et al. Pembrolizumab in patients with advanced hepatocellular carcinoma previously treated with sorafenib (KEYNOTE-224): a non-randomised, open-label phase 2 trial. *Lancet Oncol.* 2018;19(7):940–952.
633. Finn RS, Qin S, Ikeda M, Galle PR, Ducreux M, Kim TY, et al. Atezolizumab plus Bevacizumab in Unresectable Hepatocellular Carcinoma. *N. Engl. J. Med.* 2020;382(20):1894–1905.
634. Qin S, Ren Z, Meng Z, Chen Z, Chai X, Xiong J, et al. Camrelizumab in patients with previously treated advanced hepatocellular carcinoma: a multicentre, open-label, parallel-group, randomised, phase 2 trial. *Lancet Oncol.* 2020;21(4):571–580.
635. Takayama T, Sekine T, Makuuchi M, Yamasaki S, Kosuge T, Yamamoto J, et al. Adoptive immunotherapy to lower postsurgical recurrence rates of hepatocellular carcinoma: a randomised trial. *Lancet.* 2000;356(9232):802–807.
636. Lee JH, Lee JH, Lim YS, Yeon JE, Song TJ, Yu SJ, et al. Adjuvant immunotherapy with autologous cytokine-induced killer cells for hepatocellular carcinoma. *Gastroenterology.* 2015;148(7):1383–1391 e6.
637. Yu X, Zhao H, Liu L, Cao S, Ren B, Zhang N, et al. A randomized phase II study of autologous cytokine-induced killer cells in treatment of hepatocellular carcinoma. *J. Clin. Immunol.* 2014;34(2):194–203.
638. Lee JH, Lee JH, Lim YS, Yeon JE, Song TJ, Yu SJ, et al. Sustained efficacy of adjuvant immunotherapy with cytokine-induced killer cells for hepatocellular carcinoma: an extended 5-year follow-up. *Cancer Immunol. Immunother.* 2019;68(1):23–32.
639. Guo M, Zhang H, Zheng J, Liu Y. Glypican-3: a New Target for Diagnosis and Treatment of Hepatocellular Carcinoma. *J. Cancer.* 2020;11(8):2008–2021.
640. Sawada Y, Yoshikawa T, Ofuji K, Yoshimura M, Tsuchiya N, Takahashi M, et al. Phase II study of the GPC3-derived peptide vaccine as an adjuvant therapy for hepatocellular carcinoma patients. *Oncoimmunology.* 2016;5(5):e1129483.
641. Sawada Y, Yoshikawa T, Nobuoka D, Shirakawa H, Kuronuma T, Motomura Y, et al. Phase I trial of a glypican-3-derived peptide vaccine for advanced hepatocellular carcinoma: immunologic evidence and potential for improving overall survival. *Clin. Cancer Res.* 2012;18(13):3686–3696.

642. Fuchs CS, Doi T, Jang RW, Muro K, Satoh T, Machado M, et al. Safety and Efficacy of Pembrolizumab Monotherapy in Patients With Previously Treated Advanced Gastric and Gastroesophageal Junction Cancer: phase 2 Clinical KEYNOTE-059 Trial. *JAMA Oncol.* 2018;4(5):e180013.
643. Overman MJ, McDermott R, Leach JL, Lonardi S, Lenz H-J, Morse MA, et al. Nivolumab in patients with metastatic DNA mismatch repair-deficient or microsatellite instability-high colorectal cancer (CheckMate 142): an open-label, multicentre, phase 2 study. *Lancet Oncol.* 2017;18(9):1182–1191.
644. Morse MA, Overman MJ, Hartman L, Khoukaz T, Brutcher E, Lenz HJ, et al. Safety of Nivolumab plus Low-Dose Ipilimumab in Previously Treated Microsatellite Instability-High/Mismatch Repair-Deficient Metastatic Colorectal Cancer. *Oncologist.* 2019;24(11):1453–1461.
645. El-Khoueiry AB, Sangro B, Yau T, Crocenzi TS, Kudo M, Hsu C, et al. Nivolumab in patients with advanced hepatocellular carcinoma (CheckMate 040): an open-label, non-comparative, phase 1/2 dose escalation and expansion trial. *Lancet North Am. Ed.* 2017;389(10088):2492–2502.
646. Zhu AX, Finn RS, Edeline J, Cattan S, Ogasawara S, Palmer D, et al. Pembrolizumab in patients with advanced hepatocellular carcinoma previously treated with sorafenib (KEYNOTE-224): a non-randomised, open-label phase 2 trial. *Lancet Oncol.* 2018;19(7):940–952.
647. Royal RE, Levy C, Turner K, Mathur A, Hughes M, Kammula US, et al. Phase 2 Trial of Single Agent Ipilimumab (Anti-CTLA-4) for Locally Advanced or Metastatic Pancreatic Adenocarcinoma. *J. Immunother.* 2010;33(8):828–833.
648. Kamath SD, Kalyan A, Kircher S, Nimeiri H, Fought AJ, Benson 3rd A, et al. Ipilimumab and Gemcitabine for Advanced Pancreatic Cancer: a Phase Ib Study. *Oncologist.* 2020;25(5):e808–ee15.
649. Sharma P, Dirix L, Vos FYFLD, Allison JP, Decoster L, Zaucha R, et al. Efficacy and tolerability of tremelimumab in patients with metastatic pancreatic ductal adenocarcinoma. *J. Clin. Oncol.* 2018;36(4_suppl):470.
650. O'Reilly EM, Oh DY, Dhani N, Renouf DJ, Lee MA, Sun W, et al. Durvalumab With or Without Tremelimumab for Patients With Metastatic Pancreatic Ductal Adenocarcinoma: a Phase 2 Randomized Clinical Trial. *JAMA Oncol.* 2019.
651. Weiss GJ, Blaydorn L, Beck J, Bornemann-Kolatzki K, Urnovitz H, Schutz E, et al. Phase Ib/II study of gemcitabine, nab-paclitaxel, and pembrolizumab in metastatic pancreatic adenocarcinoma. *Invest. New Drugs.* 2018;36(1):96–102.
652. Alexandrov LB, Nik-Zainal S, Wedge DC, Aparicio SA, Behjati S, Biankin AV, et al. Signatures of mutational processes in human cancer. *Nature.* 2013;500(7463):415–421.
653. Yamamoto K, Venida A, Yano J, Biancur DE, Kakiuchi M, Gupta S, et al. Autophagy promotes immune evasion of pancreatic cancer by degrading MHC-I. *Nature.* 2020;581(7806):100–105.
654. Principe DR, Park A, Dorman MJ, Kumar S, Viswakarma N, Rubin J, et al. TGFbeta Blockade Augments PD-1 Inhibition to Promote T-Cell-Mediated Regression of Pancreatic Cancer. *Mol. Cancer Ther.* 2019;18(3):613–620.
655. Janson C, Jung H, Ertl L, Liu S, Dang T, Zeng Y, et al. Abstract 5655: inhibition of CCR2 potentiates checkpoint inhibitor immunotherapy in murine model of pancreatic cancer. *Cancer Res.* 2017;77(13 Supplement):5655.
656. Jiang H, Hegde S, Knolhoff BL, Zhu Y, Herndon JM, Meyer MA, et al. Targeting focal adhesion kinase renders pancreatic cancers responsive to checkpoint immunotherapy. *Nat. Med.* 2016;22(8):851–860.
657. Nakata B, Wang YQ, Yashiro M, Nishioka N, Tanaka H, Ohira M, et al. Prognostic value of microsatellite instability in resectable pancreatic cancer. *Clin. Cancer Res.* 2002;8(8):2536–2540.
658. Marabelle A, Le DT, Ascierto PA, Giacomo AMD, Jesus-Acosta AD, Delord J-P, et al. Efficacy of Pembrolizumab in Patients With Noncolorectal High Microsatellite Instability/Mismatch Repair–Deficient Cancer: results From the Phase II KEYNOTE-158 Study. *J. Clin. Oncol.* 2020;38(1):1–10.
659. Lemery S, Keegan P, Pazdur R. First FDA Approval Agnostic of Cancer Site - When a Biomarker Defines the Indication. *N. Engl. J. Med.* 2017;377(15):1409–1412.
660. Ho WJ, Jaffee EM, Zheng L. The tumour microenvironment in pancreatic cancer — Clinical challenges and opportunities. *Nat. Rev. Clin. Oncol.* 2020.
661. Jaffee EM, Hruban RH, Biedrzycki B, Laheru D, Schepers K, Sauter PR, et al. Novel allogeneic granulocyte-macrophage colony-stimulating factor-secreting tumor vaccine for pancreatic cancer: a phase I trial of safety and immune activation. *J. Clin. Oncol.* 2001;19(1):145–156.

662. Lutz E, Yeo CJ, Lillemoe KD, Biedrzycki B, Kobrin B, Herman J, et al. A lethally irradiated allogeneic granulocyte-macrophage colony stimulating factor-secreting tumor vaccine for pancreatic adenocarcinoma. A Phase II trial of safety, efficacy, and immune activation. *Ann. Surg.* 2011;253(2):328–335.
663. Laheru D, Lutz E, Burke J, Biedrzycki B, Solt S, Onners B, et al. Allogeneic granulocyte macrophage colony-stimulating factor-secreting tumor immunotherapy alone or in sequence with cyclophosphamide for metastatic pancreatic cancer: a pilot study of safety, feasibility, and immune activation. *Clin. Cancer Res.* 2008;14(5):1455–1463.
664. Le DT, Brockstedt DG, Nir-Paz R, Hampl J, Mathur S, Nemunaitis J, et al. A live-attenuated Listeria vaccine (ANZ-100) and a live-attenuated Listeria vaccine expressing mesothelin (CRS-207) for advanced cancers: phase I studies of safety and immune induction. *Clin. Cancer Res.* 2012;18(3):858–868.
665. Le DT, Wang-Gillam A, Picozzi V, Greten TF, Crocenzi T, Springett G, et al. Safety and survival with GVAX pancreas prime and Listeria Monocytogenes-expressing mesothelin (CRS-207) boost vaccines for metastatic pancreatic cancer. *J. Clin. Oncol.* 2015;33(12):1325–1333.
666. Le DT, Picozzi VJ, Ko AH, Wainberg ZA, Kindler H, Wang-Gillam A, et al. Results from a Phase IIb, Randomized, Multicenter Study of GVAX Pancreas and CRS-207 Compared with Chemotherapy in Adults with Previously Treated Metastatic Pancreatic Adenocarcinoma (ECLIPSE Study). *Clin. Cancer Res.* 2019;25(18):5493–5502.
667. Middleton G, Silcocks P, Cox T, Valle J, Wadsley J, Propper D, et al. Gemcitabine and capecitabine with or without telomerase peptide vaccine GV1001 in patients with locally advanced or metastatic pancreatic cancer (TeloVac): an open-label, randomised, phase 3 trial. *Lancet Oncol.* 2014;15(8):829–840.
668. Abou-Alfa GK, Chapman PB, Feilchenfeldt J, Brennan MF, Capanu M, Gansukh B, et al. Targeting mutated K-ras in pancreatic adenocarcinoma using an adjuvant vaccine. *Am. J. Clin. Oncol.* 2011;34(3):321–325.
669. Ho WJ, Jaffee EM, Zheng L. The tumour microenvironment in pancreatic cancer - clinical challenges and opportunities. *Nat. Rev. Clin. Oncol.* 2020.
670. Fagin JA, Wells Jr SA. Biologic and Clinical Perspectives on Thyroid Cancer. *N. Engl. J. Med.* 2016;375(11):1054–1067.
671. American Cancer Society. Cancer Facts & Figs. 2020. 2020 [Available from: https://www.cancer.org/research/cancer-facts-statistics/all-cancer-facts-Figs./cancer-facts-Figs.-2020.html.
672. French JD, Kotnis GR, Said S, Raeburn CD, McIntyre Jr RC, Klopper JP, et al. Programmed death-1+ T cells and regulatory T cells are enriched in tumor-involved lymph nodes and associated with aggressive features in papillary thyroid cancer. *J. Clin. Endocrinol. Metab.* 2012;97(6):E934–E943.
673. Shi RL, Qu N, Luo TX, Xiang J, Liao T, Sun GH, et al. Programmed Death-Ligand 1 Expression in Papillary Thyroid Cancer and Its Correlation with Clinicopathologic Factors and Recurrence. *Thyroid.* 2017;27(4):537–545.
674. Chowdhury S, Veyhl J, Jessa F, Polyakova O, Alenzi A, MacMillan C, et al. Programmed death-ligand 1 overexpression is a prognostic marker for aggressive papillary thyroid cancer and its variants. *Oncotarget.* 2016;7(22):32318–32328.
675. Fadia M, Fookeerah P, Ali S, Shadbolt B, Greenaway T, Perampalam S. PD-L1 expression in papillary thyroid cancer with and without lymphocytic thyroiditis: a cross sectional study. *Pathology (Phila).* 2020;52(3):318–322.
676. Mehnert JM, Varga A, Brose MS, Aggarwal RR, Lin C-C, Prawira A, et al. Safety and antitumor activity of the anti–PD-1 antibody pembrolizumab in patients with advanced, PD-L1–positive papillary or follicular thyroid cancer. *BMC Cancer.* 2019;19(1):196.
677. Prando A, Prando P, Prando D. Urothelial Cancer of the Renal Pelvicaliceal System: unusual Imaging Manifestations. *Radiographics.* 2010;30(6):1553–1566.
678. Warren AY, Harrison D. WHO/ISUP classification, grading and pathological staging of renal cell carcinoma: standards and controversies. *World J. Urol.* 2018;36(12):1913–1926.
679. Schottenfeld D, Fraumeni Jr JF. *Cancer Epidemiology and Prevention*: Oxford University Press; 2006.
680. Capitanio U, Montorsi F. Renal cancer. *Lancet.* 2016;387(10021):894–906.
681. Kamat AM, Hahn NM, Efstathiou JA, Lerner SP, Malmström PU, Choi W, et al. Bladder cancer. *Lancet.* 2016;388(10061):2796–2810.

682. Parkin DM. The global burden of urinary bladder cancer. *Scand. J. Urol. Nephrol. Suppl.* 2008(218):12–20.
683. Smith ND, Prasad SM, Patel AR, Weiner AB, Pariser JJ, Razmaria A, et al. Bladder Cancer Mortality in the United States: a Geographic and Temporal Analysis of Socioeconomic and Environmental Factors. *J. Urol.* 2016;195(2):290–296.
684. Pelucchi C, La Vecchia C. Alcohol, coffee, and bladder cancer risk: a review of epidemiological studies. *Eur. J. Cancer Prev.* 2009;18(1):62–68.
685. Hashim D, Boffetta P. Occupational and environmental exposures and cancers in developing countries. *Ann Glob Health.* 2014;80(5):393–411.
686. Cumberbatch MG, Windsor-Shellard B, Catto JW. The contemporary landscape of occupational bladder cancer within the United Kingdom: a meta-analysis of risks over the last 80 years. *BJU Int.* 2017;119(1):100–109.
687. Purdue MP, Hutchings SJ, Rushton L, Silverman DT. The proportion of cancer attributable to occupational exposures. *Ann. Epidemiol.* 2015;25(3):188–192.
688. Sanli O, Dobruch J, Knowles MA, Burger M, Alemozaffar M, Nielsen ME, et al. Bladder cancer. *Nat. Rev. Dis. Primers.* 2017;3:17022.
689. Babjuk M, Burger M, Compérat E, Gontero P, Mostafid AH, Palou J, et al. EAU Guidelines on Non-muscle-invasive Bladder Cancer (TaT1 and CIS) 2020. *European Association of Urology Guidelines 2020 Edition. Presented At the EAU Annual Congress Amsterdam 2020.* Arnhem, The Netherlands: European Association of Urology Guidelines Office; 2020.
690. Witjes JA, Bruins M, Cathomas R, Compérat E, Cowan NC, Gakis G, et al. *EAU Guidelines on Muscle-invasive and Metastatic Bladder Cancer 2020. European Association of Urology Guidelines 2020 Edition. Presented At the EAU Annual Congress Amsterdam 2020.* Arnhem, The Netherlands: European Association of Urology Guidelines Office; 2020.
691. Chipollini J, da Costa WH, Werneck da Cunha I, de Almeida E Paula F, Guilherme O Salles P, Azizi M, et al. Prognostic value of PD-L1 expression for surgically treated localized renal cell carcinoma: implications for risk stratification and adjuvant therapies. *Ther Adv Urol.* 2019;11:1756287219882600.
692. Flaifel A, Xie W, Braun DA, Ficial M, Bakouny Z, Nassar AH, et al. PD-L1 Expression and Clinical Outcomes to Cabozantinib, Everolimus, and Sunitinib in Patients with Metastatic Renal Cell Carcinoma: analysis of the Randomized Clinical Trials METEOR and CABOSUN. *Clin. Cancer Res.* 2019;25(20):6080.
693. Motzer RJ, Escudier B, McDermott DF, George S, Hammers HJ, Srinivas S, et al. Nivolumab versus Everolimus in Advanced Renal-Cell Carcinoma. *N. Engl. J. Med.* 2015;373(19):1803–1813.
694. Motzer RJ, Rini BI, McDermott DF, Arén Frontera O, Hammers HJ, Carducci MA, et al. Nivolumab plus ipilimumab versus sunitinib in first-line treatment for advanced renal cell carcinoma: extended follow-up of efficacy and safety results from a randomised, controlled, phase 3 trial. *Lancet Oncol.* 2019;20(10):1370–1385.
695. Lu Y, Song Y, Xu Y, Ou N, Liang Z, Hu R, et al. The prevalence and prognostic and clinicopathological value of PD-L1 and PD-L2 in renal cell carcinoma patients: a systematic review and meta-analysis involving 3,389 patients. *Transl Androl Urol.* 2020;9(2):367–381.
696. Şenbabaoğlu Y, Gejman RS, Winer AG, Liu M, Van Allen EM, de Velasco G, et al. Tumor immune microenvironment characterization in clear cell renal cell carcinoma identifies prognostic and immunotherapeutically relevant messenger RNA signatures. *Genome Biol.* 2016;17(1):231.
697. Siska PJ, Beckermann KE, Mason FM, Andrejeva G, Greenplate AR, Sendor AB, et al. Mitochondrial dysregulation and glycolytic insufficiency functionally impair CD8 T cells infiltrating human renal cell carcinoma. *JCI Insight.* 2017;2(12).
698. Kandalaft LE, Motz GT, Busch J, Coukos G. Angiogenesis and the tumor vasculature as antitumor immune modulators: the role of vascular endothelial growth factor and endothelin. *Curr. Top. Microbiol. Immunol.* 2011;344:129–148.
699. Giraldo NA, Becht E, Pagès F, Skliris G, Verkarre V, Vano Y, et al. Orchestration and Prognostic Significance of Immune Checkpoints in the Microenvironment of Primary and Metastatic Renal Cell Cancer. *Clin. Cancer Res.* 2015;21(13):3031–3040.
700. Funakoshi T, Lee CH, Hsieh JJ. A systematic review of predictive and prognostic biomarkers for VEGF-targeted therapy in renal cell carcinoma. *Cancer Treat. Rev.* 2014;40(4):533–547.

701. Turajlic S, Litchfield K, Xu H, Rosenthal R, McGranahan N, Reading JL, et al. Insertion-and-deletion-derived tumour-specific neoantigens and the immunogenic phenotype: a pan-cancer analysis. *Lancet Oncol.* 2017;18(8):1009–1021.
702. Zhang C, Li Z, Qi F, Hu X, Luo J. Exploration of the relationships between tumor mutation burden with immune infiltrates in clear cell renal cell carcinoma. *Ann. Transl. Med.* 2019;7(22):648.
703. Nakanishi J, Wada Y, Matsumoto K, Azuma M, Kikuchi K, Ueda S. Overexpression of B7-H1 (PD-L1) significantly associates with tumor grade and postoperative prognosis in human urothelial cancers. *Cancer Immunol. Immunother.* 2007;56(8):1173–1182.
704. Inman BA, Sebo TJ, Frigola X, Dong H, Bergstralh EJ, Frank I, et al. PD-L1 (B7-H1) expression by urothelial carcinoma of the bladder and BCG-induced granulomata: associations with localized stage progression. *Cancer.* 2007;109(8):1499–1505.
705. Huang Y, Zhang SD, McCrudden C, Chan KW, Lin Y, Kwok HF. The prognostic significance of PD-L1 in bladder cancer. *Oncol. Rep.* 2015;33(6):3075–3084.
706. Wang B, Pan W, Yang M, Yang W, He W, Chen X, et al. Programmed death ligand-1 is associated with tumor infiltrating lymphocytes and poorer survival in urothelial cell carcinoma of the bladder. *Cancer Sci.* 2019;110(2):489–498.
707. Breyer J, Wirtz RM, Otto W, Erben P, Worst TS, Stoehr R, et al. High PDL1 mRNA expression predicts better survival of stage pT1 non-muscle-invasive bladder cancer (NMIBC) patients. *Cancer Immunol. Immunother.* 2018;67(3):403–412.
708. Bellmunt J, Mullane SA, Werner L, Fay AP, Callea M, Leow JJ, et al. Association of PD-L1 expression on tumor-infiltrating mononuclear cells and overall survival in patients with urothelial carcinoma. *Ann. Oncol.* 2015;26(4):812–817.
709. Sweis RF, Spranger S, Bao R, Paner GP, Stadler WM, Steinberg G, et al. Molecular Drivers of the Non-T-cell-Inflamed Tumor Microenvironment in Urothelial Bladder Cancer. *Cancer Immunol. Res.* 2016;4(7):563–568.
710. Horn T, Laus J, Seitz AK, Maurer T, Schmid SC, Wolf P, et al. The prognostic effect of tumour-infiltrating lymphocytic subpopulations in bladder cancer. *World J. Urol.* 2016;34(2):181–187.
711. Parodi A, Traverso P, Kalli F, Conteduca G, Tardito S, Curto M, et al. Residual tumor micro-foci and overwhelming regulatory T lymphocyte infiltration are the causes of bladder cancer recurrence. *Oncotarget.* 2016;7(6):6424–6435.
712. Loskog A, Ninalga C, Paul-Wetterberg G, de la Torre M, Malmström PU, Tötterman TH. Human bladder carcinoma is dominated by T-regulatory cells and Th1 inhibitory cytokines. *J. Urol.* 2007;177(1):353–358.
713. Yang G, Shen W, Zhang Y, Liu M, Zhang L, Liu Q, et al. Accumulation of myeloid-derived suppressor cells (MDSCs) induced by low levels of IL-6 correlates with poor prognosis in bladder cancer. *Oncotarget.* 2017;8(24):38378–38388.
714. Merino DM, McShane LM, Fabrizio D, Funari V, Chen S-J, White JR, et al. Establishing guidelines to harmonize tumor mutational burden (TMB): in silico assessment of variation in TMB quantification across diagnostic platforms: phase I of the Friends of Cancer Research TMB Harmonization Project. *J. Immunother. Cancer.* 2020;8(1):e000147.
715. Lv J, Zhu Y, Ji A, Zhang Q, Liao G. Mining TCGA database for tumor mutation burden and their clinical significance in bladder cancer. *Biosci. Rep.* 2020;40(4):BSR20194337.
716. Motzer RJ, Tannir NM, McDermott DF, Arén Frontera O, Melichar B, Choueiri TK, et al. Nivolumab plus Ipilimumab versus Sunitinib in Advanced Renal-Cell Carcinoma. *N. Engl. J. Med.* 2018;378(14):1277–1290.
717. Motzer RJ, Escudier B, George S, Hammers HJ, Srinivas S, Tykodi SS, et al. Nivolumab versus everolimus in patients with advanced renal cell carcinoma: updated results with long-term follow-up of the randomized, open-label, phase 3 CheckMate 025 trial. *Cancer.* 2020.
718. Motzer RJ, Penkov K, Haanen J, Rini B, Albiges L, Campbell MT, et al. Avelumab plus Axitinib versus Sunitinib for Advanced Renal-Cell Carcinoma. *N. Engl. J. Med.* 2019;380(12):1103–1115.
719. Rini BI, Plimack ER, Stus V, Gafanov R, Hawkins R, Nosov D, et al. Pembrolizumab plus Axitinib versus Sunitinib for Advanced Renal-Cell Carcinoma. *N. Engl. J. Med.* 2019;380(12):1116–1127.
720. Rini BI, Powles T, Atkins MB, Escudier B, McDermott DF, Suarez C, et al. Atezolizumab plus bevacizumab versus sunitinib in patients with previously untreated metastatic renal cell carci-

noma (IMmotion151): a multicentre, open-label, phase 3, randomised controlled trial. *Lancet.* 2019;393(10189):2404–2415.

721. McDermott DF, Choueiri TK, Motzer RJ, Aren OR, George S, Powles T, et al. CheckMate 214 post-hoc analyses of nivolumab plus ipilimumab or sunitinib in IMDC intermediate/poor-risk patients with previously untreated advanced renal cell carcinoma with sarcomatoid features. *J. Clin. Oncol.* 2019;37(15_suppl):4513.
722. McDermott DF, Lee J-L, Ziobro M, Gafanov RA, Matveev VB, Suárez C, et al. First-line pembrolizumab (pembro) monotherapy for advanced non-clear cell renal cell carcinoma (nccRCC): results from KEYNOTE-427 cohort B. *J. Clin. Oncol.* 2019;37(7_suppl):546.
723. Koshkin VS, Barata PC, Zhang T, George DJ, Atkins MB, Kelly WJ, et al. Clinical activity of nivolumab in patients with non-clear cell renal cell carcinoma. *J. Immunother. Cancer.* 2018;6(1):9.
724. Callea M, Albiges L, Gupta M, Cheng SC, Genega EM, Fay AP, et al. Differential Expression of PD-L1 between Primary and Metastatic Sites in Clear-Cell Renal Cell Carcinoma. *Cancer Immunol. Res.* 2015;3(10):1158–1164.
725. Noguchi T, Ward JP, Gubin MM, Arthur CD, Lee SH, Hundal J, et al. Temporally Distinct PD-L1 Expression by Tumor and Host Cells Contributes to Immune Escape. *Cancer Immunol. Res.* 2017;5(2):106–117.
726. McDermott DF, Huseni MA, Atkins MB, Motzer RJ, Rini BI, Escudier B, et al. Clinical activity and molecular correlates of response to atezolizumab alone or in combination with bevacizumab versus sunitinib in renal cell carcinoma. *Nat. Med.* 2018;24(6):749–757.
727. Choueiri TK, Albiges L, Haanen JBAG, Larkin JMG, Uemura M, Pal SK, et al. Biomarker analyses from JAVELIN Renal 101: avelumab + axitinib (A+Ax) versus sunitinib (S) in advanced renal cell carcinoma (aRCC). *J. Clin. Oncol.* 2019;37(15_suppl):101.
728. Rini BI, Plimack ER, Stus V, Gafanov R, Hawkins R, Nosov D, et al. Pembrolizumab plus Axitinib versus Sunitinib for Advanced Renal-Cell Carcinoma. *N. Engl. J. Med.* 2019;380(12):1116–1127.
729. Motzer RJ, Escudier B, McDermott DF, George S, Hammers HJ, Srinivas S, et al. Nivolumab versus Everolimus in Advanced Renal-Cell Carcinoma. *N. Engl. J. Med.* 2015;373(19):1803–1813.
730. Rini BI, Stenzl A, Zdrojowy R, Kogan M, Shkolnik M, Oudard S, et al. IMA901, a multipeptide cancer vaccine, plus sunitinib versus sunitinib alone, as first-line therapy for advanced or metastatic renal cell carcinoma (IMPRINT): a multicentre, open-label, randomised, controlled, phase 3 trial. *Lancet Oncol.* 2016;17(11):1599–1611.
731. Bentebibel SE, Hurwitz ME, Bernatchez C, Haymaker C, Hudgens CW, Kluger HM, et al. A First-in-Human Study and Biomarker Analysis of NKTR-214, a Novel IL2Rβγ-Biased Cytokine, in Patients with Advanced or Metastatic Solid Tumors. *Cancer Discov.* 2019;9(6):711–721.
732. Bristol Myers Squibb and Exelixis Announce Positive Topline Results from Pivotal Phase 3 CheckMate -9ER Trial Evaluating Opdivo® (nivolumab) in Combination with CABOMETYX® (cabozantinib) in Previously Untreated Advanced Renal Cell Carcinoma 2020 [Available from: https://ir.exelixis.com/news-releases/news-release-details/bristol-myers-squibb-and-exelixis-announce-positive-topline.
733. Bellmunt J, de Wit R, Vaughn DJ, Fradet Y, Lee J-L, Fong L, et al. Pembrolizumab as Second-Line Therapy for Advanced Urothelial Carcinoma. *N. Engl. J. Med.* 2017;376(11):1015–1026.
734. Powles T, Durán I, van der Heijden MS, Loriot Y, Vogelzang NJ, De Giorgi U, et al. Atezolizumab versus chemotherapy in patients with platinum-treated locally advanced or metastatic urothelial carcinoma (IMvigor211): a multicentre, open-label, phase 3 randomised controlled trial. *Lancet.* 2018;391(10122):748–757.
735. Galsky MD, Arija JÁ A, Bamias A, Davis ID, De Santis M, Kikuchi E, et al. Atezolizumab with or without chemotherapy in metastatic urothelial cancer (IMvigor130): a multicentre, randomised, placebo-controlled phase 3 trial. *Lancet.* 2020;395(10236):1547–1557.
736. Rosenberg JE, Hoffman-Censits J, Powles T, van der Heijden MS, Balar AV, Necchi A, et al. Atezolizumab in patients with locally advanced and metastatic urothelial carcinoma who have progressed following treatment with platinum-based chemotherapy: a single-arm, multicentre, phase 2 trial. *Lancet.* 2016;387(10031):1909–1920.
737. United States Food and Drug Administration (FDA). FDA limits the use of Tecentriq and Keytruda for some urothelial cancer patients. 2018 [Available from: https://www.fda.gov/drugs/resources-information-approved-drugs/fda-limits-use-tecentriq-and-keytruda-some-urothelial-cancer-patients.

738. Balar AV, Galsky MD, Rosenberg JE, Powles T, Petrylak DP, Bellmunt J, et al. Atezolizumab as first-line treatment in cisplatin-ineligible patients with locally advanced and metastatic urothelial carcinoma: a single-arm, multicentre, phase 2 trial. *Lancet North Am. Ed.* 2017;389(10064):67–76.
739. Kamat AM, Bellmunt J, Galsky MD, Konety BR, Lamm DL, Langham D, et al. Society for Immunotherapy of Cancer consensus statement on immunotherapy for the treatment of bladder carcinoma. *J. Immunother. Cancer.* 2017;5(1):68.
740. Apolo AB, Ellerton JA, Infante JR, Agrawal M, Gordon MS, Aljumaily R, et al. Avelumab treatment for metastatic urothelial carcinoma in the phase Ib JAVELIN Solid Tumor Study: updated safety and efficacy analysis with ≥two years of follow-up. *J. Clin. Oncol.* 2019;37(7_suppl):425.
741. Sharma P, Retz M, Siefker-Radtke A, Baron A, Necchi A, Bedke J, et al. Nivolumab in metastatic urothelial carcinoma after platinum therapy (CheckMate 275): a multicentre, single-arm, phase 2 trial. *Lancet Oncol.* 2017;18(3):312–322.
742. Powles T, O'Donnell PH, Massard C, Arkenau HT, Friedlander TW, Hoimes CJ, et al. Efficacy and Safety of Durvalumab in Locally Advanced or Metastatic Urothelial Carcinoma: updated Results From a Phase 1/2 Open-label Study. *JAMA Oncol.* 2017;3(9):e172411.
743. Balar AV, Castellano D, O'Donnell PH, Grivas P, Vuky J, Powles T, et al. First-line pembrolizumab in cisplatin-ineligible patients with locally advanced and unresectable or metastatic urothelial cancer (KEYNOTE-052): a multicentre, single-arm, phase 2 study. *Lancet Oncol.* 2017;18(11):1483–1492.
744. Balar AV, Kulkarni GS, Uchio EM, Boormans J, Mourey L, Krieger LEM, et al. Keynote 057: phase II trial of Pembrolizumab (pembro) for patients (pts) with high-risk (HR) nonmuscle invasive bladder cancer (NMIBC) unresponsive to bacillus calmette-guérin (BCG). *J. Clin. Oncol.* 2019;37(7_suppl):350.
745. United States Food and Drug Administration (FDA). FDA grants accelerated approval to enfortumab vedotin-ejfv for metastatic urothelial cancer 2019 [Available from: https://www.fda.gov/drugs/resources-information-approved-drugs/fda-grants-accelerated-approval-enfortumab-vedotin-ejfv-metastatic-urothelial-cancer.
746. McLaughlin CC, Wu XC, Jemal A, Martin HJ, Roche LM, Chen VW Incidence of noncutaneous melanomas in the U.S. Cancer. 2005;103(5):1000-7.
747. Schadendorf D, van Akkooi ACJ, Berking C, Griewank KG, Gutzmer R, Hauschild A, et al. Melanoma. *Lancet North Am. Ed.* 2018;392(10151):971–984.
748. Scolyer RA, Long GV, Thompson JF. Evolving concepts in melanoma classification and their relevance to multidisciplinary melanoma patient care. *Mol Oncol.* 2011;5(2):124–136.
749. Hodi FS, O'Day SJ, McDermott DF, Weber RW, Sosman JA, Haanen JB, et al. Improved Survival with Ipilimumab in Patients with Metastatic Melanoma. *N. Engl. J. Med.* 2010;363(8):711–723.
750. Rogers HW, Weinstock MA, Feldman SR, Coldiron BM. Incidence Estimate of Nonmelanoma Skin Cancer (Keratinocyte Carcinomas) in the US Population, 2012. *JAMA Dermatol.* 2015;151(10):1081–1086.
751. Rubin AI, Chen EH, Ratner D. Basal-Cell Carcinoma. *N. Engl. J. Med.* 2005;353(21):2262–2269.
752. Madan V, Lear JT, Szeimies R-M. Non-melanoma skin cancer. *Lancet North Am. Ed.* 2010;375(9715):673–685.
753. Brantsch KD, Meisner C, Schönfisch B, Trilling B, Wehner-Caroli J, Röcken M, et al. Analysis of risk factors determining prognosis of cutaneous squamous-cell carcinoma: a prospective study. *Lancet Oncol.* 2008;9(8):713–720.
754. Cassarino DS, DeRienzo DP, Barr RJ. Cutaneous squamous cell carcinoma: a comprehensive clinicopathologic classification. Part One. *J. Cutan. Pathol.* 2006;33(3):191–206.
755. American Cancer Society. Key Statistics for Merkel Cell Carcinoma 2018. [Available from: https://www.cancer.org/cancer/merkel-cell-skin-cancer/about/key-statistics.html.
756. Kaufman HL, Russell J, Hamid O, Bhatia S, Terheyden P, D'Angelo SP, et al. Avelumab in patients with chemotherapy-refractory metastatic Merkel cell carcinoma: a multicentre, single-group, open-label, phase 2 trial. *Lancet Oncol.* 2016;17(10):1374–1385.
757. Nghiem PT, Bhatia S, Lipson EJ, Kudchadkar RR, Miller NJ, Annamalai L, et al. PD-1 Blockade with Pembrolizumab in Advanced Merkel-Cell Carcinoma. *N. Engl. J. Med.* 2016;374(26):2542–2552.
758. Migden MR, Khushalani NI, Chang ALS, Lewis KD, Schmults CD, Hernandez-Aya L, et al. Cemiplimab in locally advanced cutaneous squamous cell carcinoma: results from an open-label, phase 2, single-arm trial. *Lancet Oncol.* 2020;21(2):294–305.

759. Migden MR, Rischin D, Schmults CD, Guminski A, Hauschild A, Lewis KD, et al. PD-1 Blockade with Cemiplimab in Advanced Cutaneous Squamous-Cell Carcinoma. *N. Engl. J. Med.* 2018;379(4):341–351.
760. Grob JJ, Gonzalez R, Basset-Seguin N, Schachter J, Vornicova O, Bauman JR, et al. KEYNOTE-629: phase 2 study of pembrolizumab for recurrent/metastatic or locally advanced unresectable cutaneous squamous cell carcinoma (cSCC). *J. Clin. Oncol.* 2019;37(15_suppl):TPS9598.
761. Taube JM, Anders RA, Young GD, Xu H, Sharma R, McMiller TL, et al. Colocalization of inflammatory response with B7-h1 expression in human melanocytic lesions supports an adaptive resistance mechanism of immune escape. *Sci. Transl. Med.* 2012;4(127):127ra37.
762. Morrison C, Pabla S, Conroy JM, Nesline MK, Glenn ST, Dressman D, et al. Predicting response to checkpoint inhibitors in melanoma beyond PD-L1 and mutational burden. *J. Immunother. Cancer.* 2018;6(1):32.
763. Madore J, Vilain RE, Menzies AM, Kakavand H, Wilmott JS, Hyman J, et al. PD-L1 expression in melanoma shows marked heterogeneity within and between patients: implications for anti-PD-1/PD-L1 clinical trials. *Pigment Cell Melanoma Res.* 2015;28(3):245–253.
764. Obeid JM, Erdag G, Smolkin ME, Deacon DH, Patterson JW, Chen L, et al. PD-L1, PD-L2 and PD-1 expression in metastatic melanoma: correlation with tumor-infiltrating immune cells and clinical outcome. *Oncoimmunology.* 2016;5(11):e1235107.
765. Spranger S, Bao R, Gajewski TF. Melanoma-intrinsic β-catenin signalling prevents anti-tumour immunity. *Nature.* 2015;523(7559):231–235.
766. Waaler J, Mygland L, Tveita A, Strand MF, Solberg NT, Olsen PA, et al. Tankyrase inhibition sensitizes melanoma to PD-1 immune checkpoint blockade in syngeneic mouse models. *Communications Biology.* 2020;3(1):196.
767. Chen G, Huang AC, Zhang W, Zhang G, Wu M, Xu W, et al. Exosomal PD-L1 contributes to immunosuppression and is associated with anti-PD-1 response. *Nature.* 2018;560(7718):382–386.
768. Ugurel S, Schadendorf D, Horny K, Sucker A, Schramm S, Utikal J, et al. Elevated baseline serum PD-1 or PD-L1 predicts poor outcome of PD-1 inhibition therapy in metastatic melanoma. *Ann. Oncol.* 2020;31(1):144–152.
769. Hemon P, Jean-Louis F, Ramgolam K, Brignone C, Viguier M, Bachelez H, et al. MHC class II engagement by its ligand LAG-3 (CD223) contributes to melanoma resistance to apoptosis. *J. Immunol.* 2011;186(9):5173–5183.
770. Camisaschi C, De Filippo A, Beretta V, Vergani B, Villa A, Vergani E, et al. Alternative activation of human plasmacytoid DCs in vitro and in melanoma lesions: involvement of LAG-3. *J. Invest. Dermatol.* 2014;134(7):1893–1902.
771. Tirosh I, Izar B, Prakadan SM, Wadsworth MH, Treacy D, Trombetta JJ, et al. Dissecting the multicellular ecosystem of metastatic melanoma by single-cell RNA-seq. *Science.* 2016;352(6282):189.
772. Erdag G, Schaefer JT, Smolkin ME, Deacon DH, Shea SM, Dengel LT, et al. Immunotype and Immunohistologic Characteristics of Tumor-Infiltrating Immune Cells Are Associated with Clinical Outcome in Metastatic Melanoma. *Cancer Res.* 2012;72(5):1070.
773. Cancer Genome Atlas N. Genomic Classification of Cutaneous Melanoma. *Cell.* 2015;161(7):1681–1696.
774. Tumeh PC, Harview CL, Yearley JH, Shintaku IP, Taylor EJM, Robert L, et al. PD-1 blockade induces responses by inhibiting adaptive immune resistance. *Nature.* 2014;515(7528):568–571.
775. Alexandrov LB, Nik-Zainal S, Wedge DC, Aparicio SAJR, Behjati S, Biankin AV, et al. Signatures of mutational processes in human cancer. *Nature.* 2013;500(7463):415–421.
776. Zhu B, Tang L, Chen S, Yin C, Peng S, Li X, et al. Targeting the upstream transcriptional activator of PD-L1 as an alternative strategy in melanoma therapy. *Oncogene.* 2018;37(36):4941–4954.
777. Cerezo M, Guemiri R, Druillennec S, Girault I, Malka-Mahieu H, Shen S, et al. Translational control of tumor immune escape via the eIF4F–STAT1–PD-L1 axis in melanoma. *Nat. Med.* 2018;24(12):1877–1886.
778. Eggermont AMM, Chiarion-Sileni V, Grob J-J, Dummer R, Wolchok JD, Schmidt H, et al. Prolonged Survival in Stage III Melanoma with Ipilimumab Adjuvant Therapy. *N. Engl. J. Med.* 2016;375(19):1845–1855.

779. Eggermont AMM, Chiarion-Sileni V, Grob JJ, Dummer R, Wolchok JD, Schmidt H, et al. Ipilimumab versus placebo after complete resection of stage III melanoma: long-term follow-up results the EORTC 18071 double-blind phase 3 randomized trial. *J. Clin. Oncol.* 2019;37(15_suppl):2512.
780. Weber J, Mandala M, Del Vecchio M, Gogas HJ, Arance AM, Cowey CL, et al. Adjuvant Nivolumab versus Ipilimumab in Resected Stage III or IV Melanoma. *N. Engl. J. Med.* 2017;377(19):1824–1835.
781. Eggermont AMM, Blank CU, Mandala M, Long GV, Atkinson V, Dalle S, et al. Adjuvant Pembrolizumab versus Placebo in Resected Stage III Melanoma. *N. Engl. J. Med.* 2018;378(19):1789–1801.
782. Eggermont AM, Blank CU, Mandalà M, Long GV, Atkinson V, Dalle S, et al. Pembrolizumab versus placebo after complete resection of high-risk stage III melanoma: new recurrence-free survival results from the EORTC 1325-MG/Keynote 054 double-blinded phase III trial at three-year median follow-up. *J. Clin. Oncol.* 2020;38(15_suppl):10000.
783. Amaria RN, Reddy SM, Tawbi HA, Davies MA, Ross MI, Glitza IC, et al. Neoadjuvant immune checkpoint blockade in high-risk resectable melanoma. *Nat. Med.* 2018;24(11):1649–1654.
784. Huang AC, Orlowski RJ, Xu X, Mick R, George SM, Yan PK, et al. A single dose of neoadjuvant PD-1 blockade predicts clinical outcomes in resectable melanoma. *Nat. Med.* 2019;25(3):454–461.
785. Robert C, Thomas L, Bondarenko I, O'Day S, Weber J, Garbe C, et al. Ipilimumab plus Dacarbazine for Previously Untreated Metastatic Melanoma. *N. Engl. J. Med.* 2011;364(26):2517–2526.
786. Ascierto PA, Del Vecchio M, Robert C, Mackiewicz A, Chiarion-Sileni V, Arance A, et al. Ipilimumab 10 mg/kg versus ipilimumab 3 mg/kg in patients with unresectable or metastatic melanoma: a randomised, double-blind, multicentre, phase 3 trial. *Lancet Oncol.* 2017;18(5):611–622.
787. Ribas A, Kefford R, Marshall MA, Punt CJ, Haanen JB, Marmol M, et al. Phase III randomized clinical trial comparing tremelimumab with standard-of-care chemotherapy in patients with advanced melanoma. *J. Clin. Oncol.* 2013;31(5):616–622.
788. Robert C, Long GV, Brady B, Dutriaux C, Maio M, Mortier L, et al. Nivolumab in previously untreated melanoma without BRAF mutation. *N. Engl. J. Med.* 2015;372(4):320–330.
789. Weber JS, D'Angelo SP, Minor D, Hodi FS, Gutzmer R, Neyns B, et al. Nivolumab versus chemotherapy in patients with advanced melanoma who progressed after anti-CTLA-4 treatment (CheckMate 037): a randomised, controlled, open-label, phase 3 trial. *Lancet Oncol.* 2015;16(4):375–384.
790. Larkin J, Minor D, D'Angelo S, Neyns B, Smylie M, Miller Jr WH, et al. Overall Survival in Patients With Advanced Melanoma Who Received Nivolumab Versus Investigator's Choice Chemotherapy in CheckMate 037: a Randomized, Controlled, Open-Label Phase III Trial. *J. Clin. Oncol.* 2018;36(4):383–390.
791. Weber JS, Gibney G, Sullivan RJ, Sosman JA, Slingluff Jr CL, Lawrence DP, et al. Sequential administration of nivolumab and ipilimumab with a planned switch in patients with advanced melanoma (CheckMate 064): an open-label, randomised, phase 2 trial. *Lancet Oncol.* 2016;17(7):943–955.
792. Larkin J, Chiarion-Sileni V, Gonzalez R, Grob JJ, Cowey CL, Lao CD, et al. Combined Nivolumab and Ipilimumab or Monotherapy in Untreated Melanoma. *N. Engl. J. Med.* 2015;373(1):23–34.
793. Wolchok JD, Chiarion-Sileni V, Gonzalez R, Rutkowski P, Grob JJ, Cowey CL, et al. Overall Survival with Combined Nivolumab and Ipilimumab in Advanced Melanoma. *N. Engl. J. Med.* 2017;377(14):1345–1356.
794. Postow MA, Chesney J, Pavlick AC, Robert C, Grossmann K, McDermott D, et al. Nivolumab and ipilimumab versus ipilimumab in untreated melanoma. *N. Engl. J. Med.* 2015;372(21):2006–2017.
795. Hodi FS, Chesney J, Pavlick AC, Robert C, Grossmann KF, McDermott DF, et al. Combined nivolumab and ipilimumab versus ipilimumab alone in patients with advanced melanoma: 2-year overall survival outcomes in a multicentre, randomised, controlled, phase 2 trial. *Lancet Oncol.* 2016;17(11):1558–1568.
796. Ribas A, Puzanov I, Dummer R, Schadendorf D, Hamid O, Robert C, et al. Pembrolizumab versus investigator-choice chemotherapy for ipilimumab-refractory melanoma (KEYNOTE-002): a randomised, controlled, phase 2 trial. *Lancet Oncol.* 2015;16(8):908–918.
797. Hamid O, Puzanov I, Dummer R, Schachter J, Daud A, Schadendorf D, et al. Final analysis of a randomised trial comparing pembrolizumab versus investigator-choice chemotherapy for ipilimumab-refractory advanced melanoma. *Eur. J. Cancer.* 2017;86:37–45.

798. Schachter J, Ribas A, Long GV, Arance A, Grob JJ, Mortier L, et al. Pembrolizumab versus ipilimumab for advanced melanoma: final overall survival results of a multicentre, randomised, open-label phase 3 study (KEYNOTE-006). *Lancet*. 2017;390(10105):1853–1862.
799. Robert C, Schachter J, Long GV, Arance A, Grob JJ, Mortier L, et al. Pembrolizumab versus Ipilimumab in Advanced Melanoma. *N. Engl. J. Med.* 2015;372(26):2521–2532.
800. Zimmer L, Livingstone E, Hassel JC, Fluck M, Eigentler T, Loquai C, et al. Adjuvant nivolumab plus ipilimumab or nivolumab monotherapy versus placebo in patients with resected stage IV melanoma with no evidence of disease (IMMUNED): a randomised, double-blind, placebo-controlled, phase 2 trial. *Lancet*. 2020;395(10236):1558–1568.
801. Gutzmer R, Stroyakovskiy D, Gogas H, Robert C, Lewis K, Protsenko S, et al. Atezolizumab, vemurafenib, and cobimetinib as first-line treatment for unresectable advanced BRAF(V600) mutation-positive melanoma (IMspire150): primary analysis of the randomised, double-blind, placebo-controlled, phase 3 trial. *Lancet*. 2020;395(10240):1835–1844.
802. Ribas A, Lawrence D, Atkinson V, Agarwal S, Miller WH, Carlino MS, et al. Combined BRAF and MEK inhibition with PD-1 blockade immunotherapy in BRAF-mutant melanoma. *Nat. Med.* 2019;25(6):936–940.
803. Tawbi HA, Forsyth PA, Algazi A, Hamid O, Hodi FS, Moschos SJ, et al. Combined Nivolumab and Ipilimumab in Melanoma Metastatic to the Brain. *N. Engl. J. Med.* 2018;379(8):722–730.
804. Long GV, Atkinson V, Lo S, Sandhu S, Guminski AD, Brown MP, et al. Combination nivolumab and ipilimumab or nivolumab alone in melanoma brain metastases: a multicentre randomised phase 2 study. *Lancet Oncol.* 2018;19(5):672–681.
805. Liu D, Schilling B, Liu D, Sucker A, Livingstone E, Jerby-Arnon L, et al. Integrative molecular and clinical modeling of clinical outcomes to PD1 blockade in patients with metastatic melanoma. *Nat. Med.* 2019;25(12):1916–1927.
806. Rodig SJ, Gusenleitner D, Jackson DG, Gjini E, Giobbie-Hurder A, Jin C, et al. MHC proteins confer differential sensitivity to CTLA-4 and PD-1 blockade in untreated metastatic melanoma. *Sci. Transl. Med.* 2018;10(450):eaar3342.
807. Schalper KA, Carleton M, Zhou M, Chen T, Feng Y, Huang S-P, et al. Elevated serum interleukin-8 is associated with enhanced intratumor neutrophils and reduced clinical benefit of immune-checkpoint inhibitors. *Nat. Med.* 2020;26(5):688–692.
808. Eggermont AM, Chiarion-Sileni V, Grob JJ, Dummer R, Wolchok JD, Schmidt H, et al. Adjuvant ipilimumab versus placebo after complete resection of high-risk stage III melanoma (EORTC 18071): a randomised, double-blind, phase 3 trial. *Lancet Oncol.* 2015;16(5):522–530.
809. Andtbacka RHI, Kaufman HL, Collichio F, Amatruda T, Senzer N, Chesney J, et al. Talimogene Laherparepvec Improves Durable Response Rate in Patients With Advanced Melanoma. *J. Clin. Oncol.* 2015;33(25):2780–2788.
810. Andtbacka RHI, Ross M, Puzanov I, Milhem M, Collichio F, Delman KA, et al. Patterns of Clinical Response with Talimogene Laherparepvec (T-VEC) in Patients with Melanoma Treated in the OPTiM Phase III Clinical Trial. *Ann. Surg. Oncol.* 2016;23(13):4169–4177.
811. Chesney J, Puzanov I, Collichio F, Singh P, Milhem MM, Glaspy J, et al. Randomized, Open-Label Phase II Study Evaluating the Efficacy and Safety of Talimogene Laherparepvec in Combination With Ipilimumab Versus Ipilimumab Alone in Patients With Advanced, Unresectable Melanoma. *J. Clin. Oncol.* 2018;36(17):1658–1667.
812. Chesney J, Puzanov I, Collichio F, Milhem MM, Hauschild A, Chen L, et al. Patterns of response with talimogene laherparepvec in combination with ipilimumab or ipilimumab alone in metastatic unresectable melanoma. *Br. J. Cancer.* 2019;121(5):417–420.
813. Ives NJ, Suciu S, Eggermont AMM, Kirkwood J, Lorigan P, Markovic SN, et al. Adjuvant interferon-α for the treatment of high-risk melanoma: an individual patient data meta-analysis. *Eur. J. Cancer.* 2017;82:171–183.
814. Tarhini AA, Lee SJ, Hodi FS, Rao UNM, Cohen GI, Hamid O, et al. United States Intergroup E1609: a phase III randomized study of adjuvant ipilimumab (3 or 10 mg/kg) versus high-dose interferon-α2b for resected high-risk melanoma. *J. Clin. Oncol.* 2019;37(15_suppl):9504.

815. Garbe C, Amaral T, Peris K, Hauschild A, Arenberger P, Bastholt L, et al. European consensus-based interdisciplinary guideline for melanoma. Part 2: treatment - Update 2019. *Eur. J. Cancer.* 2020;126:159–177.
816. Bright R, Coventry BJ, Eardley-Harris N, Briggs N. Clinical Response Rates From Interleukin-2 Therapy for Metastatic Melanoma Over 30 Years' Experience: a Meta-Analysis of 3312 Patients. *J. Immunother. (Hagerstown, Md : 1997).* 2017;40(1):21–30.
817. Byers BA, Temple-Oberle CF, Hurdle V, McKinnon JG. Treatment of in-transit melanoma with intra-lesional interleukin-2: a systematic review. *J. Surg. Oncol.* 2014;110(6):770–775.
818. Naing A, Wong DJ, Infante JR, Korn WM, Aljumaily R, Papadopoulos KP, et al. Pegilodecakin combined with pembrolizumab or nivolumab for patients with advanced solid tumours (IVY): a multicentre, multicohort, open-label, phase 1b trial. *Lancet Oncol.* 2019;20(11):1544–1555.
819. Hu Q, Ye X, Qu X, Cui D, Zhang L, Xu Z, et al. Discovery of a novel IL-15 based protein with improved developability and efficacy for cancer immunotherapy. *Sci. Rep.* 2018;8(1):7675.
820. Morton DL, Eilber FR, Holmes EC, Hunt JS, Ketcham AS, Silverstein MJ, et al. BCG immunotherapy of malignant melanoma: summary of a seven-year experience. *Ann. Surg.* 1974;180(4):635–643.
821. Tan JK, Ho VC. Pooled analysis of the efficacy of bacille Calmette-Guerin (BCG) immunotherapy in malignant melanoma. *J. Dermatol. Surg. Oncol.* 1993;19(11):985–990.
822. Vidal D. Topical imiquimod: mechanism of action and clinical applications. *Mini Rev. Med. Chem.* 2006;6(5):499–503.
823. Besser MJ, Shapira-Frommer R, Treves AJ, Zippel D, Itzhaki O, Hershkovitz L, et al. Clinical responses in a phase II study using adoptive transfer of short-term cultured tumor infiltration lymphocytes in metastatic melanoma patients. *Clin. Cancer Res.* 2010;16(9):2646–2655.
824. Andersen R, Donia M, Ellebaek E, Borch TH, Kongsted P, Iversen TZ, et al. Long-Lasting Complete Responses in Patients with Metastatic Melanoma after Adoptive Cell Therapy with Tumor-Infiltrating Lymphocytes and an Attenuated IL2 Regimen. *Clin. Cancer Res.* 2016;22(15):3734–3745.
825. Nguyen LT, Saibil SD, Sotov V, Le MX, Khoja L, Ghazarian D, et al. Phase II clinical trial of adoptive cell therapy for patients with metastatic melanoma with autologous tumor-infiltrating lymphocytes and low-dose interleukin-2. *Cancer Immunol. Immunother.* 2019;68(5):773–785.
826. American Cancer Society. Treatment of Melanoma Skin Cancer, by Stage. 2020 [Available from: https://www.cancer.org/cancer/melanoma-skin-cancer/treating/by-stage.html.
827. Garbe C, Amaral T, Peris K, Hauschild A, Arenberger P, Bastholt L, et al. European consensus-based interdisciplinary guideline for melanoma. Part 1: diagnostics – Update 2019. *Eur. J. Cancer.* 2020;126:141–158.
828. Gershenwald JE, Scolyer RA, Hess KR, Sondak VK, Long GV, Ross MI, et al. Melanoma staging: evidence-based changes in the American Joint Committee on Cancer eighth edition cancer staging manual. *CA Cancer J. Clin.* 2017;67(6):472–492.
829. Chandra RA, Wilhite TJ, Balboni TA, Alexander BM, Spektor A, Ott PA, et al. A systematic evaluation of abscopal responses following radiotherapy in patients with metastatic melanoma treated with ipilimumab. *Oncoimmunology*. 2015;4(11):e1046028.
830. Ott PA, Hu Z, Keskin DB, Shukla SA, Sun J, Bozym DJ, et al. An immunogenic personal neoantigen vaccine for patients with melanoma. *Nature*. 2017;547(7662):217–221.
831. Burningham Z, Hashibe M, Spector L, Schiffman JD. The Epidemiology of Sarcoma. *Clin Sarcoma Res*. 2012;2(1):14.
832. Tawbi HA, Burgess M, Bolejack V, Van Tine BA, Schuetze SM, Hu J, et al. Pembrolizumab in advanced soft-tissue sarcoma and bone sarcoma (SARC028): a multicentre, two-cohort, single-arm, open-label, phase 2 trial. *Lancet Oncol.* 2017;18(11):1493–1501.
833. American Cancer Society. Survival rates for soft tissue sarcoma. 2020 [Available from: https://www.cancer.org/cancer/soft-tissue-sarcoma/detection-diagnosis-staging/survival-rates.html.
834. Orth MF, Buecklein VL, Kampmann E, Subklewe M, Noessner E, Cidre-Aranaz F, et al. A comparative view on the expression patterns of PD-L1 and PD-1 in soft tissue sarcomas. *Cancer Immunology, Immunotherapy.* 2020;69(7):1353–1362.
835. Park HK, Kim M, Sung M, Lee SE, Kim YJ, Choi YL. Status of programmed death-ligand 1 expression in sarcomas. *J. Transl. Med.* 2018;16(1):303.

836. Kim JR, Moon YJ, Kwon KS, Bae JS, Wagle S, Kim KM, et al. Tumor infiltrating PD1-positive lymphocytes and the expression of PD-L1 predict poor prognosis of soft tissue sarcomas. *PLoS ONE*. 2013;8(12):e82870.
837. Bertucci F, Finetti P, Perrot D, Leroux A, Collin F, Le Cesne A, et al. PDL1 expression is a poor-prognosis factor in soft-tissue sarcomas. *Oncoimmunology*. 2017;6(3):e1278100.
838. Kim C, Kim EK, Jung H, Chon HJ, Han JW, Shin K-H, et al. Prognostic implications of PD-L1 expression in patients with soft tissue sarcoma. *BMC Cancer*. 2016;16:434.
839. Comprehensive and Integrated Genomic Characterization of Adult Soft Tissue Sarcomas. *Cell*. 2017;171(4):950–965 e28.
840. Petitprez F, de Reyniès A, Keung EZ, Chen TW-W, Sun C-M, Calderaro J, et al. B cells are associated with survival and immunotherapy response in sarcoma. *Nature*. 2020;577(7791):556–560.
841. Keung EZ, Burgess M, Salazar R, Parra Cuentas E, Rodrigues-Canales J, Bolejack V, et al. Correlative Analyses of the SARC028 Trial Reveal an Association Between Sarcoma-Associated Immune Infiltrate and Response to Pembrolizumab. *Clin. Cancer Res.* 2020 clincanres.1824.2019.
842. Asanuma K, Nakamura T, Hayashi A, Okamoto T, Iino T, Asanuma Y, et al. Soluble programmed death-ligand 1 rather than PD-L1 on tumor cells effectively predicts metastasis and prognosis in soft tissue sarcomas. *Sci. Rep.* 2020;10(1):9077.
843. Zhu Z, Jin Z, Zhang M, Tang Y, Yang G, Yuan X, et al. Prognostic value of programmed death-ligand 1 in sarcoma: a meta-analysis. *Oncotarget*. 2017;8(35):59570–59580.
844. Machado I, López-Guerrero JA, Scotlandi K, Picci P, Llombart-Bosch A. Immunohistochemical analysis and prognostic significance of PD-L1, PD-1, and CD8+ tumor-infiltrating lymphocytes in Ewing's sarcoma family of tumors (ESFT). *Virchows. Arch.* 2018;472(5):815–824.
845. Raj S, Bui M, Gonzales R, Letson D, Antonia SJ. 1421PD - Impact of Pdl1 Expression on Clinical Outcomes in Subtypes of Sarcoma. *Ann. Oncol.* 2014;25:iv498.
846. Berghuis D, de Hooge ASK, Santos SJ, Horst D, Wiertz EJ, van Eggermond MC, et al. Reduced human leukocyte antigen expression in advanced-stage Ewing sarcoma: implications for immune recognition. *J. Pathol.* 2009;218(2):222–231.
847. Fujiwara T, Fukushi J-I, Yamamoto S, Matsumoto Y, Setsu N, Oda Y, et al. Macrophage infiltration predicts a poor prognosis for human ewing sarcoma. *Am. J. Pathol.* 2011;179(3):1157–1170.
848. Kostine M, Cleven AHG, de Miranda NFCC, Italiano A, Cleton-Jansen A-M, Bovée JVMG. Analysis of PD-L1, T-cell infiltrate and HLA expression in chondrosarcoma indicates potential for response to immunotherapy specifically in the dedifferentiated subtype. *Mod. Pathol.* 2016;29(9):1028–1037.
849. Chan JY, Zhang Z, Chew W, Tan GF, Lim CL, Zhou L, et al. Biological significance and prognostic relevance of peripheral blood neutrophil-to-lymphocyte ratio in soft tissue sarcoma. *Sci. Rep.* 2018;8(1):11959.
850. Liu B, Huang Y, Sun Y, Zhang J, Yao Y, Shen Z, et al. Prognostic value of inflammation-based scores in patients with osteosarcoma. *Sci. Rep.* 2016;6:39862.
851. Liu T, Ma Q, Zhang Y, Wang X, Xu K, Yan K, et al. Self-seeding circulating tumor cells promote the proliferation and metastasis of human osteosarcoma by upregulating interleukin-8. *Cell Death. Dis.* 2019;10(8):575.
852. Itoh H, Kadomatsu T, Tanoue H, Yugami M, Miyata K, Endo M, et al. TET2-dependent IL-6 induction mediated by the tumor microenvironment promotes tumor metastasis in osteosarcoma. *Oncogene*. 2018;37(22):2903–2920.
853. Lissat A, Joerschke M, Shinde DA, Braunschweig T, Meier A, Makowska A, et al. IL6 secreted by Ewing sarcoma tumor microenvironment confers anti-apoptotic and cell-disseminating paracrine responses in Ewing sarcoma cells. *BMC Cancer*. 2015;15:552.
854. Mori T, Sato Y, Miyamoto K, Kobayashi T, Shimizu T, Kanagawa H, et al. TNFα promotes osteosarcoma progression by maintaining tumor cells in an undifferentiated state. *Oncogene*. 2014;33(33):4236–4241.
855. Helman LJ, Meltzer P. Mechanisms of sarcoma development. *Nat. Rev. Cancer*. 2003;3(9):685–694.
856. Burgess MA, Bolejack V, Schuetze S, Van Tine BA, Attia S, Riedel RF, et al. Clinical activity of pembrolizumab (P) in undifferentiated pleomorphic sarcoma (UPS) and dedifferentiated/pleomorphic liposarcoma (LPS): final results of SARC028 expansion cohorts. *J. Clin. Oncol.* 2019;37(15_suppl):11015.

857. Ben-Ami E, Barysauskas CM, Solomon S, Tahlil K, Malley R, Hohos M, et al. Immunotherapy with single agent nivolumab for advanced leiomyosarcoma of the uterus: results of a phase 2 study. *Cancer.* 2017;123(17):3285–3290.
858. Maki RG, Jungbluth AA, Gnjatic S, Schwartz GK, D'Adamo DR, Keohan ML, et al. A Pilot Study of Anti-CTLA4 Antibody Ipilimumab in Patients with Synovial Sarcoma. *Sarcoma.* 2013;2013:168145.
859. Paoluzzi L, Cacavio A, Ghesani M, Karambelkar A, Rapkiewicz A, Weber J, et al. Response to anti-PD1 therapy with nivolumab in metastatic sarcomas. *Clin Sarcoma Res.* 2016;6:24.
860. Xie L, Xu J, Sun X, Guo W, Gu J, Liu K, et al. Apatinib plus camrelizumab (anti-PD1 therapy, SHR-1210) for advanced osteosarcoma (APFAO) progressing after chemotherapy: a single-arm, open-label, phase 2 trial. *J. Immunother. Cancer.* 2020;8(1).
861. D'Angelo SP, Mahoney MR, Van Tine BA, Atkins J, Milhem MM, Jahagirdar BN, et al. Nivolumab with or without ipilimumab treatment for metastatic sarcoma (Alliance A091401): two open-label, non-comparative, randomised, phase 2 trials. *Lancet Oncol.* 2018;19(3):416–426.
862. Wilky BA, Trucco MM, Subhawong TK, Florou V, Park W, Kwon D, et al. Axitinib plus pembrolizumab in patients with advanced sarcomas including alveolar soft-part sarcoma: a single-centre, single-arm, phase 2 trial. *Lancet Oncol.* 2019;20(6):837–848.
863. Kelly CM, Antonescu CR, Bowler T, Munhoz R, Chi P, Dickson MA, et al. Objective Response Rate Among Patients With Locally Advanced or Metastatic Sarcoma Treated With Talimogene Laherparepvec in Combination With Pembrolizumab: a Phase 2 Clinical Trial. *JAMA Oncol.* 2020;6(3):402–408.
864. Merchant MS, Bernstein D, Amoako M, Baird K, Fleisher TA, Morre M, et al. Adjuvant Immunotherapy to Improve Outcome in High-Risk Pediatric Sarcomas. *Clin. Cancer Res.* 2016;22(13):3182–3191.
865. Ghisoli M, Barve M, Mennel R, Lenarsky C, Horvath S, Wallraven G, et al. Three-year Follow up of GMCSF/bi-shRNAfurin DNA-transfected Autologous Tumor Immunotherapy (Vigil) in Metastatic Advanced Ewing's Sarcoma. *Mol. Ther.* 2016;24(8):1478–1483.
866. Finkelstein SE, Iclozan C, Bui MM, Cotter MJ, Ramakrishnan R, Ahmed J, et al. Combination of External Beam Radiotherapy (EBRT) With Intratumoral Injection of Dendritic Cells as Neo-Adjuvant Treatment of High-Risk Soft Tissue Sarcoma Patients. *Int. J. Radiat. Oncol. Biol. Phys.* 2012;82(2):924–932.
867. Kawaguchi S, Tsukahara T, Ida K, Kimura S, Murase M, Kano M, et al. SYT-SSX breakpoint peptide vaccines in patients with synovial sarcoma: a study from the Japanese Musculoskeletal Oncology Group. *Cancer Sci.* 2012;103(9):1625–1630.
868. Robbins PF, Morgan RA, Feldman SA, Yang JC, Sherry RM, Dudley ME, et al. Tumor regression in patients with metastatic synovial cell sarcoma and melanoma using genetically engineered lymphocytes reactive with NY-ESO-1. *J. Clin. Oncol.* 2011;29(7):917–924.
869. Robbins PF, Kassim SH, Tran TL, Crystal JS, Morgan RA, Feldman SA, et al. A pilot trial using lymphocytes genetically engineered with an NY-ESO-1-reactive T-cell receptor: long-term follow-up and correlates with response. *Clin. Cancer Res.* 2015;21(5):1019–1027.
870. Frampton JE. Mifamurtide: a review of its use in the treatment of osteosarcoma. *Paediatr. Drugs.* 2010;12(3):141–153.
871. Meyers PA, Schwartz CL, Krailo M, Kleinerman ES, Betcher D, Bernstein ML, et al. Osteosarcoma: a randomized, prospective trial of the addition of ifosfamide and/or muramyl tripeptide to cisplatin, doxorubicin, and high-dose methotrexate. *J. Clin. Oncol.* 2005;23(9):2004–2011.
872. Meyers PA, Schwartz CL, Krailo MD, Healey JH, Bernstein ML, Betcher D, et al. Osteosarcoma: the addition of muramyl tripeptide to chemotherapy improves overall survival–a report from the Children's Oncology Group. *J. Clin. Oncol.* 2008;26(4):633–638.
873. Wilding CP, Elms ML, Judson I, Tan A-C, Jones RL, Huang PH. The landscape of tyrosine kinase inhibitors in sarcomas: looking beyond pazopanib. *Expert Rev. Anticancer Ther.* 2019;19(11):971–991.
874. Attard G, Parker C, Eeles RA, Schröder F, Tomlins SA, Tannock I, et al. Prostate cancer. *The Lancet.* 2016;387(10013):70–82.
875. Hanna NH, Einhorn LH. Testicular Cancer — Discoveries and Updates. *N. Engl. J. Med.* 2014;371(21):2005–2016.
876. Haffner MC, Guner G, Taheri D, Netto GJ, Palsgrove DN, Zheng Q, et al. Comprehensive Evaluation of Programmed Death-Ligand 1 Expression in Primary and Metastatic Prostate Cancer. *Am. J. Pathol.* 2018;188(6):1478–1485.

877. Wu J, Lin G, Zhu Y, Zhang H, Shi G, Shen Y, et al. Low TIM3 expression indicates poor prognosis of metastatic prostate cancer and acts as an independent predictor of castration resistant status. *Sci. Rep.* 2017;7(1):8869.
878. Bou-Dargham MJ, Sha L, Sang Q-XA, Zhang J. Immune landscape of human prostate cancer: immune evasion mechanisms and biomarkers for personalized immunotherapy. *BMC Cancer.* 2020;20(1):572.
879. Keam SP, Halse H, Nguyen T, Wang M, Van Kooten Losio N, Mitchell C, et al. High dose-rate brachytherapy of localized prostate cancer converts tumors from cold to hot. *J. Immunother. Cancer.* 2020;8(1):e000792.
880. Zhang Q, Liu S, Parajuli KR, Zhang W, Zhang K, Mo Z, et al. Interleukin-17 promotes prostate cancer via MMP7-induced epithelial-to-mesenchymal transition. *Oncogene.* 2017;36(5):687–699.
881. Seol MA, Kim J-H, Oh K, Kim G, Seo MW, Shin Y-K, et al. Interleukin-7 Contributes to the Invasiveness of Prostate Cancer Cells by Promoting Epithelial–Mesenchymal Transition. *Sci. Rep.* 2019;9(1):6917.
882. The Molecular Taxonomy of Primary Prostate Cancer. *Cell.* 2015;163(4):1011–1025.
883. Robinson D, Van Allen Eliezer M, Wu Y-M, Schultz N, J L R, Mosquera J-M, et al. Integrative Clinical Genomics of Advanced Prostate Cancer. *Cell.* 2015;161(5):1215–1228.
884. Grasso CS, Wu Y-M, Robinson DR, Cao X, Dhanasekaran SM, Khan AP, et al. The mutational landscape of lethal castration-resistant prostate cancer. *Nature.* 2012;487(7406):239–243.
885. van Dessel LF, van Riet J, Smits M, Zhu Y, Hamberg P, van der Heijden MS, et al. The genomic landscape of metastatic castration-resistant prostate cancers reveals multiple distinct genotypes with potential clinical impact. *Nat. Commun.* 2019;10(1):5251.
886. Kwon ED, Drake CG, Scher HI, Fizazi K, Bossi A, van den Eertwegh AJM, et al. Ipilimumab versus placebo after radiotherapy in patients with metastatic castration-resistant prostate cancer that had progressed after docetaxel chemotherapy (CA184-043): a multicentre, randomised, double-blind, phase 3 trial. *Lancet Oncol.* 2014;15(7):700–712.
887. Beer TM, Kwon ED, Drake CG, Fizazi K, Logothetis C, Gravis G, et al. Randomized, Double-Blind, Phase III Trial of Ipilimumab Versus Placebo in Asymptomatic or Minimally Symptomatic Patients With Metastatic Chemotherapy-Naive Castration-Resistant Prostate Cancer. *J. Clin. Oncol.* 2017;35(1):40–47.
888. Gao J, Ward JF, Pettaway CA, Shi LZ, Subudhi SK, Vence LM, et al. VISTA is an inhibitory immune checkpoint that is increased after ipilimumab therapy in patients with prostate cancer. *Nat. Med.* 2017;23(5):551–555.
889. Antonarakis ES, Piulats JM, Gross-Goupil M, Goh J, Ojamaa K, Hoimes CJ, et al. Pembrolizumab for Treatment-Refractory Metastatic Castration-Resistant Prostate Cancer: multicohort, Open-Label Phase II KEYNOTE-199 Study. *J. Clin. Oncol.* 2019;38(5):395–405.
890. united States Food and Drug Administration. FDA grants accelerated approval to pembrolizumab for first tissue/site agnostic indication 2017 [Available from: https://www.fda.gov/drugs/resources-information-approved-drugs/fda-grants-accelerated-approval-pembrolizumab-first-tissuesite-agnostic-indication.
891. Abida W, Cheng ML, Armenia J, Middha S, Autio KA, Vargas HA, et al. Analysis of the Prevalence of Microsatellite Instability in Prostate Cancer and Response to Immune Checkpoint Blockade. *JAMA Oncol.* 2019;5(4):471–478.
892. Graham LS, Montgomery B, Cheng HH, Yu EY, Nelson PS, Pritchard C, et al. Mismatch repair deficiency in metastatic prostate cancer: response to PD-1 blockade and standard therapies. *PLoS ONE.* 2020;15(5):e0233260.
893. Yu EY, Piulats JM, Gravis G, Laguerre B, Arranz Arija JA, Oudard S, et al. KEYNOTE-365 cohort A updated results: pembrolizumab (pembro) plus olaparib in docetaxel-pretreated patients (pts) with metastatic castration-resistant prostate cancer (mCRPC). *J. Clin. Oncol.* 2020;38(6_suppl):100.
894. Sharma P, Pachynski RK, Narayan V, Flechon A, Gravis G, Galsky MD, et al. Initial results from a phase II study of nivolumab (NIVO) plus ipilimumab (IPI) for the treatment of metastatic castration-resistant prostate cancer (mCRPC; CheckMate 650). *J. Clin. Oncol.* 2019;37(7_suppl):142.
895. Boudadi K, Suzman DL, Anagnostou V, Fu W, Luber B, Wang H, et al. Ipilimumab plus nivolumab and DNA-repair defects in AR-V7-expressing metastatic prostate cancer. *Oncotarget.* 2018;9(47):28561–28571.

896. Bishop JL, Sio A, Angeles A, Roberts ME, Azad AA, Chi KN, et al. PD-L1 is highly expressed in Enzalutamide resistant prostate cancer. *Oncotarget*. 2015;6(1):234–242.
897. Graff JN, Beer TM, Alumkal JJ, Slottke RE, Redmond WL, Thomas GV, et al. A phase II single-arm study of pembrolizumab with enzalutamide in men with metastatic castration-resistant prostate cancer progressing on enzalutamide alone. *J. Immunother. Cancer*. 2020;8(2):e000642.
898. Kantoff PW, Schuetz TJ, Blumenstein BA, Glode LM, Bilhartz DL, Wyand M, et al. Overall survival analysis of a phase II randomized controlled trial of a Poxviral-based PSA-targeted immunotherapy in metastatic castration-resistant prostate cancer. *J. Clin. Oncol.* 2010;28(7):1099–1105.
899. Gulley JL, Borre M, Vogelzang NJ, Ng S, Agarwal N, Parker CC, et al. Phase III Trial of PROSTVAC in Asymptomatic or Minimally Symptomatic Metastatic Castration-Resistant Prostate Cancer. *J. Clin. Oncol.* 2019;37(13):1051–1061.
900. van den Eertwegh AJ, Versluis J, van den Berg HP, Santegoets SJ, van Moorselaar RJ, van der Sluis TM, et al. Combined immunotherapy with granulocyte-macrophage colony-stimulating factor-transduced allogeneic prostate cancer cells and ipilimumab in patients with metastatic castration-resistant prostate cancer: a phase 1 dose-escalation trial. *Lancet Oncol.* 2012;13(5):509–517.
901. Cappuccini F, Bryant R, Pollock E, Carter L, Verrill C, Hollidge J, et al. Safety and immunogenicity of novel 5T4 viral vectored vaccination regimens in early stage prostate cancer: a phase I clinical trial. *J. Immunother. Cancer*. 2020;8(1).
902. Kantoff PW, Higano CS, Shore ND, Berger ER, Small EJ, Penson DF, et al. Sipuleucel-T Immunotherapy for Castration-Resistant Prostate Cancer. *N. Engl. J. Med.* 2010;363(5):411–422.
903. Huber ML, Haynes L, Parker C, Iversen P. Interdisciplinary critique of sipuleucel-T as immunotherapy in castration-resistant prostate cancer. *J. Natl. Cancer Inst.* 2012;104(4):273–279.
904. United States Food and Drug Administration. PROVENGE (sipuleucel-T) 2019 [Available from: https://www.fda.gov/vaccines-blood-biologics/cellular-gene-therapy-products/provenge-sipuleucel-t.
905. Zschäbitz S, Lasitschka F, Hadaschik B, Hofheinz R-D, Jentsch-Ullrich K, Grüner M, et al. Response to anti-programmed cell death protein-1 antibodies in men treated for platinum refractory germ cell cancer relapsed after high-dose chemotherapy and stem cell transplantation. *Eur. J. Cancer*. 2017;76:1–7.
906. Shah S, Ward JE, Bao R, Hall CR, Brockstein BE, Luke JJ. Clinical Response of a Patient to Anti-PD-1 Immunotherapy and the Immune Landscape of Testicular Germ Cell Tumors. *Cancer Immunol. Res.* 2016;4(11):903–909.
907. Adra N, Einhorn LH, Althouse SK, Ammakkanavar NR, Musapatika D, Albany C, et al. Phase II trial of pembrolizumab in patients with platinum refractory germ-cell tumors: a Hoosier Cancer Research Network Study GU14-206. *Ann. Oncol.* 2018;29(1):209–214.
908. Necchi A, Giannatempo P, Raggi D, Mariani L, Colecchia M, Farè E, et al. An Open-label Randomized Phase 2 study of Durvalumab Alone or in Combination with Tremelimumab in Patients with Advanced Germ Cell Tumors (APACHE): results from the First Planned Interim Analysis. *Eur. Urol.* 2019;75(1):201–203.
909. Webb JR, Milne K, Kroeger DR, Nelson BH. PD-L1 expression is associated with tumor-infiltrating T cells and favorable prognosis in high-grade serous ovarian cancer. *Gynecol. Oncol.* 2016;141(2):293–302.
910. Wang L. Prognostic effect of programmed death-ligand 1 (PD-L1) in ovarian cancer: a systematic review, meta-analysis and bioinformatics study. *J Ovarian Res*. 2019;12(1):37.
911. Zhang L, Conejo-Garcia JR, Katsaros D, Gimotty PA, Massobrio M, Regnani G, et al. Intratumoral T Cells, Recurrence, and Survival in Epithelial Ovarian Cancer. *N. Engl. J. Med.* 2003;348(3):203–213.
912. Sato E, Olson SH, Ahn J, Bundy B, Nishikawa H, Qian F, et al. Intraepithelial CD8+ tumor-infiltrating lymphocytes and a high CD8+/regulatory T cell ratio are associated with favorable prognosis in ovarian cancer. *Proc Natl Acad Sci U S A*. 2005;102(51):18538–18543.
913. Yeku OO, Purdon TJ, Koneru M, Spriggs D, Brentjens RJ. Armored CAR T cells enhance antitumor efficacy and overcome the tumor microenvironment. *Sci. Rep.* 2017;7(1):10541.
914. Gu X, Dong M, Liu Z, Mi Y, Yang J, Zhang Z, et al. Elevated PD-L1 expression predicts poor survival outcomes in patients with cervical cancer. *Cancer Cell Int*. 2019;19(1):146.
915. Burk RD, Chen Z, Saller C, Tarvin K, Carvalho AL, Scapulatempo-Neto C, et al. Integrated genomic and molecular characterization of cervical cancer. *Nature*. 2017;543(7645):378–384.
916. Brahmer JR, Tykodi SS, Chow LQM, Hwu W-J, Topalian SL, Hwu P, et al. Safety and Activity of Anti–PD-L1 Antibody in Patients with Advanced Cancer. *N. Engl. J. Med.* 2012;366(26):2455–2465.

917. Matulonis UA, Shapira-Frommer R, Santin AD, Lisyanskaya AS, Pignata S, Vergote I, et al. Antitumor activity and safety of pembrolizumab in patients with advanced recurrent ovarian cancer: results from the phase II KEYNOTE-100 study. *Ann. Oncol.* 2019;30(7):1080–1087.
918. Marabelle A, Le DT, Ascierto PA, Di Giacomo AM, De Jesus-Acosta A, Delord J-P, et al. Efficacy of Pembrolizumab in Patients With Noncolorectal High Microsatellite Instability/Mismatch Repair–Deficient Cancer: results From the Phase II KEYNOTE-158 Study. *J. Clin. Oncol.* 2019;38(1):1–10.
919. Disis ML, Taylor MH, Kelly K, Beck JT, Gordon M, Moore KM, et al. Efficacy and Safety of Avelumab for Patients With Recurrent or Refractory Ovarian Cancer: phase 1b Results From the JAVELIN Solid Tumor Trial. *JAMA Oncol.* 2019;5(3):393–401.
920. Drew Y, de Jonge M, Hong SH, Park YH, Wolfer A, Brown J, et al. An open-label, phase II basket study of olaparib and durvalumab (MEDIOLA): results in germline <em>BRCA</em>-mutated (<em>gBRCA</em>m) platinum-sensitive relapsed (PSR) ovarian cancer (OC). *Gynecol. Oncol.* 2018;149:246–247.
921. Konstantinopoulos PA, Waggoner S, Vidal GA, Mita M, Moroney JW, Holloway R, et al. Single-Arm Phases 1 and 2 Trial of Niraparib in Combination With Pembrolizumab in Patients With Recurrent Platinum-Resistant Ovarian Carcinoma. *JAMA Oncol.* 2019;5(8):1141–1149.
922. Liu JF, Herold C, Gray KP, Penson RT, Horowitz N, Konstantinopoulos PA, et al. Assessment of Combined Nivolumab and Bevacizumab in Relapsed Ovarian Cancer: a Phase 2 Clinical Trial. *JAMA Oncol.* 2019;5(12):1731–1738.
923. Zamarin D, Burger RA, Sill MW, Powell DJ, Lankes HA, Feldman MD, et al. Randomized Phase II Trial of Nivolumab Versus Nivolumab and Ipilimumab for Recurrent or Persistent Ovarian Cancer: an NRG Oncology Study. *J. Clin. Oncol.* 2020;38(16):1814–1823.
924. Zamarin D, Walderich S, Holland A, Zhou Q, Iasonos AE, Torrisi JM, et al. Safety, immunogenicity, and clinical efficacy of durvalumab in combination with folate receptor alpha vaccine TPIV200 in patients with advanced ovarian cancer: a phase II trial. *J. Immunother. Cancer.* 2020;8(1).
925. Tanyi JL, Haas AR, Beatty GL, Stashwick CJ, O'Hara MH, Morgan MA, et al. Anti-mesothelin chimeric antigen receptor T cells in patients with epithelial ovarian cancer. *J. Clin. Oncol.* 2016;34(15_suppl):5511.
926. Koneru M, Purdon TJ, Spriggs D, Koneru S, Brentjens RJ. IL-12 secreting tumor-targeted chimeric antigen receptor T cells eradicate ovarian tumors in vivo. *Oncoimmunology.* 2015;4(3):e994446.
927. Lheureux S, Butler MO, Clarke B, Cristea MC, Martin LP, Tonkin K, et al. Association of Ipilimumab With Safety and Antitumor Activity in Women With Metastatic or Recurrent Human Papillomavirus–Related Cervical Carcinoma. *JAMA Oncol.* 2018;4(7):e173776.
928. Chung HC, Ros W, Delord J-P, Perets R, Italiano A, Shapira-Frommer R, et al. Efficacy and Safety of Pembrolizumab in Previously Treated Advanced Cervical Cancer: results From the Phase II KEYNOTE-158 Study. *J. Clin. Oncol.* 2019;37(17):1470–1478.
929. United States Food and Drug Administration. FDA approves pembrolizumab for advanced cervical cancer with disease progression during or after chemotherapy. 2018 [Available from: https://www.fda.gov/drugs/resources-information-approved-drugs/fda-approves-pembrolizumab-advanced-cervical-cancer-disease-progression-during-or-after-chemotherapy.
930. Naumann RW, Hollebecque A, Meyer T, Devlin M-J, Oaknin A, Kerger J, et al. Safety and Efficacy of Nivolumab Monotherapy in Recurrent or Metastatic Cervical, Vaginal, or Vulvar Carcinoma: results From the Phase I/II CheckMate 358 Trial. *J. Clin. Oncol.* 2019;37(31):2825–2834.
931. Maciag PC, Radulovic S, Rothman J. The first clinical use of a live-attenuated Listeria monocytogenes vaccine: a Phase I safety study of Lm-LLO-E7 in patients with advanced carcinoma of the cervix. *Vaccine.* 2009;27(30):3975–3983.
932. Basu P, Mehta A, Jain M, Gupta S, Nagarkar RV, John S, et al. A Randomized Phase 2 Study of ADXS11-001 Listeria monocytogenes-Listeriolysin O Immunotherapy With or Without Cisplatin in Treatment of Advanced Cervical Cancer. *Int. J. Gynecol. Cancer.* 2018;28(4):764–772.
933. Stevanović S, Helman SR, Wunderlich JR, Langhan MM, Doran SL, Kwong MLM, et al. A Phase II Study of Tumor-infiltrating Lymphocyte Therapy for Human Papillomavirus-associated Epithelial Cancers. *Clin. Cancer Res.* 2019;25(5):1486–1493.
934. Smyth MJ, Ngiow SF, Ribas A, Teng MW. Combination cancer immunotherapies tailored to the tumour microenvironment. *Nat. Rev. Clin. Oncol.* 2016;13(3):143.

935. Wargo JA, Reuben A, Cooper ZA, Oh KS, Sullivan RJ. Immune effects of chemotherapy, radiation, and targeted therapy and opportunities for combination with immunotherapy. *Semin. Oncol.* 2015 Elsevier.
936. Aguilera TA, Elghonaimy E, Shehade H, Rafat M, Castellini L, Jiang D, et al. Induced tumor heterogeneity reveals factors informing radiation and immunotherapy combinations. *Clin. Cancer Res.* 2020.
937. Jiang M-J, Gu D-N, Dai J-J, Huang Q, Tian L. Dark Side of Cytotoxic Therapy: chemoradiation-Induced Cell Death and Tumor Repopulation. *Trends Cancer.* 2020.
938. Hanoteau A, Newton JM, Krupar R, Huang C, Liu H-C, Gaspero A, et al. Tumor microenvironment modulation enhances immunologic benefit of chemoradiotherapy. *J. Immunother. Cancer.* 2019;7(1):1–19.
939. Derer A, Frey B, Fietkau R, Gaipl US. Immune-modulating properties of ionizing radiation: rationale for the treatment of cancer by combination radiotherapy and immune checkpoint inhibitors. *Cancer Immunology, Immunotherapy.* 2016;65(7):779–786.
940. Xu J, Luo Y, Yuan C, Han L, Wu Q, Xu L, et al. Downregulation of Nitric Oxide Collaborated with Radiotherapy to Promote Anti-Tumor Immune Response via Inducing CD8+ T Cell Infiltration. *Int J Biol Sci.* 2020;16(9):1563.
941. Takeshima T, Chamoto K, Wakita D, Ohkuri T, Togashi Y, Shirato H, et al. Local radiation therapy inhibits tumor growth through the generation of tumor-specific CTL: its potentiation by combination with Th1 cell therapy. *Cancer Res.* 2010;70(7):2697–2706.
942. Song CK, Han HD, Noh KH, Kang TH, Park YS, Kim JH, et al. Chemotherapy enhances CD8+ T cell-mediated antitumor immunity induced by vaccination with vaccinia virus. *Mol. Ther.* 2007;15(8):1558–1563.
943. Lorenzi S, Mattei F, Sistigu A, Bracci L, Spadaro F, Sanchez M, et al. Type I IFNs control antigen retention and survival of CD8α+ dendritic cells after uptake of tumor apoptotic cells leading to cross-priming. *J. Immunol.* 2011;186(9):5142–5150.
944. Schiavoni G, Sistigu A, Valentini M, Mattei F, Sestili P, Spadaro F, et al. Cyclophosphamide synergizes with type I interferons through systemic dendritic cell reactivation and induction of immunogenic tumor apoptosis. *Cancer Res.* 2011;71(3):768–778.
945. Qi S, Li H, Lu L, Qi Z, Liu L, Chen L, et al. Long-term intravital imaging of the multicolor-coded tumor microenvironment during combination immunotherapy. *Elife.* 2016;5:e14756.
946. Roses RE, Datta J, Czerniecki BJ. Radiation as immunomodulator: implications for dendritic cell-based immunotherapy. *Radiat. Res.* 2014;182(2):211–218.
947. Dovedi SJ, Melis MH, Wilkinson RW, Adlard AL, Stratford IJ, Honeychurch J, et al. Systemic delivery of a TLR7 agonist in combination with radiation primes durable antitumor immune responses in mouse models of lymphoma. *Blood, The Journal of the American Society of Hematology.* 2013;121(2):251–259.
948. Jang B-S, Kim IA A Radiosensitivity Gene Signature and PD-L1 Predict Clinical Outcome of Patients with Invasive Breast Carcinoma in The Cancer Genome Atlas (TCGA) Dataset.
949. Nesseler JP, Lee M-H, Nguyen C, Kalbasi A, Sayre JW, Romero T, et al. Tumor Size Matters—Understanding Concomitant Tumor Immunity in the Context of Hypofractionated Radiotherapy with Immunotherapy. *Cancers (Basel).* 2020;12(3):714.
950. Robert C, Thomas L, Bondarenko I, O'Day S, Weber J, Garbe C, et al. Ipilimumab plus dacarbazine for previously untreated metastatic melanoma. *N. Engl. J. Med.* 2011;364(26):2517–2526.
951. Jure-Kunkel M, Masters G, Girit E, Dito G, Lee F, Hunt JT, et al. Synergy between chemotherapeutic agents and CTLA-4 blockade in preclinical tumor models. *Cancer Immunology, Immunotherapy.* 2013;62(9):1533–1545.
952. Lynch TJ, Bondarenko I, Luft A, Serwatowski P, Barlesi F, Chacko R, et al. Ipilimumab in combination with paclitaxel and carboplatin as first-line treatment in stage IIIB/IV non–small-cell lung cancer: results from a randomized, double-blind, multicenter phase II study. *J. Clin. Oncol.* 2012;30(17):2046–2054.
953. Demaria S, Kawashima N, Yang AM, Devitt ML, Babb JS, Allison JP, et al. Immune-mediated inhibition of metastases after treatment with local radiation and CTLA-4 blockade in a mouse model of breast cancer. *Clin. Cancer Res.* 2005;11(2):728–734.
954. Twyman-Saint Victor C, Rech AJ, Maity A, Rengan R, Pauken KE, Stelekati E, et al. Radiation and dual checkpoint blockade activate non-redundant immune mechanisms in cancer. *Nature.* 2015;520(7547):373–377.

955. Page DB, Bear H, Prabhakaran S, Gatti-Mays ME, Thomas A, Cobain E, et al. Two may be better than one: PD-1/PD-L1 blockade combination approaches in metastatic breast cancer. *NPJ breast cancer.* 2019;5(1):1–9.
956. Dewan MZ, Galloway AE, Kawashima N, Dewyngaert JK, Babb JS, Formenti SC, et al. Fractionated but not single-dose radiotherapy induces an immune-mediated abscopal effect when combined with anti–CTLA-4 antibody. *Clin. Cancer Res.* 2009;15(17):5379–5388.
957. Wang W, Kryczek I, Dostál L, Lin H, Tan L, Zhao L, et al. Effector T cells abrogate stroma-mediated chemoresistance in ovarian cancer. *Cell.* 2016;165(5):1092–1105.
958. Liang H, Deng L, Hou Y, Meng X, Huang X, Rao E, et al. Host STING-dependent MDSC mobilization drives extrinsic radiation resistance. *Nat. Commun.* 2017;8(1):1–10.
959. DeNardo DG, Brennan DJ, Rexhepaj E, Ruffell B, Shiao SL, Madden SF, et al. Leukocyte complexity predicts breast cancer survival and functionally regulates response to chemotherapy. *Cancer Discov.* 2011;1(1):54–67.
960. Zeng Z, Xi Shi Y, Samudio IJ, Wang R-Y, Ling X, Frolova O, et al. Targeting the leukemia microenvironment by CXCR4 inhibition overcomes resistance to kinase inhibitors and chemotherapy in AML. *Blood, The Journal of the American Society of Hematology.* 2009;113(24):6215–6224.
961. Gonzalez-Aparicio M, Alzuguren P, Mauleon I, Medina-Echeverz J, Hervas-Stubbs S, Mancheno U, et al. Oxaliplatin in combination with liver-specific expression of interleukin 12 reduces the immunosuppressive microenvironment of tumours and eradicates metastatic colorectal cancer in mice. *Gut.* 2011;60(3):341–349.
962. Deng C, Zhang Q, Jia M, Zhao J, Sun X, Gong T, et al. Tumors and Their Microenvironment Dual-Targeting Chemotherapy with Local Immune Adjuvant Therapy for Effective Antitumor Immunity against Breast Cancer. *Advanced Science.* 2019;6(6):1801868.
963. Affara NI, Ruffell B, Medler TR, Gunderson AJ, Johansson M, Bornstein S, et al. B cells regulate macrophage phenotype and response to chemotherapy in squamous carcinomas. *Cancer Cell.* 2014;25(6):809–821.
964. Panigrahy D, Gartung A, Yang J, Yang H, Gilligan MM, Sulciner ML, et al. Preoperative stimulation of resolution and inflammation blockade eradicates micrometastases. *J. Clin. Invest.* 2019;129(7).
965. Khairallah AS, Genestie C, Auguste A, Leary A. Impact of neoadjuvant chemotherapy on the immune microenvironment in advanced epithelial ovarian cancer: prognostic and therapeutic implications. *Int. J. Cancer.* 2018;143(1):8–15.
966. Ding Z-C, Lu X, Yu M, Lemos H, Huang L, Chandler P, et al. Immunosuppressive myeloid cells induced by chemotherapy attenuate antitumor CD4+ T-cell responses through the PD-1–PD-L1 axis. *Cancer Res.* 2014;74(13):3441–3453.
967. Perelmuter VM, Tashireva LA, Savelieva OE, Denisov EV, Kaigorodova EV, Zavyalova MV, et al. Mechanisms behind prometastatic changes induced by neoadjuvant chemotherapy in the breast cancer microenvironment. *Breast Cancer: Targets and Therapy.* 2019;11:209.
968. Ma Y, Adjemian S, Mattarollo SR, Yamazaki T, Aymeric L, Yang H, et al. Anticancer chemotherapy-induced intratumoral recruitment and differentiation of antigen-presenting cells. *Immunity.* 2013;38(4):729–741.
969. Kang TH, Mao C-P, Lee SY, Chen A, Lee J-H, Kim TW, et al. Chemotherapy acts as an adjuvant to convert the tumor microenvironment into a highly permissive state for vaccination-induced antitumor immunity. *Cancer Res.* 2013;73(8):2493–2504.
970. Wu C, Tan X, Hu X, Zhou M, Yan J, Ding C. Tumor Microenvironment following Gemcitabine Treatment Favors Differentiation of Immunosuppressive Ly6Chigh Myeloid Cells. *J. Immunol.* 2020;204(1):212–223.
971. Ocadlikova D, Lecciso M, Isidori A, Loscocco F, Visani G, Amadori S, et al. Chemotherapy-induced tumor cell death at the crossroads between immunogenicity and immunotolerance: focus on acute myeloid leukemia. *Front. Oncol.* 2019;9:1004.
972. Krysko DV, Garg AD, Kaczmarek A, Krysko O, Agostinis P, Vandenabeele P. Immunogenic cell death and DAMPs in cancer therapy. *Nat. Rev. Cancer.* 2012;12(12):860–875.
973. Larionova I, Cherdyntseva N, Liu T, Patysheva M, Rakina M, Kzhyshkowska J. Interaction of tumor-associated macrophages and cancer chemotherapy. *Oncoimmunology.* 2019;8(7):1596004.
974. Galluzzi L, Buque A, Kepp O, Zitvogel L, Kroemer G. Immunological effects of conventional chemotherapy and targeted anticancer agents. *Cancer Cell.* 2015;28(6):690–714.

975. Bracci L, Schiavoni G, Sistigu A, Belardelli F. Immune-based mechanisms of cytotoxic chemotherapy: implications for the design of novel and rationale-based combined treatments against cancer. *Cell Death & Differentiation*. 2014;21(1):15–25.
976. Fucikova J, Kralikova P, Fialova A, Brtnicky T, Rob L, Bartunkova J, et al. Human tumor cells killed by anthracyclines induce a tumor-specific immune response. *Cancer Res*. 2011;71(14):4821–4833.
977. Casares N, Pequignot MO, Tesniere A, Ghiringhelli F, Roux S, Chaput N, et al. Caspase-dependent immunogenicity of doxorubicin-induced tumor cell death. *J. Exp. Med*. 2005;202(12):1691–1701.
978. Zitvogel L, Apetoh L, Ghiringhelli F, Kroemer G. Immunological aspects of cancer chemotherapy. *Nat. Rev. Immunol*. 2008;8(1):59–73.
979. Obeid M, Tesniere A, Ghiringhelli F, Fimia G, Apetoh L, Perfettini J, et al. Calreticulin exposure dictates the immunogenicity of cancer cell death. *Nat. Med*. 2007;13:54–61.
980. Pfannenstiel LW, Lam SS, Emens LA, Jaffee EM, Armstrong TD. Paclitaxel enhances early dendritic cell maturation and function through TLR4 signaling in mice. *Cell. Immunol*. 2010;263(1):79–87.
981. McDonnell AM, Lesterhuis WJ, Khong A, Nowak AK, Lake RA, Currie AJ, et al. Tumor-infiltrating dendritic cells exhibit defective cross-presentation of tumor antigens, but is reversed by chemotherapy. *Eur. J. Immunol*. 2015;45(1):49–59.
982. Boissonnas A, Licata F, Poupel L, Jacquelin S, Fetler L, Krumeich S, et al. CD8+ tumor-infiltrating T cells are trapped in the tumor-dendritic cell network. *Neoplasia (New York, NY)*. 2013;15(1):85.
983. Liu W, Fowler D, Smith P, Dalgleish A. Pre-treatment with chemotherapy can enhance the antigenicity and immunogenicity of tumours by promoting adaptive immune responses. *Br. J. Cancer*. 2010;102(1):115–123.
984. Peng J, Hamanishi J, Matsumura N, Abiko K, Murat K, Baba T, et al. Chemotherapy induces programmed cell death-ligand 1 overexpression via the nuclear factor-κB to foster an immunosuppressive tumor microenvironment in ovarian cancer. *Cancer Res*. 2015;75(23):5034–5045.
985. Khallouf H, Märten A, Serba S, Teichgräber V, Büchler MW, Jäger D, et al. 5-Fluorouracil and interferon-α immunochemotherapy enhances immunogenicity of murine pancreatic cancer through upregulation of NKG2D ligands and MHC class I. *J. Immunother*. 2012;35(3):245–253.
986. Tsuchikawa T, Miyamoto M, Yamamura Y, Shichinohe T, Hirano S, Kondo S. The immunological impact of neoadjuvant chemotherapy on the tumor microenvironment of esophageal squamous cell carcinoma. *Ann. Surg. Oncol*. 2012;19(5):1713–1719.
987. Ohtsukasa S, Okabe S, Yamashita H, Iwai T, Sugihara K. Increased expression of CEA and MHC class I in colorectal cancer cell lines exposed to chemotherapy drugs. *J. Cancer Res. Clin. Oncol*. 2003;129(12):719–726.
988. Jackaman C, Majewski D, Fox SA, Nowak AK, Nelson DJ. Chemotherapy broadens the range of tumor antigens seen by cytotoxic CD8+ T cells in vivo. *Cancer Immunology, Immunotherapy*. 2012;61(12):2343–2356.
989. Böhm S, Montfort A, Pearce OM, Topping J, Chakravarty P, Everitt GL, et al. Neoadjuvant chemotherapy modulates the immune microenvironment in metastases of tubo-ovarian high-grade serous carcinoma. *Clin. Cancer Res*. 2016;22(12):3025–3036.
990. Parra ER, Villalobos P, Behrens C, Jiang M, Pataer A, Swisher SG, et al. Effect of neoadjuvant chemotherapy on the immune microenvironment in non–small cell lung carcinomas as determined by multiplex immunofluorescence and image analysis approaches. *J. Immunother. Cancer*. 2018;6(1):48.
991. Waks AG, Stover DG, Guerriero JL, Dillon D, Barry WT, Gjini E, et al. The Immune Microenvironment in Hormone Receptor–Positive Breast Cancer Before and After Preoperative Chemotherapy. *Clin. Cancer Res*. 2019;25(15):4644–4655.
992. Shalapour S, Font-Burgada J, Di Caro G, Zhong Z, Sanchez-Lopez E, Dhar D, et al. Immunosuppressive plasma cells impede T-cell-dependent immunogenic chemotherapy. *Nature*. 2015;521(7550):94–98.
993. Takeuchi S, Baghdadi M, Tsuchikawa T, Wada H, Nakamura T, Abe H, et al. Chemotherapy-derived inflammatory responses accelerate the formation of immunosuppressive myeloid cells in the tissue microenvironment of human pancreatic cancer. *Cancer Res*. 2015;75(13):2629–2640.
994. Bruchard M, Mignot G, Derangère V, Chalmin F, Chevriaux A, Végran F, et al. Chemotherapy-triggered cathepsin B release in myeloid-derived suppressor cells activates the Nlrp3 inflammasome and promotes tumor growth. *Nat. Med*. 2013;19(1):57.

995. Kanterman J, Sade-Feldman M, Biton M, Ish-Shalom E, Lasry A, Goldshtein A, et al. Adverse immunoregulatory effects of 5FU and CPT11 chemotherapy on myeloid-derived suppressor cells and colorectal cancer outcomes. *Cancer Res.* 2014;74(21):6022–6035.
996. Suzuki E, Kapoor V, Jassar AS, Kaiser LR, Albelda SM. Gemcitabine selectively eliminates splenic Gr-1+/CD11b+ myeloid suppressor cells in tumor-bearing animals and enhances antitumor immune activity. *Clin. Cancer Res.* 2005;11(18):6713–6721.
997. Alizadeh D, Trad M, Hanke NT, Larmonier CB, Janikashvili N, Bonnotte B, et al. Doxorubicin eliminates myeloid-derived suppressor cells and enhances the efficacy of adoptive T-cell transfer in breast cancer. *Cancer Res.* 2014;74(1):104–118.
998. Vincent J, Mignot G, Chalmin F, Ladoire S, Bruchard M, Chevriaux A, et al. 5-Fluorouracil selectively kills tumor-associated myeloid-derived suppressor cells resulting in enhanced T cell–dependent antitumor immunity. *Cancer Res.* 2010;70(8):3052–3061.
999. Sevko A, Michels T, Vrohlings M, Umansky L, Beckhove P, Kato M, et al. Antitumor effect of paclitaxel is mediated by inhibition of myeloid-derived suppressor cells and chronic inflammation in the spontaneous melanoma model. *J. Immunol.* 2013;190(5):2464–2471.
1000. Kodumudi KN, Woan K, Gilvary DL, Sahakian E, Wei S, Djeu JY. A novel chemoimmunomodulating property of docetaxel: suppression of myeloid-derived suppressor cells in tumor bearers. *Clin. Cancer Res.* 2010;16(18):4583–4594.
1001. Ruffell B, Chang-Strachan D, Chan V, Rosenbusch A, Ho CM, Pryer N, et al. Macrophage IL-10 blocks CD8+ T cell-dependent responses to chemotherapy by suppressing IL-12 expression in intratumoral dendritic cells. *Cancer Cell.* 2014;26(5):623–637.
1002. Deshmukh SK, Tyagi N, Khan MA, Srivastava SK, Al-Ghadhban A, Dugger K, et al. Gemcitabine treatment promotes immunosuppressive microenvironment in pancreatic tumors by supporting the infiltration, growth, and polarization of macrophages. *Sci. Rep.* 2018;8(1):1–10.
1003. Leroi N, Lallemand F, Coucke P, Noel A, Martinive P. Impacts of ionizing radiation on the different compartments of the tumor microenvironment. *Front Pharmacol.* 2016;7:78.
1004. Wang W, Green M, Liu JR, Lawrence TS, Zou W. *CD8+ T cells in immunotherapy, radiotherapy, and chemotherapy. Oncoimmunology*: Springer; 2018:23–39.
1005. Barker HE, Paget JT, Khan AA, Harrington KJ. The tumour microenvironment after radiotherapy: mechanisms of resistance and recurrence. *Nat. Rev. Cancer.* 2015;15(7):409–425.
1006. Lauber K, Ernst A, Orth M, Herrmann M, Belka C. Dying cell clearance and its impact on the outcome of tumor radiotherapy. *Front. Oncol.* 2012;2:116.
1007. Wan C, Sun Y, Tian Y, Lu L, Dai X, Meng J, et al. Irradiated tumor cell–derived microparticles mediate tumor eradication via cell killing and immune reprogramming. *Sci. Adv.* 2020;6(13):eaay9789.
1008. Gupta A, Probst HC, Vuong V, Landshammer A, Muth S, Yagita H, et al. Radiotherapy promotes tumor-specific effector CD8+ T cells via dendritic cell activation. *J. Immunol.* 2012;189(2):558–566.
1009. Joanne Y, Lim H, Gerber SA, Murphy SP, Lord EM. Type I interferons induced by radiation therapy mediate recruitment and effector function of CD8^ sup+^ T cells. *Cancer Immunology, Immunotherapy.* 2014;63(3):259.
1010. Burnette BC, Liang H, Lee Y, Chlewicki L, Khodarev NN, Weichselbaum RR, et al. The efficacy of radiotherapy relies upon induction of type I interferon–dependent innate and adaptive immunity. *Cancer Res.* 2011;71(7):2488–2496.
1011. Jarosz-Biej M, Smolarczyk R, Cichoń T, Kułach N. Tumor Microenvironment as A "Game Changer" in Cancer Radiotherapy. *Int. J. Mol. Sci.* 2019;20(13):3212.
1012. Reits EA, Hodge JW, Herberts CA, Groothuis TA, Chakraborty M, K. Wansley E, et al. Radiation modulates the peptide repertoire, enhances MHC class I expression, and induces successful antitumor immunotherapy. *J. Exp. Med.* 2006;203(5):1259–1271.
1013. Frey B, Rubner Y, Kulzer L, Werthmöller N, Weiss E-M, Fietkau R, et al. Antitumor immune responses induced by ionizing irradiation and further immune stimulation. *Cancer Immunol. Immunother.* 2014;63(1):29–36.
1014. Wan S, Pestka S, Jubin RG, Lyu YL, Tsai Y-C, Liu LF. Chemotherapeutics and radiation stimulate MHC class I expression through elevated interferon-beta signaling in breast cancer cells. *PLoS ONE.* 2012;7(3).

1015. Demaria S, Ng B, Devitt ML, Babb JS, Kawashima N, Liebes L, et al. Ionizing radiation inhibition of distant untreated tumors (abscopal effect) is immune mediated. *International Journal of Radiation Oncology* Biology* Physics*. 2004;58(3):862–870.
1016. Rodríguez-Ruiz ME, Vanpouille-Box C, Melero I, Formenti SC, Demaria S. Immunological mechanisms responsible for radiation-induced abscopal effect. *Trends Immunol*. 2018;39(8):644–655.
1017. Ozpiskin OM, Zhang L, Li JJ. Immune targets in the tumor microenvironment treated by radiotherapy. *Theranostics*. 2019;9(5):1215.
1018. Chen M, Qiao G, Hylander BL, Mohammadpour H, Wang X-Y, Subjeck JR, et al. Adrenergic stress constrains the development of anti-tumor immunity and abscopal responses following local radiation. *Nat. Commun*. 2020;11(1):1–12.
1019. Shi L, Wang J, Ding N, Zhang Y, Zhu Y, Dong S, et al. Inflammation induced by incomplete radiofrequency ablation accelerates tumor progression and hinders PD-1 immunotherapy. *Nat. Commun*. 2019;10(1):1–13.
1020. Xu J, Escamilla J, Mok S, David J, Priceman SJ, West BL, et al. Abrogating the protumorigenic influences of tumor-infiltrating myeloid cells by CSF1R signaling blockade improves the efficacy of radiotherapy in prostate cancer. *Cancer Res*. 2013 canres. 3981.2012.
1021. Toivonen P, Kivelä T. Infiltrating macrophages in extratumoural tissues after brachytherapy of uveal melanoma. *Acta Ophthalmol. (Copenh)*. 2012;90(4):341–349.
1022. Vatner RE, Formenti SC, eds. *Myeloid-derived Cells in tumors: Effects of radiation. Seminars in Radiation Oncology*: Elsevier; 2015.
1023. Nguyen DH, Oketch-Rabah HA, Illa-Bochaca I, Geyer FC, Reis-Filho JS, Mao J-H, et al. Radiation acts on the microenvironment to affect breast carcinogenesis by distinct mechanisms that decrease cancer latency and affect tumor type. *Cancer Cell*. 2011;19(5):640–651.
1024. Kane JL, Krueger SA, Hanna A, Raffel TR, Wilson GD, Madlambayan GJ, et al. Effect of irradiation on tumor microenvironment and bone marrow cell migration in a preclinical tumor model. *International Journal of Radiation Oncology* Biology* Physics*. 2016;96(1):170–178.
1025. Chen J, Wang Z, Ding Y, Huang F, Huang W, Lan R, et al. Hypofractionated Irradiation Suppressed the Off-Target Mouse Hepatocarcinoma Growth by Inhibiting Myeloid-Derived Suppressor Cell-Mediated Immune Suppression. *Front. Oncol*. 2020;10:4.
1026. Wennerberg E, Lhuillier C, Vanpouille-Box C, Pilones KA, García-Martínez E, Rudqvist N-P, et al. Barriers to radiation-induced in situ tumor vaccination. *Front. Immunol*. 2017;8:229.
1027. Klemm F, Joyce JA. Microenvironmental regulation of therapeutic response in cancer. *Trends Cell Biol*. 2015;25(4):198–213.
1028. Chiang C-S, Fu S-Y, Wang S-C, Yu C-F, Chen F-H, Lin C-M, et al. Irradiation promotes an m2 macrophage phenotype in tumor hypoxia. *Front. Oncol*. 2012;2:89.
1029. Klug F, Prakash H, Huber PE, Seibel T, Bender N, Halama N, et al. Low-dose irradiation programs macrophage differentiation to an iNOS+/M1 phenotype that orchestrates effective T cell immunotherapy. *Cancer Cell*. 2013;24(5):589–602.
1030. Ostrand-Rosenberg S, Horn LA, Ciavattone NG. Radiotherapy both promotes and inhibits myeloid-derived suppressor cell function: novel strategies for preventing the tumor-protective effects of radiotherapy. *Front. Oncol*. 2019;9:215.
1031. Takeshima T, Pop LM, Laine A, Iyengar P, Vitetta ES, Hannan R. Key role for neutrophils in radiation-induced antitumor immune responses: potentiation with G-CSF. *Proc. Natl. Acad. Sci*. 2016;113(40):11300–11305.
1032. Filatenkov A, Baker J, Strober S. Disruption of evasive immune cell microenvironment in tumors reflects immunity induced by radiation therapy. *Oncoimmunology*. 2016;5(2):e1072673.
1033. Tamura R, Tanaka T, Morimoto Y, Kuranari Y, Yamamoto Y, Takei J, et al. Alterations of the tumor microenvironment in glioblastoma following radiation and temozolomide with or without bevacizumab. *Ann. Transl. Med*. 2020;8(6).
1034. Meads MB, Gatenby RA, Dalton WS. Environment-mediated drug resistance: a major contributor to minimal residual disease. *Nat. Rev. Cancer*. 2009;9(9):665–674.
1035. Vacchelli E, Galluzzi L, Rousseau V, Rigoni A, Tesniere A, Delahaye N, et al. Loss-of-function alleles of P2RX7 and TLR4 fail to affect the response to chemotherapy in non-small cell lung cancer. *Oncoimmunology*. 2012;1(3):271–278.

1036. Nakasone ES, Askautrud HA, Kees T, Park J-H, Plaks V, Ewald AJ, et al. Imaging tumor-stroma interactions during chemotherapy reveals contributions of the microenvironment to resistance. *Cancer Cell.* 2012;21(4):488–503.
1037. Ruffell B, Au A, Rugo HS, Esserman LJ, Hwang ES, Coussens LM. Leukocyte composition of human breast cancer. *Proc. Natl. Acad. Sci.* 2012;109(8):2796–2801.
1038. Shree T, Olson OC, Elie BT, Kester JC, Garfall AL, Simpson K, et al. Macrophages and cathepsin proteases blunt chemotherapeutic response in breast cancer. *Genes Dev.* 2011;25(23):2465–2479.
1039. Mitchem JB, Brennan DJ, Knolhoff BL, Belt BA, Zhu Y, Sanford DE, et al. Targeting tumor-infiltrating macrophages decreases tumor-initiating cells, relieves immunosuppression, and improves chemotherapeutic responses. *Cancer Res.* 2013;73(3):1128–1141.
1040. Baghdadi M, Wada H, Nakanishi S, Abe H, Han N, Putra WE, et al. Chemotherapy-induced IL34 enhances immunosuppression by tumor-associated macrophages and mediates survival of chemoresistant lung cancer cells. *Cancer Res.* 2016;76(20):6030–6042.
1041. De Beule N, De Veirman K, Maes K, De Bruyne E, Menu E, Breckpot K, et al. Tumour-associated macrophage-mediated survival of myeloma cells through STAT3 activation. *J. Pathol.* 2017;241(4):534–546.
1042. Dijkgraaf EM, Heusinkveld M, Tummers B, Vogelpoel LT, Goedemans R, Jha V, et al. Chemotherapy alters monocyte differentiation to favor generation of cancer-supporting M2 macrophages in the tumor microenvironment. *Cancer Res.* 2013;73(8):2480–2492.
1043. Yang C, He L, He P, Liu Y, Wang W, He Y, et al. Increased drug resistance in breast cancer by tumor-associated macrophages through IL-10/STAT3/bcl-2 signaling pathway. *Med. Oncol.* 2015;32(2):14.
1044. Huang W-C, Kuo K-T, Wang C-H, Yeh C-T, Wang Y. Cisplatin resistant lung cancer cells promoted M2 polarization of tumor-associated macrophages via the Src/CD155/MIF functional pathway. *J. Exp. Clin. Cancer Res.* 2019;38(1):180.
1045. Huang Z, Yin Y, Yao S, Hu Y, Feng Y, Li M, et al. The immune-microenvironment confers Chemoresistance of colorectal Cancer through macrophage-derived IL-6. *Clin. Cancer Res.* 2017.
1046. Weizman N, Krelin Y, Shabtay-Orbach A, Amit M, Binenbaum Y, Wong R, et al. Macrophages mediate gemcitabine resistance of pancreatic adenocarcinoma by upregulating cytidine deaminase. *Oncogene.* 2014;33(29):3812–3819.
1047. Zhang X, Chen Y, Hao L, Hou A, Chen X, Li Y, et al. Macrophages induce resistance to 5-fluorouracil chemotherapy in colorectal cancer through the release of putrescine. *Cancer Lett.* 2016;381(2):305–313.
1048. Zheng Y, Cai Z, Wang S, Zhang X, Qian J, Hong S, et al. Macrophages are an abundant component of myeloma microenvironment and protect myeloma cells from chemotherapy drug–induced apoptosis. *Blood, The Journal of the American Society of Hematology.* 2009;114(17):3625–3628.
1049. Zheng Y, Yang J, Qian J, Qiu P, Hanabuchi S, Lu Y, et al. PSGL-1/selectin and ICAM-1/CD18 interactions are involved in macrophage-induced drug resistance in myeloma. *Leukemia.* 2013;27(3):702–710.
1050. Fu X-T, Song K, Zhou J, Shi Y-H, Liu W-R, Shi G-M, et al. Tumor-associated macrophages modulate resistance to oxaliplatin via inducing autophagy in hepatocellular carcinoma. *Cancer Cell Int.* 2019;19(1):71.
1051. Zheng P, Chen L, Yuan X, Luo Q, Liu Y, Xie G, et al. Exosomal transfer of tumor-associated macrophage-derived miR-21 confers cisplatin resistance in gastric cancer cells. *J. Exp. Clin. Cancer Res.* 2017;36(1):53.
1052. Zhu X, Shen H, Yin X, Yang M, Wei H, Chen Q, et al. Macrophages derived exosomes deliver miR-223 to epithelial ovarian cancer cells to elicit a chemoresistant phenotype. *J. Exp. Clin. Cancer Res.* 2019;38(1):81.
1053. Challagundla KB, Wise PM, Neviani P, Chava H, Murtadha M, Xu T, et al. Exosome-mediated transfer of microRNAs within the tumor microenvironment and neuroblastoma resistance to chemotherapy. *J. Natl. Cancer Inst.* 2015;107(7).
1054. Martin OA, Anderson RL, Narayan K, MacManus MP. Does the mobilization of circulating tumour cells during cancer therapy cause metastasis? *Nat. Rev. Clin. Oncol.* 2017;14(1):32.

1055. Purbey PK, Scumpia PO, Kim PJ, Tong A-J, Iwamoto KS, McBride WH, et al. Defined sensing mechanisms and signaling pathways contribute to the global inflammatory gene expression output elicited by ionizing radiation. *Immunity*. 2017;47(3):421–434 e3.
1056. Kalbasi A, Komar C, Tooker GM, Liu M, Lee JW, Gladney WL, et al. Tumor-derived CCL2 mediates resistance to radiotherapy in pancreatic ductal adenocarcinoma. *Clin. Cancer Res.* 2017;23(1):137–148.
1057. Kang C, Jeong S-Y, Song SY, Choi EK. The emerging role of myeloid-derived suppressor cells in radiotherapy. *Radiat Oncol J.* 2020;38(1):1.
1058. Rahal OM, Wolfe AR, Mandal PK, Larson R, Tin S, Jimenez C, et al. Blocking interleukin (IL) 4-and IL13-mediated phosphorylation of STAT6 (Tyr641) decreases M2 polarization of macrophages and protects against macrophage-mediated radioresistance of inflammatory breast cancer. *International Journal of Radiation Oncology* Biology* Physics*. 2018;100(4):1034–1043.
1059. Ayoub M, Shinde-Jadhav S, Mansure JJ, Alvarez F, Connell T, Seuntjens J, et al. The immune mediated role of extracellular HMGB1 in a heterotopic model of bladder cancer radioresistance. *Sci. Rep.* 2019;9(1):1–9.
1060. Wisdom AJ, Hong CS, Lin AJ, Xiang Y, Cooper DE, Zhang J, et al. Neutrophils promote tumor resistance to radiation therapy. *Proc. Natl. Acad. Sci.* 2019;116(37):18584–18589.
1061. Kelley K, Knisely J, Symons M, Ruggieri R. Radioresistance of brain tumors. *Cancers (Basel)*. 2016;8(4):42.
1062. Miller IS, Didier S, Murray DW, Turner TH, Issaivanan M, Ruggieri R, et al. Semapimod sensitizes glioblastoma tumors to ionizing radiation by targeting microglia. *PLoS ONE*. 2014;9(5).
1063. Chen H-Y, Xu L, Li l, Liu X-X, Gao J-X, Bai Y-R. Inhibiting the CD8+ T cell infiltration in the tumor microenvironment after radiotherapy is an important mechanism of radioresistance. *Sci. Rep.* 2018;8(1):1–10.
1064. Arina A, Beckett M, Fernandez C, Zheng W, Pitroda S, Chmura SJ, et al. Tumor-reprogrammed resident T cells resist radiation to control tumors. *Nat. Commun.* 2019;10(1):1–13.
1065. Dovedi SJ, Adlard AL, Lipowska-Bhalla G, McKenna C, Jones S, Cheadle EJ, et al. Acquired resistance to fractionated radiotherapy can be overcome by concurrent PD-L1 blockade. *Cancer Res.* 2014;74(19):5458–5468.
1066. Du R, Lu KV, Petritsch C, Liu P, Ganss R, Passegué E, et al. HIF1α induces the recruitment of bone marrow-derived vascular modulatory cells to regulate tumor angiogenesis and invasion. *Cancer Cell*. 2008;13(3):206–220.
1067. Haikerwal SJ, Hagekyriakou J, MacManus M, Martin OA, Haynes NM. Building immunity to cancer with radiation therapy. *Cancer Lett.* 2015;368(2):198–208.
1068. Ebos JM. Prodding the beast: assessing the impact of treatment-induced metastasis. *Cancer Res.* 2015;75(17):3427–3435.
1069. Karagiannis GS, Condeelis JS, Oktay MH. Chemotherapy-Induced Metastasis: molecular Mechanisms, Clinical Manifestations, Therapeutic Interventions. *Cancer Res.* 2019;79(18):4567–4576.
1070. Daenen L, Houthuijzen J, Cirkel G, Roodhart J, Shaked Y, Voest E. Treatment-induced host-mediated mechanisms reducing the efficacy of antitumor therapies. *Oncogene*. 2014;33(11):1341–1347.
1071. Fremder E, Munster M, Aharon A, Miller V, Gingis-Velitski S, Voloshin T, et al. Tumor-derived microparticles induce bone marrow-derived cell mobilization and tumor homing: a process regulated by osteopontin. *Int. J. Cancer*. 2014;135(2):270–281.
1072. Paraskeva P, Ridgway P, Olsen S, Isacke C, Peck D, Darzi A. A surgically induced hypoxic environment causes changes in the metastatic behaviour of tumours in vitro. *Clin. Exp. Metastasis*. 2006;23(2):149–157.
1073. Chen L, Li J, Wang F, Dai C, Wu F, Liu X, et al. Tie2 expression on macrophages is required for blood vessel reconstruction and tumor relapse after chemotherapy. *Cancer Res.* 2016;76(23):6828–6838.
1074. Gingis-Velitski S, Loven D, Benayoun L, Munster M, Bril R, Voloshin T, et al. Host response to short-term, single-agent chemotherapy induces matrix metalloproteinase-9 expression and accelerates metastasis in mice. *Cancer Res.* 2011;71(22):6986–6996.
1075. Kozin SV, Kamoun WS, Huang Y, Dawson MR, Jain RK, Duda DG. Recruitment of myeloid but not endothelial precursor cells facilitates tumor regrowth after local irradiation. *Cancer Res.* 2010;70(14):5679–5685.

1076. Vala IS, Martins LR, Imaizumi N, Nunes RJ, Rino J, Kuonen F, et al. Low doses of ionizing radiation promote tumor growth and metastasis by enhancing angiogenesis. *PLoS ONE*. 2010;5(6).
1077. Shojaei F, Wu X, Qu X, Kowanetz M, Yu L, Tan M, et al. G-CSF-initiated myeloid cell mobilization and angiogenesis mediate tumor refractoriness to anti-VEGF therapy in mouse models. *Proc. Natl. Acad. Sci*. 2009;106(16):6742–6747.
1078. Ebos JM, Lee CR, Cruz-Munoz W, Bjarnason GA, Christensen JG, Kerbel RS. Accelerated metastasis after short-term treatment with a potent inhibitor of tumor angiogenesis. *Cancer Cell*. 2009;15(3):232–239.
1079. Kumara HMS, Feingold D, Kalady M, Dujovny N, Senagore A, Hyman N, et al. Colorectal resection is associated with persistent proangiogenic plasma protein changes: postoperative plasma stimulates in vitro endothelial cell growth, migration, and invasion. *Ann. Surg*. 2009;249(6):973–977.
1080. Wu S-Y, Chiang C-S. Distinct Role of CD11b+ Ly6G− Ly6C− Myeloid-Derived Cells on the Progression of the Primary Tumor and Therapy-Associated Recurrent Brain Tumor. *Cells*. 2020;9(1):51.
1081. Volk-Draper L, Hall K, Griggs C, Rajput S, Kohio P, DeNardo D, et al. Paclitaxel therapy promotes breast cancer metastasis in a TLR4-dependent manner. *Cancer Res*. 2014;74(19):5421–5434.
1082. Hughes R, Qian B-Z, Rowan C, Muthana M, Keklikoglou I, Olson OC, et al. Perivascular M2 macrophages stimulate tumor relapse after chemotherapy. *Cancer Res*. 2015;75(17):3479–3491.
1083. Zhang C, Yu X, Gao L, Zhao Y, Lai J, Lu D, et al. Noninvasive imaging of CD206-positive M2 macrophages as an early biomarker for post-chemotherapy tumor relapse and lymph node metastasis. *Theranostics*. 2017;7(17):4276.
1084. Zhang W, Zhu X-D, Sun H-C, Xiong Y-Q, Zhuang P-Y, Xu H-X, et al. Depletion of tumor-associated macrophages enhances the effect of sorafenib in metastatic liver cancer models by antimetastatic and antiangiogenic effects. *Clin. Cancer Res*. 2010;16(13):3420–3430.
1085. Kioi M, Vogel H, Schultz G, Hoffman RM, Harsh GR, Brown JM. Inhibition of vasculogenesis, but not angiogenesis, prevents the recurrence of glioblastoma after irradiation in mice. *J. Clin. Invest*. 2010;120(3):694–705.
1086. Martin OA, Anderson RL, Russell PA, Cox RA, Ivashkevich A, Swierczak A, et al. Mobilization of viable tumor cells into the circulation during radiation therapy. *International Journal of Radiation Oncology* Biology* Physics*. 2014;88(2):395–403.
1087. Okubo M, Kioi M, Nakashima H, Sugiura K, Mitsudo K, Aoki I, et al. M2-polarized macrophages contribute to neovasculogenesis, leading to relapse of oral cancer following radiation. *Sci. Rep*. 2016;6:27548.
1088. Ahn G-O, Tseng D, Liao C-H, Dorie MJ, Czechowicz A, Brown JM. Inhibition of Mac-1 (CD11b/CD18) enhances tumor response to radiation by reducing myeloid cell recruitment. *Proc. Natl. Acad. Sci*. 2010;107(18):8363–8368.
1089. Ahn G-O, Brown JM. Matrix metalloproteinase-9 is required for tumor vasculogenesis but not for angiogenesis: role of bone marrow-derived myelomonocytic cells. *Cancer Cell*. 2008;13(3):193–205.
1090. Russell JS, Brown JM. The irradiated tumor microenvironment: role of tumor-associated macrophages in vascular recovery. *Front Physiol*. 2013;4:157.
1091. Langenberg MH, Nijkamp MW, Roodhart JM, Snoeren N, Tang T, Shaked Y, et al. Liver surgery induces an immediate mobilization of progenitor cells in liver cancer patients: a potential role for G-CSF. *Cancer Biol. Ther*. 2010;9(9):743–748.
1092. Ma X, Wang M, Yin T, Zhao Y, Wei X. Myeloid-derived suppressor cells promote metastasis in breast cancer after the stress of operative removal of the primary cancer. *Front. Oncol*. 2019;9.
1093. Predina J, Eruslanov E, Judy B, Kapoor V, Cheng G, Wang l, et al. Changes in the local tumor microenvironment in recurrent cancers may explain the failure of vaccines after surgery. *Proc. Natl. Acad. Sci*. 2013;110(5):E415–EE24.
1094. Krall JA, Reinhardt F, Mercury OA, Pattabiraman DR, Brooks MW, Dougan M, et al. The systemic response to surgery triggers the outgrowth of distant immune-controlled tumors in mouse models of dormancy. *Sci. Transl. Med*. 2018;10(436):eaan3464.
1095. Ceelen W, Pattyn P, Mareel M. Surgery, wound healing, and metastasis: recent insights and clinical implications. *Crit. Rev. Oncol. Hematol*. 2014;89(1):16–26.

1096. Bartal I, Melamed R, Greenfeld K, Atzil S, Glasner A, Domankevich V, et al. Immune perturbations in patients along the perioperative period: alterations in cell surface markers and leukocyte subtypes before and after surgery. *Brain Behav. Immun.* 2010;24(3):376–386.
1097. Veenhof A, Sietses C, Von Blomberg B, Van Hoogstraten I, Vd Pas M, Meijerink W, et al. The surgical stress response and postoperative immune function after laparoscopic or conventional total mesorectal excision in rectal cancer: a randomized trial. *Int. J. Colorectal Dis.* 2011;26(1):53–59.
1098. Tohme S, Simmons RL, Tsung A. Surgery for cancer: a trigger for metastases. *Cancer Res.* 2017;77(7):1548–1552.
1099. Weber M, Moebius P, Büttner-Herold M, Amann K, Preidl R, Neukam F, et al. Macrophage polarisation changes within the time between diagnostic biopsy and tumour resection in oral squamous cell carcinomas—An immunohistochemical study. *Br. J. Cancer.* 2015;113(3):510–519.
1100. Alieva M, van Rheenen J, Broekman ML. Potential impact of invasive surgical procedures on primary tumor growth and metastasis. *Clin. Exp. Metastasis.* 2018;35(4):319–331.
1101. Coffelt SB, Chen Y-Y, Muthana M, Welford AF, Tal AO, Scholz A, et al. Angiopoietin 2 stimulates TIE2-expressing monocytes to suppress T cell activation and to promote regulatory T cell expansion. *J. Immunol.* 2011;186(7):4183–4190.
1102. Tham M, Khoo K, Yeo KP, Kato M, Prevost-Blondel A, Angeli V, et al. Macrophage depletion reduces postsurgical tumor recurrence and metastatic growth in a spontaneous murine model of melanoma. *Oncotarget.* 2015;6(26):22857.
1103. Polyak K, Weinberg RA. Transitions between epithelial and mesenchymal states: acquisition of malignant and stem cell traits. *Nat. Rev. Cancer.* 2009;9(4):265–273.
1104. Eyler CE, Rich JN. Survival of the fittest: cancer stem cells in therapeutic resistance and angiogenesis. *J. Clin. Oncol.* 2008;26(17):2839.
1105. Chefetz I, Alvero A, Holmberg J, Lebowitz N, Craveiro V, Yang-Hartwich Y, et al. TLR2 enhances ovarian cancer stem cell self-renewal and promotes tumor repair and recurrence. *Cell Cycle.* 2013;12(3):511–521.
1106. Jia D, Li L, Andrew S, Allan D, Li X, Lee J, et al. An autocrine inflammatory forward-feedback loop after chemotherapy withdrawal facilitates the repopulation of drug-resistant breast cancer cells. *Cell Death. Dis.* 2017;8(7):e2932.
1107. Korkaya H, Kim G-I, Davis A, Malik F, Henry NL, Ithimakin S, et al. Activation of an IL6 inflammatory loop mediates trastuzumab resistance in HER2+ breast cancer by expanding the cancer stem cell population. *Mol. Cell.* 2012;47(4):570–584.
1108. Liu L, Yang L, Yan W, Zhai J, Pizzo DP, Chu P, et al. Chemotherapy induces breast cancer stemness in association with dysregulated monocytosis. *Clin. Cancer Res.* 2018;24(10):2370–2382.
1109. Jinushi M, Chiba S, Yoshiyama H, Masutomi K, Kinoshita I, Dosaka-Akita H, et al. Tumor-associated macrophages regulate tumorigenicity and anticancer drug responses of cancer stem/initiating cells. *Proc. Natl. Acad. Sci.* 2011;108(30):12425–12430.
1110. Shibue T, Weinberg RA. EMT, CSCs, and drug resistance: the mechanistic link and clinical implications. *Nat. Rev. Clin. Oncol.* 2017;14(10):611.
1111. Mani SA, Guo W, Liao M-J, Eaton EN, Ayyanan A, Zhou AY, et al. The epithelial-mesenchymal transition generates cells with properties of stem cells. *Cell.* 2008;133(4):704–715.
1112. Liu G, Chen Y, Qi F, Jia L, Xa L, He T, et al. Specific chemotherapeutic agents induce metastatic behaviour through stromal-and tumour-derived cytokine and angiogenic factor signalling. *J. Pathol.* 2015;237(2):190–202.
1113. Timaner M, Bril R, Kaidar-Person O, Rachman-Tzemah C, Alishekevitz D, Kotsofruk R, et al. Dequalinium blocks macrophage-induced metastasis following local radiation. *Oncotarget.* 2015;6(29):27537.
1114. del Pozo Martin Y, Park D, Ramachandran A, Ombrato L, Calvo F, Chakravarty P, et al. Mesenchymal cancer cell-stroma crosstalk promotes niche activation, epithelial reversion, and metastatic colonization. *Cell Rep.* 2015;13(11):2456–2469.
1115. Liu W, Wang W, Wang X, Xu C, Zhang N, Di W. Cisplatin-stimulated macrophages promote ovarian cancer migration via the CCL20-CCR6 axis. *Cancer Lett.* 2020;472:59–69.

1116. Kuwada K, Kagawa S, Yoshida R, Sakamoto S, Ito A, Watanabe M, et al. The epithelial-to-mesenchymal transition induced by tumor-associated macrophages confers chemoresistance in peritoneally disseminated pancreatic cancer. *J. Exp. Clin. Cancer Res.* 2018;37(1):1–10.
1117. Calabrese C, Poppleton H, Kocak M, Hogg TL, Fuller C, Hamner B, et al. A perivascular niche for brain tumor stem cells. *Cancer Cell.* 2007;11(1):69–82.
1118. Hambardzumyan D, Becher OJ, Rosenblum MK, Pandolfi PP, Manova-Todorova K, Holland EC. PI3K pathway regulates survival of cancer stem cells residing in the perivascular niche following radiation in medulloblastoma in vivo. *Genes Dev.* 2008;22(4):436–448.
1119. Fernandez-L A, Squatrito M, Northcott P, Awan A, Holland EC, Taylor MD, et al. Oncogenic YAP promotes radioresistance and genomic instability in medulloblastoma through IGF2-mediated Akt activation. *Oncogene.* 2012;31(15):1923–1937.
1120. Lewis CE, Harney AS, Pollard JW. The multifaceted role of perivascular macrophages in tumors. *Cancer Cell.* 2016;30(1):18–25.
1121. Toh B, Wang X, Keeble J, Sim WJ, Khoo K, Wong W-C, et al. Mesenchymal transition and dissemination of cancer cells is driven by myeloid-derived suppressor cells infiltrating the primary tumor. *PLoS Biol.* 2011;9(9).
1122. Freisinger CM, Huttenlocher A. Live imaging and gene expression analysis in zebrafish identifies a link between neutrophils and epithelial to mesenchymal transition. *PLoS ONE.* 2014;9(11).
1123. Bockhorn M, Jain RK, Munn LL. Active versus passive mechanisms in metastasis: do cancer cells crawl into vessels, or are they pushed? *Lancet Oncol.* 2007;8(5):444–448.
1124. Martin OA, Anderson RL. *Therapy-induced Metastasis*: Springer; 2018.
1125. Kaigorodova EV, Savelieva OE, Tashireva LA, Tarabanovskaya NA, Simolina EI, Denisov EV, et al. Heterogeneity of circulating tumor cells in neoadjuvant chemotherapy of breast cancer. *Molecules.* 2018;23(4):727.
1126. Mathenge EG, Dean CA, Clements D, Vaghar-Kashani A, Photopoulos S, Coyle KM, et al. Core needle biopsy of breast cancer tumors increases distant metastases in a mouse model. *Neoplasia.* 2014;16(11):950–960.
1127. Park HJ, Griffin RJ, Hui S, Levitt SH, Song CW. Radiation-induced vascular damage in tumors: implications of vascular damage in ablative hypofractionated radiotherapy (SBRT and SRS). *Radiat. Res.* 2012;177(3):311–327.
1128. Lim SH, Spring KJ, De Souza P, MacKenzie S, Bokey L. Circulating tumour cells and circulating nucleic acids as a measure of tumour dissemination in non-metastatic colorectal cancer surgery. *European Journal of Surgical Oncology (EJSO).* 2015;41(3):309–314.
1129. Behrenbruch C, Shembrey C, Paquet-Fifield S, Mølck C, Cho H-J, Michael M, et al. Surgical stress response and promotion of metastasis in colorectal cancer: a complex and heterogeneous process. *Clin. Exp. Metastasis.* 2018;35(4):333–345.
1130. Kusukawa J, Suefuji Y, Ryu F, Noguchi R, Iwamoto O, Kameyama T. Dissemination of cancer cells into circulation occurs by incisional biopsy of oral squamous cell carcinoma. *J. Oral Pathol. Med.* 2000;29(7):303–307.
1131. Hu X, Chow LW. Fine needle aspiration may shed breast cells into peripheral blood as determined by RT-PCR. *Oncology.* 2000;59(3):217–222.
1132. Karagiannis GS, Condeelis JS, Oktay MH. Chemotherapy-induced metastasis: mechanisms and translational opportunities. *Clin. Exp. Metastasis.* 2018;35(4):269–284.
1133. Robinson BD, Sica GL, Liu Y-F, Rohan TE, Gertler FB, Condeelis JS, et al. Tumor microenvironment of metastasis in human breast carcinoma: a potential prognostic marker linked to hematogenous dissemination. *Clin. Cancer Res.* 2009;15(7):2433–2441.
1134. Harney AS, Arwert EN, Entenberg D, Wang Y, Guo P, Qian B-Z, et al. Real-time imaging reveals local, transient vascular permeability, and tumor cell intravasation stimulated by TIE2hi macrophage–derived VEGFA. *Cancer Discov.* 2015;5(9):932–943.
1135. Roussos ET, Balsamo M, Alford SK, Wyckoff JB, Gligorijevic B, Wang Y, et al. Mena invasive (MenaINV) promotes multicellular streaming motility and transendothelial migration in a mouse model of breast cancer. *J. Cell Sci.* 2011;124(13):2120–2131.

1136. Pignatelli J, Bravo-Cordero JJ, Roh-Johnson M, Gandhi SJ, Wang Y, Chen X, et al. Macrophage-dependent tumor cell transendothelial migration is mediated by Notch1/Mena INV-initiated invadopodium formation. *Sci. Rep.* 2016;6(1):1–15.
1137. Chang YS, Jalgaonkar SP, Middleton JD, Hai T. Stress-inducible gene Atf3 in the noncancer host cells contributes to chemotherapy-exacerbated breast cancer metastasis. *Proc. Natl. Acad. Sci.* 2017;114(34):E7159–E7E68.
1138. Karagiannis GS, Pastoriza JM, Wang Y, Harney AS, Entenberg D, Pignatelli J, et al. Neoadjuvant chemotherapy induces breast cancer metastasis through a TMEM-mediated mechanism. *Sci. Transl. Med.* 2017;9(397):eaan0026.
1139. Arwert EN, Harney AS, Entenberg D, Wang Y, Sahai E, Pollard JW, et al. A unidirectional transition from migratory to perivascular macrophage is required for tumor cell intravasation. *Cell Rep.* 2018;23(5):1239–1248.
1140. Sanchez LR, Borriello L, Entenberg D, Condeelis JS, Oktay MH, Karagiannis GS. The emerging roles of macrophages in cancer metastasis and response to chemotherapy. *J. Leukocyte Biol.* 2019;106(2):259–274.
1141. Oudin MJ, Barbier L, Schäfer C, Kosciuk T, Miller MA, Han S, et al. MENA confers resistance to paclitaxel in triple-negative breast cancer. *Mol. Cancer Ther.* 2017;16(1):143–155.
1142. Wyckoff JB, Wang Y, Lin EY, Li J-F, Goswami S, Stanley ER, et al. Direct visualization of macrophage-assisted tumor cell intravasation in mammary tumors. *Cancer Res.* 2007;67(6):2649–2656.
1143. Manner T-D. Paclitaxel Therapy Promotes Breast Cancer Metastasis in. *Cancer Res.* 2014;74:5421–5434.
1144. Alishekevitz D, Gingis-Velitski S, Kaidar-Person O, Gutter-Kapon L, Scherer SD, Raviv Z, et al. Macrophage-induced lymphangiogenesis and metastasis following paclitaxel chemotherapy is regulated by VEGFR3. *Cell Rep.* 2016;17(5):1344–1356.
1145. Bieniasz-Krzywiec P, Martín-Pérez R, Ehling M, García-Caballero M, Pinioti S, Pretto S, et al. Podoplanin-expressing macrophages promote lymphangiogenesis and lymphoinvasion in breast cancer. *Cell Metab.* 2019;30(5):917–936 e10.
1146. Watari K, Shibata T, Kawahara A, Sata K-I, Nabeshima H, Shinoda A, et al. Tumor-derived interleukin-1 promotes lymphangiogenesis and lymph node metastasis through M2-type macrophages. *PLoS ONE.* 2014;9(6).
1147. Pereira ER, Kedrin D, Seano G, Gautier O, Meijer EF, Jones D, et al. Lymph node metastases can invade local blood vessels, exit the node, and colonize distant organs in mice. *Science.* 2018;359(6382):1403–1407.
1148. Daenen LG, Roodhart JM, van Amersfoort M, Dehnad M, Roessingh W, Ulfman LH, et al. Chemotherapy enhances metastasis formation via VEGFR-1–expressing endothelial cells. *Cancer Res.* 2011;71(22):6976–6985.
1149. Seth R, Tai l, Falls T, de Souza CT, Bell JC, Carrier M, et al. Surgical stress promotes the development of cancer metastases by a coagulation-dependent mechanism involving natural killer cells in a murine model. *Ann. Surg.* 2013;258(1):158–168.
1150. Tohme S, Yazdani HO, Al-Khafaji AB, Chidi AP, Loughran P, Mowen K, et al. Neutrophil extracellular traps promote the development and progression of liver metastases after surgical stress. *Cancer Res.* 2016;76(6):1367–1380.
1151. Spiegel A, Brooks MW, Houshyar S, Reinhardt F, Ardolino M, Fessler E, et al. Neutrophils suppress intraluminal NK cell–mediated tumor cell clearance and enhance extravasation of disseminated carcinoma cells. *Cancer Discov.* 2016;6(6):630–649.
1152. McDonald B, Spicer J, Giannais B, Fallavollita L, Brodt P, Ferri LE. Systemic inflammation increases cancer cell adhesion to hepatic sinusoids by neutrophil mediated mechanisms. *Int. J. Cancer.* 2009;125(6):1298–1305.
1153. Spicer JD, McDonald B, Cools-Lartigue JJ, Chow SC, Giannias B, Kubes P, et al. Neutrophils promote liver metastasis via Mac-1–mediated interactions with circulating tumor cells. *Cancer Res.* 2012;72(16):3919–3927.
1154. Cools-Lartigue J, Spicer J, McDonald B, Gowing S, Chow S, Giannias B, et al. Neutrophil extracellular traps sequester circulating tumor cells and promote metastasis. *J. Clin. Invest.* 2013;123(8):3446–3458.

1155. Huh SJ, Liang S, Sharma A, Dong C, Robertson GP. Transiently entrapped circulating tumor cells interact with neutrophils to facilitate lung metastasis development. *Cancer Res.* 2010;70(14):6071–6082.
1156. Wculek SK, Malanchi I. Neutrophils support lung colonization of metastasis-initiating breast cancer cells. *Nature.* 2015;528(7582):413–417.
1157. Acharyya S, Massague J. Arresting supporters: targeting neutrophils in metastasis. *Cell Res.* 2016;26(3):273–274.
1158. Peinado H, Zhang H, Matei IR, Costa-Silva B, Hoshino A, Rodrigues G, et al. Pre-metastatic niches: organ-specific homes for metastases. *Nat. Rev. Cancer.* 2017;17(5):302–317.
1159. Liu Y, Cao X. Characteristics and significance of the pre-metastatic niche. *Cancer Cell.* 2016;30(5):668–681.
1160. Gunjal PM, Schneider G, Ismail AA, Kakar SS, Kucia M, Ratajczak MZ. Evidence for induction of a tumor metastasis-receptive microenvironment for ovarian cancer cells in bone marrow and other organs as an unwanted and underestimated side effect of chemotherapy/radiotherapy. *J Ovarian Res.* 2015;8(1):20.
1161. Rachman-Tzemah C, Zaffryar-Eilot S, Grossman M, Ribero D, Timaner M, Mäki JM, et al. Blocking surgically induced lysyl oxidase activity reduces the risk of lung metastases. *Cell Rep.* 2017;19(4):774–784.
1162. Keklikoglou I, Cianciaruso C, Güç E, Squadrito ML, Spring LM, Tazzyman S, et al. Chemotherapy elicits pro-metastatic extracellular vesicles in breast cancer models. *Nat. Cell Biol.* 2019;21(2):190–202.
1163. Raskov H, Orhan A, Salanti A, Gögenur I. Pre-metastatic niches, exosomes and circulating tumor cells Early mechanisms of tumor dissemination and the relation to surgery. *Int. J. Cancer.* 2019.
1164. Bandari SK, Purushothaman A, Ramani VC, Brinkley GJ, Chandrashekar DS, Varambally S, et al. Chemotherapy induces secretion of exosomes loaded with heparanase that degrades extracellular matrix and impacts tumor and host cell behavior. *Matrix Biol.* 2018;65:104–118.
1165. Hiratsuka S, Watanabe A, Aburatani H, Maru Y. Tumour-mediated upregulation of chemoattractants and recruitment of myeloid cells predetermines lung metastasis. *Nat. Cell Biol.* 2006;8(12):1369–1375.
1166. Shaked Y, Henke E, Roodhart JM, Mancuso P, Langenberg MH, Colleoni M, et al. Rapid chemotherapy-induced acute endothelial progenitor cell mobilization: implications for antiangiogenic drugs as chemosensitizing agents. *Cancer Cell.* 2008;14(3):263–273.
1167. Zhang H, Yu Y, Zhou L, Ma J, Tang K, Xu P, et al. Circulating tumor microparticles promote lung metastasis by reprogramming inflammatory and mechanical niches via a macrophage-dependent pathway. *Cancer Immunol. Res.* 2018;6(9):1046–1056.
1168. Feys L, Descamps B, Vanhove C, Vral A, Veldeman L, Vermeulen S, et al. Radiation-induced lung damage promotes breast cancer lung-metastasis through CXCR4 signaling. *Oncotarget.* 2015;6(29):26615.
1169. Ratajczak MZ, Jadczyk T, Schneider G, Kakar SS, Kucia M. Induction of a tumor-metastasis-receptive microenvironment as an unwanted and underestimated side effect of treatment by chemotherapy or radiotherapy. *J Ovarian Res.* 2013;6(1):95.
1170. Erler JT, Bennewith KL, Cox TR, Lang G, Bird D, Koong A, et al. Hypoxia-induced lysyl oxidase is a critical mediator of bone marrow cell recruitment to form the premetastatic niche. *Cancer Cell.* 2009;15(1):35–44.
1171. Sceneay J, Chow MT, Chen A, Halse HM, Wong CS, Andrews DM, et al. Primary tumor hypoxia recruits CD11b+/Ly6Cmed/Ly6G+ immune suppressor cells and compromises NK cell cytotoxicity in the premetastatic niche. *Cancer Res.* 2012;72(16):3906–3911.
1172. Tai l, de Souza CT, Bélanger S, Ly L, Alkayyal AA, Zhang J, et al. Preventing postoperative metastatic disease by inhibiting surgery-induced dysfunction in natural killer cells. *Cancer Res.* 2013;73(1):97–107.
1173. Chai RC, Kouspou MM, Lang BJ, Nguyen CH, van der Kraan AGJ, Vieusseux JL, et al. Molecular stress-inducing compounds increase osteoclast formation in a heat shock factor 1 protein-dependent manner. *J. Biol. Chem.* 2014;289(19):13602–13614.
1174. Rana T, Chakrabarti A, Freeman M, Biswas S. Doxorubicin-mediated bone loss in breast cancer bone metastases is driven by an interplay between oxidative stress and induction of TGFβ. *PLoS ONE.* 2013;8(10).

1175. Chai RC, McDonald MM, Terry RL, Kovačić N, Down JM, Pettitt JA, et al. Melphalan modifies the bone microenvironment by enhancing osteoclast formation. *Oncotarget*. 2017;8(40):68047.
1176. King TJ, Georgiou KR, Cool JC, Scherer MA, Ang ES, Foster BK, et al. Methotrexate chemotherapy promotes osteoclast formation in the long bone of rats via increased pro-inflammatory cytokines and enhanced NF-κB activation. *Am. J. Pathol.* 2012;181(1):121–129.
1177. Zheng H, Bae Y, Kasimir-Bauer S, Tang R, Chen J, Ren G, et al. Therapeutic antibody targeting tumor-and osteoblastic niche-derived Jagged1 sensitizes bone metastasis to chemotherapy. *Cancer Cell*. 2017;32(6):731–747 e6.
1178. Sethi N, Dai X, Winter CG, Kang Y. Tumor-derived JAGGED1 promotes osteolytic bone metastasis of breast cancer by engaging notch signaling in bone cells. *Cancer Cell*. 2011;19(2):192–205.
1179. Park SI, Liao J, Berry JE, Li X, Koh AJ, Michalski ME, et al. Cyclophosphamide creates a receptive microenvironment for prostate cancer skeletal metastasis. *Cancer Res.* 2012;72(10):2522–2532.
1180. Mulholland BS, Forwood MR, Morrison NA. Monocyte Chemoattractant Protein-1 (MCP-1/CCL2) Drives Activation of Bone Remodelling and Skeletal Metastasis. *Curr Osteoporos Rep*. 2019;17(6):538–547.
1181. Mizutani K, Sud S, McGregor NA, Martinovski G, Rice BT, Craig MJ, et al. The chemokine CCL2 increases prostate tumor growth and bone metastasis through macrophage and osteoclast recruitment. *Neoplasia (New York, NY)*. 2009;11(11):1235.
1182. Gül N, Bögels M, Grewal S, van der Meer AJ, Rojas LB, Fluitsma DM, et al. Surgery-induced reactive oxygen species enhance colon carcinoma cell binding by disrupting the liver endothelial cell lining. *Gut*. 2011;60(8):1076–1086.
1183. Gül N, Grewal S, Bögels M, Van der Bij GJ, Koppes MM, Oosterling SJ, et al. Macrophages mediate colon carcinoma cell adhesion in the rat liver after exposure to lipopolysaccharide. *Oncoimmunology*. 2012;1(9):1517–1526.
1184. Peyvandi S, Lan Q, Lorusso G, Rüegg C. Chemotherapy-induced immunological breast cancer dormancy: a new function for old drugs? *J Cancer Metastasis Treat*. 2019;5:44.
1185. Sosa MS, Bragado P, Aguirre-Ghiso JA. Mechanisms of disseminated cancer cell dormancy: an awakening field. *Nat. Rev. Cancer*. 2014;14(9):611–622.
1186. Romero I, Garrido F, Garcia-Lora AM. Metastases in immune-mediated dormancy: a new opportunity for targeting cancer. *Cancer Res.* 2014;74(23):6750–6757.
1187. Giancotti FG. Mechanisms governing metastatic dormancy and reactivation. *Cell*. 2013;155(4):750–764.
1188. Möhrmann L, Zowada MK, Strakerjahn H, Siegl C, Kopp-Schneider A, Krunic D, et al. A perivascular niche in the bone marrow hosts quiescent and proliferating tumorigenic colorectal cancer cells. *Int. J. Cancer*. 2020.
1189. Grzelak CA, Ghajar CM. Metastasis 'systems' biology: how are macro-environmental signals transmitted into microenvironmental cues for disseminated tumor cells? *Curr. Opin. Cell Biol.* 2017;48:79–86.
1190. Carlson P, Dasgupta A, Grzelak CA, Kim J, Barrett A, Coleman IM, et al. Targeting the perivascular niche sensitizes disseminated tumour cells to chemotherapy. *Nat. Cell Biol.* 2019;21(2):238–250.
1191. Clever D, Roychoudhuri R, Constantinides MG, Askenase MH, Sukumar M, Klebanoff CA, et al. Oxygen sensing by T cells establishes an immunologically tolerant metastatic niche. *Cell*. 2016;166(5):1117–1131 e14.
1192. Tjensvoll K, Oltedal S, Heikkilä R, Kvaløy JT, Gilje B, Reuben JM, et al. Persistent tumor cells in bone marrow of non-metastatic breast cancer patients after primary surgery are associated with inferior outcome. *BMC Cancer*. 2012;12(1):190.
1193. Piranlioglu R, Lee E, Ouzounova M, Bollag RJ, Vinyard AH, Arbab AS, et al. Primary tumor-induced immunity eradicates disseminated tumor cells in syngeneic mouse model. *Nat. Commun.* 2019;10(1):1–13.
1194. Lawson MA, McDonald MM, Kovacic N, Khoo WH, Terry RL, Down J, et al. Osteoclasts control reactivation of dormant myeloma cells by remodelling the endosteal niche. *Nat. Commun.* 2015;6(1):1–15.
1195. Kubo H, Mensurado S, Gonçalves-Sousa N, Serre K, Silva-Santos B. Primary tumors limit metastasis formation through induction of IL15-mediated cross-talk between patrolling monocytes and NK cells. *Cancer Immunol. Res.* 2017;5(9):812–820.

1196. Ananth AA, Tai l, Lansdell C, Alkayyal AA, Baxter KE, Angka L, et al. Surgical stress abrogates pre-existing protective T cell mediated anti-tumor immunity leading to postoperative cancer recurrence. *PLoS ONE*. 2016;11(5).
1197. Albrengues J, Shields MA, Ng D, Park CG, Ambrico A, Poindexter ME, et al. Neutrophil extracellular traps produced during inflammation awaken dormant cancer cells in mice. *Science*. 2018;361(6409):eaao4227.
1198. Li T-S, Kaneda Y, Ueda K, Hamano K, Zempo N, Esato K. The influence of tumour resection on angiostatin levels and tumour growth—An experimental study in tumour-bearing mice. *Eur. J. Cancer*. 2001;37(17):2283–2288.
1199. Retsky M, Demicheli R, Hrushesky WJ. Does surgery induce angiogenesis in breast cancer? Indirect evidence from relapse pattern and mammography paradox. *International Journal of Surgery*. 2005;3(3):179–187.
1200. Al-Sahaf O, Wang JH, Browne TJ, Cotter TG, Redmond HP. Surgical injury enhances the expression of genes that mediate breast cancer metastasis to the lung. *Ann. Surg*. 2010;252(6):1037–1043.
1201. Peeters CF, De Waal RM, Wobbes T, Westphal JR, Ruers TJ. Outgrowth of human liver metastases after resection of the primary colorectal tumor: a shift in the balance between apoptosis and proliferation. *Int. J. Cancer*. 2006;119(6):1249–1253.

# CHAPTER 5

# Immunodeficiencies

**Mona Sadeghalvad**[a,b,c], **Nima Rezaei**[a,b,c]
[a]Department of Immunology, School of Medicine, Tehran University of Medical Sciences, Tehran, Iran
[b]Research Center for Immunodeficiencies, Children's Medical Center, Tehran University of Medical Sciences, Tehran, Iran
[c]Network of Immunity in Infection, Malignancy and Autoimmunity (NIIMA), Universal Scientific Education and Research Network (USERN), Tehran, Iran

## Introduction

Immunodeficiency refers to a group of diseases in which defects in one or more molecules or cells associated with the immune system lead to defects in the development of immune responses to pathogens. Immunodeficiency includes any developmental, differentiation, proliferative, or functional defect of one or more groups of immune system components and is divided into primary and secondary immunodeficiencies. Inborn errors of immunity (IEIs) or primary immunodeficiency diseases (PIDs) are caused by genetic disorders in one or more parts of the immune system, which are also called congenital immunodeficiency diseases. Genetic mutations, polymorphisms, and multigene disorders can cause primary immunodeficiencies. On the other hand, secondary or acquired immunodeficiency diseases are not genetic disorders and are caused by infectious agents or environmental factors such as acquired immunodeficiency syndrome (AIDS), nutritional disorders, or after taking certain therapies. Immune deficiencies can lead to the development of other disorders, including autoimmunity, allergies, and cancers.[1]

Immune deficiencies increase the risk of opportunistic infections. For example, antibodies serve a critical role in the eradication of extracellular pathogens. Therefore, recurrent infections with encapsulated bacteria are a symptom of insufficient antibody generation. In addition, antibodies are an important line of defense against respiratory tract infections. Infections with staphylococci, gram-negative organisms, and fungi may indicate impaired phagocyte function or a decrease in phagocyte numbers. On the other hand, T lymphocytes and macrophages are important in detecting and eradicating intracellular infections. Thus, T cell abnormalities or macrophage deficiencies frequently predispose individuals to intracellular infections like viruses and intracellular bacteria like mycobacteria.[2,3]

Early diagnosis of immunodeficiency disorders, particularly in childhood, can be very beneficial in treating, decreasing symptoms, and reducing mortality in children. Understanding deficiency disorders, symptoms, and approaches for diagnosing them can thus be a helpful step toward the early detection of these diseases. In this chapter,

*Clinical Immunology*
DOI: https://doi.org/10.1016/B978-0-12-818006-8.00004-9

we aimed to present the types of immunodeficiency diseases, their possible diagnosis and treatment.

## Initial screening of patients with immunodeficiencies

Recurrent infections are the most common clinical manifestation of immunodeficiency in general. The patient may have up to ten respiratory infections per year. As a result, a thorough history of the patient is required to evaluate infectious diseases and other problems in order to diagnose an immunodeficiency disorder. In a patient with primary immunodeficiency, failure to thrive (FTT), upper and lower respiratory tract infections, and chronic diarrhea are common manifestations. As a result, it is critical to assess clinical manifestations in addition to laboratory diagnostic assays. Some laboratory tests, including complete blood counts (CBC) and differential (platelet volume, absolute lymphocyte count, neutrophil and eosinophil counts), immunoglobulin levels (IgG, IgM, IgA), lymphocyte subpopulations, vaccine titers, and complement assessment (e.g., CH50, AH50), are considered essential initial tests in order to screen the patients with immunodeficiencies.[4,5]

Since T cells account for roughly 70 percent of circulating lymphocytes, lymphopenia could indicate a T-cell-related deficiency. A patient who has persistent leukocytosis, particularly between infections, may have a leukocyte adhesion deficiency. Thrombocytopenia can be used to screen for Wiskott-Aldrich syndrome. Reduced immunoglobulin levels may indicate an antibody deficiency. Although these laboratory evaluations are useful for the early screening of patients, additional tests are needed to make an accurate diagnosis, which may vary for each immunodeficiency depending on the initial screening.[6,7]

## Inborn errors of immunity (IEIs)

IEIs have a genetic basis and can be caused by genetic mutations or polymorphisms in any part of the immune system. There are several types of IEIs that can be divided into different types based on the specific immunodeficiency[8,9]:

1. Immunodeficiencies related to B lymphocytes and antibodies:
   - Agammaglobulinemia (X-linked and autosomal recessive forms)
   - Hypogammaglobulinemia (selective IgA deficiency, selective IgG deficiency, common variable immunodeficiency (CVID), and ICF syndrome)
   - Hyper IgM syndrome (HIGM) (X-linked and autosomal recessive forms)
2. Immune deficiencies related to T lymphocyte/ combined immunodeficiencies:
   - Severe combined immunodeficiencies, which in turn include a group of diseases such as defects in cytokine signaling (X-linked and autosomal recessive forms), defects in nucleotide salvage pathways (ADA deficiency, PNP deficiency), defects

in V (D) J recombination (recombination activating genes (RAG)1 and RAG2 deficiency, double-stranded break repair), and defects in thymus development (Di George syndrome, FoxN1 deficiency)
- Wiskott-Aldrich Syndrome
- Ataxia-telangiectasia
- X-linked lymphoproliferative disease (XLP)
- Defects in cytotoxic T lymphocytes (CTL) and natural killer (NK) cell activation
- FoxP3 mutation
- Autoimmune Lymphoproliferative Syndrome (ALPS)

3. Defects in the innate immune system:
   - Leukocyte Adhesion Defects (LADI, LADII, LADIII)
   - Chronic Granulomatosis Disease (CGD)
   - Shwachman-Diamond syndrome
   - Kostmann syndrome
   - Hyper-IgE syndrome
   - Defects in the signaling pathways (TLRs, NF-κB, interferon (IFN)-I
   - Defects in the complement system

## Humoral immunodeficiencies

Antibodies-related defects are the most common primary immunodeficiency diseases. Among them, selective serum IgA deficiency is the most common defect. Patients with antibody deficiency are often diagnosed with recurrent infections with encapsulated bacteria that often affect the upper and lower respiratory tract. However, the severity of the infection may be low in some patients with selective IgA deficiency or in infants.[10]

## X-linked agammaglobulinemia (XLA)

### *Definition*

XLA is known as Bruton's syndrome, and it is characterized by the development of defective B lymphocytes. The cause of the disease is a deletion or mutation in the gene encoding the enzyme *Bruton tyrosine kinase* (*Btk*). The abnormal gene is located on the long arm of chromosome X. Btk is a member of the cytoplasmic tyrosine kinases and is widely expressed in the B cell lineage, including pre B cells. Btk is involved in the pre B cell signaling pathway and is essential for the proliferation of pre B cells and their maturation into B cells expressing membrane immunoglobulin. Therefore, due to a defect in this enzyme, the development of pre B cells to immature B cells in the bone marrow is impaired, resulting in decreased frequencies of B cells in the bloodstream and severe hypogammaglobulinemia.[11]

### *Clinical manifestations and diagnosis*

Most patients with XLA are healthy in the first 6–9 months of life due to the presence of maternal IgG antibodies, which are responsible for protecting the baby during this time. The disease is often seen in males. Carriers are detected by mutation analysis, and prenatal diagnosis of infected male fetuses is possible. Due to the decreased serum antibodies, encapsulated and purulent extracellular infections such as haemophilus, pneumococcus, and staphylococcus are common in these patients. Besides, patients with XLA are more susceptible to Echoviruses. Chronic fungal infections and neutropenia are also seen.

Laboratory characteristics of XLA include a decrease or absence of the number of B cells, a lack of blood group antibodies, and a decrease in the gamma band on electrophoresis. The percentage of peripheral blood B lymphocytes is less than one percent, percentage of T cell subgroups and T cell function are normal. Clinically, tonsillitis is not seen in these patients, or it is very small. Also, their lymph nodes are intangible.

In general, an XLA diagnosis should be considered if lymph node hypoplasia is observed on physical examination and the patient has low serum concentrations of IgG, IgA, IgM, and IgE with a total immunoglobulin level below 100 mg/dL. In addition, in this disorder, the level of natural antibodies against blood group antigens (isohemagglutinins) is low. Flow cytometry is an important test to determine the absence of circulating B cells.[11,12]

### *Treatment*

Treatment of XLA is done with frequent broad-spectrum antibiotics along with receiving intravenous immunoglobulin G (IVIG). IVIG is currently a common treatment option for most antibody deficits and is given by infusion weekly or every two to four weeks. Dosage and intervals might be altered based on individual clinical responses. Antibiotics such as amoxicillin and amoxicillin/clavulanate are administered to prevent infections.

## Autosomal recessive agammaglobulinemia

Similar to XLA, the number of circulating B cells falls in this disorder, resulting in a drop in all antibody isotypes in serum. There is frequently a deficiency in pre-BCR signaling, and mutations are found in the heavy chain, the *surrogate light chain 5*, the p85a subunit of *phosphatidylinositol 3-kinase* (*PI3K*), and the *BLNK* genes.[13]

## Hyper IgM syndrome (HIGM)

### *Definition*

In these patients, normal or elevated IgM levels, deficiency or absence of IgG, IgA, and IgE indicate a defect in the antibody class switching process. These patients suffer recurrent bacterial infections or are predisposed to increased autoimmunity.[14,15]

### *Classification*

There are several types of HIGM, which are discussed further below:

### Type I hyper IgM (HIgM1)

The disease is x-linked and is caused by a mutation in the gene encoding cluster of differentiation (CD)40-ligand (CD154, CD40L). CD40L is expressed on helper T cells and its interaction with CD40 on B cells is necessary for isotype switching. Therefore, in boys with this syndrome, serum levels of IgG and IgA are very low, but IgM level is normal or sometimes elevated. Besides, the number of B cells is usually normal. The patients often have severe neutropenia. The lymph nodes are usually palpable. Due to T cell deficiency and impaired cellular immunity, *pneumocystis carinii* and *cryptosporidium* are common among these patients. It has been shown that autoimmune diseases and cancer are common in these individuals.

Similar to XLA patients, boys with CD40L deficiency have recurrent purulent infections, including otitis media, sinusitis, pneumonia, and tonsillitis in the first and second years of life. These patients have a normal number of circulating B lymphocytes, but the number of CD27+ memory cells has decreased. The number of circulating T cells and the response to mitogens in-vitro is normal.[16,17]

### Hyper IgM due to the NEMO mutation

This syndrome is predominant in boys and is clinically characterized by non-sweating ectodermal dysplasia with immunodeficiency. This condition is caused by a mutation in the *IKBKG* gene that encodes NEMO. NEMO is a regulatory protein needed to activate the NF-κB transcription factor. Mutations in the coding region of the *IKBKG* are associated with EDA-ID. Most patients show abnormal antibody responses to polysaccharide antigens.[18,19]

### Type II hyper IgM (HIgM2)

The disease is an autosomal recessive form of HIGM caused by mutations in the *activation-induced cytidine deaminase* (*AID*). AID is a DNA deaminase that is required for the somatic mutation of immunoglobulin genes. Affected patients usually have a normal number of circulating B lymphocytes, but their B cells are unable to switch from IgM-secreting cells to IgG, IgA, or IgE-secreting cells. Besides, these cells are not able to produce these antibodies in vitro even when treated with cytokines.

Histological evaluation of the lymph nodes shows the presence of large germinal centers with high frequencies of B cells. These cells express IgM, IgD, and CD38, which are thought to be in a transient state that initiates somatic mutations in the variable region of their immunoglobulin genes. Deficiency of AID in these cells leads to impaired ultimate differentiation of B cells and lack of somatic mutation.

In these patients, the serum concentration of IgG, IgA, and IgE is very low, but unlike patients with CD40 ligand deficiency, the serum concentration of IgM is increased. Patients with this type of HIGM have lymphoid hyperplasia, and their disease usually begins at an older age. Most of the patients have isohemagglutinins and are less likely to develop neutropenia.[20,21]

### Type III hyper IgM (HIgM3)

This form of hyper IgM is due to mutations in the CD40 molecule with autosomal recessive inheritance. CD40 is expressed on various cells, including B cells, macrophages, and dendritic cells. Clinical manifestations often include recurrent sinus and lung infections, pneumonia, and it is usually an indistinguishable disease of HIgM3. These patients have very low IgA and IgG levels. However, the level of IgM is normal.[22,23]

### Type IV hyper igm (HIgM4)

Patients with HIGM4 have a milder HIgM syndrome than those with HIGM2, but the defective genes in the disease have not yet been identified. The *AID* gene sequence is normal, but the defective expression of *AID* is thought to account for this disease.

HIgM4 patients, like HIgM2 patients, suffer from recurrent bacterial infections throughout childhood with no opportunistic infections, showing that T cell immunity is intact. Lymphoid organ hyperplasia in HIgM4 appears to be milder than in HIgM2. Autoimmune disorders, especially, cytopenia have been reported in these patients. The presence of normal (or high) IgM levels rules out CVID, which is defined by a reduction in the blood concentration of all Ig isotypes, including IgM. However, there may be an overlap between the two diseases.[24]

### Type V hyper igm (HIgM5)

The disease is caused by a mutation in the *Uracil N-Glycosylase* (*UNG*) gene. UNG, along with AID, is involved in antibody class switching. As mentioned earlier, AID is a deaminase enzyme involved in the deamination of cytosine (C) in target DNA and its conversion to uracil (U), which is removed by UNG. Defects in these enzymes are associated with increased IgM levels and high serum levels of IgG and IgA. These patients are also prone to bacterial infections as well as lymphoid hyperplasia.[25–27]

#### *Treatment*

The only curative treatment is stem cell transplantation, and an alternative treatment is monthly IVIG injections. Although this therapy is generally used for patients with X-linked HIGM or HIgM3. Besides, in patients with severe neutropenia, the use of granulocyte colony-stimulating factor (GCSF) is beneficial.

## Selective IgA deficiency

### Definition

This disease is the most common congenital immunodeficiency disorder, which is characterized by a complete absence or reduction of serum IgA levels. On the other hand, the level of IgM or IgG antibodies is normal and sometimes increased. In these patients, there are B cells with a normal phenotype in the blood, but the differentiation of B cells into IgA-secreting plasma cells is defective. Nevertheless, the phenotype or responses of T cells are normal. Because interleukin (IL)−5 and transforming growth factor (TGF)-β cytokines play an important role in the production of IgA, the cause of the defect is thought to be a defect in the production of these cytokines. Mutations in *Transmembrane Activator and Calcium modulator and cyclophilin ligand Interactor* (*TACI*) have also been reported in some patients.

TACI is one of the receptors of cytokines called B cell activating factor (BAFF) and a proliferation-inducing ligand (APRIL). This receptor plays an important role in the differentiation and survival of plasma cells. In addition to selective IgA deficiency, it is also considered an important cause of CVID, which will be described later. IgA deficiency may also occur transiently due to side effects of some medications.[28,29]

### Clinical manifestations and diagnosis

These patients often suffer from recurrent bacterial or viral sinus-pulmonary infections or celiac disease. Of course, some patients may be completely asymptomatic. This disease often occurs with CVID. In general, these patients are highly susceptible to allergies and often suffer from respiratory, gastrointestinal, and genitourinary tract infections. It has been observed that the incidence of autoimmune diseases and malignancies has increased in these patients. Laboratory findings include decreased IgA and normal levels of IgM and IgG. The frequency and function of T cells are normal.

### Treatment

Patients with IgA deficiency are often treated with broad-spectrum antibiotics. Treatment using IVIG is not effective because this product contains IgG that these patients make naturally. In addition, because some patients have serum antibodies against IgA, these patients may produce antibodies against the transmitted IgA, which can lead to type III hypersensitivity reactions or severe anaphylactic reactions.[28,29]

## Selective IgG deficiency

### Definition

IgG is the most abundant antibody in the serum, which includes four subclasses including IgG1-IgG4. It has been proposed that IgG subclass deficiency is one of the most common types of antibody deficiency. William Terry (1968) first described IgG subclass deficiency in a patient with recurrent infections. The mechanism causing selective IgG subclass deficiency in humans is mostly unknown, but it is probably the abnormal differentiation of inactive lymphocytes in this disease. In these patients, the serum level of IgG, IgA, and IgM antibodies is normal, but the concentration of one or more subclasses of IgG is lower than normal. IgG subclass deficiency has been associated with numerous other main immunodeficiencies, including selective IgA deficiency, selective IgM deficiency, and ataxia-telangiectasia. IgG3 and IgG2 deficiency are the most common types of deficiency in the IgG subclasses in adults and children, respectively.[30–33]

### *Clinical manifestations and diagnosis*

Some patients with very low concentrations or no IgG2 also have IgA deficiency. Some patients with IgG2 deficiency also develop CVID, indicating that a lack of an IgG subclass can be a sign of broader immunodeficiency. These people sometimes have recurrent infections and sometimes have no clinical symptoms. Selective IgG2 deficiency can be associated with respiratory infections importantly meningitis and pneumococcus. Recurrent respiratory infections and lung damage were also reported in patients with selective IgA deficiency who were also IgG2 deficient. In general, selective IgG2 deficiency is associated with increased susceptibility to infections with capsulated bacterial pathogens (e.g., *Streptococcus pneumoniae*).[30–33]

### *Treatment*

IVIG replacement therapy is currently the treatment of choice for individuals with an IgG subclass deficit. In addition, antibiotics are generally administered to prevent infections.

## Common variable immunodeficiency (CVID)

### *Definition*

CVID is a group of immunodeficiency diseases characterized by a decrease in the serum level of immunoglobulins and an increase in the incidence of infections. This abnormality may be diagnosed in early childhood or late life. Its manifestations and pathogenicity are highly variable and are usually diagnosed when other primary immunodeficiency diseases are ruled out. The inheritance pattern of this disease is autosomal dominant or recessive. Of course, most CVIDs are sporadic or have autosomal dominant inheritance patterns. The B cell phenotype is normal, but plasma cells are less present in the lymph tissues, which may indicate a defect in the differentiation of B cells into antibody-producing cells. In this regard, the mutations that cause this disorder include mutations in *T cell co-stimulator inducible co-stimulatory* (*ICOS*), *TACI*, *BAFF receptor* (*BAFFR*), *CD19*, *CD20*, and *CD81*. ICOS is a marker expressed on activated T cells and by binding to its ligand called ICOSL on the B cells, leads to the production of antibodies, follicular helper T cell (TFH) differentiation, and the production of memory cells.

TACI is involved in the proliferation and differentiation of B cells and the production of antibodies. As mentioned before, the TACI defect is also involved in IgA deficiency. BAFF is a cytokine involved in B cell proliferation and antibody production. Therefore, a defect in its receptor named BAFFR is associated with a decrease in antibody production. The frequency of T cells is usually normal, although T cell function is suppressed in some patients.[34,35]

### Clinical manifestations and diagnosis

Patients with CVID are unable to produce antibodies in response to immunization or natural infection. Their lymphatic tissues and bone marrow are basically free of plasma cells. They have normal or large tonsils and lymph nodes. These people suffer from recurrent respiratory infections such as sinusitis, otitis, bronchitis, and pneumonia. Due to the lack of mucosal antibodies, these patients are prone to gastrointestinal infections caused by Giardia lamblia. These patients are also prone to autoimmune diseases such as inflammatory bowel disease, rheumatoid arthritis, and pernicious anemia. In addition, the development of malignant tumors, especially lymphomas, is associated with this disease. These patients are often treated with IVIG and antibiotics. Laboratory symptoms include normal B cell count, NK cell count, decreased IgG production, and low serum antibodies. These patients may have thrombocytopenia and neutropenia.[34,35]

### Treatment

As with other humoral immunodeficiencies, treatment for patients with CVID involves immunoglobulin replacement therapy and preventive antibiotics.

## Laboratory assays for humoral immunity deficiencies

Quantitative immunoglobulin evaluations are the most important early screening when a humoral immunity-related immunodeficiency is suspected. Serum antibody titers may be used for frequent vaccinations like diphtheria, tetanus, and pneumococcus. Antibody titers in the serum are frequently detected using enzyme-linked immunoassay (ELISA).[36,37]

Several advanced techniques can be used to evaluate a patient suspected of having a humoral immune deficiency. For example, determination of B cell phenotype by analyzing the expression of B cell markers (e.g., IgM, IgD, IgG, CD19, CD20, CD27, and CD38). In this regard, patients with CVID and XLA (or Bruton) may have lower levels of memory B cells (CD27+, IgM-, IgD-) and a low or absent circulating B cell population.[38] Genome sequencing is another method that can be used to identify a specific mutation. For example, XLA is linked to a genetic defect in the *BTK* gene, while CVID and ataxia-telangiectasia are associated with a genetic defect in the *TACI*, *BAFFR*, and *ATM* genes, respectively.[39–42] Another method for determining whether or not a patient has a humoral immunodeficiency disorder is to use Kappa-deleting recombination excision circle (KREC). KRECs are episomal DNA fragments that are produced during B lymphocyte development, particularly when the kappa light-chain genes are rearranged. KRECs can be detected in newborn blood spots using polymerase chain reaction (PCR), which can be used to screen for B cell-related deficiencies such as XLA and ataxia-telangiectasia.[43]

## Cellular immunodeficiencies and combined immunodeficiencies

There are a variety of immunodeficiency diseases in which the number and function of T cells are impaired. Immunodeficiencies related to T lymphocytes or combined immunodeficiencies are more severe than B cell and antibody deficiencies, and these patients rarely live beyond childhood. In this section, we will review types of T cell-associated or combined immunodeficiencies.

### Di george syndrome

#### *Definition*

This immunodeficiency is due to a congenital disorder in the development of the thymus epithelium, which is characterized by thymus hypoplasia or lack of thymus formation, resulting in impaired cellular immunity. The animal model of this disease is nude mice that, in addition to thymus hypoplasia, lack hair and have inherited abnormal skin epithelial cells. These patients are susceptible to viral and fungal infections and are deficient in response to thymus-dependent antigens. The disease is often caused by a deletion on chromosome 22q11. There are several genes in this area, including *TBX1*, which is known to be the main cause of Di George syndrome. It should be noted that the *FOXN1* gene mutation is also associated with an immunological defect related to an alteration of the thymic epithelial stroma. *FOXN1* mutation causes severe combined immunodeficiencies (SCID) with the phenotype of T-/lowB+NK+ and other several features involving the skin and hair.[44,45]

#### *Clinical manifestations and diagnosis*

Children with Di George syndrome may grow normally but are more susceptible to infection with opportunistic pathogens, including fungi and viruses. In addition to thymus deficiency or thymus hypoplasia, these patients could show a wide spectrum of clinical features, including hypothyroidism, cardiovascular disorders, vessel malformations, and facial dysmorphisms. Hypothyroidism is associated with decreased parathyroid hormone levels, decreased calcium absorption, as well as increased phosphorus levels. Serum immunoglobulin concentrations are usually normal, but IgA may be decreased. The number of T cells decreased, and increased levels of B cells were found. Early diagnosis of this disease is crucial and can be fatal if left untreated. Infants born with primary hypothyroidism should be screened for Di George and T cell counts.[44,45]

### Treatment

Thymus transplantation with major histocompatibility complex (MHC) compatibility could be a good therapeutic approach for patients with Di George syndrome.

## Severe combined immunodeficiencies (SCID)

SCID includes a group of immunodeficiencies caused by gene mutations that lead to defects in both B and T cells. In addition, the function of NK cells may be impaired. Affected infants have lymphopenia and develop skin infections, recurrent diarrhea, pneumonia, and otitis media in the first few months of life. Patients have a small thymus without lymphocytes and no corticomedullary region. However, histologically, the thymus epithelium is normal. In addition, there are no tonsils and lymph nodes and Peyer's patches. Infants with developmental defects are prone to opportunistic infections such as *Pneumocystis jirovecii*, *Candida albicans*, and *Epstein-Barr virus (EBV)*. Neonates have T cell lymphopenia and lack lymphocyte proliferative responses to mitogens in vitro. It is a pediatric emergency, and death usually occurs in the first year of life unless stem cell transplantation or gene therapy is performed. There are several types of SCIDs that we will discuss below. X-linked SCID is caused by mutations in the common gamma chain ($\gamma$c), and autosomal recessive SCID could be caused by mutations in several genes, including *ADA*, *PNP*, *Janus kinase 3* (*Jak3*), *IL-7R*$\alpha$, *RAG1*, *RAG2*, *Artemis*, *DNA protein kinases*, *CD3* and *CD45*.[46,47]

### SCID caused by gamma chain mutation

It is an X-linked disease and the most common form of SCID. The disease is caused by a mutation in a gene encoding $\gamma$c, an important component for signaling cytokines including IL-2, IL-4-IL-7, IL-9, 1L-15, and IL-21. Importantly, IL-7 is needed for the development of immature thymocytes, and defects in the IL-7 receptor could result in impaired development of thymocytes. In addition, IL-15 is a potent stimulus for NK cell proliferation, and its receptor uses the gamma chain for signal transduction. Therefore, a defect in the function of IL-15 leads to a deficiency of NK cells. In general, X-linked SCID is characterized by defects in the maturation of T cells, NK, and a sharp decrease in the frequency of mature T cells and NK cells. However, the number of B cells is usually normal or increased that is generally characterized by the T-*B*+NK- phenotype. Because the existence of T cells is also required for B cell responses and antibody production, humoral immunodeficiency in these patients is due to a lack of T cell help.[48,49]

### SCID caused by defects in adenosine deaminase (ADA)

This form is the second most common form of SCID after X-linked SCID. The *ADA* gene is on chromosome 20q, and its point and deletion mutations can lead to ADA defects. ADA is an enzyme involved in the deamination of adenosine to inosine as well as 2-deoxyadenosine to 2-deoxyinosine in the purine salvage pathway. ADA deficiency leads to an increase in 2-deoxyadenosine and adenosine, which have toxic effects on T cells. These patients have more severe lymphopenia than other forms of SCID, and the number of T, B, and NK cells is very low. However, the function of NK cells is normal. Pneumonia, slowed growth, chronic diarrhea, and skin rashes are the earliest symptoms of ADA deficiency.[50,51]

### SCID caused by defects in purine nucleoside phosphorylase (PNP)

This disease is another rare autosomal recessive type of SCID that is caused by a defect in the enzyme PNP. Like ADA, this enzyme is involved in the catabolism of purines (salvage pathway) and the conversion of inosine to hypoxanthine and guanosine to guanine. PNP deficiency is associated with increased deoxyguanosine and deoxyguanosine triphosphate, which causes apoptosis of T cells, and also leads to the destruction of the nervous system. The disease is characterized by recurrent infections, neurologic symptoms, and autoimmune disorders like autoimmune hemolytic anemia, autoimmune neutropenia, lupus, and idiopathic thrombocytopenia (ITP).[52–54]

### SCID caused by mutation in RAG1 and RAG2

RAG1 and RAG2 are the important enzymes involved in V(D)J recombination. Mutations in these two enzymes lead to the most severe form of SCID with the B-T-NK+ phenotype. These patients do not have B and T lymphocytes, but the frequency of NK cells is normal. These patients have leukocytosis with lymphocytosis and eosinophilia and low levels of IgG, IgA, and IgM antibodies. In addition to RAG1 and RAG2, a defect in another enzyme involved in the recombination process, called Artemis, also leads to an inability to V(D) J recombination. Children with these mutations do not have B and T lymphocytes.[55–57]

### SCID caused by defects in interleukin-7 receptor a (IL-7Ra)

It is the third most common form of SCID, characterized by a lack of T cells and a normal or increased number of B cells (phenotype T-*B*+NK+). The disease has an autosomal recessive inheritance pattern. In general, IL-7R is composed of two chains, including IL-7Ra (also known as CD127) and γc, and its expression is essential for the normal development of T cells. This receptor is involved in inducing proliferative and survival signals to thymocytes during the early stages of T cell development. Patients with mutations in the IL-7R gene are prone to recurrent infections, prolonged diarrhea, FTT, infection with *pneumocystis jirovicii*, and lymph node hypoplasia. The frequency of T cells is significantly decreased. However, the number of B cells is normal or even increased.[58,59]

### SCID caused by defects in CD45

CD45 is a membrane molecule called leukocyte common antigen that is expressed on the surface of hematopoietic cells. This molecule has tyrosine kinase activity and is involved in the stimulation of tyrosine kinases involved in the activation of T and B cells.[60–62]

### SCID caused by defects in CD3σ, CD3ε, *and* CD3ζ

*CD3σ, CD3ε, CD3ζ* are components of the T cell receptor that participate in the signal transduction of the receptor. These molecules are essential for the development of T cells inside the thymus. Thus, mutations in these genes lead to a severe deficiency of circulating mature T cells. In this form of SCID, B and T cells are normal and have a phenotype similar to IL-7Rα-SCID (phenotype T-*B*+NK+).[63–65]

### *SCID caused by defects in ZAP70*

ZAP70 deficiency is a rare autosomal recessive form of SCID caused by a mutation in the *ZAP70* gene. ZAP70 is a tyrosine kinase that plays a significant role in triggering T cell responses and T cell signal transduction. The transition from the double-positive stage (CD4+ CD8+) during T cell development in the thymus is arrested in ZAP70 deficient mice. This form of SCID is characterized by a lack of CD8+ T cells and a normal frequency of nonfunctional CD4+ T cells in the peripheral blood. Therefore, the patients are susceptible to a variety of infections, and they are fatal if untreated. The diagnosis is usually made within the first six months of life.[66–68]

### *SCID caused by defects in JAK3*

*JAK3* gene is located on chromosome 19 and encodes an enzyme, which is critical for the function of γc. JAK3 deficiency is also an autosomal recessive form of SCID, and patients are clinically similar to other patients with SCID. The patients have a similar phenotype to X-SCID patients ($T^-$ *B*+NK-). These patients have a very low number of T and NK cells and an increased percentage of B cells.[69–71]

### *SCID caused by defects in ORAI1 and STIM1*

ORAI1 and STIM1 deficiencies are other rare forms of SCID. Ca2+ influx through specific Ca2+ channels in the plasma membrane is required for lymphocyte activation. The Ca2+ release activated Ca2+ (CRAC) channel encoded by the gene ORAI1 is the most prominent Ca2+ channel in T cells. ORAI1 is triggered by the stromal interaction molecule (STIM) 1, which is found in the endoplasmic reticulum (ER) and detects the levels of accumulated Ca2+. The activation of STIM1 occurs following antigen binding to TCR when the Ca2+ stores in the ER are depleted. Subsequently, the ORAI1-CRAC channels open, leading to the entrance of Ca2+. This process is essential for lymphocyte activation. Defects in ORAI1 and STIM1 genes result in the expression of non-functional or absent ORAI1 or STIM1. This immunodeficiency is associated with muscular hypotonia, anhidrotic ectodermal dysplasia, autoimmunity, and lymphoproliferative disease. These patients' immunodeficiency is caused by significant impairment in T cell activation but not lymphocyte development.[72,73]

### SCID caused by defects in adenylate kinase 2 (Reticular dysgenesis)

The disease is an autosomal recessive form of SCID caused by a mutation in the gene encoding adenylate kinase 2 (AK2). This disorder is extremely rare, accounting for approximately 1 percent−3 percent of SCID patients. The AK2 protein regulates the amount of adenosine diphosphate, and in its absence, apoptosis of lymphoid and myeloid precursors increases. Therefore, the disease is caused by defects in the development of lymphoid and myeloid precursors. Monocytes and neutrophils have been reduced substantially. Despite the lack of monocytes, macrophages are found in normal quantities in the dermis and (abnormal) lymphoid tissues. Affected patients lacked peripheral blood lymphocytes and granulocytes, and bone marrow.[74,75]

### Treatment

The treatment of choice for patients with various types of SCID is stem cell transplantation. Enzyme replacement therapy can also be performed in patients with ADA and PNP deficiency. After stem cell transplantation, B cell function also improves due to improved T cell function. For patients with reticular dysgenesis, short-term GM-CSF treatment can alleviate the symptoms by increasing stem cell differentiation. However, this disease is fatal without bone marrow/hematopoietic stem cell transplantation because of overwhelming infections.

## Wiskott-aldrich syndrome

### Definition

The disease is X-linked and is caused by a defect in the expression of the WASP protein. The *WASP* gene is located on the short arm of the X chromosome and encodes a protein that is essential for the accumulation of actin filaments needed to form microvesicles and rearrange the cytoskeleton. This protein is expressed only in bone marrow-derived cells. Defects in this protein lead to defects in the activation and formation of synapses in lymphocytes and defective migration of all leukocytes.[76,77]

### Clinical manifestations and diagnosis

The disease is a combination of cellular and humoral deficiencies and is associated with eczema, thrombocytopenia, and immunodeficiency. The patients exhibit severe eczema and recurrent infections with purulent and opportunistic microorganisms, usually during the first year of life. *Streptococcus pneumoniae* and other bacteria with polysaccharide capsules lead to otitis media, pneumonia, meningitis, and sepsis. Platelets and leukocytes are small and do not develop normally, and have difficulty migrating. These patients have normal IgG levels and increased IgE and IgA. Because of the decreased levels of IgM, the patients have a poor response to polysaccharides. Secondary responses to protein antigens are absent or very weak. Bleeding in the first six months of life, especially in boys, and diarrhea are the first symptoms of this disease. Infections, bleeding, and malignancies associated with *EBV* are the most common causes of death.[76–79]

### *Treatment*

Splenectomy, bone marrow transplantation, IVIG, and antibiotics are treatments for this disease.

## Ataxia-telangiectasia

### *Definition*

Ataxia-telangiectasia is a complex multisystem syndrome that varies in severity and may affect both B and T cells. The disease is caused by a mutation in the *ATM* gene. *ATM* is located on the long arm of chromosome 11 and encodes a protein kinase that is involved in controlling cell cycle checkpoints and apoptosis in response to double-stranded DNA breaks. Defects in this protein lead to impaired DNA repair, chromosomal abnormalities, or impaired production of antigen receptors.[80,81]

### *Clinical manifestations and diagnosis*

This is an autosomal recessive syndrome characterized by immunological, endocrinological, neurological, cutaneous, and hepatic abnormalities. The disorder is characterized by progressive difficulty with control of movement (ataxia) that begins to develop usually at the age of 3 to 6 years. Patients are prone to bacterial infections of the upper and lower respiratory tract, multiple autoimmune disorders, chromosomal instability, and an increased incidence of cancer. The most severe manifestations of the disease, which are associated with varying degrees of humoral and cellular immunodeficiency, are cerebellar ataxia, ocular-telangiectasia, abnormal control of eye movement, and a high incidence of malignancies. Due to the important role of the ATM protein in immunoglobulin class switching, IgA and IgG are decreased. Increased levels of alpha fetoprotein (AFP) could be found in the serum after two years of age. Defects in cellular immunity could be associated with thymus hypoplasia.[80,81]

### **Treatment**

Currently, there is no treatment for this disease. However, treatment is aimed at preventing neurodegeneration, respiratory infections, and supporting immune system function. The treatments are mostly aimed at preventing and managing symptoms.

## X-linked lymphoproliferative syndrome (XLP)

### *Definition*

XLP is a rare immunodeficiency characterized by an impaired immune response to infection with *EBV*. The inability to remove *EBV* leads to severe infectious mononucleosis and is associated with the development of B cell tumors and hypogammaglobulinemia. In this disease, the decreased responses of CTL, NK, and natural killer T cells (NKT) and severe *EBV* infection with the unlimited proliferation of B cells have been found. There are two types of XLP, which are determined by the type of mutation. In XLP1, which accounts for about 80 percent of patients, there is a defect in the SLAM-associated protein (SAP). SAP is a protein that is encoded by *SH2D1A* and participates in signal transduction to stimulate T and NK cells. This protein transmits signals through the signaling lymphocytic activation molecule (SLAM). In this regard, SAP binds the SLAM protein to induce Fyn kinase and trigger cell signaling transduction. Defects in the SAP lead to a decrease in the activity of NK and T cell cells and are thus associated with increased susceptibility to viral infections. In addition, SAP is necessary for the development of helper T cells, and patients with SAP deficiency have difficulty in developing the germinal center and producing high-affinity antibodies. In XLP2, there is a defect in the gene encoding X-linked inhibitor of apoptosis (XIAP). This defect leads to increased apoptosis of T cells and NKT cells.[82,83]

### *Clinical manifestations and diagnosis*

Nearly half of patients with XLP develop severe, life-threatening mononucleosis that is characterized by pharyngitis, fever, swollen lymph nodes, splenomegaly, and hepatomegaly. Liver and bone marrow damage could result in life-threatening complications. Aplastic anemia and thrombocytopenia can also be found in XLP patients. Thrombocytopenia makes the patients more prone to excessive bleeding. The patients may develop B cell lymphomas subsequent to *EBV* exposure. These lymphomas are distinguished by the malignant transformation of abnormally proliferating B lymphocytes.[82,83]

### *Treatment*

Treatment for affected individuals identified with XLP following *EBV* exposure may include medicines to prevent opportunistic infections, such as prophylactic antibiotic therapy and IVIG administration.

## Familial homophagocytosis lymphohistocytosis syndrome (FHL)

### *Definition*

Familial homophagocytosis lymphohistocytosis syndrome (FLH) is a group of immunodeficiency disorders caused by defects in the activation of killer cells, including CTL and NK cells, inherited in an autosomal recessive pattern. Defect in perforin, which is the most important component of the CTL and NK cell granules, is the most common form of FHL. Mutations in various genes, including mutations in *RAB27* and *MUNC13*, all of which are involved in granular exocytosis, can contribute to the disease. Defects in the release of cytolytic granules lead to uncontrolled viral infections resulting in the proliferation of unfunctional CTLs producing excessive amounts of tumor necrosis factor (TNF) and IFN-$\gamma$. Subsequently, macrophages are activated by these cytokines, which can be involved in the ingestion of red blood cells (hemophagocytosis) and leukocytes.[84]

### Clinical manifestations and diagnosis

Overactivation and the excessive response of T cells and macrophages to compensate for NK and CTL cell defects are thought to lead to hemophagocytosis and lymphadenopathy. This overactivation causes fever, and damages the liver and spleen, leading to hepatomegaly and splenomegaly, respectively. In FLH, the brain may also be affected, resulting in neurological problems. The signs and symptoms of FLH commonly develop during infancy, but they can appear later in life as well. Most patients with FLH die within a few months if they do not receive therapy.[84]

### Treatment

The disease is usually fatal. However, it may be treated with immunosuppressive drugs and hematopoietic stem cell therapy.

## Autoimmune lymphoproliferative syndrome (ALPS)

### Definition

ALPS is a rare disorder with an autosomal dominant pattern characterized by uncontrolled and severe proliferation of lymphocytes accompanied by lymphoma, despite the fact that a limited percentage of cases are inherited in an autosomal recessive manner. Patients are prone to systemic autoimmune diseases and increased susceptibility to chronic viral infections. The main cause of this disease is a mutation in the gene encoding Fas (CD95). Fas is a molecule whose interaction with the Fas ligand (CD178 or FasL) expressed on activated lymphocytes is involved in cell apoptosis and the establishment of immune homeostasis. Fas defect is associated with a lack of apoptosis of hyperactive and self-reactive lymphocytes, which leads to uncontrolled proliferation of lymphocytes and eventually the development of lymphoma.[85]

### Clinical manifestations and diagnosis

Mutations in *Fas* are associated with lymphadenopathy, hepatosplenomegaly, and autoimmune cytopenia. The symptoms of this disease are due to the lack of regulation of the immune system, which causes enlargement of the lymph nodes, liver, and spleen. Affected individuals are more likely to develop lymphoma as well as other cancers. They may also suffer from a number of autoimmune illnesses, most of which cause blood cell, nerve, liver, and kidney destruction. The patients with ALPS also have skin rashes, arthritis, vasculitis, and neurological damage.[85]

### Treatment

Depending on the severity of the disorder, treatment may involve steroids or other drugs, blood transfusions, and/or splenectomy.

## Immune dysregulation- Polyendocrinopathy-enteropathy -x-linked syndrome (IPEX)

### *Definition*

Immune dysregulation- Polyendocrinopathy-Enteropathy-X-linked syndrome (IPEX), which is an X-linked disorder, is due to a mutation in the gene encoding FoxP3, a critical regulator of regulatory T (Treg) cell gene expression. FoxP3 is responsible for the suppressive ability of Tregs. Defects in this molecule lead to dysfunction of Treg lymphocytes, and as a result, active self-reactive lymphocytes penetrate the target organs and cause damage. IPEX syndrome can be fatal in infancy.[86]

### *Clinical manifestations and diagnosis*

Symptoms include skin rashes, uncontrolled diarrhea, and insulin-dependent diabetes that occurs in the first months of life. Almost all patients with IPEX syndrome have an intestinal disorder known as autoimmune enteropathy that causes severe diarrhea, which is the primary symptom of IPEX syndrome and usually manifests in the first few months of life. Autoimmune enteropathy could also result in FTT and weight loss. Due to disruption of cutaneous and mucosal barriers, dermatitis or skin irritation is common in people with IPEX syndrome. The patients might suffer from a variety of endocrine gland disorders. Type 1 diabetes mellitus, which can occur within the first few months of life, is the most frequent endocrine problem. People with IPEX syndrome may develop autoimmune thyroid dysfunction as well. However, these patients may also have other symptoms, such as thrombocytopenia, anemia, and neutropenia caused by the immune system responses.[86]

### *Treatment*

Hematopoietic stem cell transplantation is an effective treatment for this disorder. Of course, the use of immunosuppressive drugs could also be effective in the control of autoimmunity.

## Bare lymphocyte syndrome

### *Definition*

It is a rare disease characterized by defects in MHC II molecules. Because the expression of MHC II molecules is essential in the development of CD4+ T cells, a defect in this molecule leads to a decrease in CD4+ T cells. In most cases, the expression of MHC I is normal or slightly decreased. Their CTL cells are also normal. Decreased CD4+ T cells and their cytokines could lead to disruption of the interaction of CD40-CD40L, resulting in hypogammaglobulinemia. Mutations in genes such as *Class II transactivator (CIITA)*, *Regulatory Factor X5 (RFX5)*, *Regulatory Factor X Associated Ankyrin Containing Protein (RFXANK)*, and *Regulatory Factor X Associated Protein (RFXAP)* can contribute to the disease. These are transcription factors involved in the expression of the MHC II molecules.

Autosomal recessive defects in MHC I are also found, which make up less than 10 percent of cases and lead to CD8+ T cell deficiency. Mutations in the *Transporter Associated with Antigen Processing 1 (TAP1)* and *TAP2* genes are involved in this disorder. These proteins are involved in the transport of peptides from the cytosol into the ER, which ultimately leads to the assembly of MHC I molecules on the cell surface. In this disease, the number and selection process of CTLs in the thymus is impaired. Due to the presence of normal MHC II molecules, antibody production is normal.[87]

### Clinical manifestations and diagnosis

The disease usually occurs during the first year of life and is usually fatal unless treated with a bone marrow transplant. Patients with MHC II Deficiency develop persistent diarrhea, which is often caused by enterovirus and cryptosporidium infections. In addition, patients are prone to viral herpes infections, bacterial pneumonia, and sepsis. Patients with MHC II deficiency have a decreased frequency of CD4+ T cells, but CD8+ T cells are normal or increased. MHC II antigens are not detectable at the cell surface, and patients have hypogammaglobulinemia.

Patients with MHC I deficiency possess serum MHC I antigens and β2-microglobulin. However, the MHC I molecules are not detectable on the cell surface. There is a defect in CD8+ T cells, and CD4+ T cells are normal.[87]

### Treatment

As of yet, allogeneic stem cell transplantation is the only treatment that has proven to be effective. However, some patients may need IVIG therapy. The treatment for bare lymphocyte syndrome aims to alleviate the disease's symptoms, prevent infections, and improve the quality of life.

## Laboratory assays for cellular immunity deficiencies

A CBC with differential can be conducted on a patient suspected of having cellular immunodeficiency to distinguish newborns with low/absent absolute lymphocyte counts. The frequency and function of T cells can then be assessed using flow cytometry and in-vitro functional analysis. The counts of CD3, CD4, CD8, NK, and B cells can be distinguished using flow cytometry. T lymphocyte markers CD3, CD4, and CD8 are typically reduced in abnormalities associated with cellular immunity, such as Di George Syndrome. Increased frequencies of CD45RO+ T cells are reported in Omenn syndrome. CD45RA is a naïve T cell marker in neonates, but CD45RO is a memory T cell marker that can be used to identify maternal T cells.[88,89]

The cutaneous delayed-type hypersensitivity (DTH) assays are another way to examine T cell function. It is important to mention that DTH is not suggested for children under the age of 12 months. The cellular mediated memory response is identified in these assays by injecting antigens such as purified protein derivative (PPD), *Candida albicans*, and mumps into the skin. The outcome is determined by measuring cutaneous induration 48–72 h later.

Another essential test for determining T cell activity is the Lymphocyte Mitogen Assay. T cell mitogens are utilized to stimulate lymphocytes in this assay. The radiolabeled thymidine that can be integrated into the DNA of proliferating cells is used to conduct the quantification. Mitogens for T cell stimulation include phytohemagglutinin (PHA), anti-CD3 antibodies, and concanavalin (ConA). Pokeweed (PWM) can be used to trigger both T and B cell responses.[90,91]

T cell replication excision circle (TREC) is a novel test that can be used to screen infants for severe T cell lymphopenia. The use of TREC to assess patients with cellular immunodeficiencies has resulted in early diagnosis and a reduction in morbidity and mortality. TRECs are circular, non-replicating fragments of DNA created following TCR rearrangement and can be used to identify naïve T cells.[92]

Another method for detecting cellular immunity abnormalities and combined immunodeficiency, in which both the cellular and humoral immune systems are compromised, is genetic evaluation of specific genes. The genetic evaluation might be complemented with the examination of the patient's protein level. A mutation in the WAS protein (WASp), for example, is linked to WAS. Flow cytometry detection of WASp allows for quick screening for this disorder. In addition, Quantitative real-time PCR has high sensitivity and specificity for mutation identification. However, fluorescent in situ hybridization (FISH) is a newer approach for detecting gene alterations. This approach can discover deletions at 22q11 that result in Di George Syndrome.[93,94]

The causative genetic deficiencies of several phenotypes of SCID, including T-/*B*+/NK-, T-/*B*+/NK+, T-/B-/NK+, T-/B-/NK-, have been identified, which could be detected by genetic analysis and flow cytometry technique. The most common type of SCID is X-linked SCID (T-/*B*+/NK- phenotype), which is caused by a lack of the common gamma chain (CD132) or Jak3. IL-7Rα, CD3, CD45, ZAP70, and Coronin-1A deficiency are all linked to the T-/*B*+/NK+ phenotype of SCID. Gene deficiencies in *RAG1* or *RAG2*, *Artemis*, *Ligase4* (LIG4), *DNA-dependent protein kinase* (*DNA-PK* or *PRKDC*), and *Cernunnos* are linked to the T-/B-/NK+ phenotype. In addition, the T-/B-/NK- phenotype is linked to deficits in adenosine deaminase (ADA), purine nucleoside phosphorylase (PNP), and adenylate kinase 2 (AK2).[95,96]

## Innate immunity immunodeficiencies

The innate and adaptive components of the immune system collaborate to control and neutralize the numerous infections that threaten vertebrates. Although innate immunity may look unsophisticated at first glance, innate immune cells may coordinate unique immune responses to different illnesses by recognizing diverse pathogens via germline-encoded pattern recognition receptors. The innate immune system consists of immune cells and mediators, including macrophages, neutrophils, dendritic cells, NK cells and NKT cells, the complement system, cytokines, antimicrobial agents, and epithelial and mucosal barriers. Innate immunodeficiencies are a group of abnormalities characterized by defects in one or more components of the innate immune system, which will be described in detail below.[97]

## Leukocyte adhesion deficiency (LAD)

### *Definition*

Leukocyte adhesion defects include three types, LADI, LADII, and LADIII, with an autosomal recessive inheritance pattern. This disorder is rare and is characterized by defects in the adhesion and function of leukocytes. Neutrophilia is evident; however, neutrophils have defects in adhesion, movement, and function. As a result, these individuals are prone to recurrent bacterial and fungal infections.[98]

### Leukocyte adhesion deficiency i (LADI)

The disease is characterized by defects in the adhesion molecules of the beta2-integrins family. Members of this family of adhesive molecules have two chains: 1) Alpha chain that is different between the members and 2) Common beta chain. In general, the beta-integrin family consists of three groups, which are involved in the attachment of leukocytes to other cells (such as endothelial cells, in order to exit the bloodstream), as well as in the binding to pathogens and the induction of phagocytosis.[99] These include:

1. LFA1 (CD11a CD18)
2. Mac1 (CD11b CD18): also known as iC3b receptor or CR3
3. CR4 (CD11c CD18): also known as p150,95, $\alpha X\beta 2$

In patients with LADI, defects in the beta chain (CD18) lead to a decrease in the function of neutrophils in phagocytosis, chemotaxis, and diapedesis. In other words, neutrophils are unable to bind to the intercellular adhesion molecule (ICAM)−1 and ICAM-2 molecules, which are expressed on the inflamed endothelial surface due to defects in CD18, and cannot migrate to the site of infection. Hence, these patients have a disorder in response to pyogenic infections. Also, due to the impaired iC3b receptor, neutrophils are unable to detect pathogens bound to opsonin iC3b.[100]

### Leukocyte adhesion deficiency ii (LADII)

The disease is caused by a defect in the sialyl-Lewis X (sLex/CD15s). This molecule is expressed on the surface of neutrophils and is required for binding to E-selectin and P-selectin expressed on the active endothelium cells. The disease is caused by mutations in genes encoding enzymes involved in fucose metabolism, leading to the absence of fucose in the carbohydrate structure of sialyl-Lewis. In these patients, the rolling function of neutrophils is impaired, which is considered the first step in the migration of neutrophils to the site of infection. Patients with LADII have similar clinical manifestations to LADI, but the infections are milder in these patients.[101]

### Leukocyte adhesion deficiency III (LADIII)

This disease is clinically similar to LADI but has impaired inside-out signaling of integrins. There is a disruption in the activation of integrins, which is necessary for the strong attachment of leukocytes to the endothelium. In some patients, a mutation occurs in the gene encoding KINDLIN-3, which plays a role in integrin signal transduction. Due to integrin dysfunction in platelets, increased bleeding is observed in these patients.[98]

#### *Clinical manifestations and diagnosis*

Symptoms of these patients include abscesses, hepatosplenomegaly, pneumonia, delayed umbilical cord clamping, and gingivitis. Affected children are prone to recurrent bacterial infections of the skin, mouth, respiratory tract, intestinal tract, and genitals. Delay in umbilical cord clamping is often associated with infection. The presence of omphalitis is an important manifestation that differentiates patients from healthy children. Skin infections can lead to large chronic sores. Severe gingivitis can lead to premature loss of primary teeth. Patients are unable to produce pus, and the number of neutrophils in the lesions is low. Neutrophilia is one of the consequences of the disease. Diagnosis of the disease is by flow cytometry technique and measuring the marker of CD11a CD18 on the surface of neutrophils in LADI and measuring CD15 (sLex) in LADII. Patients' antibody levels are normal; however, some patients have defects in T cell-dependent responses.[98–101]

#### *Treatment*

Bone marrow transplantation is the best treatment, and the patients need supportive care, including treatment with broad-spectrum antibiotics.

## Chronic granulomatosis disease (CGD)

#### *Definition*

The disease is caused by a defect in the killing function of phagocytes and the production of antimicrobial active oxygen metabolites. More specifically, patients with CGD have a defect in one of the subunits of the enzyme called phagocyte oxidase or nicotinamide adenine dinucleotide phosphate (NADPH) oxidase. This enzyme in phagocytes plays a vital role in pathogen killing and the phagocytosis process. NADPH oxidase is composed of cytoplasmic and transmembrane subunits in phagocytes. In this regard, once the phagocyte cell is activated, three cytosolic components of this complex called $p47^{phox}$, $p67^{phox}$, and $p40^{phox}$ are transferred to the phagocyte cell membrane. Initially, $p47^{phox}$ is phosphorylated and moves to the phagosome membrane along with $p40^{phox}$ and $p67^{phox}$. Subsequently, $p47^{phox}$ binds to cytochrome B558 ($Cyt_{b558}$, a heterodimer including the $gp91^{phox}$ and $p22^{phox}$ subunits), and a complete NADPH oxidase complex is formed. The enzyme catalyzes the oxidation reaction of NADPH and initiates the production of superoxide free radicals. Superoxide is converted to hydrogen peroxide either spontaneously or by the enzyme superoxide dismutase. Defects in any of the enzyme subunits can lead to CGD. The most common form of CGD (about 65 percent of patients) is caused by a mutation in the gp91$^{phox}$ subunit. This subunit is encoded by the *CYBB* gene on the X chromosome. Other types of CGDs are autosomal recessive due to defects in the p22$^{phox}$ subunit (encoded by the *CYBA* gene on chromosome 16) or p47$^{phox}$ (encoded by the *NCF1* gene on chromosome 7) or P67 (encoded by the *NCF2* gene on chromosome 1). A small number of patients with CGD may be deficient in enzymes such as glucose-6-phosphate dehydrogenase and myeloperoxidase.[102]

IFN-γ increases transcription of the gene encoding gp91$^{phox}$ and stimulates the production of superoxide radicals by the NADPH oxidase. Today, IFN-γ therapy is used for X-linked CGD patients.[102]

#### Clinical manifestations and diagnosis

Clinical manifestations are variable; however, due to defects in the killing activity of phagocytes, recurrent and pyogenic infections increase in patients, which eventually lead to the production of granulomas, especially in childhood. Patients are more susceptible to catalase-positive bacteria and are frequently infected with infections caused by *Staphylococcus*, *Escherichia*, *Candida*, *Salmonella*, *Legionella*, and *Aspergillus*. The most common pathogen is *Staphylococcus aureus*. Patients suffering from pneumonia, hepatomegaly, osteomyelitis, recurrent and purulent skin infections, and skin abscesses, as well as abscesses in the liver, lung, and spleen. Other manifestations include colitis or chronic enteritis, and sepsis. From a laboratory point of view, these people have high erythrocyte sedimentation rate (ESR) and leukocytosis, the number and function of T cells and B cells are normal, and active oxygen mediators are not produced.[102] CGD diagnostic tests include the following:

1. Flow cytometry: Evaluation of oxidation of dihydrorhodamine (DHR)
2. Nitroblue tetrazolium or NBT: If the activity of the enzyme is normal, adding NBT to a drop of blood will stimulate the enzyme and produce a blue color. This test is less commonly used today.
3. Quantitative luminescence test

#### Treatment

Successful treatment involves hematopoietic stem cell transplantation. However, some patients have also been treated with gene therapy. Supportive therapies, including broad-spectrum antibiotics and antifungal therapy, should also be given. Corticosteroids may also be effective in treating children with granulomatous colitis or intestinal obstruction.[103]

### Chediak-higashi syndrome

#### Definition

This rare disease has an autosomal recessive inheritance pattern and is characterized by defects in granule formation and defects in phagosome-lysosome integration. The disease is caused by a mutation in a gene encoding lysosomal trafficking regulator (LYST) protein. LYST plays an important role in vesicle movement, and its deficiency leads to defects in phagosome-lysosome fusion in phagocytes, defects in melanosome formation in melanocytes, and disorders of the nervous system and platelets. Neutrophils, lymphocytes, monocytes, platelets, and melanocytes have giant lysosomes. Large abnormal granules are found in many tissues. Melanosomes are large in size, and their transport to keratinocytes and hair follicles is disrupted, leading to ocular albinism and photosensitivity. Neutrophils are impaired in phagocytosis and chemotaxis. Due to defects in the cytoplasmic granules, the killing function of NK and CTL cells can also be impaired.[104]

There is another disorder called Griscelli Syndrome, which like Chediak-higashi syndrome, is associated with a lack of regulation of lysozyme secretion and is caused by a mutation in a small GTPase molecule called Rab27a. These patients also have neutropenia, partial albinism, hypogammaglobulinemia, and a high risk of developing hemophagocytic lymphohistiocytosis (HLH) but lack giant granules in peripheral blood granulocytes. This disease has an autosomal recessive inheritance pattern, and its treatment is hematopoietic stem cell transplantation.[104]

### *Clinical manifestations and diagnosis*

These patients are characterized by recurrent infections by purulent bacteria, partial oculocutaneous albinism, and progressive peripheral neuropathy. Patients develop progressive neutropenia with dysfunction of NK cells. Abnormalities in melanosomes cause their skin and hair to lighten in color and have photophobia with nystagmus. Patients are prone to infections of the respiratory tract, mucous membranes, and skin with bacteria and fungi, especially *Staphylococcus aureus*. Neuropathy is common and usually begins in the second decade of life. Patients have prolonged bleeding due to impaired platelet aggregation. The severe phase of the disease is characterized by high fever, pancytopenia, and lymphohistiocytic infiltration of the lymph nodes, liver, and spleen, which usually results in death. The diagnosis is by observation of the presence of large inclusions in all nucleated blood cells. Patients have progressive neutropenia and abnormal neutrophil, NK, and platelet function, and impaired phagocytosis and chemotaxis of neutrophils and monocytes.[104]

### *Treatment*

Hematopoietic stem cell transplantation is an effective treatment that leads to the restoration of cell function.

## Neutropenia

### *Definition*

Neutropenia is characterized by a decrease in the absolute count of segmented neutrophils (ANC). Based on ANC, neutropenia can be divided into mild (ANC 1000 to 1500 per microliter), moderate (ANC between 500 and 1000 microliter), and severe (ANC less than 200 per microliter). Neutropenia can be innate (or inherited), acquired due to infection, medication, malnutrition, or of autoimmune origin. Neutropenia associated with other immunodeficiency diseases includes Chediac-Higashi Syndrome, Griscelli Syndrome, Cohen Syndrome, CVID, IGA Deficiency, and SCID.[105]

### *Classification*

#### Cyclic neutropenia

This rare disease is characterized by an autosomal dominant genetic pattern with fluctuations in neutrophil counts in the normal range to less than 200 per microliter at regular intervals (approximately 21 days). Clinical manifestations in the neutropenic phase include oral and gingival ulcers, gingivitis, pharyngitis, fever, and fatigue. The disease is caused by a mutation in the *neutrophil elastase gene (ELANE)* that leads to cell apoptosis. The disease is diagnosed through repeated sampling three times a week for 6 to 8 weeks.[106]

#### Treatment

Treatment for patients includes antibiotics to prevent the spread of infections, administration of GCSF, and bone marrow transplantation.

#### Severe congenital neutropenia (SCN)

This disease is also rare and is characterized by the cessation of neutrophil maturation in the promyelocyte stage in the bone marrow. It has an autosomal dominant inheritance pattern (mutation in *ELANE*) or recessive (mutation in *HAX1*, or *G6PC3*), or it may occur sporadically. The absolute neutrophil count is less than 200 per microliter. The mutation in *HAX1* 1 is known as Costman's disease and is associated with neurological defects. Patients with SCN are prone to skin infections, oral ulcers, gingivitis, pneumonia, and abscesses around the rectum. In addition, patients are at risk for myelodysplastic syndrome (MDS) associated with monosomy 7 and acute myeloid leukemia (AML). Therefore, regular monitoring of peripheral blood cells and annual bone marrow evaluation should be performed in patients.[107]

#### Treatment

Treatment for patients is similar to that for other forms of neutropenia, including administration of antibiotics, GCSF, and bone marrow transplantation.

**Shwachman-diamond syndrome.** The disease is characterized by an autosomal recessive inheritance pattern with a mutation in the *SBDS* gene that leads to a molecular defect in ribosome biogenesis. Patients have neutropenia (ANC less than 1000 per microliter), defects in neutrophil migration, and decreased neutrophil chemotaxis. The patients could present with pancreatic insufficiency, malabsorption of fats and fatty diarrhea, slow growth, bone marrow dysfunction, hematologic abnormalities, or respiratory manifestations, along with pneumonia and otitis media. In addition, patients have short stature and skeletal abnormalities and are prone to bone marrow hypoplasia, MDS, and cytogenetic abnormalities.[108,109]

**Dyskeratosis congenita.** The disease is characterized by a defect in the telomerase enzyme and the inability of the bone marrow to produce sufficient blood cells. Three types, including X-linked, autosomal dominant, and autosomal recessive, have been described. The disease is associated with bone marrow failure, nail dystrophy, abnormal skin, and oral leukoplakia. The decreased number of circulating blood cells, including red blood cells, white blood cells, and platelets, is commonly associated with bone marrow failure. Patients with dyskeratosis congenita may also have low stature, eye and dental abnormalities, and other symptoms, including pulmonary disease, gut abnormalities, and osteoporosis. X-linked dyskeratosis congenita (the classic form of the disease) is caused by mutations in the *DKC1* gene. Autosomal dominant dyskeratosis congenita could occur due to mutations in three different genes, including the telomerase RNA gene, *TERC*, the gene encoding the enzymatically active component of telomerase, *TERT*, and the *TINF2* gene, encoding the telomere-associated protein TIN2. Patients with autosomal dominant inheritance pattern generally have fewer abnormalities and symptoms that appear later in life. Autosomal recessive dyskeratosis congenita is caused by mutations in different genes, including the *NOP10 (NOLA3)* gene, the *NHP2 (NOLA2)* gene, and the *TERT* gene.[110,111]

## Treatment

The treatment of dyskeratosis congenita is focused on the specific symptoms that each person exhibits. Treatment for patients includes the administration of GCSF. Androgens may boost red blood cells, and less frequently, platelet synthesis in some patients. Hematopoietic stem cell transplantation, if a matched donor can be found, has the potential to treat the blood abnormalities associated with dyskeratosis congenital.

**Neutropenia caused by infections.** Neutropenia can occur following viral infections. In this regard, a variety of mechanisms are involved, including infection of hematopoietic precursor cells or endothelial cells, and suppression of bone marrow. Viruses that commonly cause neutropenia are as follows: Adenoviruses, enteroviruses, influenza A and B viruses, chickenpox, *Measles*, rubella, and *Hepatitis A* and *B*. Neutropenia can also occur following bacterial infections such as pertussis, brucellosis, paratyphoid, and tuberculosis, and fungal infections, including histoplasmosis. Chronic neutropenia usually follows infection with *Cytomegalovirus* (*CMV*), *HIV*, and *EBV*.[112,113]

**Drug-induced neutropenia.** Medications are a common cause of neutropenia, which often occurs in adults over the age of 65. The most common drugs that can cause neutropenia are as follows: anti-rheumatic, antithyroid, and antimicrobial drugs such as penicillin, quinine, and chloramphenicol. Drug-induced neutropenia is usually caused by immune-related mechanisms, such as forming immune complexes.

### Treatment

The most effective treatment is to stop taking the drug, and if neutropenia persists after stopping the drug, administration of GCSF can be effective.[114]

### *Clinical manifestations and diagnosis*

Patients with neutropenia have a higher risk of infections, especially with *Staphylococcus aureus* and gram-negative bacteria. The most common clinical manifestations of severe neutropenia include fever, gingivitis, sinusitis, otitis, pneumonia, abscess, and sepsis. White blood cell counts should be performed three times a week for 6 to 8 weeks to check for cyclic neutropenia. Bone marrow aspiration and biopsy are performed in patients to assess cellularity and myeloid maturation. In addition, the patients should be analyzed for leukemia and other malignancies.

## Hyper-IgE syndrome

### *Definition*

The disease is often characterized by autosomal recessive inheritance and often by a defect in the gene encoding DOCK8. A number of patients also have an autosomal dominant inheritance pattern. DOCK8 is involved in many processes, including T cell proliferation and activation, cell growth, cell binding, and adhesion.[115,116]

### *Clinical manifestations and diagnosis*

Eosinophilia, lymphopenia, T cell dysfunction are considered to be features of this disease. Patients with hyper IgE syndrome present severe atopic dermatitis, asthma, allergies, and anaphylaxis. The disease is associated with increased susceptibility to recurrent skin infections with viruses such as herpes simplex, chickenpox, and papillomavirus, as well as abscesses, pneumonia, and upper respiratory infections. Patients have elevated IgA levels and low IgM.[115,116]

### *Treatment*

Treatment includes antibiotics and, in patients with immunoglobulin deficiency, IVIG administration.

## Defects in toll-like receptor (TLR) signaling pathway

### *Definition*

TLRs are the key innate immune receptors that play critical roles in early immune system responses. They are widely expressed by both immune and non-immune cells, including dendritic cells, macrophages, B and T lymphocytes, endothelial cells, and fibroblasts, and they can recognize microbial or host-derived macromolecules. Once activated with ligands, TLRs begin the process of signal transmission resulting in enhancing innate and adaptive immune responses. To intracellular signal transduction, TLRs use myeloid differentiation factor 88 (MyD88) and the adaptor molecule IL-1 receptor-associated kinase (IRAK) complex. However, TLR3 is an exception to this rule and uses other adapters called Toll/IL-1 receptor (TIR) domain-containing adaptor–inducing interferon-β (TRIF) and the TRIF-related adaptor molecule (TRAM) to transmit the signal. TLR signaling primarily activates the mitogen-activated protein kinase (MAPK) and nuclear factor of kappa light polypeptide gene enhancer in B cells (NF-κB) signal transduction pathways, which control cell differentiation, proliferation, and survival.[117]

Several IEIs have been found in which the mediators involved in the transmission of TLR signals are impaired, which we will discuss below.

### *Classification*

### IRAK-4 and myd88 deficiency

This disease has an autosomal recessive pattern and is characterized by impaired TLR and IL-1 receptor responses. Patients are prone to invasive and recurrent bacterial infections, including *Streptococcus pneumoniae*, *Staphylococcus aureus*, and Pseudomonas *aeruginosa*, especially in infancy and early childhood. Meningitis, sepsis, cutaneous and respiratory infections are invasive infections, which could occur before the age of 2 years. The number and proliferation of T cells in response to the antigen are both normal. However, in some patients, reduced IgM+IgD+CD27+ B cells have been reported that can be associated with reduced IgM responses against bacteria.[118]

### Treatment

Prophylactic antibiotics and immunization are required, and immunoglobulin replacement treatment has been used in several patients.

### IκBα and NEMO (IKKγ) deficiency

*IκBα* and *NEMO* mutations have been inherited in autosomal dominant and X-linked manner, respectively. *IκBα* and *NEMO* have a wider role, and their defects lead to more severe complications than IRAK-4 and MyD88 defects. *IκBα* and *NEMO* deficiency could result in impaired function of both MyD88-dependent and TRIF-dependent TLR signaling. The function of TCRs and B cell receptors (BCRs), as well as TNF receptors could also be affected. Therefore, patients are prone to a broad spectrum of infections, including fungi, mycobacteria, and viruses, in addition to bacteria. The patients may develop arthritis, hemolytic anemia, inflammatory bowel disease-like colitis, and recurrent diarrhea. Anhidrotic ectodermal dysplasia (EDA-ID), which is characterized by abnormal teeth, hypohidrosis, and sparse hair, is also an X-linked recessive disorder caused by NEMO deficiency. In this disorder, the response to TLR signals as well as CD40 signals is impaired, and patients are prone to infection with encapsulated purulent bacteria, mycobacteria, *Pneumocystis jirovesi*, and viruses.[119,120]

### Treatment

Vaccinations, antibiotic prophylaxis, immunoglobulin replacement therapy, and bone marrow transplantation could be effective for patients with EDA-ID

**HOIL-1 deficiency.** HOIL-1 (RBCK1) is involved in the polyubiquitination of NEMO and NF-κB activation. HOIL-1 is one of the components of LUBAC that is involved in the conjugation of linear polyubiquitin chains onto NEMO, and therefore activation of the NF-κB signaling pathway. *HOIL-1* mutations are inherited in an autosomal recessive manner and results in impaired NF-κB transcription and cytokine production in response to TNF and IL-1β. These patients are prone to invasive bacterial infections, systemic autoinflammation, and muscular amylopectinosis. These patients' susceptibility to invasive bacterial disease is most likely due to impaired NF-κB responses. The antibody response to pneumococcal carbohydrates is reduced. The number of T and B lymphocytes is normal.[121,122]

**Deficiency in TLR3 signaling and UNC-93B.** TLR3 uses TRIF, TRAF, and TBK1 adaptor molecules to transmit the signal. Patients with autosomal recessive mutations affecting *TRIF* and autosomal dominant mutations in *TRAF* and *TBK1* are susceptible to herpes simplex virus (HSV)−1 encephalitis.

The TLRs located in the endosomes, including TLR3, 7, 8, and 9, need a protein called UNC93B, which is located in the membrane of the ER. UNC93B is essential for signaling by these types of TLRs, and mutations in it are associated with increased susceptibility to herpes encephalitis. Similarly, loss-of-function mutations in *signal transducer and activator of transcription (STAT) 1* are associated with severe viral infections, especially herpes simplex encephalitis. STAT1 is required for signal transduction by type I (IFN-α/β) and type II (IFN-γ) interferons.[123,124]

### Treatment

The treatment is generally based on the prevention of infectious diseases. Acyclovir should be used to treat *HSV* infections aggressively. The use of IFN-α in the treatment of severe acute viral infections could be beneficial.

## Defects in IFN-γ/IL-12 pathway

### *Definition*

The IFN-γ/IL-12 pathway is an important player in the immune system and is essential for controlling mycobacterial infections. IL-12, a heterodimer consisting of IL-12p40 (IL-12B) and IL-12p35 (IL-12A), is produced by activated macrophages. IL-12, by interaction with its receptor, which is a heterodimer of IL-12Rb1 and IL-12Rb2, results in T cell and NK cell activation. Activation of IL-12R leads to induction of STAT4 activation, resulting in IFN-γ production. IL-12 deficiency is associated with tuberculosis, disseminated non-tuberculous mycobacterial infections, and *Salmonella* infections. T and NK cells do not produce IFN-γ as a result of faulty IL-12R signaling.

IFN-γ by interaction with its receptors, IFN-γ receptor (IFN-γR)1 and IFN-γR2, enhances the transcription of specific genes. STAT1 is activated by the effect of IFN-γ. *IFN-γR1* mutations are more common than *IFN-γR2* mutations. It has been reported that mycobacterial infections are associated with mutations in both IFN-γ receptors.

IFN-γR1can be found in all nucleated cells. IFN-γR1 deficiency is caused by mutations with both recessive and dominant inheritance patterns. The majority of recessive IFN-γR1 deficiencies are caused by a complete loss of IFN-γR1 expression on the cell surface, resulting in a complete loss of IFN-γ responsiveness. Dominant IFN-γR1 deficiency is caused by heterozygous truncations in IFN-γR1′s cytoplasmic domain, leading to the accumulation of non-functional IFN-γR1 proteins on the cell surface. IL-12 and IL-23 receptors share the IL-12p40 subunit. As a result, patients with IL-12Rb1 deficiency also lack an important part of the IL-23R and are deficient in response to both IL-12 and IL-23.[125,126]

### Treatment

Although there is no cure for IL-12 receptor deficiency, antibiotics and antifungals can be used to treat the infections that ensue. IFN-γ has been utilized to treat patients with disseminated *bacille Calmette-Guerin* infection who had an IL-12R1 deficiency. In addition, the use of IFN-γ enhances macrophage activity.

## Defects in complement system

### Definition

The complement system is an essential component of innate immunity and consists of three major pathways, including classic, alternative, and lectin. All three pathways have a common goal and work together to eliminate the pathogen. In addition, by activating the complement system, mediators are produced that play a role in improving the innate and adaptive immune responses, including the production of opsonins (e.g., c3b, ic3b, and c4b) and anaphylatoxins (e.g., c3a, c4a, and c5a). Complement deficiencies are rare, and deficiencies in any of the components increase the risk of recurrent infections, which are described below.[127–129]

### Clinical manifestations and diagnosis

All components of the classical and alternative pathways except properdin are inherited as an autosomal dominant pattern. Properdin deficiency is an X-linked disorder.

Defects in any of the components of the classical pathway (C1, C2, and C4) lead to systemic lupus erythematosus-like disease characterized by the deposition of immune complexes in the kidneys, skin, and blood vessels. In C1 deficiency, C1q deficiency is common and is associated with increased susceptibility to lupus and glomerulonephritis. Some children develop severe infections, like sepsis and meningitis. People who are deficient in other components of C1 (C1r, C1s) also have a high risk of developing autoimmune syndromes, especially systemic lupus erythematosus.[130]

C2 deficiency is one of the most common complement system deficiencies and is associated with recurrent skin infections and lupus. These patients are prone to sepsis, especially with *pneumococcus*. C2 deficiency can be associated with a relative decrease in the level of the B factor.

C3 deficiency is associated with an increase in purulent infections. This defect leads to decreased opsonization and phagocytosis and decreased antigen clearance and uptake of immune complexes. Severe infections with *meningococcus* and *Hemophilus* are common in these patients. C4 deficiency is very rare because C4 is encoded by two genes, including *C4A* and *C4B*. The C4 defect is associated with sepsis and meningitis, and patients are prone to increased systemic lupus erythematosus. Meningococcal infections are very common in patients with C5 to C9 deficiency.[131,132]

Among the defects associated with the lectin pathway, Mannose-binding lectin (MBL) deficiency is associated with an increase in recurrent lung infections, autoimmunity, sepsis, and bacterial infections. However, patients with low levels of MBL are more likely to develop respiratory infections. MASP2 deficiency is associated with systemic lupus erythematosus-like disease and pneumonia, and Ficolin deficiency leads to recurrent pneumonia, brain abscesses, and bronchiectasis.[133]

Alternative pathway defects are rarer than classical pathway defects. Factor D and factor B deficiency are associated with gonococcal and meningococcal infections and an increased risk of bacterial infections. Properdin deficiency causes meningococcal meningitis, and patients are at high risk for other purulent infections as well as sepsis.[134,135]

In a disease called Paroxysmal Nocturnal Hemoglobinuria (PNH), which results from a defect in the enzyme needed to produce the protein glycosylphosphatidylinositol, or GPI (the *PIG-A* gene on chromosome X), red blood cells are prone to lysis by the complement system. GPI as a hook helps to attach proteins such as CD59 and CD55 to the cell membrane. These molecules act as regulators of the complement system, and their defects in patients with PNH lead to lysis of blood cells, including granulocytes, platelets, and especially red blood cells, by complement. Patients with PNH develop chronic infections and anemia.[136]

Activation of the complement system is under control, and without its regulation, it will cause severe damage to the host. Defects in complement regulators lead to continuous and uncontrolled activity of the complement system. The factor I is an essential regulator of both the classical and alternative pathways, and its deficiency is associated with the frequent conversion of C3 to C3b and the increase of purulent infections, especially meningococcal and pneumococcal infections.[137,138] Deficiency in the factor H has similar effects and leads to continuous activity of the alternative pathway. Patients are prone to meningococcal infections and other purulent infections. Also, glomerulonephritis and uremic hemolytic syndrome are common in these patients.[139]

Deficiency of C1 inhibitor (C1INH), a vital regulator of C1, leads to hereditary angioedema (HAE). This disease has an autosomal dominant inheritance pattern and is characterized by a decrease in C1INH and consequent overactivity of C1r and C1s proteases leading to increased degradation of C4 and C1 and the release of bradykinin, which causes vasodilation and local edema. HAE is not usually associated with infection or autoimmunity. However, systemic lupus erythematosus and glomerulonephritis have been reported in some patients.[140]

The CH50 test is useful in assessing complement-related diseases. In congenital defects of C1 to C8 components, CH50 is very low. Lack of I or H factors causes C3 consumption and a relative decrease in the amount of CH50. In HAE, a decrease in C2 and C4 leads to a significant decrease in CH50. Decreased C3 levels and normal C4 can indicate alternative pathway activity. Alternative pathway activity can be measured by the AH50 test.

### *Treatment*

Complement deficits do not currently have any particular treatments. Infection prevention and treatment (typically with antibiotics) are critical in the management of people with these deficits.

## References


1. Raje N, Dinakar C. Overview of Immunodeficiency Disorders. *Immunol Allergy Clin North Am*. 2015;35(4):599–623. doi:10.1016/j.iac.2015.07.001.
2. Amaya-Uribe L, Rojas M, Azizi G, Anaya JM, Gershwin ME. Primary immunodeficiency and autoimmunity: a comprehensive review. *J Autoimmun*. 2019;99:52–72. doi:10.1016/j.jaut.2019.01.011 Epub 2019 Feb 20. PMID: 30795880.
3. Cooper MD, Lanier LL, Conley ME, Puck JM. Immunodeficiency disorders. *Hematology Am Soc Hematol Educ Program*. 2003:314–330. doi:10.1182/asheducation-2003.1.314 PMID: 14633788.
4. Galal N, Ohida M, Meshaal S, Elaziz DA, Elhawary I. Targeted screening for primary immunodeficiency disorders in the neonatal period and early infancy. *Afr Health Sci*. 2019;19(1):1449–1459. doi:10.4314/ahs.v19i1.18.
5. El-Sayed ZA, Radwan N. Newborn Screening for Primary Immunodeficiencies: the Gaps, Challenges, and Outlook for Developing Countries. *Front Immunol*. 2020;10:2987. doi:10.3389/fimmu.2019.02987 PMID: 32082296; PMCID: PMC7002357.
6. Buckley RH. Humoral immunodeficiency. *Clin Immunol Immunopathol*. 1986;40(1):13–24. doi:10.1016/0090-1229(86)90065-6 PMID: 2424651.
7. Buckley RH. Primary cellular immunodeficiencies. *J Allergy Clin Immunol*. 2002;109(5):747–757. doi:10.1067/mai.2002.123617 PMID: 11994695.
8. Notarangelo L, Casanova JL, Fischer A, Puck J, Rosen F, Seger R, et al. International Union of Immunological Societies Primary Immunodeficiency diseases classification committee. Primary immunodeficiency diseases: an update. *J Allergy Clin Immunol*. 2004;114(3):677–687. doi:10.1016/j.jaci.2004.06.044 PMID: 15356576.
9. McCusker C, Upton J, Warrington R. Primary immunodeficiency. *Allergy Asthma Clin Immunol*. 2018;14(Suppl 2):61. doi:10.1186/s13223-018-0290-5 PMID: 30275850; PMCID: PMC6157160.
10. Gernez Y, Baker MG, Maglione PJ. Humoral immunodeficiencies: conferred risk of infections and benefits of immunoglobulin replacement therapy. *Transfusion (Paris)*. 2018;58 Suppl 3(Suppl 3):3056–3064. doi:10.1111/trf.15020 PMID: 30536429; PMCID: PMC6939302.

11. Lackey AE, Ahmad F. X-linked Agammaglobulinemia*StatPearls [Internet]*. Treasure Island (FL): StatPearls Publishing; 2021 2021 Jan–. PMID: 31751055.
12. El-Sayed ZA, et al. X-linked agammaglobulinemia (XLA):phenotype, diagnosis, and therapeutic challenges around the world. *World Allergy Organ J*. 2022;12(3):100018. doi:10.1016/j.waojou.2019.100018.
13. Tang P, Upton JEM, Barton-Forbes MA, Salvadori MI, Clynick MP, Price AK, et al. Autosomal Recessive Agammaglobulinemia Due to a Homozygous Mutation in PIK3R1. *J Clin Immunol*. 2018;38(1):88–95. doi:10.1007/s10875-017-0462-y Epub 2017 Nov 25. PMID: 29178053.
14. Yazdani R, Fekrvand S, Shahkarami S, Azizi G, Moazzami B, Abolhassani H, et al. The hyper IgM syndromes: epidemiology, pathogenesis, clinical manifestations, diagnosis and management. *Clin Immunol*. 2019;198:19–30. doi:10.1016/j.clim.2018.11.007 Epub 2018 Nov 13. PMID: 30439505.
15. Qamar N, Fuleihan RL. The hyper IgM syndromes. *Clin Rev Allergy Immunol*. 2014;46(2):120–130. doi:10.1007/s12016-013-8378-7 PMID: 23797640.
16. Dunn CP, de la Morena MT. X-Linked Hyper IgM Syndrome. 2007, [updated 2020 Feb 20]. In: Adam MP, Ardinger HH, Pagon RA, Wallace SE, Bean LJH, Mirzaa G, Amemiya A, editors. GeneReviews® [Internet]. Seattle (WA): University of Washington, Seattle; 1993–2021. PMID: 20301576.
17. Dunn CP, de la Morena MT. X-Linked Hyper IgM Syndrome. 2007, [Updated 2020 Feb 20]. In: Adam MP, Ardinger HH, Pagon RA, et al., editors. GeneReviews® [Internet]. Seattle (WA): University of Washington, Seattle; 1993-2021. Available from: https://www.ncbi.nlm.nih.gov/books/NBK1402/
18. Jain A, Ma CA, Liu S, Brown M, Cohen J, Strober W. Specific missense mutations in NEMO result in hyper-IgM syndrome with hypohydrotic ectodermal dysplasia. *Nat Immunol*. 2001;2(3):223–228. doi:10.1038/85277 PMID: 11224521.
19. Davies EG, Thrasher AJ. Update on the hyper immunoglobulin M syndromes. *Br J Haematol*. 2010;149(2):167–180. doi:10.1111/j.1365-2141.2010.08077.x.
20. Imai K, Zhu Y, Revy P, Morio T, Mizutani S, Fischer A, et al. Analysis of class switch recombination and somatic hypermutation in patients affected with autosomal dominant hyper-IgM syndrome type 2. *Clin Immunol*. 2005;115(3):277–285. doi:10.1016/j.clim.2005.02.003 PMID: 15893695.
21. Durandy A, Revy P, Imai K, Fischer A. Hyper-immunoglobulin M syndromes caused by intrinsic B-lymphocyte defects. *Immunol Rev*. 2005;203:67–79. doi:10.1111/j.0105-2896.2005.00222.x PMID: 15661022.
22. Al-Saud BK, Al-Sum Z, Alassiri H, Al-Ghonaium A, Al-Muhsen S, Al-Dhekri H, et al. Clinical, immunological, and molecular characterization of hyper-IgM syndrome due to CD40 deficiency in eleven patients. *J Clin Immunol*. 2013;33(8):1325–1335. doi:10.1007/s10875-013-9951-9 PMID: 24122029.
23. Leite LFB, Máximo TA, Mosca T, Forte WCN. CD40 Ligand Deficiency. *Allergol Immunopathol. (Madr.)*. 2020;48(4):409–413. doi:10.1016/j.aller.2019.08.005 Epub 2019 Dec 9. PMID: 31831191.
24. Imai K, Catalan N, Plebani A, et al. Hyper-IgM syndrome type 4 with a B lymphocyte-intrinsic selective deficiency in Ig class-switch recombination. *J Clin Invest*. 2003;112(1):136–142. doi:10.1172/JCI18161.
25. Imai K, Slupphaug G, Lee WI, Revy P, Nonoyama S, Catalan N, et al. Human uracil-DNA glycosylase deficiency associated with profoundly impaired immunoglobulin class-switch recombination. *Nat Immunol*. 2003;4(10):1023–1028. doi:10.1038/ni974 Epub 2003 Sep 7. PMID: 12958596.
26. Kavli B, Andersen S, Otterlei M, Liabakk NB, Imai K, Fischer A, et al. B cells from hyper-IgM patients carrying UNG mutations lack ability to remove uracil from ssDNA and have elevated genomic uracil. *J Exp Med*. 2005;201(12):2011–2021. doi:10.1084/jem.20050042 PMID: 15967827; PMCID: PMC2212036.
27. Durandy A, Taubenheim N, Peron S, Fischer A. Pathophysiology of B-cell intrinsic immunoglobulin class switch recombination deficiencies. *Adv Immunol*. 2007;94:275–306. doi:10.1016/S0065-2776(06)94009-7 PMID: 17560278.
28. Yel L. Selective IgA deficiency. *J Clin Immunol*. 2010;30(1):10–16. doi:10.1007/s10875-009-9357-x Epub 2010 Jan 26. PMID: 20101521; PMCID: PMC2821513.
29. Swain S, Selmi C, Gershwin ME, Teuber SS. The clinical implications of selective IgA deficiency [published correction appears in J Transl Autoimmun. 2020 Feb 25;3:100041]. *J Transl Autoimmun*. 2019;2:100025. doi:10.1016/j.jtauto.2019.100025 Published 2019 Nov 23.

30. Lacombe C, Aucouturier P, Preud'homme JL. Selective IgG1 deficiency. *Clin Immunol Immunopathol.* 1997;84(2):194–201. doi:10.1006/clin.1997.4386 PMID: 9245552.
31. Chou CC, Hsieh KH, Lin YZ, Ting CK, Wang JY. Selective IgG subclass deficiencies in patients with recurrent sinopulmonary infections: report of two cases. *Asian Pac J Allergy Immunol.* 1988;6(2):129–133 PMID: 3219160.
32. Jefferis R, Kumararatne DS. Selective IgG subclass deficiency: quantification and clinical relevance. *Clin Exp Immunol.* 1990;81(3):357–367. doi:10.1111/j.1365-2249.1990.tb05339.x PMID: 2204502; PMCID: PMC1534990.
33. Khokar A, Gupta S. Clinical and Immunological Features of 78 Adult Patients with Primary Selective IgG Subclass Deficiencies. *Arch Immunol Ther Exp (Warsz.).* 2019;67(5):325–334. doi:10.1007/s00005-019-00556-3 Epub 2019 Jul 30. PMID: 31363786.
34. Yazdani R, Habibi S, Sharifi L, Azizi G, Abolhassani H, Olbrich P, et al. Common Variable Immunodeficiency: epidemiology, Pathogenesis, Clinical Manifestations, Diagnosis, Classification, and Management. *J Investig Allergol Clin Immunol.* 2020;30(1):14–34. doi:10.18176/jiaci.0388 Epub 2019 Feb 11. PMID: 30741636.
35. Saikia B, Gupta S. Common Variable Immunodeficiency. *Indian J Pediatr.* 2016;83(4):338–344. doi:10.1007/s12098-016-2038-x Epub 2016 Feb 12. PMID: 26868026.
36. Locke BA, Dasu T, Verbsky JW. Laboratory diagnosis of primary immunodeficiencies. *Clin Rev Allergy Immunol.* 2014;46(2):154–168. doi:10.1007/s12016-014-8412-4 PMID: 24569953.
37. Goldman AS, Goldblum RM. Primary deficiencies in humoral immunity. *Pediatr Clin North Am.* 1977;24(2):277–291. doi:10.1016/s0031-3955(16)33419-8 PMID: 323802.
38. Aghamohammadi A, Farhoudi A, Moin M, et al. Clinical and immunological features of 65 Iranian patients with common variable immunodeficiency. *Clin Diagn Lab Immunol.* 2005;12:825–832.
39. Moin M, Aghamohammadi A, Farhoudi A, Pourpak Z, Rezaei N, Movahedi M, et al. X-linked agammaglobulinemia: a survey of 33 Iranian patients. *Immunol Invest.* 2004;33:81–93.
40. Mohammadi J, Liu C, Aghamohammadi A, Bergbreiter A, Du L, Lu J, et al. Novel mutations in TACI (TNFRSF13B) causing common variable immunodeficiency. *J Clin Immunol.* 2009;29:777–785.
41. Zaki-Dizaji M, Akrami SM, Abolhassani H, Rezaei N, Aghamohammadi A. Ataxia telangiectasia syndrome: moonlighting ATM. *Expert Rev Clin Immunol.* 2017;13:1155–1172.
42. Losi CG, Silini A, Fiorini C, Soresina A, Meini A, Ferrari S, et al. Mutational analysis of human BAFF receptor TNFRSF13C (BAFF-R) in patients with common variable immunodeficiency. *J Clin Immunol.* 2005;25:496–502.
43. Serana F, Chiarini M, Zanotti C, et al. Use of V(D)J recombination excision circles to identify T- and B-cell defects and to monitor the treatment in primary and acquired immunodeficiencies. *J Transl Med.* 2013;11:119.
44. Lackey AE, Muzio MR. DiGeorge Syndrome. 2021 Aug 11 *StatPearls [Internet].* Treasure Island (FL): StatPearls Publishing; 2021 PMID: 31747205.
45. McDonald-McGinn DM, Sullivan KE. Chromosome 22q11.2 deletion syndrome (DiGeorge syndrome/velocardiofacial syndrome). *Medicine (Baltimore).* 2011;90(1):1–18. doi:10.1097/MD.0b013e3182060469 PMID: 21200182.
46. Fischer A. Severe combined immunodeficiencies (SCID). *Clin Exp Immunol.* 2000;122(2):143–149. doi:10.1046/j.1365-2249.2000.01359.x PMID: 11091267; PMCID: PMC1905779.
47. Justiz Vaillant AA, Mohseni M. Severe Combined Immunodeficiency [Updated 2021 Aug 14] *StatPearls [Internet].* Treasure Island (FL): StatPearls Publishing; 2021. Available from: https://www.ncbi.nlm.nih.gov/books/NBK539762/.
48. Fugmann SD, Müller S, Friedrich W, Bartram CR, Schwarz K. Mutations in the gene for the common gamma chain (gammac) in X-linked severe combined immunodeficiency. *Hum Genet* 1998;103(6):730–731. doi:10.1007/pl00008710 PMID: 9921912.
49. Puck JM, Pepper AE, Henthorn PS, Candotti F, Isakov J, Whitwam T, et al. Mutation analysis of IL2RG in human X-linked severe combined immunodeficiency. *Blood.* 1997;89(6):1968–1977 PMID: 9058718.
50. Flinn AM, Gennery AR. Adenosine deaminase deficiency: a review. *Orphanet J Rare Dis.* 2018;13(1):65. doi:10.1186/s13023-018-0807-5 Published 2018 Apr 24.

51. Sauer AV, Morbach H, Brigida I, Ng YS, Aiuti A, Meffre E. Defective B cell tolerance in adenosine deaminase deficiency is corrected by gene therapy. *J Clin Invest*. 2012;122(6):2141–2152. doi:10.1172/JCI61788 Epub 2012 May 24. PMID: 22622038; PMCID: PMC3366410.
52. Dalal I, Grunebaum E, Cohen A, Roifman CM. Two novel mutations in a purine nucleoside phosphorylase (PNP)-deficient patient. *Clin Genet*. 2001;59(6):430–437. doi:10.1034/j.1399-0004.2001.590608.x PMID: 11453975.
53. la Marca G, Canessa C, Giocaliere E, Romano F, Malvagia S, Funghini S, et al. Diagnosis of immunodeficiency caused by a purine nucleoside phosphorylase defect by using tandem mass spectrometry on dried blood spots. *J Allergy Clin Immunol*. 2014;134(1):155–159. doi:10.1016/j.jaci.2014.01.040 Epub 2014 Apr 24. PMID: 24767876.
54. Fleischman A, Hershfield MS, Toutain S, et al. Adenosine deaminase deficiency and purine nucleoside phosphorylase deficiency in common variable immunodeficiency. *Clin Diagn Lab Immunol*. 1998;5(3):399–400. doi:10.1128/CDLI.5.3.399-400.1998.
55. Tabori U, Mark Z, Amariglio N, Etzioni A, Golan H, Biloray B, et al. Dalal I. Detection of RAG mutations and prenatal diagnosis in families presenting with either T-B- severe combined immunodeficiency or Omenn's syndrome. *Clin Genet*. 2004;65(4):322–326. doi:10.1111/j.1399-0004.2004.00227.x PMID: 15025726.
56. Gennery A Recent advances in understanding RAG deficiencies. *F1000Res*. 2019;8:F1000 Faculty Rev-148. Published 2019 Feb 4. doi:10.12688/f1000research.17056.1
57. Greenberg-Kushnir N, Lee YN, Simon AJ, Lev A, Marcus N, Abuzaitoun O, et al. A Large Cohort of RAG1/2-Deficient SCID Patients-Clinical, Immunological, and Prognostic Analysis. *J Clin Immunol*. 2020;40(1):211–222. doi:10.1007/s10875-019-00717-1 Epub 2019 Dec 14. PMID: 31838659.
58. Puel A, Ziegler SF, Buckley RH, Leonard WJ. Defective IL7R expression in T(-)B(+)NK(+) severe combined immunodeficiency. *Nat Genet*. 1998;20(4):394–397. doi:10.1038/3877 PMID: 9843216.
59. Mazzucchelli RI, Riva A, Durum SK. The human IL-7 receptor gene: deletions, polymorphisms and mutations. *Semin Immunol*. 2012;24(3):225–230. doi:10.1016/j.smim.2012.02.007.
60. Roberts JL, Buckley RH, Luo B, et al. CD45-deficient severe combined immunodeficiency caused by uniparental disomy. *Proc Natl Acad Sci. U. S. A*. 2012;109(26):10456–10461. doi:10.1073/pnas.1202249109.
61. Tasher D, Dalal I. The genetic basis of severe combined immunodeficiency and its variants. *Appl Clin Genet*. 2012;5:67–80. doi:10.2147/TACG.S18693 Published 2012 Aug 7.
62. Roberts JL, Buckley RH, Luo B, Pei J, Lapidus A, Peri S, et al. CD45-deficient severe combined immunodeficiency caused by uniparental disomy. *Proc Natl Acad Sci U S A*. 2012;109(26):10456–10461. doi:10.1073/pnas.1202249109 Epub 2012 Jun 11. PMID: 22689986; PMCID: PMC3387083.
63. Kelly J, Leonard WJ. Immune deficiencies due to defects in cytokine signaling. *Curr Allergy Asthma Rep*. 2003;3(5):396–401. doi:10.1007/s11882-003-0073-y PMID: 12906775.
64. Roberts JL, Lauritsen JP, Cooney M, Parrott RE, Sajaroff EO, Win CM, et al. T-B+NK+ severe combined immunodeficiency caused by complete deficiency of the CD3zeta subunit of the T-cell antigen receptor complex. *Blood*. 2007;109(8):3198–3206. doi:10.1182/blood-2006-08-043166 Epub 2006 Dec 14. PMID: 17170122; PMCID: PMC1852234.
65. de Saint Basile G, Geissmann F, Flori E, Uring-Lambert B, Soudais C, Cavazzana-Calvo M, et al. Severe combined immunodeficiency caused by deficiency in either the delta or the epsilon subunit of CD3. *J Clin Invest*. 2004;114(10):1512–1517. doi:10.1172/JCI22588 PMID: 15546002; PMCID: PMC525745.
66. Walkovich K, Vander Lugt M ZAP70-Related Combined Immunodeficiency. 2009, [Updated 2021 Sep 23]. In: Adam MP, Ardinger HH, Pagon RA, et al., editors. GeneReviews® [Internet]. Seattle (WA): University of Washington, Seattle; 1993-2021. Available from: https://www.ncbi.nlm.nih.gov/books/NBK20221/
67. Sharifinejad N, Jamee M, Zaki-Dizaji M, et al. Clinical, Immunological, and Genetic Features in 49 Patients With ZAP-70 Deficiency: a Systematic Review. *Front Immunol*. 2020;11:831. doi:10.3389/fimmu.2020.00831 Published 2020 May 5.
68. Elder ME. SCID due to ZAP-70 deficiency. *J Pediatr Hematol Oncol*. 1997;19(6):546–550. doi:10.1097/00043426-199711000-00014 PMID: 9407944.

69. Notarangelo LD, Mella P, Jones A, de Saint Basile G, Savoldi G, Cranston T, et al. Mutations in severe combined immune deficiency (SCID) due to JAK3 deficiency. *Hum Mutat*. 2001;18(4):255–263. doi:10.1002/humu.1188 PMID: 11668610.
70. Russell SM, Tayebi N, Nakajima H, Riedy MC, Roberts JL, Aman MJ, et al. Mutation of Jak3 in a patient with SCID: essential role of Jak3 in lymphoid development. *Science*. 1995;270(5237):797–800. doi:10.1126/science.270.5237.797 PMID: 7481768.
71. O'Shea JJ, Husa M, Li D, Hofmann SR, Watford W, Roberts JL, et al. Jak3 and the pathogenesis of severe combined immunodeficiency. *Mol Immunol*. 2004;41(6–7):727–737. doi:10.1016/j.molimm.2004.04.014 PMID: 15220007.
72. Lacruz RS, Feske S. Diseases caused by mutations in ORAI1 and STIM1. *Ann N Y Acad Sci*. 2015;1356(1):45–79. doi:10.1111/nyas.12938 Epub 2015 Oct 15. PMID: 26469693; PMCID: PMC4692058.
73. Thompson JL, Mignen O, Shuttleworth TJ. The Orai1 severe combined immune deficiency mutation and calcium release-activated Ca2+ channel function in the heterozygous condition. *J Biol Chem*. 2009;284(11):6620–6626. doi:10.1074/jbc.M808346200.
74. Pannicke U, Hönig M, Hess I, Friesen C, Holzmann K, Rump EM, et al. Reticular dysgenesis (aleukocytosis) is caused by mutations in the gene encoding mitochondrial adenylate kinase 2. *Nat Genet*. 2009;41(1):101–105. doi:10.1038/ng.265 Epub 2008 Nov 30. PMID: 19043417.
75. Ichikawa S, Prockop S, Cunningham-Rundles C, Sifers T, Conner BR, Wu S, et al. Reticular dysgenesis caused by an intronic pathogenic variant in *AK2*. *Cold Spring Harb Mol Case Stud*. 2020;6(3):a005017. doi:10.1101/mcs.a005017 PMID: 32532877; PMCID: PMC7304357.
76. Massaad MJ, Ramesh N, Geha RS. Wiskott-Aldrich syndrome: a comprehensive review. *Ann NY Acad Sci*. 2013;1285:26–43. doi:10.1111/nyas.12049 Epub 2013 Mar 25. PMID: 23527602.
77. Malik MA, Masab M. Wiskott-Aldrich Syndrome *StatPearls [Internet]*. Treasure Island (FL): StatPearls Publishing; 2021 2021 Jan–. PMID: 30969660.
78. Candotti F. Clinical Manifestations and Pathophysiological Mechanisms of the Wiskott-Aldrich Syndrome. *J Clin Immunol*. 2018;38(1):13–27. doi:10.1007/s10875-017-0453-z Epub 2017 Oct 30. PMID: 29086100.
79. Ochs HD, Filipovich AH, Veys P, Cowan MJ, Kapoor N. Wiskott-Aldrich syndrome: diagnosis, clinical and laboratory manifestations, and treatment. *Biol Blood Marrow Transplant*. 2009;15(1 Suppl):84–90. doi:10.1016/j.bbmt.2008.10.007 PMID: 19147084.
80. Greenberger S, Berkun Y, Ben-Zeev B, Levi YB, Barziliai A, Nissenkorn A. Dermatologic manifestations of ataxia-telangiectasia syndrome. *J Am Acad Dermatol*. 2013;68(6):932–936. doi:10.1016/j.jaad.2012.12.950 Epub 2013 Jan 27. PMID: 23360865.
81. Amirifar P, Ranjouri MR, Yazdani R, Abolhassani H, Aghamohammadi A. Ataxia-telangiectasia: a review of clinical features and molecular pathology. *Pediatr Allergy Immunol*. 2019;30(3):277–288. doi:10.1111/pai.13020 Epub 2019 Mar 20. PMID: 30685876.
82. Hoshino T, Kanegane H, Doki N, Irisawa H, Sakura T, Nojima Y, et al. X-linked lymphoproliferative disease in an adult. *Int J Hematol*. 2005;82(1):55–58. doi:10.1532/IJH97.05020 PMID: 16105760.
83. MacGinnitie AJ, Geha R. X-linked lymphoproliferative disease: genetic lesions and clinical consequences. *Curr Allergy Asthma Rep*. 2002;2(5):361–367. doi:10.1007/s11882-002-0068-0 PMID: 12165201.
84. Gholam C, Grigoriadou S, Gilmour KC, Gaspar HB. Familial haemophagocytic lymphohistiocytosis: advances in the genetic basis, diagnosis and management. *Clin Exp Immunol*. 2011;163(3):271–283. doi:10.1111/j.1365-2249.2010.04302.x.
85. Shah S, Wu E, Rao VK, Tarrant TK. Autoimmune lymphoproliferative syndrome: an update and review of the literature. *Curr Allergy Asthma Rep*. 2014;14(9):462. doi:10.1007/s11882-014-0462-4 PMID: 25086580; PMCID: PMC4148697.
86. Barzaghi F, Passerini L, Bacchetta R. Immune dysregulation, polyendocrinopathy, enteropathy, x-linked syndrome: a paradigm of immunodeficiency with autoimmunity. *Front Immunol*. 2012;3:211. doi:10.3389/fimmu.2012.00211 Published 2012 Jul 31.
87. Shrestha D, Szöllosi J, Jenei A. Bare lymphocyte syndrome: an opportunity to discover our immune system. *Immunol Lett*. 2012;141(2):147–157. doi:10.1016/j.imlet.2011.10.007 Epub 2011 Oct 17. PMID: 22027563.

88. Locke BA, Dasu T, Verbsky JW. Laboratory diagnosis of primary immunodeficiencies. *Clin Rev Allergy Immunol*. 2014;46:154–168.
89. Shahbazi Z, Yazdani R, Shahkarami S, Shahbazi S, et al. Genetic mutations and immunological features of severe combined immunodeficiency patients in Iran. *Immunol Lett*. 2019;216:70–78.
90. Raszka WV, Moriarty RA, Ottolini MG, Waecker NJ, et al. Delayed-type hypersensitivity skin testing in human immunodeficiency virus-infected pediatric patients. *J Pediatr*. 1996;129:245–250.
91. Ahmed AR, Blose DA. Delayed-type hypersensitivity skin testing. A review. *Arch Dermatol*. 1983;119:934–945.
92. Somech R. T-cell receptor excision circles in primary immunodeficiencies and other T-cell immune disorders. *Curr Opin Allergy Clin Immunol*. 2011;11:517–524.
93. Stewart DM, Candotti F, Nelson DL. The phenomenon of spontaneous genetic reversions in the Wiskott-Aldrich syndrome: a report of the workshop of the ESID Genetics Working Party at the XIIth Meeting of the European Society for Immunodeficiencies (ESID). *J Clin Immunol*. 2007;27:634–639.
94. Stachon AC, Baskin B, et al. Molecular diagnosis of 22q11.2 deletion and duplication by multiplex ligation dependent probe amplification. *Am J Med Genet A*. 2007;143A:2924–2930.
95. Fallah S, Mesdaghi M, Mansouri M, et al. Severe Combined Immunodeficiency: a Case Series and Review from a Tertiary Pediatric Hospital. *Iran J Allergy Asthma Immunol*. 2018;17:201–207.
96. Locke BA, Dasu T, Verbsky JW. Laboratory diagnosis of primary immunodeficiencies. *Clin Rev Allergy Immunol*. 2014;46:154–168.
97. Jung S, Gies V, Korganow AS, Guffroy A. Primary Immunodeficiencies With Defects in Innate Immunity: focus on Orofacial Manifestations. *Front Immunol*. 2020;11:1065. doi:10.3389/fimmu.2020.01065 PMID: 32625202; PMCID: PMC7314950.
98. Das J, Sharma A, Jindal A, Aggarwal V, Rawat A. Leukocyte adhesion defect: where do we stand circa 2019? *Genes Dis*. 2019;7(1):107–114. doi:10.1016/j.gendis.2019.07.012 Published 2019 Aug 7.
99. Dababneh R, Al-Wahadneh AM, Hamadneh S, Khouri A, Bissada NF. Periodontal manifestation of leukocyte adhesion deficiency type I. *J Periodontol*. 2008;79(4):764–768. doi:10.1902/jop.2008.070323 PMID: 18380573.
100. Tewari N, Mathur VP, Yadav VS, Chaudhari P Leukocyte adhesion defect-I: rare primary immune deficiency. Spec Care Dentist. 2017;37(6):309-313. doi: 10.1111/scd.12249. Epub 2017 Nov 15. PMID: 29139565.
101. Phillips ML, Schwartz BR, Etzioni A, Bayer R, Ochs HD, Paulson JC, et al. Neutrophil adhesion in leukocyte adhesion deficiency syndrome type 2. *J Clin Invest*. 1995;96(6):2898–2906. doi:10.1172/JCI118361 PMID: 8675661; PMCID: PMC186001.
102. Rosenzweig SD. Inflammatory manifestations in chronic granulomatous disease (CGD). *J Clin Immunol*. 2008;28(Suppl 1):S67–S72. doi:10.1007/s10875-007-9160-5 Epub 2008 Jan 12. PMID: 18193341.
103. Carnide EG, Jacob CA, Castro AM, Pastorino AC. Clinical and laboratory aspects of chronic granulomatous disease in description of eighteen patients. *Pediatr Allergy Immunol*. 2005;16(1):5–9. doi:10.1111/j.1399-3038.2005.00225.x PMID: 15693905.
104. Toro C, Nicoli ER, Malicdan MC, Adams DR, Introne WJ. Chediak-Higashi Syndrome. 2009 [updated 2018 Jul 5]. In: Adam MP, Ardinger HH, Pagon RA, Wallace SE, Bean LJH, Mirzaa G, Amemiya A, editors. GeneReviews® [Internet]. Seattle (WA): University of Washington, Seattle; 1993–2021. PMID: 20301751.
105. Baley JE, Stork EK, Warkentin PI, Shurin SB. Neonatal neutropenia. Clinical manifestations, cause, and outcome. *Am J Dis Child*. 1988;142(11):1161–1166. doi:10.1001/archpedi.1988.02150110039016 PMID: 3177322.
106. Lange RD, Jones JB. Cyclic neutropenia. Review of clinical manifestations and management. *Am J Pediatr Hematol Oncol*. 1981;3(4):363–367 WinterPMID: 7036779.
107. Skokowa J, Dale DC, Touw IP, Zeidler C, Welte K. Severe congenital neutropenias. *Nat Rev Dis Primers*. 2017;3:17032. doi:10.1038/nrdp.2017.32 Published 2017 Jun 8.
108. Furutani E, Shah AS, Zhao Y, Andorsky D, Dedeoglu F, Geddis A, et al. Inflammatory manifestations in patients with Shwachman-Diamond syndrome: a novel phenotype. *Am J Med Genet A*. 2020;182(7):1754–1760. doi:10.1002/ajmg.a.61593 Epub 2020 Apr 15. PMID: 32293785.

109. Erdos M, Maródi L. Shwachman-Diamond-szindróma: klinikai manifesztációk és molekuláris genetikai vizsgálatok [Shwachman-Diamond syndrome: clinical manifestations and molecular genetics]. *Orv Hetil*. 2007;148(11):513–519. doi:10.1556/OH.2007.27922 HungarianPMID: 17350924.
110. Savage SA, Alter BP. Dyskeratosis congenita. *Hematol Oncol Clin North Am*. 2009;23(2):215–231. doi:10.1016/j.hoc.2009.01.003.
111. Niewisch MR, Savage SA. An update on the biology and management of dyskeratosis congenita and related telomere biology disorders. *Expert Rev Hematol*. 2019;12(12):1037–1052. doi:10.1080/17474086.2019.1662720 Epub 2019 Sep 10. PMID: 31478401.
112. Husain EH, Mullah-Ali A, Al-Sharidah S, Azab AF. Adekile A. Infectious etiologies of transient neutropenia in previously healthy children. *Pediatr Infect Dis J*. 2012;31(6):575–577. doi:10.1097/INF.0b013e318250084a PMID: 22414904.
113. Boxer L, Dale DC. Neutropenia: causes and consequences. *Semin Hematol*. 2002;39(2):75–81. doi:10.1053/shem.2002.31911 PMID: 11957188.
114. Moore DC. Drug-Induced Neutropenia: a Focus on Rituximab-Induced Late-Onset Neutropenia. *P T*. 2016;41(12):765–768.
115. Minegishi Y, Saito M. Cutaneous manifestations of Hyper IgE syndrome. *Allergol Int*. 2012;61(2):191–196. doi:10.2332/allergolint.12-RAI-0423 Epub 2012 Mar 25. PMID: 22441639.
116. Freeman AF, Holland SM. Clinical manifestations of hyper IgE syndromes. *Dis Markers*. 2010;29(3–4):123–130. doi:10.3233/DMA-2010-0734 PMID: 21178271; PMCID: PMC3835387.
117. Maglione PJ, Simchoni N, Cunningham-Rundles C. Toll-like receptor signaling in primary immune deficiencies. *Ann NY Acad Sci*. 2015;1356(1):1–21. doi:10.1111/nyas.12763.
118. Picard C, von Bernuth H, Ghandil P, Chrabieh M, Levy O, et al. Clinical features and outcome of patients with IRAK-4 and MyD88 deficiency. *Medicine (Baltimore*. 2010;89(6):403–425. doi:10.1097/MD.0b013e3181fd8ec3 )PMID: 21057262; PMCID: PMC3103888.
119. Picard C, Casanova JL, Puel A. Infectious diseases in patients with IRAK-4, MyD88, NEMO, or IκBα deficiency. *Clin Microbiol Rev*. 2011;24(3):490–497. doi:10.1128/CMR.00001-11.
120. Israël A. The IKK complex, a central regulator of NF-kappaB activation. *Cold Spring Harb Perspect Biol*. 2010;2(3):a000158. doi:10.1101/cshperspect.a000158.
121. MacDuff DA, Baldridge MT, Qaqish AM, Nice TJ, Darbandi AD, Hartley VL, et al. HOIL1 Is Essential for the Induction of Type I and III Interferons by MDA5 and Regulates Persistent Murine Norovirus Infection. *J Virol*. 2018;92(23):e01368. doi:10.1128/JVI.01368-18 PMID: 30209176; PMCID: PMC6232484.
122. Boisson B, Laplantine E, Dobbs K, et al. Human HOIP and LUBAC deficiency underlies autoinflammation, immunodeficiency, amylopectinosis, and lymphangiectasia. *J Exp Med*. 2015;212(6):939–951. doi:10.1084/jem.20141130.
123. Koehn J, Huesken D, Jaritz M, Rot A, Zurini M, Dwertmann A, et al. Assessing the function of human UNC-93B in Toll-like receptor signaling and major histocompatibility complex II response. *Hum Immunol*. 2007;68(11):871–878. doi:10.1016/j.humimm.2007.07.007 Epub 2007 Sep 24. PMID: 18082565.
124. Conley ME. Immunodeficiency: UNC-93B gets a toll call. *Trends Immunol*. 2007;28(3):99–101. doi:10.1016/j.it.2007.01.001 Epub 2007 Jan 19. PMID: 17240194.
125. Rosenzweig SD, Holland SM. Defects in the interferon-gamma and interleukin-12 pathways. *Immunol Rev*. 2005;203:38–47. doi:10.1111/j.0105-2896.2005.00227.x PMID: 15661020.
126. Lammas DA, Casanova JL, Kumararatne DS. Clinical consequences of defects in the IL-12-dependent interferon-gamma (IFN-gamma) pathway. *Clin Exp Immunol*. 2000;121(3):417–425. doi:10.1046/j.1365-2249.2000.01284.x.
127. Tichaczek-Goska D. Deficiencies and excessive human complement system activation in disorders of multifarious etiology. *Adv Clin Exp Med*. 2012;21(1):105–114 PMID: 23214307.
128. Zipfel PF, Heinen S, Józsi M, Skerka C. Complement and diseases: defective alternative pathway control results in kidney and eye diseases. *Mol Immunol*. 2006;43(1–2):97–106. doi:10.1016/j.molimm.2005.06.015 PMID: 16026839.
129. Frank MM. Complement disorders and hereditary angioedema. *J Allergy Clin Immunol*. 2010;125(2 Suppl 2):S262–S271. doi:10.1016/j.jaci.2009.10.063 PMID: 20176263.

130. Mayilyan KR. Complement genetics, deficiencies, and disease associations. *Protein Cell.* 2012;3(7):487–496. doi:10.1007/s13238-012-2924-6 Epub 2012 Jul 10. PMID: 22773339; PMCID: PMC4875391.
131. D'Cruz D, Taylor J, Ahmed T, Asherson R, Khamashta M, Hughes GR. Complement factor 2 deficiency: a clinical and serological family study. *Ann Rheum Dis.* 1992;51(11):1254–1256. doi:10.1136/ard.51.11.1254.
132. Sanal O, Yel L, Tezcan I, Ersoy F, Berkel AI. Homozygous C2 deficiency: association with defective alternative pathway function and immunoglobulin deficiency. *Int Arch Allergy Immunol.* 1996;110(2):195–198. doi:10.1159/000237287 PMID: 8645999.
133. Eisen DP. Mannose-binding lectin deficiency and respiratory tract infection. *J Innate Immun.* 2010;2(2):114–122. doi:10.1159/000228159 Epub 2009 Jul 7. PMID: 20375630; PMCID: PMC7179718.
134. Ram S, Lewis LA, Rice PA. Infections of people with complement deficiencies and patients who have undergone splenectomy. *Clin Microbiol Rev.* 2010;23(4):740–780. doi:10.1128/CMR.00048-09.
135. Lewis LA, Ram S. Meningococcal disease and the complement system. *Virulence.* 2014;5(1):98–126. doi:10.4161/viru.26515.
136. Brodsky RA. Paroxysmal nocturnal hemoglobinuria. *Blood.* 2014;124(18):2804–2811. doi:10.1182/blood-2014-02-522128 Epub 2014 Sep 18. PMID: 25237200; PMCID: PMC4215311.
137. Alba-Domínguez M, López-Lera A, Garrido S, Nozal P, González-Granado I, Melero J, et al. Complement factor I deficiency: a not so rare immune defect: characterization of new mutations and the first large gene deletion. *Orphanet J Rare Dis.* 2012;7:42. doi:10.1186/1750-1172-7-42 PMID: 22710145; PMCID: PMC3458969.
138. Genel F, Sjöholm AG, Skattum L, Truedsson L. Complement factor I deficiency associated with recurrent infections, vasculitis and immune complex glomerulonephritis. *Scand J Infect Dis.* 2005;37(8):615–618. doi:10.1080/00365540510034536 PMID: 16138437.
139. Zipfel PF, Skerka C, Caprioli J, Manuelian T, Neumann HH, Noris M, et al. Complement factor H and hemolytic uremic syndrome. *Int Immunopharmacol.* 2001;1(3):461–468. doi:10.1016/s1567-5769(00)00047-3 PMID: 11367530.
140. Pappalardo E, Zingale LC, Terlizzi A, Zanichelli A, Folcioni A, Cicardi M. Mechanisms of C1-inhibitor deficiency. *Immunobiology.* 2002;205(4–5):542–551. doi:10.1078/0171-2985-00153 PMID: 12396014.

# CHAPTER 6

# Infection and Immunity

**Kiarash Saleki[a,b], Sepideh Razi[c,d,e], Nima Rezaei[e,f,g]**
[a]Student Research Committee, Babol University of Medical Sciences, Babol, Iran
[b]USERN Office, Babol University of Medical Sciences, Babol, Iran
[c]Cancer Immunology Project (CIP), Universal Scientific Education and Research Network (USERN), Tehran, Iran
[d]School of Medicine, Iran University of Medical Sciences, Tehran, Iran
[e]Research Center for Immunodeficiencies, Children's Medical Center, Tehran University of Medical Sciences, Tehran, Iran
[f]Department of Immunology, School of Medicine, Tehran University of Medical Sciences, Tehran, Iran
[g]Network of Immunity in Infection, Malignancy and Autoimmunity (NIIMA), Universal Scientific Education and Research Network (USERN), Tehran, Iran

## Introduction

Infectious diseases are caused by viruses, bacteria, fungi, and parasites and are a major cause of human suffering in terms of both human morbidity and mortality throughout history. The dissemination of infectious diseases was affected by various epochs in human civilization. For example, parasitic and zoonotic infections have become more prevalent after animals' domestication, while airborne infections of viral and bacterial etiology have become common after large settlements and urbanization. Throughout history, humanity was affected by large pandemics such as plague, smallpox, cholera, influenza, and Coronavirus disease 2019 (COVID-19), as well as by the more chronic infections, such as tuberculosis and syphilis. Morbidity due to infectious diseases is prevalent despite the recent advancements in diagnosis, treatment, and management protocols. World Health Organization (WHO) reported that there are 300–500 million cases of malaria, 333 million cases of sexually transmitted diseases (STDs) (e.g., syphilis, gonorrhea, chlamydia, and trichomonas), 33 million cases of the *Human immunodeficiency virus* (*HIV*)/ acquired immunodeficiency disease syndrome (AIDS), 14 million individuals infected with tuberculosis, and 3–5 million cases of cholera, worldwide.[1]

The immune response to infectious microorganisms can be classified into two main classes: innate and adaptive immune responses. These responses are inseparable. For instance, activation of innate receptors (e.g., toll-like receptors (TLRs)) leads to the release of cytokines, which results in activation of the adaptive immune system. The innate immune response to a pathogen begins when pathogen-associated molecular patterns (PAMPs) of the bacterial pathogens induce pattern recognition receptors (PRRs) of the innate immune system. The innate immune system triggers antigen-specific responses produced by the adaptive immune system. This is followed by the secretion of pro-inflammatory and anti-inflammatory factors that help contain the infection. In turn, pathogens manipulate host defense procedures (e.g., avoid phagocytosis) to survive and ultimately replicate.[2] Adaptive immunity includes antigen-specific responses that

*Clinical Immunology*
DOI: https://doi.org/10.1016/B978-0-12-818006-8.00007-4

are highly adapted to the specific pathogen and are precisely regulated through innate immune cells' crosstalk. It has evolved to provide a versatile and accurately calibrated repertoire of receptors that can differentiate self- and non-self-antigens. During maturation, naïve B and T lymphocytes go through antigen receptor gene reorganization to create a diverse repertoire comprising antigen-specific receptors that can recognize all potential antigens. After overcoming pathogen, pathogen-specific long-lived memory lymphocytes will be developed. These memory cells quickly and robustly reply to future encounters with the invading microorganism and synthesize new effector cells to contain the infection.[3] Whether an infectious microorganism is an "old acquaintance" or a newly surfaced threat, the immune system's fight against it is normally the initial line of defense it encounters. With vaccines and effective therapies often unavailable, the immune system's attempts to eradicate infectious agents or infected cells are commonly the only means to eliminate them. Deciphering the immune system in addition to the infectious microorganisms tactics to sabotage it is of key significance to the researchers and clinicians.[4]

Accurate and timely diagnosis of infection is crucial for successful and targeted treatment. However, routine microbiological recognition is inefficient and often delayed to the extent that makes it clinically impractical. The immune system is capable of a rapid, high-sensitivity, and high-specificity recognition of a broad spectrum of microbes that has been refined over millions of years of evolution. Therefore, the early immune response is likely to provide far better insight into the true nature and severity of microbial infections compared to conventional tests.[5] We briefly go over the application of immunoassays, such as enzyme and antigen assays, in different scenarios of pathogenic infection.

Emerging issues in the therapy of infections demand the development of advanced treatments targeting the innate and adaptive immune processes. For example, despite our efforts to halt the increase and spread of antimicrobial resistance, bacteria are progressively becoming less vulnerable to antimicrobial treatment, and rates of development of novel antibiotics are declining. As a result, it is necessary to explore new paradigms for anti-infective therapy. One promising approach involves the host-directed immunomodulatory treatment, whereby natural mechanisms in the host are exploited to improve treatment benefit. The goal is to activate or improve protective antimicrobial immunity while limiting inflammation-induced tissue injury.[6] The first and only human vaccine in use against a parasitic disorder is RTS, S/AS01 (Mosquirix, GlaxoSmithKline) that had suboptimal efficacy, less than 50 percent, against *Plasmodium falciparum* in children.[7] Similar scenarios apply to other infectious diseases.

The present chapter provides an overview of definition and epidemiology, molecular immunological mechanisms, immune-based diagnostics, and immunomodulating treatments for viral, bacterial, fungal, and parasitic agents that contribute to human infectious disease. Also, areas where further research is demanded have been highlighted.

## Bacterial infections

### Definition

Bacteria are single-celled pathogens without nuclear membrane, exhibit active metabolism, and divide via binary fission.[8] The bacterial cell wall is a complicated, mesh-resembling construct, which in bacteria is required for the conservation of cellular form and integrity of constructure. The cell wall is regarded as a promising target for some of our most potent antibiotics.[9] Additionally, bacterial cell wall particles can exert immune activating and cytotoxic effects and have an essential role in bacterial diseases.[10-15] To crosstalk with their surroundings, bacteria usually exhibit long proteinaceous appendices on their cellular surface, named pili or fimbriae. These non-flagellar thread-resembling constructs are polymers made up of covalently or non-covalently interconnecting pilin repeats.[16] While bacteria are present within almost all spectrums of environmental conditions, only a small proportion of the global bacteria cause infectious diseases. These infections have a significant impact on the population. Generally, bacterial infections are treated easier compared to viral infections because the armamentarium of antimicrobial therapies that target bacteria is more comprehensive. However, bacterial resistance to antimicrobials is a swiftly growing issue with significant large-scale consequences.[17] In 2021, a global epidemiological evaluation reported the global prevalence of multidrug-resistant (MDR) bacteria that was 34 percent, 95 percent CI.[31-37] The prevalence of MDR bacteria varied meaningfully between geographical regions, with the highest prevalence in Asia. Independent risk factors for infection with MDR bacteria are infection in Asia (in particular in India), antibiotics use within the 3 months prior to hospitalization, healthcare exposure, and infection site of infection. Infections that result from MDR bacteria are linked to a decreased rate of recovery, an increased risk for shock and organ failures, and an increase in-hospital mortality compared to those that result from non-MDR bacteria.[18] A recent study on MDR prevalence in cases with renal disease reported bacterial pathogens most commonly isolated were: *Escherichia coli*, *Staphylococcus aureus*, *Enterococcus faecalis*, *Pseudomonas aeruginosa*, *Candida*, *Staphylococcus epidermidis*, and *Klebsiella pneumoniae*.[19]

Bacteria are special among the prokaryotes, as a wide range of them are considered normal flora, which colonize in the host without being infectious. After being infected, the clinical infection can be detected, and solely in a trivial subset of infections do we see the clinically important infection. Bacterial infections spread in many ways. For an effective transmission, a prominent number of them should survive in the environment and arrive at a susceptible organism. Many bacteria have adapted to survive in food, soil, water, and elsewhere. Some infect vectors such as insects or animals before being transmitted to another human.

New species and variants of familiar species continue to be discovered, particularly as we intrude into new ecosystems. Both Legionnaire's disease, and Lyme disease, which are now well-known to healthcare professionals, were discovered in the 1970s. The recent increased prevalence of severely immunosuppressed patients, as a result of AIDS, the rising use of immunosuppressive chemotherapies, and treatments for transplantation of organs, tissues, and cells have amplified the population of cases highly susceptible to subtypes of bacterial diseases, which were relatively rare before.[17]

## Mechanisms

The immune response to a bacterial stimulus initiates when PAMPs of the bacterial pathogens trigger PRRs of the innate immune system. Moreover, the innate immune system activates antigen-specific responses regulated via the adaptive immune system. In turn, pathogens manipulate host defense mechanisms to survive and ultimately replicate. This is followed by the release of pro-inflammatory and anti-inflammatory agents that aim to limit infection and mediate clinical sepsis. When sepsis and signs of deteriorating organs are evident, pro-inflammatory phenomena have diminished, and a hypo-inflammatory phase takes over that is recognized via anergy of monocytes and apoptosis of T lymphocytes. The mentioned cascade of occurrences appears to vary among patients.[2] We will discuss the response to bacterial infections in two sections: innate and adaptive immunity. Also, a brief overview of immune response to infections is depicted in Fig. 6.1.

### *Innate immunity*

#### Inflammasomes

**An overview of inflammasomes** Inflammasomes are a recently explained class of proteins classically characterized for their key role in the activation of inflammation. They include a carboxy-terminal leucine-rich repeat, a central nucleotide oligomerization region, and an amino-terminal effector region that helps to categorize inflammasomes into three groups: pyrin-containing NOD-like receptors (NLRPs), CARD-containing NOD-like receptors (NLRCs), and a baculovirus inhibitor of apoptosis protein repeat (BIR) domain-containing group. Caspase-1, a proteolytic enzyme, is induced after the synthesis of inflammasomes and helps to handle pro-interleukin (IL)-1β modifications. IL-1 acts both locally and systemically[20,21] and is different from many other cytokines as its formation and secretion include a two-stage mechanism. The initial stage is the transcriptional enhancement of IL-1β as an inactive precursor (pro-IL-1β) downstream from Dectin-1 and TLR-2/4,[22] and the second stage is a proteolytic breakdown by caspase-1 secreting active IL-1β.[23] Likewise, pro-IL-18 is also cleaved by caspase-1.[24] Overall, cytokines release represents the product of complex regulatory mechanisms within the inflammasome complex.

**NLRP3** Three models of NLRP3 induction in response to microbial ligands have been suggested.[25] The channel model explains that extracellular adenosine triphosphate (ATP) from microbial pathogens induces the P2 × 7 receptor and permits the efflux of

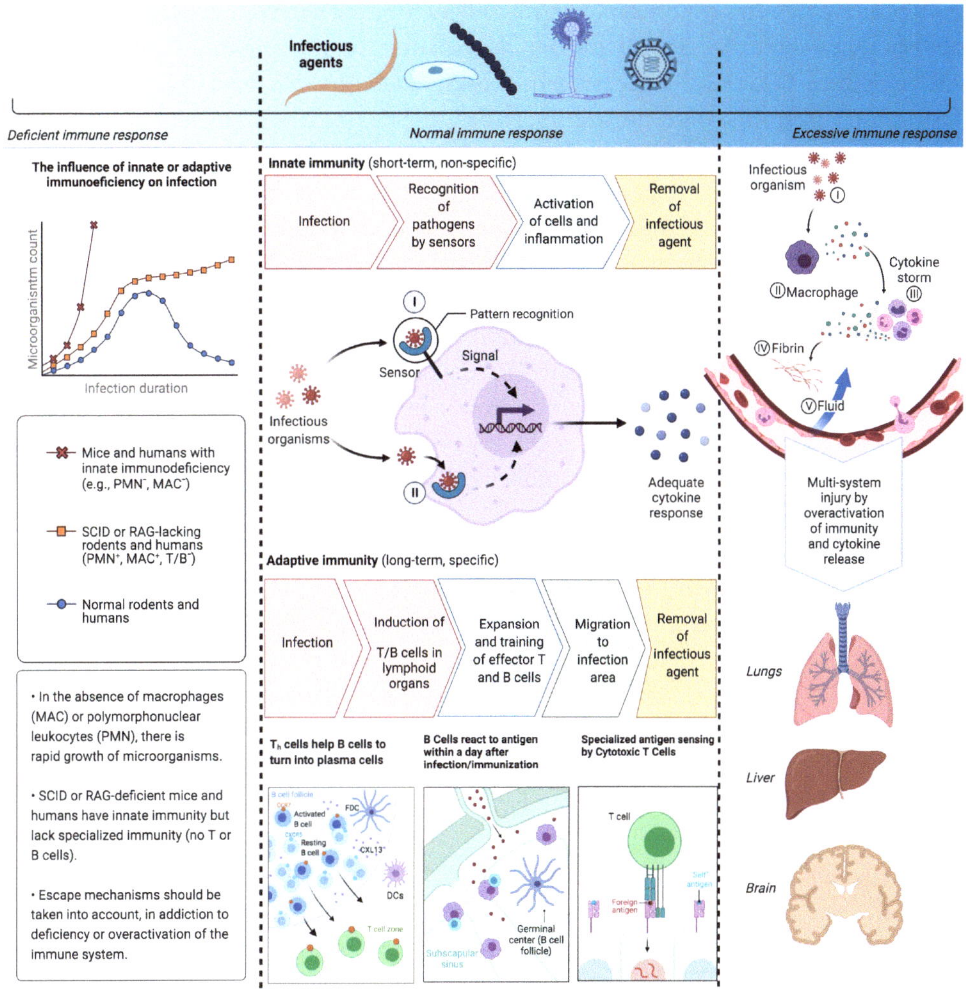


**Fig. 6.1** ***Overview of innate and adaptive immune responses to infection.***

intracellular potassium ions (K+), leading to NLRP3 induction. Also, several bacterial pore-forming toxins can induce cellular ion dysregulation and cause NLRP3 activation, such as group B Streptococcus. Also, ion imbalance via NLRP3 mediation is found in *Chlamydia pneumoniae*,[26,27] *Staphylococcus aureus*,[28] and *Streptococcus pneumoniae*.[29] Cellular induction by some bacteria is unrelated to P2 × 7R, denoting that multiple processes can modulate NLRP3 induction.[30]

Evading the lysosome after phagocytosis is a key phase during the movement of numerous pathogens, toxins, and cholesterol-dependent cytolysins. The lysosomal rupture model for NLRP3 induction postulates that the secretion of lysosomal enzymes like cathepsin B into the cell cytoplasm during lysosomal disruption results in NLRP3 induction.[25] Interestingly, prokaryotic messenger ribonucleic acid (mRNA) shed from the lysosome into the cytosol during degradation of phagocytosed live bacteria is able to induce NLRP3,[31] indicating that bacterial RNA can be a major activator of the NLRP3 inflammasome during infectious disease. Reactive oxygen species (ROS) secreted from the mitochondria is considered to be a cellular stress-triggered signal and may also trigger NLRP3 inflammasomes.[32] The ROS model relies on observations that NLRP3 is induced after mitochondrial injury and secretion of ROS.[33] This function relies on the mitochondrial voltage-dependent ion channels that enhance the transport of ions between the intermembrane area and the cell cytosol. Oxidized mitochondrial DNA (mtDNA) from mitochondria injured via bacterial infection may bind and activate NLRP3.[33] This phenomenon is negatively mediated via the anti-apoptotic protein B-cell lymphoma protein (BCL)-2, indicating a linkage between apoptosis and inflammasome induction. The concept that the NLRP3 inflammasome senses mitochondrial dysfunction could potentially help in understanding the linkage between mitochondrial damage and inflammatory disorders.[34]

New agents mediating NLRP3 induction have been recognized. For instance, guanylate-binding protein (GBP)5 and double-stranded RNA-dependent protein kinase (PKR) have been found to exert fundamental functions in NLRP3 induction. GBP5 has been displayed to react with the pyrin domain of NLRP3 and helps the oligomerization of the inflammasome.[35] Furthermore, GBP5 mediates NLRP3 activation by live bacteria, contrary to what has been observed during sterile inflammation. Infected GBP5-lacking rodents have shown elevated bacterial burdens and a more rapid disease deterioration compared to wild-type rodents. It has been reported that PKR is able to auto-phosphorylate as a result of macrophage activation by NLRP3 ligands. Activated PKR can attach to NLRP3, NLRP1b, NLRC4, and absent in melanoma (AIM)2,[36] and PKR can induce the NLRP3 inflammasome and enhance secretion of the pro-inflammatory cytokine high-mobility group protein B1 (HMGB1) when activated by a group of ligands comprising bacterial pathogens. As many of the NLRP3 activators result in inhibition of protein synthesis, it has also been shown that direct blockade of ribosomal actions, irrespective of K+ efflux, induces inflammasomes.[37] However, it is unclear how the PKR phosphorylation that precedes NLRP3 inflammasome activation is produced during infection.

A recent experiment reported that NLRP3 inflammasome regulates IL-1β synthesis in immune cells in response to *Acinetobacter baumannii* and contributes to pulmonary inflammation in mice. Findings indicated that NLRP3, apoptosis-associated speck-like protein containing a C-terminal caspase recruitment domain (ASC), and caspase-1, but not NLRC4, are required for *Acinetobacter baumannii*-triggered synthesis of IL-1β in macrophages. An inhibitor assay showed that multiple pathways, such as P2 × 7R, K+ efflux, ROS release, and release of cathepsins, contribute to IL-1β production in macrophages in response to *Acinetobacter baumannii*. IL-1β production in bronchoalveolar lavage fluid was disrupted in NLRP3-lacking and caspase-1/11-lacking rodents infected with *Acinetobacter baumannii* in comparison to that in wild-type rodents.[38] In another study, researchers investigated the NLRP3 production in the context of different T helper (Th) cytokine microenvironments and its function in response to sublytic $\alpha$-toxin activation in cases with atopic dermatitis and psoriasis compared with healthy controls. NLRP3 and caspase-1 expressions were attenuated in lesioned atopic dermatitis skin in comparison to psoriatic and healthy skin. IL-4, IL-5, and IL-13 downregulated NLRP3 and ASC, while interferon (IFN)-$\gamma$ enhanced NLRP3 in human primary keratinocytes. In monocytes, caspase-1 expression was attenuated by Th2 cytokines and enhanced by a Th1 milieu. Caspase-1-dependent IL-1$\beta$ secretion was disrupted in monocytes from cases with atopic dermatitis in comparison to cases with psoriasis and healthy controls via $\alpha$-toxin activation after priming with lipoteichoic acid.[39] This study concluded that disrupted NLRP3 function might explain how skin colonization and infection with *Staphylococcus aureus* can lead to chronic skin inflammation in atopic dermatitis.[40]

**Other NLRPs: NLRP1b, NLRP6, NLRP7, NLRP10, and NLRP12** Research on THP1 cells displayed that NLRP1 shapes a complex with CARD8, ASC, caspase-5, and caspase-1 to modify IL-1$\beta$.[41] NLRP1 is linked to IL-1$\beta$ release by muramyl-dipeptide in a BCL-2- and BCL-XL-mediated manner.[42] Also, rodent NLRP1b has been explained as a receptor for a lethal toxin from *Bacillus anthracis* in the host cytosol and plays a role in caspase-1-regulated IL-1$\beta$ release and pyroptosis.[43] NLRP6 is reported to be involved in the mediation of commensal microflora and bacterial detection.[44-46] The NLRP6 inflammasome function has come to light as NLRP6-lacking rodents showed modified gut microbiota and a predisposition for colitis following a diminish in IL-18 excretion via intestinal epithelial cells.[44] However, Anand et al.[45] presented NLRP6 as a negative mediator of innate immunity during certain bacterial infections because rodents deficient in NLRP6 were resistant to infection with *Listeria monocytogenes*, Salmonella, and *E. coli*. A preliminary study of NLRP12 (Monarch-1/PYPAF7) showed that the protein could act as an inflammasome element.[47] Complying with this, the NLRP12 inflammasome has been explained to exert a pro-inflammatory effect during bacterial infection as an important mediator of IL-1$\beta$ and IL-18 secretion. In this study, NLRP12-deficient mice were unable to control infection with a modified *Yersinia pestis* strain and had attenuated blood IL-1$\beta$ and IL-18, and amplified spleen bacterial loads.[48] Research has also proposed NLRP12 as a suppressor of colon inflammation and tumorigenesis in a dextran sodium sulfate (DSS) colitis model, by mediating dendritic cell (DCs) employment. Interestingly, Nlrp12-/- DCs display a remarkably decreased ability to transport to draining lymph nodes.[49-51] NLRP6 and NLRP12, as well as other NOD-like receptors (NLRs), can play different roles in the immune system. NLRP7 is not expressed in rodents, but human NLRP7 is linked to inflammasome actions in response to bacterial lipopeptides (TLR-2 ligands) via a small interfering (si)RNA knockdown system.[52] It has been shown that NLRC5, which is a transcriptional regulator of major histocompatibility complex (MHC) class I genes,[53] could participate in inflammasome activation during infection.[54] NLRP10 is a cytoplasmically localized protein that enhances the innate immune responses activated by the invasive bacterial pathogen *Shigella flexneri*. Researchers have shown that NLRP10 is involved in pro-inflammatory cytokine release, activated via shigella in epithelial cells and primary dermal fibroblasts by affecting p38 and nuclear factor kappa B (NF-κB) induction. This action depends on the ATPase activity of NLRP10 and its PYD subunit. NLRP10 reacts with nucleotide-binding oligomerization domain (NOD)1, an NLR that contributes to the sensing of invasive microbes, and both proteins are recruited to the bacterial entry area at the cell membrane. Furthermore, NLRP10 reacts with downstream elements of the NOD1 signaling pathway, including RIP2, TAK1, and NEMO.[55]

**NLRC4** Bacteria such as Pseudomonas, Legionella, Salmonella, Yersinia, and Listeria may trigger caspase-1 activation and IL-1β/IL-18 development by NLRC4 activation.[39, 56-58] NLRC4 is particularly triggered via a functional bacterial type III or IV secretion system (T3SS/T4SS) or flagellin.[57,58] *Salmonella typhimurium* is one of the first bacteria reported to be able to induce caspase-1 by the NLRC4-inflammasome. Mutants of *S. typhimurium* that lack the fliC and flipB genes, which encode flagellin monomers, cannot stimulate caspase-1 through NLRC4.[58] Ligands may directly attach to specific subtypes of the neuronal apoptosis inhibitor protein (NAIP) NLR class to induce the NLRC4 inflammasome. NAIP5/NAIP6 react with flagellin, while NAIP2 reacts with the T3SS rod ingredients Salmonella PrgJ and Burkholderia BsaK.[59] NLRC4/NAIP5 inflammasome stimulation is directly linked to eicosanoid secretion from resident peritoneal macrophages.[60] By intestinal mononuclear phagocytes, NLRC4 is involved in the pro-inflammatory defense processes in the intestine against foreign, but not commensal, bacteria.[61] Moreover, NLRC4 activation can be harmful to the host during infection, as the colonization of pathogenic *E. coli* develops in the intestine following antibiotic therapy, which significantly changes the ingredients of microbiota.[62] Possibly similar to NLRP3 activation by PKR, NLRC4 can be induced after phosphorylation at Ser533 via Protein Kinase C δ (PKCδ).[63] NLRC4 is also linked to other mechanisms that do not recruit IL-1β and IL-18 excretion, like the degradation and restriction of intercellular bacterial growth of Legionella pneumophila downstream of caspase-7 activation[64] and NLRC4-dependent cell death.[65] Activation of caspase-1 by the inflammasome is related to pyroptosis, a pro-inflammatory form of caspase-1-dependent cell death. NLRC4-dependent pyroptosis takes place in response to some bacterial infections, such as *Salmonella*, *Legionella pneumophila*, and *Francisella tularensis*.[66] This cell death process exerts a defensive function within the host. Activation of caspase-1 through NLRC4 by *S. typhimurium* consistently producing flagellin can result in antibacterial defenses irrespective of IL-1β and IL-18,[65] as the inflammatory cell death drove clearance of the pathogen from the surrounding tissue by neutrophil employment. Also, NLRP3 and NLRC4 assist each other in the development of a proper response against Salmonella.[66]

Some bacteria can activate multiple inflammasomes following infection, as they include ligands for multiple NLRs or Absent in melanoma 2 (AIM2). Future research should focus on deciphering how inflammasome elements cooperate for optimal host responses to pathogens. Bacterial population dynamics suggest that the NAIP/NLRC4 inflammasome particularly limits *S. typhimurium* migration from the gut to draining lymph nodes. This may be caused by NAIP/NLRC4 pathways within intestinal epithelial cells, while *S. typhimurium* escapes restriction through phagocyte NAIP/NLRC4. NLRP3 and caspase-11 also fail to restrict *S. typhimurium* from crossing the mucosa, migration to lymph nodes, and systemic dissemination. The ability of intestinal epithelial cells to drive an NAIP/NLRC4 defense can be understood by the high NAIP/NLRC4 expression in intestinal epithelial cells and the necessity for epithelium-attacking *S. typhimurium* to produce the NAIP1-6 ligands-flagella and type-III-secretion-system-1. Imaging shows both ligands are downregulated upon crossing the intestinal epithelial cells.[67]

**Absent in melanoma 2 (AIM2)** AIM2 is a cytosolic binding receptor for double-stranded DNA, known to shape an inflammasome and trigger caspase-1 in the presence of pathogens.[26] Bone marrow-derived macrophages (BMDMs) from AIM2-/- rodents lack pro-caspase-1, pro-IL-1β, and pro-IL-18 development after infection with *Listeria monocytogenes* and *Francisella tularensis*, and AIM2-lacking rodents were more sensitive to subcutaneous infection with *Francisella tularensis*, correlating to reduced serum IL-18 concentrations.[68-70]

Recent work reported the functional significance of inflammasome activity during central nervous system (CNS) infection with *Staphylococcus aureus*. Findings suggested the involvement of AIM2 based on similar disease algorithms among AIM2 and ASC knockout rodents. In addition to IL-1β, other major inflammatory mediators, such as IL-6, C-X-C chemokine ligand (CXCL)1, CXCL10, and C-C chemokine ligand (CCL)2 were markedly reduced in the CNS of AIM2 and ASC knockout mice, denoting autocrine/paracrine functions of IL-1β, as these regulators do not need inflammasome processing for secretion. These studies exhibit the role of the AIM2 inflammasome as a major molecular platform for mediating IL-1β secretion and survival during acute CNS *Staphylococcus aureus* infection.[71]

## TLRs

Current models postulate that innate immune cells sense pathogens through TLRs and other PRRs and reply quickly via secreting cytokines and antimicrobial mediators (e.g., ROS and nitric oxide (NO)). The role of TLRs in several major bacterial infections is described in the following passage.

Mycobacterium tuberculosis-activated tumor necrosis factor (TNF) release is TLR-2-dependent in vitro.[72] TLR-2, along with TLR-1 and TLR-6, regulates responses to mycobacterial lipoproteins, lipomannan, arabinose-capped lipoarabinomannan (ara-LAM), and phosphatidyl-myo-inositol mannoside (PIM). While most purified mycobacterial elements act via TLR-2, enhanced TLRs expression enables cells to reply to the whole bacilli by TLR-2 or TLR-4 in a MyD88-dependent fashion.[31,32] Still, primary mouse macrophages that express normal concentrations of TLRs detect intact mycobacteria irrespective of TLR/MyD88 pathways.[33] Moreover, mycobacterial DNA contains stimulatory CpG motifs that induce TLR-9.[27] TLR induction through mycobacterial elements results in the release of pro-inflammatory cytokines, such as TNF and IL-12, and release of NO, a byproduct with strong anti-mycobacterial activity in rodents.[34,36] These together imply that disruption in TLR signaling may lead to exacerbation of the *Mycobacterium tuberculosis* infection.

Salmonella has at least four TLR inducers: Lipopolysaccharide (LPS), bacterial lipoproteins, flagellin, and CpG DNA that induce TLR-4, TLR-2, TLR-5, and TLR-9, respectively. Cells such as macrophages and DCs can detect Salmonella via these TLRs and activate the production of cytokines that are also involved in responses to Salmonella in vitro. Injection of Salmonella or LPS directly into the blood circulation leads to shock. This finding led to the hypothesis that LPS is a main virulence element of Salmonella. C3H/HeJ rodents that display a mutation in the TLR-4 allele show increased endurance to intraperitoneal or intravenous challenge by LPS or Salmonella than the closely related C3H/HeN rodents that display a wild-type copy of TLR-4.[46] In fact, the discovery of the importance of different genetic variations in TLRs, which can affect the susceptibility of individuals to LPS, is very crucial.[73]

Staphylococci possess several TLR inducers. Bacterial lipoproteins and lipoteichoic acid serve as TLR-2/6 activators,[74-76] while CpG DNA functions via TLR-9. In addition, NOD2 detects *Staphylococcus aureus* by the recognition of peptidoglycan motifs.[26]

## Other mechanisms

**Immune evasion by bacteria after invasion** After attacking the host, there are multiple evasion processes through which bacteria dodge the immune system, such as evading the early vacuole synthesis, disruption in the early and late endocytic processes, and altering the exocytic procedures. Two brief examples are provided here.

One path to avoid the unfavorable environment resulting from the fusion with degradative enzyme-rich endocytic compartments is to swiftly evade the nascent vacuole, attack the cytoplasm and utilize the actin cytoskeleton to facilitate intracellular motility. This approach is used by *Burkholderia pseudomallei*, the causative agent of the melioidosis, *Listeria monocytogenes*, *Rickettsia rickettsii*, *Mycobacterium marinum*, and *Shigella flexneri*. *Shigella flexneri* produces invasion plasmid antigen (Ipa)B that plays an important role in host cell entrance and shows a lytic activity that is used to infiltrate the vacuolar membrane.[77]

The reaction of the nascent vacuole with early endosomes takes place 5–20 minutes following the invasion and is temporary. But vacuoles containing *Mycobacterium tuberculosis* and *Mycobacterium avium* show the features of early endosomal organelles that do not develop into late endosomal and lysosomal sections. Precisely, vacuoles that comprise mycobacteria keep the early endosomal guanosine triphosphatases (GTP)ase RAB5 while specifically leaving out the late endosomal GTPase RAB7 and the early endosome antigen 1 (EEA1), both of which are mediators of vesicular trafficking and phagosome development.[78-80]

Spirochetal bacteria *Leptospira* spp. can cause leptospirosis, a disregarded and reemerging zoonotic disorder worldwide. Infection by these agents can result in an acute and possibly fatal disease or chronic asymptomatic colonization of the bacteria in the kidney. Both subtypes of the disorder display the ability of leptospires to escape the host immune response.[81] The prominent motility of leptospires is represented by two atypical "endoflagella", which lie at poles of the bacterium and stretch within the periplasm. Their spiral form is due to the peptidoglycan mesh, shaping a thin layer in proximity to the inner membrane. The membranes are rich in lipoproteins.[82] In contrast with that of other spirochetes, the leptospiral outer membrane is enclosed by LPS.[83] Live leptospires also escape TLR-5 recognition. However, once leptospires are killed by antimicrobial peptides, leptospiral flagellins are recognized by human TLR-5 but not through rodent TLR-5.[84] Leptospires activate the NLRP3 inflammasome in both humans and rodents. In animal experiments, activation of the inflammasome requires 2-phase signaling, utilizing LPS and lipoprotein signaling by TLR-4 and TLR-2, respectively, in combination with the attenuation of a $Na+/K-$ pump, a danger protein.[85] In humans, NLRP3 induction is regulated by bacteria-activated ROS.[86] Ultimately, peptidoglycan from leptospires evades host detection via NOD1 and NOD2 and because of the lipoprotein LipL21 that is tightly linked to the peptidoglycan. Also, human but not rodent NOD1 can recognize leptospiral peptidoglycan independent of LipL21.[87]

## *Adaptive immunity*

### Cellular immunity

The adaptive immune response to a bacterial stimulus necessitates the presentation of the bacterial antigen from DCs and monocytes that act as antigen-presenting cells (APCs) to naïve T (Th0) cells. To this aim, surface elements of APCs, such as MHC class II or human leukocyte antigen (HLA)-DR and cluster of differentiation (CD)40 adhere to co-activating agents of Th0 cells, namely CD28 and CD40-ligand, respectively. This attachment triggers the production of other co-activating factors on the cell membranes of APCs, like CD80 and CD86, and as a result, facilitates the antigen presentation to Th0 cells. During this procedure, Th0 cells differentiate into four categories of functionally different T cells:

- Th1: release TNF-$\alpha$, IL-2, and IFN-$\gamma$ and prime pro-inflammatory responses to enhance bacterial phagocytosis.
- Th2: release IL-4, IL-6, and IL-10 and prime anti-inflammatory responses.
- T17: release IL-17 to recruit neutrophils and prime optimal phagocytosis.
- Regulatory T cells (Tregs): prime anti-inflammatory responses.

Differentiation of Th0 to these functionally unique subtypes is managed by the heterodimeric cytokines IL-12/IL-23, IL-27, IL-6, and transforming growth factor (TGF)-β. IL-12 and IL-23 are dimeric proteins that share a p40 peptide. Peptide p35 is present in IL-12 and peptide p19 is present in IL-23. IL-12/IL-23 is secreted by DCs and monocytes. IL-12 promotes Th1 responses. IL-23 helps IL-12 and shifts the immune system towards Th17 responses. IL-27 performs by suppressing the pro-inflammatory T17 response. IL-6 has many functions. It participates in the pro-inflammatory innate immune response and the anti-inflammatory Th2 response. The immune homeostasis mediates the balance between T17 cells and Tregs. In more detail, differentiation of Th0 cells into T17 cells requires induction of the orphan nuclear receptors, such as retinoid-related orphan receptor-γt and retinoid-related orphan receptor (ROR)-α. This is mediated through the combined action of TGF-β and IL-6. When TGF-β exists in the cell microenvironment in the absence of IL-6, the transcription factor Foxp3 is induced resulting in differentiation of Th0 cells into Tregs. On the contrary, the IL-6 triggering of Foxp3 and consequent differentiation into Tregs is suppressed.[2,88] Animal research has shown that ROR-γ is expressed in muscle, brain, heart, and skin. Moreover, expression analysis of ROR-γ homologues demonstrates that it may play a cell-type dependent role in defense against extracellular bacteria.[89]

## Humoral immunity

The clinical presentation of bacterial infection may be due to toxic molecules released by the bacteria rather than from the presence of the microorganisms themselves. Antibodies to these toxins can enable quintessential defense against infection, without directly targeting the bacteria themselves. A classic example is *Corynebacterium diphtheriae* that releases a deadly exotoxin. A newer example is the *Clostridium difficile* that releases both an enterotoxin (toxin A) and cytotoxin (toxin B). Passive immunotherapy by antibody may reduce relapse. Also, high antibody levels against toxin A and B correlate with the reduction of relapse.

Bacteria can possess virulence agents, like enzymes, which enhance dissemination within tissues. Host antibodies that disable these enzymes may have a positive effect on the clinical presentation of bacterial infection. Disabling of toxins and enzymes may stem from direct competition of antibodies and the target molecule or substrate. Competitive mechanisms may also involve the establishment or induction of structures unsuitable for the normal role of the toxin or enzyme. Also, the protection afforded by exotoxin-disabling antibodies may rely on Fcγ receptors.[90]

## Other mechanisms

**Sepsis** Sepsis is the major cause of mortality in most intensive care units. A recent meta-analysis found that patients with severe sepsis administered with usual care had a 28-day mortality of 33.2 percent.[91] Progress in comprehending the immune response to sepsis helps the development of more effective treatments. The immune response in sepsis is defined by a hyper-inflammatory stage that is followed by an immune-repressing stage. Patients fail to defeat attacking bacteria and are prone to opportunistic microorganisms during the hypo-inflammatory phase. The immune response in sepsis is outlined by elements such as co-morbidities (e.g., cancer, heart disease, and diabetes), microbial inoculums size, and the pathogen virulence. Processes that contribute to sepsis-activated immuno-suppression include apoptotic elimination of immune cells, enhanced Tregs and myeloid-derived suppressor cells (MDSCs), and cellular exhaustion. Cellular exhaustion is a phenotype defined via abnormal function, elevated programmed cell death protein (PD)-1, and reduced IL-7 receptor production on T lymphocytes.

In more detail, while both pro- and anti-inflammatory mechanisms are induced together during the onset of sepsis within the initial days, a hyper-inflammatory response usually dictates the clinical feature. The hyper-inflammatory stage has been named a "cytokine storm", which is defined by increased contents of cytokines, such as TNF-α, IL-1β, and IL-6, up to harmful levels. Rapid elimination of both innate and adaptive immune cells by apoptosis takes place to attenuate the response. During this stage, patients may experience a controlled anti-inflammatory response to improve immunological homeostasis. However, some patients may experience an uncontrolled anti-inflammatory response and enter a hypo-inflammatory stage. A prolonged hypo-inflammatory stage may lead to cellular exhaustion. During this stage, patients fail to direct proper immune responses towards microbial pathogens resulting in the reactivation of pathogens and secondary infections, mainly caused by avirulent and opportunistic pathogens.[92]

**Central nervous system infections** Bacterial involvement of the CNS is a critical condition with substantial mortality, which may lead to irreversible neurological damage in survivors. Astrocytes that make up most of the CNS glial cell population mediate the innate and adaptive immune responses in the CNS during infection and help sustain CNS homeostasis and neuronal actions. After antigen detection, astrocytes activate the innate immune response and drive an adaptive immune response to employ peripheral immune cells. The interplay of the CNS and peripheral immune system by a lymphatic system in the meninges suggests that the CNS is under continuous immunological surveillance.[93] Patrolling APCs of this immune network may enter the cervical lymph nodes after an encounter with pathogens that invaded the CNS and prime naïve T cells for differentiation. Triggered T cells can cross the blood-brain barrier with the help of intracellular adhesion molecule (ICAM)-1 and/or vascular cell adhesion protein-1 (VCAM-1).[94] Such adhesives help the astrocyte-lymphocyte interconnection, which promotes upon astrocytes contact with IFN-γ, TNF-α, IL-1β, or TLR ligands like LPS in vitro.[95] Next, employed T cells enter the CNS parenchyma and are reactivated by native APCs like astrocytes and microglia.[96]

Glial cells exert their role in bacterial involvement of the CNS through detecting bacterial molecules such as LPS and bacterial DNA via TLRs.[97] The most well-researched TLR in bacterial involvement of the CNS is TLR-2. Following exposure to the gram-positive bacterium *Staphylococcus aureus*, primary mouse astrocytes enhance TLR-2 production via the secretion of TNF-α. Furthermore, the cells produce IL-1β, CCL2, and NO, a potent antibacterial free radical[98] that triggers astrocytes.[97] These mechanisms are dampened in TLR2-/- astrocytes, indicating that they may be regulated by astroglial TLR-2 pathways.[98] Also, TLR-2 can detect *Streptococcus suis*, a bacterium that can cause meningitis.[99] TLR-2 signaling has been implicated in the activation of astrocytes in response to *Streptococcus suis*. While primary murine astrocytes do not internalize *Streptococcus suis*, contact with the bacteria promotes astroglial TLR-2 expression. This is accompanied by astrocyte induction and release of the pro-inflammatory factors. Moreover, contact with *Streptococcus suis* enhances TLR-6 transcript levels, while TLR-1 expression is not altered. TLR-1 and TLR-6 synthesize heterodimers with TLR-2. As TLR-2/TLR-1 and TLR-2/TLR-6 signaling evoke special cellular responses, the specific amplification in TLR-6 expression could shape the inflammatory reaction of astrocytes.[100] Astroglial TLR-2 may play a role in the involvement of the CNS via Brucella, a gram-negative bacterium that can cause neurobrucellosis and neurological impairments.[101] It should be noted that clinical-radiologic relation in neurobrucellosis ranges from normal radiographic findings accompanied by a positive clinical presentation to different imaging irregularities (e.g., white matter lesions in periventricular and subcortical areas) that denote either an inflammatory response, an immunological response, or a vascular injury.[102,103] Other than endothelial cells,[104] Brucella induces astrocytes and the secretion of cytokines, chemokines, and matrix metalloproteinases (MMPs).[105] The results of a study in monkeys infected with *Brucella melitensis* showed that TLR-2 immune sensitivity and the number of TLR-2-positive astrocytes were amplified in the white matter of subcortical areas. This was accompanied by astrocyte hypertrophy and complication of cell branching.[106] The importance of the alterations found in astrocytes in response to Brucella infections is unknown. We refer the readers to the literature review by Li et al. for more details.[107]

An intriguing scenario for the immune response against CNS infections is within craniectomy settings. Prevalence of infection after craniotomy is 1 percent-3 percent, with about half related to *Staphylococcus aureus*. Such infections represent a major difficulty for pharmacotherapy because of the antibiotic resistance of biofilm and special immunological features of the CNS. Previous studies have shown a major role in innate immune responses during *Staphylococcus aureus* craniotomy infection. Animal research carried out on rodents has detected the role of TLR-2 and its adaptor protein, MyD88, in defense against infection by *Staphylococcus aureus* during craniotomy biofilm infection. Noteworthy is that the immune responses provoked during *Staphylococcus aureus* craniotomy infection are different from peripheral biofilm infection, suggesting a role for niche-specific determinants in *Staphylococcus aureus* biofilm-leukocyte crosstalk.[108]

**MicroRNAs** MicroRNAs, small non-coding RNAs with historically unchanged sequences, are synthesized in different cells, having important roles in both normal and pathologic mechanisms. Recent research has suggested that microRNAs have important roles in bacterial infections via regulating inflammatory responses, tissue reorganization, cellular infiltration, and innate and adaptive immunity. Here, we discuss the example of Helicobacter pylori, and for detailed information regarding other pathogens, refer the readers to the recent review by Zhou et al.[109]

Infection of gastric epithelial cells by Helicobacter pylori may change the expression of microRNAs, such as let-7,[110-112] microRNA-30b,[113] microRNA-210,[114] microRNA-1289,[115] microRNA-4270,[116] microRNA-152/microRNA-200b,[117] microRNA-155,[118-120] microRNA-16,[121] microRNA-376,[122] and microRNA-146a.[123]

Of the numerous microRNAs that contribute to gastric inflammation, adenocarcinoma development, and immune checkpoint control, microRNA-155 is special as its enhanced expression is regarded as a major biomarker of chronic gastric inflammation that makes patients more prone to gastric carcinogenesis. MicroRNA-155 is prominently produced in B and T lymphocytes and in monocytes/macrophages present in chronic gastric inflammation. Of note, microRNA-155 was shown to suppress the expression of some mismatch repair (MMR) genes, including *MLH1*, *MSH2*, and *MSH6*. *MMR* gene sequences are included in the human DNA and function as repair utilities that detect and rectify the mistakes made during cell replication.[124] Immune checkpoints are mediators of the immune system that avert the immune system from the non-selective invasion of self-antigens. Although this is essential to avoid autoimmune reactions, it also diminishes the ability of the immune system to eradicate or suppress cancerous cells. Cancerous cells exploit immune checkpoint pathways as the main process of immune resistance. Provoking immune checkpoints requires ligand-receptor interactions. Therefore, blocking these immune checkpoints permits antitumor defense to continue. In addition, this approach is among the most robust methods of inducing therapeutic antitumor immunity.[125] In tumor-penetrating microRNA-155-lacking CD8+ T cells, antibodies attacking immune checkpoint proteins reinstated the expression of derepressed microRNA-155 targets, suggesting that microRNA-155 could regulate overlapping mechanisms to enhance antitumor immunity. Therefore, it may be clinically valuable that gastric pathologies influenced by microRNA-155 are a consequence of its overexpression.[126] Histological analysis has found higher microRNA-155 concentrations in gastric mucosal tissue specimens of patients positive for Helicobacter pylori. Attachment areas for NF-κB and activator protein-1 (AP-1) have been detected within the BIC/microRNA-155 promoter. Indeed, these factors are required for the activation of microRNA-155 after Helicobacter pylori infection in gastric epithelial cells. The expression of microRNA-155 can also be affected by Foxp3 in T cells infected by Helicobacter pylori.[119] Other than the NF-κB pathway in BMDMs, an increase in microRNA-155 may rely on the Helicobacter pylori class IV excretion system (T4SS).[118] Certain microRNA-155-affected mRNAs, comprising tumor protein p53-inducible nuclear protein 1 (TP53INP1), tetraspanin 14 (Tspan14), lipin 1 (Lpin1), phorbol-12-myristate-13-acetate-induced protein 1 (Pmaip1), protein kinase (cAMP-dependent, catalytic) inhibitor alpha (PKIα), IκB kinase ε (IKK-ε), Sma- and Mad-related protein 2 (SMAD2), and Fas-associated death domain protein (FADD), have been related to proapoptotic and immune responses.[127]

MicroRNAs play a role in escape from phagocytosis that may explain the long-life coexistence of Helicobacter pylori and the human host. It has been recently reported that during Helicobacter pylori infection, phagocytic cells present with high Helicobacter pylori loads as opposed to bacterial clearance. It has been shown that Helicobacter pylori influences the antigen presentation of macrophages by mediating the expression of the immune receptor CD300E via microRNA-4270. In these cells, Helicobacter pylori remains in "megasomes", large constructs that are formed as a result of the homotypic fusion of phagosomes, dodging the phagocytic elimination. One possible mechanism is achieved with the help of microRNA-4270. MicroRNA-4270 targets the most increased gene, the immune receptor CD300E, which its production depends on Helicobacter pylori infection. CD300E promotes the pro-inflammatory actions of macrophages. Also, it affects macrophages' expression and presentation of MHC class II on the cell membrane without altering phagocytosis. This influence restrains the effector T cells from provoking the killing mechanisms of macrophages that could act as a survival condition for the bacteria.[116]

Helicobacter pylori infection suppresses microRNA-375 expression in the gastric tissue. Attenuation of microRNA-375 provokes the Janus kinase (JAK)2-signal transducer and activator of transcription (STAT)3 signaling, resulting in the secretion of IL-6, IL-10, and vascular endothelial growth factor (VEGF). These lead to immature differentiation of DCs and the development of gastric cancer.[122]

## Diagnosis

Precise and early diagnosis of bacterial infection is essential for effectual and targeted therapy. Still, routine microbiological detection (e.g., diagnosis via culture) is sometimes inadequate and slow to the extent that makes it clinically unsuitable. The immune system can quickly carry out the recognition of a versatile range of pathogens with significant sensitivity and specificity. This process has been optimized by evolution throughout history.[5] Here, we briefly go over the application of immunoassays in different scenarios of bacterial infection.

### *Helicobacter pylori*

In line with current guidelines, the European Helicobacter pylori Study Group suggested that at the primary-care level, detection of Helicobacter pylori infection in dyspeptic cases younger than 45 years presenting without severe symptoms is carried out via less invasive approaches, like the urea breath test or serological tests. But, patients with predisposing factors for gastric malignancies should be examined by endoscopy. At the specialist level, both non-invasive methods (e.g., urea breath test and serological assays) and invasive methods using biopsy samples (e.g., culture, histology, rapid urease test, and polymerase chain reaction (PCR)) can be selected. Helicobacter pylori infection activates local and systemic antibody responses. The systemic immune response classically exhibits a temporary increase in Helicobacter pylori-associated immunoglobulin (Ig)M antibodies and precedes with an increase in IgG and IgA antibodies, which continues throughout the course of the disease. Because IgM antibodies against Helicobacter pylori are detected only temporarily, they are unhelpful for the serological detection of Helicobacter pylori. Hence, diagnostic assays have been invented for the recognition of IgG/IgA antibodies in serum, saliva, and urine samples. Diagnosis of Helicobacter pylori-associated IgA/IgG antibodies in saliva has provided insufficient sensitivity and specificity. Although tests for recognition of IgG antibodies against Helicobacter pylori in urine have been found to be both sensitive and specific, major serological diagnostic tests are serum-based.[128-135] Enzyme Immunoassay (EIA) is the main assay utilized for serological evaluation of Helicobacter pylori infection. Many studies have assessed the diagnostic robustness of commercial EIAs for recognition of Helicobacter pylori infection.[136-142] Most of these assays include acid glycine extracts, nonionic detergent extracts, or otherwise somewhat purified antigens. These EIAs mainly recognize IgG antibodies for Helicobacter pylori. The sensitivity and specificity of the various commercial tests range from about 60 percent to 100 percent,[139] with the majority of tests having values above 85 percent.[143]

Helicobacter pylori serology evaluation has been shown to be beneficial for screening symptomatic inner-city children. Serum IgG antibody test, fecal antigen test, and rapid urease test were evaluated in a recent study. The serum Helicobacter pylori antibody test exhibited promising sensitivity (88.4 percent, CI 95 percent, 74.9–96.1) and specificity (93.4 percent, CI 95 percent, 89.1–96.3).[144]

More recently, the diagnostic value of four Helicobacter pylori serological tools was examined, with stool antigen assay as the gold standard. Serological tools examined included Rapid Immunochromatographic Hexagon, Helicoblot 2.1, an EIA IgG kit, and an EIA IgA kit. Stool and blood specimens were collected from 162 healthy individuals (control) and 60 type 2 diabetes mellitus cases. The diagnostic value of the four serological detection tools was influenced by gender, age, health status, and ethnicity of the subjects. For the healthy group, the Helicoblot 2.1 kit displayed the best performance (area under the curve (AUC) = 0.85; $p < 0.05$, accuracy = 86.4 percent), followed by EIA IgG (AUC = 0.75; $p < 0.05$, accuracy = 75.2 percent). The Rapid Hexagon and EIA IgA kits showed unfavorable diagnostic values. For the type 2 diabetes mellitus group, the kits H2.1 and EIA IgG had the highest performances, with accuracies of 96.5 percent and 93.1 percent, respectively.[145]

## *Yersinia*

Yersiniosis is a foodborne disease that results from infection by *Yersinia enterocolitica* or *Yersinia pseudotuberculosis*. While yersiniosis is usually self-limiting, certain individuals can experience chronic infections, including reactive arthritis, glomerulonephritis, and myocarditis, and should receive antibiotics.[146] Interestingly, "reactive arthritis" was first mentioned by clinicians from Finland in 1969 who described the disease as sterile arthritis after infection with *Y. enterocolitica.*[147]

An indirect hemagglutination test (IHA) was among the initial serological assays[148] and is still being used. In IHA, erythrocytes are exposed to heated bacterial extracts. Antibodies to different *Y. enterocolitica* or *Y. pseudotuberculosis* serotypes, or biotypes, or serogroups interact with antigens, resulting in clumping. IHA and complement fixation detect IgM antibodies as these are 10-valent compared to 2-valent IgG-class antibodies. Generally, when the immune responses are started, IgM antibodies that interact with LPS will rise first. This reply precedes a class switch and the formation of IgA and IgG antibodies against protein constructs. These tests cannot differentiate recent infection from past exposure unless IgM is disabled through pre-treatment sample because IgM and IgG can react in IHA or complement fixation. Agglutination assays are sensitive. However, their specificity could be suboptimal if a crude extract antigen is employed. For example, sera from brucellosis cases could react with particles sensitized with the *Y. enterocolitica* serotype O:9 antigen. Discrimination of these bacteria can be performed through EIA or immunoblot, recognizing antibodies against plasmid-encoded Yersinia-related outer membrane proteins (OMPs).[8] Notably, the result of a single agglutination assay may have poor diagnostic performance.[149] In Tanzania, by microagglutination, *Y. enterocolitica* antibodies to the serotype O:3 were detected in 2.6 percent of children and 0.9 percent of healthy individuals, and to the serotype O:9 in 5.3 percent and 2.3 percent, respectively.[150] But, in places where eating pork is more common, seropositivity among normal subjects could also see a rise. By EIA and immunoblot, the seropositivity to Yersinia antigens was detected 19 percent-31 percent and 33 percent-43 percent in Finnish and German healthy subjects, respectively.[151] By Immunoblot, IgA antibodies to a 36-kDa protein were present in 18/19 reactive arthritis cases in comparison with 8/17 with non-arthritic yersiniosis cases. These antibodies remained positive for 8–12 months.[152] Despite this substantial variance, these antibodies may not be a marker for the diagnosis of Yersinia-induced reactive arthritis.[153,154] The deciphering of clinical significance for persisting IgG/IgA antibodies to various antigens is still debated.[155] In recent research, the correlation between the positivity for Yersinia IgA and formalinized complete bacteria "OH" antigens, and arthritis was ruled out when antibodies to plasmid-encoded antigens were explored in patients during a 10-year follow-up. It was concluded that neither IgA nor IgG persistence has a visible influence on the clinical course.[156]

It is clinically most important to know whether Yersinia actually persists. What explains "chronic *Y. enterocolitica* infection", clinically?[157,158] During latent infection, why is it not possible to display bacterial activation by any type of immunosuppression? Chronic infection is explained as the combination of a negative culture accompanied by a lack of agglutinins and positivity for IgA/IgG antibodies to 36 and 46 kDa virulence-related factors evaluated through immunoblot. Understandably, antibody persistence is not the same as infection persistence, the question mentioned earlier.[159] *Y. enterocolitica* O:3 remains for multiple weeks in primary cultures of human synovial cells or fibroblasts,[160,161] but these experimental models do not represent the complex model of the multiple systems within the human body. Bacterial LPS, heat shock protein (HSP),[162] and the 16S ribosomal RNA molecules were recognized in patients with *Y. enterocolitica* O:3 induced reactive arthritis,[158] but alive Yersinia in any body compartment has not been found.

Information regarding the pathogenesis of infections caused by Yersinia has been expanded, and multiple adhesion components have been reported.[163] The most vital adhesives are invasin (Inv), YadA (Yersinia adhesion A, formerly named Yop1), which is the main adhesin, and Ail. Also, there are various other molecules, like YeuB, that activate immunological responses. Upon acute infection, all classes of antibodies towards YeuB, Ail, YadA, and Inv are formed rapidly with the maximum titers on the second and third weeks. These antibodies were more common in cases with gastroenteritis in comparison to cases with reactive arthritis.[164] Yad in *Y. enterocolitica* displays collagen attaching activity. However, Yad in *Y. pseudotuberculosis* attaches mostly to fibronectin.[163] Both subtypes are involved in reactive arthritis (it has been reported that only *Y. pseudotuberculosis* serotypes O:1a and O:3 can induce reactive arthritis).[165]

A new Western blot assay has been developed by Yersinia OMPs as antigens for the detection of Yersinia antibodies as a substitute for the complement fixation assay. The clinical agreement, sensitivity, and specificity were assessed via evaluating 19 positive and 21 negative serum specimens via the complement fixation assay, western blot assay, and enzyme-linked immunosorbent assay (ELISA). In this research, the western blot assay was the reference test. The agreement, sensitivity, and specificity of the complement fixation approach were 61 percent, 26 percent, and 95 percent, respectively, and these values for the ELISA reached 89 percent, 95 percent, and 82 percent, respectively. The amount of Yersinia antibodies in 50 healthy subjects was 6 percent for IgG, 2 percent for IgA, and 2 percent for IgM. Sera positive for *Bartonella henselae*, Brucella, *Chlamydia pneumoniae*, and *Rickettsia rickettsii* antibodies exhibited cross-reactivity via the western blot assay. The strongest cross-reactivity was reported with *Borrelia burgdorferi*, and 5 of 11 (45 percent) samples showed cross-reactivity via the IgM test. Together, this western blot assay demonstrated good performance and proved to be more sensitive than the complement fixation assay, and it can be a useful substitute to the complement fixation test. It is important to take the cross-reactivity into account, in particular with *Borrelia burgdorferi* that is associated with oligoarthritis (or pauciarthritis, defined as the involvement of four or fewer joints) resembling reactive arthritis. The diagnosis of reactive arthritis should be made according to the clinical presentation and by serological evaluation of the infectious etiology.[166]

Fraction 1 (F1) antigen in *Y. pestis* plays a role in suppressing phagocytosis[167] and can be used as a diagnostic test. In a recent work, a novel subtype of F1 antigen was produced and purified. Different anti-F1 monoclonal antibodies (mAbs) were also produced. To assess the performance of the produced *Y. pestis* F1 test strip, the F1 protein/*Y. pestis* was spiked into emulated clinical samples like the human serum, mouse bronchoalveolar lavage fluids, and mouse blood to mimic a natural infection state. Moreover, this approach was applied to recognize the *Y. pestis* in the environment-collected rodents to assess the practical performance of the test. Using this mAb-based-lateral flow assay (LFA) technique, 4 ng/ml of recombinant F1 protein and 103 colony forming unit (CFU)/ml of *Y. pestis* could be recognized within 10 mins that is at least 10-folds more than that of the polyclonal antibody format. While different Yersinia subtypes were exposed to the strips, only the *Y. pestis* subtype prompted a positive signal, and this indicates the high efficiency and specificity of the mAb-based F1 tests.[168]

While early infections can be detected by direct methods, chronic infections can solely be recognized via serological assays. Using a serological approach, which can discriminate between infections, with *Y. enterocolitica* and *Y. pseudotuberculosis* is demanded because the antibiotic therapy of these bacteria is different. Conventional immunoassays do not differentiate these subtypes. An assay that enables this discrimination is Mikrogen's strip assay, in which separation of the two Yersinia depends on two novel bacterial elements, MyfA and PsaA, corresponding to *Y. enterocolitica* and *Y. pseudotuberculosis*, respectively. Researchers reported that the two Yersinia subtypes cultured in conditions that resemble the normal route of infection produce other surface antigens, which can be used to differentiate them.[146]

### *Salmonella*

Salmonella infections more commonly result in reactive arthritis, compared to Campylobacter infections.[169-172] The initial serodiagnostic assay for Salmonella was proposed in 1896 by Widal after it was found that the sera of typhoid cases clustered formalin-fixed bacteria from the host.[173] Such bacterial preparations keep the O-antigen and the Flagella intact. The test has been improved multiple times.[174] The timeline for the development and assessment of this assay has been reviewed by Chart et al.[175] In the first version of the test, sera from cases who presented with fever were combined with a suspension of eliminated *S. typhi* bacteria. If the antibodies (agglutinins) towards bacterial constructs were detected, agglutination of the cell suspension took place. Currently, this assay helps to support the diagnosis of reactive arthritis. The assay can differentially show antibodies towards O-, H-, or Vi-antigens. Anti-O IgM antibodies rise first, anti-H IgG antibodies are produced with a delay and can last, and anti-Vi antibodies can recognize carriers.[176] The slide test improves on the Widal test when the serum and cell suspension are combined and clumps are scored. A more robust modification is carried out in tubes or microwells and demands an incubation phase. The Widal assay can exhibits false interaction due to variability in antigen production, too early collection of the specimen, or technical problems of analysis, and it has unfavorable standardization and reproducibility. False-positive interaction may be prevalent because of intrinsic cross-reactivity by malaria and Enterobacteria. In a Nigerian population who had a positive malaria smear, were not vaccinated for *S. typhi*, and whose stool specimens were negative for *S. typhi*, the Widal test was positive in titers 1:40, 1:80, and 1:160 in 85 percent, 12 percent, and 3 percent, respectively. The parallel values for cases without malaria were 45 percent, 15 percent, and 10 percent.[177] These results warn against selecting only a single finding to evaluate Salmonella serology. Indeed, classically, all assays based on the evaluation of antibody titers compared acute and convalescent sera. All assays are interpretable only if the diagnostic performance of the assay for the specific laboratory is determined.[178] While the Widal assay has faced decreasing popularity,[176] more recent tests for IgM/IgG antibody recognition provide suboptimal performance when assayed on the specimen of cases with verified typhoid fever.[179]

IHA employs erythrocytes sensitized with the Salmonella O-antigen. The sensitivity of this method reaches 62 percent, and its specificity is 98.2 percent. Countercurrent immunoelectrophoresis utilize the depiction of a precipitation band of antigen-antibody complexes. This method shows a sensitivity somewhat similar to the Widal assay.[176]

A new approach to studying Salmonella serology has been developed. In this approach, extracted LPS and flagellar antigens from four strains each are employed and exposed to the gels for sodium dodecyl sulfate polyacrylamide gel electrophoresis (SDS-PAGE) and immunoblot. The interacting antibodies are recognized via polyvalent anti-human antibodies. This approach permits the depiction of bands against LPS and flagellin on separate gels, and the combination of bands allows judgment for the positivity for special antibodies and the infectious agent. The authors found that all cases with culture-verified salmonellosis produced anti-LPS antibodies. Conversely, humoral response to flagellar "d" antigens was found in only 67 percent of cases.[175]

Evaluation of antibodies to LPS of salmonellae other than *S. typhi* is normally performed, in particular in *S. typhimurium* or *Salmonella enteritidis* infections, the two principal subtypes that cause gastroenteritis in Europe. In cases with salmonellosis, the LPS antibodies were found to be similar to antigens obtained from phenolic or trichloro acid isolation, but in the control subjects, these antibodies were very common.[180]

In a recent project, EIA for the detection and measurement of serum IgM, IgG, and IgA antibodies to salmonella was produced with commercial LPSs of *S. typhimurium* and *S. enteritidis* combined as antigen. Among 130 sera from cases with culture-confirmed Salmonella infections, 115 (88.5 percent) were detected by this test. However, the Widal assay was positive in solely 50 (38.5 percent) patients. This method provided a remarkable advance in the serological detection of acute salmonella infections, and it recognizes antibodies towards the salmonellae of groups B and D that account for 70 percent of culture-detectable salmonellosis cases. As well, antibodies against other salmonellae are detected. This EIA is valuable for the post-infection diagnosis of salmonella antibodies when extraction of the pathogen is usually not plausible.[181]

A recent study characterized the local immune responses of adult patients during acute peritoneal dialysis-related peritonitis via multicolor flow cytometry and multiplex ELISA and explained the immunological patterns relative to standard biological culture findings and to clinical presentations. The authors found local "immune fingerprints" that are unique for pathogens exist in peritoneal dialysis cases on the day of clinically acute peritonitis and can discriminate among culture-negative, gram-positive, and gram-negative epochs of infection. Humoral and cellular patterns with the highest suitability for the establishment of disease-specific immune fingerprints comprise the local concentrations of IL-1β, IL-10, IL-22, TNF-α, and CXCL10 along with the frequency of local γδ T cells and the ratio of neutrophils and monocytes/macrophages within total peritoneal cells population. This study highlights the suitability of utilizing immune fingerprints to facilitate the production of point-of-care assays that will enable high-performance diagnosis of infection, targeted antibiotic treatments, and clinical management of the infection.[5]

### *Shigella*

Infection with *Shigella* spp. causes bacillary dysentery and general and mucosal antibody responses. Shigella is an important etiology for diarrhea globally, with different subtypes: *Shigella flexneri*, *Shigella dysenteriae*, *Shigella sonnei* (highly prevalent), and *Shigella boydii*. The immune response to Shigella targets different antigens, such as LPS and the Ipa proteins, and is able to provide a short-term, serotype-restricted defense. Conventionally, Shigella-associated antibody responses are assessed by ELISA. While ELISA is a useful immunological assay, restricted specimen volume and assay costs often make its utilization difficult for immunological assaying of multiple antigens. Therefore, multiplexed immunoassays to assess Shigella-associated antibody responses have been developed to overwhelm these problems. This new test concurrently assays specific antibody titers for six Shigella antigens, comprising three serotype-restricted LPS preparations and three preserved protein antigens in a Luminex™-dependent system. Coupling methods were enhanced to covalently interconnect recombinant Ipa proteins (IpaB, IpaC, and IpaD) and purified LPS from *Shigella sonnei*, *Shigella flexneri 2a*, and *Shigella dysenteriae-1* to unique bead sets. The antigen-attached beads sustained their interactions with mAbs for 6 weeks (protein) to 3 months (LPS). The performance of the Luminex assay matched an ELISA to a considerable extent, with the multiplexed assay providing a wider dynamic range. Comparable levels of antigen-specific reactivity were achieved in monoplex or multiplex formats denoting negligible interference. The correlation between the ELISA and the multiplexed test, as well as the repeatability and reproducibility of the test were remarkable.[182]

In a recent study, samples from Sri Lankan cases with dysentery were assayed for IgM antibodies towards the LPSs of *Shigella dysenteriae-1* and *E. coli O157:H7*. Using ELISA and immunoblotting, 59/113 cases displayed serum antibodies solely to the LPS of

*Shigella dysenteriae-1*. Four specimens from one case were found to have serum antibodies against the LPSs of both *Shigella dysenteriae-1* and *E. coli O157:H7*. Antibodies to the LPS of *Shigella dysenteriae-1* were also detected in 16 specimens from 25 children in Sri Lanka. One of these children also had antibodies against the LPS of *E. coli O157:H7*. Evaluation of 16 specimens from seemingly healthy children in the United Kingdom displayed antibodies against the LPS of *Shigella dysenteriae-1* solely in one sample, with a travel history to Pakistan. These data suggest that the isolation of *Shigella dysenteriae-1* is still the best test for the detection of bacillary dysentery. Serological testing for *Shigella dysenteriae-1* could aid as an adjunct to cultural methods and requires thorough validation, particularly in regions with endemic Shigella.[183]

Interestingly, diagnostic assays for Shigella can help the development of vaccines. Many attempts are directed towards the Shigella LPS-based vaccines, as O antigen-specific conjugate vaccines are immunogenic and efficient. Immunization with Shigella vaccines comprising LPS can provoke antibodies that are able to eliminate Shigella in a serotype-specific fashion. As a result, to help vaccine research for Shigella, scientists developed a serum bactericidal assay (SBA) specific for three Shigella serotypes that evaluates elimination of target bacteria at multiple serum dilutions wherein exogenous complements are present. The SBA is high-throughput but utilizes simple technologies and easily accessible reagents. The SBA was assessed by serum specimens with bactericidal antibodies against *Shigella flexneri 2a*, *Shigella flexneri 3a*, and *Shigella sonnei*. Purified LPS of a homologous subtype, but not a heterologous serotype, suppressed bacterial killing. For these subtypes, assessment of diagnostic accuracy detected median intra-assay precision to be 13.3 percent and median inter-assay precision to be 19 percent to 30 percent.[184]

### *Campylobacter*

Campylobacter serology is very inconsistent. For instance, in 40 diarrheal patients in whom *Campylobacter jejuni* was extracted, the seropositivity was detected in 82 percent, 62 percent, and 38 percent of cases by immunofluorescence, complement fixation, and agglutination methods, respectively. By means of matched sera samples from 15 patients, a 4-fold or greater increase in titers was detected in only 5 patients.[185] In a comparative exploration among the complement fixation and western blot, the seropositivity with complement fixation was 88.6 percent and 28.5 percent for infected cases and blood donors, respectively. Seven immunoreactive antigens (14–67 kDa) were recognized, among which 29, 37, and 43 kDa were detected by 86 percent, 84 percent, and 91 percent of infected cases, respectively.[186] During the early 1980s, EIA-dependent approaches were discovered.[172,187,188] One EIA utilized heated and sonicated crude antigen preparations from six *Campylobacter jejuni* subtypes, and another utilized a single *Campylobacter jejuni* subtype. In the second assay, the common antigen was produced via acid isolation that was cross-reactive among different *Campylobacter jejuni* and

*Campylobacter coli* strains. In a third EIA, the acid extract was produced by three subtypes. The acid extract tests have been utilized for regular detection of Campylobacter infections since then. Two immunodominant antigens were detected in the acid isolate as 30 and 60 kDa.[188] However, it could be presumed that it was a combination of several water-soluble proteins. These EIAs were assessed by human and immunized rabbits' sera.[187] IgM/IgG antibodies were found in solely 73 percent and 52 percent, respectively. The seroprevalence to the antigen, Acid extract from a C. pylori, in normal individuals' blood specimens are related directly to age, with the prevalence of 60 percent, 42 percent, and 21 percent for the age class of 56–65 years for IgG, IgA, and IgM, respectively.[189] These findings describe how a single positive result should be viewed. First, IgM antibodies may remain detectable. Diagnosis of acute infection based on a single serum sample is therefore inaccurate. Second, serological assessment is more reliable in younger individuals. During the initial emergence of EIAs in the 1980s, an EIA based on a combination of LPS from two subtypes was also produced, which performed with 70 percent sensitivity when matched serum specimens were evaluated. When formalin-treated complete bacteria were employed, IgG/IgM antibodies from cases with recent *Campylobacter jejuni/coli enteritis* were found in 82 percent and 77 percent, respectively, whereas antibodies were found in 5 percent of normal individuals' blood specimens. Sera from small children displayed low reactivities. Intriguingly, in a comparative exploration, improved diagnostic performance was attained with sonicated complete cell and ultracentrifuged sonicate compared to acid glycine isolate.[190] More recently, an EIA to recognize antibodies against a heat-stable antigen was explained. The researchers assessed more than 600 sera specimens from 210 cases with recent infections and established that IgG, IgA, and IgM EIA sensitivities were 71 percent, 60 percent, and 80 percent, respectively, with a specificity of 90 percent. It was found that IgG antibodies remained for a minimum of 4.5 months with significant inter-subject variation, while for IgM/IgA antibodies decline of immune response was detected within 2 months from the onset of the disease.

A recent study explored the normal serum response to an acute Campylobacter infection and the diagnostic performance of anti-Campylobacter antibodies in detecting recent Campylobacter infection. After acute infection, all types of antibodies were increased in most, but not in all cases. This preceded declining antibody levels, which did not stabilize at baseline titers. 16 percent of enteritis patients did not show an increase in concentrations, and 9 percent of cases had high concentrations of antibodies 20 months after infection. The ELISA used was reported to be highly specific for the recognition of Campylobacter antibodies.[165,191]

Another serological test that predicts accurately active *Campylobacter pylori* infection in the human stomach has been verified via serum specimens from 189 cases that were evaluated by endoscopy in Sydney. This study used ELISA with a sensitivity of 100 percent and a specificity of 94 percent. A significant part of the assay was the inclusion of a simple absorption phase with *Campylobacter jejuni* for those sera whose findings are near the cut-off value for positivity. This has been shown to be especially useful in epidemiological research in populations that have been exposed to *Campylobacter jejuni* consistently.[192]

Lately, several immunogenic antigens in Campylobacter have been explained. The main immunodominant antigen is flagellin, the subunit protein of flagella. Moreover, major outer membrane proteins (MOMPs), periplasmic-related membrane proteins PEB1 (28 kDa), and PEB3 (30 kDa), as well as 47 and 84 kDa proteins are immune-activating. New approaches recognize antibodies against multiple recombinant proteins of Campylobacter (e.g., MOMP, PEB4, PEB2, PEB1 OMP18, and P39) by a line blot approach or traditional ELISA.

Interestingly, Campylobacter infection can lead to reactive arthritis and involvement of the nervous system, such as Guillain-Barré syndrome and Miller Fisher syndrome. In pediatric patients with Guillain-Barré syndrome, diagnosis based on recombinant antigens produces superior specificity compared to assays utilizing thermostable and complete cell antigens.[193] This has not been found for reactive arthritis. It has been reported that in Guillain-Barré syndrome, the antibodies against nerve GM1b gangliosides cross-react with the lipooligosaccharide of Campylobacter. This could suggest that Campylobacter serology for Guillain-Barré syndrome may require distinct antigen preparations compared to methods for reactive arthritis.[165] Guillain-Barré syndrome, also regarded as Acute Inflammatory Demyelinating Polyneuropathy, is an autoimmune polyradiculoneuropathy that may be developed after certain infections. The most frequent preceding microorganisms are *Campylobacter jejuni*, with *cytomegalovirus* (*CMV*) in second place. Still, over 40 percent of Guillain-Barré syndrome cases cannot be ascribed to inducing agents. This could be because of the inadequacies of the serological assays utilized for diagnosing infections, particularly for *Campylobacter jejuni*. In a recent work exploring 36 cases with acute Guillain-Barré syndrome, standard serological approaches detected the inducing viral or bacterial organisms solely in 25 percent of patients. Nevertheless, by a robustly specific ELISA assay based on two recombinant outer antigens encoded by *Campylobacter jejuni* genes *Cj0017* (P39) and *Cj0113* (*P18*), the authors reported serological positivity for a preceding *Campylobacter jejuni* in 80.6 percent of the cases but in solely 3.5 percent of the controls. It can be suggested that the role of *Campylobacter jejuni* in inducing Guillain-Barré syndrome has been largely underappreciated.[194] Serological biomarkers of recent infection by *Campylobacter jejuni* in cases with Guillain-Barré syndrome were investigated in the state of Piauí, Brazil, from 2014 to 2016. In this study, pre-treatment serum specimens from 63 Guillain-Barré syndrome patients were assayed via IgM ELISA for *Campylobacter jejuni*. *Campylobacter jejuni* IgM antibodies were found in 17 percent (11/63) of the specimens. Surprisingly, this study found no relation between IgM positivity for *Campylobacter jejuni* and diarrhea.[195] Establishment of a proper linkage between *Campylobacter jejuni* and

Guillain-Barré syndrome in different populations with high-performance universal assay warrants further research.

For *Mycobacterium tuberculosis*, the readers are referred to the summary provided by Steingart et al. that compared the performance of available serological assays.[196]

## Treatment

Despite attempts to stop the rise in antimicrobial resistance, bacteria constantly become less prone to antimicrobial treatments as time passes by, and rates of discovery for new antibiotics are declining. As a result, it is vital to investigate new models for antimicrobial treatment. A robust method is host-directed immunoregulatory treatments, by which natural processes in the host are taken advantage of to optimize the therapeutic usage. The goal is to start or improve defensive antimicrobial immunity while limiting inflammation-induced tissue damage.[6] Here, we summarize several immune-regulating treatments for bacterial infections that target immune receptors (e.g., TLRs, NLRs), immune checkpoints, mAbs, and cytokines. For further detail, the readers are referred to the recent work by McCulloch et al.[197]

### *Targeting innate immune receptors*

#### TLR modulating therapies

The TLR family of PRRs in humans comprises ten transmembrane proteins. Each subclass of the TLR family recognizes specific classes of ligands and is situated either on the cell surface or in the endosomal section. The cell surface TLRs usually detect signature elements of microbial cell envelopes or flagella. For example, TLR-4 and accessory proteins detect LPS, TLR-2 in conjunction with TLR-1/TLR-6 detects lipoteichoic acid and different lipopeptides, and TLR-5 detects flagellin. Endosomal TLRs mainly recognize microbial nucleic acids. For instance, TLR-3 detects double-stranded RNA, TLR-7 and TLR-8 attach to single-stranded RNA, and TLR-9 detects microbial DNA with unmethylated CpG. motifs. Other than the mentioned microbial ligands, TLRs detect endogenous ligands, usually called damage-associated molecular patterns (DAMPs) or alarmins, such as HMGB1, S100A8-S100A9, HSPs, uric acid, heparin, DNA, and purine metabolites. These molecular algorithms are probably misnamed, as they represent very distinct elements from microbial signatures and possibly exert their effects via distinct processes or attachment regions. The reaction of microbial signature elements with TLRs induces the activation of signal transduction processes, like the mitogen-activated protein kinase (MAPK) and NF-κB pathways, leading to the induction of innate immune cells. This helps the secretion of pro-inflammatory elements and enhances the induction of antimicrobial effector actions. The importance of TLR pathways in antimicrobial protection is depicted via the fact that polymorphisms in the TLR pathways network have been related to flaws in the management of human bacterial infections. There are two plausible approaches for the regulation of TLR-related responses, and both scenarios use elements that usually act similar to natural ligands. Agonists have an adjuvant influence on the innate immune processes, enhancing protective responses while potentially promoting inflammation. Moreover, antagonists may suppress immune processes and hazardous inflammation, which are either associated with infection or the result of modified immune reactions with the bacterial microbiota (named dysbiosis). However, antagonists can also suppress defensive processes.[198-200] Some examples of TLR-modulating therapies that have been investigated in animal models include macrophage-activating lipopeptide-2 (MALP-2) that utilizes TLR-2 to target *Streptococcus pneumoniae*, monophosphoryl lipid A (MPL) that utilizes TLR-4 to target *Listeria monocytogenes*, and Pam2CSK4 and ODN2395 that utilize TLR-2/TLR-9 to target *Streptococcus pneumoniae*, *Pseudomonas aeruginosa*, Bacillus anthrax, and *Staphylococcus aureus*. For a detailed review, please refer to the recent publication by Mifsud et al.[201]

## NOD-like receptors modulating therapies

NLRs are a family of cytoplasmic innate immune receptors that detect both microbial and endogenous alarm signals to induce inflammation and exert antimicrobial functions. In this family, NOD1 and NOD2 sense peptidoglycan products from the bacterial cell wall to induce NF-κB and MAPK signaling. Distinct subunits of these bacterial cell wall products, named muropeptides, are necessary for the induction of NOD1 and NOD2. NOD1 senses diaminopimelate (DAP) of muropeptides that are mainly found in gram-negative pathogens, while NOD2 senses muramyl dipeptide, which is present in all bacteria. DAP, along with the d-amino acids that form the main peptides of peptidoglycan, exists solely in bacteria, establishing its place as a special signature to alert the host about microbial infections. Another member of this group, NLRP3, senses both microbial and endogenous alarm signals, resulting in the synthesis of the caspase-1-dependent inflammasome and subsequently, the breakdown of pro-IL-1β and pro-IL-18 to their functional, excreted shapes. The stimulation of innate immunity by NLR induction is vital for provoking acquired immunity, and NLR inducers like muropeptides have the ability to be utilized as vaccine adjuvants. Furthermore, there is a potential to use immunomodulation by NLRs as an anti-infective approach. NLR agonists have been used mainly to improve both innate and adaptive immune responses. For instance, the NLRP3 agonist alum is the most widely utilized adjuvant for vaccines, but its mechanism of action, in addition to whether its actions in vivo demand NLRP3 induction or not, remains unclear. It should be considered that alum is a poor activator of Th1 immunity. Also, activation of NOD2 via muramyl dipeptide, a main component of Freund's complete adjuvant, along with activation of other NLRs, leads to adaptive immune activation with a shift in favor of Th2 immunity. This has led to the design of second-generation adjuvants that mix alum with other additives, usually TLR agonists, to improve overall potential.[200,202,203] Recent progress in the production of antigen candidates brings new hope for vaccines targeting *Neisseria meningitidis* serogroup B and other respiratory microorganisms, such as *Streptococcus pneumoniae*. Effective adjuvants will be needed to expedite this process, and the well-established role of NLRP3 in protection against pneumococcus suggests that NLRP3-activating adjuvants may be beneficial.[204]

### *Targeting immune checkpoints*

#### Programmed cell death protein (PD)-1

Immune cells such as adaptive lymphocytes (e.g., T and B cells) and innate lymphocytes (e.g., natural killer (NK) cells and innate lymphoid cells) exert major roles in the management and elimination of infection through killing infected cells and release of inflammatory elements that promote myeloid bactericidal responses. However, trigger elements produced during infection can result in an increase in immune regulatory checkpoints. When taking the evolutionary significance of these mechanisms into account, such as the principal T cell checkpoint suppressive mechanism, PD-1/ programmed death ligand (PD-L)1, it should be noted that they can stop overactivation of the immune response that can result in harmful influences like exacerbated inflammation and tissue damage. For instance, increased PD-1 expression on T cells during *Mycobacterium tuberculosis* infection seems vital, but other pathogenic bacteria can utilize immunomodulatory mechanisms to escape from the immune system, and suppression of these mechanisms may present as a suitable approach in restoring immune actions to fight disease. Among these bacteria, Burkholderia can induce chronic infection via intrinsic multi-resistance to antibiotics, making infection hard to treat with a significant risk of mortality. Some small-colony subtypes of *Burkholderia pseudomallei* enhance PD-1 on innate and adaptive immune cells in animal models of infection. Also, *Burkholderia pseudomallei* enhanced PD-L1expression on human neutrophils in an in vitro setting that simulates infection, can suppress PD-1+ T cell proliferation and IFN-$\gamma$ release. Such PD-1/ PD-L1 processes potentially result in the chronicity of infection, and suppressing this mechanism could enhance bacterial elimination in this challenging infection. In a similar manner, it has been reported that infection with Helicobacter pylori results in enhanced PD-1 expression on T cells[23] and increased PD-L1 expression on epithelial cells. PD-L1 suppression in an in vitro model of Helicobacter pylori infection led to enhanced CD4+ T cell-regulated release of IL-2, a principal proliferation and survival element for lymphocytes. This increase in PD-1/PD-L1 has been found to be a major inducer of premalignant lesions during the development of Helicobacter pylori-triggered gastric cancer. Also, suppression of the PD-1/PD-L1 mechanism reduces susceptibility to bacterial infection related to acute liver injury and chronic liver disease, by improving Kupffer cell function.[197,205-207]

### T cell immunoglobulin and mucin domain-containing protein 3 (Tim-3)

While anti-PD1 therapy is likely excluded during tuberculosis infection, suppression of T cell immunoglobulin and mucin domain-containing protein 3 (Tim-3) is more suitable. Similar to PD-1, Tim-3 is an immune checkpoint protein produced on T and NK cells, and its attachment to its ligand, galectin-9, leads to the production of a suppressive signal. *Mycobacterium tuberculosis* infection has been reported to be able to enhance Tim-3 expression on both human and rodent T cells. In human CD8+ T cells, Tim-3 production is related to attenuated IFN-γ release, degranulation, and proliferation ex vivo, which could be recovered through treatment with an anti-Tim-3 suppressing antibody.[30] It has been shown that in a rodent model of tuberculosis, Tim-3 is enhanced on CD4+ and CD8+ T cells. In recent research, Tim-3 knockout mice and anti-Tim-3 suppressing antibodies were selected to exhibit that Tim-3 is a suitable treatment target, as it is involved in the chronicity of bacterial infection. Although this experiment focused on T cells, it did not reject the possible contribution of Tim-3 mechanisms in NK cells. NK cells from cases with latent or active tuberculosis infection showed enhanced Tim-3 production that was inversely related to IFN-γ release in response to IL-12, a major activator of IFN-γ. Once again, this suppression could be derepressed in vitro by Tim-3- inhibiting antibody. Currently, the involvement of Tim-3 upregulation on NK cells in a rodent model of tuberculosis has not been evaluated yet, and it remains an area for future research.[197,208]

### *Cytokine modulation therapies*

Cytokines are important messenger elements that regulate the actions of immune cells. Clinical trials have found therapy by regulation of cytokines for the management of sepsis and several other possible bacterial infections. Type I and III IFNs are vital for defense against respiratory viruses. Nevertheless, respiratory viruses play a role in coinfection with *Streptococcus pneumoniae*, the most common cause of bacterial pneumonia. In ex vivo settings, these IFNs suppress IL-1β production during secondary *Streptococcus pneumoniae* infection. This leads to an attenuated granulocyte-macrophage colony-stimulating factor (GM-CSF) release, a cytokine vital for optimal functions of alveolar macrophages. Suppression of both type I and III IFN pathways via blockade of IFN receptor I- and III-associated tyrosine kinase 2 (Tyk2) can recover the IL-1β/GM-CSF axis pathway and result in attenuation of bacterial burdens ex vivo. Although this information implicates that inhibition of this pathway may be a treatment method for reinstating immunity in bacterial pneumonia, how this would influence subsequent immunity to viral infection is still unclear. Intriguingly, IFN-sensitive macrophages are linked to a shift from latent to active pulmonary tuberculosis, and type I IFNs have been reported to be involved in the pathogenesis of tuberculosis infection, also via the suppression of IL-1 pathways. This highlights the potential role of Tyk2 inhibitors in tuberculosis infection. In tuberculosis, IFN-triggered loss of IL-1 unsettles immunity by attenuating lung prostaglandin (PG)E2 concentrations, and therapeutically restoring

PGE2 can recover immune function when the IFN/IL-1 balance is skewed in favor of disease. This inflammatory crosstalk is an interesting topic, which deserves further research to develop therapeutics helping to recover antibacterial immune system actions.[197,209,210]

### *mAbs*

mAbs are being tested for the therapy of bacterial infections. Antibodies play an important role in immunomodulation during tuberculosis. The latent phase of infection is characterized by amplified Fc-regulated immune effector function and macrophages that eliminate intracellular pathogens, denoting the defensive actions of these antibodies. Although currently, the development of immunizing mAbs against *Mycobacterium tuberculosis* has been unsuccessful, some engineered mAbs for *Pseudomonas aeruginosa* and *Staphylococcus aureus* have surpassed preclinical research and are being tested in clinical trials. MEDI3902 (AstraZeneca PLC), a bispecific IgG1 antibody affecting the PcrV protein (host cell cytotoxicity) and Psl exopolysaccharide (colonization and tissue adherence) of *Pseudomonas aeruginosa*, is being developed as a prophylactic candidate for pneumonia in the at-risk population (NCT02696902). In addition, the targets are preserved within isolates of *Pseudomonas aeruginosa* throughout the globe, potentially leading to wide coverage. AR-301 (Aridis Pharmaceuticals), a mAb with alpha-toxin disabling potential, protected against alpha toxin-regulated host cell injury when used as an adjunctive treatment in patients with methicillin-resistant Staphylococcus aureus (MRSA) pneumonia (NCT03816956). Moreover, MEDI4893 (AstraZeneca PLC), a long-acting mAb targeting alpha-toxin was effective as a preventive treatment for *Staphylococcus aureus* infection in addition to achieving sustained serum concentrations following intravenous therapy of healthy subjects and is now being tested in a phase II clinical trial (NCT02296320).[211]

## Fungal infections

### Definition

Globally, about a billion are affected by skin, nail, and hair fungal infections, multiple 10's of millions by mucosal candidiasis, and over 150 million individuals by critical fungal diseases that have a key influence on their lives or are deadly. Severity ranges from asymptomatic-mild mucocutaneous infections to possibly life-threatening systemic involvements. Also, mortality due to fungal etiology is about the same as for tuberculosis and over 3 times higher than malaria.[212-218] Mortality among infected cases may reach 75 percent to 100 percent, offering a serious challenge to clinicians.[219] Usually, fungi are disseminated all over the planet, and humans are exposed via inhaling spores or small yeast cells. Common fungi include *Aspergillus fumigatus*, *Cryptococcus neoformans*, and the thermally dimorphic fungi (e.g., *Histoplasma capsulatum*, *Blastomyces dermatitidis*,

*Paracoccidioides brasiliensis*, *Coccidioides immitis*, *Penicillium marneffei*, and *Sporothrix schenckii*). Some fungi are fortuitous microorganisms in humans, inducing superficial, subcutaneous, and systemic diseases. Fungi usually lead to systemic or deep-rooted infection by direct inhalation of them into the lung or through invasion of an injured area. The rest, like *Candida albicans*, are commensal inhabitants of the gastrointestinal tract and skin, which under certain circumstances may multiply and transport into the blood, for instance, when introduced into the body by medical tools like vascular catheters. Indeed, over 250 fungal subtypes cause human infections. About 80 percent of these infections result from Candida species. Throughout the ages, *Candida albicans* has been the most prevalent and underlies most Candida infections. Additional subtypes such as *Candida tropicalis, Candida glabrata,* and *Candida krusei* make up for most of the remainder, and the prevalence of such subtypes is on the rise. Another major fungal etiology of human infections is the Aspergillus subtype that makes up for 15 percent-20 percent of infections. More infrequent but of rising prevalence, human mycoses include blastomycoses, coccidioidomycoses, cryptococcosis, histoplasmosis, and sporotrichosis.[220] Socioeconomic status, geoecological features, and the rising number of at-risk subjects are the main factors of disparity in the prevalence of fungal disease throughout the globe. The prevalence of local and systemic fungal infections is rising at a concerning pace. This is because of the progress in clinical medicine that has led to the rise in critically ill, immunosuppressed, hospitalized patients. The *HIV* epidemic and other disorders of the immune system have also extended this rising high-risk population in both developed and underdeveloped regions globally, like tuberculosis, chronic obstructive pulmonary disease, asthma, and malignancies.[221] A number of fungi can produce clinical diseases in the otherwise healthy population, but many subtypes are harmful solely when the host is weakened, like conditions mentioned earlier.[222]

As a matter of fact, as the population of immunosuppressed individuals has grown (e.g., subsequent to the elevated frequency of malignancies, chemotherapy, organ transplantation, and autoimmune disorders), so has the prevalence of fungal disorders.[223, 224] It has been suggested that global warming will introduce new fungal infections to mammals.[225]

Fungi are heterotrophic eukaryotes that are traditionally and morphologically categorized into yeast and filamentous subtypes (e.g., molds). A number of fungi are dimorphic, living as either yeasts or molds based on environmental conditions (e.g., temperature). Exploration of these eukaryotes has been inspired by their unique and intriguing biology, their numerous beneficial products (e.g., cheese, antibiotics), their utilization as experimental models for molecular biology, and their significance as animal and plant pathogens.

Fungi are very skillful at recognizing their neighboring and replying to signals, which enhance their survival in changing environments. Hence, they can communicate with plants, animals, and humans in different ways, establishing symbiotic, commensal, latent, or pathogenic relations. They can colonize most niches within the human body by specific reorganizing methods that make them able to adjust to environmental circumstances, fight for nutrient resources, and manage or even exploit "stresses" produced by host immunoprotective processes.[226-228] Genomic and transcriptomic methods have displayed a connection among fungal metabolism, morphogenesis, and the response to stress in adjustment to the host environment.[226] Such adjustments can amplify pathogen virulence while simultaneously helping the development of treatments by providing therapeutic targets.[229] As discussed, fungi are linked to a versatile range of diseases in humans and animals, varying in severity from acute self-limiting pulmonary presentations and cutaneous lesions in immunocompetent individuals to inflammatory disorders and potentially deadly infections in immunocompromised cases. A number of fungal subtypes (e.g., *Pneumocystis jiroveci*)[230] and commensal fungi like *Malassezia* spp. and *Candida albicans* have changed during evolution together with their mammalian hosts throughout history. This suggests the existence of complex mechanisms of immune surveillance in the host and of sophisticated fungal strategies to antagonize immunity.

The above discussion denotes that fungal infections may represent a noteworthy paradigm in clinical immunology, as they can stem from either a suboptimal recognition via the immune system or overexcitation of the pro-inflammatory response. Investigation in this field is moving into an interesting period of transition from exploring the molecular and cellular underpinnings of fungal virulence to outlining the cellular and molecular processes that preserve immune homeostasis with fungi. The fine line between these two research areas is quintessential to our knowledge of tissue homeostasis and its potential breakdown in fungal disease. Recent research in immune responses to fungi highlights that functionally separate mechanisms have undergone evolution to achieve the most favorable host-fungus reactions in mammals (e.g., immunity to fungal infections).[231] In this light, the immune system does not dismiss commensal or ubiquitous fungi, and therefore, a precise balance among pro- and anti-inflammatory signals is vital to obtain a sustainable host-fungus relation, and the interruption in this process can have infectious complications. Further, the host immune response to fungi includes two major components: resistance (the potential to decrease fungal burden) and tolerance (the potential to restrict the host damage caused via the immune response or alternative processes). Both abilities are historically preserved in plants and vertebrates.[232] Understanding the interplay between them may allow us to define how fungi have adjusted to the mammalian immune system and to translate this information into novel medical diagnostics and treatments. Below, important fungal infections are briefly explained in the context of immunity.

### Respiratory allergy

Respiratory fungal infection is a critical clinical issue, particularly in cases with weakened immune functions. Endemic fungi, Pneumocystis, Cryptococcus, and Aspergillus are the main pulmonary fungal microorganisms that can lead to life-threatening invasive diseases.[233] Asthma prevalence is high and continues to rise in developed countries. Research has related deteriorating asthma with contact to subtypes of Aspergillus, Alternaria, Cladosporium, and Penicillium. In adults, mold sensitivity has been linked to more severe asthma and increased hospital and intensive care admissions and mortality. Also, in children, it is related to increased bronchial reactivity.[231] Aspergillus mold is one of the most prevalent fungal subtypes that can adequately sporulate through shedding conidia in the air. The produced airborne conidia are tiny enough (2–3 μm) to reach human airways and lung alveoli, leading to a spectrum of conditions, such as lethal infections in immunocompromised individuals and atopic patients with asthma allergies.[234,235] In healthy individuals, inhaled conidia are engulfed by alveolar macrophages and killed in a phagocyte oxidase-dependent manner.[236-238] In immunocompromised patients, incomplete elimination of inhaled fungal conidia leads to germination and assault on tissues via fungal hyphae.[239]

Cryptococcosis results from Cryptococcus contact with the respiratory system following the inhalation of airborne microorganisms. As a subtype of Cryptococcus, *Cryptococcus neoformans* is disseminated widely, especially in soil and avian habitats. The most critical outcome of Cryptococcus infection is cryptococcal meningitis. *Cryptococcus neoformans* and *Cryptococcus gattii* can disseminate from the lung to attack the brain by crossing the blood-brain barrier. The fungal cells straightly enter the blood-brain barrier through endothelial cells on the blood vessels of the CNS via a "Trojan horse" approach, which helps the transfer of phagocytes.[240] *Cryptococcus neoformans* could persist in the CNS, where large-scale colonization and tissue damage could take place despite the protective mechanisms recruited by the host.[241]

### *Skin diseases*

The skin can be a means of entrance for fungal infections when the epithelial barricade is violated. Superficial fungal diseases are not severe. However, they may disseminate to other areas of the body or, occasionally, to other individuals. More critically, but less commonly, they can turn into invasive types. Although not lethal, infections like onychomycosis can have a severe influence on an individual' life quality and self-image.[221] Hence, treatment of local fungal infections to avoid the risk of dissemination should be sought after early. While Malassezia yeasts are considered a part of the physiological microbiota, they have been linked to certain diseases affecting the human skin, such as Pityriasis Versicolor, folliculitis, seborrhoeic dermatitis and dandruff, atopic dermatitis, and psoriasis. Chronic mucocutaneous candidiasis, a primary immunodeficiency (PID) in which the immune system cannot eliminate yeasts, is an uncontrollable clinical display of *Candida albicans* infection.[231]

### *Recurrent vulvovaginal candidiasis*

Recurrent vulvovaginal candidiasis is a widespread mucosal infection caused by saprophytic and opportunistic yeasts of the Candida genus, which can influence up to 75 percent of females of child-bearing age. There are multiple predisposing factors, such as antibiotics and oral contraceptive consumption, hormone replacement therapy (HRT), pregnancy, and uncontrolled diabetes mellitus. Regardless of progress in treatment strategies, vulvovaginal candidiasis stays a major problem globally, with a significant associated cost and a considerable potential for drug resistance.[231] Recurrent vulvovaginal candidiasis leads to worse quality of life and elevated healthcare-related costs. It has been long thought that vulvovaginal candidiasis is the result of insufficient host protection against Candida colonization, a situation found in PIDs related to continuous fungal infections and insufficient clearance. Newer investigations put forth the hypothesis that an overt and disproportionate local mucosal reaction of the immune system, and not a deficient host response to Candida colonization, can cause vulvovaginal candidiasis. Both animal and human studies highlight that the immunological profile varies among recurrent vulvovaginal candidiasis patient subclasses. While defects in the immune response to fungal infections represent a limited number of cases, most present with an exaggerated pro-inflammatory response against Candida colonization and attack, which might be occurring because of the host's genetic context. Notably, in contrast to what was thought (recurrent vulvovaginal candidiasis is an immunodeficiency), an acute immune response has been found in cases infected via minimal fungal loads.[242] Because of this, Candida by itself cannot predict disease. In this sense, a mixture of genetic research in recurrent vulvovaginal candidiasis cases and paired controls combined with immunological information is required to demonstrate the function of the acquired immunity and unlock the elements that contribute to vaginal mucosal protective processes after Candida infection.[243]

### *Inflammatory bowel disease (IBD)*

The gastrointestinal tract utilizes a system of tolerance and well-balanced inflammation to restrict the response to dietary or pathogen-associated antigens of the gut. Mucosal homeostasis emerges from a very dynamic equipoise among host defensive immunity and regulatory processes. When this complicated system is interrupted in a genetically high-risk individual, it could lead to the development of inflammatory bowel disease (IBD). Antibodies towards *Saccharomyces cerevisiae* are found in a subgroup of cases with Crohn's disease (a type of IBD) and are associated with *Candida albicans* colonization. These findings show that a change in sensing of *Candida albicans* colonization may result in abnormal immune responses in IBD.[231] The fungal microbiota of the patients with IBD might be different from healthy individuals. For example, an elevated Basidiomycota/Ascomycota proportion, a reduced proportion of *Saccharomyces cerevisiae*, and an elevated proportion of *Candida albicans* have been reported in patients with IBD compared to the healthy individuals. This study also reported disease-specific changes in diversity, highlighting that a Crohn's disease-specified gut microenvironment may be beneficial to fungi at the cost of bacteria. The analysis of bacterial and fungal microbiota uncovered a dense and homogenous interconnection network in healthy subjects but a significantly deranged network in IBD patients, denoting the presence of disease-specific inter-kingdom changes.[244] A systematic review investigated fungal infections in IBD and took 14 studies with data on 1524 cases into account. The most prevalent fungal infections in cases with IBD resulted from Candida subtypes and the most highly-reported area of Candida infection was the gastrointestinal tract. Current studies support that fungal infections usually happen within 12 months of IBD therapy and within 6 months when anti-TNF-α agents are utilized.[245]

### *Invasive fungal infections*

Invasive fungal infections comprise nosocomial and device-related infections, which are found in cases with hematological diseases or after solid organ or hematopoietic stem cell transplantation (HSCT). In a tertiary care center that includes a significant number of patients who are immunocompromised, a wide variety of fungal pathogens exists. The most prevalent clinically influential fungal pathogens in resource-rich healthcare settings are *Aspergillus* spp. and *Candida* spp. Invasive aspergillosis is a major cause of infectious morbidity and death in cases that are profoundly immunocompromised. Invasive aspergillosis is mostly found in patients with profound and prolonged neutropenia, HSCT, or solid (particularly lung) organ transplantation. Moreover, invasive aspergillosis is commonly found in cases who are severely ill and are in intensive care units, and it might also be found in a variety of scenarios where there is a critical underlying injury to the lung (e.g., near drowning and post-influenza).[246] Invasive candidiasis is another infection, which is deadly in certain patient populations. Candidemia is mostly seen in patients who are critically ill and non-neutropenic. There is a declining prevalence in patients with neutropenia that may be related to the increased utilization of anti-fungal treatments and other helpful actions in these cases. The predisposing factors for invasive candidiasis include the use of an intravenous catheter or total parenteral nutrition. The most prevalent pathogenic cause of invasive candidiasis is *Candida albicans*. Alternative causes comprise *Candida glabrata* (usually displays resistance to fluconazole), *Candida parapsilosis* (displays decreased susceptibility to echinocandins), *Candida krusei* (resistant to fluconazole), and *Candida tropicalis* (the major cause of invasive candidiasis in Indians).[247] Worldwide, *Cryptococcus neoformans* is a major cause of infectious morbidity and death, with approximate yearly mortality of 600000.[248] Physicians could face a versatile range of rather scarce and hard-to-manage pathogens such as Mucorales (e.g., *Rhizopus* spp.), hyalohyphomycetes (e.g., *Fusarium* and *Scedosporium* spp.), and phaeohyphomycosis (e.g., *Alternaria* spp. and *Cladophialophora bantiana*). These organisms are usually hard-to-treat and demand special care.[247] The agricultural utilization of fungicides may be involved in drug resistance in cases with deadly invasive fungal infections. Invasive fungal infections have also been found in cases that are not at-risk, like cases with H1N1 influenza virus or *Mycobacterium tuberculosis* infection and individuals who are treated with TNF.[231]

## Mechanisms

We discuss the mechanisms of immune response to fungal infections in two sections: innate immune response by inflammasomes, TLRs, and C-type lectin receptors (CLRs), and adaptive immune response by T and B lymphocytes. It should be noted that role of these components is at times inseparable. For instance, TLRs and CLRs bridge the innate and adaptive immune responses.

### *Innate immunity*

#### Inflammasomes

Caspase-1 helps the maturation of pro-IL-1 and pro-IL-18 into IL-1 and IL-18, respectively. However, IL-18 does not seem to exert a significant role in fungal immunity compared to IL-1. Host responses to a number of fungal pathogens such as *Candida albicans* infections,[22,249] Fusarium species causing ocular keratitis,[250] and Histoplasma capsulatum pulmonary disease[251] depend on IL-1 receptor pathways (that can be activated by both IL-1$\alpha$ and IL-1$\beta$),

The initial data regarding the role of NLRP3 in anti-fungal protection was produced using a rodent model of oral candidiasis in which NLRP3 deficit led to enhanced vulnerability to mucosal candidiasis, along with the ensuing spread of infections.[22] NLRP3 is critical for protection in intravenous models of Candida stimulation.[252] The exact element of Candida that is necessary for inducing the NLRP3 inflammasome is to be determined, but multiple yeast cell wall concoctions, such as curdlan,[253] zymosan, and mannan[254] have been found to be able to induce NLRP3, and a recent report detected released aspartic proteases from Candida as proficient in activating IL-1$\beta$ secretion through NLRP3.[255]

Aspergillus hyphal particles, contrary to spores, summon the NLRP3 inflammasome to regulate IL-1$\beta$ secretion from monocytes.[256] In a recent article, pathways proposed for NLRP3 inflammasome activation, namely, cathepsin B activity, K+ efflux, and ROS production, were all needed for the inflammasome induction triggered by *Microsporum canis*. Syk, Dectin-1, and Card9 were reported to be involved in *Microsporum canis*-triggered IL-1$\beta$ secretion by the mediation of pro-IL-1$\beta$ production. Of high significance is the finding that the *Microsporum canis*-triggered production of IL-1$\beta$ relies on the NLRP3 inflammasome in vivo.[257] In spite of numerous studies, the molecular basis of NLRP3 activation has not been deciphered yet. In a recent article, it was found that internalization and lysosomal injury, a feature of crystalline inducers, were vital for Candida-regulated IL-1$\beta$ secretion from macrophages.[255] However, a contrasting analysis identified no obvious role for lysosomal injury in response to Candida in DCs.[252] Further research should decipher whether these variations are attributed to different Candida subtypes or stem from different mechanisms of inflammasome induction in these two cell types. For Aspergillus, it was reported that K+ efflux and ROS production were needed for IL-1$\beta$ secretion from perpetuated monocytes.[256] These processes were also found to be crucial for human peripheral blood mononuclear cell (PBMC) IL-1β release in response to Candida.[255] Only a few experiments have been carried out on the function of the rest of the inflammasomes in fungal immunity. A non-canonical inflammasome using caspase-8 was found to be induced directly by downstream from Dectin-1 in response to *Candida albicans* and did not depend on phagocytosis.[258] Additionally, NLRC4 (initially named IPAF) has been well-researched for its actions in inflammatory responses to common bacterial microorganisms[259] and was recently shown to be able to control a tissue-specific defensive response to *Candida albicans*.[260] Another inflammasome studied in fungal infection is NLRP10, which was reported to have little influence on the excretion of IL-1β in response to Candida but the death rate was enhanced in Nlrp10-/- rodents after intravenous challenge due to vast kidney injury and revoked Th1 and Th17 responses.[261]

## TLRs

The accurate molecular nature of fungal PAMPs that induce specific TLRs is difficult to pinpoint because of the cooperative mechanisms of TLR recognition and the plasticity of the cell wall in fungi. Despite that fungal PAMPs are sensed through certain TLR subclasses (e.g., TLR-2/1, TLR-4, TLR-3, TLR-2/6, TLR-7, and TLR-9), they are not the principal receptors propelling the elimination of fungi. Fungal PAMPs that are expressed on the cell surface have been described for *Candida albicans*, but they are mostly unidentified for the rest of fungi. For *Candida albicans*, mutants with special cell wall flaws have helped the characterization of PAMPs. As cell wall mutations usually diminish virulence or activate compensatory modification of the cell wall ingredients,[262] changes in immune responses against these mutants should be considered carefully. Cell wall ingredients trigger TLRs. For instance, TLR-2 senses fungal β-glucans of multiple fungal subtypes.[263] Additionally, it particularly reacts with phospholipo-mannans (PLMs) and linear beta-1,2-oligomannoside constructs of *Candida albicans*.[264] TLR-2 is triggered via currently incognito ligands that exist on conidia and hyphae of *Aspergillus Fumigatus*.[265] TLR-2/TLR-1 and TLR-2/TLR-6 heterodimers act as receptors for the glucuronoxylomannan (GXM) element of *Cryptococcus neoformans*.[266] Of note, *Aspergillus fumigatus* induces rodent but not human TLR-2/6 heterodimers, while TLR-2/1 heterodimers sense *Aspergillus fumigatus* both in humans and rodents.[267] This is a good instance of variations among humans and mice in fungal detection. TLR-4 is triggered after ligation of *Candida albicans* O-linked mannans[268] and *Cryptococcus neoformans* GXM.[269] Ligands for TLR-4 are present as well on *Aspergillus fumigatus* conidia but not hyphae.[265]

Because microbial pathogens mainly carry different classes of PAMPs, their detection may involve the parallel or consecutive induction of multiple PRRs from several subclasses. Cooperation among PRRs and interplay among their signaling mechanisms can improve the specificity and coverage of PAMP detection and, as a result, potentiates the host response.[270] TLR-2 converts signals as a heterodimer employing TLR-1/TLR-6.[271] *Candida albicans* is especially detected via TLR-2 following anti-fungal therapy, which modifies the cell wall.[272] Also, it has been reported that the administration of anti-fungal treatments can improve the potential of *Candida albicans* or *Aspergillus fumigatus* to induce TLR production in human polymorphonuclear cells (PMNs).[273] These findings highlight that in addition to their direct fungicidal features, anti-fungal treatments can help the recognition of harmful microorganisms by the host, and ultimately, expedite clearance.

Mammalian PRRs sense not only PAMPs but also damaged host cell elements, like nucleic acids and alarmins, together recognized as DAMPs. In fact, nucleic acids shed from fungi within the phagosome mediate the host's immune response during infection. TLR-3 is triggered by double-stranded RNA of *Aspergillus fumigatus* conidia in respiratory epithelial cells.[274] Single-stranded RNAs of *Candida* spp. are TLR-7 ligands in rodent bone-marrow DCs.[275] TLR-9-regulated recognition of fungal genomic DNA (gDNA) seems to be preserved in various fungal subtypes,[275] and the employment of TLR-9 to fungi-containing phagosome is observed with certain fungal species.[276] Recognition of gDNA of *Aspergillus fumigatus* and *Cryptococcus neoformans* takes place at non-methylated CpG motifs.[277] On the contrary, TLR-9 recognition of Candida gDNA is probably not limited to such motifs.[278]

Despite the detection of unique signaling processes that dampen responses to either PAMPs or DAMPs,[279] the unanticipated intersection of the molecular mechanisms that contribute to the recognition of PAMPs and DAMPs outlines the question of whether and how the host immune system differentiate between these two kinds of molecular algorithms. The respective contributions of PAMPs and DAMPs to inflammation, immune balance, and restorative processes during infection are not deciphered completely. Still, a process has recently been suggested that may enable the host to separate PAMP- and DAMP-triggered immune responses. The alarmin S100B manages this mechanism by the spatiotemporal interconnection of signals from TLRs and the receptor for advanced glycation end-products (RAGE).[280] By attachment of fungal TLR-2 ligands to nucleic acids, S100B initially suppresses TLR-2-activated inflammation during fungal pneumonia and then induces intracellular TLR-3 and TLR-9 to activate its own transcriptional downregulation.[279,280]

## CLRs

CLRs are proteins within the cellular membrane that attach to carbohydrates through preserved extracellular C-type lectin-resembling regions. CLRs are glycosylated type II transmembrane receptors with single carbohydrate recognition domains (CRD) in their extracellular C-termini.[281] CLRs class comprises over 1000 proteins and is categorized into 17 subclasses by construct and regional formations. CLRs are produced in myeloid cells and exert major functions in host protection against fungal infections via driving acquired immunity. On attachment to ligand, CLRs activate cellular responses via triggering the release of cytokines and ROS by the Syk/CARD9 signaling pathway resulting in fungal destruction. Because of explorations on the CLRs, the underpinnings of the anti-mycotic immunity are being deciphered.[282] Dectin-1 and Dectin-2 are two instances where CLRs exert a role in the anti-fungal immune response. Dectin-1 is the first recognized and is the best-defined CLR that is involved in anti-mycotic immunity.[283] Contrary to the rest of CLRs, Dectin-1 includes HemITAM in its cytoplasmic N-terminus that is preserved in many mammals, such as primates and rodents. This receptor is mostly produced in innate immune cells, such as macrophages, DCs, neutrophils, monocytes, and γδ T cells in rodents and humans. It is also present in human microglia and eosinophils. Dectin-1 was first cloned as a lectin unique to DCs that triggers CD4+ T cell to multiply by an unknown endogenous ligand,[284] while later, Dectin-1 was reported to be able to attach to β-Glucans that are key fungal cell wall elements found in human-consumable mushrooms, seaweeds, and baker's yeasts, and in pathogenic and commensal fungi.[285] Dectin-2 was first cloned as a CLR unique to DCs with Dectin-1, but it is produced in multiple DC subtypes and in macrophages and monocytes. Dectin-2 comprises an EPN (Glu-Pro-Asn) motif, a putative Ca2+-dependent mannose-attaching amino acid sequence in its C-terminal extracellular CRD. Since Dectin-2 has no discovered signaling motifs in its smaller cytoplasmic domain, it demands the ITAM bearing Fc receptor g chain (FcRg) for signal conversion and induction.[286] Experiments utilizing glycan arrays showed that Dectin-2 attaches to mannose-rich constructs from a versatile range of microorganisms, such as fungi, parasites, bacteria, and mammals.[287] Furthermore, *Candida albicans* has mannose-rich-type N-glycan cell wall constructs named a-mannans that include polycarbohydrate backbones of a-1,6-connected mannose subunit, along with a-1,2-connected polymannose side chains. The a-mannans of *Candida albicans* are plentifully produced in the outermost sections of cell walls, and mannose detection is considered the initial step in the ensuing innate immune responses. As predicted, Dectin-2-lacking rodents showed remarkably higher mortality rates after systemic *Candida albicans* infection.[288] Also, the significance of Dectin-2 in anti-mycotic immunity has been displayed for Malassezia, *Aspergillus fumigatus*, and *Candida glabrata*, in vivo.[289,290] While no fungal infections have been related to Dectin-2 polymorphisms in humans, impairments of the signaling element CARD9 resulted in critical candidiasis in experiments on both rodents and humans, highlighting that Dectin-2 or Dectin-1 accompanied by CARD9-associated CLRs are involved in anti-mycotic immunity.[291]

### *Adaptive immunity*

#### Cellular immunity

The adaptive immunity, particularly that of T cells, exerts important actions in the anti-mycotic host response.[231] To induce anti-mycotic T cells, innate PRRs on APCs sample fungal PAMPs and activate a mixture of key cytokines and co-activating agents, which will drive the differentiation of naïve T cells into Th subtypes.[122] After detection of fungi, PRRs and signaling pathways activate a plethora of cytokines. A number of these cytokines drive Th differentiation.[292] To keep our overview concise, we limit the discussion to PRRs and signaling mechanisms triggering cytokines, which result in differentiation of naïve T cells into special Th subsets. The differentiation of Th1 and Th17 CD4+ T cells is particularly important for the anti-fungal immunity as these cells synthesize pro-inflammatory cytokines like IFN-γ and IL-17 that are identified to recruit and activate phagocytes to eliminate fungi. Despite that IL-17 is usually linked to CD4+ Th17 cells, lately, there has been rising attention toward the significance of innate lymphoid resources of IL-17.[293,294] These resources include natural killer T (NKT) cells, γδ T cells, CD4-CD8-T cell receptor (TCR)β+ cells, and "natural" Th17 cells that do not demand activation through a special antigen and are hence considered innate. However, such innate "type 17" cells share some features with Th17 cells, for example, they produce C-C chemokine receptor (CCR)6, IL-7Rα, IL-23R, and the master transcription factor ROR-γt but they may not always demand a TCR for their development as some cell types have been recognized in Rag1-/- rodents that lack acquired immunity.[295-297]

## Humoral immunity

Data on the contribution of antibodies against fungi infection are very limited. Experiments on the sera showed that though many clonal isotypes of antibodies were present during fungi infection, only a limited number of the isotypes were immunoprotective. The ability to produce mAbs against fungal antigens made it possible for researchers to inquire if particular clonally derived antibodies could confer protection. Most notable is that for many clinically significant fungi, most importantly *Cryptococcus neoformans* and *Candida albicans*, antibodies exert immunoprotection in adoptive transfer experiments. Also, antibodies defend against intracellular pathogens like fungal microorganisms (e.g., *Histoplasma capsulatum*) and bacteria (e.g., *Listeria monocytogenes*, and *Mycobacterium tuberculosis*).[297-304] A hurdle for establishing a valid humoral response by vaccines, is that it is vital to verify that only defensive antibodies are increased. Contrastingly, antibodies as immunotherapy have a wide application and can show robust effectiveness. Currently, most of the defensive antibodies explained detect surface elements that comprise, but are not restricted to, the capsule of cryptococcus, mannotriose and β-glucan of *Candida albicans*, β-glucan of *Aspergillus fumigatus*, HSP-60 and histones of *Histoplasma capsulatum*, and kexin and glycoprotein 120 of *Pneumocystis* murina .[305,306] As a result, there seem to be no shared targets, as of yet, that cover the different subtypes of fungi. An intriguing candidate may be β-glucan. However, a number of fungi like *Histoplasma capsulatum* have developed processes to conceal the surface production of this carbohydrate.[305,307,308]

### *Other mechanisms*

### Interconnecting the innate and adaptive immunity

Provoking the innate immune system by the activation of PRRs lays the foundation to establish a robust adaptive immune response.[309,310] DCs interconnect innate and adaptive immune systems through modulating the T cell response after PRR-dependent cytokine release. DCs are able to prime naïve T cells to produce long-term memory against infectious organisms. T cell priming through DCs takes place via the presentation of pathogen-related antigen on MHC class I or MHC class II proteins for the priming of CD8+ or CD4+ T cells, respectively, other than via the expression of co-activating agents for TCR activation. Following maturation, DCs enhance the production of co-activating agents, and they display high concentrations of PRRs on the cell surface for direct reaction with pathogens by means of signal transduction from PRRs to T cells.[310,311] After the activation of T cells, the response is described as Treg, Th1, Th2, or Th17 according to different patterns of cytokine release by Th CD4+ T cells. As a result, DCs can determine the fate of the immune response, making them both paramount to stabilize immunity and a suitable target as a vaccine candidate against pathogenic fungi.[312]

## Diagnosis

Ultimate clinical diagnosis of invasive fungi relies on detection of a particular fungus from the sample or microscopic proof of fungi with characteristic morphological properties (e.g., encapsulated *Cryptococcus neoformans* cells in cryptococcosis). But, in case these methods are inaccessible, other tools should be utilized. Evaluation of host antibody responses provides this supplementary data for the clinical diagnosis of invasive fungi. While serologic assays have been used for several decades for diagnosis of some fungal infections,[313-315] antibody tests have been rarely used for the diagnosis of invasive candidiasis, invasive aspergillosis, and cryptococcosis.[313,316,317] The poor diagnostic performance of antibody evaluation in the case of these infections stems from that antibodies usually exist in colonized, but uninfected subjects[315] and that critically immunocompromised subjects may produce weak specific antibody responses. Interestingly though, evaluation of host antibody responses is commonly performed for the detection of endemic fungal infections that are usually hard to diagnose through conventional approaches, like culture and staining methods. Conventional serologic tests present restrictions, in particular when crude cocktails of antigens are used as reagents. These restrictions include cross-interactions between various subtypes, the existence of antibodies against prevalent environmental or commensal organisms, and no systematization of antigens and methods for measuring antibodies. This section will review the recent developments and the problems associated with serologic assays for fungal infection, with special attention directed towards the endemic mycoses.[318]

### Candidiasis

The clinical diagnosis and treatment of invasive candidiasis are major challenges for the specialists. Although timely diagnosis and therapy are correlated with a more favorable prognosis, apart from subjects with positive blood cultures or tissue/fluid biopsy, candidiasis diagnosis is not specific and sensitive, and it depends on many factors. Therefore, there exists a demand for specific biomarkers in this infection. Lately, novel serodiagnostic tests, such as *Candida albicans* germ-tube antibodies or$^{1,3}$-beta-D-glucan recognition and molecular approaches for the detection of unique fungal DNA, have been produced with disputed outcomes in critical care conditions. One of the key properties for diagnosis is the assessment of risk factors for infection, which will identify patients in need of preventive or empirical treatment. Clinical scores are calculated according to such risk factors. As of now, the combined use of predictive methods and non-culture immunological approaches may be a valuable blueprint for improving the detection and prognosis of invasive fungal infections in critically ill cases.[319] A novel immunological method of detecting systemic candida was developed by EIA to detect IgG antibodies against cell wall-attached and cytoplasmic candida antigens. Measuring antibodies in crude sera specimens by EIA, utilizing all of these antigenic extracts was highly specific (98 percent-100 percent), while the sensitivity of the method was poor (3.5 percent-17.8 percent). Interestingly, adsorption of sera with latex microspheres laced with purified Candida mannan to specifically dismiss anti-mannan antibodies before performing EIA enhanced the diagnostic efficiency of this test.[320]

### Blastomycosis

Initial serologic assays for blastomycosis were classically based on antibodies against *Blastomyces dermatitidis* A antigen, which was achieved via permitting Blastomyces yeast cell walls to go through autolysis in neutral buffer.[321,322] The titer of IgG antibody against *Blastomyces dermatitidis* A antigen is associated with infection activity, and this antibody could be found even over 12 months after complete therapy.[323] WI-1 is a 120-kDa protein in the external cell wall of *Blastomyces dermatitidis*, which has been purified and employed as a target in immunological diagnosis.[109,189] Antibodies against WI-1 can be found earlier than antibodies against A antigen, they can be sustained for a longer period, and their level drops to small or unnoticeable levels within 6 months following illness onset in cases with resolution or successful treatment of disease.[324,325]

### Coccidiomycosis

Serologic detection of coccidioidomycosis depends on the assessment of antibodies to two *Coccidioides immitis* proteins, the tube precipitin (TP) and the complement fixation antigens. Antibodies against TP have been related to primary acute infection and are considered to be IgM. Complement fixation antibodies are sustained during the chronic systematic stage of the infection and have been reported to be mainly IgG.[326] Complement fixation antibodies may not exist in immunocompromised or immunosuppressed cases, like AIDS patients,[327-329] highlighting that this method may have little clinical usage in such clinical scenarios.

### Histoplasmosis

Culture usually necessitates a 2- to 4-week incubation interval until the fungus can be detected, while diagnostic antibody assays put forward a quick and efficient substitute to microbiological tools.

Prior to the 1970s, the most significant resource of antigens in evaluating antibody responses in histoplasmosis cases was histoplasmin that was produced using filtrates of mycelial-stage cultures of *Histoplasma capsulatum* raised in artificial media.[330] Histoplasmin comprises unique *Histoplasma capsulatum* H and M antigens along with C antigen. Antibodies towards the H antigen are produced during active histoplasmosis,[331] whereas antibodies towards M antigens may be produced in both active and chronic histoplasmosis and are the earliest to emerge upon becoming serologically positive.[332]

Antigens obtained from the filtrate of mycelial-stage cultures of *Histoplasma capsulatum* contain elements, which cross-react with antibodies to other fungal subtypes.[333] Hence, glycosylated and nonglycosylated subtypes of M antigens were analyzed, and cross-reactivity with serum from aspergillosis, blastomycosis, coccidioidomycosis, and paracoccidioidomycosis cases was ruled out when M antigen was administered with periodate.[334,335] Moreover, a modified antigen corresponding to a 60-kDa native *Histoplasma capsulatum* antigen was recognized in the sera from all histoplasmosis cases and in the sera from none of the control subjects.[336] Researchers cloned and sequenced H antigen and reported similarities to β-glucosidases that are found outside cells. But, the performance of modified H as a diagnostic reagent has not been assayed. The antibody may be unrecognizable in *HIV* cases, possibly because of disrupted antibody synthesis.[337,338] In such conditions, antigen sensing assays reviewed in the following section may be better suited for the diagnosis of such infections.

### Paracoccidioidomycosis

The time is needed to separate Paracoccidioides brasiliensis from clinical specimens, and making a definitive diagnosis renders a barrier to timely diagnosis. Serological tests are helpful for timely diagnosis and depend on the recognition of antibody responses against *Paracoccidioides brasiliensis*. However, antibody responses are hard to recognize in AIDS cases infected by paracoccidioidomycosis. On the contrary, they are beneficial in cases without AIDS who are infected by paracoccidioidomycosis, in particular in cases of systematic infection.[339] Anti-*Paracoccidioides brasiliensis* IgG titers are commonly amplified in recently confirmed paracoccidioidomycosis cases, and these titers have been shown to be suitable biomarkers for screening cases with either the acute or chronic type of the illness and monitoring responses to therapy.[340-342]

### *Penicillinosis*

Penicillinosis cases have increased levels of antibodies towards *Penicillium marneffei*, and antibodies have been found even in immunocompromised (e.g., AIDS) cases.[343] Yet, immunoassays utilizing either unprocessed antigens or complete fungal cell have shortcomings. Therefore, efforts have been made to improve immunological tests.

Scientists cloned a *Penicillium marneffei* gene which encodes a robustly antigenic cell wall mannoprotein, Mp1p,[344] and showed antibodies against Mp1p via immunoprecipitation in *Penicillium marneffei*-inoculated guinea pigs as well as in penicilliosis patients. Another assay that utilized the purified modified Mp1p protein in an ELISA antibody assay recognized 14/17 (82 percent) *HIV* cases with penicilliosis. Also, the specificity of this assay appeared to be promising and no false-positive interactions were found in serum specimens from healthy subject, typhoid fever cases, or tuberculosis cases.[345] Although these studies showed good performance with the purified recombinant Mp1p protein, longitudinal studies are needed before the usage of this method can be generalized in clinical practice.[318]

### *Mucormycosis*

Currently, there are no standard serological assays for the detection of mucormycosis, but a number of allergens have been explained that may have potential as antigens in developing novel serological assays.[346] Immunohistochemistry assays aid histomorphologic diagnosis by differentiating mucormycosis and aspergillosis. Several verified mucormycosis cases with positive galactomannan had histopathology in line with aspergillosis and gastrointestinal mucormycosis. Approximately one-fourth of these cases were infected simultaneously with aspergillosis, as diagnosed by PCR.[347]

## Treatment

The reduced burden of fungal diseases in cases with balanced immune response has been taken as valid evidence that intact immunity can easily resist fungal infections.[348] Modifying the immune system components to recover deficient host immune responses and thus, increasing the effectiveness of anti-mycotic treatments is a promising approach to ameliorate the prognosis of fungal disease.[349] Therefore, the concept of immunoregulation covers a versatile spectrum of therapies targeted at tackling patients' immune system to attain management, stabilization, and plausible elimination of disease.[350,351] As can be found below, many immunoregulatory approaches have been clinically tested for the therapy of fungal infections.

### *Adoptive T-cell therapy*

Adoptive T-cell therapy includes acquiring T cells from a patient or donor's blood sample, triggering the cells to proliferate and expand in an in vitro setting, and subsequently re-injecting the cells back into the patient. Utilizing Aspergillus-exclusive CD4+ T cells separated from the spleens of immunized rodents that were re-activated in vitro were protective and extended the life of mice.[352] In a clinical study by Perruccio et al., ten haploidentical stem cell transplant subjects with evidence of invasive aspergillosis were administered with a single infusion of $1 \times 10^5$–$1 \times 10^6$ cells/kg of expanded donor-obtained anti-Aspergillus T cell clones, and 9/10 patients eradicated the pathogen within $7.8 \pm 3.4$ weeks.[353]

### Chimeric antigen receptor (CAR) T-cells

Chimeric Antigen Receptors (CARs) are synthetically produced receptors that are inserted into the composition of T cells. The CAR modification permits T cells to carry out their killing duty without needing to bind other receptors.[354] Dectin-1, a receptor of the innate immune system that is not produced on T cells, has been aimed for CAR therapy. β-glucan, the ligand for Dectin-1, is a polysaccharide detected on the exterior of some fungi.[355] Researchers produced a CAR T-cell adjusting the fungal receptor Dectin-1 for Aspergillus to induce T cells by chimeric CD28 and CD3-ζ. In this experiment, the Dectin-CAR was induced by β-glucan, and the proliferation of *Aspergillus fumigatus* was suppressed.[356] CAR T-cells are one of the most valuable immune-regulating treatment methods. MHC unlimited antigen detection is the principal benefit of CAR T-cell treatment. Lately, repurposing T cells via CAR T-cell treatment has become an important field for further investigation in the battle against infections and hematological cancers. Nevertheless, this method may prompt cytokine release syndrome and neurotoxicity.[357,358] Also, the autologous production of an adequate amount of CAR T-cells may require multiple weeks that might be slow in acute clinical conditions, such as invasive fungi.[359] Allogeneic CAR T-cell therapy, however, may bring about readily accessible products with reduced cost, and it can also be appropriate for a large number of patients as opposed to autologous CAR T-cell treatment in which each therapy must be performed separately for each case. Still, allogeneic CAR T-cells can cause lethal graft versus host disease (GVHD), and these allogeneic T cells may also be quickly removed via the host immune response, restricting their purposed activity.[360]

### Granulocyte transfusion

In the 1950s, Brecher et al. reported that granulocytes infused to neutropenic canines emigrated to regions of infection.[361] Since that time, various researches back the effectiveness of granulocyte transfusion for invasive fungi. Diaz et al. discussed that most children with granulocyte impairments or critical neutropenia who were treated with granulocyte transfusion exhibited an immune reaction to invasive fungi.[362] Moreover, among pediatric hematopoietic stem cell receivers who were transfused with granulocyte, half of the cases with invasive fungal involvement exhibited radiological improvement. Granulocyte transfusion, along with granulocyte colony-stimulating factors (G-CSFs), resulted in an overall response rate (ORR) of 50 percent-90 percent in patients with invasive fungi.[363] Nonetheless, the transfusion of granulocyte is restricted because of low granulocyte amounts, poor quality, and limited lifetime of the granulocytes.[364] A supplementary method to whole recombinant yeast immunization utilizes nanoparticles in targeting antigens. Nanoparticles are internalized particularly by DCs because of their sub-micron size and can be more uniquely aimed towards DCs via adding DC receptor (e.g., Dec 205) modulating antibodies or DCs receptor ligands to their surface. Nanoparticle regulated targeting of DCs enables the bundling of defined antigen or antigens with an adjuvant and a DCs receptor targeting molecule, permitting accurate delivery to DCs. The superiority of this method was recently reported by a DEC205 F(ab')2 fragment laced nanoparticle comprising TLR-3, TLR-7, and TLR-8 ligands along with OVA antigen.[365] This work highlighted that nanoparticles can convey vaccine antigens to DCs efficiently and that when antigen and adjuvant are conveyed in parallel, promising immune responses with restricted toxicity can be activated. In a sense, the targeting nanoparticle packed with antigen and adjuvant starts to mimic the fungal vaccine target itself.[366]

### DCs therapy

DCs sense fungi by PRRs and process fungal antigens. Activated DCs secrete cytokines and chemokines, emigrate to the lymph nodes, and display antigens to special T cells that, in turn, are induced and primed.[367] In this method, DCs may be induced with fungal antigens ex vivo and infused into the subject. Such DCs activate immunoprotection against the fungus because of the induction of fungus-exclusive T cells.[366] In an in vivo study, DCs which had been transduced with IL-12 and triggered by *Aspergillus fumigatus* were injected into neutropenic rodents, and the DCs treatment led to decreased mortality and fungal burden because of a prominent Th1 response.[368] After subcutaneous injection of a *Blastomyces dermatitidis* vaccine, DEC205-producing skin-extracted DCs emigrated to the skin draining lymph node in a CCR7-dependent manner, presented the model antigen expressed by the fungus, and activated CD4+ T cells.[369]

### NK cell therapy

NK cell treatment exerts an immunoprotective role against a versatile range of fungal infections, such as *Aspergillus fumigatus*, *Cryptococcus neoformans*, *Rhizopus oryzae*, *Candida albicans, Paracoccidioides brasiliensis*, and *Mucorales*. For example, in allogeneic stem cell transplantation cases, enhanced NK cell levels were related to better control of invasive aspergillosis. NK cells produce IFN-$\gamma$ and soluble agents such as GM-CSF and regulated on activation, normal T cell expressed and secreted (RANTES), both of which enhance the host immune reactions through the activation of phagocytosis and T cells, respectively.[370-372]

### *Granulocyte colony-stimulating factor (G-CSF) and granulocyte-macrophage colony-stimulating factor (GM-CSF)*

G-CSF and GM-CSF cannot improve invasive fungi-associated prevalence and death, but they can help to quicken the recuperation of the patient. During chemotherapy-triggered febrile neutropenia, G-CSF is routinely prescribed. G-CSF shortens the duration of neutropenia and the hospitalization period during febrile neutropenia episodes, but its usage did not clearly affect infection-associated death in febrile neutropenia.[373] A recent Cochrane Database Systematic Review on the usage of G-CSF and GM-CSF in febrile neutropenia highlighted similar outcomes.[374] The study explained that there was a reduced duration of neutropenia, quicker resolution of fever, and reduced duration for empiric antibiotic use, and treatment with the colony-stimulating agents did not have an effect on total death rates, as well as fungus-associated death. However, a stage IV randomized clinical study investigated the influence of preventive therapy of 206 allogenic HSCT receivers with G-CSF, GM-CSF, or both, and researchers detected invasive fungi-associated death rate after 600 days to be reduced in the GM-CSF, G-CSF + GM-CSF subgroups when compared to the G-CSF-only subgroup (the values for mentioned groups were 1.47 percent, 1.45 percent, and 11.59 percent, respectively). The findings of this study may warrant further research utilizing preventive GM-CSF, with or without G-CSF, to attenuate invasive fungi-associated death. Regarding invasive fungal infections prevalence, studies showed no dissimilarity when G-CSF or GM-CSF was prophylactically administered with antimycotics in patients with allogeneic or autologous HSCT.[375,376] On an individual patient level, GM-CSF has exerted highly favorable outcomes. For instance, Chen et al. (2017) reported success when GM-CSF was used as an adjunct therapy to treat Aspergillus ventriculitis. In this experiment, GM-CSF was given in parallel with voriconazole, amphotericin B, and caspofungin. The function of GM-CSF in this scenario was found remarkable, considering that fungal ventriculitis has a significant death rate of 67 percent with traditional therapy. In a patient with *Scedosporium apiospermum* with inadequate success with voriconazole treatment, favorable outcomes were found after switching to the micafungin infusion in parallel with GM-CSF.[377]

### *Cytokine therapy*

Fortifying the immunity via cytokine-mediating treatments is another method to defend against fungal infections. Neutropenia makes cancer patients receiving corticosteroids susceptible to invasive fungi. Cytokines will reduce the duration of neutropenia by enhancing the phagocytic and cidal activities of neutrophils, monocytes, and macrophages.[378] Cytokines used as immunoregulatory elements in fungal infection comprise CSFs, IFN-$\gamma$, TNF-$\alpha$, and ILs. IFN-$\gamma$ treatment enhances the anti-mycotic activity via amplifying the number of macrophages and neutrophils.[351,379]

# Parasitic infections

## Definition

Despite current treatments, over 2 billion individuals are affected by infections with parasites that are responsible for significant mortality.[380] Among parasites, intestinal parasitic infections are endemic globally and have been described as constituting the most significant single global cause of the disease.[381,382] About 3.5 billion individuals are influenced by intestinal parasitic infections around the world, of them, 450 million are affected by a wide range of intestinal parasitic infections.[383,384] According to a worldwide approximation, 895 million individuals are affected by soil-transmitted helminths (STHs), as about 447 million, 290 million, and 229 million cases suffer from *Ascaris lumbricoides*, *Trichuris trichiura*, and hookworms, respectively.[385] On the contrary, intestinal protozoa are less prevalent compared to STHs, as about 184 million, 104 million, and 64 million people are affected by *Giardia lamblia*, *Entamoeba histolytica*, and *Cryptosporidium* spp., respectively.[386] Intestinal parasitic infections are a major issue in low- and middle-income regions and are associated with poverty, illiteracy, suboptimal hygiene, lack of access to drinkable water, along with hot and humid tropical climates.[387,388] Intestinal parasitic infections can lead to chronic diseases, including iron deficiency anemia, growth retardation, and digestive problems, such as diarrhea, flatulence, anorexia, nausea, vomiting, and abdominal discomfort. These clinical sequels are usually found in high-risk populations (e.g., immunosuppressed patients, children, and pregnant women).[389-391]

Parasites are classically categorized into three groups: protozoa, helminths, and ectoparasites.[392] The most significant protozoal parasites comprise Plasmodium species (leading to malaria), *Entamoeba histolytica* (leading to amebiasis), Leishmania species (leading to leishmaniasis), and Trypanosoma species (leading to sleeping sickness and Chagas' disease). The most important helminthic parasites comprise nematodes like *Ascaris lumbricoides*, trematodes like *Schistosoma mansoni* (leading to schistosomiasis), and cestodes or tapeworms like *Taenia solium* (leading to taeniasis).[393] Most parasites that cause disease in humans are eukaryotes with significant size differences, and life cycle complexity. They include unicellular protozoan and multi-cellular metazoans, like worms, which spend part or all of their life cycles in a host that is able to establish a wide range of anti-pathogen immune responses.

Parasitic infections denote an important immunological paradigm. Most parasites, by the nature of their contact with the immune system, produce prominent immune response. The immune response may be pathogenic like hypersensitivity, immune-regulated fibrosis, and circulating immune complexes. Better studying these immune responses helps to diagnose and treat parasitic infections.[394] Also, parasites have acquired special methods of defending against the immune system, such as changing their antigenic coat and triggering immunosuppression. Such advanced biological mechanisms of parasites can lead to the development of chronic illnesses.[395] Parasitic infections and the host's immune responses are contributed to the host-parasite reciprocal evolutionary changes and the parasite's complicated life cycle. Each period of the life cycle leads to different interactions with the immune system,[396,397] which despite outstanding progress, have not been clearly determined.[398,399] One of the major functions of any parasite is to promote its dissemination to a new host. For most air-borne pathogens (e.g., respiratory viruses and bacteria), the limited time for the infection that is provided by acute infection is sufficient for their dissemination. Sterilizing immunity is defined by a state in which the immune system can stop a pathogen from multiplying within the body.[400] Blood and tissue parasites that rely on an invertebrate host for cyclical transmission (e.g., *African trypanosomes*, *Plasmodium* spp., *Leishmania* spp., *Trypanosoma cruzi*, and filarial or schistosome worms) postpone the establishment of sterilizing immunity to extend the period during which they can spread through a vector or intermediate host. Hence, it is comprehendible that most parasites utilize methods such as active (e.g., phagocytosis) and passive (e.g., being concealed within the immune-privileged parts like the CNS and the eye) immune escape processes to prevent their removal by the immune system.[401]

It may be beneficial to exemplify evading phagocytosis as an advanced escape mechanism used by multiple harmful parasites to human health and its relevance to clinical treatment of infection. Phagocytes are involved in both innate and adaptive immunity and denote an important paradigm in the immunology of parasites.[402]

In 1883, Elie Metchnikoff initially explained phagocytes and phagocytosis. At the time, it was assumed that phagocytosis is mainly carried out in animals and is related to homeostasis, nutrition, and tissue reabsorption. Subsequently, Metchnikoff explained how this mechanism could also defend against harmful organisms.[403] "Infection, a struggle between two organisms" was the heading Metchnikoff chose for his initial lecture given in 1891,[404] a title that precisely explained the advanced interconnection between an evolutionary perspective of the host immune system and infectious microorganisms. After 130 years, the hard part is to understand optimal treatments for infectious diseases resulting from microorganisms, which select phagocytes as hosts for infection, multiplying, and sustaining of themselves.

The immune escape mechanisms are clinically important as they complicate the treatment of parasitic infections. It is only in the light of such immunological parasitic mechanisms that efforts should test immune-based therapies, such as immunotherapy or preventive vaccination (e.g., efforts to extract "host-defending" antigens in parasitic infections can help vaccine development). The example of phagocytosis mentioned earlier is employed by certain species (e.g., Leishmania). Leishmaniasis is a vector-borne infection with versatile clinical presentations, which are a result of the intersection of the parasite subtypes and the host immune feedback.[405] During infection by the intracellular parasite Leishmania, the disease raises major challenges for therapy and prophylaxis because of advanced processes it utilizes to escape the immune system, enabling it to affect the very same cells recruited by the immune system to eliminate the parasite.[406,

[407] From the 1970s onwards, Leishmania parasites are regarded as phagosomal microorganisms that occupy and multiply in phagocytes.[408–411] Currently, we recognize that even a single Leishmania parasite disseminated by a sandfly bite is adequate to cause infection,[412,413] verifying material explained in this chapter that innate processes of immunity are not adequate to confer protection and that the development of acquired immune feedback, regulated chiefly by Th1 cells, is necessary to induce phagocytic cells.[414] Overall, how this parasite has matured to survive against the innate immune system of the host and exploit T-cell immunity and induce and sustain clinical infection suggests the importance of underlying immunological mechanisms, and may be a guidance to develop better treatments.[415] Also, macrophages biology can be exploited by other parasites, such as Yersinia and Shigella through Yops protein and IpaB, respectively.[416,417]

Taken together, compared to other classes of microorganisms, parasite classes are versatile in their biological systems and mechanisms, producing special imbalanced immune responses or obligating these pathogens to develop immune escape mechanisms. The epidemiology, life cycle, clinical presentation, treatment, and diagnosis of parasitic infections relate to immunity within the context of these underlying immunological mechanisms.

## Mechanisms

### *Innate immunity*

#### Inflammasomes

Although generally the function of NLRC4, AIM2, and NLRP12 during parasitic infections is not clear, the function of NLRP1 and NLRP3 has been investigated more extensively in parasitic infections, such as significant protozoan and helminthic infections that were mentioned earlier, as well as ectoparasite-related pathogens. Here, we detail the role of inflammasomes in Leishmaniosis as an essential example and refer the authors to elegant reviews by Carvalho and Zamboni, and Celias et al. on the role of inflammasomes in protozoa and helminths, respectively.[418–421]

While the activation of inflammasome-dependent cytokines after infection, like IL-1β and IL-1α, has been found in early studies,[422] it was not until 2013 that the first explanation of the molecular processes of inflammasome induction after Leishmania infection were explained.[423] Through the utilization of various subtypes of Leishmania, it was shown that all these subtypes could activate IL-1β secretion via macrophages' inflammasome components, such as NLRP3, ASC, and caspase-1. After phagocytosis, parasites activate the CLR, and Dectin-1. This activates a Syk-dependent signaling pathway that leads to ROS production, which results in NLRP3 induction after *Leishmania amazonensis* infection.[424] The Leishmania lipophosphoglycan (LPG) can induce caspase-11 and the noncanonical NLRP3 inflammasome.[425] By utilizing macrophages genetically lacking caspase-11, highly purified LPG, and parasites lacking a transferase, which is crucial for LPG anchoring in the membrane (*Leishmania major* Lpg1-/-), it was shown that caspase-11 is induced via different Leishmania subtypes and their corresponding LPGs enhance pore formation, cell death, NLRP3 induction, and IL-1β secretion when delivered in the cytoplasm of macrophages. This work also shows that the amastigote kind of the parasite that exhibits little concentrations of LPG on its surface leads to lower inflammasome triggering in comparison with promastigote forms. Also, that amastigotes disrupt NLRP3 induction in macrophages via targeting histone H3.[426] NLRP3 induction is important to the course of the Leishmania infection. But, while some researchers proposed a defensive function for NLRP3 during Leishmaniasis, others have found a deleterious function for this inflammasome to the host. These variations may be justified by the use of various parasite subtypes, strains, and different mouse backgrounds.[427] For instance, by inducing *Leishmania amazonensis* infection in C57BL/6 rodents, it was found that NLRP3 exerts a key function in parasite killing and lesion healing.[428,429] On the contrary, researchers utilizing C57BL/6 and *Leishmania braziliensis*[16] or the nonhealing *Leishmania major* Seidman strain[17] found a harmful function for NLRP3, acting in favor of parasite chronicity and lesion expansion.[430,431] Similarly, studies carried out in cases infected by *Leishmania braziliensis* have reported a positive correlation between inflammasome activation and the infection severity.[432,433]

Regarding the role of NOD receptors, currently, there is no conclusive relation with parasites, but as their nature may suggest, they may be involved in intracellular detection of intracellular parasites, as Finney et al.[434] put forth in their evaluation of the inflammatory actions regulated via NOD receptors in cerebral malaria.

### TLRs

There are limited articles reporting the role of TLRs in the detection of parasites. However, they have been involved in different responses against parasites, like TLR-2 on DCs and its attachment to lysophosphatidylserine of *Schistosoma mansoni* and Tc-52 or glycophosphatidylinositol (GPI) anchors of *Trypanosoma cruzi*. In the former parasite, the interaction activates the Th2 response, and in the later parasite, Th1 response. This polar immune response may be associated with the collaboration of TLR-2 with TLR-1 and TLR-6.[435] Also, GPI anchor proteins from *Trypanosoma cruzi*, *Plasmodium falciparum*, and *Toxoplasma gondii* seem to activate the release of TNF via macrophages through TLR.[436] TLR-9 senses unmethylated CpG motifs in bacterial DNA content of phagosomes, and it has been reported that protozoal DNA comprising CpG motifs is adequate to induce a TLR-9-response of host cells.[437] The induction of TLRs could result in complications related to parasitic infections, like anemia and nephritis that result from autoantibodies in malaria.[438]

### Other mechanisms

**Other innate immune receptors** PAMPs have been identified in human parasitic pathogens, which are detected via PRR of various kinds. However, none has been found that is specific for parasites, as those receptors are also employed via other microorganisms.[420,439]

Other than inflammasomes and TLRs, several extracellular classical PRRs have been related to the detection of parasites. For instance, from collectins, the mannose-binding lectin (MBL)[440,441] attaches mannose-rich LPG of Leishmania and *Plasmodium falciparum* proteins on affected erythrocytes,[442,443] *Trypanosoma cruzi* amastigotes,[444,445] *Schistosoma mansoni*,[446] and all *Trichinella spiralis* developmental phases.[447] Moreover, pentraxins that act as classical human receptors act as opsonins when adhered to their ligand. One member of the pentraxin family, the C-reactive protein (CRP), attaches to elements of Leishmania LPG and enhances via opsonization of infiltrated parasites in macrophages.[448] Additionally, CRP attaches to Plasmodium sporozoites and thereby defends the host against its hepatocyte attack.[449] Also, CRP contributes to the natural resistance to *Schistosoma mansoni* infection.[450] Various C- type lectins produced on the external surface of macrophages and DCs have been related to parasite detection. From them, the macrophage mannose receptor has been found to be able to enhance the permissive entrance of *Trypanosoma cruzi* amastigotes into macrophages, and DC-exclusive ICAM-3- grabbing non-integrin receptor (DC-SIGN) on DCs attaches with high affinity to schistosomes via Lewis x[451] and amastigotes and promastigotes of Leishmania by mannose-capped LPG.[452-454] Alternative C-type lectins, the calcium-dependent galactose-attaching proteins, named intelectins, are produced via paneth cells and goblet cells and have as well been indicated in the detection of gastrointestinal helminths, along with in the reaction with the surface of parasites to avoid binding to host surfaces.[455] Among the scavenger receptors, CD-36, a type B-scavenger receptor, helps the attachment to PfEMP1 that permits the phagocytosis of *Plasmodium falciparum*-infected erythrocytes through macrophages, and it has been shown that this attachment mediates the actions of DCs.[456,457] Complement receptor, CR3, which has a multifaceted function in the innate immune response like other members of its PRR family, is the gateway to multiple intracellular pathogens, such as *Leishmania major*, where it was recently explained to be quintessential in avoiding the advancement of lesions during the course of infection.[458]

### *Adaptive immunity*

The role of cellular and humoral immunity is extensive in protozoan and helminthic parasitic infections. Here, we exemplify a few protozoan species and refer the readers to comprehensive expert reviews on the topic.[439]

### Cellular immunity

In Th1 responses to protozoa, IFN-γ release by CD4+ T cells and CD8+ T cells results in the triggering of effector processes to effectively eradicate parasites, like macrophages activation to destroy phagocytosed parasites (e.g., *Trypanosoma cruzi*).[459] This point is very important as many protozoa escape the humoral immunity via infiltrating the macrophages, such as Toxoplasma[460] or Leishmania.[461,462]

It has been found that cellular immune response rather than antibody production is crucial for resistance to protozoa with intracellular phases, such as the Plasmodium pre-erythrocytic phase.[463,464] The versatile clinical presentations of malaria have been explained via defining the contradicting poles of T cell immune responses. In the rodent model, a Th1 immune response is related to low numbers of Leishmania parasites in lesions, while a Th2 immune response has been related to uncontrolled parasite outgrowth.[465]

Moreover, IFN-γ induces Th1 cells' development through triggering of the transcription factor T-bet generation and blocks Th2 cytokine release by inhibition of the transcription factor GATA-3 expression by T-bet.[466] Moreover, IFN-γ enhances the expression of MHC class I to help detection and killing via CD8+ T cells and MHC class II molecules to facilitate the presentation of antigens to CD4+ T cells.[462]

Cellular immunity affects humoral immunity in parasitic infections. For instance, IFN activates the switch to special classes of Igs, such as IgG2a, and suppresses isotype switching to IL-4 dependent Igs, like IgE and IgG1.[467] The most typical example of the defensive role of Th1 responses at the expense of Th2 is Leishmania infection. While this applies to cutaneous leishmaniasis, this is to be determined in visceral leishmaniasis.[468] Th1 responses are defined, other than IFN-γ release, by the induction of cytotoxic T lymphocyte (CTL)-regulated cell lysis, despite that the significance of these cells in the protection against protozoa results from their IFN-producing potential rather than to its lytic activity, such as in toxoplasmosis.[469] However, CD8+ T cells protect against malaria through demolishing Plasmodium sporozoites-infected hepatocytes. Overstreet et al.[470] reported that memory CD8+ T cells incapable of producing perforin, FasL, or IFN-γ, separately, could defend against the liver stage in any of the three cases. This highlights that the effector actions of memory CD8+ T cells are because of a mixture of the cytotoxic/cytolytic processes and IFN release. However, any of these is indispensable in the presence of others. The function of CD8+ T cells seems necessary for the immune response to Plasmodium sporozoites.[463,464,471] Cellular responses towards the erythrocytic phase of malaria have also been explained,[472] but, while the role of CD4+ T cells is evidently vital, it has not been determined if CD8+ T cells are indispensable,[473] and yet, CD8+ T cells have been related to the immunopathology of cerebral malaria.[474]

The involvement of CD8+ T cells in Chagas′ disease is important for the management of infection, to the extent that *Trypanosoma cruzi* infection has been highlighted as a model for CD8+ T cells-regulated vaccine design for intracellular pathogens. Indeed, knowledge of the importance of CD8+ T cell responses in protozoan infections is leading to the exploration of parasite epitopes that strongly activate CD8+ T cells to design efficient vaccines.[475,476]

## Humoral immunity

Even though antibodies are not probably the chief control process in parasitic infections with intracellular phases, they increase in response to all protozoal infections such as Leishmania,[477] *Trypanosoma cruzi*,[478] *Toxoplasma gondii*,[479] and Plasmodium.[480] In addition, in African trypanosomes, which is caused by *Trypanosoma brucei* (extracellular parasite), the significance of various immunoglobulins has been found. It has been reported that IgGs play a more important role than IgMs in infection management, despite that IgM concentrations are high. Also, it has been found that different subclasses of IgGs are produced at each phase of infection based on the detected antigen (although the immunodominant antigen is probably the variable surface glycoprotein (VSG)).[481-484] As a result, although the synthesis of Igs is not always the major effector process, they are contributed to the immune response to various parasitic protozoa.

The roles of antibodies in response to protozoa are miscellaneous. For instance, direct lysis through antibodies (e.g., for *Trypanosoma cruzi* infection[485]) and complement-regulated lysis (e.g., for Plasmodium gametocytes and *Trypanosoma cruzi* trypomastigotes[485,486]) has been explained. While previous research showed the role of cellular immunity is more prominent in malaria, in a recent work, authors reported instances in human, canine, and some rodent models of leishmaniasis that exhibit a direct relation between high anti-parasite antibody responses and uncontrolled parasite outgrowth. The spectral character of malaria infection may be caused by quantitative and qualitative variations in the antibodies, which are synthesized during infection. In human visceral leishmaniasis, a reduction in anti-parasite antibody titers could predict disease resolution. As a result, rather than defining this disease as a simple Th1/Th2 dichotomy, the authors showed that clinical leishmaniasis relies on the degree of humoral immunity, with high IgG predicting a higher chance for chronicity of the infection.[465]

### *Immune escape mechanisms*

Immune escape mechanisms are explained here, through the lens of the parasites, in two passive and active sections. However, these mechanisms can also be categorized into innate and adaptive changes in the immunity of the host.[439]

### Passive

Parasites can conceal from the immune system via attacking immune-privileged tissues, including the CNS and the eye.[487] Moreover, several parasitoids lay their eggs within tissue like the fat tissue, which is not screened prominently via the host's immune system. Parasites may become undetectable to the immune system. For instance, this may be attained through protecting surface elements as soon as they are opsonized via the host's immune system (e.g., in Plasmodium[488]). Parasites are also able to alter their surface character. The cellular and humoral immunity of the vertebrate's immune system sense special epitopes, and the parasite evades this detection by altering its antigenic outer layer during infection. Usually, parasites contain surface variants that are sequentially expressed. For instance, *Plasmodium falciparum* has kept about 60 variants, and *Trypanosoma brucei* has a few hundred,[489-491] and antigenic differences are recognized from bacteria (phase shift[492,493]) and nematodes.[494] Parasites can also escape through mutation of their epitopes, and they outsmart the immune system.[495] The parasites can be transiently inactivated, and as a result, they can dodge the immune system (i.e., quiescence). This characteristic of parasites is like some bacteria that can also go quiescent with limited or no metabolic activity and no cellular replication, and by this mechanism, they prevent inhibition through antibiotics, which target cell division.[496] Furthermore, viruses like herpes simplex virus (HSV) are able to enter a state of latency during which the formation of viral proteins is significantly diminished.[497]

### Active

The most important class of immune escape mechanisms denote active interference with the host's immune responses. Particularly, parasites usually disrupt the regulatory relations that orchestrate the different branches of immune protection. However, parasites also disrupt the fundamental actions of the host's cells. To this aim, parasites synthesize molecules that can inhibit or modulate special phases in the host's immune response, along with general cellular actions that are important for host defense (e.g., cell motility). These regulatory elements are positioned differently.

## Diagnosis

### Falcon assay screening test-elisa (FAST-ELISA)

The Falcon assay screening test-ELISA (FAST-ELISA) comprises the utilization of artificial peptides to assess antibody responses to an antigen.[498] In the late 20th century, this approach was used to diagnose malaria, fasciolosis, schistosomiasis, and taeniasis.[499-502] In 2011, an assessment of FAST-ELISA compared to standard ELISA to diagnose human fasciolosis was performed. The sensitivity, specificity, positive, and negative predictive values were reported as 97.2 percent, 100 percent, 94.6 percent, and 95.6 percent for both assays, and the results showed that FAST-ELISA had a similar and good performance in detecting the infection.[503] However, this approach has some downsides similar to most serological assays. For instance, antibodies against a peptide of one parasite can cross-react with proteins from other subtypes. Also, antibodies produced against a peptide may react only in specific tests, and certain regions of a peptide may be more immunogenic compared to others. Therefore, more research on the utilization of the FAST-ELISA for the detection of parasitic infections is needed.

#### *Dot-ELISA*

The major difference between the standard ELISA and the dot-ELISA is the surface of attachment for the antigen. In the dot-ELISA, the plastic plate is substituted by nitrocellulose or other paper membranes with a low amount of specimen volume. The attachment matrix significantly enhances the diagnostic performance of the test via decreasing the attachment of nonspecific proteins observed when plastic-attaching matrices are utilized. The methodology resembles that of the immunoblot. First, the dotted membrane is incubated with an antigen-exclusive antibody and then with an enzyme-conjugated anti-antibody. Adding a precipitable, chromogenic substrate results in the synthesis of a colored dot on the membrane that is visible.[2] The advantages of this approach include high speed of the test, cost-effectiveness, and that it can be easily performed and interpreted. Because of these, throughout these years, the dot-ELISA has been routinely employed for the diagnosis of human and animal parasitic infections, such as amebiasis, babesiosis, fascioliasis, cutaneous and visceral leishmaniasis, cysticercosis, echinococcosis, malaria, schistosomiasis, toxocariasis, toxoplasmosis, trichinosis, and trypanosomiasis.[504] Recently, the dot-ELISA has been utilized to diagnose *Fasciola gigantica*, *Haemonchus contortus*, *Theileria equi*, *Trypanosoma cruzi*, and *Trypanosoma brucei*. The researchers showed that the dot-ELISA had higher diagnostic performance compared to the ELISA in the recognition of anti-neurofilament and anti-galactocerebrosides antibodies in cerebrospinal fluid of patients infected with African trypanosomes. The better diagnostic performance of the dot-ELISA was attributed to the nitrocellulose membrane. Importantly, this test was proved to be reproducible in the field.[505-509]

### *Rapid diagnostic tests (RDTs)*

Rapid diagnostic tests (RDTs) are depended on immunochromatographic antigen recognition. These tests have been utilized in numerous diagnostic facilities as an aid to microscopy for the detection of malaria. In RDTs, soluble proteins are captured through binding with capture antibodies embedded on a nitrocellulose strip. A small amount of blood specimen is administered to the strip and eluted from the nitrocellulose strip via adding multiple drops of buffer, which included a labeled antibody. Then, the antigen-antibody complex will be visible directly from the membrane. After the use of the first RDTs, significant enhancement has been made to this approach, making the utilization of RDTs practical in rural areas. RDTs are currently quick, stable at temperatures as high as 40 °C, easy to perform, and cost-effective. Because of these reasons, they are better than the conventional microscopic methods. RDTs are useful in the diagnosis of *Plasmodium falciparum* and *Plasmodium vivax* infections but cannot be utilized to diagnose *Plasmodium malariae* and *Plasmodium ovale* infections. Additionally, they are not practical for detecting very poor-density infections. In this case, methods based on PCR remain optimal strategy. There are over 80 RDTs for the diagnosis of either histidine-rich protein (HRP) unique to *Plasmodium falciparum* or species-exclusive isotypes of lactate dehydrogenase (LDH).[49] Nevertheless, as Murray et al.[510] showed, only 23 have fulfilled the WHO's criteria for international marketing. Malaria RDTs have lately been utilized in African regions to help avoid misdiagnosis of malaria infections and to consequently decrease the practice of presumptive therapy. Indeed, the tendency to treat slide-negative samples with antimalarials is still a prevalent phenomenon. This results in issues for the patients' health care and also unnecessarily increases the cost of treatment with the more expensive malaria drugs, such as sulfadoxine/pyrimethamine and artemisinin-dependent regimens. Ultimately, excessive drug use may facilitate the development of drug-resistant strains.[510-512]

### *Luciferase immunoprecipitation system (LIPS)*

LIPS is an adjusted ELISA-dependent test. In this assay, serum comprising antigen-exclusive antibodies may be recognized via assessment of light production. Indeed, an antigen of choice is fused to the enzyme reporter Renilla luciferase (Ruc) and expressed as a Ruc-fusion in mammalian cells to permit mammalian-exclusive posttranslational alterations. The crude protein isolate is then exposed to the test serum along with protein A/G beads. While incubating with the serum, the Ruc-antigen fusion is stabilized on the A/G beads, which permits the antigen-exclusive antibody to be calculated via washing the beads and adding coelenterazine substrate and evaluating light production.[513] Lately, LIPS has been effectively used for the detection of sera specimens from cases infected with *Strongyloides stercoralis* (by a Ruc-NIE fusion)[134] and *Loa loa* (by a Ruc-LlSXP-1 fusion).[514] Certain benefits of the LIPS technology comprise its rapidity and accuracy in recognizing infected cases. Sensitivity is enhanced through the utilization of mammalian cells that express fusion antigens, clear of bacterial proteins contamination. Additionally, low backgrounds are produced in comparison with the ELISA. This helps the differentiation of negative and positive specimens. Also, the Strongyloides LIPS utilizing the NIE antigen exhibit higher specificity compared to ELISA because no cross-reactivity is present with serum from filarial-infected patients.[515] A normal LIPS test can be conducted in about 2.5 hours. A study showed 100 percent specificity and sensitivity are attainable by conducting a LIPS test based on the *Loa loa* SXP-1 antigen with a very small degree of cross-reactivity with some *Onchocerca volvulus* and *Wuchereria bancrofti*-infected patient sera. Also, cross-reactivity was decreased by reducing the incubation period of a normal LIPS test. A considerable proportion of the *Onchocerca volvulus* sera specimen that were positive by the LIPS test, were negative by this 15-minute LIPS assay, named QLIPS. In addition, it was reported that blood obtained via finger-prick (contaminated with red blood cells and other elements) did not disrupt the LIPS test.[514]

Immune-based diagnostic assays have a number of important restrictions. Parasitic infections like amebiasis, cryptosporidiosis, filariasis, giardiasis, malaria, cysticercosis, schistosomiasis, and African trypanosomiasis still do not have commercially- or Food and Drug Administration (FDA)- verified antibody diagnostics with a favorable performance. Laboratory findings lack consistency because of the type of antigen preparation utilized (e.g., crude, recombinant purified, adult worm, and egg) and also because of the use of non-standardized test processes. Also, cross-reactivity that causes false-positive and misdiagnosis is an issue, especially in areas where multiple parasites are endemic. While a number of parasites in South America share similar epitopes, coinfection with *Trypanosoma cruzi* and Leishmania subtypes is rather prevalent.[516] Similarly, in Africa, the issue of cross-reactivity among filarial and other helminth antigens is present.[514]

Additionally, it is vital to note that it is difficult for antibody-diagnostic assays to differentiate between the past and current active infections.[517] Moreover, antibody-recognition assays cannot be utilized in parasitic infections that do not raise significant antibody responses. This has been found in certain individuals who are carriers for Echinococcus cysts[518] or during cutaneous leishmaniasis.[519] Also, for the diagnosis of African trypanosomiasis, these assays are of restricted use as seroconversion takes place only after the initiation of clinical symptoms.[83] Overall, these highlight a need to improve available diagnostic tools.

## Treatment

### *Leishmaniasis*

Leishmaniasis is the most-researched parasitic infection in the sense of the number of immunotherapy trials for its therapy. The first attempt to vaccinate humans against leishmaniasis employing dead leishmanial promastigote preparation was done in 1939. It investigated the influence of vaccine injection containing killed dermotropic *Leishmania* spp. and phenol on cutaneous leishmaniasis infections. Beneficial influences of suspension of killed leishmanial promastigote concoction (the proposed vaccine) were observed against the infection.[520,521] The first human clinical trial against leishmaniasis was conducted in 1940s, using the suspension of promastigotes, which achieved a decrease by 80 percent in the incidence of the disease. After inoculation, researchers reported no adverse events and that the Montenegro skin test stayed negative.[520] After that, other studies continued to experiment immunotherapy in localized cutaneous leishmaniasis via dead promastigotes and bacillus Calmette-Guerin, and in mucosal leishmaniasis via dead promastigote complete antigen, with the efficiency of 76 percent[522] to 94 percent,[523] respectively. Vaccination is a safer and more suitable option and a practical preventive tool in American cutaneous leishmaniasis. However, it could be beneficial for the therapy of mucosal leishmaniasis in specific cases as well.[520] While these vaccines are advised, they have unspecified concoction, are hard to standardize, and have the potential of inducing noxious local or systemic unwanted influences. Therefore, it appears implausible to be administered routinely.[524,525] The mixture of a single-strain *Leishmania amazonensis* dead promastigote crude antigen vaccine accompanied by a half dose administration of meglumine antimoniate is greatly efficient for the therapy of American cutaneous leishmaniasis.[525] Immunotherapy by crude productions of Leishmania antigen, with or without bacillus Calmette-Guerin, is advised and used with success in therapy of mucosal leishmaniasis, and clearly displayed healing in some cases with the infection.[520,522,523,526,527] The vaccine with a regimen of antigen, in combination with standard chemotherapy, was found to be an effective approach for therapy of drug-resistant mucosal leishmaniasis. This approach also displays mild systemic complications like fever, headache, malaise, and somnolence in the first therapy. Local reactions of the injection area like redness and edema can take place and resemble leishmanin skin-test induration. However, vivid granulomatous reactions are absent. The local reaction occurs in the first, second, and third doses of immunotherapy. Drug-resistant mucosal leishmaniasis has been successfully treated with antigens thiol-specific antioxidant, Leishmania major stress-inducible protein-1, Leishmania elongation initiation factor, Leishmania HSP83, and GM-CSF.[524] The effective role of Leishmania complete antigen in the facilitation of healing of cutaneous leishmaniasis and mucosal leishmaniasis and also its less serious adverse events has been shown.[523,526,527] Adverse events mostly take place when the vaccine is utilized along with bacillus Calmette-Guerin.[523,527] Immunotherapy is widely practiced for canine visceral leishmaniasis. The fucose mannose ligand (FML)-vaccine provided a good effect on curing visceral leishmaniasis in non-symptomatic dogs infected in the lab via *Leishmania donovani* and *Leishmania chagasi*. As well, this vaccine resulted in an enhancement in CD8+ lymphocytes proportion in the peripheral blood of dogs.[528] Fucose mannose ligand (*Leishmania donovani* FML)-saponin inoculation led to an elevation in various FML-neutralizing antibodies in visceral leishmaniasis in an experimentally infected rodent model. The delayed type of hypersensitivity response, known as type IV hypersensitivity, against promastigote lysate (DTH) and the in vitro proliferative response of ganglion cells against FML antigen were reported. Moreover, a reduction in liver parasitic load was found in 94.7 percent of FML-vaccine-administered rodents.[529]

Immunotherapeutic influences of heat-treated dead Leishmania crude antigen accompanied by live bacillus Calmette-Guerin are correlated with T cell responses by Th1 and release of IFN-γ. T cell response by antigen-driven IFN-γ release alone does not result in immunopathology in mucocutaneous leishmaniasis. As a result, triggering the Th1 response in cases with American cutaneous leishmaniasis does not end with immunopathology.[530]

Overall, the triumphant utilization of immune-based therapies for cutaneous leishmaniasis made this approach an outstanding alternative for chemotherapy in single-lesion cutaneous leishmaniasis in which chemotherapy is not advised because of the development of drug resistance and also in severe infections, like diffuse cutaneous leishmaniasis and/or leprosy/*HIV* and Leishmania co-infections.[520] Enhancement of Th1 response and also the absence of Th2 response are contributed to resistance to Leishmania infection.[531-533] Immunotherapy is an efficient, safe, and cheap approach for therapy of cutaneous leishmaniasis of humans and visceral leishmaniasis of animals.[523, 526, 528-530]

## *Cryptosporidiosis*

Protozoan parasite Cryptosporidium is the cause of cryptosporidial diarrhea in both animals and humans.[534] Cryptosporidiosis is not common.[535-537] it is a benign infection of humans that generally continues for two weeks, but in some unique conditions, it may progress into a dangerous disease. For instance, it is difficult to cure the infection in immunocompromised/immunosuppressed cases, individuals who have been diagnosed with *HIV*/AIDS or received organ transplantation.[534] Chemotherapy for cryptosporidiosis has restricted efficacy in the therapy of the infection, and that made scientists establish valid reasoning for immunological experiments of Cryptosporidium with recombinant vaccine utilizing the live or attenuated parasite.[538] Researches performed in animals showed an efficient influence of hyperimmune bovine colostrum, paromomycin, and nitazoxanide for the treatment of Cryptosporidium infections.[539-543]

Passive and active immunotherapeutic approaches are useful strategies for immunizing against cryptosporidiosis.[544] Passive immunotherapy with antibodies for Cryptosporidium infection is an approach of therapy that has been performed experimentally and clinically. Many studies in this area have been started in the last years, namely on utilization of hyperimmune or by-nature-immune bovine colostrum comprising the colostral antibody, antibodies from chicken egg yolk, mAbs, and antibodies from human plasma that are administrated orally. Most articles have applied oral administration method of treating or preventing of this protozoan infection. Different antibody preparations have been evaluated in animals and humans and proved partial efficiency.[545] *Cryptosporidium parvum*-targeting antibodies in hyperimmune bovine colostrum have curative influences on cryptosporidiosis. These antibodies differentiate sporozoite, oocyst, and merozoite antigens. Also, they sense phase-specific antigens. Following incubation of hyperimmune antibodies with sporozoites, they undergo detectable morphologic changes and are characterized by forthcoming production and secretion of sporozoite membranous surface antibody-antigen complexes. The interaction counteracts the infectivity of sporozoites.[546] In the lab-infected nude rodent model, the intestinal-infection score is attenuated when administered with disabling mAbs (mAb 17.41). Disabling mAbs against sporozoite and merozoite external antigens disable the infectivity of sporozoites[547] and attenuate oocyst release and the infection score in the gall bladder.[546] Bovine immune colostrum attenuates intestinal development score of *Cryptosporidium parvum* to about half in rodents.[540] Several recognized antigens of *Cryptosporidium parvum* that are recognized by antibodies comprise gp15/45/60(Cpgp40/15),[548] CP15,[549] Gp900,[550] TRAP-C1,[551] and COWP.[552] Some known antigens of *Cryptosporidium parvum*, which are identified by antibodies, are suggested to play a role in host immune response.[544] Defense against cryptosporidiosis would be obtained via designing a vaccine against *Cryptosporidium* spp., which if done, would have several beneficial influences, particularly and most importantly on immunocompromised cases that are at risk of developing chronic infection. It has been shown that a suitable method in the therapy of Cryptosporidium infection in immunocompromised cases is passive immunotherapy by antibodies targeted towards merozoites and sporozoites of *Cryptosporidium parvum*, released into the gastrointestinal lumen.[544,553]

### Malaria

Glycosylphosphatidylinositol (GPI) is a glycolipid antigen of *Plasmodium* spp., which can activate the oversecretion of TNF-α and IL-1 and is potentially involved in the malarial pathophysiology, such as cerebral malaria. GPI from malaria parasite can be an important candidate to raise mAbs and subsequently can disable the toxicity of extracts of the parasite. Indeed, GPI of parasitic origin can be utilized as a target for immunotherapies.[554] A robust immunotherapeutic approach to malaria is cytotoxic T lymphocyte-associated protein (CTLA)-4 suppression. T cells exhaustion is a routine immune escape process in tumors and long-lasting infections. It is a condition of T cell impairment that occurs during chronic infections and cancer and is characterized by abnormal effector function, consistent production of suppressive receptors, and a transcriptional condition, different from that of functional effector or memory T cells.[555] Moreover, the exhaustion process may involve the loss of the cells. Recent research on malaria has investigated the PD-1 process that regulates the exhaustion of T cells. These explorations have reported exhaustion of CD4+ T cells and an underappreciated role for CD8+ T cells in provoking sterilizing immunity against blood-stage malaria. Interestingly, this underappreciation is due to that PD-1 is responsible for up to a 95 percent decrease in quantity and functional capability of parasite-exclusive CD8+ T cells. The concept of T cell exhaustion during malaria justifies the lack of sterile immunity after the clearance of acute infection. These data will be relevant to upcoming malaria-vaccine development.[556] mAb 7H8 is an IgM mAb against a protein of *Plasmodium* spp. This antibody attaches to Pf93, which is a special antigen of *Plasmodium falciparum*. mAb 7H8 is suitable for immune-based diagnostic assays and therapies of malaria in humans and other animals.[557]

### Trypanosomiasis

Designing a vaccine against the infection is a hard and complex duty, as the parasite can activate many different processes, making the host immune system incapable to fully eliminate the infection.[558,559] Immunotherapy can enhance the efficiency of the anti-parasite treatments, and as a result, reduce the severity of chronic infections like deadly Chagas' disease.[560,561] Optimal immunotherapy towards American trypanosomiasis would cover these agents that activate lymphocytes to function in concordant immune responses, such as antibody release, cytotoxic function to induce moieties of the parasite, and cytokines to mediate the immune response against the parasite.[558,562] *Trypanosoma cruzi* produces GPI that is an activator of IL-12 release. During the Chagas' disease, IL-12 and GPI activate NKT cells to direct a defensive response. In fact, NKT cells are involved in defensive immune responses against this infection.[563,564] For efficient immunotherapy against *Trypanosoma cruzi* infection, the importance of polyclonal lymphocyte responses right after the infections, and the inadequate immune homeostasis that they induce, are the most significant restrictions. It is believed that immunotherapy can provoke sustained immunity against *Trypanosoma cruzi*, if it includes agents that can neutralize non-specific immune responses.[558] In addition to American trypanosomiasis, African trypanosomiasis exists. Bloodstream subtypes of African trypanosomes are enclosed with a high-density packed defensive coat comprising over 107 clones ofVSG agents.[565] Similar to the situation with malaria, Trypanosomiasis is affected by PD-1 and CD8+ T cells.[566]

The transcription of *VSG* genes takes place at a telomere of the chromosomes surrounding the *VSG* expression areas.[567] Since solely one expression area can function at any given time, no more than one of the VSG molecules is presented on the surface coat of the parasite, resulting in the identical exhibition of the surface coat.[565] Additionally, because antibody response is raised solely to this special antigenic subtype, which is being expressed, a switch in VSG production would result in the triggering of the antibody response. Subsequently, this could smooth the path for immune exhaustion because of the persisting need to induce the immune response to multiple VSG-expressing clones. Trypanosomes can manage *VSG* gene production via disabling a functional expression site and enabling a formerly silent expression region, and by reorganization of the *VSG* genes chiefly via reciprocal recombination and gene conversion.[568-570] Researches indicated polyclonal induction of CD8+ T cells via *Trypanosoma brucei*-derived T lymphocyte triggering factor (TLTF) could lead to the massive release of IFN-γ, which is responsible for profound immunosuppression and susceptibility to the infection.[571] Research conducted by Wei and Tabel presented that the advantageous influence of anti-CD25 therapy in rodents with *Trypanosoma* congolense infection vanished after they were emptied of CD8+ T cells,[572] indicating that CD8+ T cells could be immunoprotective during *Trypanosoma* congolense infection. Therefore, the role of CD8+ T cells in African trypanosomiasis still remains controversial.[573]

### *Toxoplasmosis*

Toxoplasmosis is a benign condition of humans and other warm-blooded animals that results from a zoonotic protozoan *Toxoplasma gondii*, which is of the phylum Apicomplexa.[574,575] The worldwide prevalence of toxoplasmosis is rather significant.[576,577]

It has been reported that transfer of the spleen or serum and lymph node cells of guinea pigs, which were immunized against the RH strain of *Toxoplasma gondii*, can lead to a partial defense of symptomatic infection in receiver guinea pigs. This observation is due to the decrease in the spread or replication of Toxoplasma from the inoculation spot to other different systems of immunotherapy recipients. The same extent of partial immunity against systemic toxoplasmosis occurs in animals treated with suspensions of cells enriched with immune T cells. However, the immune cells exposed to a mAb raised against guinea pig T cells and complement lose their ability to transport resistance.[578]

### *Trichomoniasis*

Trichomoniasis is an infection that results from *Trichomonas vaginalis* that is a usual cause of vaginitis.[579] Lactobacillus vaccine, Solco Trichovac, has a beneficial effect on trichomoniasis that may result from cross-reactivity of vaccine-activated antibodies with *Trichomonas vaginalis*.[580] The Solco Trichovac is a lactobacillus vaccine that displayed a dramatic positive influence on trichomoniasis. The effectiveness ratio has been found 90 percent[581] and 80 percent[582] in vaccinology experiments. Immunotherapy of trichomoniasis has several benefits compared to metronidazole, such as the preventive influence of vaccines on patients in terms of reinfection and recurrence.[581] There is a study on metronidazole and immunotherapy resistant trichomoniasis in two cases that the parasites lasted following a high-dosage metronidazole injection. On such limited occasions, the immunotherapy by Lactobacillus failed.[583] Ultimately, more research by well-designed clinical trials assessing repurposed vaccines is warranted.

### *Schistosomiasis*

*Schistosoma* spp. are flatworms and underlying etiology of schistosomiasis, which is a parasitic disease that, after malaria, is of the highest public health importance. The prevalence of the illness is approximated to be over 200 million cases and 100000 deaths yearly.[584]

Granulomatous response against ova of Schistosoma that are entrapped within the host's liver contributes to fibrosis. Treating with IL-12 and Schistosoma egg averts the development of pulmonary granuloma. Treatment with eggs and IL-12 leads to partial suppression of granuloma formation. This treatment significantly decreases the tissue fibrosis caused as a result of natural *Schistosoma mansoni* infection. This achievement is an example of a vaccination effort in which the pathogenesis of infection is averted, but not the infection itself. This is occurring through the replacement of Th2 cytokine response, characterized by Schistosoma infection immune response, with Th1 that is activated by IL-12.[585]

IL-13 is functionally similar to IL-4,[586] and it shares similar receptor subunits with IL-4. Hence, it has the same function in the pathogenesis of schistosomiasis. Therapy with IL-13 (sIL-13R$\alpha$2-Fc) prevents the development of hepatic fibrosis in rodents when infected by *Schistosoma mansoni*.[587]

Administering of rodents by *Schistosoma mansoni* in the lab with a mAb raised against IL-4 inhibits the formation of granuloma in the lung, but not the formation of hepatic granuloma. Anti-IL-4 therapy significantly attenuates the collagen accumulation within the liver. IL-4 has a key role in the activation of the Th2 response in rodents infected with *Schistosoma mansoni* and, as a result, is involved in the formation of hepatic fibrosis.[588-590] These data open new horizons for the development of new therapies targeted at the patients' clinical condition, and demonstrate a need for novel treatments to eradicate the Schistosoma infection.

## Viral infections

## Definition

The global severity and incidence of viral sepsis are increasing over time. However, sepsis-linked mortality is declining.[591-594] A new systematic review and meta-analysis[591] demonstrated a 26 percent and 270 per 100000 person-years mortality and global incidence of hospital-treated sepsis in adults, respectively, in the last ten years. Generalizing these numbers to the globe denotes estimates of 5.3 million deaths and 19.4 million sepsis patients annually. Another worldwide study[595] found mortality and incidence of 9 percent-20 percent and 22 per 100000 person-years sepsis in pediatric populations (between 4 weeks and 20 years of age), respectively. The mortality and incidence of neonatal sepsis (Sepsis-2 classification, for the comparative description of sepsis classifications, refer to the recent article by Poutsiaka et al.[596]) were 11 percent-19 percent and 2202 in 100000 living childbirths, respectively.[597]

Viruses are intracellular parasites that abuse cells for their own replication and spread. Despite being highly cytotoxic, viral infections rarely cause human mortality. Mortality usually happens while viruses undergo zoonotic transmission (e.g., *HIV* or Ebola), when the viral antigens change drastically (i.e., influenza viruses), or when the immune system is weakened. One of the most bizarre viruses that causes mortality in humans is *HIV*. However, *HIV* initiates a slow death that gives the virus enough time for distribution in the species. Although adults can well tolerate viral infections, critical clinical presentations or death could occur in infants or neonates, especially if they are lacking passive immunity. These data result from the increasing wealth of immunological tools, such as tetramers of MHC and transgenic animal models, and have gained incremental efficiency and sensitivity to identify the immune mechanisms of antiviral resistance. Mostly, there are substantial variations in hosts' immunological resistance mechanisms against the virus, and the effect of each mechanism varies enormously depending on the viral entrance, replication, and spreading within the host.[598]

The viruses must tackle many barriers to reach out human tissues. The most effective barriers comprise mechanical ones. For example, mucosal surfaces and the skin are in line with the acidic environment of the gut. Several usual human viruses infect and invade through the gut comprising enteric adenoviruses, *Hepatitis A virus* (*HAV*), and *Rotavirus* that are distributed through close contact or polluted water and food. Respiratory viruses that are spread by droplets and close contact consist of coronaviruses, influenza viruses, *Measles virus*, rhinoviruses, respiratory syncytial virus (RSV), and varicella-zoster virus (VZV). Numerous herpes viruses attack the mucosa or skin, such as VZV and HSV. HSV can infect the eye, genital and oral mucosa, and skin through scratches and small cuts. Herpesviruses, like *CMV* and *Epstein-Barr virus* (*EBV*), attack the mucosa. *CMV* can also spread through mother-borne or blood transfusions in rare instances. *Human papillomavirus* (*HPV*) attacks mucosa and skin and causes cell transformation, resulting in cervical cancer and warts. Also, viruses such as the *Semliki Forest virus* and *West Nile virus* can enter by the means of the skin through insects. *Hepatitis B virus* (*HBV*) and *HIV* are good examples of sexually spreadable viruses. *Hepatitis C virus* (*HCV*), *HBV* and *HIV* are also blood-borne through blood transfusions and needles. Due to viral receptor distribution, most human viruses can only infect specific tissues. Viruses usually utilize two receptors. For instance, *HIV* uses CCR5 and CD4 co-receptor. After binding to their receptors, viruses might enter the cell by being fused with lipid membrane or endocytosis and access the cytoplasm or nucleus by being fused with the vesicular membrane (e.g., in HSV and *HIV* that are enveloped viruses), or alternatively, cross the cell membrane or cause the endocytic vesicle to lyse when they are in the cytoplasm (*Norwalk virus* and poliovirus that are non-enveloped viruses).[599] Viruses then use the host cell's functions and their own specialized proteins to multiplicate at high rates inside the cell. When they replicate excessively inside the cell, lots of viruses lyse the cell to enable the liberation of new infectious virions (such as the poliovirus, poxviruses, and herpes viruses). Some viruses bud through the cell membrane in the absence of cell death to get liberated (e.g., influenza virus and *HIV*).

However, by entering the body, viruses confront various innate defensive mechanisms and trigger adaptive immunity. Adaptive immunity stops the viral infection from becoming clinically evident. Considering the fundamental role of immunity in viral infections, manipulating the immune system for their treatment and management is beneficial. However, many challenges still should be overcome (e.g., development of vaccines for chronic infections by *HCV* and *HIV*[600]).

## Mechanisms

The viruses and relevant intermediates could be detected through numerous innate immune receptors on the cell surface or within the cell. Numerous innate immune receptors can mediate immune response in viral infections, such as inflammasomes, TLRs, retinoic acid-inducible gene I (RIG-I, also known as DDX58). The endosomal TLRs (TLR-8, TLR-3, TLR-9, and TLR-7) normally take part in the detection of virus infections through recognition of double-stranded RNAs and viral nucleic acids.[601] The viral DNA is recognized by NLRs, whereas viral or genomic RNA is detected by cytoplasmic RIG-I-like receptors.[602] In summary, pro-inflammatory cytokines and IFNs are the results of innate immunity receptors activation in line with signals recruiting and activating cells engaged in initiation of adaptive immunity and inflammation. The innate immune patterns established after the virus entry could predict the infection outcome. The persistence of viruses induces innate cells such as NK cells, macrophages, and DCs to release anti-inflammatory proteins such as TGF-β and IL-10. For example, DCs derived from mice infected with *Lymphocytic choriomeningitis virus* (*LCMV*) produce high amounts of IL-10,[603] and also monocytes derived from patients infected with *HCV*, *HIV*, or *HBV* release IL-10.[604-606] The interface between RSV and plasmacytoid DCs (pDCs) in the lungs is vital since the removal of pDCs before infection leads to an immunopathological response in them.[607] The viruses interfering with innate defenses could cause a detrimental reaction.

## *Innate immunity*
### Inflammasomes

The evidence on the role of inflammasomes in viral infections is comprehensive. An up-to-date discussion of major examples for each inflammasome component has been provided in this section, and for further details, readers can refer to the article by Chen and Ichinohe.[608]

Research has confirmed the viral activation of NLRP3 by influenza virus, encephalomyocarditis virus, *Human rhinovirus*, RSV, *HCV*, *Japanese encephalitis virus*, Sendai virus, Rift valley fever virus, *Dengue virus*, *West Nile virus*, HSV-1, *Vesicular stomatitis virus*, vaccinia virus Ankara, and *Rabies virus*,[609-624] NLRP1 by *LCMV*,[625] AIM2 by *Vaccinia virus*,[69,626] and RIG-1 by influenza virus and *Vesicular stomatitis virus*.[627,628]

**NLRP3** The most well-known viral inducer of NLRP3 is the influenza virus. Influenza virus activates the development of caspase-1 and the excretion of IL-1β in BMDMs and bone marrow-derived dendritic cells (BMDCs) isolated from wild-type rodents, contrary to what has been observed in BMDMs or BMDCs extracted from NLRP3- or caspase-1-lacking rodents. Amplified IL-1β production has been reported in bronchoalveolar lavage fluid of wild-type rodents, contrary to bronchoalveolar lavage fluid of Nlrp3-/-, Casp1-/-, or Asc-/- rodents following infection by the influenza virus. Production of NLRP3 inflammasome elements is elevated in the lung tissue of wild-type rodents after intranasal infection by the influenza virus. Ca-074-Me (that blocks lysosomal cathepsin B) and N-acetyl-L-cysteine or (2R,4R)-4-aminopyrrolidine-2,4-dicarboxylate (APDC) (that block the formation of ROS) block the influenza virus-triggered elevation of IL-1β. Influenza virus triggering of the NLRP3 inflammasome is believed to take place via influenza virus RNA and its non-contractual element PB1-F2. These can be potentially explained by the lysosomal rupture and ROS models. Transfecting viral RNA into wild-type BMDMs activates the amplification of IL-1β. However, this has not been observed in Nlrp3-/- or Casp1-/- BMDMs. The viral RNA analogs poly(I:C) and single-stranded GU-rich RNA (ssRNA40) also activate IL-1β release. The amount of IL-1β in bronchoalveolar lavage fluid from PB1-F2-lacking mutant (ΔPB1-F2) influenza virus-infected rodents is remarkably few, compared to bronchoalveolar lavage fluid isolates of wild-type virus-challenged rodents. Administering with a PB1-F2 C-terminal peptide activates IL-1β secretion in rodents bronchoalveolar lavage fluid, human peripheral blood mononuclear cells (hPBMCs), and wild-type BMDMs, contrary to what has been observed in BMDMs isolated from NLRP3-, ASC-, or caspase-1-lacking rodents. Latrunculin A suppresses phagocytosis, prevents PB1-F2 peptide-activated IL-1β release by BMDMs. In conclusion, such findings denote that PB1-F2 accumulates in phagosomes to additionally activate the secretion of IL-1β by the NLRP3 inflammasome during infection by the influenza virus. A new study showed that the production of the influenza virus proton-exclusive ion channel M2 protein in the acidic trans-Golgi network induces the NLRP3 inflammasome. Infection by wild-type influenza virus triggers the secretion of IL-1β and IL-18 from BMDMs. As well, transduction of BMDMs and BMDCs primed by LPS via a recombinant *Lentivirus* producing the M2 protein triggers the NLRP3 inflammasome. Histidine 37 that lies in the transmembrane domain of the M2 element is crucial for the proton-specific functionality of the M2 elements. Transduction of BMDMs and BMDCs primed by LPS / poly(I:C) via a *Lentivirus* that produces H37G (a mutant M2 protein) is two times as potent as transduction with a *Lentivirus* that produces wild-type M2 protein, in activating the secretion of IL-1β. Moreover, exposing wild-type influenza virus-infected BMDMs to monensin (a Na+/H+ antiporter within the trans-Golgi nexus) more potently activates the secretion of IL-1β and amplifies localization of the M2 protein in the Golgi apparatus. Brefeldin A dismantles the Golgi apparatus, inhibits the secretion of IL-1β, and triggers the M2 element to accumulate in the endoplasmic reticulum (ER). Because of this, the intracellular accumulation and biological ion channel functions of the M2 element are a major influence in NLRP3 inflammasome induction.[610-612,629-631] It should be noted that inflammasomes, in particular NLRP3, are an important mechanism of immune escape targeted by different viral components, such as the influenza virus NS1 protein, *Measles virus*, and paramyxoviruses (e.g., Sendai virus and *Nipah virus*) V protein. These elements suppress NLRP3 inflammasome triggering through reaction with NLRP3, subsequently reducing the excretion of IL-1β.[632-635]

**NLRP1.** Similar to NLRP3, NLRP1 is involved in immunological escape by viruses. The *Vaccinia virus* B-cell chronic lymphocytic leukemia (CLL)/lymphoma 2 (BCL2) homolog protein F1L assists viruses in evading the immunity of the host. The F1L element reacts with NLRP1, but not with NLRP3, through its N-terminal area. The function and level of developed caspase-1 and the secretion of IL-1β are higher in F1L-deficient mutant *Vaccinia virus*-infected THP-1 cells compared to wild-type *Vaccinia virus* or other viral protein-deficient cells infected by mutant *Vaccinia virus*. Infection by F1L-deficient mutant *Vaccinia virus* or mutant *Vaccinia virus* harboring mutant F1L (that does not attach to NLRP1) displays less virulence compared to wild-type *Vaccinia virus* in rodents. The reaction between F1L and NLRP1 potentially influences the structural alteration of NLRP1 that is essential in NLRP1 inflammasome induction. Further studies should explore inducers as well as mechanisms of induction of the NLRP1 inflammasome in the context of viral infection.[636,637]

**AIM2** *Vaccinia virus* double-stranded DNA-activated development of caspase-1 is AIM2-dependent and it does not depend on NLRP3. As a result, AIM2 straightly reacts with double-stranded DNA through its HIN200 region. It then reacts with ASC by its PYD to employ caspase-1 to shape the AIM2 inflammasome. AIM2 is also vital for infection via murine cytomegalovirus (mCMV) compared to infection by HSV-1. mCMV-triggered induction of developed IL-1β and caspase-1 is inhibited in Aim2-/- BMDCs and IL-18 production is inhibited in mCMV-affected Asc-/- and Aim2-/-

rodents. Inhibition of IL-18 because of ASC or AIM2 deficiency leads to a decrease in the level of IFN-γ-releasing NK cells and an elevation in the mCMV viral load. Such data show the significance of the AIM2 inflammasome in virus-activated innate immune response.[69,626] Whether mCMV is a robust model for human disease or not has been explained in the review article by Fisher and Lloyd in 2021.[638] Interestingly, a recent article showed that HSV-1 VP22 suppresses AIM2-dependent inflammasome induction to make possible efficient viral multiplication.[639] Moreover, a study showed HPV-16 DNA can trigger IL-1β and IL-18 secretion by the AIM2 inflammasome in healthy human keratinocytes. While *HPV* DNA could not activate IFN-β in keratinocytes, IFN-β excretion was found when AIM2 was inhibited. Additionally, inhibiting IFI16 amplifies HPV-16 DNA-activated release of IL-1β, contrary to IL-18. Such observations indicate an interplay between IFI16 and AIM2 in the immune response to *HPV* DNA.[640] AIM2 inflammasome has been found to be an important factor for influenza-triggered lung damage and death.[641]

**TLRs** In the spleen of rodents infected by mCMV, viral clearance relies on TLR2-related IFN-α/IFN-β, and IL-18 release, which can affect NK cell multiplication.[642]

TLR3-dependent responses could lead to poor clinical outcomes based on the subtype of viruses like *West Nile virus*, which is a single-stranded RNA from *Flaviviridae* class, or influenza A virus that is a single-stranded RNA virus from *Orthomyxoviridae* class. After recognition of *West Nile virus*, TLR3-dependent inflammatory responses consisting of TNF-α receptor 1 pathways, essential for the blood-brain barrier, aid the viral entry into the CNS of rodents with consequent deadly encephalitis.[643]

Influenza A virus-infected TLR3-/- rodents have an advantage to influenza A virus infection, with decreased levels of inflammatory mediators, declined CD8+ T cell infiltration, and extended survival, probably because of the existence of an imbalanced TLR3-dependent CD8+ T cell response that could bring about prolonged respiratory damage.[644]

TLR4 senses RSV via the F protein, activating IL-6 secretion.[645] A defensive function of TLR4 has been presented in multiple other viral infections like *Kaposi's sarcoma-related herpesvirus* (*KSHV*) or *Vaccinia virus*, even though some articles corroborate that TLR4 can enhance viral dissemination, such as in infection by MMVT. MMVT is a virus that can be spread by breast milk. It initially invades B cells in Peyer's patches of the gastrointestinal system. MMVT Env proteins may attach to TLR4 and activate the development of BMDCs, enhancing the levels of co-activating molecules, TNF-α, IL-6, and IL-12p40. Of note, the reaction of MMVT with DCs through TLR4 helps the progression of infection by promoting the production of the viral cell entrance protein CD71.[646]

TLR7 and TLR8 usually recognize endocytosed viruses with single-stranded RNA genomes and promote the formation of IFNs and pro-inflammatory factors. In rodents,

TLR7 function is well-characterized, while TLR8 might not be functional. TLR7 activation in pDCs leads to cross-priming promotion and induction of high levels of type I IFNs, regulating type I Th1 responses and B cells isotype switching, as it occurs upon activation with influenza A virus or synthetic oligoribonucleotides simulating *HIV* genomic sequence.[647]

TLR10 binds double-stranded RNA in endosomal compartments and negatively regulates the type I IFN response by reducing phosphorylation of IRF7. Also, in vitro production of TLR10 withdraws double-stranded RNA from TLR3 attachment and promotes the production of SARM1, a negative mediator for TLR3 mechanisms.[648]

The role of TLRs in viral infection has been reviewed in further detail in other comprehensive articles.[649-651]

### *Adaptive immunity*

### Cellular immunity

Adaptive immune cells can worsen tissue damage by destroying cells. Virus-infected cells could straightly be destroyed by T cells that release cytokines such as TNF. In infection by some viruses such as *HBV* and *HCV*, the liver is mainly damaged by the elimination of infected cells by CD8+ T cells.[652,653] The reaction of various types of CD4+ T cells organizes a tissue-insulting inflammatory response that could become chronic against persisting viruses. The cell subsets usually involved are Th1 cells, but Th17 cells might exacerbate inflammatory reactions in influenza virus, *HIV*, and *HCV* infections.[652-656] In reactions caused by Th17 cells, neutrophils are also engaged, becoming a major source of tissue-insulting proteins. Th2 cells rarely related to inflammatory reactions in viral infections could cause such reactions in severe lung RSV infection.[657]

### Humoral immunity

Efficient vaccination for some viruses, including measles, chickenpox, and rubella, in childhood, shows the significance of defensive antibodies, and currently, vaccines in clinical practice rely on the production of neutralizing antibodies but not solely on T cell-modulated immunity.[658] Worthy of note is that all current vaccines, which are clinically effective rely on neutralizing antibody responses.[659] While cytotoxic lymphocytes can destroy infected cells, antibodies have the ability to both destroy infected cells and avert harmful viruses from invading a cell (neutralization). Placental transfer of defensive IgG antibodies from mother to newborns is an outstanding "demonstration by nature" of the efficiency of humoral immunity. It has been shown that agammaglobulinemia or hypogammaglobulinemia children are less prone to critical viral infections compared to children with deficient cellular immunity. Based on this data, it has been debated that T cells are more significant than B cells in antiviral immunity. This interpretation neglects the quintessential role of Th cells not solely for cellular but also for humoral immune response, particularly the production of memory B cells and long-lasting plasma cells. Following *Orthopoxvirus* infection, T cells are necessary for the activation of humoral memory in primary responses and become of secondary significance in secondary responses when neutralizing antibodies exert a major function in defense against reinfection.[660] Ultimately, the significance of humoral immunity in antiviral responses can be understood better based on several reports that evaluated the induction and maintenance of specific T and B cell responses and resulting antiviral titers. It has been reported that antiviral antibodies can provide substantial defense, even where CD4+ or CD8+ T cells have been depleted before viral (re-)infection.[661]

## Diagnosis

### *Advanced serological immunoassays*

The immunoassays are mainly considered antibody/antigen-dependent assays. Quantifying antibodies such as IgG are favorably utilized as diagnostic markers. The antibodies or antigens are coated with conjugated labels such as radioactive isotopes, metals, and fluorescent tags. A diagnostic approach towards chronic hepatitis C infection (CHC) determines specific antibodies to *HCV* (anti-HCV) (indirect tests) and can characterize, detect, or quantify parts of *HCV* viral particles. It can also determine *HCV* RNA and central antigen (direct tests). Measuring *HCV* central antigen as a single-step process has been vital. As a result, in order to assess the execution of central antigen quantifying in analyzing CHC and how it is affected by associated *HIV* or *HBV* viruses, cross-sectional confirmation tests, like *HCV* antigen quantitation as a single-step process in analyzing CHC in Cameroon was intended to shorten the diagnostic procedure.[662] It is worth noting that a newly developed complex microsphere immunoassay (MIA) holds diagnosis strength to confine viral envelope protein that conjures up being strong cross-sensitive antibodies to other flaviviruses and differencing ability of viral non-structural proteins NS1 and NS5. Remarkably, this serological test needs to be used for quick clinical detection of *Zika virus* and/or dengue viral infections in screening for immune reactions in vaccine clinical studies.[663] It is remarkable that oral fluid is a non-invasive biological sample that can employ pathogen-concrete antibodies and achieve the potential for a substitute for blood-borne test procedures. As a result, a saliva-ordered oral fluid immunological test has been developed to evaluate past and present *Hepatitis E virus* (*HEV*) infections by non-destructive sampling methods. The sensitivity and specificity of this test were similar to serum-borne ELISAs. This salivary test could enhance our understanding of the ecological and natural science of *HEV*.[664] Analyzing the *Zika virus* continues to be a major challenge, as the discovery of viral RNA is only possible a few days after the beginning of symptoms. Vice versa, novel high-throughput image-based fluorescent deactivation by the method to establish the identity of *Zika virus* has been thoroughly assessed and have reported greater sensitivity than Plaque reduction neutralization test (PRNT) and MAC-ELISA, respectively. The present test might use clinical diagnostics, clinical studies, and serological prevalence studies of *Zika virus* illness.[665] Determination of serum *HEV* antigen is considered a delicate and auspicious biomarker for *HEV* antigen diagnostics with *HEV* RNA in both acute and chronic genotypes. An antigen test has been recently assessed and it has been reported that it can diagnose *HEV* genotypes with greater sensitivity than commercial anti-*HEV* IgM and *HEV* RNA ELISA assays.[666] Nevertheless, current research on RSV has been developing Luciferase Immunological Precipitation Systems (LIPS) test to determine IgG antibodies against human RSV G-Glycoprotein. Furthermore, human RSV G-Glycoprotein functions as a biological indicator for natural exposure or vaccination. RSV genes encoding native and mutant G (mG) proteins from subgroups A and B strains were cloned, expressed in luciferase-tagged proteins, and tested individually to spot anti-RSV-G specific IgG antibodies using a high-throughput luciferase immunological precipitation system (LIPS-G). It is worth noting that RSV mAbs and polyclonal antisera are bound in LIPS-$G_A$ and/or -$G_B$ tests.[667] Diagnoses of *Zika virus* and *Dengue virus* diseases versus the viral envelope protein and non-structural proteins were developed by using the *Flavivirus* MIA. Nevertheless, MIA cannot diagnose more recently from past infections, which constitutes a key diagnosis struggle. Thus, in the last report, an IgG-based tendency test has been developed for its diagnosis that can distinguish recent *Zika* and past *Dengue virus* illnesses. This test was found helpful in patients with a high risk of Zika comorbidities and women who are pregnant. Also, follow-up of the immune response in vaccine clinical studies is possible by using this test.[668] Sequentially, in order to design a serological diagnosis of *Zika virus*-IgA and *Zika virus*-IgG, tendency tests were assessed to distinguish Zika infections in need of viremia. These tests eased interpretation of low tendency of IgG and IgA findings, and improved the serological diagnostic of *Zika virus*.[669] In a different study, homologous proteins of diverse flaviviruses showed a high degree of sequence individuality, mostly inside subgroups. This has led to widespread immunologic cross-responsiveness. As a result, a relative unfolding of the intricate B cell responses versus *Zika virus* and other flaviviruses was reflected by testing with a microarray chip-based high-resolution serology prepared from intersecting peptides covering the entire amino acid sequence of *Zika virus* genomic polyprotein. Furthermore, with the emergence of this test, several infections such as yellow fever, dengue, West Nile virus, and tick-borne encephalitis shall have been diagnosed with it.[670]

### *ELISA-based detection*

Enzymes are comprehensive tools to diagnose the virus and have different applications, such as enzyme immune assay and ELISA. Enzyme immune assay has various applications, such as micro-particle immune assay (MEIA), fluorescence polarization immune assay (FPIA), and chemiluminescent immune assay (CLIA). Enzyme immune tests work via antigen-antibody interaction on conjugate tags like fluorescent tags and chemiluminescent tags, which are complemented with surfaces such as polarized light and fluorescent substrates. A highly sensitive colorimetric test is known as a magnetic nano(e)zyme-linked immunosorbent assay (MagLISA), wherein silica-peeled magnetic nanobeads (MagNBs) and gold nanoparticles were collected to monitor influenza A virus up to femtogram per milliliter concentration.[671] Sensitive and specific determination of *Crimean-Congo hemorrhagic fever virus* (*CCHFV*) was developed using specific IgM and IgG antibodies in human sera using recombinant *CCHFV* nucleoprotein as antigen in μ-capture and IgG immune complex (IC) ELISA tests.[672] Recently, truncated forms of *Hendra* and *Nipah virus* G proteins in line with full-length *Nipah virus* nucleocapsid (N) protein were utilized for the determination of *Hendra* and *Nipah virus*-specific antibodies in pigs. These recombinant proteins have been expressed through diverse expressing systems, and an indirect ELISA has been developed for determination.[673] A rapid diagnosis platform in the colorimetric difference determination of *Dengue virus* and *Chikungunya virus* viral illnesses was recently developed with a probability to manipulate clinical diagnoses of acute febrile diseases in resource-restricted hospitals. This platform primarily enables consistent and correct multiplexed determination of *Chikungunya* and *Dengue* IgM/IgG antibodies in human clinical specimens within a short period.[674]

### Immunofluorescence-based immunodetection

Immunofluorescence is widely used for the rapid detection of viral illnesses in clinics began in the early 1970s. Immunofluorescence is used to diagnose viral antigens and virus-specific IgG/IgA/IgM antibodies in clinical samples. In this method, fluorescein-labeled antibodies to stain samples that contain certain viral antigens were applied for ultraviolet illumination. New genetically modified *Rabies virus* that expresses green fluorescent protein (rRV-GFP) is a faster, simpler, and cheaper detector for quantifying virus-neutralizing antibodies in blood serum. This method streamlined the multistep Rapid Fluorescent Focus Inhibition Test (RFFIT) process by removing the immunological staining step.[675,676]

### mAb-based immunodetection

Creating diagnostic and treatment platforms with aptamer technology is no doubt a possible approach to viral illnesses. However, the oligonucleotide aptamers, potentially an alternative to mAb-based determination, could be aimed against any protein in the infected cells, and all components of viral particles are considered to be potential new diagnosis molecules against viral hepatitis. These aptamers can be a beneficial replacement for the mAbs in the foreseeable future.[677,678]

### Hemagglutination inhibition (HI) assay

Some viruses such as *Adenovirus*, *Dengue virus*, *Measles virus*, rubella virus, and influenza virus have hemagglutinin antigens on their surfaces, which can bind to red blood cells (RBCs) and agglutinate them termed hemagglutination (HA). The suppression of the capability of the viruses to agglutinate RBCs is used to develop hemagglutination inhibition (HI) test. In the HI test, the sequentially diluted serum specimen is prepared in a microtiter plate. Then, a certain amount of viral hemagglutinin will be added. Finally, proper RBCs will be added. Lack of HA suggests a positive response. This is concluded by tilting the microtiter plate, which permits free RBCs to stream. The dilution speed at which complete suppression of agglutination of RBCs took place is being recorded. The HI titer, thus, is mutual for the last serum dilution that completely inhibits HA.[679-681] The HI test has been used for serological monitoring of influenza A (H1N1) pdm09 virus[682] and *Measles virus*.[683] In a study, HI assay was employed to test the efficacy of the pandemic flu vaccine.[684] A verification study using sera from 79 RT-qPCR-confirmed cases and 176 sera from an unexposed population showed that the HI assay has high sensitivity (92 percent) and specificity (91 percent) for the determination of human infection with the 2009 pandemic H1N1 virus.[685,686]

## Treatment

### *Interferons*

From the very mid-1930s, scientists have acknowledged that in certain circumstances, one virus could interfere with another. In 1957, Isaacs and Lindenman made a sharp breakthrough, which explained the mechanism of resistance. They found that virus-contaminated cells can secrete a protein known as IFN that, when added to the normal cells in culture, protects against viral infection. There are three types of IFN: $\alpha$, $\beta$, and $\gamma$. IFN-$\alpha$ is generated by leukocytes, IFN-$\beta$ is released mainly by fibroblasts, and IFN-$\gamma$ is secreted by triggered lymphocytes. IFNs tend to show species specificity (mouse cell IFN will protect mouse cells much more than human cells) and are suppressive for numerous viruses. For years, it was impossible to obtain adequate quantities of IFNs to carry out important studies. However, genetically modified DNA technology and cell culture technology have resulted in the manufacturing of an adequate supply of IFNs, resulting in the conduction of large clinical trials. IFN-$\alpha$ has proven to be effective on a limited number of viral illnesses of humans like chronic hepatitis B and C and chronic condylomata acuminata. Moreover, IFNs have been effective in treating other diseases. For example, IFN-$\alpha$ has proven to be effective in treating hairy cell leukemia and AIDS-related Kaposi's sarcoma in the select group of patients, IFN-$\beta$ has been shown to be useful for relapsing-remitting multiple sclerosis, and IFN-$\gamma$ has been reported to be able to reduce the incidence and severity of serious infections related to chronic granulomatosis.[687]

### *Cellular therapies*

During the last few years, there has been an overwhelming body of research, which shows cellular immune therapies can overturn the advancement of hematological malignancies and can as well be an advantageous treatment option for deadly viral diseases. Although it is well-known that the expansion and adoptive transfer of virus-exclusive T cells from the non-infected donor can be an efficient approach to manage viral multiplication, recent evidence highlights that this is not feasible when donors are seronegative or are subsequently unreachable. Lately, researchers have reported robust expansion of virus-exclusive T cells from seropositive stem cell transplant receivers of a seronegative graft with an active viral infection and the long-term reconstitution of antiviral immunity after their adoptive transport. Moreover, this treatment approach has been expanded for different agents such as *CMV*, *EBV*, *Adenovirus*, and BK polyoma-virus. This solution can be used to quickly expand different pathogens-exclusive T cells that can be used for adoptive immunotherapy. Ultimately, novel tests to screen T cell immunity have been designed that will enable the detection of at-risk transplant subjects. These subjects could develop virus-related complications after transplantation and can be administered with adoptive T cell treatment as a prophylactic measure.[688]

### Vaccines

Vaccination has been the most effective method of avoiding viral illnesses. Although intentional contact with virulent viruses such as *Smallpox* (syn. variolation) has been long acknowledged as an efficient, though the hazardous, technique of prevention, the whole concept of vaccination was commonly introduced by Edward Jenner in 1798 to help protect people against smallpox. A century later, the idea was proven by Louis Pasteur to have broader uses and, most particularly, could be used to avoid rabies. With the discovery of cell culture methods in the 1950s, the second age of vaccination was presented, and numerous live-attenuated virus and deactivated-virus vaccines were developed. Lately, the field of vaccines has seen the deployment of several novel "new generation" vaccines manufactured through various forms of genetically modified DNA and relevant technologies. When live-weakened and deactivated virus vaccines of the second generation are yet the "workhorses" of the veterinary profession, new generation vaccines are now supplementing and, evermore, substituting them. There are a few significant differences among the vaccination of men and animals. Financial constraints are normally of less importance for human use than animal medicine. There is also greater agreement regarding the safety and efficacy of vaccines used in humans than animal vaccines and superior mechanisms responsible for reporting probable adverse reactions related to the use of special products. Internationally, the WHO leads persuasion in human vaccine utilization and holds several programs that have no counterparts for animal vaccine utilization in its counterpart agencies, the food, and agriculture organization and the Office International des Epizooties (OIE; syn. the World Organization for Animal Health). Additionally, in countries, greater freedom is permitted in the production and utilization of vaccines for veterinary diseases than is permitted by national regulators for human vaccines. Before the latest emergence of new breed vaccines based on genetically-modified DNA technology, there were just two main strategies in the manufacture of virus vaccines: one using live-toned-down (syn. modified-live) viral strains and the other using chemically deactivated (syn. killed) virus formulations. Live-attenuated virus vaccines multiplicate in the target cells and boost the number of antigens presented to the host immune system. There are crucial advantages in this method since the multiplication of virus simulates infection, host immune reaction is more similar to that happening following natural infection than occurs with inactivated or a few subunit vaccines. When deactivated virus vaccines are manufactured, the chemical or physical treatment used to eradicate infection may be harmful enough to lessen the immunogenicity of the virus, especially inductions of viral-specific cell-mediated immune reactions. Thus, deactivated vaccines often cause immune reactions to be narrower in the antigenic spectrum, shorter in duration, weaker in cell-mediated and mucosal immune responses, and possibly less effective in inducing sterilizing immunity. However, very effective and safe deactivated vaccines are readily available and most used. Most vaccines produced in larger scales to be used in animals still include an either live-attenuated or deactivated virus. Nevertheless, the new-generation vaccines developed through genetically-modified DNA technologies provide substantial enhancements and probable benefits of both their safety and efficacy. A notable range of such vaccines has recently been produced, a growing number of which are now in industrial manufacturing.[689]

## References


1. Straif-Bourgeois S, Ratard R, Kretzschmar M. Infectious Disease Epidemiology. *Handbook of Epidemiology*. 2014:2041–2119.
2. Giamarellos-Bourboulis EJ, Raftogiannis M. The immune response to severe bacterial infections: consequences for therapy. *Expert Rev Anti Infect Ther*. 2012;10(3):369–380.
3. Mirzaei HR. Adaptive Immunity*Reference Module in Biomedical Sciences*: Elsevier; 2020.
4. Lazar T. Immunology of Infectious Diseases. *Emerg Infect Dis*. 2002;8(11):1362–1363.
5. Lin CY, Roberts GW, Kift-Morgan A, Donovan KL, Topley N, Eberl M. Pathogen-specific local immune fingerprints diagnose bacterial infection in peritoneal dialysis patients. *J Am Soc Nephrol*. 2013;24(12):2002–2009.
6. Hancock REW, Nijnik A, Philpott DJ. Modulating immunity as a therapy for bacterial infections. *Nat Rev Microbiol*. 2012;10(4):243–254.
7. Skwarczynski M, Chandrudu S, Rigau-Planella B, Islam MT, Cheong YS, Liu G, et al. Progress in the Development of Subunit Vaccines against Malaria. *Vaccines*. 2020;8(3):373.
8. Baron S, Fons M, Albrecht T. *Viral Pathogenesis*. 4th edition: Medical Microbiology; 1996.
9. Schneider T, Sahl H-G. An oldie but a goodie–cell wall biosynthesis as antibiotic target pathway. *Int J Med Microbiol*. 2010;300(2-3):161–169.
10. Goldman WE, Klapper D, Baseman J. Detection, isolation, and analysis of a released Bordetella pertussis product toxic to cultured tracheal cells. *Infect Immun*. 1982;36(2):782–794.
11. Fleming TJ, Wallsmith DE, Rosenthal RS. Arthropathic properties of gonococcal peptidoglycan fragments: implications for the pathogenesis of disseminated gonococcal disease. *Infect Immun*. 1986;52(2):600–608.
12. Royet J, Gupta D, Dziarski R. Peptidoglycan recognition proteins: modulators of the microbiome and inflammation. *Nat Rev Immunol*. 2011;11(12):837–851.
13. Sorbara MT, Philpott DJ. Peptidoglycan: a critical activator of the mammalian immune system during infection and homeostasis. *Immunol Rev*. 2011;243(1):40–60.

14. Jutras BL, Lochhead RB, Kloos ZA, Biboy J, Strle K, Booth CJ, et al. Borrelia burgdorferi peptidoglycan is a persistent antigen in patients with Lyme arthritis. *Proc Natl Acad Sci*. 2019;116(27):13498–13507.
15. Dörr T, Moynihan PJ, Mayer C. Editorial: Bacterial Cell Wall Structure and Dynamics. *Frontiers in Microbiology*. 2019;10(2051).
16. Lukaszczyk M, Pradhan B, Remaut H. The biosynthesis and structures of bacterial pili. *Bacterial cell walls and membranes*. 2019:369–413.
17. Doron S, Gorbach SL. Bacterial Infections: Overview. *International Encyclopedia of Public Health*. 2008:273–282.
18. Piano S, Singh V, Caraceni P, Maiwall R, Alessandria C, Fernandez J, et al. Epidemiology and Effects of Bacterial Infections in Patients With Cirrhosis Worldwide. *Gastroenterology*. 2019;156(5):1368–1380 e10.
19. Bono L, Li Cavoli G, Verde MS, Sodano C, Tortorici C, Ferrantelli A, et al. Prevalence of bacterial pathogens and their emerging resistance patterns in patients with renal diseases. *Diálisis y Trasplante*. 2015;36(2):78–82.
20. Roh MS, Moldawer LL, Ekman LG, Dinarello CA, Bistrian BR, Jeevanandam M, et al. Stimulatory effect of interleukin-1 upon hepatic metabolism. *Metabolism*. 1986;35(5):419–424.
21. Gauldie J, Sauder DN, McAdam KP, Dinarello CA. Purified interleukin-1 (IL-1) from human monocytes stimulates acute-phase protein synthesis by rodent hepatocytes in vitro. *Immunology*. 1987;60(2):203–207.
22. Hise AG, Tomalka J, Ganesan S, Patel K, Hall BA, Brown GD, et al. An essential role for the NLRP3 inflammasome in host defense against the human fungal pathogen Candida albicans. *Cell Host Microbe*. 2009;5(5):487–497.
23. Wilson KP, Black JA, Thomson JA, Kim EE, Griffith JP, Navia MA, et al. Structure and mechanism of interleukin-1 beta converting enzyme. *Nature*. 1994;370(6487):270–275.
24. Pedra JH, Sutterwala FS, Sukumaran B, Ogura Y, Qian F, Montgomery RR, et al. ASC/PYCARD and caspase-1 regulate the IL-18/IFN-gamma axis during Anaplasma phagocytophilum infection. *J Immunol*. 2007;179(7):4783–4791.
25. Davis BK, Wen H, Ting JP-Y. The inflammasome NLRs in immunity, inflammation, and associated diseases. *Annu Rev Immunol*. 2011;29:707–735.
26. He X, Mekasha S, Mavrogiorgos N, Fitzgerald KA, Lien E, Ingalls RR. Inflammation and fibrosis during Chlamydia pneumoniae infection is regulated by IL-1 and the NLRP3/ASC inflammasome. *J Immunol*. 2010;184(10):5743–5754.
27. Shimada K, Crother TR, Karlin J, Dagvadorj J, Chiba N, Chen S, et al. Oxidized mitochondrial DNA activates the NLRP3 inflammasome during apoptosis. *Immunity*. 2012;36(3):401–414.
28. Kebaier C, Chamberland RR, IC Allen, Gao X, Broglie PM, Hall JD, et al. Staphylococcus aureus α-hemolysin mediates virulence in a murine model of severe pneumonia through activation of the NLRP3 inflammasome. *J Infect Dis*. 2012;205(5):807–817.
29. McNeela EA, Burke A, Neill DR, Baxter C, Fernandes VE, Ferreira D, et al. Pneumolysin activates the NLRP3 inflammasome and promotes proinflammatory cytokines independently of TLR4. *PLoS Pathog*. 2010;6(11):e1001191.
30. Petrilli V, Papin S, Dostert C, Mayor A, Martinon F, Tschopp J. Activation of the NALP3 inflammasome is triggered by low intracellular potassium concentration. *Cell Death & Differentiation*. 2007;14(9):1583–1589.
31. Sander LE, Davis MJ, Boekschoten MV, Amsen D, Dascher CC, Ryffel B, et al. Detection of prokaryotic mRNA signifies microbial viability and promotes immunity. *Nature*. 2011;474(7351):385–389.
32. Zhou R, Tardivel A, Thorens B, Choi I, Tschopp J. Thioredoxin-interacting protein links oxidative stress to inflammasome activation. *Nat Immunol*. 2010;11(2):136–140.
33. Zhou R, Yazdi AS, Menu P, Tschopp J. A role for mitochondria in NLRP3 inflammasome activation. *Nature*. 2011;469(7329):221–225.
34. Beal MF. Mitochondria, oxidative damage, and inflammation in Parkinson's disease. *Annals-New York Academy of Sciences*. 2003;991:120–131.
35. Shenoy AR, Wellington DA, Kumar P, Kassa H, Booth CJ, Cresswell P, et al. GBP5 promotes NLRP3 inflammasome assembly and immunity in mammals. *Science*. 2012;336(6080):481–485.
36. Lu B, Nakamura T, Inouye K, Li J, Tang Y, Lundbäck P, et al. Novel role of PKR in inflammasome activation and HMGB1 release. *Nature*. 2012;488(7413):670–674.

37. Vyleta ML, Wong J, Magun BE. Suppression of ribosomal function triggers innate immune signaling through activation of the NLRP3 inflammasome. *PLoS One*. 2012;7(5):e36044.
38. Kang MJ, Jo SG, Kim DJ, Park JH. NLRP 3 inflammasome mediates interleukin-1β production in immune cells in response to Acinetobacter baumannii and contributes to pulmonary inflammation in mice. *Immunology*. 2017;150(4):495–505.
39. Case CL, Roy CR. Asc modulates the function of NLRC4 in response to infection of macrophages by Legionella pneumophila. *MBio*. 2011;2(4):e00117–e00121.
40. Niebuhr M, Baumert K, Heratizadeh A, Satzger I, Werfel T. Impaired NLRP 3 inflammasome expression and function in atopic dermatitis due to Th2 milieu. *Allergy*. 2014;69(8):1058–1067.
41. Martinon F, Burns K, Tschopp J. The inflammasome: a molecular platform triggering activation of inflammatory caspases and processing of proIL-β. *Mol Cell*. 2002;10(2):417–426.
42. Bruey J-M, Bruey-Sedano N, Luciano F, Zhai D, Balpai R, Xu C, et al. Bcl-2 and Bcl-XL regulate proinflammatory caspase-1 activation by interaction with NALP1. *Cell*. 2007;129(1):45–56.
43. Terra JK, Cote CK, France B, Jenkins AL, Bozue JA, Welkos SL, et al. Cutting edge: resistance to Bacillus anthracis infection mediated by a lethal toxin sensitive allele of Nalp1b/Nlrp1b. *J Immunol*. 2010;184(1):17–20.
44. Elinav E, Strowig T, Kau AL, Henao-Mejia J, Thaiss CA, Booth CJ, et al. NLRP6 inflammasome regulates colonic microbial ecology and risk for colitis. *Cell*. 2011;145(5):745–757.
45. Anand PK, Malireddi RS, Lukens JR, Vogel P, Bertin J, Lamkanfi M, et al. NLRP6 negatively regulates innate immunity and host defence against bacterial pathogens. *Nature*. 2012;488(7411):389–393.
46. Chen GY, Liu M, Wang F, Bertin J, Núñez G. A functional role for Nlrp6 in intestinal inflammation and tumorigenesis. *J Immunol*. 2011;186(12):7187–7194.
47. Wang L, Manji GA, Grenier JM, Al-Garawi A, Merriam S, Lora JM, et al. PYPAF7, a novel PYRIN-containing Apaf1-like protein that regulates activation of NF-κB and caspase-1-dependent cytokine processing. *J Biol Chem*. 2002;277(33):29874–29880.
48. Vladimer GI, Weng D, Paquette SWM, Vanaja SK, Rathinam VA, Aune MH, et al. The NLRP12 inflammasome recognizes Yersinia pestis. *Immunity*. 2012;37(1):96–107.
49. Allen IC, Wilson JE, Schneider M, Lich JD, Roberts RA, Arthur JC, et al. NLRP12 suppresses colon inflammation and tumorigenesis through the negative regulation of noncanonical NF-κB signaling. *Immunity*. 2012;36(5):742–754.
50. Arthur JC, Lich JD, Ye Z, IC Allen, Gris D, Wilson JE, et al. Cutting edge: NLRP12 controls dendritic and myeloid cell migration to affect contact hypersensitivity. *J Immunol*. 2010;185(8):4515–4519.
51. Zaki MH, Vogel P, Malireddi RS, Body-Malapel M, Anand PK, Bertin J, et al. The NOD-like receptor NLRP12 attenuates colon inflammation and tumorigenesis. *Cancer Cell*. 2011;20(5):649–660.
52. Khare S, Dorfleutner A, Bryan NB, Yun C, Radian AD, de Almeida L, et al. An NLRP7-containing inflammasome mediates recognition of microbial lipopeptides in human macrophages. *Immunity*. 2012;36(3):464–476.
53. Meissner TB, Li A, Biswas A, Lee K-H, Liu Y-J, Bayir E, et al. NLR family member NLRC5 is a transcriptional regulator of MHC class I genes. *Proc Natl Acad Sci*. 2010;107(31):13794–13799.
54. Davis BK, Roberts RA, Huang MT, Willingham SB, Conti BJ, Brickey WJ, et al. Cutting edge: NLRC5-dependent activation of the inflammasome. *J Immunol*. 2011;186(3):1333–1337.
55. Lautz K, Damm A, Menning M, Wenger J, Adam AC, Zigrino P, et al. NLRP 10 enhances S higella-induced pro-inflammatory responses. *Cell Microbiol*. 2012;14(10):1568–1583.
56. Miao EA, Ernst RK, Dors M, Mao DP, Aderem A. Pseudomonas aeruginosa activates caspase 1 through Ipaf. *Proc Natl Acad Sci*. 2008;105(7):2562–2567.
57. Zhao Y, Yang J, Shi J, Gong Y-N, Lu Q, Xu H, et al. The NLRC4 inflammasome receptors for bacterial flagellin and type III secretion apparatus. *Nature*. 2011;477(7366):596–600.
58. Miao EA, Mao DP, Yudkovsky N, Bonneau R, Lorang CG, Warren SE, et al. Innate immune detection of the type III secretion apparatus through the NLRC4 inflammasome. *Proc Natl Acad Sci*. 2010;107(7):3076–3080.
59. Kofoed EM, Vance RE. Innate immune recognition of bacterial ligands by NAIPs determines inflammasome specificity. *Nature*. 2011;477(7366):592–595.
60. von Moltke J, Trinidad NJ, Moayeri M, Kintzer AF, Wang SB, van Rooijen N, et al. Rapid induction of inflammatory lipid mediators by the inflammasome in vivo. *Nature*. 2012;490(7418):107–111.

61. Franchi L, Kamada N, Nakamura Y, Burberry A, Kuffa P, Suzuki S, et al. NLRC4-driven production of IL-1β discriminates between pathogenic and commensal bacteria and promotes host intestinal defense. *Nat Immunol.* 2012;13(5):449–456.
62. Ayres JS, Trinidad NJ, Vance RE. Lethal inflammasome activation by a multidrug-resistant pathobiont upon antibiotic disruption of the microbiota. *Nat Med.* 2012;18(5):799–806.
63. Qu Y, Misaghi S, Izrael-Tomasevic A, Newton K, Gilmour LL, Lamkanfi M, et al. Phosphorylation of NLRC4 is critical for inflammasome activation. *Nature.* 2012;490(7421):539–542.
64. Akhter A, Gavrilin MA, Frantz L, Washington S, Ditty C, Limoli D, et al. Caspase-7 activation by the Nlrc4/Ipaf inflammasome restricts Legionella pneumophila infection. *PLoS Pathog.* 2009;5(4):e1000361.
65. Miao EA, Leaf IA, Treuting PM, Mao DP, Dors M, Sarkar A, et al. Caspase-1-induced pyroptosis is an innate immune effector mechanism against intracellular bacteria. *Nat Immunol.* 2010;11(12):1136–1142.
66. Miao EA, Rajan JV, Aderem A. Caspase-1-induced pyroptotic cell death. *Immunol Rev.* 2011;243(1):206–214.
67. Hausmann A, Böck D, Geiser P, Berthold DL, Fattinger SA, Furter M, et al. Intestinal epithelial NAIP/NLRC4 restricts systemic dissemination of the adapted pathogen Salmonella Typhimurium due to site-specific bacterial PAMP expression. *Mucosal immunology.* 2020;13(3):530–544.
68. Fernandes-Alnemri T, Yu J-W, Juliana C, Solorzano L, Kang S, Wu J, et al. The AIM2 inflammasome is critical for innate immunity to Francisella tularensis. *Nat Immunol.* 2010;11(5):385–393.
69. Rathinam VA, Jiang Z, Waggoner SN, Sharma S, Cole LE, Waggoner L, et al. The AIM2 inflammasome is essential for host defense against cytosolic bacteria and DNA viruses. *Nat Immunol.* 2010;11(5):395–402.
70. Jones JW, Kayagaki N, Broz P, Henry T, Newton K, O'Rourke K, et al. Absent in melanoma 2 is required for innate immune recognition of Francisella tularensis. *Proc Natl Acad Sci.* 2010;107(21):9771–9776.
71. Hanamsagar R, Aldrich A, Kielian T. Critical role for the AIM 2 inflammasome during acute CNS bacterial infection. *J Neurochem.* 2014;129(4):704–711.
72. Drennan MB, Nicolle D, Quesniaux VJF, Jacobs M, Allie N, Mpagi J, et al. Toll-Like Receptor 2-Deficient Mice Succumb to Mycobacterium tuberculosis Infection. *Am J Pathol.* 2004;164(1):49–57.
73. Henao-Mejia J, Elinav E, Jin C, Hao L, Mehal WZ, Strowig T, et al. Inflammasome-mediated dysbiosis regulates progression of NAFLD and obesity. *Nature.* 2012;482(7384):179–185.
74. Ali SR, Timmer AM, Bilgrami S, Park EJ, Eckmann L, Nizet V, et al. Anthrax toxin induces macrophage death by p38 MAPK inhibition but leads to inflammasome activation via ATP leakage. *Immunity.* 2011;35(1):34–44.
75. Kovarova M, Hesker PR, Jania L, Nguyen M, Snouwaert JN, Xiang Z, et al. NLRP1-dependent pyroptosis leads to acute lung injury and morbidity in mice. *J Immunol.* 2012;189(4):2006–2016.
76. Ceballos-Olvera I, Sahoo M, Miller MA, Ld Barrio, Re F. Inflammasome-dependent pyroptosis and IL-18 protect against Burkholderia pseudomallei lung infection while IL-1β is deleterious. *PLoS Pathog.* 2011;7(12):e1002452.
77. High N, Mounier J, Prevost MC, Sansonetti PJ. IpaB of Shigella flexneri causes entry into epithelial cells and escape from the phagocytic vacuole. *EMBO J.* 1992;11(5):1991–1999.
78. Diacovich L, Gorvel J-P. Bacterial manipulation of innate immunity to promote infection. *Nat Rev Microbiol.* 2010;8(2):117–128.
79. Fratti RA, Backer JM, Gruenberg J, Corvera S, Deretic V. Role of phosphatidylinositol 3-kinase and Rab5 effectors in phagosomal biogenesis and mycobacterial phagosome maturation arrest. *J Cell Biol.* 2001;154(3):631–644.
80. Philips JA. Mycobacterial manipulation of vacuolar sorting. *Cell Microbiol.* 2008;10(12):2408–2415.
81. Santecchia I, Ferrer MF, Vieira ML, Gómez RM, Werts C. Phagocyte Escape of Leptospira: The Role of TLRs and NLRs. *Front Immunol.* 2020;11(2596).
82. Haake DA, Zückert WR. Spirochetal lipoproteins in pathogenesis and immunity. *Spirochete biology: the post genomic era.* 2017:239–271.
83. Werts C. Interaction of leptospira with the innate immune system. *Spirochete Biology: The Post Genomic Era.* 2017:163–187.

84. Holzapfel M, Bonhomme D, Cagliero J, Vernel-Pauillac F, Fanton d'Andon M, Bortolussi S, et al. Escape of TLR5 Recognition by Leptospira spp.: A Rationale for Atypical Endoflagella. *Front Immunol.* 2020;11:2007.
85. Lacroix-Lamandé S, d'Andon MF, Michel E, Ratet G, Philpott DJ, Girardin SE, et al. Downregulation of the Na/K-ATPase pump by leptospiral glycolipoprotein activates the NLRP3 inflammasome. *J Immunol.* 2012;188(6):2805–2814.
86. Li S, Wang M, Ojcius DM, Zhou B, Hu W, Liu Y, et al. Leptospira interrogans infection leads to IL-1β and IL-18 secretion from a human macrophage cell line through reactive oxygen species and cathepsin B mediated-NLRP3 inflammasome activation. *Microbes Infect.* 2018;20(4):254–260.
87. Ratet G, Santecchia I, Fanton d'Andon M, Vernel-Pauillac F, Wheeler R, Lenormand P, et al. LipL21 lipoprotein binding to peptidoglycan enables Leptospira interrogans to escape NOD1 and NOD2 recognition. *PLoS Pathog.* 2017;13(12):e1006725.
88. O'Dwyer MJ, Mankan AK, White M, Lawless MW, Stordeur P, O'Connell B, et al. The human response to infection is associated with distinct patterns of interleukin 23 and interleukin 27 expression. *Intensive Care Med.* 2008;34(4):683–691.
89. Monte MM, Wang T, Costa MM, Harun NO, Secombes CJ. Cloning and expression analysis of two ROR-γ homologues (ROR-γa1 and ROR-γa2) in rainbow trout Oncorhynchus mykiss. *Fish Shellfish Immunol.* 2012;33(2):365–374.
90. Greenspan NS, Cavacini LA. 15 - Immunoglobulin Function. In: Rich RR, Fleisher TA, Shearer WT, Schroeder HW, Frew AJ, Weyand CM, eds. *Clinical Immunology.* Fifth Edition London: Elsevier; 2019:223–233 e1.
91. Stevenson EK, Rubenstein AR, Radin GT, Wiener RS, Walkey AJ. Two decades of mortality trends among patients with severe sepsis: a comparative meta-analysis*. *Crit Care Med.* 2014;42(3):625–631.
92. Boomer JS, Green JM, Hotchkiss RS. The changing immune system in sepsis: is individualized immuno-modulatory therapy the answer?. *Virulence.* 2014;5(1):45–56.
93. Louveau A, Smirnov I, Keyes TJ, Eccles JD, Rouhani SJ, Peske JD, et al. Structural and functional features of central nervous system lymphatic vessels. *Nature.* 2015;523(7560):337–341.
94. Gimenez MA, Sim JE, Russell JH. TNFR1-dependent VCAM-1 expression by astrocytes exposes the CNS to destructive inflammation. *J Neuroimmunol.* 2004;151(1-2):116–125.
95. Carpentier PA, Begolka WS, Olson JK, Elhofy A, Karpus WJ, Miller SD. Differential activation of astrocytes by innate and adaptive immune stimuli. *Glia.* 2005;49(3):360–374.
96. Geyer S, Jacobs M, Hsu NJ. Immunity Against Bacterial Infection of the Central Nervous System: An Astrocyte Perspective. *Front Mol Neurosci.* 2019;12:57.
97. Geyer S, Jacobs M, Hsu N-J. Immunity Against Bacterial Infection of the Central Nervous System: An Astrocyte Perspective. *Frontiers in Molecular Neuroscience.* 2019;12(57).
98. Phulwani NK, Esen N, Syed MM, Kielian T. TLR2 Expression in Astrocytes Is Induced by TNF-α- and NF-κB-Dependent Pathways. *J Immunol.* 2008;181(6):3841–3849.
99. Graveline R, Segura M, Radzioch D, Gottschalk M. TLR2-dependent recognition of Streptococcus suis is modulated by the presence of capsular polysaccharide which modifies macrophage responsiveness. *Int Immunol.* 2007;19(4):375–389.
100. Zheng H, Domínguez Punaro MC, Segura M, Lachance C, Rivest S, Xu J, et al. Toll-like receptor 2 is partially involved in the activation of murine astrocytes by Streptococcus suis, an important zoonotic agent of meningitis. *J Neuroimmunol.* 2011;234(1):71–83.
101. Guven T, Ugurlu K, Ergonul O, Celikbas AK, Gok SE, Comoglu S, et al. Neurobrucellosis: clinical and diagnostic features. *Clin Infect Dis.* 2013;56(10):1407–1412.
102. Al-Sous MW, Bohlega S, Al-Kawi MZ, Alwatban J, McLean DR. Neurobrucellosis: clinical and neuroimaging correlation. *AJNR Am J Neuroradiol.* 2004;25(3):395–401.
103. Martínez-Chamorro E, Muñoz A, Esparza J, MaJ Muñoz, Giangaspro E. Focal cerebral involvement by neurobrucellosis: pathological and MRI findings. *Eur J Radiol.* 2002;43(1):28–30.
104. Ferrero MC, Bregante J, Delpino MV, Barrionuevo P, Fossati CA, Giambartolomei GH, et al. Proinflammatory response of human endothelial cells to Brucella infection. *Microbes Infect.* 2011;13(10):852–861.
105. Miraglia MC, Scian R, Samartino CG, Barrionuevo P, Rodriguez AM, Ibañez AE, et al. Brucella abortus induces TNF-α-dependent astroglial MMP-9 secretion through mitogen-activated protein kinases. *Journal of Neuroinflammation.* 2013;10(1):819.

106. Lee K, Chiu K, Sansing H, Didier P, Ficht T, Arenas-Gamboa A, et al. Aerosol-induced brucellosis increases TLR-2 expression and increased complexity in the microanatomy of astroglia in rhesus macaques. *Frontiers in Cellular and Infection Microbiology*. 2013;3(86).
107. Li L, Acioglu C, Heary RF, Elkabes S. Role of astroglial toll-like receptors (TLRs) in central nervous system infections, injury and neurodegenerative diseases. *Brain Behav Immun*. 2021;91:740–755.
108. de Morais SD, Kak G, Menousek JP, Kielian T. Immunopathogenesis of Craniotomy Infection and Niche-Specific Immune Responses to Biofilm. *Front Immunol*. 2021;12(45).
109. Zhou X, Li X. Wu M. miRNAs reshape immunity and inflammatory responses in bacterial infection. *Signal Transduction and Targeted Therapy*. 2018;3(1):14.
110. Fassan M, Saraggi D, Balsamo L, Cascione L, Castoro C, Coati I, et al. Let-7c down-regulation in Helicobacter pylori-related gastric carcinogenesis. *Oncotarget*. 2016;7(4):4915.
111. Teng G-g, Wang W-h, Dai Y, Wang S-j, Chu Y-x, Li J. Let-7b is involved in the inflammation and immune responses associated with Helicobacter pylori infection by targeting Toll-like receptor 4. *PLoS One*. 2013;8(2):e56709.
112. Hayashi Y, Tsujii M, Wang J, Kondo J, Akasaka T, Jin Y, et al. CagA mediates epigenetic regulation to attenuate let-7 expression in Helicobacter pylori-related carcinogenesis. *Gut*. 2013;62(11):1536–1546.
113. Tang B, Li N, Gu J, Zhuang Y, Li Q, Wang H-G, et al. Compromised autophagy by MIR30B benefits the intracellular survival of Helicobacter pylori. *Autophagy*. 2012;8(7):1045–1057.
114. Kiga K, Mimuro H, Suzuki M, Shinozaki-Ushiku A, Kobayashi T, Sanada T, et al. Epigenetic silencing of miR-210 increases the proliferation of gastric epithelium during chronic Helicobacter pylori infection. *Nat Commun*. 2014;5(1):1–11.
115. Zhang Y-M, Noto JM, Hammond CE, Barth JL, Argraves WS, Backert S, et al. Helicobacter pylori-induced posttranscriptional regulation of HK-ATPase α-subunit gene expression by miRNA. *American Journal of Physiology-Gastrointestinal and Liver Physiology*. 2014;306(7):G606–GG13.
116. Pagliari M, Munari F, Toffoletto M, Lonardi S, Chemello F, Codolo G, et al. Helicobacter pylori Affects the Antigen Presentation Activity of Macrophages Modulating the Expression of the Immune Receptor CD300E through miR-4270. *Front Immunol*. 2017;8(1288).
117. Xie G, Li W, Li R, Wu K, Zhao E, Zhang Y, et al. Helicobacter pylori promote B7-H1 expression by suppressing miR-152 and miR-200b in gastric cancer cells. *PLoS One*. 2017;12(1):e0168822.
118. Koch M, Mollenkopf HJ, Klemm U, Meyer TF. Induction of microRNA-155 is TLR- and type IV secretion system-dependent in macrophages and inhibits DNA-damage induced apoptosis. *Proc Natl Acad Sci U S A*. 2012;109(19):E1153–E1162.
119. Fassi Fehri L, Koch M, Belogolova E, Khalil H, Bolz C, Kalali B, et al. Helicobacter pylori induces miR-155 in T cells in a cAMP-Foxp3-dependent manner. *PLoS One*. 2010;5(3):e9500.
120. Oertli M, Engler DB, Kohler E, Koch M, Meyer TF, Müller A. MicroRNA-155 is essential for the T cell-mediated control of Helicobacter pylori infection and for the induction of chronic Gastritis and Colitis. *J Immunol*. 2011;187(7):3578–3586.
121. Shiotani A, Murao T, Kimura Y, Matsumoto H, Kamada T, Kusunoki H, et al. Identification of serum miRNAs as novel non-invasive biomarkers for detection of high risk for early gastric cancer. *Br J Cancer*. 2013;109(9):2323–2330.
122. Zhang Z, Chen S, Fan M, Ruan G, Xi T, Zheng L, et al. Helicobacter pylori induces gastric cancer via down-regulating miR-375 to inhibit dendritic cell maturation. *Helicobacter*. 2021;26(4):e12813.
123. Liu Z, Wang D, Hu Y, Zhou G, Zhu C, Yu Q, et al. MicroRNA-146a negatively regulates PTGS2 expression induced by Helicobacter pylori in human gastric epithelial cells. *J Gastroenterol*. 2013;48(1):86–92.
124. Salem ME, Bodor JN, Puccini A, Xiu J, Goldberg RM, Grothey A, et al. Relationship between MLH1, PMS2, MSH2 and MSH6 gene-specific alterations and tumor mutational burden in 1057 microsatellite instability-high solid tumors. *Int J Cancer*. 2020;147(10):2948–2956.
125. Darvin P, Toor SM, Nair VS, Elkord E. Immune checkpoint inhibitors: recent progress and potential biomarkers. *Exp Mol Med*. 2018;50(12):1–11.
126. Prinz C, Weber D. MicroRNA (miR) dysregulation during Helicobacter pylori-induced gastric inflammation and cancer development: critical importance of miR-155. *Oncotarget*. 2020;11(10):894–904.

127. Saito Y, Suzuki H, Tsugawa H, Imaeda H, Matsuzaki J, Hirata K, et al. Overexpression of miR-142-5p and miR-155 in gastric mucosa-associated lymphoid tissue (MALT) lymphoma resistant to Helicobacter pylori eradication. *PLoS One*. 2012;7(11):e47396.
128. Luzza F, Oderda G, Maletta M, Imeneo M, Mesuraca L, Chioboli E, et al. Salivary immunoglobulin G assay to diagnose Helicobacter pylori infection in children. *J Clin Microbiol*. 1997;35(12):3358–3360.
129. Fallone CA, Elizov M, Cleland P, Thompson JA, Wild GE, Lough J, et al. Detection of Helicobacter pylori infection by saliva IgG testing. *Am J Gastroenterol*. 1996;91(6):1145–1149.
130. Loeb MB, Riddell RH, James C, Hunt R, Smaill FM. Evaluation of Salivary Antibodies to Detect Infection with *Helicobacter pylori*. *Can J Gastroenterol*. 1997;11:294081.
131. Christie JM, McNulty CA, Shepherd NA, Valori RM. Is saliva serology useful for the diagnosis of Helicobacter pylori?. *Gut*. 1996;39(1):27–30.
132. Simor AE, Lin E, Saibil F, Cohen L, Louie M, Pearen S, et al. Evaluation of enzyme immunoassay for detection of salivary antibody to Helicobacter pylori. *J Clin Microbiol*. 1996;34(3):550–553.
133. Luzza F, Oderda G, Maletta M, Imeneo M, Mesuraca L, Chioboli E, et al. Salivary immunoglobulin G assay to diagnose Helicobacter pylori infection in children. *J Clin Microbiol*. 1997;35(12):3358–3360.
134. Alemohammad MM, Foley TJ, Cohen H. Detection of immunoglobulin G antibodies to Helicobacter pylori in urine by an enzyme immunoassay method. *J Clin Microbiol*. 1993;31(8):2174–2177.
135. Katsuragi K, Noda A, Tachikawa T, Azuma A, Mukai F, Murakami K, et al. Highly Sensitive Urine-Based Enzyme-Linked Immunosorbent Assay for Detection of Antibody to Helicobacter pylori. *Helicobacter*. 1998;3(4):289–295.
136. Meijer BC, Thijs JC, Kleibeuker JH, AAv Zwet. Berrelkamp RJ. Evaluation of eight enzyme immunoassays for detection of immunoglobulin G against Helicobacter pylori. *J Clin Microbiol*. 1997;35(1):292–294.
137. Talley NJ, Kost L, Haddad A, Zinsmeister AR. Comparison of commercial serological tests for detection of Helicobacter pylori antibodies. *J Clin Microbiol*. 1992;30(12):3146–3150.
138. van Doorn LJ, Henskens Y, Nouhan N, Verschuuren A, Vreede R, Herbink P, et al. The efficacy of laboratory diagnosis of Helicobacter pylori infections in gastric biopsy specimens is related to bacterial density and vacA, cagA, and iceA genotypes. *J Clin Microbiol*. 2000;38(1):13–17.
139. Laheij RJF, Straatman H, Jansen JBMJ, Verbeek ALM. Evaluation of Commercially Available*Helicobacter pylori*Serology Kits: a Review. *Journal of Clinical Microbiology*. 1998;36(10):2803–2809.
140. Lerang F, Moum B, Mowinckel P, Haug J, Ragnhildstveit E, Berge T, et al. Accuracy of seven different tests for the diagnosis of Helicobacter pylori infection and the impact of H2-receptor antagonists on test results. *Scand J Gastroenterol*. 1998;33(4):364–369.
141. Van de Wouw B, de Boer WA, Jansz AR, Roymans R, Staals A. Comparison of three commercially available enzyme-linked immunosorbent assays and biopsy-dependent diagnosis for detecting Helicobacter pylori infection. *J Clin Microbiol*. 1996;34(1):94–97.
142. Granberg C, Mansikka A, Lehtonen OP, Kujari H, Grönfors R, Nurmi H, et al. Diagnosis of Helicobacter pylori infection by using pyloriset EIA-G and EIA-A for detection of serum immunoglobulin G (IgG) and IgA antibodies. *J Clin Microbiol*. 1993;31(6):1450–1453.
143. Herbrink P, van Doorn LJ. Serological methods for diagnosis of Helicobacter pylori infection and monitoring of eradication therapy. *Eur J Clin Microbiol Infect Dis*. 2000;19(3):164–173.
144. Chart H, Cheasty T. The serodiagnosis of human infections with Yersinia enterocolitica and Yersinia pseudotuberculosis. *FEMS Immunology & Medical Microbiology*. 2006;47(3):391–397.
145. Biranjia-Hurdoyal SD, Seetulsingh-Goorah SP. Performances of Four Helicobacter pylori Serological Detection Kits Using Stool Antigen Test as Gold Standard. *PLoS One*. 2016;11(10):e0163834.
146. Wielkoszynski T, Moghaddam A, Bäckman A, Broden J, Piotrowski R, Mond-Paszek R, et al. Novel diagnostic ELISA test for discrimination between infections with Yersinia enterocolitica and Yersinia pseudotuberculosis. *Eur J Clin Microbiol Infect Dis*. 2018;37(12):2301–2306.
147. Ahvonen P, Sievers K, Aho K. Arthritis associated with Yersinia enterocolitica infection. *Acta Rheumatol Scand*. 1969;15(3):232–253.
148. MÆLand JA, Digranes A. Common Enterobacterial Antigen in Yersinia Enterocolitica. *Acta Pathologica Microbiologica Scandinavica Section B Microbiology*. 1975;83B(4):382–386.

149. Maeland JA, Digranes A. Human serum antibodies against heat-stable antigens from Yersinia enterocolitica. *Acta Pathol Microbiol Scand B*. 1975;83(5):451–456.
150. MHALU FS, MYRMEL H, DIGRANES A, OEDING P. Antibodies to Yersinia enterocolitica in a healthy population in Tanzania. *APMIS*. 1988;96(1-6):377–378.
151. Mäki-Ikola O, Heesemann J, Toivanen A, Granfors K. High frequency ofYersinia antibodies in healthy populations in Finland and Germany. *Rheumatol Int*. 1997;16(6):227–229.
152. Ståhlberg TH, Heesemann J, Granfors K, Toivanen A. Immunoblot analysis of IgM, IgG, and IgA responses to plasmid encoded released proteins ofYersinia enterocolitica in patients with or without yersinia triggered reactive arthritis. *Ann Rheum Dis*. 1989;48(7):577–581.
153. Granfors K. Measurement of immunoglobulin M (IgM), IgG, and IgA antibodies against Yersinia enterocolitica by enzyme-linked immunosorbent assay: persistence of serum antibodies during disease. *Journal of Clinical Microbiology*. 1979;9(3):336–341.
154. Bitzan M, Häck HJ, Mauff G. Yersinia enterocolitica serodiagnosis: A dual role of specific IgA. Evaluation of microagglutination and ELISA. *Zentralblatt für Bakteriologie, Mikrobiologie und Hygiene Series A: Medical Microbiology, Infectious Diseases, Virology, Parasitology*. 1987;267(2):194–205.
155. Lahesmaa-Rantala R, Heesemann J, Lehtonen OP, Granfors K, Toivanen A. Avidity of antibodies against released proteins ofYersinia spp: comparison of patients with or without reactive arthritis. *Ann Rheum Dis*. 1989;48(12):1003–1006.
156. Herrlinger JD, Asmussen JU. Long term prognosis in yersinia arthritis: clinical and serological findings. *Ann Rheum Dis*. 1992;51(12):1332–1334.
157. Hoogkamp-Korstanje JAA, de Koning J, Heesemann J. Persistence ofYersinia enterocolitica in man. *Infection*. 1988;16(2):81–85.
158. Hill Gaston JS, Cox C, Granfors K. Clinical and experimental evidence for persistent Yersinia infection in reactive arthritis. *Arthritis & Rheumatism*. 1999;42(10):2239–2242.
159. Tuuminen T, Palomäki P, Paavonen J. The use of serologic tests for the diagnosis of chlamydial infections. *J Microbiol Methods*. 2000;42(3):265–279.
160. Huppertz HI, Heesemann J. Experimental Yersinia infection of human synovial cells: persistence of live bacteria and generation of bacterial antigen deposits including "ghosts," nucleic acid-free bacterial rods. *Infect Immun*. 1996;64(4):1484–1487.
161. Huppertz HI, Heesemann J. Effect of cytokines on invasion and survival ofYersinia in primary human fibroblasts. *Med Microbiol Immunol (Berl)*. 1999;187(3):157–164.
162. Granfors K, Merilahti-Palo R, Luukkainen R, Möttönen T, Lahesmaa R, Probst P, et al. Persistence ofYersinia antigens in peripheral blood cells from patients with Yersinia enterocolitica O:3 infection with or without reactive arthritis. *Arthritis & Rheumatism*. 1998;41(5):855–862.
163. Leo JC, Skurnik M. Adhesins of Human Pathogens from the Genus Yersinia. In: Linke D, Goldman A, eds. *Bacterial Adhesion: Chemistry, Biology and Physics*. Dordrecht: Springer Netherlands; 2011:1–15.
164. Rastawicki W. [Humoral response to recombinant YeuB, Ail, YadA and Inv proteins ofYersinia enterocolitica in patients with yersiniosis]. *Med Dosw Mikrobiol*. 2009;61(1):21–32.
165. Tuuminen T, Lounamo K, Leirisalo-Repo M. A Review of Serological Tests to Assist Diagnosis of Reactive Arthritis: Critical Appraisal on Methodologies. *Front Immunol*. 2013;4(418).
166. Rawlins ML, Gerstner C, Hill HR, Litwin CM. Evaluation of a Western Blot Method for the Detection of *Yersinia*Antibodies: Evidence of Serological Cross-Reactivity between *Yersinia*Outer Membrane Proteins and *Borrelia burgdorferi*. *Clinical and Vaccine Immunology*. 2005;12(11):1269–1274.
167. Du Y, Rosqvist R, Ak Forsberg. Role of fraction 1 antigen ofYersinia pestis in inhibition of phagocytosis. *Infect Immun*. 2002;70(3):1453–1460.
168. Hsu H-L, Chuang C-C, Liang C-C, Chiao D-J, Wu H-L, Wu Y-P, et al. Rapid and sensitive detection of Yersinia pestis by lateral-flow assay in simulated clinical samples. *BMC Infectious Diseases*. 2018;18(1):402.
169. Townes JM, Angulo FJ. Reactive Arthritis after Enteric Infections in the United States: The Problem of Definition. *Clin Infect Dis*. 2010;50(2):247–254.
170. Hannu T. Reactive arthritis. *Best Practice & Research Clinical Rheumatology*. 2011;25(3):347–357.
171. Pope JE, Krizova A, Garg AX, Thiessen-Philbrook H, Ouimet JM. Campylobacter reactive arthritis: a systematic review. *Semin Arthritis Rheum*. 2007;37(1):48–55.

172. Kaldor J, Pritchard H, Serpell A, Metcalf W. Serum antibodies in Campylobacter enteritis. *J Clin Microbiol*. 1983;18(1):1–4.
173. FW. Sero-diagnosis of typhoid fever. *Bull Mem Soc Med Hop Paris*. 1896;13:561–566.
174. Felix A, Bensted HJ. Proposed standard agglutinating sera for typhoid and paratyphoid A and B fevers. *Bull World Health Organ*. 1954;10(6):919–926.
175. Chart H, Cheasty T, de Pinna E, Siorvanes L, Wain J, Alam D, et al. Serodiagnosis of Salmonella enterica serovar Typhi and S. enterica serovars Paratyphi A, B and C human infections. *J Med Microbiol*. 2007;56(Pt 9):1161–1166.
176. John W, Salih H. The laboratory diagnosis of enteric fever. *The Journal of Infection in Developing Countries*. 2008;2(06).
177. Ley B, Mtove G, Thriemer K, Amos B, von Seidlein L, Hendriksen I, et al. Evaluation of the Widal tube agglutination test for the diagnosis of typhoid fever among children admitted to a rural hdospital in Tanzania and a comparison with previous studies. *BMC Infectious Diseases*. 2010;10(1):180.
178. Olopoenia LA, King AL. Widal agglutination test – 100 years later: still plagued by controversy. *Postgrad Med J*. 2000;76(892):80–84.
179. Siba V, Horwood PF, Vanuga K, Wapling J, Sehuko R, Siba PM, et al. Evaluation of serological diagnostic tests for typhoid fever in Papua New Guinea using a composite reference standard. *Clin Vaccine Immunol*. 2012;19(11):1833–1837.
180. Rastawicki W, Rokosz N, Jagielski M. [Comparison of usefulness of lipopolysaccharides extracted by phenol and trichloroacetic acid from Salmonella Typhimurium and Enteritidis for serodiagnosis of salmonelosis]. *Med Dosw Mikrobiol*. 2011;63(1):65–71.
181. Isomaki O, Vuento R, Granfors K. Serological diagnosis of salmonella infections by enzyme immunoassay. *The Lancet*. 1989;333(8652):1411–1414.
182. Kaminski RW, Clarkson K, Kordis AA, Oaks EV. Multiplexed immunoassay to assess Shigella-specific antibody responses. *J Immunol Methods*. 2013;393(1-2):18–29.
183. de Silva DG, Candy DC, Mendis LN, Chart H, Rowe B. Serological diagnosis of infection by Shigella dysenteriae-1 in patients with bacillary dysentery. *J Infect*. 1992;25(3):273–278.
184. Nahm MH, Yu J, Weerts HP, Wenzel H, Tamilselvi CS, Chandrasekaran L, et al. Development, Interlaboratory Evaluations, and Application of a Simple, High-Throughput Shigella Serum Bactericidal Assay. *mSphere*. 2018;3(3).
185. Watson K, Kerr E. Comparison of agglutination, complement fixation and immunofluorescence tests in Campylobacter jejuni infections. *Epidemiology & Infection*. 1982;88(2):165–171.
186. Tuuminen T, Lounamo K, Leirisalo-Repo M. A review of serological tests to assist diagnosis of reactive arthritis: critical appraisal on methodologies. *Front Immunol*. 2013;4:418.
187. Rautelin H, Kosunen TU. An acid extract as a common antigen in Campylobacter coli and Campylobacter jejuni strains. *J Clin Microbiol*. 1983;17(4):700–701.
188. Blaser MJ, Duncan DJ. Human serum antibody response to Campylobacter jejuni infection as measured in an enzyme-linked immunosorbent assay. *Infect Immun*. 1984;44(2):292–298.
189. Kosunen T, Höök J, Rautelin H, Myllylä G. Age-dependent increase of Campylobacter pylori antibodies in blood donors. *Scand J Gastroenterol*. 1989;24(1):110–114.
190. Hirschl A, Pletschette M, Hirschl M, Berger J, Stanek G, Rotter M. Comparison of different antigen preparations in an evaluation of the immune response to Campylobacter pylori. *Eur J Clin Microbiol Infect Dis*. 1988;7(4):570–575.
191. Taylor BV, Williamson J, Luck J, Coleman D, Jones D, McGregor A. Sensitivity and specificity of serology in determining recent acute Campylobacter infection. *Intern Med J*. 2004;34(5):250–258.
192. Mitchell HM, Lee A, Berkowicz J, Borody T. The use of serology to diagnose active Campylobacter pylori infection. *Med J Aust*. 1988;149(11-12):604–609.
193. Rokosz N, Rastawicki W, Jagielski M. Hetkowska-Abramczyk Z. Detection of antibodies to Campylobacter jejuni in pediatrics patients with Gullain-Barré syndrome using different antigen preparations. *Med Dosw Mikrobiol*. 2011;63(3):255–261.
194. Schmidt-Ott R, Schmidt H, Feldmann S, Brass F, Krone B, Gross U. Improved serological diagnosis stresses the major role of Campylobacter jejuni in triggering Guillain-Barré syndrome. *Clin Vaccine Immunol*. 2006;13(7):779–783.

195. Souza CO, Vieira MACS, Batista FMA, Eulálio KD, Neves JMM, Sá LC, et al. Serological Markers of Recent Campylobacter jejuni Infection in Patients with Guillain-Barré Syndrome in the State of Piauí, Brazil, 2014-2016. *Am J Trop Med Hyg*. 2018;98(2):586–588.
196. Steingart KR, Ramsay A, Dowdy DW, Pai M. Serological tests for the diagnosis of active tuberculosis: relevance for India. *Indian J Med Res*. 2012;135(5):695–702.
197. McCulloch TR, Wells TJ, Souza-Fonseca-Guimaraes F. Towards efficient immunotherapy for bacterial infection. *Trends Microbiol*. 2021.
198. Medzhitov R, Preston-Hurlburt P, Janeway CA. A human homologue of the Drosophila Toll protein signals activation of adaptive immunity. *Nature*. 1997;388(6640):394–397.
199. Ferwerda B, McCall MB, Verheijen K, Kullberg B-J, Van Der Ven AJ, Van der Meer JW, et al. Functional consequences of toll-like receptor 4 polymorphisms. *Mol Med*. 2008;14(5):346–352.
200. Hancock RE, Nijnik A, Philpott DJ. Modulating immunity as a therapy for bacterial infections. *Nat Rev Microbiol*. 2012;10(4):243–254.
201. Mifsud EJ, Tan ACL, Jackson DC. TLR Agonists as Modulators of the Innate Immune Response and Their Potential as Agents Against Infectious Disease. *Front Immunol*. 2014;5:79.
202. Werts C, Rubino S, Ling A, Girardin SE, Philpott DJ. Nod-like receptors in intestinal homeostasis, inflammation, and cancer. *J Leukocyte Biol*. 2011;90(3):471–482.
203. Fritz JH, Le Bourhis L, Sellge G, Magalhaes JG, Fsihi H, Kufer TA, et al. Nod1-mediated innate immune recognition of peptidoglycan contributes to the onset of adaptive immunity. *Immunity*. 2007;26(4):445–459.
204. Lavelle EC, McNaughton A, McNeela E. NLRP3 in protective immunity and vaccination against respiratory infection. *Expert Rev Vaccines*. 2011;10(3):255–257.
205. Das S, Suarez G, Beswick EJ, Sierra JC, Graham DY, Reyes VE. Expression of B7-H1 on gastric epithelial cells: its potential role in regulating T cells during Helicobacter pylori infection. *J Immunol*. 2006;176(5):3000–3009.
206. Shen B, Qian A, Lao W, Li W, Chen X, Zhang B, et al. Relationship between Helicobacter pylori and expression of programmed death-1 and its ligand in gastric intraepithelial neoplasia and early-stage gastric cancer. *Cancer management and research*. 2019;11:3909.
207. Triantafyllou E, Gudd CL, Mawhin M-A, Husbyn HC, Trovato FM, Siggins MK, et al. PD-1 blockade improves Kupffer cell bacterial clearance in acute liver injury. *J Clin Invest*. 2021;131(4).
208. Wang X, Cao Z, Jiang J, Li Y, Dong M, Ostrowski M, et al. Elevated expression of Tim-3 on CD8 T cells correlates with disease severity of pulmonary tuberculosis. *J Infect*. 2011;62(4):292–300.
209. Mayer-Barber KD, Yan B. Clash of the Cytokine Titans: counter-regulation of interleukin-1 and type I interferon-mediated inflammatory responses. *Cellular & molecular immunology*. 2017;14(1):22–35.
210. Mayer-Barber KD, Andrade BB, Oland SD, Amaral EP, Barber DL, Gonzales J, et al. Host-directed therapy of tuberculosis based on interleukin-1 and type I interferon crosstalk. *Nature*. 2014;511(7507):99–103.
211. Ramamurthy D, Nundalall T, Cingo S, Mungra N, Karaan M, Naran K, et al. Recent advances in immunotherapies against infectious diseases. *Immunotherapy Advances*. 2020;1(1).
212. Brown GD, Denning DW, Gow NA, Levitz SM, Netea MG, White TC. Hidden killers: human fungal infections. *Sci Transl Med*. 2012;4(165):165rv13.
213. Denning DW. Minimizing fungal disease deaths will allow the UNAIDS target of reducing annual AIDS deaths below 500 000 by 2020 to be realized. *Philosophical Transactions of the Royal Society B: Biological Sciences*. 2016;371(1709):20150468.
214. Armstrong-James D, Meintjes G, Brown GD. A neglected epidemic: fungal infections in HIV/AIDS. *Trends Microbiol*. 2014;22(3):120–127.
215. Guinea J, Torres-Narbona M, Gijón P, Muñoz P, Pozo F, Peláez T, et al. Pulmonary aspergillosis in patients with chronic obstructive pulmonary disease: incidence, risk factors, and outcome. *Clin Microbiol Infect*. 2010;16(7):870–877.
216. Marr KA, Carter RA, Boeckh M, Martin P, Corey L. Invasive aspergillosis in allogeneic stem cell transplant recipients: changes in epidemiology and risk factors. *Blood, The Journal of the American Society of Hematology*. 2002;100(13):4358–4366.
217. Limper AH, Adenis A, Le T, Harrison TS. Fungal infections in HIV/AIDS. *Lancet Infect Dis*. 2017;17(11):e334–ee43.

218. Bongomin F, Gago S, Oladele RO, Denning DW. Global and Multi-National Prevalence of Fungal Diseases-Estimate Precision. *J Fungi (Basel)*. 2017;3(4):57.
219. Meyers J, ed. *Fungal Infections in Bone Marrow Transplant Patients*: Seminars in oncology; 1990.
220. Parsons PE, Wiener-Kronish JP, Berra L, Stapleton RD. *Critical Care Secrets E-Book*: Elsevier Health Sciences; 2018.
221. Garber G. An overview of fungal infections. *Drugs*. 2001;61(1):1–12.
222. Groll A, Shah P, Mentzel C, Schneider M, Just-Nuebling G, Huebner K. Trends in the postmortem epidemiology of invasive fungal infections at a university hospital. *J Infect*. 1996;33(1):23–32.
223. Pappas PG. Opportunistic fungi: a view to the future. *Am J Med Sci*. 2010;340(3):253–257.
224. Vinh DC, Sugui JA, Hsu AP, Freeman AF, Holland SM. Invasive fungal disease in autosomal-dominant hyper-IgE syndrome. *J Allergy Clin Immunol*. 2010;125(6):1389–1390.
225. Garcia-Solache MA, Casadevall A. Global warming will bring new fungal diseases for mammals. *MBio*. 2010;1(1):e00061–e00070.
226. Brown AJ, Odds FC, Gow NA. Infection-related gene expression in Candida albicans. *Curr Opin Microbiol*. 2007;10(4):307–313.
227. Cooney NM, Klein BS. Fungal adaptation to the mammalian host: it is a new world, after all. *Curr Opin Microbiol*. 2008;11(6):511–516.
228. Hube B. Fungal adaptation to the host environment. *Curr Opin Microbiol*. 2009;12(4):347–349.
229. Richie DL, Hartl L, Aimanianda V, Winters MS, Fuller KK, Miley MD, et al. A role for the unfolded protein response (UPR) in virulence and antifungal susceptibility in Aspergillus fumigatus. *PLoS Pathog*. 2009;5(1):e1000258.
230. Cushion MT, Smulian AG, Slaven BE, Sesterhenn T, Arnold J, Staben C, et al. Transcriptome of Pneumocystis carinii during fulminate infection: carbohydrate metabolism and the concept of a compatible parasite. *PLoS One*. 2007;2(5):e423.
231. Romani L. Immunity to fungal infections. *Nat Rev Immunol*. 2011;11(4):275–288.
232. Schneider DS, Ayres JS. Two ways to survive infection: what resistance and tolerance can teach us about treating infectious diseases. *Nat Rev Immunol*. 2008;8(11):889–895.
233. Li Z, Lu G, Meng G. Pathogenic Fungal Infection in the Lung. *Front Immunol*. 2019;10:1524.
234. Latgé J-P. Aspergillus fumigatus and aspergillosis. *Clin Microbiol Rev*. 1999;12(2):310–350.
235. Yaguchi T. Basic mycology 1. The genus Aspergillus. *Medical Mycology Journ*. 2011;52(3):193–197.
236. Ibrahim-Granet O, Philippe B, Boleti H, Boisvieux-Ulrich E, Grenet D, Stern M, et al. Phagocytosis and intracellular fate of Aspergillus fumigatus conidia in alveolar macrophages. *Infect Immun*. 2003;71(2):891–903.
237. Mouyna I, Sarfati J, Recco P, Fontaine T, Henrissat B, Latgé J-P. Molecular characterization of a cell wall-associated ß (1-3) endoglucanase of Aspergillus fumigatus. *Med Mycol*. 2002;40(5):455–464.
238. Bernard M, Mouyna I, Dubreucq G, Debeaupuis J-P, Fontaine T, Vorgias C, et al. Characterization of a cell-wall acid phosphatase (PhoAp) in Aspergillus fumigatusThe GenBank accession number for the A. fumigatus PHOA sequence reported in this paper is AF462065. *Microbiology*. 2002;148(9):2819–2829.
239. Latgé J-P. The pathobiology of Aspergillus fumigatus. *Trends Microbiol*. 2001;9(8):382–389.
240. Kronstad JW, Attarian R, Cadieux B, Choi J, D'souza CA, Griffiths EJ, et al. Expanding fungal pathogenesis: Cryptococcus breaks out of the opportunistic box. *Nat Rev Microbiol*. 2011;9(3):193–203.
241. Blasi E, Barluzzi R, Mazzolla R, Bistoni F. Differential host susceptibility to intracerebral infections with Candida albicans and Cryptococcus neoformans. *Infect Immun*. 1993;61(8):3476–3481.
242. Black CA, Eyers FM, Russell A, Dunkley ML, Clancy RL, Beagley KW. Acute neutropenia decreases inflammation associated with murine vaginal candidiasis but has no effect on the course of infection. *Infect Immun*. 1998;66(3):1273–1275.
243. Rosati D, Bruno M, Jaeger M, Ten Oever J, Netea MG. Recurrent Vulvovaginal Candidiasis: An Immunological Perspective. *Microorganisms*. 2020;8(2):144.
244. Sokol H, Leducq V, Aschard H, Pham H-P, Jegou S, Landman C, et al. Fungal microbiota dysbiosis in IBD. *Gut*. 2017;66(6):1039–1048.
245. Stamatiades GA, Ioannou P, Petrikkos G, Tsioutis C. Fungal infections in patients with inflammatory bowel disease: A systematic review. *Mycoses*. 2018;61(6):366–376.
246. Meersseman W, Vandecasteele SJ, Wilmer A, Verbeken E, Peetermans WE, Van Wijngaerden E. Invasive aspergillosis in critically ill patients without malignancy. *Am J Respir Crit Care Med*. 2004;170(6):621–625.

247. Hope W, Natarajan P, Goodwin L. Invasive fungal infections. *Clin Med (Lond)*. 2013;13(5):507–510.
248. Park BJ, Wannemuehler KA, Marston BJ, Govender N, Pappas PG. Chiller TM. Estimation of the current global burden of cryptococcal meningitis among persons living with HIV/AIDS. *AIDS*. 2009;23(4):525–530.
249. Bellocchio S, Montagnoli C, Bozza S, Gaziano R, Rossi G, Mambula SS, et al. The contribution of the Toll-like/IL-1 receptor superfamily to innate and adaptive immunity to fungal pathogens in vivo. *J Immunol*. 2004;172(5):3059–3069.
250. Tarabishy AB, Hise AG, Traboulsi EI. Ocular manifestations of the autoinflammatory syndromes. *Ophthalmic Genet*. 2012;33(4):179–186.
251. Deepe J, George S, McGuinness M. Interleukin-1 and host control of pulmonary histoplasmosis. *J Infect Dis*. 2006;194(6):855–864.
252. Gross O, Poeck H, Bscheider M, Dostert C, Hannesschläger N, Endres S, et al. Syk kinase signalling couples to the Nlrp3 inflammasome for anti-fungal host defence. *Nature*. 2009;459(7245):433–436.
253. Kumar H, Kumagai Y, Tsuchida T, Koenig PA, Satoh T, Guo Z, et al. Involvement of the NLRP3 inflammasome in innate and humoral adaptive immune responses to fungal beta-glucan. *J Immunol*. 2009;183(12):8061–8067.
254. Lamkanfi M, Malireddi RK, Kanneganti TD. Fungal zymosan and mannan activate the cryopyrin inflammasome. *J Biol Chem*. 2009;284(31):20574–20581.
255. Pietrella D, Pandey N, Gabrielli E, Pericolini E, Perito S, Kasper L, et al. Secreted aspartic proteases of Candida albicans activate the NLRP3 inflammasome. *Eur J Immunol*. 2013;43(3):679–692.
256. Saïd-Sadier N, Padilla E, Langsley G, Ojcius DM. Aspergillus fumigatus stimulates the NLRP3 inflammasome through a pathway requiring ROS production and the Syk tyrosine kinase. *PLoS One*. 2010;5(4):e10008.
257. Mao L, Zhang L, Li H, Chen W, Wang H, Wu S, et al. Pathogenic fungus Microsporum canis activates the NLRP3 inflammasome. *Infect Immun*. 2014;82(2):882–892.
258. Gringhuis SI, Kaptein TM, Wevers BA, Theelen B, van der Vlist M, Boekhout T, et al. Dectin-1 is an extracellular pathogen sensor for the induction and processing of IL-1β via a noncanonical caspase-8 inflammasome. *Nat Immunol*. 2012;13(3):246–254.
259. Suzuki T, Franchi L, Toma C, Ashida H, Ogawa M, Yoshikawa Y, et al. Differential regulation of caspase-1 activation, pyroptosis, and autophagy via Ipaf and ASC in Shigella-infected macrophages. *PLoS Pathog*. 2007;3(8):e111.
260. Tomalka J, Ganesan S, Azodi E, Patel K, Majmudar P, Hall BA, et al. A novel role for the NLRC4 inflammasome in mucosal defenses against the fungal pathogen Candida albicans. *PLoS Pathog*. 2011;7(12):e1002379.
261. Joly S, Ma N, Sadler JJ, Soll DR, Cassel SL, Sutterwala FS. Cutting edge: Candida albicans hyphae formation triggers activation of the Nlrp3 inflammasome. *J Immunol*. 2009;183(6):3578–3581.
262. Murciano C, Moyes DL, Runglall M, Islam A, Mille C, Fradin C, et al. Candida albicans cell wall glycosylation may be indirectly required for activation of epithelial cell proinflammatory responses. *Infect Immun*. 2011;79(12):4902–4911.
263. Sorgi CA, Secatto A, Fontanari C, Turato WM, Belangér C, de Medeiros AI, et al. Histoplasma capsulatum cell wall {beta}-glucan induces lipid body formation through CD18, TLR2, and dectin-1 receptors: correlation with leukotriene B4 generation and role in HIV-1 infection. *J Immunol*. 2009;182(7):4025–4035.
264. Jouault T, Ibata-Ombetta S, Takeuchi O, Trinel PA, Sacchetti P, Lefebvre P, et al. Candida albicans phospholipomannan is sensed through toll-like receptors. *J Infect Dis*. 2003;188(1):165–172.
265. Netea MG, Warris A, Van der Meer JW, Fenton MJ, Verver-Janssen TJ, Jacobs LE, et al. Aspergillus fumigatus evades immune recognition during germination through loss of toll-like receptor-4-mediated signal transduction. *J Infect Dis*. 2003;188(2):320–326.
266. Fonseca FL, Nohara LL, Cordero RJ, Frases S, Casadevall A, Almeida IC, et al. Immunomodulatory effects of serotype B glucuronoxylomannan from Cryptococcus gattii correlate with polysaccharide diameter. *Infect Immun*. 2010;78(9):3861–3870.
267. Rubino I, Coste A, Le Roy D, Roger T, Jaton K, Boeckh M, et al. Species-specific recognition of Aspergillus fumigatus by Toll-like receptor 1 and Toll-like receptor 6. *J Infect Dis*. 2012;205(6):944–954.

268. Netea MG, Gow NA, Munro CA, Bates S, Collins C, Ferwerda G, et al. Immune sensing of Candida albicans requires cooperative recognition of mannans and glucans by lectin and Toll-like receptors. *J Clin Invest*. 2006;116(6):1642–1650.
269. Shoham S, Huang C, Chen JM, Golenbock DT, Levitz SM. Toll-like receptor 4 mediates intracellular signaling without TNF-alpha release in response to Cryptococcus neoformans polysaccharide capsule. *J Immunol*. 2001;166(7):4620–4626.
270. van de Veerdonk FL, Kullberg BJ, van der Meer JW, Gow NA, Netea MG. Host-microbe interactions: innate pattern recognition of fungal pathogens. *Curr Opin Microbiol*. 2008;11(4):305–312.
271. Ozinsky A, Underhill DM, Fontenot JD, Hajjar AM, Smith KD, Wilson CB, et al. The repertoire for pattern recognition of pathogens by the innate immune system is defined by cooperation between toll-like receptors. *Proc Natl Acad Sci U S A*. 2000;97(25):13766–13771.
272. Roeder A, Kirschning CJ, Schaller M, Weindl G, Wagner H, Korting HC, et al. Induction of nuclear factor- kappa B and c-Jun/activator protein-1 via toll-like receptor 2 in macrophages by antimycotic-treated Candida albicans. *J Infect Dis*. 2004;190(7):1318–1326.
273. Salvenmoser S, Seidler MJ, Dalpke A, Müller FM. Effects of caspofungin, Candida albicans and Aspergillus fumigatus on toll-like receptor 9 of GM-CSF-stimulated PMNs. *FEMS Immunol Med Microbiol*. 2010;60(1):74–77.
274. Beisswenger C, Hess C, Bals R. Aspergillus fumigatus conidia induce interferon-β signalling in respiratory epithelial cells. *Eur Respir J*. 2012;39(2):411–418.
275. Biondo C, Signorino G, Costa A, Midiri A, Gerace E, Galbo R, et al. Recognition of yeast nucleic acids triggers a host-protective type I interferon response. *Eur J Immunol*. 2011;41(7):1969–1979.
276. Kasperkovitz PV, Khan NS, Tam JM, Mansour MK, Davids PJ, Vyas JM. Toll-like receptor 9 modulates macrophage antifungal effector function during innate recognition of Candida albicans and Saccharomyces cerevisiae. *Infect Immun*. 2011;79(12):4858–4867.
277. Tanaka M, Ishii K, Nakamura Y, Miyazato A, Maki A, Abe Y, et al. Toll-like receptor 9-dependent activation of bone marrow-derived dendritic cells by URA5 DNA from Cryptococcus neoformans. *Infect Immun*. 2012;80(2):778–786.
278. Miyazato A, Nakamura K, Yamamoto N, Mora-Montes HM, Tanaka M, Abe Y, et al. Toll-like receptor 9-dependent activation of myeloid dendritic cells by Deoxynucleic acids from Candida albicans. *Infect Immun*. 2009;77(7):3056–3064.
279. DAMPs Bianchi ME. PAMPs and alarmins: all we need to know about danger. *J Leukocyte Biol*. 2007;81(1):1–5.
280. Sorci G, Giovannini G, Riuzzi F, Bonifazi P, Zelante T, Zagarella S, et al. The danger signal S100B integrates pathogen–and danger–sensing pathways to restrain inflammation. *PLoS Pathog*. 2011;7(3):e1001315.
281. Zelensky AN, Gready JE. The C-type lectin-like domain superfamily. *FEBS J*. 2005;272(24):6179–6217.
282. Shiokawa M, Yamasaki S, Saijo S. C-type lectin receptors in anti-fungal immunity. *Curr Opin Microbiol*. 2017;40:123–130.
283. Gantner BN, Simmons RM, Canavera SJ, Akira S, Underhill DM. Collaborative induction of inflammatory responses by dectin-1 and Toll-like receptor 2. *J Exp Med*. 2003;197(9):1107–1117.
284. Ariizumi K, Shen G-L, Shikano S, Xu S, Ritter R, Kumamoto T, et al. Identification of a novel, dendritic cell-associated molecule, dectin-1, by subtractive cDNA cloning. *J Biol Chem*. 2000;275(26):20157–20167.
285. Brown GD, Gordon S. A new receptor for β-glucans. *Nature*. 2001;413(6851):36–37.
286. Sato K, Yang X-l, Yudate T, Chung J-S, Wu J, Luby-Phelps K, et al. Dectin-2 is a pattern recognition receptor for fungi that couples with the Fc receptor γ chain to induce innate immune responses. *J Biol Chem*. 2006;281(50):38854–38866.
287. McGreal EP, Rosas M, Brown GD, Zamze S, Wong SY, Gordon S, et al. The carbohydrate-recognition domain of Dectin-2 is a C-type lectin with specificity for high mannose. *Glycobiology*. 2006;16(5):422–430.
288. Saijo S, Ikeda S, Yamabe K, Kakuta S, Ishigame H, Akitsu A, et al. Dectin-2 recognition of α-mannans and induction of Th17 cell differentiation is essential for host defense against Candida albicans. *Immunity*. 2010;32(5):681–691.

289. Ishikawa T, Itoh F, Yoshida S, Saijo S, Matsuzawa T, Gonoi T, et al. Identification of distinct ligands for the C-type lectin receptors Mincle and Dectin-2 in the pathogenic fungus Malassezia. *Cell host & microbe*. 2013;13(4):477–488.
290. Ifrim DC, Bain JM, Reid DM, Oosting M, Verschueren I, Gow NA, et al. Role of Dectin-2 for host defense against systemic infection with Candida glabrata. *Infect Immun*. 2014;82(3):1064–1073.
291. Shiokawa M, Yamasaki S, Saijo S. C-type lectin receptors in anti-fungal immunity. *Curr Opin Microbiol*. 2017;40:123–130.
292. Bourgeois C, Majer O, Frohner IE, Tierney L, Kuchler K. Fungal attacks on mammalian hosts: pathogen elimination requires sensing and tasting. *Curr Opin Microbiol*. 2010;13(4):401–408.
293. Cua DJ, Tato CM. Innate IL-17-producing cells: the sentinels of the immune system. *Nat Rev Immunol*. 2010;10(7):479–489.
294. Spits H, Artis D, Colonna M, Diefenbach A, Di Santo JP, Eberl G, et al. Innate lymphoid cells—a proposal for uniform nomenclature. *Nat Rev Immunol*. 2013;13(2):145–149.
295. Spits H, Artis D, Colonna M, Diefenbach A, Di Santo JP, Eberl G, et al. Innate lymphoid cells–a proposal for uniform nomenclature. *Nat Rev Immunol*. 2013;13(2):145–149.
296. Drummond RA, Gaffen SL, Hise AG, Brown GD. Innate Defense against Fungal Pathogens. *Cold Spring Harb Perspect Med*. 2014;5(6):a019620.
297. Cua DJ, Tato CM. Innate IL-17-producing cells: the sentinels of the immune system. *Nat Rev Immunol*. 2010;10(7):479–489.
298. Dromer F, Charreire J, Contrepois A, Carbon C, Yeni P. Protection of mice against experimental cryptococcosis by anti-Cryptococcus neoformans monoclonal antibody. *Infect Immun*. 1987;55(3):749–752.
299. Mukherjee J, Nussbaum G, Scharff MD. Casadevall A. Protective and nonprotective monoclonal antibodies to Cryptococcus neoformans originating from one B cell. *J Exp Med*. 1995;181(1):405–409.
300. Mukherjee J, Pirofski LA, Scharff MD, Casadevall A. Antibody-mediated protection in mice with lethal intracerebral Cryptococcus neoformans infection. *Proc Nat Acad Sci USA*. 1993;90(8):3636–3640.
301. Han Y, Cutler JE. Antibody response that protects against disseminated candidiasis. *Infect Immun*. 1995;63(7):2714–2719.
302. Nosanchuk JD, Steenbergen JN, Shi L, Deepe Jr GS, Casadevall A. Antibodies to a cell surface histone-like protein protect against Histoplasma capsulatum. *J Clin Invest*. 2003;112(8):1164–1175.
303. Edelson BT, Cossart P, Unanue ER. Cutting edge: paradigm revisited: antibody provides resistance to Listeria infection. *J Immunol*. 1999;163(8):4087–4090.
304. Teitelbaum R, Glatman-Freedman A, Chen B, Robbins JB, Unanue E, Casadevall A, et al. A mAb recognizing a surface antigen of Mycobacterium tuberculosis enhances host survival. *Proc Natl Acad Sci*. 1998;95(26):15688–15693.
305. Feldmesser M. Prospects of vaccines for invasive aspergillosis. *Med Mycol*. 2005;43(7):571–587.
306. Rappleye CA, Eissenberg LG, Goldman WE. Histoplasma capsulatum α-(1, 3)-glucan blocks innate immune recognition by the β-glucan receptor. *Proc Natl Acad Sci*. 2007;104(4):1366–1370.
307. Casadevall A, Feldmesser M, L-a Pirofski. Induced humoral immunity and vaccination against major human fungal pathogens. *Curr Opin Microbiol*. 2002;5(4):386–391.
308. Zheng M, Shellito JE, Marrero L, Zhong Q, Julian S, Ye P, et al. CD4+ T cell–independent vaccination against Pneumocystis carinii in mice. *J Clin Invest*. 2001;108(10):1469–1474.
309. Steinman RM, Hemmi H. Dendritic cells: translating innate to adaptive immunity. *From innate immunity to immunological memory*. 2006:17–58.
310. Pasare C, Medzhitov R. Toll-like receptors: linking innate and adaptive immunity. *Microbes Infect*. 2004;6(15):1382–1387.
311. Manicassamy S, Pulendran B. Modulation of adaptive immunity with Toll-like receptors. *Semin Immunol*. 2009;21(4):185–193.
312. Wüthrich M, Deepe Jr GS, Klein B. Adaptive immunity to fungi. *Annu Rev Immunol*. 2012;30:115–148.
313. Burnie JP. Developments in the serological diagnosis of opportunistic fungal infections. *J Antimicrob Chemother*. 1991;28(Suppl A):23–33.
314. Hamilton AJ. Serodiagnosis of histoplasmosis, paracoccidioidomycosis and penicilliosis marneffei; current status and future trends. *Med Mycol*. 1998;36(6):351–364.

315. Walsh TJ, Chanock SJ. Diagnosis of invasive fungal infections: advances in nonculture systems. *Curr Clin Top Infect Dis*. 1998;18:101–153.
316. de Repentigny L, Reiss E. Current trends in immunodiagnosis of candidiasis and aspergillosis. *Rev Infect Dis*. 1984;6(3):301–312.
317. Haynes KA, Latge JP, Rogers TR. Detection of Aspergillus antigens associated with invasive infection. *J Clin Microbiol*. 1990;28(9):2040–2044.
318. Yeo SF, Wong B. Current status of nonculture methods for diagnosis of invasive fungal infections. *Clin Microbiol Rev*. 2002;15(3):465–484.
319. Pemán J, Zaragoza R. Current diagnostic approaches to invasive candidiasis in critical care settings. *Mycoses*. 2010;53(5):424–433.
320. Navarro D, Monzonis E, López-Ribot JL, Sepúlveda P, Casanova M, Nogueira JM, et al. Diagnosis of systemic candidiasis by enzyme immunoassay detection of specific antibodies to mycelial phase cell wall and cytoplasmic candidal antigens. *Eur J Clin Microbiol Infect Dis*. 1993;12(11):839–846.
321. Green JH, Harrell WK, Johnson JE, Benson R. Isolation of an antigen from Blastomyces dermatitidis that is specific for the diagnosis of blastomycosis. *Curr Microbiol*. 1980;4(5):293–296.
322. Hurst SF, Kaufman L. Western immunoblot analysis and serologic characterization of Blastomyces dermatitidis yeast form extracellular antigens. *J Clin Microbiol*. 1992;30(12):3043–3049.
323. Bradsher RW, Pappas PG. Detection of specific antibodies in human blastomycosis by enzyme immunoassay. *South Med J*. 1995;88(12):1256–1259.
324. Klein BS, Vergeront JM, Kaufman L, Bradsher RW, Kumar UN, Mathai G, et al. Serological tests for blastomycosis: assessments during a large point-source outbreak in Wisconsin. *J Infect Dis*. 1987;155(2):262–268.
325. Klein BS, Vergeront JM, Disalvo AF, Kaufman L, Davis JP. Two outbreaks of blastomycosis along rivers in Wisconsin: isolation of Blastomyces dermatitidis from riverbank soil and evidence of its transmission along waterways. *Am Rev Respir Dis*. 1987;136(6):1333–1338.
326. Pappagianis D, Zimmer BL. Serology of coccidioidomycosis. *Clin Microbiol Rev*. 1990;3(3):247–268.
327. Roberts CJ. Coccidioidomycosis in acquired immune deficiency syndrome: depressed humoral as well as cellular immunity. *Am J Med*. 1984;76(4):734–736.
328. Bronnimann DA, Adam RD, Galgiani JN, Habib MP, Petersen EA, Porter B, et al. Coccidioidomycosis in the acquired immunodeficiency syndrome. *Ann Intern Med*. 1987;106(3):372–379.
329. Antoniskis D, Larsen RA, Akil B, Rarick MU, Leedom JM. Seronegative disseminated coccidioidomycosis in patients with HIV infection. *AIDS*. 1990;4(7):691–693.
330. Pine L. Histoplasma antigens: their production, purification and uses. *Contrib Microbiol Immunol*. 1977;3:138–168.
331. Flor A, Estivill D, Pérez R, Ordeig J, Ramos F, Bel JS, et al. Histoplasmosis pulmonar aguda en un viajero español a Nicaragua: ejemplo de enfermedad importada. *Rev Iberoam Micol*. 2003;20:24–28.
332. Reiss E, Knowles J, Bragg S, Kaufman L. Monoclonal antibodies against the M-protein and carbohydrate antigens of histoplasmin characterized by the enzyme-linked immunoelectrotransfer blot method. *Infect Immun*. 1986;53(3):540–546.
333. Kaufman L, Kovacs J, Reiss E. Clinical immunomycology. In: de Macario, Folds JD, Lane HC, Nakamura RM, eds. *Manual of Clinical Laboratory Immunology*. 5th ed Washington, DC: American Society for Microbiology; 1997:575–583.
334. Zancope-Oliveira R, Bragg S, Reiss E, Peralta J. Immunochemical analysis of the H and M glycoproteins from Histoplasma capsulatum. *Clin Diagn Lab Immunol*. 1994;1(5):563–568.
335. Zancopé-Oliveira R, Bragg S, Reiss E, Wanke B, Peralta J. Effects of histoplasmin M antigen chemical and enzymatic deglycosylation on cross-reactivity in the enzyme-linked immunoelectrotransfer blot method. *Clin Diagn Lab Immunol*. 1994;1(4):390–393.
336. Chandrashekar R, Curtis K, Rawot B, Kobayashi G, Weil G. Molecular cloning and characterization of a recombinant Histoplasma capsulatum antigen for antibody-based diagnosis of human histoplasmosis. *J Clin Microbiol*. 1997;35(5):1071–1076.
337. Deepe Jr GS, Durose GG. Immunobiological activity of recombinant H antigen from Histoplasma capsulatum. *Infect Immun*. 1995;63(8):3151–3157.
338. Hamilton A. Serodiagnosis of histoplasmosis, paracoccidioidomycosis and penicilliosis marneffei; current status and future trends. *Med Mycol*. 1998;36(6):351–364.

339. Restrepo AM. Immune response to Paracoccidioides brasiliensis in human and animal hosts. *Curr Top Med Mycol*. 1988:239–277.
340. Cano LE, Brummer E, Stevens DA, Restrepo A. An evaluation of the enzyme-linked immunoabsorbent assay (ELISA) for quantitation of antibodies to Paracoccidioides brasiliensis. *J Med Vet Mycol*. 1986;24(6):467–475.
341. Bueno J, Mendes-Giannini MJS, Del Negro G, Assis C, Takiguti C, Shikanai-Yasuda M. IgG, IgM and IgA antibody response for the diagnosis and follow-up of paracoccidioidomycosis: comparison of counterimmunoelectrophoresis and complement fixation. *J Med Vet Mycol*. 1997;35(3):213–217.
342. Bougnoux M-E, Dupont C, Mateo J, Saulnier P, Faivre V, Payen D, et al. Serum is more suitable than whole blood for diagnosis of systemic candidiasis by nested PCR. *J Clin Microbiol*. 1999;37(4):925–930.
343. Viviani M, Tortorano A, Rizzardini G, Quirino T, Kaufman L, Padhye A, et al. Treatment and serological studies of an Italian case of penicilliosis marneffei contracted in Thailand by a drug addict infected with the human immunodeficiency virus. *Eur J Epidemiol*. 1993;9(1):79–85.
344. Cao L, Chan C-m, Lee C, Sai-yin Wong S, Yuen K-y. MP1 encodes an abundant and highly antigenic cell wall mannoprotein in the pathogenic fungus Penicillium marneffei. *Infect Immun*. 1998;66(3):966–973.
345. Cao L, Chen DL, Lee C, Chan CM, Chan KM, Vanittanakom N, et al. Detection of specific antibodies to an antigenic mannoprotein for diagnosis of Penicillium marneffei penicilliosis. *J Clin Microbiol*. 1998;36(10):3028–3031.
346. Cao L, Chen D-L, Lee C, Chan C-M, Chan K-M, Vanittanakom N, et al. Detection of specific antibodies to an antigenic mannoprotein for diagnosis of Penicillium marneffei penicilliosis. *J Clin Microbiol*. 1998;36(10):3028–3031.
347. Choi S, Song JS, Kim JY, Cha HH, Yun JH, Park JW, et al. Diagnostic performance of immunohistochemistry for the aspergillosis and mucormycosis. *Mycoses*. 2019;62(11):1006–1014.
348. Gellin B, Modlin JF, Casadevall A, L-a Pirofski. Adjunctive immune therapy for fungal infections. *Clin Infect Dis*. 2001;33(7):1048–1056.
349. Segal BH, Kwon-Chung J, Walsh TJ, Klein BS, Battiwalla M, Almyroudis NG, et al. Immunotherapy for fungal infections. *Clin Infect Dis*. 2006;42(4):507–515.
350. Sam QH, Yew WS, Seneviratne CJ, Chang MW, Chai LYA. Immunomodulation as therapy for fungal infection: are we closer?. *Frontiers in microbiology*. 2018;9:1612.
351. Ademe M. Immunomodulation for the Treatment of Fungal Infections: Opportunities and Challenges. *Frontiers in cellular and infection microbiology*. 2020;10:469.
352. Deo SS, Gottlieb DJ. Adoptive T-cell therapy for fungal infections in haematology patients. *Clinical & translational immunology*. 2015;4(8):e40.
353. Perruccio K, Tosti A, Burchielli E, Topini F, Ruggeri L, Carotti A, et al. Transferring functional immune responses to pathogens after haploidentical hematopoietic transplantation. *Blood*. 2005;106(13):4397–4406.
354. Meiliana A, Dewi NM, Wijaya A. Cancer immunotherapy: a review. *The Indonesian Biomedical Journal*. 2016;8(1):1–20.
355. Lauruschkat CD, Einsele H, Loeffler J. Immunomodulation as a therapy for Aspergillus infection: current status and future perspectives. *Journal of Fungi*. 2018;4(4):137.
356. Kumaresan PR, Manuri PR, Albert ND, Maiti S, Singh H, Mi T, et al. Bioengineering T cells to target carbohydrate to treat opportunistic fungal infection. *Proc Natl Acad Sci U S A*. 2014;111(29):10660–10665.
357. Kochenderfer JN, Dudley ME, Feldman SA, Wilson WH, Spaner DE, Maric I, et al. B-cell depletion and remissions of malignancy along with cytokine-associated toxicity in a clinical trial of anti-CD19 chimeric-antigen-receptor-transduced T cells. *Blood*. 2012;119(12):2709–2720.
358. Brudno JN, Kochenderfer JN. Toxicities of chimeric antigen receptor T cells: recognition and management. *Blood*. 2016;127(26):3321–3330.
359. Neelapu SS, Locke FL, Bartlett NL, Lekakis LJ, Miklos DB, Jacobson CA, et al. Axicabtagene Ciloleucel CAR T-Cell Therapy in Refractory Large B-Cell Lymphoma. *N Engl J Med*. 2017;377(26):2531–2544.
360. Depil S, Duchateau P, Grupp SA, Mufti G, Poirot L. Off-the-shelf' allogeneic CAR T cells: development and challenges. *Nat Rev Drug Discov*. 2020;19(3):185–199.

361. Brecher G, Wilbur KM, Cronkite EP. Transfusion of separated leukocytes into irradiated dogs with aplastic marrows. *Proc Soc Exp Biol Med*. 1953;84(1):54–56.
362. Díaz R, Soundar E, Hartman SK, Dreyer Z, Teruya J, Hui S-KR. Granulocyte transfusions for children with infection and neutropenia or granulocyte dysfunction. *Pediatr Hematol Oncol*. 2014;31(5):425–434.
363. West KA, Gea-Banacloche J, Stroncek D, Kadri SS. Granulocyte transfusions in the management of invasive fungal infections. *Br J Haematol*. 2017;177(3):357–374.
364. Estcourt LJ, Stanworth SJ, Hopewell S, Doree C, Trivella M, Massey E. Granulocyte transfusions for treating infections in people with neutropenia or neutrophil dysfunction. *Cochrane Database Syst Rev*. 2016;4(4):CD005339.
365. Tacken PJ, Zeelenberg IS, Cruz LJ, van Hout-Kuijer MA, van de Glind G, Fokkink RG, et al. Targeted delivery of TLR ligands to human and mouse dendritic cells strongly enhances adjuvanticity. *Blood, The Journal of the American Society of Hematology*. 2011;118(26):6836–6844.
366. Roy René M, Klein Bruce S. Dendritic Cells in Antifungal Immunity and Vaccine Design. *Cell Host & Microbe*. 2012;11(5):436–446.
367. Bozza S, Perruccio K, Montagnoli C, Gaziano R, Bellocchio S, Burchielli E, et al. A dendritic cell vaccine against invasive aspergillosis in allogeneic hematopoietic transplantation. *Blood*. 2003;102(10):3807–3814.
368. Shao HJ, Chen L, Su YB. DNA fragment encoding human IL-1beta 163-171 peptide enhances the immune responses elicited in mice by DNA vaccine against foot-and-mouth disease. *Vet Res Commun*. 2005;29(1):35–46.
369. Ersland K, Wüthrich M, Klein BS. Dynamic interplay among monocyte-derived, dermal, and resident lymph node dendritic cells during the generation of vaccine immunity to fungi. *Cell Host Microbe*. 2010;7(6):474–487.
370. Stuehler C, Kuenzli E, Jaeger VK, Baettig V, Ferracin F, Rajacic Z, et al. Immune reconstitution after allogeneic hematopoietic stem cell transplantation and association with occurrence and outcome of invasive aspergillosis. *J Infect Dis*. 2015;212(6):959–967.
371. Wang R, Jaw JJ, Stutzman NC, Zou Z, Sun PD. Natural killer cell-produced IFN-γ and TNF-α induce target cell cytolysis through up-regulation of ICAM-1. *J Leukocyte Biol*. 2012;91(2):299–309.
372. Schneider A, Blatzer M, Posch W, Schubert R, Lass-Flörl C, Schmidt S, et al. Aspergillus fumigatus responds to natural killer (NK) cells with upregulation of stress related genes and inhibits the immunoregulatory function of NK cells. *Oncotarget*. 2016;7(44):71062.
373. Clark OA, Lyman GH, Castro AA, Clark LG, Djulbegovic B. Colony-stimulating factors for chemotherapy-induced febrile neutropenia: a meta-analysis of randomized controlled trials. *J Clin Oncol*. 2005;23(18):4198–4214.
374. Mhaskar R, Clark OAC, Lyman G, Botrel TEA, Paladini LM, Djulbegovic B. Colony-stimulating factors for chemotherapy-induced febrile neutropenia. *Cochrane Database of Systematic Reviews*. 2014(10).
375. Wan L, Zhang Y, Lai Y, Jiang M, Song Y, Zhou J, et al. Effect of granulocyte-macrophage colony-stimulating factor on prevention and treatment of invasive fungal disease in recipients of allogeneic stem-cell transplantation: a prospective multicenter randomized phase IV trial. *J Clin Oncol*. 2015;33(34):3999–4006.
376. Hovi L, Saarinen-Pihkala U, Vettenranta K, Saxen H. Invasive fungal infections in pediatric bone marrow transplant recipients: single center experience of 10 years. *Bone Marrow Transplant*. 2000;26(9):999–1004.
377. Goldman C, Akiyama MJ, Torres J, Louie E, Meehan SA. Scedosporium apiospermum infections and the role of combination antifungal therapy and GM-CSF: A case report and review of the literature. *Medical mycology case reports*. 2016;11:40–43.
378. Winn RM, Gil-Lamaignere C, Roilides E, Simitsopoulou M, Lyman CA, Maloukou A, et al. Selective effects of interleukin (IL)-15 on antifungal activity and IL-8 release by polymorphonuclear leukocytes in response to hyphae of Aspergillus species. *J Infect Dis*. 2003;188(4):585–590.
379. Stevens DA, Brummer E, Clemons KV. Interferon- gamma as an antifungal. *J Infect Dis*. 2006;194(Suppl 1):S33–S37.
380. Maizels RM, Yazdanbakhsh M. Immune regulation by helminth parasites: cellular and molecular mechanisms. *Nat Rev Immunol*. 2003;3(9):733–744.

381. Mehraj V, Hatcher J, Akhtar S, Rafique G, Beg MA. Prevalence and factors associated with intestinal parasitic infection among children in an urban slum of Karachi. *PLoS One*. 2008;3(11):e3680.
382. Taghipour A, Olfatifar M, Rostami A, Foroutan M, Vasigala V, Norouzi M. Intestinal parasites in hemodialysis patients from developing countries: A systematic review and meta-analysis. *Hemodialysis International*. 2020;24(1):12–21.
383. Bethony J, Brooker S, Albonico M, Geiger SM, Loukas A, Diemert D, et al. Soil-transmitted helminth infections: ascariasis, trichuriasis, and hookworm. *Lancet North Am Ed*. 2006;367(9521):1521–1532.
384. Watkins BM. Drugs for the control of parasitic diseases: current status and development. *Trends Parasitol*. 2003;19(11):477–478.
385. James SL, Abate D, Abate KH, Abay SM, Abbafati C, Abbasi N, et al. Global, regional, and national incidence, prevalence, and years lived with disability for 354 diseases and injuries for 195 countries and territories, 1990–2017: a systematic analysis for the Global Burden of Disease Study 2017. *Lancet North Am Ed*. 2018;392(10159):1789–1858.
386. Kirk MD, Pires SM, Black RE, Caipo M, Crump JA, Devleesschauwer B, et al. World Health Organization estimates of the global and regional disease burden of 22 foodborne bacterial, protozoal, and viral diseases, 2010: a data synthesis. *PLoS Med*. 2015;12(12):e1001921.
387. Taghipour A, Javanmard E, Haghighi A, Mirjalali H, Zali MR. The occurrence of Cryptosporidium sp., and eggs of soil-transmitted helminths in market vegetables in the north of Iran. *Gastroenterology and hepatology from bed to bench*. 2019;12(4):364.
388. Pereira A, Alencar M, Cohen S, Souza-Júnior P, CECCHETTO F, Mathias L, et al. The influence of health education on the prevalence of intestinal parasites in a low-income community of Campos dos Goytacazes, Rio de Janeiro State, Brazil. *Parasitology*. 2012;139(6):791–801.
389. Mahmud MA, Spigt M, Bezabih AM, Dinant G-J, Velasco RB. Associations between intestinal parasitic infections, anaemia, and diarrhoea among school aged children, and the impact of hand-washing and nail clipping. *BMC research notes*. 2020;13(1):1–6.
390. Taghipour A, Javanmard E, Mirjalali H, Haghighi A, Tabarsi P, Sohrabi MR, et al. Blastocystis subtype 1 (allele 4); predominant subtype among tuberculosis patients in Iran. *Comp Immunol Microbiol Infect Dis*. 2019;65:201–206.
391. Tsoka-Gwegweni JM, Ntombela N. A double load to carry: parasites and pregnancy. *Southern African Journal of Infectious Diseases*. 2014;29(2):52–55.
392. Garcia LS. Classification of human parasites, vectors, and similar organisms. *Clin Infect Dis*. 1999;29(4):734–736.
393. Varki A, Cummings RD, Esko JD, Stanley P, Hart GW, Aebi M, et al. Essentials of Glycobiology [internet]. 2015.
394. Davidson RA. Immunology of parasitic infections. *Med Clin North Am*. 1985;69(4):751–758.
395. Pearce EJ, Sher A. Mechanisms of immune evasion in schistosomiasis. *Contrib Microbiol Immunol*. 1987;8:219–232.
396. Anthony RM, Rutitzky LI, Urban Jr JF, Stadecker MJ, Gause WC. Protective immune mechanisms in helminth infection. *Nat Rev Immunol*. 2007;7(12):975–987.
397. MacDonald AS, Araujo MI, Pearce EJ. *Immunology of Parasitic Helminth Infections Infection and Immunity*. 2002;70(2):427–433.
398. Tedla MG, Every AL, Scheerlinck J-PY. Investigating immune responses to parasites using transgenesis. *Parasites & Vectors*. 2019;12(1).
399. Brindley PJ, Mitreva M, Ghedin E, Lustigman S. Helminth genomics: The implications for human health. *PLoS Negl Trop Dis*. 2009;3(10):e538.
400. Stevenson FK, Genova GD, Ottensmeier C, Savelyeva N. Chapter 11 - Cancer Vaccines. In: Prendergast GC, Jaffee EM, eds. *Cancer Immunotherapy*. Burlington: Academic Press; 2007:183–204.
401. Yazdanbakhsh M, Sacks DL. Why does immunity to parasites take so long to develop?. *Nat Rev Immunol*. 2010;10(2):80–81.
402. Schmid-Hempel P. Immune defence, parasite evasion strategies and their relevance for 'macroscopic phenomena' such as virulence. *Philos Trans R Soc Lond B Biol Sci*. 2009;364(1513):85–98.
403. Merien FA. Journey with Elie Metchnikoff: From Innate Cell Mechanisms in Infectious Diseases to Quantum Biology. *Front Public Health*. 2016;4:125.
404. Metchnikoff E. Lectures on the comparative pathology of inflammation delivered at the Pasteur Institute in 1891: Рипол Классик; 1893.

405. Burza S, Croft SL, Boelaert M. Leishmaniasis. *Lancet*. 2018;392(10151):951–970.
406. Hohman LS, Peters NC. CD4(+) T Cell-Mediated Immunity against the Phagosomal Pathogen Leishmania: Implications for Vaccination. *Trends Parasitol*. 2019;35(6):423–435.
407. Sacks D, Sher A. Evasion of innate immunity by parasitic protozoa. *Nat Immunol*. 2002;3(11):1041–1047.
408. Alexander J, Vickerman K. Fusion of host cell secondary lysosomes with the parasitophorous vacuoles of Leishmania mexicana-infected macrophages. *J Protozool*. 1975;22(4):502–508.
409. Chang KP, Dwyer DM. Multiplication of a human parasite (Leishmania donovani) in phagolysosomes of hamster macrophages in vitro. *Science*. 1976;193(4254):678–680.
410. Chang KP, Dwyer DM. Leishmania donovani. Hamster macrophage interactions in vitro: cell entry, intracellular survival, and multiplication of amastigotes. *J Exp Med*. 1978;147(2):515–530.
411. Lewis DH, Peters W. The resistance of intracellular Leishmania parasites to digestion by lysosomal enzymes. *Ann Trop Med Parasitol*. 1977;71(3):295–312.
412. Carneiro MB, Hohman LS, Egen JG, Peters NC. Use of two-photon microscopy to study Leishmania major infection of the skin. *Methods*. 2017;127:45–52.
413. Peters NC, Egen JG, Secundino N, Debrabant A, Kimblin N, Kamhawi S, et al. In vivo imaging reveals an essential role for neutrophils in leishmaniasis transmitted by sand flies. *Science*. 2008;321(5891):970–974.
414. Scott P, Natovitz P, Coffman RL, Pearce E, Sher A. Immunoregulation of cutaneous leishmaniasis. T cell lines that transfer protective immunity or exacerbation belong to different T helper subsets and respond to distinct parasite antigens. *J Exp Med*. 1988;168(5):1675–1684.
415. Carneiro MB, Peters NC. The Paradox of a Phagosomal Lifestyle: How Innate Host Cell-Leishmania amazonensis Interactions Lead to a Progressive Chronic Disease. *Front Immunol*. 2021;12(3468).
416. Hornef MW, Wick MJ, Rhen M, Normark S. Bacterial strategies for overcoming host innate and adaptive immune responses. *Nat Immunol*. 2002;3(11):1033–1040.
417. Hilbi H, Zychlinsky A, Sansonetti P. Macrophage apoptosis in microbial infections. *Parasitology*. 1997;115(7):79–87.
418. Celias DP, Motrán CC, Cervi L. Helminths turning on the NLRP3 inflammasome: pros and cons. *Trends Parasitol*. 2020;36(2):87–90.
419. de Carvalho RV, Zamboni DS. Inflammasome activation in response to intracellular protozoan parasites. *Trends Parasitol*. 2020;36(5):459–472.
420. Chavarría-Smith J, Vance RE. The NLRP 1 inflammasomes. *Immunol Rev*. 2015;265(1):22–34.
421. Shaw DK, McClure EE, Wang X, Pedra JHF. Deviant Behavior: Tick-Borne Pathogens and Inflammasome Signaling. *Vet Sci*. 2016;3(4):27.
422. Delfino D, Chiofalo MS, Riggio G, Angelici MC, Gramiccia M, Gradoni L, et al. Induction of interleukin 1α in murine macrophages infected in vitro with different species and strains of Leishmania. *Microb Pathog*. 1995;18(2):73–80.
423. Lima-Junior DS, Costa DL, Carregaro V, Cunha LD, Silva AL, Mineo TW, et al. Inflammasome-derived IL-1β production induces nitric oxide–mediated resistance to Leishmania. *Nat Med*. 2013;19(7):909–915.
424. Lima-Junior DS, Mineo TW, Calich VL, Zamboni DS. Dectin-1 activation during Leishmania amazonensis phagocytosis prompts Syk-dependent reactive oxygen species production to trigger inflammasome assembly and restriction of parasite replication. *J Immunol*. 2017;199(6):2055–2068.
425. de Carvalho RV, Andrade WA, Lima-Junior DS, Dilucca M, de Oliveira CV, Wang K, et al. Leishmania lipophosphoglycan triggers caspase-11 and the non-canonical activation of the NLRP3 inflammasome. *Cell Rep*. 2019;26(2):429–437 e5.
426. Lecoeur H, Prina E, Rosazza T, Kokou K, N'Diaye P, Aulner N, et al. Targeting macrophage histone H3 modification as a Leishmania strategy to dampen the NF-κB/NLRP3-Mediated inflammatory response. *Cell Rep*. 2020;30(6):1870–1882 e4.
427. Zamboni DS, Sacks DL. Inflammasomes and Leishmania: in good times or bad, in sickness or in health. *Curr Opin Microbiol*. 2019;52:70–76.
428. Chaves MM, Sinflorio DA, Thorstenberg ML, Martins MDA, Moreira-Souza ACA, Rangel TP, et al. Non-canonical NLRP3 inflammasome activation and IL-1β signaling are necessary to L. amazonensis control mediated by P2X7 receptor and leukotriene B4. *PLoS Pathog*. 2019;15(6):e1007887.

429. de Carvalho RV, Silva AL, Santos LL, Andrade WA, de Sá KS, Zamboni DS. Macrophage priming is dispensable for NLRP3 inflammasome activation and restriction of Leishmania amazonensis replication. *J Leukocyte Biol*. 2019;106(3):631–640.
430. Novais FO, Carvalho AM, Clark ML, Carvalho LP, Beiting DP, Brodsky IE, et al. CD8+ T cell cytotoxicity mediates pathology in the skin by inflammasome activation and IL-1β production. *PLoS Pathog*. 2017;13(2):e1006196.
431. Charmoy M, Hurrell BP, Romano A, Lee SH, Ribeiro-Gomes F, Riteau N, et al. The Nlrp3 inflammasome, IL-1β, and neutrophil recruitment are required for susceptibility to a nonhealing strain of Leishmania major in C57BL/6 mice. *Eur J Immunol*. 2016;46(4):897–911.
432. Gupta G, Santana AK, Gomes CM, Turatti A, Milanezi CM, Bueno Filho R, et al. Inflammasome gene expression is associated with immunopathology in human localized cutaneous leishmaniasis. *Cell Immunol*. 2019;341:103920.
433. Santos D, Campos TM, Saldanha M, Oliveira SC, Nascimento M, Zamboni DS, et al. IL-1β production by intermediate monocytes is associated with immunopathology in cutaneous leishmaniasis. *J Invest Dermatol*. 2018;138(5):1107–1115.
434. Muhangi L, Woodburn P, Omara M, Omoding N, Kizito D, Mpairwe H, et al. Associations between mild-to-moderate anaemia in pregnancy and helminth, malaria and HIV infection in Entebbe. *Uganda Transactions of the Royal Society of Tropical Medicine and Hygiene*. 2007;101(9):899–907.
435. McGuinness DH, Dehal PK. Pleass RJ. Pattern recognition molecules and innate immunity to parasites. *Trends Parasitol*. 2003;19(7):312–319.
436. Denkers EY, Butcher BA, Del Rio L, Bennouna S. Neutrophils, dendritic cells and Toxoplasma. *Int J Parasitol*. 2004;34(3):411–421.
437. Brown WC, Corral RS. Stimulation of B lymphocytes, macrophages, and dendritic cells by protozoan DNA. *Microbes Infect*. 2002;4(9):969–974.
438. Daniel-Ribeiro CT, Zanini G. Autoimmunity and malaria: what are they doing together?. *Acta Trop*. 2000;76(3):205–221.
439. Tormo N, del Remedio Guna M, Teresa Fraile M, Dolores Ocete M, Garcia A, Navalpotro D, et al. Immunity to Parasites. *Current Immunology Reviews*. 2011;7(1):25–43.
440. Turner MW. Mannose-binding lectin: the pluripotent molecule of the innate immune system. *Immunol Today*. 1996;17(11):532–540.
441. Green PJ, Feizi T, Stoll MS, Thiel S, Prescott A, McConville MJ. Recognition of the major cell surface glycoconjugates of Leishmania parasites by the human serum mannan-binding protein. *Mol Biochem Parasitol*. 1994;66(2):319–328.
442. Klabunde J, Uhlemann A-C, Tebo AE, Kimmel J, Schwarz RT, Kremsner PG, et al. Recognition of Plasmodium falciparum proteins by mannan-binding lectin, a component of the human innate immune system. *Parasitol Res*. 2002;88(2):113–117.
443. Garred P, Nielsen MA, Kurtzhals JA, Malhotra R, Madsen HO, Goka BQ, et al. Mannose-binding lectin is a disease modifier in clinical malaria and may function as opsonin for Plasmodium falciparum-infected erythrocytes. *Infect Immun*. 2003;71(9):5245–5253.
444. Kahn S, Wleklinski M, Aruffo A, Farr A, Coder D, Kahn M. Trypanosoma cruzi amastigote adhesion to macrophages is facilitated by the mannose receptor. *J Exp Med*. 1995;182(5):1243–1258.
445. Kahn SJ, Wleklinski M, Ezekowitz R, Coder D, Aruffo A, Farr A. The major surface glycoprotein of Trypanosoma cruzi amastigotes are ligands of the human serum mannose-binding protein. *Infect Immun*. 1996;64(7):2649–2656.
446. Klabunde J, Berger J, Jensenius JC, Klinkert M-Q, Zelck UE, Kremsner PG, et al. Schistosoma mansoni: adhesion of mannan-binding lectin to surface glycoproteins of cercariae and adult worms. *Exp Parasitol*. 2000;95(4):231–239.
447. Gruden-Movsesijan A, Petrovic M, Sofronic-Milosavljevic L. Interaction of mannan-binding lectin with Trichinella spiralis glycoproteins, a possible innate immune mechanism. *Parasite Immunol*. 2003;25(11-12):545–552.
448. Culley FJ, Harris RA, Kaye PM, McAdam K. Raynes JG. C-reactive protein binds to a novel ligand on Leishmania donovani and increases uptake into human macrophages. *J Immunol*. 1996;156(12):4691–4696.
449. Pied S, Nussler A, Pontent M, Miltgen F, Matile H, Lambert P, et al. C-reactive protein protects against preerythrocytic stages of malaria. *Infect Immun*. 1989;57(1):278–282.

450. Bout D, Joseph M, Pontet M, Vorng H, Deslee D, Capron A. Rat resistance to schistosomiasis: platelet-mediated cytotoxicity induced by C-reactive protein. *Science*. 1986;231(4734):153–156.
451. van Die I, van Vliet SJ, Nyame AK, Cummings RD, Bank CM, Appelmelk B, et al. The dendritic cell–specific C-type lectin DC-SIGN is a receptor for Schistosoma mansoni egg antigens and recognizes the glycan antigen Lewis x. *Glycobiology*. 2003;13(6):471–478.
452. Appelmelk BJ, van Die I, van Vliet SJ, Vandenbroucke-Grauls CM, Geijtenbeek TB, van Kooyk Y. Cutting edge: carbohydrate profiling identifies new pathogens that interact with dendritic cell-specific ICAM-3-grabbing nonintegrin on dendritic cells. *J Immunol*. 2003;170(4):1635–1639.
453. Colmenares M, Corbí AL, Turco SJ, Rivas L. The dendritic cell receptor DC-SIGN discriminates among species and life cycle forms of Leishmania. *J Immunol*. 2004;172(2):1186–1190.
454. Colmenares Ma, Puig-Kröger A, Pello OM, Corbí AL, Rivas L. Dendritic Cell (DC)-specific Intercellular Adhesion Molecule 3 (ICAM-3)-grabbing Nonintegrin (DC-SIGN, CD209), a C-type Surface Lectin in Human DCs, Is a Receptor for LeishmaniaAmastigotes. *J Biol Chem*. 2002;277(39):36766–36769.
455. Perrigoue JG, Marshall FA, Artis D. On the hunt for helminths: innate immune cells in the recognition and response to helminth parasites. *Cell Microbiol*. 2008;10(9):1757–1764.
456. Patel SN, Serghides L, Smith TG, Febbraio M, Silverstein RL, Kurtz TW, et al. CD36 mediates the phagocytosis of Plasmodium falciparum–infected erythrocytes by rodent macrophages. *J Infect Dis*. 2004;189(2):204–213.
457. Urban BC, Roberts DJ. Malaria, monocytes, macrophages and myeloid dendritic cells: sticking of infected erythrocytes switches off host cells. *Curr Opin Immunol*. 2002;14(4):458–465.
458. Carter CR, Whitcomb JP, Campbell JA, Mukbel RM, McDowell MA. Complement receptor 3 deficiency influences lesion progression during Leishmania major infection in BALB/c mice. *Infect Immun*. 2009;77(12):5668–5675.
459. Hoft DF, Schnapp AR, Eickhoff CS, Roodman ST. Involvement of CD4+ Th1 cells in systemic immunity protective against primary and secondary challenges with Trypanosoma cruzi. *Infect Immun*. 2000;68(1):197–204.
460. Morisaki JH, Heuser JE, Sibley LD. Invasion of Toxoplasma gondii occurs by active penetration of the host cell. *J Cell Sci*. 1995;108(6):2457–2464.
461. Suzuki E, Tanaka AK, Toledo MS, Takahashi HK, Straus AH. Role of β-D-galactofuranose in Leishmania major macrophage invasion. *Infect Immun*. 2002;70(12):6592–6596.
462. Handman E, Bullen DV. Interaction of Leishmania with the host macrophage. *Trends Parasitol*. 2002;18(8):332–334.
463. Doolan D, Martinez-Alier N. Immune response to pre-erythrocytic stages of malaria parasites. *Curr Mol Med*. 2006;6(2):169–185.
464. Romero P, Maryanski JL, Corradin G, Nussenzweig RS, Nussenzweig V, Zavala F. Cloned cytotoxic T cells recognize an epitope in the circumsporozoite protein and protect against malaria. *Nature*. 1989;341(6240):323–326.
465. Goncalves R, Christensen SM, Mosser DM. Humoral immunity in leishmaniasis – Prevention or promotion of parasite growth?. *Cytokine: X*. 2020;2(4):100046.
466. Usui T, Preiss JC, Kanno Y, Yao ZJ, Bream JH, O'Shea JJ, et al. T-bet regulates Th1 responses through essential effects on GATA-3 function rather than on IFNG gene acetylation and transcription. *J Exp Med*. 2006;203(3):755–766.
467. Finkelman F, Katona I, Mosmann T, Coffman R. IFN-gamma regulates the isotypes of Ig secreted during in vivo humoral immune responses. *J Immunol*. 1988;140(4):1022–1027.
468. Tripathi P, Singh V, Naik S. Immune response to leishmania: paradox rather than paradigm. *FEMS Immunology & Medical Microbiology*. 2007;51(2):229–242.
469. Denkers EY, Gazzinelli RT. Regulation and function of T-cell-mediated immunity during Toxoplasma gondii infection. *Clin Microbiol Rev*. 1998;11(4):569–588.
470. Overstreet MG, Cockburn IA, Chen YC, Zavala F. Protective CD8+ T cells against Plasmodium liver stages: immunobiology of an 'unnatural'immune response. *Immunol Rev*. 2008;225(1):272–283.
471. Mueller A-K, Deckert M, Heiss K, Goetz K, Matuschewski K, Schlüter D. Genetically Attenuated Plasmodium berghei Liver Stages Persist and Elicit Sterile Protection Primarily via CD8 T Cells. *Am J Pathol*. 2007;171(1):107–115.

472. H. FELL A, CURRIER J, F. GOOD M. Inhibition of Plasmodium falciparum growth in vitro by CD4+ and CD8+ T cells from non-exposed donors. *Parasite Immunol*. 1994;16(11):579–586.
473. Perlmann P. Malaria and the immune system in humans. *Malaria Immonology*. 2002:229–242.
474. Miyakoda M, Kimura D, Yuda M, Chinzei Y, Shibata Y, Honma K, et al. Malaria-Specific and Nonspecific Activation of CD8$^{+}$T Cells during Blood Stage of <em>Plasmodium berghei</em>Infection. *J Immunol*. 2008;181(2):1420–1428.
475. Martin DL, Weatherly DB, Laucella SA, Cabinian MA, Crim MT, Sullivan S, et al. CD8+ T-Cell Responses to Trypanosoma cruzi Are Highly Focused on Strain-Variant trans-Sialidase Epitopes. *PLoS Pathog*. 2006;2(8):e77.
476. Miyahira Y. Trypanosoma cruzi infection from the view of CD8+ T cell immunity — An infection model for developing T cell vaccine. *Parasitol Int*. 2008;57(1):38–48.
477. Abass EM, Mansour D, el Harith A. Demonstration of agglutinating anti-Leishmania antibodies in lymph node aspirate for confirmation of kala-azar serodiagnosis. *J Med Microbiol*. 2007;56(9):1256–1258.
478. Cordeiro FD, Martins-Filho OA, Rocha MODC, Adad SJ, Corrêa-Oliveira R, Romanha AJ. Anti-Trypanosoma cruzi Immunoglobulin G1 Can Be a Useful Tool for Diagnosis and Prognosis of Human Chagas' Disease. *Clinical Diagnostic Laboratory Immunology*. 2001;8(1):112–118.
479. Couper KN, Roberts CW, Brombacher F, Alexander J, Johnson LL. Toxoplasma gondii-Specific Immunoglobulin M Limits Parasite Dissemination by Preventing Host Cell Invasion. *Infect Immun*. 2005;73(12):8060–8068.
480. Beck HP, Felger I, Genton B, Alexander N, al-Yaman F, Anders RF, et al. Humoral and cell-mediated immunity to the Plasmodium falciparum ring-infected erythrocyte surface antigen in an adult population exposed to highly endemic malaria. *Infect Immun*. 1995;63(2):596–600.
481. Magez S, Schwegmann A, Atkinson R, Claes F, Drennan M, De Baetselier P, et al. The Role of B-cells and IgM Antibodies in Parasitemia, Anemia, and VSG Switching in Trypanosoma brucei–Infected Mice. *PLoS Pathog*. 2008;4(8):e1000122.
482. Schopf LR, Filutowicz H, Bi X-J, Mansfield JM. Interleukin-4-Dependent Immunoglobulin G1 Isotype Switch in the Presence of a Polarized Antigen-Specific Th1-Cell Response to the Trypanosome Variant Surface Glycoprotein. *Infect Immun*. 1998;66(2):451–461.
483. Diffley P. Trypanosoma brucei: Immunogenicity of the variant surface coat glycoprotein of virulent and avirulent subspecies. *Exp Parasitol*. 1985;59(1):98–107.
484. Mansfield JM, Radwanska M, Magez S, Michel A, Stijlemans B, Geuskens M, et al. Comparative Analysis of Antibody Responses against HSP60, Invariant Surface Glycoprotein 70, and Variant Surface Glycoprotein Reveals a Complex Antigen-Specific Pattern of Immunoglobulin Isotype Switching during Infection by *Trypanosoma brucei*. *Infect Immun*. 2000;68(2):848–860.
485. Almeida IC, Milani SR, Gorin PA, Travassos LR. Complement-mediated lysis of Trypanosoma cruzi trypomastigotes by human anti-alpha-galactosyl antibodies. *J Immunol*. 1991;146(7):2394–2400.
486. Healer J, McGuinness D, Hopcroft P, Haley S, Carter R, Riley E. Complement-mediated lysis of Plasmodium falciparum gametes by malaria-immune human sera is associated with antibodies to the gamete surface antigen Pfs230. *Infect Immun*. 1997;65(8):3017–3023.
487. Bhopale G. Pathogenesis of toxoplasmosis. *Comp Immunol Microbiol Infect Dis*. 2003;26(4):213–222.
488. Bloom BR. Games parasites play: how parasites evade immune surveillance. *Nature*. 1979;279(5708):21–26.
489. Frank SA. *Immunology and Evolution of Infectious Disease*: Princeton University Press; 2020.
490. Sacks D, Sher A. Evasion of innate immunity by parasitic protozoa. *Nat Immunol*. 2002;3(11):1041–1047.
491. Turner C. A perspective on clonal phenotypic (antigenic) variation in protozoan parasites. *Parasitology*. 2002;125(7):S17–S23.
492. Barbour AG, Dai Q, Restrepo BI, Stoenner HG, Frank SA. Pathogen escape from host immunity by a genome program for antigenic variation. *Proc Natl Acad Sci*. 2006;103(48):18290–18295.
493. Van Der Woude MW, Bäumler AJ. Phase and antigenic variation in bacteria. *Clin Microbiol Rev*. 2004;17(3):581–611.
494. Blaxter M, Page A, Rudin W, Maizels R. Nematode surface coats: actively evading immunity. *Parasitol Today*. 1992;8(7):243–247.

495. Kent SJ, Fernandez CS, Dale CJ, Davenport MP. Reversion of immune escape HIV variants upon transmission: insights into effective viral immunity. *Trends Microbiol*. 2005;13(6):243–246.
496. Lewis K. Persister cells, dormancy and infectious disease. *Nat Rev Microbiol*. 2007;5(1):48–56.
497. Kapadia SB, Levine B, Speck SH, Virgin IV HW. Critical role of complement and viral evasion of complement in acute, persistent, and latent γ-herpesvirus infection. *Immunity*. 2002;17(2):143–155.
498. Hancock K, Tsang VC. Development and optimization of the FAST-ELISA for detecting antibodies to Schistosoma mansoni. *J Immunol Methods*. 1986;92(2):167–176.
499. Campbell G, Aley S, Ballou W, Hall T, Hockmeyer W, Hollingdale M, et al. *Use of Synthetic and Recombinant Peptides in the Study of Host-Parasite Interactions in the Malarias*: NAVAL MEDICAL RESEARCH INST BETHESDA MD; 1987.
500. Hillyer GV, de Galanes MS, Rodriguez-Perez J, Bjorland J, de Lagrava MS, Guzman SR, et al. Use of the Falcon™ assay screening test-enzyme-linked immunosorbent assay (FAST-ELISA) and the enzyme-linked immunoelectrotransfer blot (EITB) to determine the prevalence of human fascioliasis in the Bolivian altiplano. *Am J Trop Med Hyg*. 1992;46(5):603–609.
501. Ko R, Ng T. Evaluation of excretory/secretory products of larval Taenia solium as diagnostic antigens for porcine and human cysticercosis. *J Helminthol*. 1998;72(2):147–154.
502. Maddison SE. The present status of serodiagnosis and seroepidemiology of schistosomiasis. *Diagn Microbiol Infect Dis*. 1987;7(2):93–105.
503. Rahimi MT, Ashrafi K, Koosha S, Abdi J, Rokni MB. Evaluation of Fast-ELISA versus standard-ELISA to diagnose human fasciolosis. 2011.
504. Pappas MG. Recent applications of the Dot-ELISA in immunoparasitology. *Vet Parasitol*. 1988;29(2-3):105–129.
505. Courtioux B, Bisser S, M'belesso P, Ngoungou E, Girard M, Nangouma A, et al. Dot enzyme-linked immunosorbent assay for more reliable staging of patients with human African trypanosomiasis. *J Clin Microbiol*. 2005;43(9):4789–4795.
506. Kumar N, Ghosh S, Gupta S. Early detection of Fasciola gigantica infection in buffaloes by enzyme-linked immunosorbent assay and dot enzyme-linked immunosorbent assay. *Parasitol Res*. 2008;103(1):141–150.
507. Prasad A, Nasir A, Singh N.
Detection of anti–Haemonchus contortus antibodies in sheep by dot-ELISA with immunoaffinity purified fraction of ES antigen during prepatency. 2008.
508. Carrasco HJ, Torrellas A, García C, Segovia M, Feliciangeli MD. Risk of Trypanosoma cruzi I (Kinetoplastida: Trypanosomatidae) transmission by Panstrongylus geniculatus (Hemiptera: Reduviidae) in Caracas (metropolitan district) and neighboring states. *Venezuela International Journal for Parasitology*. 2005;35(13):1379–1384.
509. Kumar S, Kumar R, Gupta A, Dwivedi S. Passive transfer of Theileria equi antibodies to neonate foals of immune tolerant mares. *Vet Parasitol*. 2008;151(1):80–85.
510. Murray CK, Gasser Jr RA, Magill AJ, Miller RS. Update on rapid diagnostic testing for malaria. *Clin Microbiol Rev*. 2008;21(1):97–110.
511. Drakeley C, Reyburn H. Out with the old, in with the new: the utility of rapid diagnostic tests for malaria diagnosis in Africa. *Trans R Soc Trop Med Hyg*. 2009;103(4):333–337.
512. Shokoples SE, Ndao M, Kowalewska-Grochowska K, Yanow SK. Multiplexed real-time PCR assay for discrimination of Plasmodium species with improved sensitivity for mixed infections. *J Clin Microbiol*. 2009;47(4):975–980.
513. Burbelo PD, Goldman R, Mattson TL. A simplified immunoprecipitation method for quantitatively measuring antibody responses in clinical sera samples by using mammalian-produced Renilla luciferase-antigen fusion proteins. *BMC Biotech*. 2005;5(1):1–10.
514. Burbelo PD, Ramanathan R, Klion AD, Iadarola MJ, Nutman TB. Rapid, novel, specific, high-throughput assay for diagnosis of Loa loa infection. *J Clin Microbiol*. 2008;46(7):2298–2304.
515. Ramanathan R, Burbelo PD, Groot S, Iadarola MJ, Neva FA, Nutman TB. A luciferase immunoprecipitation systems assay enhances the sensitivity and specificity of diagnosis of Strongyloides stercoralis infection. *J Infect Dis*. 2008;198(3):444–451.
516. AdC Vexenat, Santana JM, Teixeira AR. Cross-reactivity of antibodies in human infections by the kinetoplastid protozoa Trypanosoma cruzi, Leishmania chagasi and Leishmania (Viannia) braziliensis. *Revista do Instituto de Medicina Tropical de São Paulo*. 1996;38(3):177–185.

517. Singh B. Molecular methods for diagnosis and epidemiological studies of parasitic infections. *Int J Parasitol*. 1997;27(10):1135–1145.
518. Moro P, Schantz PM. Echinococcosis: a review. *Int J Infect Dis*. 2009;13(2):125–133.
519. CDC A. *Parasites–Leishmaniasis*: Center for Disease Control and Prevention; 2013.
520. Genaro O, de Toledo VP, da Costa CA, Hermeto MV, Afonso LC, Mayrink W. Vaccine for prophylaxis and immunotherapy. *Brazil Clin Dermatol*. 1996;14(5):503–512.
521. Mayrink W, Botelho AC, Magalhães PA, Batista SM, Lima Ade O, Genaro O, et al. Immunotherapy, immunochemotherapy and chemotherapy for American cutaneous leishmaniasis treatment. *Rev Soc Bras Med Trop*. 2006;39(1):14–21.
522. Mayrink W, Magalhaes PA, Michalick MS, da Costa CA, Lima Ade O, Melo MN, et al. Immunotherapy as a treatment of American cutaneous leishmaniasis: preliminary studies in Brazil. *Parassitologia*. 1992;34(1-3):159–165.
523. Convit J, Castellanos PL, Rondon A, Pinardi ME, Ulrich M, Castes M, et al. Immunotherapy versus chemotherapy in localised cutaneous leishmaniasis. *Lancet*. 1987;1(8530):401–405.
524. Badaro R, Lobo I, Munos A, Netto EM, Modabber F, Campos-Neto A, et al. Immunotherapy for drug-refractory mucosal leishmaniasis. *J Infect Dis*. 2006;194(8):1151–1159.
525. Machado-Pinto J, Pinto J, da Costa CA, Genaro O, Marques MJ, Modabber F, et al. Immunochemotherapy for cutaneous leishmaniasis: a controlled trial using killed Leishmania (Leishmania) amazonensis vaccine plus antimonial. *Int J Dermatol*. 2002;41(2):73–78.
526. Convit J, Castellanos PL, Ulrich M, Castés M, Rondón A, Pinardi ME, et al. Immunotherapy of localized, intermediate, and diffuse forms of American cutaneous leishmaniasis. *J Infect Dis*. 1989;160(1):104–115.
527. Convit J, Ulrich M, Zerpa O, Borges R, Aranzazu N, Valera M, et al. Immunotherapy of american cutaneous leishmaniasis in Venezuela during the period 1990-99. *Trans R Soc Trop Med Hyg*. 2003;97(4):469–472.
528. Borja-Cabrera GP, Cruz Mendes A, Paraguai de Souza E, Hashimoto Okada LY, de ATFA, Kawasaki JK, et al. Effective immunotherapy against canine visceral leishmaniasis with the FML-vaccine. *Vaccine*. 2004;22(17-18):2234–2243.
529. Santos WR, Aguiar IA, Paraguai de Souza E, de Lima VM, Palatnik M. Palatnik-de-Sousa CB. Immunotherapy against murine experimental visceral leishmaniasis with the FML-vaccine. *Vaccine*. 2003;21(32):4668–4676.
530. Cabrera M, Blackwell JM, Castes M, Trujillo D, Convit J, Shaw MA. Immunotherapy with live BCG plus heat killed Leishmania induces a T helper 1-like response in American cutaneous leishmaniasis patients. *Parasite Immunol*. 2000;22(2):73–79.
531. Barral-Netto M, da Silva JS, Barral A, Reed S. Up-regulation of T helper 2 and down-regulation of T helper 1 cytokines during murine retrovirus-induced immunodeficiency syndrome enhances susceptibility of a resistant mouse strain to Leishmania amazonensis. *Am J Pathol*. 1995;146(3):635–642.
532. Holaday BJ, Sadick MD, Wang ZE, Reiner SL, Heinzel FP, Parslow TG, et al. Reconstitution of Leishmania immunity in severe combined immunodeficient mice using Th1- and Th2-like cell lines. *J Immunol*. 1991;147(5):1653–1658.
533. Verwaerde C, Thiam K, Delanoye A, Fernandez-Gomez R, D'Halluin J, Auriault C. Systemic delivery of an adenovirus expressing EBV-derived vIL-10 in mice infected with Schistosoma mansoni or Leishmania amazonensis: controversial effects on the development of pathological parameters. *Eur Cytokine Netw*. 1999;10(2):161–170.
534. Fayer R, Xiao L. *Cryptosporidium and Cryptosporidiosis*: CRC press; 2007.
535. Jafari R, Gharibi Z, Fallah M. The prevalence of cryptosporidium infection among renal transplanted patients in Hamadan city, West of Iran. *Avicenna Journal of Clinical Microbiology and Infection*. 2014;1(1):19570.
536. Jafari R, Maghsood AH, Fallah M. Prevalence of Cryptosporidium infection among livestock and humans in contact with livestock in Hamadan district, Iran, 2012. *J Res Health Sci*. 2012;13(1):86–89.
537. Jafari R, Maghsood AH, Safari M, Latifi M, Fallah M. Comparison of fecal antigen detection using enzyme linked immunosorbent assay with the auramine phenol staining method for diagnosis of human cryptosporidiosis. *Jundishapur J Microbiol*. 2015;8(2):e16470.
538. Santín M, Trout J, Fayer R, Xiao L. Cryptosporidium and cryptosporidiosis. 2008.

539. Fayer R, Ellis W. Paromomycin is effective as prophylaxis for cryptosporidiosis in dairy calves. *J Parasitol.* 1993;79(5):771–774.
540. Jenkins MC, O'Brien C, Trout J, Guidry A, Fayer R. Hyperimmune bovine colostrum specific for recombinant Cryptosporidium parvum antigen confers partial protection against cryptosporidiosis in immunosuppressed adult mice. *Vaccine.* 1999;17(19):2453–2460.
541. Perryman LE, Kapil SJ, Jones ML, Hunt EL. Protection of calves against cryptosporidiosis with immune bovine colostrum induced by a Cryptosporidium parvum recombinant protein. *Vaccine.* 1999;17(17):2142–2149.
542. Theodos CM, Griffiths JK, D'Onfro J, Fairfield A, Tzipori S. Efficacy of nitazoxanide against Cryptosporidium parvum in cell culture and in animal models. *Antimicrob Agents Chemother.* 1998;42(8):1959–1965.
543. Tzipori S, Rand W, Griffiths J, Widmer G, Crabb J. Evaluation of an animal model system for cryptosporidiosis: therapeutic efficacy of paromomycin and hyperimmune bovine colostrum-immunoglobulin. *Clin Diagn Lab Immunol.* 1994;1(4):450–463.
544. Boulter-Bitzer JI, Lee H, Trevors JT. Molecular targets for detection and immunotherapy in Cryptosporidium parvum. *Biotechnol Adv.* 2007;25(1):13–44.
545. Crabb JH. Antibody-based immunotherapy of cryptosporidiosis. *Adv Parasitol.* 1998;40:121–149.
546. Riggs MW, Cama VA, Leary Jr HL, Sterling CR. Bovine antibody against Cryptosporidium parvum elicits a circumsporozoite precipitate-like reaction and has immunotherapeutic effect against persistent cryptosporidiosis in SCID mice. *Infect Immun.* 1994;62(5):1927–1939.
547. Bjorneby JM, Hunsaker BD, Riggs MW, Perryman LE. Monoclonal antibody immunotherapy in nude mice persistently infected with Cryptosporidium parvum. *Infect Immun.* 1991;59(3):1172–1176.
548. Cevallos AM, Zhang X, Waldor MK, Jaison S, Zhou X, Tzipori S, et al. Molecular cloning and expression of a gene encoding Cryptosporidium parvum glycoproteins gp40 and gp15. *Infect Immun.* 2000;68(7):4108–4116.
549. Jenkins MC, Fayer R. Cloning and expression of cDNA encoding an antigenic Cryptosporidium parvum protein. *Mol Biochem Parasitol.* 1995;71(1):149–152.
550. Petersen C, Gut J, Doyle PS, Crabb JH, Nelson RG, Leech JH. Characterization of a >900,000-M(r) Cryptosporidium parvum sporozoite glycoprotein recognized by protective hyperimmune bovine colostral immunoglobulin. *Infect Immun.* 1992;60(12):5132–5138.
551. Spano F, Putignani L, Naitza S, Puri C, Wright S, Crisanti A. Molecular cloning and expression analysis of a Cryptosporidium parvum gene encoding a new member of the thrombospondin family1Note: Nucleotide sequence data reported in this paper are available in the GenBank™ data base under the accession numbers AF017267 (cp/ZAP.4) and U42213 (Cw.TC1).1. *Mol Biochem Parasitol.* 1998;92(1):147–162.
552. Fayer R, Morgan U, Upton SJ. Epidemiology of Cryptosporidium: transmission, detection and identification. *Int J Parasitol.* 2000;30(12):1305–1322.
553. Petersen C, Gut J, Doyle PS, Crabb JH, Nelson RG, Leech JH. Characterization of a >900,000-M(r) Cryptosporidium parvum sporozoite glycoprotein recognized by protective hyperimmune bovine colostral immunoglobulin. *Infect Immun.* 1992;60(12):5132–5138.
554. Schofield L, Vivas L, Hackett F, Gerold P, Schwarz RT, Tachado S. Neutralizing monoclonal antibodies to glycosylphosphatidylinositol, the dominant TNF-alpha-inducing toxin of Plasmodium falciparum: prospects for the immunotherapy of severe malaria. *Ann Trop Med Parasitol.* 1993;87(6):617–626.
555. Wherry EJ. T cell exhaustion. *Nat Immunol.* 2011;12(6):492–499.
556. Wykes MN, Horne-Debets JM, Leow C-Y, Karunarathne DS. Malaria drives T cells to exhaustion. *Frontiers in microbiology.* 2014;5:249.
557. Taylor DW. Monoclonal antibodies to a pan-malarial antigen. *Google Patents;.* 1991.
558. Chamond N, Coatnoan N, Minoprio P. Immunotherapy of Trypanosoma cruzi infections. *Curr Drug Targets Immune Endocr Metabol Disord.* 2002;2(3):247–254.
559. de Souza W, de Carvalho TM, Barrias ES. Review on Trypanosoma cruzi: Host Cell Interaction. *Int J Cell Biol.* 2010;2010.
560. Kumar S, Tarleton RL. Antigen-specific Th1 but not Th2 cells provide protection from lethal Trypanosoma cruzi infection in mice. *J Immunol.* 2001;166(7):4596–4603.
561. Tarleton RL, Grusby MJ, Zhang L. Increased susceptibility of Stat4-deficient and enhanced resistance in Stat6-deficient mice to infection with Trypanosoma cruzi. *J Immunol.* 2000;165(3):1520–1525.

562. Camargo EP. Perspectives of vaccination in Chagas disease revisited. *Mem Inst Oswaldo Cruz*. 2009;104(Suppl 1):275–280.
563. Duthie MS, Wleklinski-Lee M, Smith S, Nakayama T, Taniguchi M, Kahn SJ. During Trypanosoma cruzi infection CD1d-restricted NK T cells limit parasitemia and augment the antibody response to a glycophosphoinositol-modified surface protein. *Infect Immun*. 2002;70(1):36–48.
564. Wilson MT, Singh AK, Van Kaer L. Immunotherapy with ligands of natural killer T cells. *Trends Mol Med*. 2002;8(5):225–231.
565. Baral TN. Immunobiology of African trypanosomes: need of alternative interventions. *J Biomed Biotechnol*. 2010;2010.
566. Olivera GC, Vetter L, Tesoriero C, Del Gallo F, Hedberg G, Basile J, et al. Role of T cells during the cerebral infection with Trypanosoma brucei. *PLoS Negl Trop Dis*. 2021;15(9):e0009764.
567. Pays E, Lips S, Nolan D, Vanhamme L, Pérez-Morga D. The VSG expression sites of Trypanosoma brucei: multipurpose tools for the adaptation of the parasite to mammalian hosts. *Mol Biochem Parasitol*. 2001;114(1):1–16.
568. Borst P, Ulbert S. Control of VSG gene expression sites. *Mol Biochem Parasitol*. 2001;114(1):17–27.
569. Pays E, Guyaux M, Aerts D, Van Meirvenne N, Steinert M. Telomeric reciprocal recombination as a possible mechanism for antigenic variation in trypanosomes. *Nature*. 1985;316(6028):562–564.
570. Pays E, Van Assel S, Laurent M, Darville M, Vervoort T, Van Meirvenne N, et al. Gene conversion as a mechanism for antigenic variation in trypanosomes. *Cell*. 1983;34(2):371–381.
571. Bakhiet M, Olsson T, Edlund C, HÖJeberg B, Holmberg K, Lorentzhn J, et al. A Trypanosoma brucei brucei-Derived Factor that Triggers CD8+ Lymphocytes to Interferon-γ Secretion: Purification, Characterization and Protective Effects In Vivo by Treatment with a Monoclonal Antibody against the Factor. *Scand J Immunol*. 1993;37(2):165–178.
572. Wei G, Tabel H. Regulatory T Cells Prevent Control of Experimental African Trypanosomiasis. *J Immunol*. 2008;180(4):2514–2521.
573. Onyilagha C, Uzonna JE. Host Immune Responses and Immune Evasion Strategies in African Trypanosomiasis. *Front Immunol*. 2019;10(2738).
574. Galvan-Ramirez Mde L, Troyo R, Roman S, Calvillo-Sanchez C, Bernal-Redondo R. A systematic review and meta-analysis of Toxoplasma gondii infection among the Mexican population. *Parasit Vectors*. 2012;5:271.
575. Zhou P, Chen Z, Li HL, Zheng H, He S, Lin RQ, et al. Toxoplasma gondii infection in humans in China. *Parasit Vectors*. 2011;4:165.
576. Jafari R, Sadaghian M, Safari M. Seroprevalence of Toxoplasma gondii infection and related risk factors in Tabriz City, Iran, 2008. *J Res Health Sci*. 2012;12(2):119–121.
577. Rasouli S, Sadaghian M, Jafari R. Prevalence of human toxoplasmosis and related risk factors using Electrochemiluminescence (ECLIA) method in West Azarbaijan Province, Iran, 2010. *Int J Biosci*. 2014;4(8):124–130.
578. Pavia CS. Protection against experimental toxoplasmosis by adoptive immunotherapy. *J Immunol*. 1986;137(9):2985–2990.
579. Schwebke JR, Trichomoniasis Burgess D. *Clin Microbiol Rev*. 2004;17(4):794–803 Table of contents.
580. Gombosová A, Demes P, Valent M. Immunotherapeutic effect of the lactobacillus vaccine, Solco Trichovac, in trichomoniasis is not mediated by antibodies cross reacting with Trichomonas vaginalis. *Genitourin Med*. 1986;62(2):107–110.
581. Bonilla-Musoles F. Immunotherapy in vaginal trichomoniasis–therapeutic and prophylactic effects of the vaccine SolcoTrichovac. *Gynakol Rundsch*. 1984;24(Suppl 3):63–69.
582. Karkut G. [Effect of lactobacillus immunotherapy on genital infections in women (Solco Trichovac/Gynatren)]. *Geburtshilfe Frauenheilkd*. 1984;44(5):311–314.
583. van der Weiden RM, van der Meijden WI, Bogchelman DH, Polderman AM. Treatment failure in trichomoniasis and persistence of the parasite after Lactobacillus immunotherapy; two case reports. *Eur J Obstet Gynecol Reprod Biol*. 1990;34(1-2):171–178.
584. Jenkins-Holick DS, Kaul TL. Schistosomiasis. *Urol Nurs*. 2013;33(4):163–170.
585. Wynn TA, Cheever AW, Jankovic D, Poindexter RW, Caspar P, Lewis FA, et al. An IL-12-based vaccination method for preventing fibrosis induced by schistosome infection. *Nature*. 1995;376(6541):594–596.
586. de Vries JE. The role of IL-13 and its receptor in allergy and inflammatory responses. *J Allergy Clin Immunol*. 1998;102(2):165–169.

587. Chiaramonte MG, Donaldson DD, Cheever AW, Wynn TA. An IL-13 inhibitor blocks the development of hepatic fibrosis during a T-helper type 2-dominated inflammatory response. *J Clin Invest*. 1999;104(6):777–785.
588. Cheever AW, Williams ME, Wynn TA, Finkelman FD, Seder RA, Cox TM, et al. Anti-IL-4 treatment of Schistosoma mansoni-infected mice inhibits development of T cells and non-B, non-T cells expressing Th2 cytokines while decreasing egg-induced hepatic fibrosis. *J Immunol*. 1994;153(2):753–759.
589. Kaplan MH, Whitfield JR, Boros DL, Grusby MJ. Th2 cells are required for the Schistosoma mansoni egg-induced granulomatous response. *J Immunol*. 1998;160(4):1850–1856.
590. Yousofi Darani H, Yousefi M, Safari M, Jafari R. Parasites and immunotherapy: with or against?. *J Parasit Dis*. 2016;40(2):217–226.
591. Fleischmann C, Scherag A, Adhikari NK, Hartog CS, Tsaganos T, Schlattmann P, et al. Assessment of Global Incidence and Mortality of Hospital-treated Sepsis. Current Estimates and Limitations. *Am J Respir Crit Care Med*. 2016;193(3):259–272.
592. Martin GS, Mannino DM, Eaton S, Moss M. The epidemiology of sepsis in the United States from 1979 through 2000. *N Engl J Med*. 2003;348(16):1546–1554.
593. Meyer N, Harhay MO, Small DS, Prescott HC, Bowles KH, Gaieski DF, et al. Temporal Trends in Incidence, Sepsis-Related Mortality, and Hospital-Based Acute Care After Sepsis. *Crit Care Med*. 2018;46(3):354–360.
594. Vincent JL, Lefrant JY, Kotfis K, Nanchal R, Martin-Loeches I, Wittebole X, et al. Comparison of European ICU patients in 2012 (ICON) versus 2002 (SOAP). *Intensive Care Med*. 2018;44(3):337–344.
595. Fleischmann-Struzek C, Goldfarb DM, Schlattmann P, Schlapbach LJ, Reinhart K, Kissoon N. The global burden of paediatric and neonatal sepsis: a systematic review. *Lancet Respir Med*. 2018;6(3):223–230.
596. Poutsiaka DD, Porto MC, Perry WA, Hudcova J, Tybor DJ, Hadley S, et al. Prospective Observational Study Comparing Sepsis-2 and Sepsis-3 Definitions in Predicting Mortality in Critically Ill Patients. *Open Forum Infectious Diseases*. 2019;6(7):ofz271.
597. Lin G-L, McGinley JP, Drysdale SB, Pollard AJ. Epidemiology and Immune Pathogenesis of Viral Sepsis. *Front Immunol*. 2018;9(2147).
598. SN M, BT R. Immune responses to viruses. *Clin Immunol*. 2008:421–431. doi:10.1016/B978-0-323-04404-210027-2 Epub 2009.
599. Marsh M, Helenius A. Virus entry: open sesame. *Cell*. 2006;124(4):729–740.
600. Berzofsky JA, Ahlers JD, Belyakov IM. Strategies for designing and optimizing new generation vaccines. *Nat Rev Immunol*. 2001;1(3):209–219.
601. Pichlmair A. Reis e Sousa C. Innate recognition of viruses. *Immunity*. 2007;27(3):370–383.
602. Iwasaki A, Medzhitov R. Toll-like receptor control of the adaptive immune responses. *Nat Immunol*. 2004;5(10):987–995.
603. Brooks DG, Trifilo MJ, Edelmann KH, Teyton L, McGavern DB, Oldstone MB. Interleukin-10 determines viral clearance or persistence in vivo. *Nat Med*. 2006;12(11):1301–1309.
604. Brady MT, MacDonald AJ, Rowan AG, Mills KH. Hepatitis C virus non-structural protein 4 suppresses Th1 responses by stimulating IL-10 production from monocytes. *Eur J Immunol*. 2003;33(12):3448–3457.
605. Brockman MA, Kwon DS, Tighe DP, Pavlik DF, Rosato PC, Sela J, et al. IL-10 is up-regulated in multiple cell types during viremic HIV infection and reversibly inhibits virus-specific T cells. *Blood*. 2009;114(2):346–356.
606. Hyodo N, Nakamura I, Imawari M. Hepatitis B core antigen stimulates interleukin-10 secretion by both T cells and monocytes from peripheral blood of patients with chronic hepatitis B virus infection. *Clin Exp Immunol*. 2004;135(3):462–466.
607. Smit JJ, Rudd BD, Lukacs NW. Plasmacytoid dendritic cells inhibit pulmonary immunopathology and promote clearance of respiratory syncytial virus. *J Exp Med*. 2006;203(5):1153–1159.
608. Chen IY, Ichinohe T. Response of host inflammasomes to viral infection. *Trends Microbiol*. 2015;23(1):55–63.
609. Ichinohe T, Yamazaki T, Koshiba T, Yanagi Y. Mitochondrial protein mitofusin 2 is required for NLRP3 inflammasome activation after RNA virus infection. *Proc Natl Acad Sci*. 2013;110(44):17963–17968.

610. Allen IC, Scull MA, Moore CB, Holl EK, McElvania-TeKippe E, Taxman DJ, et al. The NLRP3 inflammasome mediates in vivo innate immunity to influenza A virus through recognition of viral RNA. *Immunity*. 2009;30(4):556–565.
611. Ichinohe T, Pang IK, Iwasaki A. Influenza virus activates inflammasomes via its intracellular M2 ion channel. *Nat Immunol*. 2010;11(5):404–410.
612. McAuley JL, Tate MD, MacKenzie-Kludas CJ, Pinar A, Zeng W, Stutz A, et al. Activation of the NLRP3 inflammasome by IAV virulence protein PB1-F2 contributes to severe pathophysiology and disease. *PLoS Pathog*. 2013;9(5):e1003392.
613. Ito M, Yanagi Y, Ichinohe T. Encephalomyocarditis virus viroporin 2B activates NLRP3 inflammasome. 2012.
614. Rajan JV, Rodriguez D, Miao EA, Aderem A. The NLRP3 inflammasome detects encephalomyocarditis virus and vesicular stomatitis virus infection. *J Virol*. 2011;85(9):4167–4172.
615. Chen W, Xu Y, Li H, Tao W, Xiang Y, Huang B, et al. HCV genomic RNA activates the NLRP3 inflammasome in human myeloid cells. *PLoS One*. 2014;9(1):e84953.
616. Delaloye J, Roger T, Steiner-Tardivel Q-G, Le Roy D, Knaup Reymond M, Akira S, et al. Innate immune sensing of modified vaccinia virus Ankara (MVA) is mediated by TLR2-TLR6, MDA-5 and the NALP3 inflammasome. *PLoS Pathog*. 2009;5(6):e1000480.
617. Ermler ME, Traylor Z, Patel K, Schattgen SA, Vanaja SK, Fitzgerald KA, et al. Rift Valley fever virus infection induces activation of the NLRP3 inflammasome. *Virology*. 2014;449:174–180.
618. Johnson KE, Chikoti L, Chandran B. Herpes simplex virus 1 infection induces activation and subsequent inhibition of the IFI16 and NLRP3 inflammasomes. *J Virol*. 2013;87(9):5005–5018.
619. Kaushik DK, Gupta M, Kumawat KL, Basu A. NLRP3 inflammasome: key mediator of neuroinflammation in murine Japanese encephalitis. *PLoS One*. 2012;7(2):e32270.
620. Negash AA, Ramos HJ, Crochet N, Lau DT, Doehle B, Papic N, et al. IL-1β production through the NLRP3 inflammasome by hepatic macrophages links hepatitis C virus infection with liver inflammation and disease. *PLoS Pathog*. 2013;9(4):e1003330.
621. Park S, Juliana C, Hong S, Datta P, Hwang I, Fernandes-Alnemri T, et al. The mitochondrial antiviral protein MAVS associates with NLRP3 and regulates its inflammasome activity. *J Immunol*. 2013;191(8):4358–4366.
622. Ramos HJ, Lanteri MC, Blahnik G, Negash A, Suthar MS, Brassil MM, et al. IL-1β signaling promotes CNS-intrinsic immune control of West Nile virus infection. *PLoS Pathog*. 2012;8(11):e1003039.
623. Triantafilou K, Kar S, Vakakis E, Kotecha S, Triantafilou M. Human respiratory syncytial virus viroporin SH: a viral recognition pathway used by the host to signal inflammasome activation. *Thorax*. 2013;68(1):66–75.
624. Wu M-F, Chen S-T, Yang A-H, Lin W-W, Lin Y-L, Chen N-J, et al. CLEC5A is critical for dengue virus–induced inflammasome activation in human macrophages. *Blood, The Journal of the American Society of Hematology*. 2013;121(1):95–106.
625. Masters SL, Gerlic M, Metcalf D, Preston S, Pellegrini M, O'Donnell JA, et al. NLRP1 inflammasome activation induces pyroptosis of hematopoietic progenitor cells. *Immunity*. 2012;37(6):1009–1023.
626. Hornung V, Ablasser A, Charrel-Dennis M, Bauernfeind F, Horvath G, Caffrey DR, et al. AIM2 recognizes cytosolic dsDNA and forms a caspase-1-activating inflammasome with ASC. *Nature*. 2009;458(7237):514–518.
627. Pothlichet J, Meunier I, Davis BK, Ting JP, Skamene E, von Messling V, et al. Type I IFN triggers RIG-I/TLR3/NLRP3-dependent inflammasome activation in influenza A virus infected cells. *PLoS Pathog*. 2013;9(4):e1003256.
628. Poeck H, Bscheider M, Gross O, Finger K, Roth S, Rebsamen M, et al. Recognition of RNA virus by RIG-I results in activation of CARD9 and inflammasome signaling for interleukin 1β production. *Nat Immunol*. 2010;11(1):63–69.
629. Ichinohe T, Lee HK, Ogura Y, Flavell R, Iwasaki A. Inflammasome recognition of influenza virus is essential for adaptive immune responses. *J Exp Med*. 2009;206(1):79–87.
630. Kanneganti T-D, Body-Malapel M, Amer A, Park J-H, Whitfield J, Franchi L, et al. Critical role for Cryopyrin/Nalp3 in activation of caspase-1 in response to viral infection and double-stranded RNA. *J Biol Chem*. 2006;281(48):36560–36568.

631. Thomas PG, Dash P, Aldridge Jr JR, Ellebedy AH, Reynolds C, Funk AJ, et al. The intracellular sensor NLRP3 mediates key innate and healing responses to influenza A virus via the regulation of caspase-1. *Immunity*. 2009;30(4):566–575.
632. Komune N, Ichinohe T, Ito M, Yanagi Y. Measles virus V protein inhibits NLRP3 inflammasome-mediated interleukin-1β secretion. *J Virol*. 2011;85(24):13019–13026.
633. Moriyama M, Chen I-Y, Kawaguchi A, Koshiba T, Nagata K, Takeyama H, et al. The RNA-and TRIM25-binding domains of influenza virus NS1 protein are essential for suppression of NLRP3 inflammasome-mediated interleukin-1β secretion. *J Virol*. 2016;90(8):4105–4114.
634. Komatsu T, Tanaka Y, Kitagawa Y, Koide N, Naiki Y, Morita N, et al. Sendai virus V protein inhibits the secretion of interleukin-1β by preventing NLRP3 inflammasome assembly. *J Virol*. 2018;92(19):e00842–e00848.
635. Zhao C, Zhao W. NLRP3 Inflammasome—A Key Player in Antiviral Responses. *Front Immunol*. 2020;11(211).
636. Faustin B, Lartigue L, Bruey J-M, Luciano F, Sergienko E, Bailly-Maitre B, et al. Reconstituted NALP1 inflammasome reveals two-step mechanism of caspase-1 activation. *Mol Cell*. 2007;25(5):713–724.
637. Gerlic M, Faustin B, Postigo A, Yu EC-W, Proell M, Gombosuren N, et al. Vaccinia virus F1L protein promotes virulence by inhibiting inflammasome activation. *Proc Natl Acad Sci*. 2013;110(19):7808–7813.
638. Fisher MA, Lloyd ML. A Review of Murine Cytomegalovirus as a Model for Human Cytomegalovirus Disease-Do Mice Lie?. *Int J Mol Sci*. 2020;22(1):214.
639. Maruzuru Y, Ichinohe T, Sato R, Miyake K, Okano T, Suzuki T, et al. Herpes Simplex Virus 1 VP22 Inhibits AIM2-Dependent Inflammasome Activation to Enable Efficient Viral Replication. *Cell Host & Microbe*. 2018;23(2):254–265 e7.
640. Reinholz M, Kawakami Y, Salzer S, Kreuter A, Dombrowski Y, Koglin S, et al. HPV16 activates the AIM2 inflammasome in keratinocytes. *Arch Dermatol Res*. 2013;305(8):723–732.
641. Zhang H, Luo J, Alcorn JF, Chen K, Fan S, Pilewski J, et al. AIM2 Inflammasome Is Critical for Influenza-Induced Lung Injury and Mortality. *J Immunol*. 2017;198(11):4383–4393.
642. Szomolanyi-Tsuda E, Liang X, Welsh RM, Kurt-Jones EA, Finberg RW. Role for TLR2 in NK cell-mediated control of murine cytomegalovirus in vivo. *J Virol*. 2006;80(9):4286–4291.
643. Wang T, Town T, Alexopoulou L, Anderson JF, Fikrig E, Flavell RA. Toll-like receptor 3 mediates West Nile virus entry into the brain causing lethal encephalitis. *Nat Med*. 2004;10(12):1366–1373.
644. Goffic RL, Balloy V, Lagranderie M, Alexopoulou L, Escriou N, Flavell R, et al. Detrimental contribution of the Toll-like receptor (TLR) 3 to influenza A virus–induced acute pneumonia. *PLoS Pathog*. 2006;2(6):e53.
645. Kurt-Jones EA, Popova L, Kwinn L, Haynes LM, Jones LP, Tripp RA, et al. Pattern recognition receptors TLR4 and CD14 mediate response to respiratory syncytial virus. *Nat Immunol*. 2000;1(5):398–401.
646. Burzyn D, Rassa JC, Kim D, Nepomnaschy I, Ross SR, Piazzon I. Toll-like receptor 4-dependent activation of dendritic cells by a retrovirus. *J Virol*. 2004;78(2):576–584.
647. Diebold SS. Recognition of viral single-stranded RNA by Toll-like receptors. *Adv Drug Deliv Rev*. 2008;60(7):813–823.
648. Lee SM-Y, Yip T-F, Yan S, Jin D-Y, Wei H-L, Guo R-T, et al. Recognition of double-stranded RNA and regulation of interferon pathway by toll-like receptor 10. *Front Immunol*. 2018;9:516.
649. Mabrey FL, Morrell ED, Wurfel MM. TLRs in COVID-19: How they drive immunopathology and the rationale for modulation. *Innate Immunity*. 2021:17534259211051364.
650. Lester SN, Li K. Toll-like receptors in antiviral innate immunity. *J Mol Biol*. 2014;426(6):1246–1264.
651. Sartorius R, Trovato M, Manco R, D'Apice L, De Berardinis P. Exploiting viral sensing mediated by Toll-like receptors to design innovative vaccines. *npj Vaccines*. 2021;6(1):127.
652. Guidotti LG, Rochford R, Chung J, Shapiro M, Purcell R, Chisari FV. Viral clearance without destruction of infected cells during acute HBV infection. *Science*. 1999;284(5415):825–829.
653. Rehermann B. Hepatitis C virus versus innate and adaptive immune responses: a tale of coevolution and coexistence. *J Clin Invest*. 2009;119(7):1745–1754.
654. Bermejo-Martin JF, Ortiz de Lejarazu R, Pumarola T, Rello J, Almansa R, Ramírez P, et al. Th1 and Th17 hypercytokinemia as early host response signature in severe pandemic influenza. *Crit Care*. 2009;13(6):R201.

655. Favre D, Lederer S, Kanwar B, Ma ZM, Proll S, Kasakow Z, et al. Critical loss of the balance between Th17 and T regulatory cell populations in pathogenic SIV infection. *PLoS Pathog*. 2009;5(2):e1000295.
656. Rowan AG, Fletcher JM, Ryan EJ, Moran B, Hegarty JE, O'Farrelly C, et al. Hepatitis C virus-specific Th17 cells are suppressed by virus-induced TGF-beta. *J Immunol*. 2008;181(7):4485–4494.
657. Culley FJ, Pennycook AM, Tregoning JS, Hussell T, Openshaw PJ. Differential chemokine expression following respiratory virus infection reflects Th1- or Th2-biased immunopathology. *J Virol*. 2006;80(9):4521–4527.
658. Zinkernagel RM, Hengartner H. Protective 'immunity'by pre-existent neutralizing antibody titers and preactivated T cells but not by so-called 'immunological memory. *Immunol Rev*. 2006;211(1):310–319.
659. Letvin NL. Correlates of immune protection and the development of a human immunodeficiency virus vaccine. *Immunity*. 2007;27(3):366–369.
660. Edghill-Smith Y, Golding H, Manischewitz J, King LR, Scott D, Bray M, et al. Smallpox vaccine–induced antibodies are necessary and sufficient for protection against monkeypox virus. *Nat Med*. 2005;11(7):740–747.
661. Dörner T, Radbruch A. Antibodies and B Cell Memory in Viral Immunity. *Immunity*. 2007;27(3):384–392.
662. Duchesne L, Njouom R, Lissock F, Tamko-Mella GF, Rallier S, Poiteau L, et al. HCV Ag quantification as a one-step procedure in diagnosing chronic hepatitis C infection in Cameroon: the ANRS 12336 study. *J Int AIDS Soc*. 2017;20(1):21446.
663. Wong SJ, Furuya A, Zou J, Xie X, Dupuis 2nd AP, Kramer LD, et al. A Multiplex Microsphere Immunoassay for Zika Virus Diagnosis. *EBioMedicine*. 2017;16:136–140.
664. Pisanic N, Rahman A, Saha SK, Labrique AB, Nelson KE, Granger DA, et al. Development of an oral fluid immunoassay to assess past and recent hepatitis E virus (HEV) infection. *J Immunol Methods*. 2017;448:1–8.
665. Koishi AC, Suzukawa AA, Zanluca C, Camacho DE, Comach G. Duarte Dos Santos CN. Development and evaluation of a novel high-throughput image-based fluorescent neutralization test for detection of Zika virus infection. *PLoS Negl Trop Dis*. 2018;12(3):e0006342.
666. Zhang H, Rao H, Wang Y, Wang J, Kong X, Ji Y, et al. Evaluation of an antigen assay for diagnosing acute and chronic hepatitis E genotype 4 infection. *J Gastroenterol Hepatol*. 2019;34(2):458–465.
667. Crim RL, Kumari S, Jayanti P, Audet S, Kulkarni A, Beeler J. Development of Luciferase Immunoprecipitation Systems (LIPS) Assay to Detect IgG Antibodies against Human Respiratory Syncytial Virus G-Glycoprotein. *Vaccines (Basel)*. 2019;7(1).
668. Furuya AKM, Hunt D, George KS, Dupuis 2nd AP, Kramer LD, Shi PY, et al. Use of the immunoglobulin G avidity assay to differentiate between recent Zika and past dengue virus infections. *Clin Sci (Lond)*. 2019;133(7):859–867.
669. Amaro F, Sánchez-Seco MP, Vázquez A, Alves MJ, Zé-Zé L, Luz MT, et al. The Application and Interpretation of IgG Avidity and IgA ELISA Tests to Characterize Zika Virus Infections. *Viruses*. 2019;11(2).
670. Hansen S, Hotop SK, Faye O, Ndiaye O, Böhlken-Fascher S, Pessôa R, et al. Diagnosing Zika virus infection against a background of other flaviviruses: Studies in high resolution serological analysis. *Sci Rep*. 2019;9(1):3648.
671. Oh S, Kim J, Tran VT, Lee DK, Ahmed SR, Hong JC, et al. Magnetic Nanozyme-Linked Immunosorbent Assay for Ultrasensitive Influenza A Virus Detection. *ACS Appl Mater Interfaces*. 2018;10(15):12534–12543.
672. Emmerich P, Mika A, von Possel R, Rackow A, Liu Y, Schmitz H, et al. Sensitive and specific detection of Crimean-Congo Hemorrhagic Fever Virus (CCHFV)-Specific IgM and IgG antibodies in human sera using recombinant CCHFV nucleoprotein as antigen in μ-capture and IgG immune complex (IC) ELISA tests. *PLoS Negl Trop Dis*. 2018;12(3):e0006366.
673. Fischer K, Diederich S, Smith G, Reiche S, Pinho Dos Reis V, Stroh E, et al. Indirect ELISA based on Hendra and Nipah virus proteins for the detection of henipavirus specific antibodies in pigs. *PLoS One*. 2018;13(4):e0194385.
674. Wang R, Ongagna-Yhombi SY, Lu Z, Centeno-Tablante E, Colt S, Cao X, et al. Rapid Diagnostic Platform for Colorimetric Differential Detection of Dengue and Chikungunya Viral Infections. *Anal Chem*. 2019;91(8):5415–5423.

675. Qin P, Park M, Alfson KJ, Tamhankar M, Carrion R, Patterson JL, et al. Rapid and Fully Microfluidic Ebola Virus Detection with CRISPR-Cas13a. *ACS Sens*. 2019;4(4):1048–1054.
676. Qin S, Volokhov D, Rodionova E, Wirblich C, Schnell MJ, Chizhikov V, et al. A new recombinant rabies virus expressing a green fluorescent protein: A novel and fast approach to quantify virus neutralizing antibodies. *Biologicals*. 2019;59:56–61.
677. PV B, G MS, AMVN P, M M, K SK, NNR R, et al. Advanced Immunotechnological Methods for Detection and Diagnosis of Viral. *Dynamics of Immune Activation in Viral Diseases*. 2019:261–275 Nov 5.
678. Mirian M, Khanahmad H, Darzi L, Salehi M, Sadeghi-Aliabadi H. Oligonucleotide aptamers: potential novel molecules against viral hepatitis. *Res Pharm Sci*. 2017;12(2):88–98.
679. Kindt TJ, Goldsby RA, Osborne BA, Kuby J. *Kuby Immunology*: Macmillan; 2007.
680. Mather S, Scott S, Temperton N, Wright E, King B, Daly J. Current progress with serological assays for exotic emerging/re-emerging viruses. *Future Virol*. 2013;8(8):745–755.
681. Souf S. Recent advances in diagnostic testing for viral infections. *Bioscience Horizons: The International Journal of Student Research*. 2016;9.
682. Alladi CSH, Jagadesh A, Prabhu SG, Arunkumar G. Hemagglutination Inhibition Antibody Response Following Influenza A(H1N1)pdm09 Virus Natural Infection: A Cross-Sectional Study from Thirthahalli, Karnataka, India. *Viral Immunol*. 2019;32(5):230–233.
683. Numazaki K. Study on assays for the detection of serum antibodies to measles from children and its standardization. *International Journal of Pediatrics and Neonatal Care*. 2015;1:108.
684. Noah DL, Hill H, Hines D, White EL, Wolff MC. Qualification of the hemagglutination inhibition assay in support of pandemic influenza vaccine licensure. *Clin Vaccine Immunol*. 2009;16(4):558–566.
685. Reta DH, Tessema TS, Ashenef AS, Desta AF, Labisso WL, Gizaw ST, et al. Molecular and Immunological Diagnostic Techniques of Medical Viruses. *International Journal of Microbiology*. 2020;2020:8832728.
686. Veguilla V, Hancock K, Schiffer J, Gargiullo P, Lu X, Aranio D, et al. Sensitivity and specificity of serologic assays for detection of human infection with 2009 pandemic H1N1 virus in U.S. populations. *J Clin Microbiol*. 2011;49(6):2210–2215.
687. Goldenthal KL, Midthun K, Zoon KC. Control of Viral Infections and Diseases. In: Baron S, ed. *Medical Microbiology*. Galveston (TX): University of Texas Medical Branch at Galveston Copyright © 1996, The University of Texas Medical Branch at Galveston; 1996.
688. Khanna R, Smith C. Cellular immune therapy for viral infections in transplant patients. *Indian J Med Res*. 2013;138(5):796.
689. Chapter 4 - Antiviral Immunity and Prophylaxis. In: MacLachlan NJ, Dubovi EJ, eds. *Fenner's Veterinary Virology*. Fourth Edition San Diego: Academic Press; 2011:75–99.

# CHAPTER 7

# Transplantation

**Melina Farshbafnadi[a,b], Sepideh Razi[b,c,d], Nima Rezaei[d,e,f]**
[a]School of Medicine, Tehran University of Medical Sciences, Tehran, Iran
[b]Cancer Immunology Project (CIP), Universal Scientific Education and Research Network (USERN), Tehran, Iran
[c]School of Medicine, Iran University of Medical Sciences, Tehran, Iran
[d]Research Center for Immunodeficiencies, Children's Medical Center, Tehran University of Medical Sciences, Tehran, Iran
[e]Department of Immunology, School of Medicine, Tehran University of Medical Sciences, Tehran, Iran
[f]Network of Immunity in Infection, Malignancy and Autoimmunity (NIIMA), Universal Scientific Education and Research Network (USERN), Tehran, Iran

## Introduction

From more than a century ago, successful attempts of transplanting tissues, including human skin and cornea, have been recorded.[1] However, it was not until December 23, 1954, that doctor Joseph Murray performed the first successful renal transplant on genetically identical twins.[2] Ever since that day, organ transplant has revolutionized modern medicine. Although initially organ transplant was only considered as a clinical experiment, it is now widely regarded as a regular and valid practice. Furthermore, organ transplant is currently a critical therapeutic option for many patients with terminal organ failure. Liver transplantation was established a few years following renal transplantation. After that, several attempts were made for the transplantation of other organs, including the heart, pancreas, and lung. However, the patients' survival rates were not favorable initially.[1,3,4] When it was discovered that cyclosporine has promising immunomodulatory effects, it was soon implemented into the immunosuppressive regimens of organ transplantation, increasing the 1-year graft survival rates to more than 89 percent in patients with renal transplantation and 70 percent in patients with heart and liver transplantation. However, such regimens led to notable complications, including neurotoxicity, nephrotoxicity, opportunistic infection, de novo diabetes, and B cell lymphoma.[1]

In the early 60s, hematopoietic stem cell transplantation (HSCT) was developed to cure hematologic malignancies and congenital and acquired disorders of the hematopoietic system. HSCT is an operation that leads to the substitution of the hematopoiesis and immune system of the recipient with donor cells. HSCT can be obtained from the bone marrow, mobilized peripheral stem cells, and placental blood. HSCT is either autologous in which cells are harvested from the patient and reinfused to the patient or allogeneic in which cells are yielded from a donor who can be related or unrelated to the recipient.[5] Patients undergoing HSCT require certain conditioning regimens prior to transplantation to lessen the disease burden and bestow adequate immunoablation to impede graft rejection.[6]

*Clinical Immunology*
DOI: https://doi.org/10.1016/B978-0-12-818006-8.00008-6

Although transplantation has significantly improved the length and quality of life of several patients with end-stage diseases, it is not without fault. The immune system within the body, both humoral and cell-mediated, which is designed to protect the body from foreign antigens, may act against the transplanted organ and induce rejection. This can cause catastrophic problems for the patients and be fatal.[7] However, immunosuppressive regimens are being developed to be administered to patients following kidney transplantation and are utilized to impede graft rejection and ameliorate unfavorable complications, including infection, malignancy, and drug toxicity.[8] Graft versus host disease (GVHD) is yet another complication that can happen following transplantation. It is a multifaceted syndrome that occurs following recognition of genetically different tissues of the host by donor T cells. The degree of histocompatibility variation between the donor and the recipient plays an important role in preventing GVHD.[9,10] Potential organ donors and recipients should be evaluated prior to transplantation to minimize the risks associated with transplantation and improve the outcomes. Also, infectious disease screening is performed to identify major infections that can jeopardize transplant outcomes.[4]

This chapter explores different types of transplantations, the immunopathogenesis of transplantation, the process of matching the donor and the recipient, pre-transplantation conditioning, and complications after transplant, and ways to manage them.

## Solid organ transplantation (SOT)

### Sources

#### *Autologous/allogeneic*

Autotransplantation is an important surgical procedure in which the problematic organ is harvested from its original place and inserted back into the same location or another location after the patient and/or the organ is at a better state.[11–14]

Allogeneic transplantation is a procedure in which a genetically different organ (allograft) of the same species is harvested from a deceased or live donor and transferred to the recipients.[15,16]

#### *Deceased/live donor*

Organs needed for transplantation can be obtained from deceased or live donors. Deceased donors can be classified into two categories: donation after brain death (DBD) and donation after cardiac death (DCD). Donors in the DBD category are donors who experienced primary brain death. However, the heart circulation and respiration are functional or are externally preserved by medical procedures. A donor that does not qualify for brain death but in whom the heart stopped or is unfunctional before harvesting the organ is classified as DCD.[17]

## Kidney transplantation

Kidney transplant is a routine procedure for treating end-stage chronic renal failure and is linked to better patient survival and quality of life. This procedure includes surgery in which the failed kidney is replaced by a healthy kidney from a living or dead donor.[18,19] The demand for donated kidneys continues to rise, which outmatches the supply. As a result, the number of days spent on the waiting list for kidney transplants increases rapidly, especially for the patients who have extremely reactive human leukocyte antigen (HLA)-specific alloantibodies.[20] To compensate for this ever-growing demand for organ, the types of donors used has increased, and donors could be either alive or dead.[21] Over the decades, the survival rates for transplanted kidneys have improved progressively as a result of better immunosuppression, hemodialysis, and continuous ambulatory peritoneal dialysis that could prepare patients for transplantation before the procedure.[22,23]

Comprehensive physical examination, detailed medical history, and laboratory testing are required for assessing renal transplant candidates. Psychiatric disorders are related to unfavorable results. On the contrary, strong family and social support, good insight, spirituality, and being able to cope with various stressors are associated with a better prognosis. The main cause of mortality in post kidney transplantation is cardiovascular disease. For this reason, cardiovascular screening is an important part of the transplant assessment process. All of the patients should also be evaluated for latent or active infections, and a history of immunization is also required to ascertain the adequacy of immunization before transplantation. Because of the use of immunosuppressants, kidney transplant patients are at greater risk for developing malignancies. For patients with a history of cancer, consulting an oncologist is preferred. Screening for assessing the risk of coagulation is also of importance. Although a history of thromboembolism does not prohibit transplantation, a history of considerable venous thrombosis that involves inferior vena cava, iliac vein, or both may preclude transplantation. Some centers consider obesity a contraindication to transplantation as it involves a greater risk of post-transplant complications.[24] The majority of transplant centers refrain from accepting smokers for transplantation and instruct smokers to give up smoking prior to transplantation as smokers are twice more likely to develop cardiac incidents and malignancy following transplantation. Due to the scarcity of organs, most patients are placed on the waiting list and are not allowed to undergo transplantation until the glomerular filtration rate (GFR) is less than 15 mL/min/1.73 $m^2$.[25]

Kidney grafts can be harvested from both live and deceased donors. Kidney donors can be selected according to standard criteria donor (SCD) or expanded criteria donor (ECD). SCD is a 35-year-old man without a history of hypertension or diabetes whose cause of death is a motor vehicle accident.[17] In ECD criteria, either of the following terms should be applied: 1) donor age more than or equal to 60 years, or 2) donor age 50 to 59 years with at least 2 of the following criteria: serum creatinine more than 1.5 mg/dL, death due to cerebrovascular accident, and history of hypertension.[26] Graft survivals are more favorable in living donor transplantations compared with deceased donor transplantations. 1-year survival is greater than 90 percent in both types of transplantation. However, 5-year survival is approximately 80 percent and 65 percent in live-donor transplantation and deceased donor transplantation, respectively.[25]

HLA matching has always been a controversial area in kidney transplantation. Geography is a key factor to take into consideration. In bigger countries, there would be increased cold ischemia time (CIT) if the dead donor organ has to travel long distances compared with smaller countries such as the United Kingdom that HLA matching is focused on.[27] A study published by the United Network for Organ Sharing (UNOS) registry in the United States of America of a cohort from 1987 to 1998 demonstrated that HLA mismatch did not result in notable variation in kidney allograft survival of patients younger than 21 years of age.[28] Another cohort in the novel immunosuppression era that examined the impacts of HLA matching and donor age in patients younger than 21 years old concluded that increased age in dead donor but not living donor transplant and increased HLA mismatches for both dead and living donor transplants decreases the allograft survival. However, the results were not statistically notable.[29] A recent study examining the whole cohort from 1987 to 2016 found a linear relationship between each HLA mismatch and allograft failure in both living and dead donor transplantations in patients under 18 years old, with the relation being more significant in the living donor group.[30] Class I HLA antigen mismatches were demonstrated to be associated with clinical outcomes in living donor kidney transplantation in earlier studies. This association was not significant in dead donor kidney transplantation. After HLA-DR antigens discovery, the role of HLA antigen mismatches on dead donor transplantations was observed.[31] ABO blood group antigens have also been considered in kidney transplantation. However, studies suggest that the association may not be significant.[32] In conclusion, the ultimate verdict for the type of transplant and a reasonable amount of HLA mismatches relies on the condition of the recipient, although HLA matching seems to be useful for very long-term aftermaths. Increased waiting times and complications accompanying end-stage kidney disease and dialysis are important factors to consider.[27]

Kidney transplant patients who have increased serum creatinine or proteinuria are suspected to have undergone rejection. A kidney biopsy is needed to confirm rejection, which is challenging, expensive, unsuitable, invasive, and risky. To overcome this challenge, several immune biomarkers are needed to help detect rejection rapidly.[33] Donor-specific antibodies (DSA) are an early biomarker of acute antibody-mediated rejection (AMR). However, the pathogenicity of DSAs relies on properties such as isotype (immunoglobulin (Ig)M versus IgG), class specificity (HLA class I versus class II), antigenic specificity, strength, IgG subclass, and complement binding capacity.[34] The AlloSure test measures circulating donor-derived cell-free deoxyribonucleic acid (dd-cfDNA) in transplant patients, which indicates injury as rejection includes cell death in the allograft.[34] Several other tests such as urinary chemokines, complement *C3* gene polymorphism, allogeneic B cell and B cell-activating factor assay, peripheral blood gene expression assay, the kidney biopsy gene expression assay, and plasma endothelial microparticles are used to detect AMR.[33] Several biomarkers have also been used to detect T-cell-mediated rejection (TCMR). ImmuKnow assay measures ATP generation by the mitogen-stimulated cluster of differentiation (CD)4+ lymphocytes, which are associated with rejection prediction.[33] Peripheral blood and leukocytes gene expression assay, Allograft gene expression assay, Allogeneic circulating T cell assays, single nucleotide polymorphisms, peripheral blood microRNAs, urinary cell mRNA, urinary microRNAs, urinary chemokines, urine proteomics/peptidomics, TruGraf test, and PleximarkTx test are another helpful test used to determine TCMR.[33]

Using calcineurin inhibitor-based immunosuppression has reduced T cell-mediated graft rejection. However, antibody-mediated graft injury and rejection are on the rise. In 30 percent−50 percent of acute rejection incidents and more than 60 percent of late graft failures, antibodies are to blame. Acute graft rejection happens days to weeks after transplantation, and the risk is highest in the first three months.[35] Acute T-cell-mediated and antibody-mediated kidney transplant rejections have different histopathologic characteristics. Interstitial infiltration and tubulitis with intimal endarteritis are observed in TCMR and thrombotic microangiopathy, neutrophil, and macrophage margination in capillaries and often inside glomeruli are characteristics of acute AMR.[36] After suspecting acute kidney rejection, treatment should begin with a 3-day usage of intravenous methylprednisolone, and simultaneously serum creatinine levels should be tested. Treatment with intravenous corticosteroids should be started if the patients experience similar rejection incidents.[35] Hyperacute rejection is an immensely uncommon happening caused by excessive levels of antibodies against antigens on the endothelium of glomeruli and microvasculature of the donated kidney that develops within seconds of implantation and results in complement activation, platelet accumulation, and endothelial necrosis. However, recent developments in detecting DSAs and advanced cross-matching approaches have significantly prevented this phenomenon.[15]

Graft failure that occurs over 1 year after kidney transplantation is considered chronic kidney transplant rejection (CKTR). CKTR could be cell-mediated or antibody-mediated and generally happens due to inadequate immunosuppression. Acute rejection is also associated with a higher risk of CKTR. Delayed graft function, immunosuppressive medication toxicity, recurrence of primary kidney disease, diabetes, hypertension, and hyperlipidemia are other risk factors associated with CKTR.[37]

Amid transplantation, induction therapy, a T-lymphocyte-depleting agent, or an interleukin (IL)−2 inhibitor is used to treat the patients, and maintenance immunosuppression is started in the hospital and maintained throughout the life of the allograft. T cell activation and proliferation have a 3-signal approach. Signal 1 initiates the calcineurin pathway and IL-2 (T cell growth factor) transcription. Signal 2 enables the expression of IL-2 and other cytokines. IL-2 stimulation, in turn, results in signal 3, which activates the mammalian target of rapamycin (mTOR). Calcineurin inhibitors (CNIs) affect signal 1 and interfere with T cell proliferation. Corticosteroids suppress nuclear factor kappa B (NF-κB), which is required for the expression of several cytokines that play important roles in T cell activation. Mycophenolic acid, which inhibits the inosine monophosphate dehydrogenase (IMPDH) enzyme, is the active metabolite for mycophenolate mofetil. Mycophenolic acid suppresses T cell proliferation and downregulates the expression of adhesion molecules leading to inhibition of lymphocytes from binding to vascular endothelial cells and preventing them from gaining access to the rejection site. mTOR inhibitors and Belatacept are also other forms of immunosuppressive agents that are used post-transplantation. Careful screening of drug levels is important as many of the immunosuppressive drugs have a restricted therapeutic window. As time passes from transplantation, target levels for different immunosuppressive agents become lower. However, these levels are also influenced by side effects, infectious and malignancy complications, underlying renal disease, and time from transplantation. Kidney function should also be screened as long as the transplanted kidney is used. In the first month, it should be screened two times a week, and it should be diminished slowly over the first year. However, laboratory values should never be monitored less than every 3 months. 30 percent to 50 percent of renal transplant recipients have a glomerular disease, which has led to end-stage renal disease (ESRD). Glomerulonephritis occurrence is 5 percent at first year, 22 percent at five years, and 42 percent at 10 years after transplantation. Glomerular hyperfiltration, reflux nephropathy, drug exposures, and viral infections result in secondary focal segmental glomerulosclerosis (FSGS), and primary FSGS can be familial or idiopathic. Mutations in podocyte proteins can lead to familial FSGS. Patients who have FSGS recurrence in the first-year post-transplantation have more than an 80 percent chance of recurrence in future grafts. Careful screening of urine protein-creatinine ratio right after transplantation is necessary for the detection of early recurrence. The usual treatment for recurrence is timely recruitment of plasmapheresis and preservation of high-dose CNI therapy. 40 percent to 50 percent of transplant recipients experience membranous nephropathy (MN), and graft failure from recurrence in 10 years occurs in 10 percent to 15 percent of the patients. CNIs, steroid, and alkylating agents have demonstrated favorable results in the treatment of recurrent MN. 20 percent of ESRD in kidney transplant patients happens due to IgA nephropathy (IgAN). Microscopic hematuria, proteinuria, and slow deterioration of kidney function are a few of the clinical manifestations. Membranoproliferative glomerulonephritis (MPGN) is linked to viral infections (such as *Hepatitis C virus* (*HCV*) and *Hepatitis B virus* (*HBV*)), autoimmune disorders, and monoclonal gammopathies. The existence of HLA-B8 and -DR3, living-related donors, and previous graft loss from the recurrent disease are risk factors for recurrence. 15 percent of graft loss at 10 years is because of recurrence. Antineutrophil cytoplasmic antibody-associate glomerulonephritis is a comparatively rare cause of ESRD.

Postponing kidney transplantation until the disease is inactive is suggested. Lupus nephritis is a notable cause of ESRD in transplant patients. In about 30 percent of transplant patients, histologic recurrence has been reported. It has been suggested that the disease should be inactive for 6 to 9 months prior to transplantation to decrease the risk for recurrent lupus nephritis and morbidity. Urinary tract infections (UTIs) are widespread complications that occur after transplantation. Usage of foley catheters or ureteral stents can be the reason for developing UTIs in the early post-transplantation period. In addition, diabetes and bladder outlet congestion due to enlarged prostate can result in urinary stasis and UTIs. Sexually active women should be advised on urinating after sex and personal hygiene. A medical examination is required to detect any possible anatomic defect in patients with recurrent UTIs. Present immunosuppressants mostly inhibit T cell activation, which is mostly responsible for cellular rejection. However, these cells play an important role in repressing malignancies and viral and fungal infections as well. Furthermore, viral infections can impose great risks after transplantation. Infection with *Cytomegalovirus (CMV)* is usual in transplant patients, mostly if the donor is seropositive and the recipient is seronegative. Diarrhea, fever, malaise, pulmonary symptoms, and leukopenia are common manifestations of the disease. Annual influenza vaccines are suggested. However, usage of any form of the live vaccine is not recommended, which is an inhibitory factor for transplant patients who wish to travel to other countries. About 80 percent of adults have been exposed to polyoma (BK virus) throughout their lives, and about 20 percent of transplant patients develop BK viremia after transplantation. Currently, there is no known antiviral therapy for the BK virus, which makes reducing immunosuppression the only potent therapy. Transplant recipients are more likely to suffer from severe influenza disease, which is problematic. Transplantation candidates must be examined for tuberculosis prior to transplantation. Patients with positive tuberculosis should be examined for active disease and should be treated for active or latent tuberculosis. Fungal infections in kidney transplant patients can be deadly. *Aspergillus* and *mucormycosis* have long been linked to increased morbidity and mortality. The main treatment is the noticeable decrease in immunosuppression.[15]

Non-melanoma skin cancer is the most widespread malignancy after transplantation. The risk of developing squamous cell skin cancer is also increased among transplant patients. If the patient is experiencing recurrent skin cancers, it is better to switch to mTOR inhibitors. Renal cell cancers are more common among transplant recipients. Women of child-bearing age who want to become pregnant should consult with their physicians. The most favorable plot for conception is to be at least 1 year after transplantation, and the use of azathioprine instead of mycophenolate from 3 months before conception is suggested, and the patient should have a stable GFR, controlled blood pressure, and no notable proteinuria.[15]

Transplant outcomes have undergone significant transformation throughout time. From 1986 to 1999 and after 2000 to a lesser extent, transplant results have improved. These improvements were more apparent in the short-term outcomes compared with long-term outcomes. The significant change in graft survival that occurred between 1986 and 1999 was concurrent with the implementation of the progressively strong and original immunosuppressive regimens that led to a reduction in the risk of acute rejection. Other alterations such as improved management of high blood pressure, anemia, high serum cholesterol, and high serum glucose, a more uniformed histological assessment of kidney biopsies, improved donor care, better kidney storing and conserving, modernized distribution methods and crossmatching approaches, improved identification, prophylaxis, and handling of infections, improved handling of cardiovascular and urological hurdles, and other factors led to better transplantation results prior to the year 2000. Age until 55 years is indirectly associated with the risk of graft failure as younger patients are more likely to experience graft failure following transplantation than older kidney recipients.[38] The state of the patient before transplantation is an important contributing factor to graft outcome. Patients with pre-transplantation malignancy are more likely to experience malignancy reoccurrence and have increased overall mortality compared with patients who do not have pre-transplantation malignancy.[39]

## Liver transplantation

Liver transplantation has advanced significantly over the last decades. Thomas E Starzl performed the first orthotopic liver transplant on a 3-year-old patient with biliary atresia.[40] Currently, the only treatment choice for end-stage liver disease, acute fulminant hepatic failure, hepatocellular carcinoma, hilar cholangiocarcinoma, and many metabolic disorders is a liver transplant. Recent improvements in surgical techniques, perioperative care, and post-transplantation therapies have increased the overall success of the liver transplant and patient survival.[41]

The demand for liver transplantation is on the rise. However, the number of donors does not increase at the same rate.[41] To compensate for the shortcoming of donors, using liver allografts from non-heart-beating donors started in the early 90s.[42] Unfortunately, overall graft survival rates of DCD are significantly lower than those of DBD donors. However, there are several risk factors that if controlled, can improve the overall survival rates. Previous liver transplant, being on life-support, being hospitalized or in an intensive care unit (ICU), having received dialysis, having serum creatinine value > 2.0 mg/dL, and being older than 60 years are recipient characteristics that have harmful effects on transplant outcomes. Minimal donor warm ischemia time (DWIT) or CIT under 10 h reduces the effects of ischemic injury and improves the DBDs' graft survival.[43] Prior to liver transplantation, hypothermic perfusion can help decelerate the cellular metabolism and elongate the time liver can be functional without oxygen.[44] Favorable outcomes of hypothermic perfusion have been observed in allografts from DCD and DBD donors.[45–48] Constant delivery of required nutrients and oxygen to the organ in order to preserve cellular metabolism using a normothermic perfusion setup is more appealing.[49] This method allows secure transplantation of liver allografts and liver function assessment throughout the pre-implantation period.[50] Henri Bismuth proposed the method of graft size reduction in the 1980s to use adult donor grafts for pediatric recipients.[40] However, to avoid sacrificing the remnant liver, Rudolf Pichlamyr pioneered split liver transplantation (SLT) in 1988. This method enables the transplant of one donor liver into one pediatric and one adult recipient.[51] All these efforts were made to decrease the waitlist mortality.

The donor and recipient should either be ABO identical or compatible to minimize humoral and cellular rejection.[52] However, in hopeless situations when an ABO-compatible organ is unavailable, an ABO-incompatible liver can be used.[53,54] Blood group-O is generally considered a universal donor, and in acute settings, O-group grafts are considered for all patients of all blood groups. However, transplantation of O-group grafts to recipients with A, B, and AB blood groups can cause hemolysis. This happens because donor lymphocytes moved to the recipient's body during transplantation produce antibodies against A and B antigens on the red blood cell (RBC) of the patient.[55] About 10 percent of people with blood group A express lesser A antigens on their RBCs and are subtyped as A2. A2 grafts can be used for recipients with O and B blood groups.[56] As opposed to ABO blood groups, Rhesus (Rh) factor is not normally considered significant in matching organs for transplantation.[57] As mentioned earlier, HLA matching has long been considered for kidney transplantation. However, evidence is still lacking surrounding the relevance of HLA matching in liver transplantation, and it is not routinely used for matching liver grafts.[58] GVHD is a rare complication after liver transplant, which happens in about 0.5 percent−1 percent of the patients. However, it is highly fatal due to hemorrhage, sepsis, and multiple organ failure.[58,59]

Long-term outcomes of liver transplantation need to be improved. The main reasons for long-term mortality after liver transplantation include allograft failure, cardiovascular events, infection, malignancy, and renal failure.[60] Long-term use of immunosuppressive drugs is linked to such outcomes, and minimizing the usage of such medications is important.[41] Under attentive and strict supervision, withdrawal of immunosuppressive drugs is safe in patients who have received a liver transplant 2 years prior.[61]

## Heart transplantation

Christian Barnard performed the first heart transplant in 1967.[62] In the beginning, the results were not sufficient, and there were high mortality rates. However, cyclosporine was discovered at the end of the 1970s, which helped decrease rejection rates.[63] Patients with serious indications of heart failure, intractable angina, and rhythm disturbances can be considered for heart transplantation. However, due to the advancements in medicine, the definition of end-stage heart disease is not constant, and the health status of many patients that are considered for heart transplantation has undergone improvements by using the new methods. Therefore, they do not need heart transplantation.[64] The patient's mental and emotional status is also important for the transplantation process.[65] As it is difficult to determine end-stage heart disease, the transplant team should thoroughly inspect the patient to propose the ultimate management plan.[64] Important heart diseases such as angina pectoris, myocardial infarction, prior coronary bypass surgery, moderate to severe valvular disease, cardiomyopathy, and important arrhythmias are the only definite contraindication for heart donation. Other indefinite contraindications include untreated sepsis, malignancies, and active infections.[64] The gold standard for early diagnosis of rejection is by endomyocardial biopsy, which is regularly performed in the beginning stages of transplantation as the patients are mostly asymptomatic.[66] The most important reason for early death after heart transplant are primary graft failure and infection that account for approximately 12 percent of deaths in the first month and 29 percent of deaths between the first month and the first year.[67] It is important for the transplanted heart to produce the required cardiac output in the primary stage after surgery and is one of the most crucial factors determining transplant outcome. Following reperfusion, severe inflammatory responses in the area near the graft result in tissue acidosis, severe reduction of adenosine triphosphate (ATP), membrane impairment, and secretion of hydrolytic enzymes. As a result, ischemic damage may lead to irreversible or reversible impairment to the myocytes, which results in delayed recovery of the transplanted organ. The occurrence of early graft dysfunction is from 2 percent to 28 percent with about 30 percent death rate that depends on several factors, including increased right atrial pressure of the recipient, being older than 60 years old, diabetes, inotropic support, donor older than 40 years old, and duration of ischemia. With the development of potent immunosuppressive regimens, allograft rejection has diminished. However, approximately 5 percent, 10 percent, 11 percent, and 2 percent of deaths during month 1, month 1 to 12, month 12 to 36, and month 36 onward, respectively, are due to graft rejection.[68]

## Lung transplantation

Lung transplantation is an approved therapy for individuals with end-stage pulmonary disease. In 1963, James Hardy performed the first lung transplantation on a lung cancer patient. However, the patient died 18 days after the transplant due to renal failure. Stanford University team performed the first successful cardiopulmonary transplant in 1981. Later in 1983, the first isolated lung transplant was conducted in a patient with idiopathic pulmonary fibrosis at the University of Toronto.[69,70] Over the years, the lung transplantation field has progressed significantly.[71]

As there are several risks involved, the process of patient selection is strict so that the patient has a greater chance of long-term survival. Absolute contraindications of lung transplantation for recipients include a history of neoplasm treated in the last two years, lung cancer, cardiac dysfunction unrelated to pulmonary disease, notable organic impairment of any other organs, hepatitis B and C infection without treatment, active pulmonary tuberculosis, addiction to tobacco, alcohol, and narcotics, usage of psychoactive substances in the past six months, having a serious psychiatric disease without control, and lack of dedication to the suggested medical plan.[70] Donor and recipient should also be matched based on ABO blood groups.[72] Over the long run, survival is jeopardized by chronic lung allograft dysfunction and bronchiolitis obliterans syndrome (BOS), which is the main risk factor for late death. It has been reported that mortality rates have decreased in patients diagnosed with BOS who received azithromycin in time. Patients that have undergone lung transplantation are at higher risk of infection, which can lead to death. The average survival in lung transplant recipients is 5.8 years that is less than that of other SOT recipients.[73]

## Other

Other forms of transplantation are also being performed. Islet transplantation has long been an attractive solution for regaining glucose homeostasis in patients who have lost β-cells because of autoimmune reaction of type 1 diabetes, or from surgical resection, or pancreatic fibrosis in pancreatogenic forms of diabetes. Islet autotransplantation is used in patients with acute and chronic pancreatitis, trauma to the pancreas, or neoplasm of the pancreas. In such patients, total pancreatectomy is required, and then the patients' own islets are transplanted into the liver to improve diabetes caused by pancreatectomy.[74] Patients with type 1 diabetes or any cause of insulin-deficient diabetes who have problematic hypoglycemia are considered for islet allotransplantation, which results in excellent glycemic control and improved quality of life.[74,75] Kidney and islet transplantations are sometimes done simultaneously in diabetic patients to protect the transplanted kidney from the reappearance of diabetic nephropathy.[76] Immunosuppression with T lymphocyte-depleting agents such as thymoglobulin, a humanized monoclonal antibody against the cell surface glycoprotein CD52, and alemtuzumab, and T lymphocyte inhibitory agents that block IL-2 receptor such as basiliximab is required for islet allotransplantation.[77–81]

One of the main causes of reversible blindness is corneal blindness, which can be reverted back to normal with the transplantation of a healthy cornea donor.[82] Due to the lack of vasculature, it is the most successful organ transplantation in the human body. The first successful keratoplasty was performed by Zirm in 1905.[83] The main cause of failure is allograft rejection, which is associated with the existence of high-risk features, the most important being corneal neovascularization.[84] HLA and ABO matching is not required. However, Class I HLA matching is favored in recent studies for high-risk corneal transplantations.[85]

The skin graft is one of the most necessary techniques in plastic surgery and dermatology. In 1869, Reverdin performed the first skin autotransplantation. Since then, several pioneers have attempted to make the outcomes of skin grafting better.[86] In 1929, Brown et al. found the split-thickness skin grafting technique and distinguished between full-thickness, intermediate-thickness, and epidermal grafts and depicted the benefits and drawbacks of each method, which set the foundation of skin grafting that is still being used.[86] Split-thickness grafts include a portion of the dermis and can endure regions with less vascularity and are more likely to undergo contracture. The full-thickness graft consists of the entire dermis and demands a better vascular bed to survive. However, it is less likely to go through contracture.[87] HLA-A and -B matching improves skin graft survival.[88] However, it is not routinely done in practice due to internal immunosuppressive effects of severe burns, which preserve the unmatched skin from rejection. The graft will ultimately be rejected. However, it acts as a short-term barrier to prevent infections. To achieve better results aesthetically, the site of the donated skin should have compatible consistency, thickness, color, and texture.[86]

## Hematopoietic stem cell transplantation (HSCT)

HSCT is the most widely used cellular immunotherapy in which the hematopoietic stem cells of any donor type and any source are utilized to substitute the patient's hematopoietic system.[89]

## Indications

HSCT may be beneficial for many disorders. Currently, the general indications for the HSCT procedure are different in adults and children and should be discussed separately.

### *Adults*

#### Acute myeloid leukemia (AML)

Acute myeloid leukemia (AML) is the most frequent indication for allogeneic HSCT in Europe, and adult patients with AML should always be considered for HSCT. However, whether or not they should receive HSCT depends on the interplay between the risk of disease relapse and the risk of mortality post-transplantation.[90] Recently, other factors such as cytogenetics refined by molecular markers and somatic mutations play important roles in determining risk for acute leukemia in addition to white blood cell (WBC) count and response to induction therapy.[91,92] Furthermore, better evaluation of risk factors and comorbidities have also contributed to improved outcomes and decreased mortality.[93] After prognosis calculation, patients should be evaluated for autologous HSCT in first complete remission (CR1). If patients are positive for minimal residual disease (MRD), they may be candidates for allogeneic HSCT.[94] Patients who do not reach CR1 after one induction course should also be considered to receive allogeneic HSCT. Patients who receive an allogeneic or an autologous HSCT in CR1 have a significantly higher relapse-free survival compared with patients receiving chemotherapy.[93]

#### Acute lymphoblastic leukemia (ALL)

Acute lymphoblastic leukemia (ALL) is the second most common indication for allogeneic HSCT. A large proportion of adult patients with ALL have molecular targets for MRD evaluation and MRD can be utilized to determine various risk groups. However,

MRD is not appropriate at any time and the relevance depends on the particular prior therapy.[95]

## Chronic myeloid leukemia (CML)

Since the usage of tyrosine kinase inhibitors (TKIs) in patients with chronic myeloid leukemia (CML), allogeneic HSCT is not suggested as the first-line treatment following CML diagnosis. When first-line TKI therapy is not successful, second-line TKI therapy should be commenced. In case of failure of second-line TKI therapy, the search for a suitable related or unrelated donor should start as soon as possible. Furthermore, depending on the ABL mutation examination and risk scores, the patient should proceed to HSCT.[93]

## Myeloproliferative disorders other than CML

Currently, the only possible cure for patients with myeloproliferative disorders is HSCT except for polycythemia vera and essential thrombocytopenia patients that are not suggested to undergo allogeneic HSCT unless the disease has advanced to myelofibrosis or secondary leukemia.[96,97]

## Myelodysplastic syndromes (MDS)

The treatment of choice for adult myelodysplastic syndromes (MDS) patients is allogeneic HSCT, and if the treatment is done prior to disease advancement or in CR following chemotherapy, the chance of long-term disease-free survival is suitable.[98] If the number of blast cells is less than 5 percent at the time of transplantation, allogeneic HSCT will result in better outcomes. In patients with overabundant blast cells, intensive chemotherapy or hypomethylating agents are regularly utilized before transplantation. However, the beneficial effects of such treatments before transplantation on the post-transplant outcomes are yet to be proven by controlled studies. Whether or not the patient should proceed with allogeneic HSCT depends on the risk of the disease and the risk of the transplantation, which is predicted by the European Society for Blood and Marrow Transplantation (EBMT) risk score.[99]

## Chronic lymphocytic leukemia (CLL)

Chronic lymphocytic leukemia (CLL) management had undergone significant changes after the establishment of signaling pathway inhibitors (PI) like Bruton's TKI, ibrutinib, the phosphatidylinositol-3-kinase inhibitor, idelalisib, and the BCL2-inhibitor, venetoclax.[100] Patients who do not respond to both chemoimmunotherapy and PI should be assessed for cellular therapies such as chimeric antigen receptor (CAR)-T cell therapy and allogeneic HSCT. Patients who are diagnosed with CLL and MDS simultaneously and those with aggressive alteration in CLL should be considered for HSCT irrespective of the treatment stage of their CLL.[101]

## Lymphomas

The development of two categories for CR1 was the most prominent improvement regarding lymphoma. It is split into "true" CR1, which is achieving first CR directly by standard first-line therapy, and "first" CR, which is attained by one or more salvage therapies after initial induction failure.[93]

### Diffuse large B cell lymphoma (DLBCL)

The standard treatment for patients that experience a chemosensitive relapse of diffuse large B cell lymphoma (DLBCL) following first-line therapy and chemosensitive relapse of DLBCL after the failure of the previous autograft is still autologous HSCT.[102–107]

### Follicular lymphoma

Autologous HSCT might be an alternative choice in patients with chemosensitive high-grade alteration of follicular lymphoma if they had previously undergone systemic therapy for follicular lymphoma (particularly if it contained immunochemotherapy).[93]

### Waldenström's macroglobulinemia (lymphoplasmacytic lymphoma with IgM gammopathy; WM)

As there are more potent new therapeutic options available for Waldenström's macroglobulinemia (lymphoplasmacytic lymphoma with IgM gammopathy; WM) such as rituximab, purine analogs, proteasome inhibitors, and kinase inhibitors, utilizing autologous HSCT as first-line therapy is controversial and not advocated outside of clinical trial settings.[108] However, usage of allogeneic HSCT is supported as a clinical option for younger patients with aggressive or high-risk types of WM.[93]

### Mantle cell lymphoma (MCL)

Ibrutinib has been an accepted salvage treatment for patients with relapsed or refractory mantle cell lymphoma (MCL).[109] Available data does not recommend HSCT in patients with MCL in CR1.[93]

### T cell lymphomas

Peripheral T cell lymphomas generally have a very poor prognosis, and allogeneic HSCT is an effective therapeutic option in patients with relapsed and refractory disease and is suggested as standard care for patients with chemosensitive relapse.[110]

### Hodgkin lymphoma

HSCT is the standard care for Hodgkin lymphoma patients with chemosensitive relapse. It should be autologous in patients who previously received an autograft and allogeneic in patients with a prior unsuccessful autograft.[93]

### Multiple myeloma (MM)

Currently, first-line autologous HSCT remains the standard treatment for recently diagnosed multiple myeloma (MM) patients.[93]

### Systemic immunoglobulin-light-chain amyloidosis

High-dose therapy along with autologous HSCT is beneficial to patients with systemic immunoglobulin-light-chain amyloidosis without severe heart failure.[111] Allogeneic HSCT might be taken into consideration in younger patients who did not respond or relapsed following autologous HSCT and were administered at least one alternative drug.[93]

### Acquired severe aplastic anemia

The standard treatment for adult acquired severe aplastic anemia patients is HLA-identical sibling allogeneic HSCT with worse results in patients older than 40 years old. Along with age, evaluation of comorbidities is also important. To decrease the chance of chronic GVHD, all patients should undergo T cell depletion with anti-thymocyte globulin (ATG) or alemtuzumab. Matched unrelated allogeneic HSCT is considered as first-line therapy in severe aplastic anemia patients younger than 18 years.[93]

### Constitutional severe aplastic anemia

Allogeneic HSCT is the only treatment capable of restoring the normal hematopoiesis in patients with constitutional severe aplastic anemia.[93]

### Solid tumors

Autologous HSCT ameliorates progression-free survival (PFS) in breast cancer. The standard treatment for patients with germ cell tumors that do not respond to platinum-based chemotherapy or have relapsed is high-dose therapy and autologous HSCT.[93]

### Autoimmune diseases

HSCT has long been considered as a treatment option for patients with autoimmune diseases. Patients with severe autoimmune disease resistant to standard therapy are considered for autologous and allogeneic HSCT. Autologous HSCT is utilized in multiple sclerosis, systemic sclerosis, Crohn's disease, and systemic lupus erythematosus, and allogeneic HSCT has been mostly used in pediatric patients, especially those with refractory autoimmune cytopenia and juvenile idiopathic arthritis.[93]

#### *Children and adolescents*

More than 20 percent of all allogeneic HSCTs are performed on children and adolescents. Transplant complications are related to the vulnerability of the developing child, organ development dysfunction, growth retardation, delayed hormonal development, and increased risk for malignancies in congenital disorders with chromosomal breakage syndromes. High-resolution HLA matching for unrelated donors, conditioning regimens, and palliative care for infectious and non-infectious complications have improved, which resulted in lower mortality and further supported the use of allogeneic HSCT in the early stages of non-malignant indications.[93]

### Acute myeloid leukemia (AML)

Childhood AML is a rare and heterogeneous disease with heterogeneous behavior. The cure and survival rates have increased due to rigorous chemotherapy, especially in patients with positive prognostic markers. Consequently, allogeneic HSCT is the standard treatment for high- and very high-risk patients in CR1. However, it is not recommended as a first-line treatment in low-risk patients(112–115). Children who undergo AML relapse and achieve the second CR are considered for allogeneic HSCT. Children with high- and very-high-risk AML in CR1 are considered for autologous HSCT if a well-matched allogeneic donor is not available.[116]

### Acute lymphoblastic leukemia (ALL)

The standard treatment for high-risk ALL patients in CR1 and those in CR2 or later is allogeneic HSCT from a matched sibling or a well-matched unrelated donor.[93] The most critical prognostic factor for distinguishing high and very-high ALL is MRD

### Chronic myeloid leukemia (CML)

Allogeneic HSCT is not suggested as the first-line treatment of CML in children and adolescents. However, in the case of treatment, patients with failure or relapse after receiving salvage second-generation TKI treatment and advanced-stage CML are candidates to receive allogeneic HSCT as the standard treatment.[117–119]

### MDS and juvenile myelomonocytic leukemia

The treatment of choice for pediatric patients with primary MDS, including juvenile myelomonocytic leukemia and secondary AML is allogeneic HSCT from a sibling or a well-matched unrelated donor.[117–119]

### Lymphoma

Almost all children and adolescents with Hodgkin and non-Hodgkin lymphoma (NHL) are treated with multidrug chemotherapy. Patients with the lingering disease following repeated therapy by the current chemotherapy protocols, patients with early NHL relapses, and patients without adequate response or relapse of anaplastic lymphoma kinase- (ALK) positive anaplastic large cell lymphoma are eligible for HSCT.[93]

### Inherited diseases

**Primary immunodeficiencies (PID)** Primary immunodeficiencies (PID) refers to a group of genetic disorders characterized by the increased risk of infections, auto-immunity, and malignancies, which are resulted from incapable or malfunctioning innate or adaptive immune system. Allogeneic HSCT is a treatment option in pediatric patients with PID.[93] Severe combined immunodeficiency (SCID) is a pediatric emergency, and patients should receive allogeneic HSCT from a well-matched related or unrelated donor rapidly, which could increase the survival rates to more than 90 percent when performed shortly after birth.[120–122] Most of the T-lymphocyte immunodeficiencies, including CD40 ligand deficiency, and Wiskott-Aldrich syndrome, phagocyte disorders such as leukocyte adhesion deficiency, and chronic granulomatous diseases, hemophagocytic syndromes, including familial lymphohistiocytosis, and a growing number of other immunodeficiencies can be cured with allogeneic HSCT. A pre-transplantation conditioning regimen is required. Survival is not significantly different between HLA-identical family donors and HLA-matched unrelated donors.[123–127]

**Metabolic diseases** Most of the metabolic diseases that lead to HSCT are lysosomal storage diseases that depend on the transference of enzymes from donor-derived blood cells to the reticuloendothelial system and solid organs. Recently, the HSCT outcomes have advanced by adjusted transplant strategies.[93]

**Hemoglobinopathies** Treatment of choice for pediatric patients with severe β-thalassemia is allogeneic HSCT from a healthy related sibling or a related cord blood. If an HLA-matched related donor is not accessible, a well-matched unrelated donor is considered as an option.[93]

**Osteopetrosis** Malignant infantile osteopetrosis is a rare genetic type of skeletal dysplasia that typically presents in infancy and is characterized by osteoclast deficiency, which leads to elevated bone density, pancytopenia from medullary obliteration, cranial nerve compression, and pathologic features. Allogeneic HSCT is suggested as a potent treatment option.[93]

**Acquired severe aplastic anemia and inherited bone marrow failure syndromes** The standard first-line therapy for pediatric patients diagnosed with acquired severe aplastic anemia is allogeneic HSCT from an HLA-matched related donor.[93]

**Solid tumors** Generally, allogeneic HSCT in pediatric patients should only be examined within clinical trial settings. However, HSCT can be used after high-dose chemotherapy as a clinical option and a part of the front-line treatment.[93]

**Autoimmune diseases** Autologous and allogeneic HSCTs are viewed as a clinical choice for pediatric patients diagnosed with autoimmune diseases.[128–130] Pediatric patients diagnosed with inflammatory arthritis and other autoimmune diseases such as systemic sclerosis, systemic lupus erythematosus, vasculitis, and polymyositis-dermatomyositis can be considered for autologous HSCT.[131]

## Sources

### *Autologous/allogeneic/syngeneic*

There are three main types of HSCT: autologous, allogeneic, and syngeneic. In autologous HSCT, the stem cells are gathered from the patient and are returned back to the patient at another time. In allogeneic hemopoietic stem cell transplantation, the cells are harvested from a different individual, either related or unrelated, and are infused into the patient.[89] A well-matched unrelated donor is an unrelated donor that is 10 out of 10 or 8 out of 8 identical according to HLA high-resolution typing for class I (HLA-A, -B, -C) and II (HLA-DRB1, -DQB1). A mismatched unrelated donor is an unrelated adult donor that is not matched in a minimum of one antigen or allele at HLA-A, -B, -C, or -DR. The outcomes of all HLA mismatches are not the same.[132–134] In syngeneic HSCT, hematopoietic stem cells are harvested from one identical twin and infused into the other identical twin.[135]

### *Peripheral blood/bone marrow/umbilical cord blood/amniotic fluid*

There are different candidates for stem cell therapy. Originally, stem cells were harvested from bone marrow. In addition, peripheral blood is a new source of stem cells that is being used more and more as it seems to reduce the risk of relapse.[136] Patients receiving stem cells from peripheral blood have better recovery rates compared with patients who received stem cells from the bone marrow.[137] Human umbilical cord blood has been proven to be incredibly effective, at least in certain situations. These cells can be obtained when an infant is born and can be reserved. Cord blood contains mesenchymal stem cells that can differentiate into all tissues.[138] These cells have an important role in providing a crucial microenvironment for hematopoiesis and can be used during HSCT to facilitate hematopoietic recuperation.[139] Also, amniotic fluid is a new source of mesenchymal stem cells that can be utilized in transplantation settings.[140]

## Establishment process

### *Homing/engraftment/repopulation/reconstitution*

Successful transplantation of hematopoietic stem cells relies on the effective homing, engraftment, and repopulation of the stem cells in the bone marrow. Stem cell homing occurs using the bloodstream to the bone marrow. For engraftment to occur, first, the transplanted hematopoietic stem cells need to interact with the sinusoidal endothelial cells of the bone marrow. Furthermore, the E- and P-selectin that are expressed on the bone marrow sinusoids bind to glycosylated ligands on hematopoietic stem cells and migrate through the endothelium.[141] Engraftment is defined as the series of actions by which hematopoietic stem cells reach free bone marrow recesses where they are able to find the most favorable circumstances in which they can survive and proliferate to produce all of the subtypes of the hematopoietic cells. Engraftment is usually considered the first three days in a row that the peripheral blood neutrophil count is sustained at more than 500 × $10^6$/L. Engraftment is mostly influenced by the source of the graft and the conditioning regimen of HSCT. Sometimes, following stem cell transplantation during neutrophil recovery, patients experience a clinical condition presented by fever, rash, pulmonary edema, weight gain, liver and renal dysfunction, and/or encephalopathy called engraftment syndrome. It has been suggested that this condition is caused by a proinflammatory circumstance resulting from the release of various cytokines and other mediators of inflammation. Engraftment syndrome is self-limited, and there is no need for therapy. However, if the fever is higher than 39 °C and is not caused by an infection and it has presentations associated with vascular leak like pulmonary edema, corticosteroids are administered until the symptoms are resolved.[137] After the engraftment process, the hematopoietic stem cells repopulate the bone marrow that was previously ablated.[142] Following HSCT, the immune system undergoes reconstitution. The innate immunity experiences reconstitution first, followed by adaptive immunity. Monocytes followed by neutrophils are the first cells to return to normal condition. Two weeks after transplantation, more than 80 percent of circulating dendritic cells (DCs) are of donor origin. Seven to eight weeks after transplantation, NK cells reconstitution occurs. B cells and T cells are the last types of cells, which undergo reconstitution.[143]

## Transplantation immunopathogenesis

### The role of cellular immunity

#### *T cell expansion and repertoire formation*

The traditional T cell feedback to alloantigen is crucial for evaluating short and long-term results for solid organ transplants. Alloantigen can be detected through at least two routes (Fig. 7.1). The direct pathway is temporary and accounts for acute rejection. The indirect pathway lasts longer and leads to chronic rejection.[144] In the direct pathway, which was long considered the main pathway responsible for rejection, CD4+ T cells detect the major histocompatibility complex (MHC) class II, and CD8+ T cells recognize MHC class I alloantigens that are on the surface of donor antigen-presenting cells (APCs).[145] In order to explain this phenomenon, passenger leukocyte theory was suggested. Allograft rejection is stimulated when donor DCs that have relocated to the host's secondary lymphoid tissues are recognized through the direct pathway.[146–149] The indirect pathway was proposed when allografts that did not have passenger leukocytes still underwent rejection offering the idea that alloantigen could also be detected traditionally. There are several mismatched major and minor histocompatibility antigens on the cells' surface of transplanted organs, which could result in the production of large numbers of variable allopeptide epitopes. These epitopes are able to be recognized through the indirect pathway. The role of the indirect pathway has been enhanced more and more in allogeneic organ rejection.[144] Intact antigens can move between different cell types, which can indicate that T cells of the direct pathway may recognize

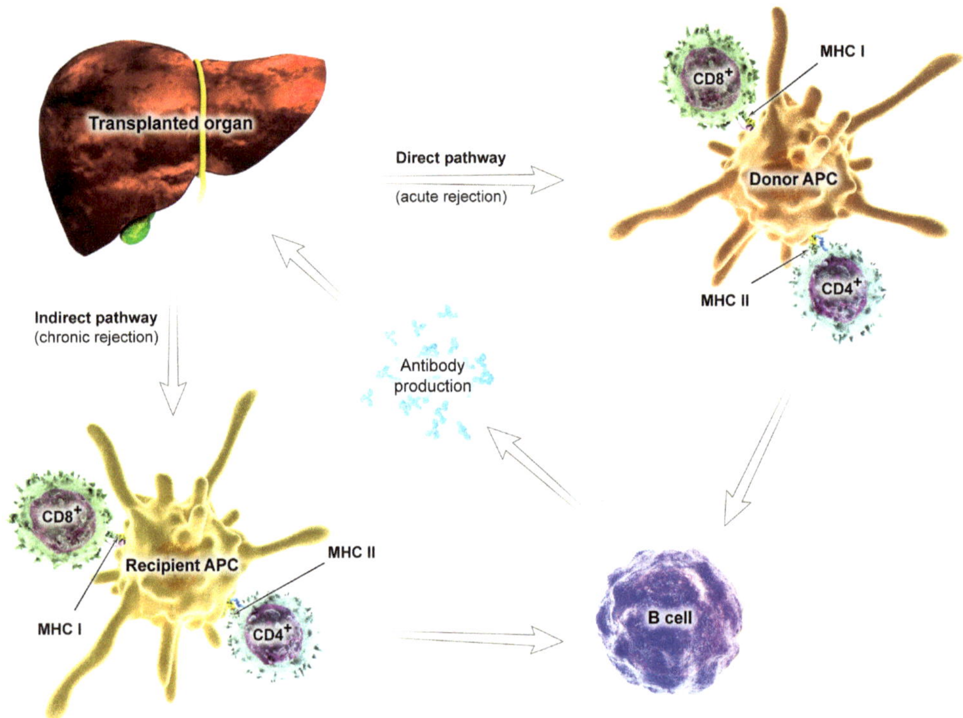


**Fig. 7.1** ***The role of T cells in antigen presentation.*** 1) Direct pathway: Donor antigen-presenting cells (APCs) present alloantigen to T cells of the recipient. 2) Indirect pathway: Recipient APCs present alloantigen of the donor organ to the recipient T cells.

intact alloantigens that are presented on DCs, which is called the semi-direct pathway. Although hard to prove, it has gained support from the migration of alloantigen to DCs.[150–153]

In the direct pathway, CD4+ T cell responses are restricted to the first few weeks following transplantation and it was suggested that its length depends on the lifespan of the donor DC proportion in mouse models.[154–157] A few human studies also demonstrated the brief lifespan of CD4 T cell stimulation through the direct pathway.[154,158–160] The response of CD4+ T cell through indirect pathway against processed alloantigen can be longer than those through direct pathway against intact alloantigen. Several animal studies have proposed the possible contribution of the indirect pathway CD4+ T cell response to the development and maintenance of chronic allograft rejection.[161–164] The duration of indirect responses against MHC class I allopeptide is longer lasting than indirect responses against MHC class II allopeptide, which was as brief as the direct pathway and only detectable during the first week following transplantation.[144] The main mechanism for prompting direct pathway CD8+ T cell alloimmunity is presenting intact MHC class I alloantigen by migrating donor DCs. However, differentiation of naïve CD8+ T cells depends on aid from stimulated CD4+ T cells.[144]

### *Notch signaling*

Notch is a fundamental extremely preserved signaling pathway that constitutes the cell signaling foundation of multi-cellular organisms by affecting cell fate and, as a result, morphogenesis. The final signals channeled by the Notch receptor are significantly pleiotropic and can greatly influence differentiation, proliferation, and apoptosis. It is not surprising that disorders in this pathway may result in diseases and can potentially be a therapeutic aim of treatment.[165] Notch has been acknowledged as a crucial component in early T cell evolution for a long time.[166,167] In vitro studies showed that Notch signaling regulates T helper (Th)1 differentiation. Notch1 and Notch2 receptors are also crucial for some models of Th1 polarization. The suggested functions of Notch signaling in immunity has a wide range. However, the exact procedures of these effects are still unclear.[168]

The role of Notch signaling in the establishment of alloimmune injury caused by GVHD following allogeneic HSCT has been defined with the help of mouse models. GVHD is a major complication that patients can face following allogeneic HSCT as a result of the recognition of the transplant patient antigens by naïve donor T cells.[168] Impeding the Notch signaling pathway in mature T cells can protect against GVHD. In MHC-mismatched and matched allogeneic HSCT patients, those receiving Notch-deprived T cells can have extended GVHD-free survival. These T cells that are deprived of Notch have deficiencies in several cytokines, including interferon (IFN)-$\gamma$, tumor necrosis factor (TNF)-$\alpha$, IL-2, IL-17, and IL-4. Although inhibiting Notch only had insignificant effects on allogeneic T cells' proliferation, it notably increases regulatory T cells (Tregs) proliferation.[169–171] In conclusion, Notch signaling has demonstrated promising results in the treatment of GVHD. Notch signaling has also been associated with solid organ rejection. Inhibiting Notch signaling seems to be beneficial in allograft HSCT as in heart transplant patients, pan-Notch blocking in mature T cells increases the allograft survival. Notch signaling using Dll1/4 ligands is suggested to have crucial roles in the regulation of solid organ rejection. Overall, Notch signaling is an important component in alloimmune responses that lead to GVHD and solid organ rejection. Treatments aimed at Notch signaling in animal models have proved to be beneficial, making it a potential therapeutic option in the future.[168]

### *Treg activation*

Tregs are cells that express CD4 and CD25 molecules and FOXP3, which is a transcription factor crucial for their evolution and function.[172,173] Tregs can be classified based on their source into thymic-derived (tTregs) naturally occurring and peripherally derived Tregs (pTregs), which can be discerned by their Treg-specific demethylated region.[174] Tregs are known for their ability to modulate the immune system. However, their function is not carried by only one mechanism, and it is believed that several mechanisms are involved in harmony to orchestrate immune modulation. T lymphocytes' existence and reproduction depend on IL-2. Tregs express IL-2 receptor, CD25, which can attract

IL-2s, making them unavailable for T lymphocytes.[172] Another mechanism involves the cytotoxic T lymphocyte-associated antigen (CTLA)−4 molecules that are on the surface of Tregs and have a higher affinity to CD80/86 costimulatory molecules than the proinflammatory CD28 molecule that effector T cells express. This can inhibit the activation of effector T cells.[175] Lymphoproliferative disorders and severe T-cell-directed autoimmune diseases have been linked to CTLA-4 deficiencies.[174] Studies also demonstrated the role of Tregs in the suppression of immune responses in cancer, chronic infection, and allogeneic transplantations.[176] CD4+ CD25+ Tregs were shown to have roles in tolerance induction as the infusion of allogeneic blood in the rat produced CD4+ T cells that could inhibit anti-donor responses.[177] It was later observed that naïve CD4+ CD25+*T* cells could impede allogeneic skin graft rejection and autoimmune responses. However, CD4+ CD25- T cells could not produce the same effect.[178] The exact mechanisms, which Tregs utilize to induce allograft tolerance is still not clear. However, some of the mechanisms are absolutely necessary for allograft induction in mice. Tregs preserve immune homeostasis in mice utilizing IL-10 and CTLA-4 to a certain extent.[176] Therefore, it did not come as a surprise that CD4+ CD25+ Tregs from mice provided tolerance to heart allografts using IL-10-dependent pathways.[179,180] Furthermore, inhibiting CTLA-4 impedes graft tolerance that was induced by CD4+ CD25+ Tregs.[180] These properties have made scientists use Tregs in transplantation settings.

### Memory T cells

When our bodies reencounter specific antigens, the responses tend to be stronger and quicker. These responses are crucial for infections, vaccinations, and tumor immunosurveillance. However, in the context of transplantation, such memory immune responses that are directed against donor antigens can be dangerous and lead to unfavorable graft outcomes.[181] When previous exposure to alloantigen has not occurred, 1 percent to 10 percent of memory T cells are able to act against MHC molecules utilizing a direct allorecognition pathway in experimental settings.[181,182] It is possible that these memory cells are produced when peptides from other antigens are presented by MHC molecules and can imitate complexes by allogeneic MHC molecules that are attached to other peptides.[183] An example can be sensitization to allo-MHC molecule HLA-B4402 because of antigen mimicry after *Epstein-Barr virus* (*EBV*) infection in HLA-B8+ patients.[184,185] Memory T cells can be produced from prior exposure to alloantigen through previous transplants, pregnancies, and blood transfusions.[181] Different mechanisms mediate the contribution of memory T cells in allograft rejection. Memory T cells can turn into effector cells after reactivating. They can also aid in strong stimulation of donor-reactive effector CD8+ T cells that can induce rejection.[186] It is currently acknowledged that detection of memory T cells is associated with worse outcomes, and alloreactive memory T cells can speed up the process of allograft rejection and impede tolerance.[181]

### *Natural killer T cells*

Natural killer T (NKT) cells comprise a small proportion of T lymphocytes (<1 percent) that can recognize glycolipids presented by a molecule like MHC class I known as CD1d.[187] After NKT cells activation, they can regulate the fast and sustained production of a series of cytokines that can affect innate and acquired immunity.[188] As CD1d molecules are not polymorphic as opposed to MHC molecules, it is unclear whether or not NKT cells can detect alloantigen directly.[189]

Following transplantation, nonspecific inflammation produces an environment of cytokines that may stimulate NKT cells. Furthermore, NKT cells may prompt rejection or tolerance according to their reaction to such stimuli. IFN-γ secreted from NKT cells was shown to regulate graft injury by recruiting neutrophils in islet transplantation. Although these reports exist, more studies suggest the inhibitory role of NKT cells in transplantation.[190] Invariant natural killer T (iNKT) cells are a small proportion of lymphocytes that are defined by Vα14-Jα18 invariant T cell receptors. Following activation by α-GalCer, they rapidly excrete immense quantities of cytokines such as IFN-γ and IL-2, and Th2 cytokines, including IL-4 and IL-10.[187] It has been acknowledged that iNKT cells are required for promoting and/or sustaining tolerance in transplantation.[187]

## The role of humoral immunity

The humoral immunity involved in allografts can be divided into two principal branches: adaptive B cell immunity and innate B cell immunity. Producing high-affinity antibodies that react to foreign antigens of the donor cells (predominantly MHC class I and II molecules) with the help of T cells is the foundation of adaptive B cell immunity. Innate B cell immunity employs pre-existing antibodies against ABO blood group antigens and xenoantibodies, including IgM, which react to Ga1 α−1, 3 Gal Xenoantibodies have some common characteristics with "natural antibodies" (Nabs), which are immunoglobulins present in animals and humans. Although Nabs were discovered more than half a century ago, their exact function is still unclear, which may be due to the absence of specificity as they are reactive to numerous, supposedly irrelevant, antigenic patterns. Nabs are mostly detected as IgM and to a lesser extent, IgG. However, this equilibrium can unsettle in certain pathological states.[191]

### *Innate B cells/natural Abs*

The role of Nabs in transplantation was only observed in xenotransplantation or ABO mismatched transplantation. Previously produced Nabs in the host powerfully respond to xeno- or allogeneic carbohydrate determinants on donor cell surfaces, which results in hyperacute rejection. Increased serum quantities of IgG Nabs were reported in renal transplant patients with AMR. Furthermore, Nabs may trigger complement to deposit C4d on target cells in vitro, which proposes the possibility of a similar role in vivo.[192] Elevated levels of IgG Nabs prior to transplantation were also associated with lower survival rates following renal transplantation in non-sensitized patients.[193] There also is an extremely notable relation between the elevation in levels of Nabs following transplantation and graft loss.[194] Although Nabs are independently linked to decreased graft survival when there is a lack of DSA, when DSA and Nabs both exist, the occurrence of graft loss is at its highest.[192–194]

Complex immune infiltrates are widespread during rejection in the renal and cardiac allograft. B cells can be largely found in these infiltrates, even in TCMR.[195–208] B cells have many functions other than antibody secretion. It is extremely likely that CD20+ innate B cells have a different function from CD20- Cd138+ plasma cells, which secrete Nabs. However, their roles are yet to be understood, and there are three principal hypotheses taken into consideration: innate B cells become triggered following detecting damage-associated molecular patterns (DAMPs) and secrete pro-inflammatory cytokines and chemokines that heighten the local immune reaction, antigens being presented to infiltrating T cells by B cells, and immunomodulatory capabilities comparable to that of regulatory B cells (Bregs) producing IL-10.[191] However, future examinations are needed to discover the exact function of these cells during rejection for them to be considered as preventative or therapeutic options.

### *Donor specific antibodies (DSA)*

Detecting antibodies for the possible donor before transplantation is extremely useful. Different levels of antibodies can have different results. Low levels of antibodies may predict AMR, whereas increased levels of antibodies may result in hyperacute rejection. De novo DSAs may also be produced following transplantation.[209] Major histocompatibility loci were discovered by utilizing DSAs, thus making them sensitive and specific to MHC antigens.[210,211] Following organ transplantation, some of these antigens may not trigger humoral immunity, or if they do, they may be absorbed into the graft, making them undetectable. This can make it hard to discern if the lack of response is from the absorption of antibodies or not. Second transplants with no cross-match have a higher risk of rejection compared with primary transplants presenting the idea that sensitization does not depend on the production of DSAs.[209] Interestingly, the result of transplantation in patients who were undergoing secondary transplantation did not differ if the donated kidneys shared similar antigens or not.[212] If DSAs can be measured before or in the early stages of rejection, the process of rejection can be prevented or neutralized. These antigens can also help evaluate the effectiveness of immunosuppressive therapies.[209] It is important to understand to what degree the detected antibodies constitute the antibodies that can harm the graft. The antibodies that get absorbed into the graft probably have more affinity and pathogenicity than those that stay in the blood.[213] Either antigen alongside co-stimulation or inflammation triggers antibody creation. When it is stimulated by antigen, tolerance or a long-term state of non-reactivity can be prompted. However, if it is inflammation that has triggered antibody production, immunity or immunodeficiency can be prompted.[213–216] Therefore, it is currently not clear that measuring DSAs demonstrates immunity or inflammation.[209] The field of DSA is very attractive in transplantation settings and presents diagnostic, preventative, and therapeutic opportunities.

### *Anti-donor memory B cells*

Most of the research revolving around humoral responses to the transplanted organ has emphasized circulating antibodies and plasma cells that excrete them. Naïve B cells are activated after interaction with specific antigens with simultaneous signals from specialized CD4+ T cells and experience clonal expansion and differentiate into distinctive B cell types. B cells have to differentiate into plasma cells to gain antibody secretion ability. Memory B cells are generated when the triggered B cells inhibit their activation and become quiescent.[217] Zachary et al. were the first group to identify alloreactive B cells from peripheral blood utilizing HLA tetramers (tet). Tets are streptavidin-biotin complexes that consist of four peptide-loaded HLA molecules bonded to a fluorescent protein. These B cells are specified using flow cytometry, which permits instant and sensitive measurement of the patient's B cell reaction to the intended MHS antigen. CD27 and CD38 were employed to detect the tet+ memory B cells and plasma cells, respectively. Surprisingly, there was not a significant relationship between the number of CD27+ tet+ memory B cells or CD38+ tet+ plasma cells and the equivalent HLA mismatch for prior transplantation. However, in patients who were DSA-negative before transplantation and were among the tet+ B cells, the prevalence of CD27+ cells was increased.[218,219] These findings indicate the existence of memory B cells in sensitized patients and their considerable resistance to the regularly used immunosuppressive regimens prior to transplantation. It is important to note that pathogen-specific memory B cells are crucial for the long-term survival of the patients and such cells have to be maintained under the immunosuppressive regimen.[217]

## The role of NK cells, DCs, neutrophils, macrophages, and toll-like receptors

Innate immunity is progressively regarded as a crucial component in transplantation that not only is involved in inflammation in the early period following transplantation but also affects the differentiation of the cells of adaptive immunity that can lead to rejection or tolerance.[220] Monocytes which comprise 5 percent−10 percent of the WBCs of the peripheral circulation can arise from a myeloid progenitor and can turn into DCs or macrophages.[221] It has been increasingly suggested that monocytes may have an important part in allograft rejection. Renal transplant recipients with glomeruli infiltrated by monocytes have an increased risk of adverse kidney function at 1, 2, and 4 years after transplantation. In addition, glomerular monocyte infiltration is correlated with C4d accumulation. At the time of rejection, monocyte-derived cytokines also increase.[222] Furthermore, monocytes and macrophages are demonstrated to be adequate to prompt rejection when the adaptive immune system is depleted that without maintenance immunosuppression, all of the patients undergo acute rejection with immense infiltration of triggered monocytes.[223] Macrophages have phagocytic functions and can be classified into pro-inflammatory (M1) and anti-inflammatory (M2) subtypes. M1 subtype is active during rejection by phagocytosis, antigen-presentation to CD4+ T cells, and manufacturing pro-inflammatory cytokines such as IL-1β, IL-12, IL-18, IFN-λ, and TNF-α.[224,225] These actions are able to prompt naïve T cell differentiation and maintain the responses of memory cells.[226] These findings lead to the assumption that macrophages and monocytes may play an important role in graft rejection.

DCs are a crucial part of the innate immune system that connects innate and adaptive immunity.[227] During pro-inflammatory states, when pathogen-associated molecular patterns (PAMPs) are recognized by pattern-recognition receptors, DC maturation is prompted, which enables change from innate to adaptive immunity. Classically, it was thought that following transplantation, the graft attracts immature circulating DCs with a cascade of pro-inflammatory chemokines and cytokines. These DCs are APCs for MHC class II molecules of donor cells.[220] After DCs activation, they upregulate C—C chemokine receptor (CCR)7 that leads to them transferring to secondary lymphoid tissues in which they start cognate detection of MHC peptides by a particular type of T cells.[220] DCs can be classified into two major subgroups: myeloid or conventional DCs (mDCs) and plasmacytoid DCs (pDCs). mDCs produce elevated levels of IL-12 and can trigger proliferation and alloreaction of effector T cells. Furthermore, pDCs promote Tregs differentiation and maturation.[228] They also seem to take part in peripheral T cell tolerance.[220] Utilizing pharmacologically altered tolerogenic DCs (TolDCs) to impede autoimmune disease and graft rejection has been reported.[229,230] These contradictory effects of DCs seem to arise from the disparity in the expression of surface co-stimulatory ligands and the manufacture of cytokines, which are both crucial for the maturation and polarization of T cells.[228,231] TolDCs have reduced the number of MHC molecules, CD80 and CD86, which makes them physiologically immune to the maturation signal from stimulating DAMPs. They also do not produce cytokines that differentiate T cells into Th1 or Th2 phenotypes, and therefore, they are incapable of triggering effector T cells.[220] Although DCs have not have been an attractive target for graft rejection and tolerance, they seem to be involved in the process of transplantation.

Although NK cells arise from the lymphoid cell line, their immune functions depend on a separate network of receptors. Their activation process is controlled by the equilibrium between activating and inhibitory receptors.[232] The involvement of NK cells in allograft rejection remains debatable. In naïve mice that have undergone transplantation, NK cells play an important role in allograft rejection. Due to the lack of self MHC molecules on cells of the transplanted organs, NK cells become activated. However, traditionally animal studies demonstrated that eradication of NK cells does not affect rejection.[233–235] More recently, it was observed in a transplant from C57BL/6 to BALB/c mouse that eradication of NK cells inhibited rejection, which contrasts previous observations.[234] NK cells infiltrated the graft while the transplanted organ underwent rejection in stringent Rag-1-deficient mice, which lacked mature T and B cells. These observations indicate the role of NK cells in case of lack of T cells.[236] NK cells have direct cytotoxic functions that are mostly regulated by perforins and granzymes, which have been demonstrated to be biomarkers of rejection.[232,237] Conversely, it has been observed in some animal models that tolerance induction in allograft requires perforin-dependent NK cells.[238] There is convincing evidence indicating that NK cells enhance alloimmune responses that seem to be not sufficient to prompt rejection in humans. However, there is a need for more evidence to implement therapies directed at NK cells to prevent rejection.[220]

Neutrophils are an important player in the innate immune system. Along with monocytes, they are the first cells to respond to inflammation prompted by ischemic reperfusion injury after organ transplantation.[239,240] Neutrophils contribute to monocyte and macrophage chemotaxis by producing cytokines such as IFN-γ on site. Furthermore, they can produce and send out chemokine ligands, which trigger the maturation of DCs present at the site of inflammation by upregulating CD40, 46, and 86 on DCs.[241,242] Neutrophils also aid in T cell maturation by interacting with DCs causing them to produce more IL-12.[241–243] Neutrophils have several capabilities and are involved in both innate and adaptive immunity activation.[220] Traditionally, observing neutrophils in the graft was linked to bacterial infection. However, it has been proposed that alloimmune and non-alloimmune responses could be prompted by T cell co-localization with neutrophils and that this co-localization is not only restricted to the effector phase of the inflammation.[244] Like NK cells, neutrophils appear to be involved in allograft rejection. However, treatment options only targeting neutrophils may not be effective, and they should be in combination with T cell-directed therapies to inhibit rejection or induce tolerance.[220]

Toll-like receptors (TLRs) were discovered in 1996 in the drosophila fly, and until now, 10 operative TLRs have been detected in humans. Many leukocytes express these receptors, including monocytes, macrophages, DCs, neutrophils, T cells, and B cells.[220] Other cells, such as endothelial and epithelial cells of solid organs, also express these receptors.[245] The most widespread intracellular signaling pathway that is comprised of TLR activation occurs after a microbial agent joins TLR, which results in the universal adaptor protein MyD88 stimulation. Following MyD88 activation, a phosphorylation cascade takes place that results in the excretion of NF-κB. The final outcome is the activation of activator protein-1 (AP-1), interferon regulator factor 3, and other transcription factors that increase the expression of genes such as cytokines IL-6, IL-12, and TNF-α that are involved in inflammation.[220] Findings of studies show that ischemic-related injury is regulated by the interaction of DAMPs with TLRs.[245–247] In a mice model of graft rejection, a totally MHC-mismatched kidney mouse who lacked MyD88 experienced donor antigen-specific tolerance, which impeded acute and chronic rejection.[248] MyD88 insufficiency elevates the equilibrium of Tregs to Th17 cells, and in turn, induces tolerance.[220] Furthermore, TLRs and their role as a target in transplantation are still under research.

## The role of complement activation

The complement system comprises one of the first members of immunity. It was once accepted that complement proteins were exclusively functioning against microbial agents. Surprisingly, this view was later changed after the realization of the contribution of the complement system to many inflammatory diseases.[249,250] Classical, lectin and alternate pathways are the three pathways of activation of the complement system. The fundamental of the alternate pathway, which is the oldest pathway and is in charge of 80 percent–90 percent of the whole complement activation, is pattern recognition molecule, including properdin. This pathway is prompted after PAMPs and DAMPs on alien and injured cells are recognized.[249] The classical pathway, which depends on antibodies, was the first pathway that was discovered. Mannose-binding lectin and ficolins in the lectin pathway act as pattern recognition molecules that primarily attach to carbohydrate patterns.[250] It is widely acknowledged that the complement system has crucial roles during tissue injury, which includes ischemic-related injury after SOT.[251] The complement pathway, especially the lectin pathway, utilizes C5a, anaphylatoxin excretion, and leukocyte employment for neoepitope identification, opsonization, amplification, and regulation of the cellular response.[252] C5a has a crucial part in the chemotaxis of innate and T cells, up-regulation of cell adhesion molecules (CAMs), and P-selectin and von Willebrand factor secretion by endothelial cells.[253] In mice with elevated amounts of C5a and C3a, the need for CD40/CD154 appears to be avoided in the interplay between CD4+ and CD8+ T cells resulting in the induction of alloimmune responses.[254] C5a and C3a send direct signals to T cells using responses from C5a and C3a receptors, moderating natural Treg activity.[255] Furthermore, complement proteins injure allogeneic grafts through oxidative stress, the buildup of remains, and chronic complement stimulation, which sustains a disruptive cycle of injury.[251–253] As a novel solid-phase assay was developed for detecting anti-HLA antibodies, it was proposed that complement binding can be utilized to foretell the antibodies that are damaging to the graft. The complement system has also been a matter of interest as a therapeutic option in allograft rejection mainly due to the commercialization of eculizumab, which is an anti-C5a agent. This drug was first produced for paroxysmal nocturnal hemoglobinuria. Eculizumab impedes the development of the membrane attack complex, and it has also been utilized in transplantation to prevent AMR in sensitized kidney transplant patients who have an affirmative cross-match against the donated organ.[220] The complement system is obviously a new realm in transplantation immunology, and it is very likely that novel therapeutic options based on this system will be evolved to inhibit rejection.

## The role of cytokine level and polymorphisms

Cytokines are important messengers that partake in the innate immune system. The immune signals between the cells of innate and adaptive immunity are regulated and enhanced by cytokines.[256] The exact mechanism through which cytokines affect graft rejection is yet to be understood. However, recently there have been several publications on cytokines and their effects in transplantation. It is recognized that depending on the environment that cytokines exist, the pro- and anti-inflammatory cytokines can encourage or impede rejection.[257,258] IL-1β, TNF-α, and IL-6 are among the cytokines that have recently attained attention. Mononuclear phagocytes manufacture pro-inflammatory cytokines such as IL-1β and TNF-α that are mostly involved in triggering monocytes, neutrophils, and endothelial cells in order to create CAMs and chemokines. IL-1β, which is mainly excreted by activated cells, starts and maintains inflammation by prompting the production of IL-2, IL-6, TNF-α, TNF-β.[259] It also has an important part in supporting leukocyte migration into damaged tissues and intensifies the expression of CAMs on endothelial cells and leukocytes.[220] There have been a few reports of utilizing anti-cytokine therapies against IL-1β and TNF-α in transplantation settings, such as the routine use of anti-TNF-α in islet transplantation in some centers.[78,260] Inflammation can be efficiently restrained in rheumatoid arthritis patients by a recombinant antagonist of the human IL-1 receptor named Anakinra.[261] IL-6 is mainly secreted by APCs, fibroblasts, and endothelial cells and is a pro-inflammatory cytokine involved in T cell differentiation. IL-6 deficiency in mice leads to decreased production of IFN-γ at the time of allograft rejection.[262] In mice with extremely immunogenic skin allograft, tolerance is induced when the co-stimulatory blockade is combined with a lack of IL-6 and TNF-α.[263] In conclusion, anti-cytokine therapeutic options are slowly becoming implemented into the treatment plans of transplant patients.

## Matching

## HLA compatibility

All human cells express molecules on their surface that are considered foreign antigens by other individuals' immune system. Successful transplantation of human organs requires histocompatibility methods to find a suitable donor.[264] In 1930, the first major histocompatibility antigen was discovered in mice.[265] However, it was not until 1952 when HLA-A2m, which is a human MHC, was identified.[266] The MHC is a 3.6 million base genomic sequence on the short arm of chromosome 6 (Fig. 7.2).[267] MHC encodes many genes, including the six original HLA genes, which help regulate the immune system and have basic roles in cellular functions.[268] MHC molecules present unfamiliar peptides on their surface to T cells so that the activation of antigen-specific host defense mechanism is ensured.[266] MHC molecules are extremely heterogeneous, which provide the immune system the ability to fight against various foreign pathogens.[266] However, these molecules can cause problems in patients who have undergone transplantation. The survival of transplanted organs from a sibling with identical HLA is far higher than those from lesser matched relatives or well-matched cadavers.[269] HLA matching has since been an important part of transplantation. Molecular methods have enabled clinicians to analyze the recipient and donor characteristics and calculate the allograft failure risk. A single HLA mismatch increases the risk of graft failure by 13 percent, and six HLA mismatches increase the risk by 64 percent.[270] HLA antigens are classified as class I (HLA-A, -B, -C) and class II (HLA-DR, -DQ, -DP) molecules. HLA class I molecules can be found on the surface of all nucleated cells. However, HLA class II molecules can only be found on B cells, APCs, and activated microvascular endothelial cells.[271] HLA-DR matching has a significant correlation with the transplantation

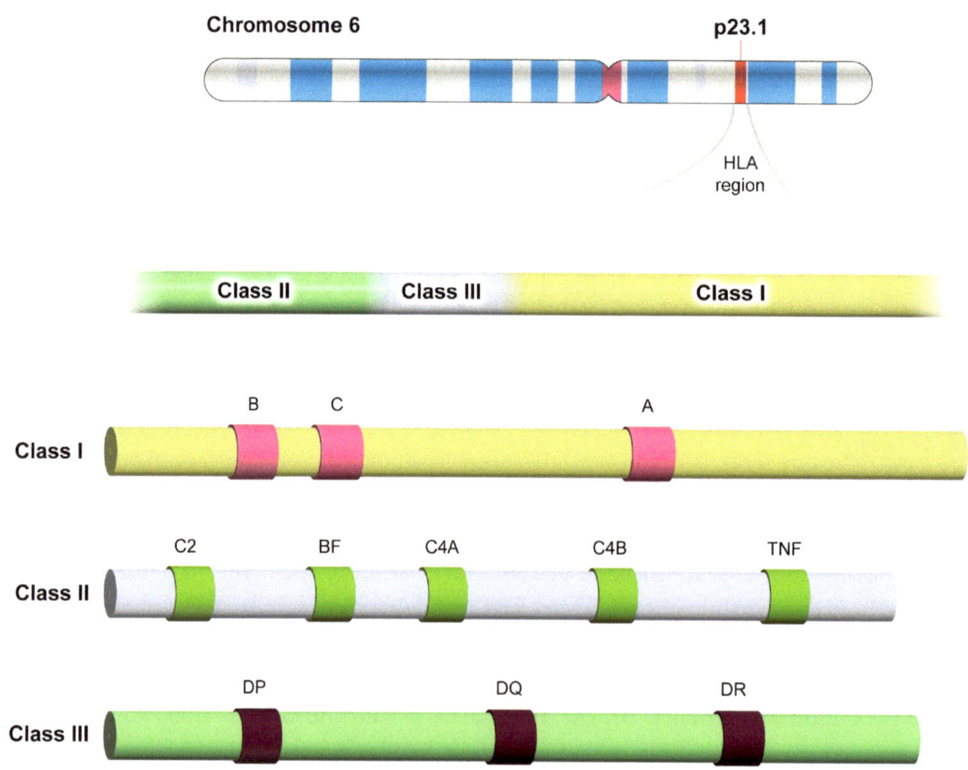


**Fig. 7.2** ***Chromosome 6 which contains major histocompatibility complex.***

outcome, and its effect is as strong as that of HLA-A and -B together.[272] HLA-DQ and -DP mismatches are generally better tolerated. However, the inclusion of these mismatches into the matching process can help to predict the outcome more accurately.[273] Any presentation of HLA antigens can result in HLA sensitization, which can adversely affect the result of or access to transplantation.[266] Therefore, it is important to match histocompatibility before an organ transplant. Sera, including antibodies for various kinds of HLA antigen specificities, are used for serologic typing. When the cell surface antigen and serum antibody are matched, cellular death takes place. Serologic typing provides fast results and can differentiate "null" HLA alleles, which are not expressed on the cell surface but can be detected on the DNA sequence. As HLA proteins are encoded by DNA regions, molecular typing methods such as sequence-specific primer PCR (SSP), sequence-specific oligonucleotide probes (SSOP), and direct DNA sequencing are also becoming popular.[264]

## Desensitization

Patients who produce DSAs because of pregnancy, blood product transfusions, or prior transplants face a significant obstacle to transplantation as a result of sensitization to HLAs.[274] They are difficult to match, have poor transplant rates, and are at increased risk of acute and chronic AMR incidents after transplantation.[275] Desensitization therapies made an appearance in the 1980s when donor-specific blood transfusion (DST) was conducted for HLA desensitization with poor outcomes. However, in the mid-1990s, HLA antibody desensitization with intravenous immunoglobulin (IVIG) was developed that introduced a new era in transplantation. IVIG is a complicated product extracted from the gamma globulin portion of pooled human plasma that is utilized as a therapeutic option for various disorders. In this therapy, broad-acting mechanisms such as neutralization of circulating antibodies, inhibition of B and T cell proliferation using interactions with Fc receptors, alteration of cytokine production, and down-regulation of complement are used to regulate auto- and allo-immune responses. This has a strong immunomodulatory impact and is broadly utilized for desensitization in patients experiencing AMR.[276,277] Rituximab is a chimeric anti-CD20 (anti-B cell) monoclonal antibody that binds to CD20 and marks the cell for obliteration and thus depletes CD20+ B cells (not plasma cells) in the bone marrow, spleen, and lymph nodes.[278–280] Rituximab has been integrated with desensitization guidelines over the years. The inclusion of two weekly doses of rituximab to a high-dose IVIG regimen in sensitized patients has significantly reduced panel reactive antibodies and improved transplant outcomes.[281] Bortezomib is a selective inhibitor of the 26S proteasome that prevents antibody production from plasma cells, regulates apoptosis of these cells, and reduces the number of bone marrow-derived plasma cells.[282–286] Most studies demonstrate encouraging results of bortezomib for HLA desensitization. However, further studies have to be designed to better understand its effects.[276]

## Tolerance induction

In the 1940s, Gibson and Medawar demonstrated that the underlying mechanism for graft rejection has an immunological basis, and that the body has the same reaction to the foreign graft as it has to the invading bacteria and viruses.[287] One of the methods to make the graft immunologically acceptable for the host is tolerance induction. Laboratory experiments demonstrated that if mammals and birds are sufficiently exposed to foreign homologous tissue cells in their fetal life, they do not initiate an immunological response against the tissue, and if they develop a reaction, it is limited.[288] Bone marrow transplantation following full-body myeloablative radiation has made skin grafts in mice aged 2 to 8 months successful.[289] However, radiating the whole body to repel the host immune system is toxic and can be even lethal.[290]

In transplant immunology, tolerance can be full immunological tolerance, or operational tolerance, or immunosuppression minimization (also known as prope tolerance).[291] Several animal studies have shown immunological tolerance. However, being completely unreactive towards donor tissue is difficult to display.[291–296] Operational tolerance is explained as a survival of an allograft for more than 1 year without signs of immunosuppression. Tolerance has been implemented using bone marrow transplantation, more targeted stimulation, and transfer of immune regulatory cells that reconstructs the immune system.[297]

A person in whom genetically diverse tissues or cells exists simultaneously without causing immunological reactions is called a chimera. It was long believed that such an individual does not exist naturally until red cell chimerism was discovered in Freemartin cattle.[298] Years later, Balner et al. demonstrated that after transient mixed chimerism, persistent skin allograft tolerance was possible.[299] The exact circumstances under which this transient state took place were not properly understood. Later, it was shown that the usage of anti-T cell antibodies to deplete peripheral T cells and further selectively radiating the thymus to destroy thymic T cells allows for stable mixed allogeneic chimerism in animals.[290] These tactics were used as the foundation for preclinical tolerance experiments. Reduced-dose total body irradiation (TBI), thymic irradiation, anti-T cell antibody treatment, splenectomy, donor bone marrow transplantation, and a brief cyclosporine treatment resulted in tolerance to renal allografts. Although donor and recipients were MHS incompatible, results were successful, with about 70 percent of the recipients having a normal renal function, and graft survival were between 4 and 70 months.[298,300] The first successful study on the utilization of mixed chimerism-based tolerance in human renal transplantation without the permanent use of immunosuppression was reported in 2008 by Kawai et al.[301] It was accidentally discovered in kidney transplant patients who had to be withdrawn from immunosuppression.[301]

The most effective methods for tolerance induction to date are mixed chimerism-based strategies. However, they are not without medical and management challenges, and selective utilization of regulatory immune components should be focused on.[297] Donor-derived DCs are originally known as the main initiators of rejection. However, evidence shows that such DCs, especially immature or semi-mature DCs, may be able to regulate alloimmune reactions. Systemic administration of immature donor DCs in mice can hinder alloimmune responses directed by T cells when anti-rejection therapy is not present and, thus, elongating the graft survival.[302] Transfer of CD86-silenced but CD80-sufficient DCs notably improves rat-to-mouse islet transplantation outcomes.[303] pDCs have an important role in preserving peripheral immune tolerance. This capacity may stem from their ability to prepare naïve T cells to express IL-10.[304] The DCs may also unintentionally promote tolerance by either inhibiting reactive T cells or prompting regulatory cells. DCs also have several other immune regulations: IL-4, IL-10, IL-27, and transforming growth factor (TGF)-β expression, T cell mediating enzyme, indoleamine 2,3-dioxygenase (IDO) expression, and ATP and adenosine destruction.[305]

One of the most established mechanisms of peripheral immune tolerance in T cell regulation can be implemented by direct removal of T cells, co-stimulatory blockade, and production of Tregs.[297] Utilizing ATG in the clinical setting has shown the importance of direct destruction of alloreactive T cells to avoid short-term rejection of graft loss.[306,307] Animal and non-human primate models have demonstrated that T cell reduction has elongated the survival of allogeneic grafts. Such studies prove that T cell depletion is helpful but not enough for tolerance induction.[78,308,309] CTLA-4 immunoglobulin can impede signaling using CD28:B7 and inhibit T cell-APC interaction. It has demonstrated promising results in tolerance induction and in mice models of heart and islet transplantation, it has provided graft tolerance.[310–312] CD40 and CD40L antibodies have shown promising results in non-human primate islet transplant recipients.[313] However, in large animal models of kidney and heart transplantation, anti-CD40L was not comparably successful, and there were significant amounts of anti-donor antibodies detected.[314,315] Bleselumab is a fully human anti-CD40 monoclonal antibody that impedes humoral and cellular immunity by obstructing CD40-CD154 interaction between T cells, B cells, and APCs. Bleselumab is well-tolerated and is not linked to any notable short- or long-term side effects. However, its usage does not significantly change graft survival.[316,317]

Utilizing Tregs to induce tolerance is a crucial part of transplant immunology. Tregs were originally known as CD4+ T cells with increased expression of CD25. Afterward, the *Foxp3* gene was found to be the main regulator in Treg cell development.[318] Tregs can inhibit immune functions with different approaches: CTLA-4-mediated inhibition of APC function, IL-2 depletion, and immunosuppressive cytokines and metabolites production.[319] Tregs are currently considered a pivotal element in cell therapy and aids in the controlling of graft rejection.[320] Several tolerance induction protocols such as costimulatory blockade and mixed chimerism Tregs have demonstrated that tolerance and better graft outcomes are linked to an increase in Tregs along with temporary T cell depletion and CD28:B7 inhibition and CD40:CD40L co-stimulation.[321–324] Integrated treatment with IL-2 and mutant IL-15 or IL-2 and anti-IL2 can change the proportion of Tregs to T effector cells, which have yielded Treg-dependent tolerance to the skin, cardiac, and islet allografts.[325,326] It is important to use a suitable type and dose of the immunosuppressive drugs to guarantee the welfare of the patient in the case of failure of the cell therapy. However, it should not be damaging to the transferred CD8+ Treg cells.[327] For example, it was recently demonstrated that mycophenolic acid inhibits Treg proliferation as opposed to rapamycin, which induces Treg proliferation.[328] CNIs are also damaging to the persistence of CD4+ Tregs in patients up to a year post renal transplantation.[329–332]

The exact role of B cells in immune regulation is not yet fully understood. However, recently, Bregs have been recognized as prominent regulators of homeostasis, autoimmunity prevention, and experimental tumor induction. The mechanism by which Bregs suppress the immune system is multifaceted with IL-10 and TGF-,β.[297] Other factors have also been demonstrated to have possible roles in Breg-mediated tolerance induction, including CD45RB, MHCII, transporter antigen presentation (TAP) CD40, intercellular adhesion molecule (ICAM), lymphocyte function-associated antigen (LFA), and B7. However, it is still being heavily researched.[333–337] CD45 is a transmembrane protein that is required for lymphocyte development and activation. It also influences the general responsiveness of the adaptive immune system to antigenic stimulation. Therefore, it could be a target for immunosuppression in autoimmune and transplant models. Anti-CD45RB treatment in mice that received heart transplants demonstrated the B cell-dependent pathway of tolerance induction in which the B cells have direct interaction with T cells.[338] Most of the animals receiving heart transplants treated with anti-CD45RB survived as opposed to the control group that rejected the graft rapidly. This B-cell-dependent tolerance declined with the age of the animal, which indicates that Breg activity is a part of the active immune regulation.[297] The T cell immunoglobulin and mucin domain (TIM) family proteins are effective costimulatory molecules in T cell activation. Recent studies showed that anti-TIM-1 solitarily did not lengthen the survival of islet allografts, whereas anti-CD45RB alone elongated the long-term survival in 40 percent of the recipients. Interestingly, the combination of these two antibodies culminated in 100 percent long-term graft survival.[339]

## Pre-transplantation conditioning

### Hematopoietic stem cell transplantation

Patients with malignant diseases that undergo HCT need preparative or conditioning regimens to produce adequate immunosuppression to impede graft rejection and decrease the tumor burden. These goals have been originally attained by total body irradiation (TBI) and chemotherapeutic agents.[6] There are three classes of conditioning regimens: myeloablative (high intensity), reduced intensity (intermediate intensity), and non-myeloablative (low intensity) conditioning derived from the myelosuppressive effect. Such conditioning regimens will lead to extended, generally irreversible pancytopenia except if hematopoiesis is restored after infusion of hematopoietic stem cells. Although myeloablative conditioning has increased toxicity, it reduces the risk of relapse and increases disease control significantly. However, only patients younger than 55 years old and with no notable comorbidities are suitable for this conditioning.[89]

### *High-dose conditioning regimens*

The widely used regimen in patients with hematologic malignancies that are opted for autologous or allogeneic HSCT is high-intensity TBI-based regimens that have immunosuppressive features, are effective against most leukemias and lymphomas, and are able to reach sanctuary regions (areas in which it is difficult to get sufficient concentration of chemotherapy). Generally, increased doses of TBI decrease the risk of relapse. However, TBI increases the risk of deadly gastrointestinal, hepatic, and pulmonary toxicities, secondary malignancies, and weakened growth and development in children. Delivered dose, dose rate fractionation, the interval between fractions, and the source of radiation can also affect the antineoplastic and toxic effects of TBI. Fractionation tends to decrease organ toxicity because an increased percentage of unimpaired repair mechanisms are maintained in normal tissues compared with leukemic cells. Multiple fractions a day (hyperfractionation) leads to reduced occurrence of interstitial pneumonitis from 50 percent to 4 percent. Currently, most TBI schedules are either fractioned or hyperfractioned.[6] High-dose chemotherapy-based regimens have been evolved in autologous and allogeneic settings to substitute TBI with other chemotherapeutic agents to minimize short- and long-term toxicities linked to high-dose TBI, particularly in patients who have undergone radiation therapy before. Alkylating agents are the central component of these regimens because of their acceptable toxicity and their impact on non-dividing tumor cells.[6]

### *Reduced-intensity and non-myeloablative conditioning regimens*

Studies in the late 1970s and early 1980s suggested that patients developing GVHD following allogeneic HCST had better relapse-free survival and that GVHD had anti-leukemic effects. It was recognized that allogeneic hematopoietic cells preserved patients from hematologic toxicity of high-dose conditioning regimens and played a role in curing the malignant disease through immunologic effects of GVHD.[340–342] Reduced relapse rates were also reported in unmodified grafts compared with autologous, syngeneic, and T cell-depleted grafts.[343–345] These outcomes resulted in the establishment of reduced-intensity and non-myeloablative regimens, which are a possible choice for patients who were not eligible for high-dose conditioning, such as older and medically weak patients.[6] Generally, such regimens produce different levels of primary mixed donor-host chimerism.[346] The difference in levels of chimerism results from the severity of the conditioning regimen, the degree of HLA divergence between donor and host, graft composition, and other factors. However, the complete donor chimerism establishes quickly following reduced-intensity regimens that utilize more myelosuppressive drug combinations. Also, reaching full donor engraftment needs months while lower intensity, non-myeloablative conditioning regimens are employed. Donor T cell chimerism has a direct relationship with grafted T cells, CD14+ cells, NK cells, and CD34+ cells numbers. This relationship is more evident in non-myeloablative settings.[347]

## Common reduced-intensity conditioning regimens

Studies conducted by MD Anderson Cancer Center used reduced-intensity conditioning with melphalan/purine analog combination in patients that were not suitable for the traditional myeloablative conditioning regimen.[348,349] The group also used a combination of various doses of melphalan with purine analogs (fludarabine or cladribine) in patients with high-risk AML and MDS experiencing allogeneic HCST. The significance of such regimens lies in non-relapse mortality (NRM) rates rather than complete remission with 2 years survival of 23 percent and 40 percent in patients with active disease with and without circulating blasts at the time of transplant, respectively. However, an update on the study showed increased 4-year overall survival and PFS.[350,351] Combination of fludarabine, oral busulfan, and ATG in younger patients with hematologic malignancies along with genetic disorders who are undergoing HSCT from HLA-identical siblings resulted in partial or complete donor chimerism in all 26 patients except 2. All of the patients experienced complete neutropenia, and 13 patients experienced sinusoidal obstruction syndrome indicating the vigorous nature of the regimen.[352] A regimen of fludarabine, cytarabine, and amsacrine, followed by 4-Gy TBI, ATG, and cyclophosphamide after 3 days of rest along with early donor lymphocyte infusion demonstrated encouraging outcomes for high-risk AML and MDS patients.[353] Additional studies showed the beneficial effects of substituting TBI with busulfan in this regimen.[354,355] Clofarabine, a second-generation purine nucleoside analog with inherent anti-leukemic effects, has shown to have beneficial effects when added to reduced-intensity conditioning regimens with an alkylating or TBI for allogeneic HSCT.[356,357]

## Common non-myeloablative regimens

In a study, a low-dose, 2-Gy TBI-dependent conditioning regimen combined with 90 $mg/m^2$ fludarabine to elevate pre-transplantation T cell immunosuppression was used. Cyclosporine and mycophenolate mofetil were also utilized for peri-transplant immunosuppression.[358] A newer study evaluated the outcomes of 1092 patients undergone HLA-matched related or unrelated donors with a conditioning regimen consisting of 2-Gy TBI either with or without 90 $mg/m^2$ fludarabine. The major reason for treatment failure was relapsing with a 34.5 percent 5-year relapse-dependent death rate. The 5-year NRM rate was 24 percent, which was mostly observed in patients with a previous history of GVHD.[359] The MD Anderson Cancer Center produced a non-myeloablative regimen, including 90 mg/m$^2$ of fludarabine and 2250 mg/m$^2$ along with peri-transplant rituximab that appeared to encourage preserved long-term clinical and molecular remission in patients who were diagnosed with relapsed, chemosensitive follicular lymphoma.[360] Another group also used this regimen in patients with relapsed or primary refractory B cell NHL who were not suitable for myeloablative conditioning due to physician decision, old age, deficient performance status, end-organ inadequacy, remarkable comorbidities, or recent high-dose therapy and autologous stem cell transplantation. This study reported good tolerability of the regimen and showed favorable results.[361] The Stanford team also produced a new regimen, including 8–12 Gy total lymphoid irradiation over 11 days and ATG given over 5 days according to murine studies to promote the presence of NK cells that inhibit GVHD but sustain graft versus tumor (GVT) effects. This regimen led to decrease rates of acute GVHD in primary reports. Anti-tumor activity was apparent, and survival rates were favorable in patients diagnosed with lymphoid malignancies and acute leukemia.[362–364]

### *Radioimmunotherapy-based regimens*

Most leukemias and lymphomas are extremely sensitive to irradiation, and increased doses of external TBI significantly decrease the risk of relapse following allogeneic HCST. The downside of irradiation is increased toxicity as it can harm normal organs.[365,366] To minimize the toxic effects of irradiation, targeted radiotherapy with radiolabeled monoclonal antibodies were developed, working towards the delivery of more doses of radiation to the tumor site and simultaneously decreasing the exposure of normal organs to radiation. To have a suitable biodistribution of a radiolabeled monoclonal antibody, there is a need to find an excellent antigen that is homogenously expressed on the tumor cells' surface and is not expressed on normal cells.[367–369] NHL cells are ideal targets for radioimmunotherapy due to their significant sensitivity to irradiation and the expression of lineage-specific antigens. I-tositumomab (Bexxar) and Y-ibritumomab (Zevalin) are two anti-CD20 radioimmunoconjugates that are the food and drug administration (FDA)-approved for treating relapsed, refractory, or transformed follicular lymphoma.[370,371] High-dose I-tositumomab showed promising results when used in conditioning regimen after autologous HSCT in excessively pretreated B cell NHL patients older than 60 years old.[372] Combining standard doses of I-tositumomab and high-dose BEAM (Carmustine + Etoposide + Cytarabine + Melphalan) after autologous HSCT and administering them to patients with chemotherapy-refractory or B cell NHL that have relapsed multiple times was relatively effective and safe.[373,374] The CD45 antigen, also known as the common leukocyte antigen, is expressed on the surface of all hematopoietic cells, excluding platelets and mature red cells. Also, it can be detected in 85 percent to 90 percent of AML and ALL.[6] Several studies have shown promising results with the inclusion of the 131I-anti-CD45 antibody in the conditioning regimens of AML and ALL patients before allogeneic HSCT.[375–377] However, further studies need to be conducted to find an efficient way to incorporate radioimmunotherapy in the conditioning regimens of patients undergoing HSCT to elevate their chances of survival.

## Complications

### Graft failure

Graft failure is a rarely occurring complication that happens following allogeneic HSCT that has a poor prognosis. Patients who face graft failure have higher mortality compared with those with persistent engraftment of donor cells. Graft failure is a condition that hematopoietic cells do not undergo engraftment following HSCT. Graft failure can be divided into primary and secondary forms. The primary graft failure is diagnosed by the lack of engraftment within the first month following transplantation with no proof of disease relapse, whereas secondary graft failure occurs when the formerly functioning graft is lost, which leads to cytopenia that involves more than one blood cell lineage.[137]

### Graft rejection

#### *Antibody-mediated rejection (AMR)*

Although desensitization protocols are effective, AMR still continues to exist as a crucial reason for graft failure in patients with DSAs. Treatment options such as plasmapheresis and high-dose IVIG have demonstrated promising results in the prevention and treatment of AMR. Antibodies that detect HLAs and incompatible ABO blood group antigens have been linked to AMR and graft failure. Although DSA-sensitized patients are at higher risk of AMR, de novo DSAs can also evolve early or late following transplantation.[378] Recently, the roles of antibodies other than HLA antibodies in graft rejection and injury have been scrutinized. It is demonstrated that patients with non-HLA antibodies are more likely to experience rejection compared with patients who do not develop non-HLA antibodies. Non-HLA antibodies also seem to appear or reappear in relation to allograft rejection or infection.[379] Main effector cells of rejection following MHC-mismatched bone marrow transplantation have been known to be NK cells for a long time. However, it has been shown that NK cells also play a role in SOT as the suppression of NK cells leads to long-term allograft survival. AMR is thought to be mainly induced by effector functions of the Fc particle of DSA.[380] After the detection of C4d in transplant biopsy, the association of AMR and complement-mediated reactions were acknowledged. Ever since a consensus diagnostic criterion was developed for acute and chronic AMR that incorporated circulating DSA and C4d accumulation in the graft. The ligation of the C1 complex to HLA antigen, which is bound to DSA, activates the classical complement pathway that eventually results in the development of the membrane attack complex (C5b-C9) that causes direct damage to the graft. This reaction usually occurs against the antigens residing on the vascular endothelium that is responsible for the histological pattern of acute microvascular injury, including glomerulitis and peritubular capillaritis, and chronic vascular injury, which includes transplant glomerulopathy. C4d, which is a remnant of C4 following degeneration, continues to covalently bind to the site of complement activation and can be detected for weeks.[378] Diagnosing acute and chronic AMR is important. AMR can be diagnosed using serological markers such as the detection of serum DSAs in the kidney, pancreas, liver, and lung transplantation.[381–385] Table 7.1 summarizes the criteria for diagnosing acute and chronic AMR following kidney, liver, heart, lung, and pancreas transplantation. AMR can present as several phenotypes. Before the development of crossmatch testing and successful immunosuppressive therapy, as a result of pre-existing DSA, hyperacute rejection was prevalent. Hyperacute rejection is exhibited as instant allograft dysfunction. However, this phenotype was abolished after the establishment of crossmatch procedures. The development of effective immunosuppression directed at T cells made AMR significantly contribute to the development of acute and chronic allograft rejection. Acute AMR develops in previously sensitized patients and chronic AMR occurs following the production of de novo DSAs more than a year after transplantation.[386]

### *T cell-mediated rejection (TCMR)*

Acute TCMR needs the existence of T cell infiltration for diagnosis, which is linked to proof of parenchymal damage, including tubulitis and arteritis.[389] It was once thought that the mechanism of tissue damage in TCMR results from the direct elimination of donor cells by cytotoxic molecules such as perforin, granzymes A and B, granulysin, and Fas ligand. Currently, it is accepted that TCMR is an inflammatory reaction inside the interstitium of the transplanted organ tissues.[390]

## GVHD

GVHD is a harmful immunologic occurrence seen after allogeneic HSCT.[391] Less commonly, it can occur after blood products transfusion, SOTs, and autologous HSCT.[392–394] GVHD happens in 40 percent to 60 percent of patients receiving HSCT. This disease can be deadly, with a mortality rate of approximately 15 percent.[391] GVHD is a complex illness, which involves several organs, needs management from multiple specialties, has acute and chronic demonstrations, and has several therapeutic possibilities.[395] Organs that may be affected include lungs, hepatobiliary system, musculoskeletal system, gastrointestinal tract, and skin.

The mechanism by which GVHD occurs differs in the acute type from the chronic type. The acute GVHD happens in between 20 percent to 70 percent of the patients and has 3 steps. The first step occurs before the infusion of the donor cells. Before

**Table 7.1** The criteria for diagnosing acute and chronic AMR following kidney, liver, heart, lung, and pancreas transplantation.

| Organ | Criteria for AMR diagnosis |
|---|---|
| Kidney[387,388] | Fordefinite acute AMR diagnosis, it is required that all of the following criteria be present:<br>**1.** Histological proof of graft damage with at least one of the succeeding: microvascular inflammation, intimal or transmural arteritis, acute thrombotic microangiopathy, or acute tubular injury when there are no other apparent reasons<br>**2.** Proof of antibody interactions with vascular endothelium with at least one of the succeeding: linear C4d staining in peritubular capillaries, moderate microvascular inflammation in case of lack of recurrent or de novo glomerulonephritis, elevated expression of gene transcripts in the biopsy tissue<br>**3.** Detecting circulating DSA mostly anti-HLA antibody (C4d staining can replace DSA)<br>For definite chronic AMR diagnosis, it is required that all of the following criteria be present:<br>**1.** Morphologic evidence of chronic tissue damage including more than one of the subsequent presentations: Transplant glomerulopathy, severe peritubular capillary basement membrane multilayering, and arterial intimal fibrosis of recent emergence eliminating other possible justifications<br>**2.** Same as criterion 2 for acute AMR<br>**3.** Same as criterion 3 for acute AMR |
| Liver[383] | Fordefinite acute AMR diagnosis, it is required that all of the following criteria be present:<br>**1.** Histopathological pattern of injury: portal microvascular endothelial cell hypertrophy, portal capillary and inlet venule dilation, monocytic eosinophilic, and neutrophilic portal microvasculitis, portal edema, ductular reaction, usual presence of cholestasis, edema and periportal hepatocyte necrosis especially in ABO-incompatible allografts, and variable active lymphocytic and/or necrotizing arteritis<br>**2.** Positive DSA<br>**3.** C4d deposition<br>**4.** Exclusion of other probable reasons<br>For probable chronic AMR diagnosis, it is required that all of the following criteria be present:<br>**1.** Histopathological pattern of injury:portal and/or perivenular inflammation with the interface and/or perivenular necro-inflammatory activity and at least moderate portal/periportal, sinusoidal, and/or perivenular fibrosis<br>**2.** Positive circulating DSA<br>**3.** C4d positive<br>**4.** Exclusion of other probable reasons |

| Organ | Criteria for AMR diagnosis |
|---|---|
| Heart[385] | Not all of the criteria are required for a definitive diagnosis.<br>1. Morphological proof of tissue damage<br>2. C4d deposition<br>3. Microvascular inflammation<br>4. Immune cell infiltration<br>5. Existence of circulating DSA |
| Lung[381] | 1. Existence of circulating DSA<br>2. Positive C4d peritubular capillary staining<br>3. Allograft dysfunction<br>4. Other histopathologic changes<br>5. Exclusion of other causes<br>Definite AMR: when all of the criteria are present<br>Probable AMR: lacks 1 criterion or other reasons have not been ruled out yet<br>Possible AMR: lacks 2 of the criteria |
| Pancreas[382] | Fordefinite acute AMR diagnosis, it is required that all of the following criteria be present:<br>1. Positive circulating DSA<br>2. Morphological proof of tissue damage (interacinar inflammation/capillaritis, acinar cell damage swelling/necrosis/apoptosis/dropout, vasculitis, thrombosis)<br>3. Positive C4d |

HSCT, the patient's tissues are already harmed as a result of several factors, including the underlying disease and its treatment, infection, drugs, and irradiation utilized in the conditioning phase.[9,396] This step results in elevated expression of MHC antigens and adhesion molecules, which lead to enhanced identification of the host's alloantigens by the donor T cells.[391] In the second step, donor T cells are activated by the APCs of the host as early as 12 h after HSCT. Inflammatory cytokines and microbial-derived molecules such as bacterial lipopolysaccharides (LPS) are taken into account as "danger signals" that aid the process of T cell activation. Stimulated NK cells can deplete host APCs and result in GVHD suppression. Activated T cells secrete cytokines that are categorized into Th1, which secretes IL-2 and IFN-α, and Th2, which secretes IL-4, IL-5, IL-10, and IL-13. DCs can change T cell function, which can lead to the following effects: increased cytokine secretion, decomposition of target cells by Fas/FasL interaction, and secretion of monocyte chemo-attractant protein (MCP)−1, which results in the employment of macrophages.[396] In the last step, cytotoxic effector T cells move to target organs and lead to tissue injury through molecular attractants and receptor interactions. Soluble inflammatory mediators act simultaneously and result in the full spectrum of detrimental consequences that can be seen in acute GVHD.[391,396] The main target organs of acute GVHD are the skin, liver, and gastrointestinal tract. Early clinical manifestations of the skin are pruritus, dysesthesias, and subtle macular erythema and edema. Furthermore, folliculocentric or morbilliform eruption occurs that commonly start on the trunk and merge gradually. Nikolsky sign, represented by epidermal denudation, is a harbinger of a more dangerous disease. Although these symptoms may suggest GVHD, it is important to differentiate between GVHD, drug interactions, and infectious exanthema.[9] Treatment and prevention of acute GVHD should interfere with the three-step pathophysiologic cycle of acute GVHD. Corticosteroids are usually included in the first line of treatment for acute GVHD, which show successful results in about 50 percent of the patients.[397]

30 percent to 70 percent of allogeneic HSCT patients experience chronic GVHD, which endangers the survival and quality of life of the patients. Chronic GVHD affects both the organs affected in acute GVHD as well as any other organ systems such as oral, esophageal, musculoskeletal, joint, fascial, ocular and lymphohematopoietic systems, hair and nails, and genital tissues.[398,399] Chronic GVHD can be divided into three phases. The first step occurs when the patient undergoes tissue injury, which is followed by early inflammation. It has been observed that areas of the cell damage caused by local pressure, exposure to sunlight, restricted irradiation, or reactivation of varicella-zoster can provoke localized, cutaneous chronic GVHD. The second phase is chronic inflammation, thymic injury, and B cell and T cell immunity dysregulation. Following tissue damage, IL-1β and IL-6 are released, which induce Th17-cell differentiation that leads to chronic inflammation. The final phase includes tissue repair with fibrosis. Also, macrophage activation has been observed in this phase.[400] In about 75 percent of the patients, skin is involved, and with lower frequency, the oral mucosa, liver, and eye.[9] Based on the NIH Consensus Development Project, poikiloderma, lichen planuse-like eruptions, lichen sclerosus-like lesions, morphea-like sclerosis, and deep sclerosis/fasciitis indicate chronic GVHD and do not need a biopsy specimen for diagnosis.[401] Nail alterations happen in about 50 percent of the patients with chronic GVHD and are distinguished by dystrophy, thickening, thinning, onycholysis, vertical ridging, and pterygium. Mucous membrane disease is also observed in chronic GVHD, and symptoms include dry mouth and oral pain, mainly with spicy food.[9]

Biomarkers are being researched to help in clinical and histopathological diagnosing as well as evaluating the response to treatment. Several biomarkers have been studied in clinical trials, including elafin, B cell-activating factor, chemokine receptors such as C-X-C chemokine ligand (CXCL)10 and CXCL11, T cell immunoglobulin and mucin-domain-containing-3, IL-6, and soluble tumor necrosis factor receptor 1 (sTNFR1).[402–404] However, implementing them in clinical settings should be further investigated.

The number of allogeneic HSCT is on the rise, and it is important to find effective therapies to treat acute and chronic GVHD. Treating acute and chronic GVHD is challenging as it mostly depends on preventive procedures and modifying treatment according to responses.[391] Generally localized acute and chronic GVHD are limited to the epidermis and have a suitable reaction to topical therapies like corticosteroids and CNIs.[405–407] Corticosteroids are the first-line therapy for the GVHD, and if failed, it is suggested to add a second-line agent such as photopheresis, mycophenolate mofetil, mTOR inhibitors, and Janus kinase (JAK) inhibitors.[391] Utilizing corticosteroids is challenging as they can have multiple fatal side effects such as diabetes, hypertension, osteoporosis, myopathy, and avascular necrosis. Current second-line treatments have unfavorable response rates and can result in worse outcomes, so better treatment options should be developed.[408]

## Change in immunosurveillance

### *Malignancies*

De novo malignancies are one of the leading late complications in transplant patients due to immunosuppression and other transplant-related and traditional risk factors. In comparison to the general population, the overall prevalence of de novo malignancies is 2- to 4- fold more in all SOT recipients. Immunosuppression inhibits immunosurveillance mechanisms and directly impairs host DNA resulting in carcinogenesis. Another mechanism that can potentially lead to malignancy is the enhancement of the effects of pro-oncogenic viruses, such as *human herpesvirus (HHV)−8* for Kaposi sarcoma, *EBV* for the post-transplantation lymphoproliferative disorder (PTLD), and *human papillomavirus (HPV)* for oropharyngeal and anogenital carcinomas. Lung transplant recipients are at greater risk for head and neck carcinoma in comparison to other SOT recipients. In addition, the most frequent solid organ tumor in lung and renal transplant recipients is lung cancer.[409]

### *Lymphoproliferative disease (LPD)*

PTLDs are disorders described by abnormal proliferation of lymphoid that occurs following the external immunosuppression after SOT or HSCT. Heterogenous pathology is observed in transplant recipients who experience PTLD, and the patients have diverse clinical manifestations.[410] The first incident of PTLD was reported in 1968.[411] However, it was not until 1984 that the term PTLD came into existence.[412] SOT recipients are about 10-fold more likely to develop lymphoma than the general population. Viruses are the cause of most PTLDs. However, the occurrence of *EBV*-negative PTLD is far higher than the occurrence of classic lymphoma in the general population.[412] PTLDs demonstrate a wide range of abnormal lymphoproliferations. However, the most frequent and lethal types arise from *EBV* infection of the transplant recipient's B cells.[413] Although *EBV* infection is generally harmless in healthy immunocompetent individuals, it has been linked to infectious mononucleosis, nasopharyngeal carcinoma, and Burkitt lymphoma. A significant number of transplant patients undergo immunosuppression and are *EBV*-positive. However, only a few patients develop PTLD, which shows other underlying factors that are beyond chronic immunosuppression. Managing PTLD needs a disease-specific approach. First-line therapy includes decreasing immunosuppression, and if it is not fully successful, treatment with rituximab is needed. If required, chemotherapy should also be included.[410]

## Infections

A broad range of possible pathogens can contaminate immunocompromised recipients. A great number of them are uncommon in healthy people. Infections can be diagnosed by other subtle laboratory or radiographic abnormalities. Antimetabolites are linked to reduced leukocyte counts and reduced maximum temperature. Some infections, including peritonitis, do not result in fever or localizing signals. The risk of infection depends on two factors: The epidemiologic exposures of the patient and the organ donor, and the patient's state of immunosuppression.[414]

The collection of microorganisms in tissues and on body surfaces is called the microbiome. The microbiome of the transplant recipient has several sources: previous colonization of mucosal surfaces, latent infections, infections from the organ donor, and newly acquired community-derived or nosocomial exposures. In transplant patients, these microbial complexes are affected by immunosuppression, infectious exposures, antimicrobial therapies, metabolic disorders, and surgery, which can influence graft outcomes.[415] However, further research is needed to examine the relationship between the microbiome and immunity in allograft recipients.

Post-transplant preventative strategies can be determined by screening the donor and recipient microbiologic profile. Such plans are personalized and include interventions such as prescribing isoniazid that can treat the patients for latent tuberculosis and Ivermectin for *Strongyloides stercoralis*, vaccinating seronegative recipients, and empiric antifungal treatment in lung recipients. After evaluating the risk of infection, antiviral treatment for the herpesvirus is decided.[416,417]

A number of donor-derived infections may manifest decades after primary exposure. Donor colonization may amplify susceptibility to graft damage, rejection, and drug toxicity. It is better to treat active infections before transplantation. Patients who are immunosuppressed and have not completed the treatment course of the infection often relapse.[418] With a standardized immunosuppressive regimen, most usual infections happen in a fairly foreseeable pattern based on the time elapsed since transplantation which reflects the altering risk factors over time: surgery/hospitalization, immunosuppression, the emergence of latent infections, and community exposure.[419]

Quick and specific diagnosis in transplant patients is required to start specific antimicrobial therapy as soon as possible and avoid drug toxicities.[414] *CMV* is a prominent microorganism in transplant patients. Characteristics of *CMV* infection differ depending on the site of infection and antiviral susceptibility.[420] Latent *CMV* infections are mostly reserved in monocytes and affect the innate immune responses to microorganisms such as *Pneumocystis* and *Aspergillus*. *CMV* replicates in all transplanted organs and vessels in fibroblasts, epithelial, endothelial, and other parenchymal cells. Without preventative measures, infection is most common 1 to 6 months following transplantation depending on the organ, the immunosuppressive regimen, and the host's immune status.[414] Viremia and symptomatic infections are infrequent while the patient is under potent antiviral preventive treatment. However, it can happen after the termination of such measures.[421] The standard therapy for *CMV* is a minimum of 2–3 weeks of intravenous ganciclovir or valganciclovir treatment.[414] *EBV* is a gamma herpesvirus, which is highly prevalent and is present in over 90 percent of adults and about 50 percent of people by age 5 in developed countries. In immunocompromised people, infection manifests as a childhood febrile respiratory illness or as infectious mononucleosis of young adults with fever, lymphadenopathy, hepatosplenomegaly, and hepatitis. After transplantation, *EBV* seronegative individuals are at risk for primary infection, which is linked to a significantly elevated chance of PTLDs.[422,423] The *EBV*-linked disease has various clinical manifestations that make the diagnosis process difficult. Other pathogens such as polyomaviruses, *HPV*, fungal infections, *Candida* spp., *Aspergillus* spp., *Cryptococcus* spp., *Strongyloides stercoralis*, Pneumonitis and Pneumocystis infections, and *Pneumocystis jiroveci* pneumonia are also important in transplant patients and need to be treated and prevented accordingly.[414]

## Autoimmune diseases

There have been infrequent cases of autoimmune presentations following allogeneic HSCT. Autoimmunity cascade begins with the donor cell infusion. The most usual autoimmune manifestation after allogeneic HSCT is hematologic autoimmune cytopenias (AICs). AICs can be divided into different subtypes according to the affected lineages and include autoimmune hemolytic anemia (AIHA), immune thrombocytopenic purpura (ITP), Evans syndrome (AIHA and ITP). Non-malignant disease and utilizing donor grafts from nonrelatives are significantly linked to AIC in children. The probable underlying mechanism of autoimmunity after HSCT is the lack of functional T cells, especially Tregs, which results in incapability to inhibit B cell proliferation following HSCT. AICs usually manifest while the thymus is not fully recovered from transplant-related injuries indicating the possible role of peripheral tolerance in preventing autoimmunity. The pathophysiology of AICs is yet to be fully established. However, it seems that AIHA is mostly caused by donor immune reactions against donor erythrocytes. HLA matching has a higher priority than ABO matching making ABO mismatch inevitable in some cases of HSCT, which is linked to hindered engraftment and other complications. However, AIHA differs from ABO mismatch. The therapy course for AIHA is mostly treatment with IVIG or steroids, rituximab monotherapy, and other approaches. ITP following allogeneic HSCT is slightly more likely to happen in children compared with adults. However, it is not common, and the pathophysiology is not fully understood.

Other non-hematologic autoimmune disorders may occur after allogeneic HSCT, such as autoimmune thyroid disease (AITD), neurological autoimmune and GVHD manifestations after AHSCT in children, and skin autoimmune GVHD-associated manifestations after allogeneic HSCT. AITD mostly includes Hashimoto thyroiditis and Graves' disease and is mediated by antibodies against thyroid antigens. Neurological autoimmune manifestations can involve both the peripheral and central nervous systems (PNS/CNS). PNS manifestations include Guillain-Barre syndrome (GBS), neuromuscular junction, and myasthenia gravis. CNS immune manifestations include cerebrovascular, stroke-like presentations, encephalopathy with resultant seizures, and demyelination. Vitiligo is a rare occurrence, which is usually seen with acute or chronic GVHD following AHSCT.[424]

## Organ-dependent complications

### Kidney transplantation

Complications following kidney transplantation can be classified into 8 groups. Arterial vascular complications, venous vascular complications, graft dysfunction, urological complications, hernia, neoplasm, and recurrent native renal disease. Arterial vascular complications include renal artery stenosis, renal transplant infarction, arteriovenous fistula, and pseudoaneurysm.[425] Transplant renal artery stenosis is normally a belated occurrence and is the most widespread vascular hurdle in kidney transplantation. This may be straightly linked to the surgical strategy, and its normal location is at the anastomosis or the proximal donor artery. This complication is more common in living donor allografts compared with cadaveric allografts.[426–428] Although renal artery thrombosis is a scarce occurrence, it can be damaging in patients who experience it. This is an early occurrence and often time results in graft loss.[429] About 10 percent of the patients that undergo biopsy experience arteriovenous fistula. Transplant renal vein thrombosis is a venous vascular complication. It is an infrequent occurrence that mostly happens within the first two weeks following transplantation. It is accompanied by abrupt oliguria, allograft pain, and swelling.[425] Urinoma, calculi, and transplant obstruction are some of the urological complications. Undergoing ureteroneocystostomy can prevent these complications.[430–432]

### Liver transplantation

As liver has a dual blood supply that includes the portal vein and the hepatic artery. Liver transplantation requires several vascular anastomoses that can lead to complications at the sites of the anastomoses. Hepatic artery thrombosis, stenosis, and pseudoaneurysm are arterial complications and are more widespread than venous complications. Stenosis or occlusion of the portal vein, hepatic vein, and inferior vena cava are venous complications. Thrombosis of the hepatic artery is the most dangerous and the most common complication of the vasculature that affects 2 percent−14 percent of the patients. It is also the main reason for graft failure and death. Biliary complications are also widespread phenomena, which mostly occur in the first 6 to 12 months following transplantation. Up to 20 percent of the patients experience biliary complications, including stricture, biliary leak, cholangitis, sphincter of Oddi dysfunction, and stone disease.[433]

### *Heart transplantation*

It is necessary to assess the function of left and right ventricles following cardiac transplantations. Left ventricular systolic dysfunction may indicate deficient heart condition or hyperacute rejection. Right ventricular dysfunction may be due to increased pulmonary vascular resistance, severe volume overload, reduced preload, or deficient conservation of the transplanted organ. Conservative therapeutic options are utilized in most patients. However, some may require extra aid. Tricuspid regurgitation is the most frequent valvular complication that 19 percent to 84 percent of transplant patients undergo. Most patients are treated with diuretics, and a few of them may need to be managed surgically. Mitral regurgitation is a mild vulvar complication that happens in more than half of the patients and usually does not need intervention.[434]

## Allergies

In 1997, the development of the first food allergy after combined kidney and liver transplantation was reported. The donor had passed away because of cardiorespiratory arrest after an anaphylactic reaction after eating a peanut. One out of the two recipients developed a new food allergy to peanuts 3 months following transplantation.[435] There have been reports of developing food allergies in recipients after SOT. Furthermore, there have been reports of food allergy development after SOT from donors with no documented history of prior food allergy.[436–438] Food allergies are IgE-mediated hypersensitivity responses after exposure to proteins of the food. There are many suggested mechanisms for developing allergies after transplantation, which include the passive transfer of donor IgE to the recipient, and more frequently, loss of tolerance to food proteins after organ transplantation. Most food allergies develop after liver transplantation. However, the passive transfer of food allergies may happen following any organ transplant, which includes lymphoid tissue. It is important to test organ donors prior to transplantation to predict the risk of developing new food allergies after organ transplantation.[439] However, additional research is needed to better understand the mechanism of developing de novo food allergies in transplant recipients.

## Other complications

Hepatic Veno-occlusive disease (VOD) is a condition, which manifests as a sudden increase in weight, ascites, painful hepatomegaly, and jaundice, and it primarily occurs following allogeneic HSCT. However, it has rarely been reported following reduced-intensity conditioning and after exposure to hepatotoxic chemotherapies.[440] The most prominent occurrence that leads to VOD appears to be damage to sinusoidal endothelial cells and hepatocytes by high-dose alkylating chemotherapy conditioning regimens.[441] Irradiation also generates the same sort of harm. The release of local cytokines triggers the induction of cell adhesion molecules on endothelial cells that leads to cell injury and disconnection and activates the coagulation pathway.[442] Fibrinolytic pathway induction results in fibrosis of sinusoids accompanied by perivascular hepatocyte necrosis and venular occlusion.[441] Early accurate diagnosis and risk evaluation is important to initiate effective treatment rapidly to prevent the progression of the disease.[442]

Transplant recipients undergo a series of complex procedures before, during, and after transplantation. These complicated procedures put patients at an increased risk of neurological disorders. Early complications usually happen in patients with organ or graft dysfunction and can also happen following toxicity from the many medications that patients are exposed to. The most frequent manifestation of neurological disorder is encephalopathy, which includes delirium, lethargy, and coma. Postoperative encephalopathy mostly originates from systemic toxic-metabolic causes. However, other factors such as strokes and infections may also be involved. Seizures occur in 5 percent–10 percent of transplant patients, generally near the acute postoperative stage. They can happen with or without encephalopathy and share many similar etiological traits. Treatment and prognosis depend on the exact cause of the seizure.[443] Organ transplant recipients have an increased chance of acquiring opportunistic infections, which can regularly involve the CNS. Recently, cases of opportunistic infections have dropped due to effective prophylactic regimens. Neurological presentations of viral infections include limbic encephalitis-like syndrome, rhombencephalitis, ventriculitis, myelitis, vascular involvement, and a multisystem PTLD, which may involve the CNS. Bacterial infections such as nocardiosis, *Listeria monocytogenes*, and *Mycobacterium tuberculosis* may also involve the nervous system. High-dose corticosteroids are the main risk factor for nocardiosis, and brain abscess is the most frequent clinical manifestation. *Listeria monocytogenes* infection may also result in meningitis or meningoencephalitis that is manifested with fever, headache, altered mental status, and seizures. *Mycobacterium tuberculosis* includes symptoms such as fever and altered mental status. Fungal and protozoan infections may also cause neurological symptoms.[444] Neurological complications after organ transplantation are diverse and may involve the CNS or PNS. Neurological presentations after organ transplantation are challenging to medical specialists and require further investigation.

## Post-transplantation therapy

Patients undergo maintenance immunosuppression starting from the hospital, and it is resumed throughout the life of the allograft.[15] Immunosuppressive drugs mostly target T cell-mediated responses. As previously mentioned, three signals are needed to activate T cells. Impeding these signals is the aim of immunosuppression that results in stable, long-term allograft tolerance.[445] Immunosuppression has undergone a lot of changes throughout the years. In the beginning, the success of immunosuppression was dependent on HLA matching, as most successful transplants were between HLA-identical siblings that did not require immunosuppression. Treatment options were corticosteroids,

6-mercaptopurine, and radiation.[446] Following the observation that allograft survival in dogs was prolonged by azathioprine, it was blended into the immunosuppressive regimens in humans.[447] Azathioprine extended the graft survival rates by about 60 percent. After the introduction of cyclosporine, rejection rates decreased to less than 50 percent, and graft survivals increased to more than 85 percent. After that, the current era of therapy started with the acceptance of tacrolimus, mycophenolate mofetil, rabbit ATG (rATG), and IL-2 receptor blockers such as basiliximab and daclizumab. Incorporating these therapeutic options increased graft survival rates to 95 percent and decreased the one-year rejection rate to 10 percent−15 percent. When opting for an immunosuppression regimen for a patient, the main aim is to balance the advantages of preventing rejection and the side effects of undergoing immunosuppression. This has to be evaluated individually and is not necessarily the same in different patients.[445]

## Maintenance therapy

Maintenance immunosuppressive therapy is used to impede rejection and maintain allograft function. The most favorable combination out of the six distinct maintenance therapies that exist (CNIs, azathioprine, mycophenolic acid, mTOR-inhibitors, prednisone, and belatacept) is being researched in clinical trials. Due to the complex nature of T cell activation, it is beneficial to use a combination of therapies compared with a single therapy. Another advantage of combination therapy is that a decreased dose of each therapy is needed, and therefore, drug-specific toxicity is alleviated.[445] CNIs are immunosuppressive agents that inhibit the second signal of T cell activation. CNIs attach to particular receptors that lead to inhibition of calcineurin. Cyclosporine and tacrolimus are two of the first CNIs to be introduced as immunosuppressants.[448] CNIs have strongly affected allograft results, particularly when combined with azathioprine or mycophenolic acid.[449–451] Patients treated with tacrolimus demonstrated decreased rates of rejection compared to patients treated with cyclosporine. These observations have made regimens, including tacrolimus and mycophenolate mofetil with or without prednisone (gold standard). However, toxicity related to CNIs has led to trials with contemporary immunosuppression that strives for lesser exposure to tacrolimus. There are three different approaches for CNI-sparing: minimization, when blood levels of CNIs are diluted to lesser than normal blood levels and are utilized de novo combined with supplementary therapy, elimination, when CNIs are originally prescribed at a standard or reduced dose along with supplementary therapy and then gradually diminished, which is in many times substituted with a less toxic agent, and avoidance, where CNIs are entirely evaded.[445] Mycophenolate mofetil and its active form, mycophenolic acid, are reversible purine synthase inhibitors that can inhibit the proliferation of T cells and B cells by inhibiting the third signal of cell activation.[452] Mycophenolate mofetil is an immunosuppressive agent that does not cause nephrotoxicity, making it beneficial for patients with renal dysfunction who require reduced doses of CNIs. Mycophenolate mofetil also has demonstrated beneficial effects in immunosuppressive regimens when it is combined with CNIs, and corticosteroid elimination is favorable.[453] Azathioprine, which is a purine synthase inhibitor, is one of the earliest immunosuppressants that was used in SOT. For a long time, it was incorporated as the sole immunosuppressant in maintenance regimens, and subsequently, it was utilized along with CNIs. When tacrolimus was introduced, the demand for azathioprine was diminished, and later it was substituted with mycophenolic acid when a second immunosuppressant was required.[448]

## Prophylaxis

Induction therapy is a rigorous perioperative preventative immunosuppression that is utilized to impede acute cellular rejection in the initial months after transplantation.[448] Induction therapy was presented as intravenous injection of high-dose corticosteroids during the transplantation and in the initial days after surgery to impede elevated rates of rejection. It is generally combined with at least another immunosuppressive drug. Although the dose of the corticosteroid administered varies, it is typically 500 or 1000 mg of methylprednisolone, which will be quickly decreased to 10 to 20 mg a day. The main hindrance to the usage of corticosteroids is their side effects. Delirium, infections, hypertension, hyperlipidemia, diabetes, and obesity are a few of the adverse effects. Arising in the 1980s, T-cell-directed antibodies, OKT3 (muromonab-CD3), equine ATG, and Minnesota anti-lymphocyte globulin (MALG) antibodies were produced to treat acute rejection. Hyperglycemia, diabetes, and *CMV* infection occur less commonly when patients are administered with antibodies compared to when they are administered corticosteroids.[447,448] These antibodies also reduce the required dose of other accompanying immunosuppressive drugs, including corticosteroids and CNIs that can attenuate the side effects associated with these agents.[454] Two groups of antibodies are used in induction immunosuppression: T cell-depleting and non-depleting antibodies.[455] T cell-depleting antibodies can be classified into polyclonal and monoclonal antibodies. ATGs are polyclonal antibodies that act against human T cells and their precursors (thymocytes). Equine ATG (eATG) is originated from the equine, and rATG is originated from the rabbit. In organ transplantation, one of the most frequently utilized drugs for antibody induction is rATG.[448] rATG is better in preventing acute renal rejection compared to eATG.[456] Alemtuzumab is a humanized rat monoclonal antibody that acts against CD52 receptors, which is expressed on all blood mononuclear cells.[457] It is a potent agent that can deplete cells and has been used in bone marrow transplantation, several autoimmune diseases, and organ transplantation. Using it in organ transplantation leads to decreased risk of rejection. It has been mostly experienced in renal transplantation. However, other forms of transplantation have demonstrated comparable outcomes.[458] IL-2Ras, which are humanized non-depleting monoclonal antibodies, attach to IL-2 receptors that are expressed on the surface of T cells leading to inhibition of T cell proliferation. IL-2Ras are utilized in patients who

**Table 7.2** Summary of drugs, their classification, and indication.

| Agent | Brand name | Classification | Indication |
|---|---|---|---|
| Methylprednisolone[460] | Medrol | Corticosteroid | Induction, Rejection, Maintenance |
| Tacrolimus[461] | Prograf, Astagraf | CNI | Maintenance |
| Cyclosporine[462] | Neoral, Sandimmune, Genraf | CNI | Maintenance |
| Mycophenolate mofetil[463] | Cellcept, Myfortic | Inosine monophosphate dehydrogenase inhibitor | Maintenance |
| Azathioprine[464] | Imuran | Purine synthase inhibitor | Maintenance |
| Sirolimus[465] | Rapamune | Macrolide, mTOR inhibitor | Maintenance, Rejection |
| Everolimus[466] | Afinitor | Kinase inhibitor, mTOR inhibitor | Maintenance, Rejection |
| Muromonab-CD3[467] | OKT3 | Monoclonal antibody | Induction, Steroid resistant Rejection |
| Alemtuzumab[468] | Campath-1H | Monoclonal antibody | Maintenance, Induction, Acute rejection |
| ATG[469] | Thymoglobulin, ATGAM | Polyclonal antibody | Induction, Steroid resistant Rejection |
| Daclizumab[470] | Zenapax | IL-2Ra, monoclonal antibody | Induction, Steroid resistant rejection |
| Basiliximab[471] | Simulect | IL-2Ra, monoclonal antibody | Induction |

must avoid or reduce the dose of an accompanying immunosuppressant.[459] A summary of drugs, their classification, and indication are presented in Table 7.2.

## Future directions and concluding remarks

Over the past few years, the field of transplantation has revolutionized. SOT has transformed from an experimental method to an acknowledged and definitive therapeutic option for patients experiencing end-stage organ failure. SOT has developed rapidly and consists of liver, kidney, islet, heart, and lung transplants. Novel developments in surgical techniques have enabled a more effective multi-organ transplantation with fewer complications and reduced ischemic injury occurrence. Immunosuppression has also been revolutionized, making it very successful in inhibiting the host immune system and improving long-term graft survival. Currently, the barrier existing in the field of SOT is the ever-increasing demand for donated organs.

Immunomodulation has currently gained attention in the field of translation, and much of the ongoing research focuses on it. Rejection is carried by complex signaling molecules and cellular and humoral immunity. These immune responses are what these researchers try to minimize by impeding parts of these mechanisms. The Notch signaling pathway is one of the interesting targets of this researches. It has been demonstrated in animal models of transplantation that inhibiting Notch signaling can decrease allograft rejection and GVHD. The ideal outcome in organ transplantation is reaching operational tolerance in which the patient does not require maintenance immunosuppression. This can reduce the toxicity and side effects that result from immunosuppression, including the increased risk for infections and malignancies. The incorporation of hematopoietic stem cells has been promising in a few human cases and many animal models. Receiving bone marrow transplant simultaneously with SOT has helped the patient to reach the state of complete immunosuppression withdrawal. Utilizing biomaterial carriers to induce tolerance is also another method for immunomodulation. Micro and nanomaterial carriers are potential immunomodulators that are able to communicate with APCs, T cells, B cells, and other parts of the immune system and impact them.

As previously mentioned, shortage of organs is a serious hurdle in transplantation as increased waiting-list time can negatively affect the outcomes of transplantation. Many of the patients die due to long waiting-list durations. Many other patients that have undergone transplantation do not show optimum results as they were not in a suitable state prior to transplantation. To minimize such problems, the field of xenotransplantation that is transplanting organs from other animals into a human recipient is being researched. Islet cells, hearts, livers, lungs, and kidneys are being massively researched into as possible transplantable organs from animals to humans. The initial reactions to xenotransplantation were not positive as there were concerns related to innate and humoral-mediated rejection and viral infections. Gene editing utilizing clustered regularly interspaced short palindromic repeats (CRISPR)/Cas9 system has addressed these issues. CRISPR/Cas9 enables researchers to eliminate multiple genes that encode the antigens that are targeted by the immune system. Human immunodeficiency virus drugs can also prevent patients from acquiring viral infections from animals. However, xenotransplantation is yet to be incorporated into clinical settings.

HSCT is also another branch in transplantation that has made ground-breaking development in the treatment of many malignant and nonmalignant disorders. It has also introduced the notion of stem cell therapy and immunotherapy as an approach against cancer. The triumph of utilizing HSCT for hematologic malignancies depends on its capacity to treat patients with rigorous chemoradiotherapy and from the powerful graft versus leukemia effect (GVL) effect that stems from donor immunity. Furthermore, HSCT has been a therapeutic option for many nonmalignant hematologic diseases by providing donor-derived hematopoiesis and immunity. Developments in HLA typing, conditioning regimens, supportive care, and understanding the nature of host versus graft and graft versus host responses have minimized the side effects of both autologous and allogeneic HSCT. Incorporation of reduced-intensity regimens allows lesser toxicity while achieving the desirable graft versus tumor state. Potent cell-based therapies have been developed to decrease the occurrence of GVHD and thus decrease mortality and morbidity. Progressions of haploidentical HSCT have made prompt access to donors in patients with severe malignancies. Gene editing tools, including CRISPR/Cas9 and transcription activator-like effector nucleases (TALEN) can delete endogenous T cell receptor and HLA genes. This can result in the elimination of alloreactivity and reduced immunogenicity of third-party T cells.

## References


1. Linden PK. History of Solid Organ Transplantation and Organ Donation. *Crit Care Clin.* 2009;25(1):165–184.
2. Merrill JP, Murray JE, Harrison JH, Guild WR. Successful homotransplantation of the human kidney between identical twins. *J Am Med Assoc.* 1956;160(4):277–282.
3. Ordikhani F, Pothula V, Sanchez-Tarjuelo R, Jordan S, Ochando J. Macrophages in Organ Transplantation. *Front Immunol.* 2020;11:582939.
4. Malinis M, Boucher HW. Screening of donor and candidate prior to solid organ transplantation—Guidelines from the American Society of Transplantation Infectious Diseases Community of Practice. *Clin Transplant.* 2019;33(9):e13548.
5. Barriga F, Ramírez P, Wietstruck A, Rojas N. Hematopoietic stem cell transplantation: clinical use and perspectives. *Biol Res.* 2012;45(3):307–316.
6. Gyurkocza B, Sandmaier BM. Conditioning regimens for hematopoietic cell transplantation: one size does not fit all. *Blood.* 2014;124(3):344–353.
7. Cozzi E, Colpo A, De Silvestro G. The mechanisms of rejection in solid organ transplantation. *Transfusion and apheresis science : official journal of the World Apheresis Association : official journal of the European Society for Haemapheresis.* 2017;56(4):498–505.
8. Jasiak NM, Park JM. Immunosuppression in solid-organ transplantation essentials and practical tips. *Crit Care Nurs Q.* 2016;39(3):227–240.
9. Hymes SR, Alousi AM, Cowen EW. Graft-versus-host disease: part I. Pathogenesis and clinical manifestations of graft-versus-host disease. *J Am Acad Dermatol.* 2012;66(4):515.e1–515.e18.
10. Socié G, Blazar BR. Acute graft-versus-host disease: from the bench to the bedside. *Blood.* 2009;114(20):4327–4336.
11. Alameddine M, Moghadamyeghaneh Z, Yusufali A, Collazo AM, Jue JS, Zheng I, et al. Kidney Autotransplantation: between the Past and the Future. *Curr Urol Rep.* 2018;19(3):7.
12. Salama M, Woodruff TK. New advances in ovarian autotransplantation to restore fertility in cancer patients. *Cancer Metastasis Rev.* 2015;34(4):807–822.
13. Shindo Y, Kanak MA. Total pancreatectomy with islet autotransplantation: recent updates and outcomes. *Curr Opin Organ Transplant.* 2017;22(5):444–451.
14. Jiang F, Xu L, Yuan F, Huang J, Lu X. Lung autotransplantation technique in the treatment for central lung cancer of upper lobe. *Journal of thoracic oncology : official publication of the International Association for the Study of Lung Cancer.* 2008;3(6):609–611.
15. Voora S, Adey DB. Management of Kidney Transplant Recipients by General Nephrologists: core Curriculum 2019. *American journal of kidney diseases : the official journal of the National Kidney Foundation.* 2019;73(6):866–879.
16. Chinen J, Buckley RH Transplantation immunology: solid organ and bone marrow. The Journal of allergy and clinical immunology. 2010 Feb;125(2 Suppl 2):S324-35.

17. Rao PS, Ojo A. The alphabet soup of kidney transplantation: SCD, DCD, ECD–fundamentals for the practicing nephrologist. *Clinical journal of the American Society of Nephrology : CJASN*. 2009;4(11):1827–1831.
18. Port FK, Wolfe RA, Mauger EA, Berling DP, Jiang K. Comparison of Survival Probabilities for Dialysis Patients vs Cadaveric Renal Transplant Recipients. *JAMA*. 1993;270(11):1339–1343.
19. Valderrabano F, Jofre R, Lopez-Gomez JM. Quality of life in end-stage renal disease patients. *Am J Kidney Dis*. 2001;38(3):443–464.
20. Vo AA, Peng A, Toyoda M, Kahwaji J, Cao K, Lai CH, et al. Use of intravenous immune globulin and rituximab for desensitization of highly HLA-sensitized patients awaiting kidney transplantation. *Transplantation*. 2010;89(9):1095–1102.
21. Voora S, Adey DB. Management of Kidney Transplant Recipients by General Nephrologists: core Curriculum 2019. *Am J Kidney Dis*. 2019;73(6):866–879.
22. Donnelly PK, Lennard TW, Proud G, Taylor RM, Henderson R, Fletcher K, et al. Continuous ambulatory peritoneal dialysis and renal transplantation: a five year experience. *British Medical Journal (Clinical research ed)*. 1985;291(6501):1001–1004.
23. O'Donoghue D, Manos J, Pearson R, Scott P, Bakran A, Johnson R, et al. Continuous Ambulatory Peritoneal Dialysis and Renal Transplantation: a Ten-Year Experience in a Single Center. *Perit Dial Int*. 1992 Apr 1;12(2):242–249.
24. Pham P-T, Pham P-A, Pham P-C, Parikh S, Danovitch G. Evaluation of adult kidney transplant candidates. *Semin Dial*. 2010;23(6):595–605.
25. Augustine J. Kidney transplant: new opportunities and challenges. *Cleve Clin J Med*. 2018;85(2):138–144.
26. Querard A-H, Foucher Y, Combescure C, Dantan E, Larmet D, Lorent M, et al. Comparison of survival outcomes between Expanded Criteria Donor and Standard Criteria Donor kidney transplant recipients: a systematic review and meta-analysis. Transplant international : *official journal of the European Society for Organ Transplantation*. 2016;29(4):403–415.
27. Kim JJ, Fuggle SV, Marks SD. Does HLA matching matter in the modern era of renal transplantation? *Pediatr Nephrol*. 2021;36(1):31–40.
28. Gjertson DW, Cecka JM. Determinants of long-term survival of pediatric kidney grafts reported to the United Network for Organ Sharing kidney transplant registry. *Pediatr Transplant*. 2001;5(1):5–15.
29. Foster BJ, Dahhou M, Zhang X, Platt RW, Hanley JA. Relative importance of HLA mismatch and donor age to graft survival in young kidney transplant recipients. *Transplantation*. 2013;96(5):469–475.
30. Williams RC, West LJ, Opelz G. The Risk of Failure With HLA Mismatch and Recipient Age in First Pediatric (<18 years) Kidney Transplants. *Transplant Direct*. 2018;4(7):e365.
31. Sypek M, Kausman J, Holt S, Hughes P. HLA Epitope Matching in Kidney Transplantation: an Overview for the General Nephrologist. *American journal of kidney diseases : the official journal of the National Kidney Foundation*. 2018;71(5):720–731.
32. Ng MSY, Ullah S, Wilson G, McDonald S, Sypek M, Mallett AJ. ABO blood group relationships to kidney transplant recipient and graft outcomes. *PLoS One*. 2020;15(7):e0236396.
33. Singh N, Samant H, Hawxby A, Samaniego MD. Biomarkers of rejection in kidney transplantation. *Curr Opin Organ Transplant*. 2019;24(1):103–110.
34. Filippone EJ, Farber JL. The Humoral Theory of Transplantation: epitope Analysis and the Pathogenicity of HLA Antibodies. *J Immunol Res*. 2016;2016:5197396.
35. J Vaillant AA, M S, F BM. Acute Transplantation Rejection. In Treasure Island (FL); 2021.
36. Baldwin 3rd WM, Valujskikh A, Fairchild RL. Mechanisms of antibody-mediated acute and chronic rejection of kidney allografts. *Curr Opin Organ Transplant*. 2016;21(1):7–14.
37. Hassanein M, Augustine JJ Chronic Kidney Transplant Rejection. In Treasure Island (FL); 2021.
38. Coemans M, Süsal C, Döhler B, Anglicheau D, Giral M, Bestard O, et al. Analyses of the short- and long-term graft survival after kidney transplantation in Europe between 1986 and 2015. *Kidney Int*. 2018;94(5):964–973.
39. Chiu H-F, Chung M-C, Chung C-J, Yu T-M, Shu K-H, Wu M-J. Prognosis of Kidney Transplant Recipients With Pretransplantation Malignancy: a Nationwide Population-Based Cohort Study in Taiwan. *Transplant Proc*. 2016;48(3):918–920.
40. Starzl TE, Marchioro TL, Vonkaulla KN, Hermann G, Brittain RS, Waddell WR. Homotransplantation of the Liver in Humans. *Surgery, gynecology & obstetrics*. 1963;117:659–676.

41. Jadlowiec CC, Taner T. Liver transplantation: current status and challenges. *World journal of gastroenterology*. 2016;22(18):4438–4445.
42. Casavilla A, Ramirez C, Shapiro R, Nghiem D, Miracle K, Bronsther O, et al. Experience with liver and kidney allografts from non-heart-beating donors. *Transplantation*. 1995;59(2):197–203.
43. Mateo R, Cho Y, Singh G, Stapfer M, Donovan J, Kahn J, et al. Risk factors for graft survival after liver transplantation from donation after cardiac death donors: an analysis of OPTN/UNOS data. *American journal of transplantation : official journal of the American Society of Transplantation and the American Society of Transplant Surgeons*. 2006;6(4):791–796.
44. Belzer FO, BS A, Gulyassy PF, Powell M. Successful seventeen-hour preservation and transplantation of human-cadaver kidney. *N Engl J Med*. 1968;278(11):608–610.
45. Guarrera JV, Henry SD, Samstein B, Reznik E, Musat C, Lukose TI, et al. Hypothermic machine preservation facilitates successful transplantation of "orphan" extended criteria donor livers. *American journal of transplantation : official journal of the American Society of Transplantation and the American Society of Transplant Surgeons*. 2015;15(1):161–169.
46. Dutkowski P, Polak WG, Muiesan P, Schlegel A, Verhoeven CJ, Scalera I, et al. First Comparison of Hypothermic Oxygenated PErfusion Versus Static Cold Storage of Human Donation After Cardiac Death Liver Transplants: an International-matched Case Analysis. *Annals of surgery*. 2015;262(5):761–764.
47. Dutkowski P, Schlegel A, de Oliveira M, Müllhaupt B, Neff F. Clavien P-A. HOPE for human liver grafts obtained from donors after cardiac death. *J Hepatol*. 2014;60(4):765–772.
48. Henry SD, Nachber E, Tulipan J, Stone J, Bae C, Reznik L, et al. Hypothermic machine preservation reduces molecular markers of ischemia/reperfusion injury in human liver transplantation. *American journal of transplantation : official journal of the American Society of Transplantation and the American Society of Transplant Surgeons*. 2012;12(9):2477–2486.
49. Brockmann J, Reddy S, Coussios C, Pigott D, Guirriero D, Hughes D, et al. Normothermic perfusion: a new paradigm for organ preservation. *Ann Surg*. 2009;250(1):1–6.
50. Neuhaus P, Blumhardt G. Extracorporeal liver perfusion: applications of an improved model for experimental studies of the liver. *Int J Artif Organs*. 1993;16(10):729–739.
51. Pichlmayr R, Ringe B, Gubernatis G, Hauss J, Bunzendahl H. [Transplantation of a donor liver to 2 recipients (splitting transplantation)–a new method in the further development of segmental liver transplantation]. *Langenbecks Arch Chir*. 1988;373(2):127–130.
52. Raut V, Uemoto S. Management of ABO-incompatible living-donor liver transplantation: past and present trends. *Surg Today*. 2011;41(3):317–322.
53. Mendes M, Ferreira AC, Ferreira A, Remédio F, Aires I, Cordeiro A, et al. ABO-incompatible liver transplantation in acute liver failure: a single Portuguese center study. *Transplant Proc*. 2013;45(3): 1110–1115.
54. Srinivas Reddy M, Wilson C, Torpey N, Manas DM. ABO incompatible liver transplantation: a case of immediate need. *Transplant international : official journal of the European Society for Organ Transplantation. England*. 2007;20:904–905.
55. Waid TH, Lucas BA, Thompson JS, Brown S, Moore D, Amlot P, et al. Treatment of acute cellular kidney allograft rejection with T10B9.1A-31A anti T-cell monoclonal antibody. *Transplant Proc*. 1989;21(1 Pt 2):1778–1784.
56. Kluger MD, Guarrera JV, Olsen SK, Brown RSJ, Emond JC, Cherqui D. Safety of blood group A2-to-O liver transplantation: an analysis of the United Network of Organ Sharing database. *Transplantation*. 2012;94(5):526–531.
57. Bryan CF, Mitchell SI, Lin HM, Nelson PW, Shield 3rd CF, Luger AM, et al. Influence of the Rh (D) blood group system on graft survival in renal transplantation. *Transplantation*. 1998;65(4):588–592.
58. Reddy MS, Varghese J, Venkataraman J, Rela M. Matching donor to recipient in liver transplantation: relevance in clinical practice. *World J Hepatol*. 2013;5(11):603–611.
59. Kohler S, Pascher A, Junge G, Sauer IM, Nagy M, Schönemann C, et al. Graft versus host disease after liver transplantation - a single center experience and review of literature. *Transplant international : official journal of the European Society for Organ Transplantation*. 2008;21(5):441–451.
60. Watt KDS, Pedersen RA, Kremers WK, Heimbach JK, Charlton MR. Evolution of causes and risk factors for mortality post-liver transplant: results of the NIDDK long-term follow-up study. *American journal of transplantation : official journal of the American Society of Transplantation and the American Society of Transplant Surgeons*. 2010;10(6):1420–1427.

61. Assy N, Adams PC, Myers P, Simon V, Minuk GY, Wall W, et al. Randomized controlled trial of total immunosuppression withdrawal in liver transplant recipients: role of ursodeoxycholic acid. *Transplantation*. 2007;83(12):1571–1576.
62. Barnard CN. The operation. A human cardiac transplant: an interim report of a successful operation performed at Groote Schuur Hospital, Cape Town. *S Afr Med J*. 1967;41(48):1271–1274.
63. Mangini S, Alves BR, Silvestre OM, Pires PV, Pires LJT, Curiati MNC, et al. Heart transplantation: review. *Einstein (Sao Paulo)*. 2015;13(2):310–318.
64. de Jonge N, Kirkels JH, Klöpping C, Lahpor JR, Caliskan K, Maat APWM, et al. Guidelines for heart transplantation. *Netherlands heart journal : monthly journal of the Netherlands Society of Cardiology and the Netherlands Heart Foundation*. 2008;16(3):79–87.
65. Swedberg K, Cleland J, Dargie H, Drexler H, Follath F, Komajda M, et al. Guidelines for the diagnosis and treatment of chronic heart failure: executive summary (update 2005): the Task Force for the Diagnosis and Treatment of Chronic Heart Failure of the European Society of Cardiology. *Eur Heart J*. 2005;26(11):1115–1140.
66. Brasileira de Cardiologia S. II Diretriz Brasileira de Transplante Cardíaco. *Arq Bras Cardiol*. 2010;94(1):e16–e76.
67. Lund LH, Edwards LB, Kucheryavaya AY, Dipchand AI, Benden C, Christie JD, et al. The Registry of the International Society for Heart and Lung Transplantation: thirtieth Official Adult Heart Transplant Report–2013; focus theme: age. *The Journal of heart and lung transplantation : the official publication of the International Society for Heart Transplantation*. 2013;32(10):951–964.
68. Potena L, Zuckermann A, Barberini F. Aliabadi-Zuckermann A. Complications of Cardiac Transplantation. *Curr Cardiol Rep*. 2018;20(9):73.
69. Unilateral Lung Transplantation for Pulmonary Fibrosis. *N Engl J Med*. 1986;314(18):1140–1145.
70. Afonso Júnior JE, Werebe E dC, Carraro RM, Teixeira RH dO B, Fernandes LM, Abdalla LG, et al. Lung transplantation. *Einstein (São Paulo)*. 2015;13(2):297–304.
71. Dabak G, Şenbaklavacı Ö. History of Lung Transplantation. *Turkish thoracic journal. 2016/04/01*. 2016;17(2):71–75.
72. Demir A, Coosemans W, Decaluwé H, De Leyn P, Nafteux P, Van Veer H, et al. Donor-recipient matching in lung transplantation: which variables are important? *Eur J Cardiothorac Surg*. 2014;47(6):974–983.
73. Costa J, Benvenuto LJ, Sonett JR. Long-term outcomes and management of lung transplant recipients. *Best practice & research Clinical anaesthesiology*. 2017;31(2):285–297.
74. Shapiro AMJ, Pokrywczynska M, Ricordi C. Clinical pancreatic islet transplantation. *Nat Rev Endocrinol*. 2017;13(5):268–277.
75. Choudhary P, Rickels MR, Senior PA, Vantyghem M-C, Maffi P, Kay TW, et al. Evidence-informed clinical practice recommendations for treatment of type 1 diabetes complicated by problematic hypoglycemia. *Diabetes Care*. 2015;38(6):1016–1029.
76. Rickels MR, Stock PG, de Koning EJP, Piemonti L, Pratschke J, Alejandro R, et al. Defining outcomes for β-cell replacement therapy in the treatment of diabetes: a consensus report on the Igls criteria from the IPITA/EPITA opinion leaders workshop. *Transplant international : official journal of the European Society for Organ Transplantation*. 2018;31(4):343–352.
77. O'Connell PJ, Holmes-Walker DJ, Goodman D, Hawthorne WJ, Loudovaris T, Gunton JE, et al. Multicenter Australian trial of islet transplantation: improving accessibility and outcomes. *American journal of transplantation : official journal of the American Society of Transplantation and the American Society of Transplant Surgeons*. 2013;13(7):1850–1858.
78. Hering BJ, Kandaswamy R, Ansite JD, Eckman PM, Nakano M, Sawada T, et al. Single-donor, marginal-dose islet transplantation in patients with type 1 diabetes. *JAMA*. 2005;293(7):830–835.
79. Hering BJ, Clarke WR, Bridges ND, Eggerman TL, Alejandro R, Bellin MD, et al. Phase 3 Trial of Transplantation of Human Islets in Type 1 Diabetes Complicated by Severe Hypoglycemia. *Diabetes Care*. 2016;39(7):1230–1240.
80. Brooks AM, Walker N, Aldibbiat A, Hughes S, Jones G, de Havilland J, et al. Attainment of metabolic goals in the integrated UK islet transplant program with locally isolated and transported preparations. *American journal of transplantation : official journal of the American Society of Transplantation and the American Society of Transplant Surgeons*. 2013;13(12):3236–3243.
81. Nijhoff MF, Engelse MA, Dubbeld J, Braat AE, Ringers J, Roelen DL, et al. Glycemic Stability Through Islet-After-Kidney Transplantation Using an Alemtuzumab-Based Induction Regimen

and Long-Term Triple-Maintenance Immunosuppression. *American journal of transplantation : official journal of the American Society of Transplantation and the American Society of Transplant Surgeons.* 2016;16(1):246–253.
82. Singh R, Gupta N, Vanathi M, Tandon R. Corneal transplantation in the modern era. *Indian J Med Res.* 2019;150(1):7–22.
83. Zirm EK. Eine erfolgreiche totale Keratoplastik (A successful total keratoplasty). 1906. *Refract Corneal Surg.* 1989;5(4):258–261.
84. Di Zazzo A, Kheirkhah A, Abud TB, Goyal S, Dana R. Management of high-risk corneal transplantation. *Surv Ophthalmol.* 2017;62(6):816–827.
85. van Essen TH, Roelen DL, Williams KA, Jager MJ. Matching for Human Leukocyte Antigens (HLA) in corneal transplantation - to do or not to do. *Prog Retin Eye Res.* 2015;46:84–110.
86. Shimizu R, Kishi K. Skin graft. *Plast Surg Int.* 2012;2012:563493.
87. Ragnell A. The secondary contracting tendency of free skin grafts. An experimental investigation on animals. *Br J Plast Surg.* 1952;5(1):6–24.
88. Jonker M, Hoogeboom J, van Leeuwen A, Koch CT, van Oud Alblas D, van Rood JJ. Influence of matching for HLA-DR antigens on skin graft survival. *Transplantation.* 1979;27(2):91—94.
89. Balassa K, Danby R, Rocha V. Haematopoietic stem cell transplants: principles and indications. *British journal of hospital medicine (London, England : 2005).* 2019;80(1):33–39.
90. Cornelissen JJ, Blaise D. Hematopoietic stem cell transplantation for patients with AML in first complete remission. *Blood.* 2016;127(1):62–70.
91. Papaemmanuil E, Gerstung M, Bullinger L, Gaidzik VI, Paschka P, Roberts ND, et al. Genomic Classification and Prognosis in Acute Myeloid Leukemia. *N Engl J Med.* 2016;374(23):2209–2221.
92. Döhner H, Estey E, Grimwade D, Amadori S, Appelbaum FR, Büchner T, et al. Diagnosis and management of AML in adults: 2017 ELN recommendations from an international expert panel. *Blood.* 2017;129(4):424–447.
93. Duarte RF, Labopin M, Bader P, Basak GW, Bonini C, Chabannon C, et al. Indications for haematopoietic stem cell transplantation for haematological diseases, solid tumours and immune disorders: current practice in Europe, 2019. *Bone Marrow Transplant.* 2019;54(10):1525–1552.
94. Balsat M, Renneville A, Thomas X, de Botton S, Caillot D, Marceau A, et al. Postinduction Minimal Residual Disease Predicts Outcome and Benefit From Allogeneic Stem Cell Transplantation in Acute Myeloid Leukemia With NPM1 Mutation: a Study by the Acute Leukemia French Association Group. *Journal of clinical oncology : official journal of the American Society of Clinical Oncology.* 2017;35(2):185–193.
95. Gupta V, Richards S, Rowe J. Allogeneic, but not autologous, hematopoietic cell transplantation improves survival only among younger adults with acute lymphoblastic leukemia in first remission: an individual patient data meta-analysis. *Blood.* 2013;121(2):339–350.
96. Alchalby H, Zabelina T, Stübig T, van Biezen A, Bornhäuser M, Di Bartolomeo P, et al. Allogeneic stem cell transplantation for myelofibrosis with leukemic transformation: a study from the Myeloproliferative Neoplasm Subcommittee of the CMWP of the European Group for Blood and Marrow Transplantation. *Biology of blood and marrow transplantation : journal of the American Society for Blood and Marrow Transplantation.* 2014;20(2):279–281.
97. Kröger N, Holler E, Kobbe G, Bornhäuser M, Schwerdtfeger R, Baurmann H, et al. Allogeneic stem cell transplantation after reduced-intensity conditioning in patients with myelofibrosis: a prospective, multicenter study of the Chronic Leukemia Working Party of the European Group for Blood and Marrow Transplantation. *Blood.* 2009;114(26):5264–5270.
98. Kröger N. Allogeneic stem cell transplantation for elderly patients with myelodysplastic syndrome. *Blood.* 2012;119(24):5632–5639.
99. de Witte T, Bowen D, Robin M, Malcovati L, Niederwieser D, Yakoub-Agha I, et al. Allogeneic hematopoietic stem cell transplantation for MDS and CMML: recommendations from an international expert panel. *Blood.* 2017;129(13):1753–1762.
100. Dreger P, Ghia P, Schetelig J, van Gelder M, Kimby E, Michallet M, et al. High-risk chronic lymphocytic leukemia in the era of pathway inhibitors: integrating molecular and cellular therapies. *Blood.* 2018;132(9):892–902.
101. Cwynarski K, van Biezen A, de Wreede L, Stilgenbauer S, Bunjes D, Metzner B, et al. Autologous and allogeneic stem-cell transplantation for transformed chronic lymphocytic leukemia (Richter's syndrome): a retrospective analysis from the chronic lymphocytic leukemia subcommittee of the

chronic leukemia working party and lymphoma working. *Journal of clinical oncology : official journal of the American Society of Clinical Oncology*. 2012;30(18):2211–2217.
102. Gisselbrecht C, Schmitz N, Mounier N, Singh Gill D, Linch DC, Trneny M, et al. Rituximab maintenance therapy after autologous stem-cell transplantation in patients with relapsed CD20(+) diffuse large B-cell lymphoma: final analysis of the collaborative trial in relapsed aggressive lymphoma. *Journal of clinical oncology : official journal of the American Society of Clinical Oncology*. 2012;30(36):4462–4469.
103. Ghielmini M, Vitolo U, Kimby E, Montoto S, Walewski J, Pfreundschuh M, et al. ESMO Guidelines consensus conference on malignant lymphoma 2011 part 1: diffuse large B-cell lymphoma (DLBCL), follicular lymphoma (FL) and chronic lymphocytic leukemia (CLL). *Annals of oncology : official journal of the European Society for Medical Oncology*. 2013;24(3):561–576.
104. Mounier N, Canals C, Gisselbrecht C, Cornelissen J, Foa R, Conde E, et al. High-dose therapy and autologous stem cell transplantation in first relapse for diffuse large B cell lymphoma in the rituximab era: an analysis based on data from the European Blood and Marrow Transplantation Registry. *Biology of blood and marrow transplantation : journal of the American Society for Blood and Marrow Transplantation*. 2012;18(5):788–793.
105. van Kampen RJW, Canals C, Schouten HC, Nagler A, Thomson KJ, Vernant J-P, et al. Allogeneic stem-cell transplantation as salvage therapy for patients with diffuse large B-cell non-Hodgkin's lymphoma relapsing after an autologous stem-cell transplantation: an analysis of the European Group for Blood and Marrow Transplantation Registry. *Journal of clinical oncology : official journal of the American Society of Clinical Oncology*. 2011;29(10):1342–1348.
106. Rigacci L, Puccini B, Dodero A, Iacopino P, Castagna L, Bramanti S, et al. Allogeneic hematopoietic stem cell transplantation in patients with diffuse large B cell lymphoma relapsed after autologous stem cell transplantation: a GITMO study. *Ann Hematol*. 2012;91(6):931–939.
107. Glass B, Hasenkamp J, Wulf G, Dreger P, Pfreundschuh M, Gramatzki M, et al. Rituximab after lymphoma-directed conditioning and allogeneic stem-cell transplantation for relapsed and refractory aggressive non-Hodgkin lymphoma (DSHNHL R3): an open-label, randomised, phase 2 trial. *Lancet Oncol*. 2014;15(7):757–766.
108. Buske C, Leblond V. How to manage Waldenstrom's macroglobulinemia. *Leukemia*. 2013;27(4):762–772.
109. Sureda A, Bader P, Cesaro S, Dreger P, Duarte RF, Dufour C, et al. Indications for allo- and auto-SCT for haematological diseases, solid tumours and immune disorders: current practice in Europe, 2015. *Bone Marrow Transplant*. 2015;50(8):1037–1056.
110. Schmitz N, Nickelsen M, Altmann B, Ziepert M, Bouabdallah K, Gisselbrecht C, et al. Allogeneic or autologous transplantation as first-line therapy for younger patients with peripheral T-cell lymphoma: results of the interim analysis of the AATT trial. *J Clin Oncol*. 2015;33(15_suppl):8507 May 20.
111. Dispenzieri A, Kyle RA, Lacy MQ, Therneau TM, Larson DR, Plevak MF, et al. Superior survival in primary systemic amyloidosis patients undergoing peripheral blood stem cell transplantation: a case-control study. *Blood*. 2004;103(10):3960–3963.
112. Niewerth D, Creutzig U, Bierings MB, Kaspers GJL. A review on allogeneic stem cell transplantation for newly diagnosed pediatric acute myeloid leukemia. *Blood*. 2010;116(13):2205–2214.
113. Burke MJ, Wagner JE, Cao Q, Ustun C, Verneris MR. Allogeneic hematopoietic cell transplantation in first remission abrogates poor outcomes associated with high-risk pediatric acute myeloid leukemia. *Biology of blood and marrow transplantation : journal of the American Society for Blood and Marrow Transplantation*. 2013;19(7):1021–1025.
114. Klusmann J-H, Reinhardt D, Zimmermann M, Kremens B, Vormoor J, Dworzak M, et al. The role of matched sibling donor allogeneic stem cell transplantation in pediatric high-risk acute myeloid leukemia: results from the AML-BFM 98 study. *Haematologica*. 2012;97(1):21–29.
115. Creutzig U, Zimmermann M, Bourquin J-P, Dworzak MN, Kremens B, Lehrnbecher T, et al. Favorable outcome in infants with AML after intensive first- and second-line treatment: an AML-BFM study group report. *Leukemia*. 2012;26(4):654–661.
116. Hasle H A critical review of which children with acute myeloid leukaemia need stem cell procedures. British journal of haematology. 2014 Jul;166(1):23–33.
117. Suttorp M, Eckardt L, Tauer JT, Millot F. Management of chronic myeloid leukemia in childhood. *Curr Hematol Malig Rep*. 2012;7(2):116–124.

118. Suttorp M, Yaniv I, Schultz KR. Controversies in the treatment of CML in children and adolescents: tKIs versus BMT? Biology of blood and marrow transplantation : *journal of the American Society for Blood and Marrow Transplantation*. 2011;17(1 Suppl):S115–S122.
119. de la Fuente J, Baruchel A, Biondi A, de Bont E, Dresse M-F, Suttorp M, et al. Managing children with chronic myeloid leukaemia (CML). *Br. J. Haematol.* 2014 Oct 1;167(1):33–47.
120. Brown L, Xu-Bayford J, Allwood Z, Slatter M, Cant A, Davies EG, et al. Neonatal diagnosis of severe combined immunodeficiency leads to significantly improved survival outcome: the case for newborn screening. *Blood*. 2011;117(11):3243–3246.
121. Pai S-Y, Logan BR, Griffith LM, Buckley RH, Parrott RE, Dvorak CC, et al. Transplantation outcomes for severe combined immunodeficiency, 2000-2009. *The New England journal of medicine*. 2014;371(5):434–446.
122. Haddad E, Logan BR, Griffith LM, Buckley RH, Parrott RE, Prockop SE, et al. SCID genotype and 6-month posttransplant CD4 count predict survival and immune recovery. *Blood*. 2018;132(17):1737–1749.
123. Moratto D, Giliani S, Bonfim C, Mazzolari E, Fischer A, Ochs HD, et al. Long-term outcome and lineage-specific chimerism in 194 patients with Wiskott-Aldrich syndrome treated by hematopoietic cell transplantation in the period 1980-2009: an international collaborative study. *Blood*. 2011;118(6):1675–1684.
124. Güngör T, Teira P, Slatter M, Stussi G, Stepensky P, Moshous D, et al. Reduced-intensity conditioning and HLA-matched haemopoietic stem-cell transplantation in patients with chronic granulomatous disease: a prospective multicentre study. *Lancet*. 2014;383(9915):436–448.
125. Ngwube A, Hanson IC, Orange J, Rider NL, Seeborg F, Shearer W, et al. Outcomes after Allogeneic Transplant in Patients with Wiskott-Aldrich Syndrome. Biology of blood and marrow transplantation : *journal of the American Society for Blood and Marrow Transplantation*. 2018;24(3):537–541.
126. Ferrua F, Galimberti S, Courteille V, Slatter MA, Booth C, Moshous D, et al. Hematopoietic stem cell transplantation for CD40 ligand deficiency: results from an EBMT/ESID-IEWP-SCETIDE-PIDTC study. *J. Allergy Clin. Immunol.* 2019;143(6):2238–2253.
127. Gennery AR, Slatter MA, Grandin L, Taupin P, Cant AJ, Veys P, et al. Transplantation of hematopoietic stem cells and long-term survival for primary immunodeficiencies in Europe: entering a new century, do we do better? *J. Allergy Clin. Immunol.* 2010;126(3):602–611.
128. Snowden JA, Badoglio M, Labopin M, Giebel S, McGrath E, Marjanovic Z, et al. Evolution, trends, outcomes, and economics of hematopoietic stem cell transplantation in severe autoimmune diseases. *Blood advances*. 2017;1(27):2742–2755.
129. Kelsey PJ, Oliveira M-C, Badoglio M, Sharrack B, Farge D, Snowden JA. Haematopoietic stem cell transplantation in autoimmune diseases: from basic science to clinical practice. *Current research in translational medicine*. 2016;64(2):71–82.
130. Alexander T, Farge D, Badoglio M, Lindsay JO, Muraro PA, Snowden JA. Hematopoietic stem cell therapy for autoimmune diseases - Clinical experience and mechanisms. *J. Autoimmun.* 2018;92:35–46.
131. Burman J, Kirgizov K, Carlson K, Badoglio M, Mancardi GL, De Luca G, et al. Autologous hematopoietic stem cell transplantation for pediatric multiple sclerosis: a registry-based study of the Autoimmune Diseases Working Party (ADWP) and Pediatric Diseases Working Party (PDWP) of the European Society for Blood and Marrow Transplan. *Bone Marrow Transplant.* 2017;52(8):1133–1137.
132. Ferrara GB, Bacigalupo A, Lamparelli T, Lanino E, Delfino L, Morabito A, et al. Bone marrow transplantation from unrelated donors: the impact of mismatches with substitutions at position 116 of the human leukocyte antigen class I heavy chain. *Blood*. 2001;98(10):3150–3155.
133. Pidala J, Wang T, Haagenson M, Spellman SR, Askar M, Battiwalla M, et al. Amino acid substitution at peptide-binding pockets of HLA class I molecules increases risk of severe acute GVHD and mortality. *Blood*. 2013;122(22):3651–3658.
134. Lee SJ, Klein J, Haagenson M, Baxter-Lowe LA, Confer DL, Eapen M, et al. High-resolution donor-recipient HLA matching contributes to the success of unrelated donor marrow transplantation. *Blood*. 2007;110(13):4576–4583.
135. del Campo L, León NG, Palacios DC, Lagana C, Tagarro D. Abdominal complications following hematopoietic stem cell transplantation. *Radiographics*. 2014;34(2):396–412.

136. Pidala J, Anasetti C, Kharfan-Dabaja MA, Cutler C, Sheldon A, Djulbegovic B. Decision Analysis of Peripheral Blood versus Bone Marrow Hematopoietic Stem Cells for Allogeneic Hematopoietic Cell Transplantation. *Biology of Blood and Marrow Transplantation*. 2009;15(11):1415–1421.
137. Hutt D. *Engraftment, Graft Failure, and Rejection*. In: Kenyon M, Babic A, eds.: Cham (CH); 2018:259–270.
138. Edwards RG, Hollands P. Will stem cells in cord blood, amniotic fluid, bone marrow and peripheral blood soon be unnecessary in transplantation? *Reprod. Biomed. Online*. 2007;14(3):396–401.
139. Chao Y-H, Wu H-P, Chan C-K, Tsai C, Peng C-T, Wu K-H. Umbilical Cord-Derived Mesenchymal Stem Cells for Hematopoietic Stem Cell Transplantation. In: Shahrokhi S, ed. Umbilical Cord-Derived Mesenchymal Stem Cells for Hematopoietic Stem Cell Transplantation. *Journal of Biomedicine and Biotechnology*. 2012;2012:759503.
140. In 't Anker PS, Scherjon SA, Kleijburg-van der K C, Noort WA, Claas FHJ, Willemze R, et al. Amniotic fluid as a novel source of mesenchymal stem cells for therapeutic transplantation102: Blood. United States; 2003:1548–1549 Vol.
141. Chute JP. Stem cell homing. *Curr. Opin. Hematol*. 2006;13(6):399–406.
142. Lapidot T, Kollet O. The brain-bone-blood triad: traffic lights for stem-cell homing and mobilization. *Hematology American Society of Hematology Education Program*. 2010;2010:1–6.
143. Elfeky R, Lazareva A, Qasim W, Veys P. Immune reconstitution following hematopoietic stem cell transplantation using different stem cell sources. *Expert Rev Clin Immunol*. 2019;15(7):735–751.
144. Siu JHY, Surendrakumar V, Richards JA, Pettigrew GJ. T cell Allorecognition Pathways in Solid Organ Transplantation. *Front Immunol*. 2018;9:2548.
145. Ali JM, Bolton EM, Bradley JA, Pettigrew GJ. Allorecognition pathways in transplant rejection and tolerance. *Transplantation*. 2013;96(8):681–688.
146. Elkins WL, Guttmann RD. Pathogenesis of a local graft versus host reaction: immunogenicity of circulating host leukocytes. *Science (New York, NY)*. 1968;159(3820):1250–1251.
147. Talmage DW, Dart G, Radovich J, Lafferty KJ. Activation of transplant immunity: effect of donor leukocytes on thyroid allograft rejection. *Science (New York, NY)*. 1976;191(4225):385–388.
148. Larsen CP, Morris PJ, Austyn JM. Migration of dendritic leukocytes from cardiac allografts into host spleens. A novel pathway for initiation of rejection. *J. Exp. Med*. 1990;171(1):307–314.
149. Lakkis FG, Arakelov A, Konieczny BT, Inoue Y. Immunologic "ignorance" of vascularized organ transplants in the absence of secondary lymphoid tissue. *Nat. Med*. 2000;6(6):686–688.
150. Joly E, Hudrisier D. What is trogocytosis and what is its purpose? *Nature immunology. United States*. 2003;4:815.
151. Knight SC, Iqball S, Roberts MS, Macatonia S, Bedford PA. Transfer of antigen between dendritic cells in the stimulation of primary T cell proliferation. *Eur. J. Immunol*. 1998;28(5):1636–1644.
152. Wykes M, Pombo A, Jenkins C, MacPherson GG. Dendritic cells interact directly with naive B lymphocytes to transfer antigen and initiate class switching in a primary T-dependent response. *Journal of immunology (Baltimore, Md : 1950)*. 1998;161(3):1313–1319.
153. Russo V, Zhou D, Sartirana C, Rovere P, Villa A, Rossini S, et al. Acquisition of intact allogeneic human leukocyte antigen molecules by human dendritic cells. *Blood*. 2000;95(11):3473–3477.
154. Baker RJ, Hernandez-Fuentes MP, Brookes PA, Chaudhry AN, Cook HT, Lechler RI. Loss of direct and maintenance of indirect alloresponses in renal allograft recipients: implications for the pathogenesis of chronic allograft nephropathy. *Journal of immunology (Baltimore, Md : 1950)*. 2001;167(12):7199–7206.
155. Ali JM, Negus MC, Conlon TM, Harper IG, Qureshi MS, Motallebzadeh R, et al. Diversity of the CD4 T Cell Alloresponse: the Short and the Long of It. *Cell Rep*. 2016;14(5):1232–1245.
156. Haynes LD, Jankowska-Gan E, Sheka A, Keller MR, Hernandez-Fuentes MP, Lechler RI, et al. Donor-specific indirect pathway analysis reveals a B-cell-independent signature which reflects outcomes in kidney transplant recipients. *American journal of transplantation : official journal of the American Society of Transplantation and the American Society of Transplant Surgeons*. 2012;12(3):640–648.
157. Kreisel D, Krasinskas AM, Krupnick AS, Gelman AE, Balsara KR, Popma SH, et al. Vascular endothelium does not activate CD4+ direct allorecognition in graft rejection. *Journal of immunology (Baltimore, Md : 1950)*. 2004;173(5):3027–3034.
158. Ciubotariu R, Liu Z, Colovai AI, Ho E, Itescu S, Ravalli S, et al. Persistent allopeptide reactivity and epitope spreading in chronic rejection of organ allografts. *J. Clin. Invest*. 1998;101(2):398–405.

159. Hornick PI, Mason PD, Baker RJ, Hernandez-Fuentes M, Frasca L, Lombardi G, et al. Significant frequencies of T cells with indirect anti-donor specificity in heart graft recipients with chronic rejection. *Circulation*. 2000;101(20):2405–2410.
160. Stanford RE, Ahmed S, Hodson M, Banner NR. RoM LA rfiailtrwobronchiolitis. *American journal of transplantation : official journal of the American Society of Transplantation and the American Society of Transplant Surgeons*. 2003;3(6):736–742.
161. Richards DM, Dalheimer SL, Ehst BD, Vanasek TL, Jenkins MK, Hertz MI, et al. Indirect minor histocompatibility antigen presentation by allograft recipient cells in the draining lymph node leads to the activation and clonal expansion of CD4+ T cells that cause obliterative airways disease. *Journal of immunology (Baltimore, Md : 1950)*. 2004;172(6):3469–3479.
162. Lee RS, Yamada K, Houser SL, Womer KL, Maloney ME, Rose HS, et al. Indirect recognition of allopeptides promotes the development of cardiac allograft vasculopathy. *Proc. Natl. Acad. Sci. U.S.A.* 2001;98(6):3276–3281.
163. Honjo K, X Y X, Kapp JA. Bucy RP. Evidence for cooperativity in the rejection of cardiac grafts mediated by CD4 TCR Tg T cells specific for a defined allopeptide. *American journal of transplantation : official journal of the American Society of Transplantation and the American Society of Transplant Surgeons*. 2004;4(11):1762–1768.
164. Honjo K, yan X X, Bucy RP. CD4+ T-cell receptor transgenic T cells alone can reject vascularized heart transplants through the indirect pathway of alloantigen recognition. *Transplantation*. 2004;77(3):452–455.
165. Louvi A, Artavanis-Tsakonas S. Notch and disease: a growing field. *Semin. Cell Dev. Biol.* 2012;23(4):473–480.
166. Pui JC, Allman D, Xu L, DeRocco S, Karnell FG, Bakkour S, et al. Notch1 expression in early lymphopoiesis influences B versus T lineage determination. *Immunity*. 1999;11(3):299–308.
167. Radtke F, Wilson A, Stark G, Bauer M, van Meerwijk J, MacDonald HR, et al. Deficient T cell fate specification in mice with an induced inactivation of Notch1. *Immunity*. 1999;10(5):547–558.
168. Radojcic V, Maillard I. Notch Signaling and Alloreactivity. *Transplantation*. 2016;100(12):2593–2600.
169. Zhang Y, Sandy AR, Wang J, Radojcic V, Shan GT, Tran IT, et al. Notch signaling is a critical regulator of allogeneic CD4+ T-cell responses mediating graft-versus-host disease. *Blood*. 2011;117(1):299–308.
170. Sandy AR, Chung J, Toubai T, Shan GT, Tran IT, Friedman A, et al. T cell-specific notch inhibition blocks graft-versus-host disease by inducing a hyporesponsive program in alloreactive CD4+ and CD8+ T cells. *Journal of immunology (Baltimore, Md : 1950)*. 2013;190(11):5818–5828.
171. Tran IT, Sandy AR, Carulli AJ, Ebens C, Chung J, Shan GT, et al. Blockade of individual Notch ligands and receptors controls graft-versus-host disease. *J. Clin. Invest.* 2013;123(4):1590–1604.
172. Liu W, Putnam AL, Xu-yu Z, Szot GL, Lee MR, Zhu S, et al. CD127 expression inversely correlates with FoxP3 and suppressive function of human CD4+ T reg cells. *Journal of Experimental Medicine*. 2006 Jul 3;203(7):1701–1711.
173. Bluestone JA, Buckner JH, Fitch M, Gitelman SE, Gupta S, Hellerstein MK, et al. Type 1 diabetes immunotherapy using polyclonal regulatory T cells. *Sci Transl Med*. 2015;7(315) Nov 25315ra189 LP-315ra189.
174. Safinia N, Grageda N, Scottà C, Thirkell S, Fry LJ, Vaikunthanathan T, et al. Cell therapy in organ transplantation: our experience on the clinical translation of regulatory T cells. *Front Immunol*. 2018;9(FEB):354.
175. Mellor AL, Munn DH. Ido expression by dendritic cells: tolerance and tryptophan catabolism. *Nature Reviews Immunology*. 2004;4(10):762–774.
176. Juvet SC, Whatcott AG, Bushell AR, Wood KJ. Harnessing regulatory T cells for clinical use in transplantation: the end of the beginning. *American journal of transplantation : official journal of the American Society of Transplantation and the American Society of Transplant Surgeons*. 2014;14(4):750–763.
177. Hall BM, Pearce NW, Gurley KE, Dorsch SE. Specific unresponsiveness in rats with prolonged cardiac allograft survival after treatment with cyclosporine. III. Further characterization of the CD4+ suppressor cell and its mechanisms of action. *J. Exp. Med.* 1990;171(1):141–157.
178. Bushell A, Morris PJ, Wood KJ. Transplantation tolerance induced by antigen pretreatment and depleting anti-CD4 antibody depends on CD4+ T cell regulation during the induction phase of the response. *Eur. J. Immunol.* 1995;25(9):2643–2649.

179. Hara M, Kingsley CI, Niimi M, Read S, Turvey SE, Bushell AR, et al. IL-10 is required for regulatory T cells to mediate tolerance to alloantigens in vivo. *Journal of immunology (Baltimore, Md : 1950)*. 2001;166(6):3789–3796.
180. Kingsley CI, Karim M, Bushell AR, Wood KJ. CD25+CD4+ regulatory T cells prevent graft rejection: CTLA-4- and IL-10-dependent immunoregulation of alloresponses. *Journal of immunology (Baltimore, Md : 1950)*. 2002;168(3):1080–1086.
181. Benichou G, Gonzalez B, Marino J, Ayasoufi K, Valujskikh A. Role of Memory T Cells in Allograft Rejection and Tolerance. *Front Immunol*. 2017;8:170.
182. Lombardi G, Sidhu S, Daly M, Batchelor JR, Makgoba W, Lechler RI. Are primary alloresponses truly primary? *Int. Immunol*. 1990;2(1):9–13.
183. Lechler R, Lombardi G. Structural aspects of allorecognition. *Curr. Opin. Immunol*. 1991;3(5):715–721.
184. Pantenburg B, Heinzel F, Das L, Heeger PS, Valujskikh A. T cells primed by Leishmania major infection cross-react with alloantigens and alter the course of allograft rejection. *Journal of immunology (Baltimore, Md : 1950)*. 2002;169(7):3686–3693.
185. Amir AL, D'Orsogna LJA, Roelen DL, van Loenen MM, Hagedoorn RS, de Boer R, et al. Allo-HLA reactivity of virus-specific memory T cells is common. *Blood*. 2010;115(15):3146–3157.
186. Chen Y, Heeger PS, Valujskikh A. In vivo helper functions of alloreactive memory CD4+ T cells remain intact despite donor-specific transfusion and anti-CD40 ligand therapy. *Journal of immunology (Baltimore, Md : 1950)*. 2004;172(9):5456–5466.
187. Hirai T, Ishii Y, Ikemiyagi M, Fukuda E, Omoto K, Namiki M, et al. A Novel Approach Inducing Transplant Tolerance by Activated Invariant Natural Killer T Cells With Costimulatory Blockade. *American Journal of Transplantation*. 2014 Mar 1;14(3):554–567.
188. Kawano T, Cui J, Koezuka Y, Toura I, Kaneko Y, Motoki K, et al. CD1d-restricted and TCR-mediated activation of valpha14 NKT cells by glycosylceramides. *Science (New York, NY)*. 1997;278(5343):1626–1629.
189. Balk SP, Bleicher PA, Terhorst C. Isolation and characterization of a cDNA and gene coding for a fourth CD1 molecule. *Proceedings of the National Academy of Sciences of the United States of America*. 86; 1989:252–256.
190. Jukes J-P, Wood KJ, Jones ND. Natural Killer T Cells: a Bridge to Tolerance or a Pathway to Rejection? *Transplantation*. 2007;84(6).
191. Zorn E. New insights on innate B-cell immunity in transplantation. *Xenotransplantation*. 2018;25(3):139–148.
192. Porcheray F, Fraser JW, Gao B, McColl A, DeVito J, Dargon I, et al. Polyreactive antibodies developing amidst humoral rejection of human kidney grafts bind apoptotic cells and activate complement. *American journal of transplantation : official journal of the American Society of Transplantation and the American Society of Transplant Surgeons*. 2013;13(10):2590–2600.
193. Gao B, Moore C, Porcheray F, Rong C, Abidoglu C, DeVito J, et al. Pretransplant IgG reactivity to apoptotic cells correlates with late kidney allograft loss. *American journal of transplantation : official journal of the American Society of Transplantation and the American Society of Transplant Surgeons*. 2014;14(7):1581–1591.
194. See SB, Aubert O, Loupy A, Veras Y, Lebreton X, Gao B, et al. Post-Transplant Natural Antibodies Associate with Kidney Allograft Injury and Reduced Long-Term Survival. *Journal of the American Society of Nephrology : JASN*. 2018;29(6):1761–1770.
195. B W M 3rd, MK H, Valujskikh A, Fairchild RL. B cells in cardiac transplants: from clinical questions to experimental models. *Semin. Immunol*. 2012;24(2):122–130.
196. Hippen BE, DeMattos A, Cook WJ, Kew 2nd CE, Gaston RS. Association of CD20+ infiltrates with poorer clinical outcomes in acute cellular rejection of renal allografts. *American journal of transplantation : official journal of the American Society of Transplantation and the American Society of Transplant Surgeons*. 2005;5(9):2248–2252.
197. Ferdman J, Porcheray F, Gao B, Moore C, DeVito J, Dougherty S, et al. Expansion and somatic hypermutation of B-cell clones in rejected human kidney grafts. *Transplantation*. 2014;98(7):766–772.
198. Huibers MMH, Gareau AJ, Vink A, Kruit R, Feringa H, Beerthuijzen JMT, et al. The composition of ectopic lymphoid structures suggests involvement of a local immune response in cardiac allograft vasculopathy. *The Journal of heart and lung transplantation : the official publication of the International Society for Heart Transplantation*. 2015;34(5):734–745.

199. Thaunat O, Patey N, Caligiuri G, Gautreau C, Mamani-Matsuda M, Mekki Y, et al. Chronic rejection triggers the development of an aggressive intragraft immune response through recapitulation of lymphoid organogenesis. *Journal of immunology (Baltimore, Md : 1950)*. 2010;185(1):717–728.
200. Thaunat O, Field A-C, Dai J, Louedec L, Patey N, Bloch M-F, et al. Lymphoid neogenesis in chronic rejection: evidence for a local humoral alloimmune response. *Proceedings of the National Academy of Sciences of the United States of America*. 102; 2005:14723–14728.
201. Martins HL, Silva C, Martini D, Noronha IL. Detection of B lymphocytes (CD20+) in renal allograft biopsy specimens. *Transplant. Proc.* 2007;39(2):432–434.
202. Zarkhin V, Kambham N, Li L, Kwok S, Hsieh S-C, Salvatierra O, et al. Characterization of intra-graft B cells during renal allograft rejection. *Kidney Int.* 2008;74(5):664–673.
203. Thaunat O, Patey N, Morelon E, Michel J-B, Nicoletti A. Lymphoid neogenesis in chronic rejection: the murderer is in the house. *Curr. Opin. Immunol.* 2006;18(5):576–579.
204. Zarkhin V, Li L, Sarwal M. To B or not to B?" B-cells and graft rejection. *Transplantation. United States*. 2008;85:1705–1714.
205. Wehner JR, Fox-Talbot K, Halushka MK, Ellis C, Zachary AA, Baldwin 3rd WM. B cells and plasma cells in coronaries of chronically rejected cardiac transplants. *Transplantation*. 2010;89(9):1141–1148.
206. Kayler LK, Lakkis FG, Morgan C, Basu A, Blisard D, Tan HP, et al. Acute cellular rejection with CD20-positive lymphoid clusters in kidney transplant patients following lymphocyte depletion. *American journal of transplantation : official journal of the American Society of Transplantation and the American Society of Transplant Surgeons*. 2007;7(4):949–954.
207. Doria C, di Francesco F, Ramirez CB, Frank A, Iaria M, Francos G, et al. The presence of B-cell nodules does not necessarily portend a less favorable outcome to therapy in patients with acute cellular rejection of a renal allograft. *Transplant. Proc.* 2006;38(10):3441–3444.
208. Tsai EW, Rianthavorn P, Gjertson DW, Wallace WD, Reed EF, Ettenger RB. CD20+ lymphocytes in renal allografts are associated with poor graft survival in pediatric patients. *Transplantation*. 2006;82(12):1769–1773.
209. Platt JL, Cascalho M. Donor specific antibodies after transplantation. *Pediatr Transplant*. 2011;15(7):686–690.
210. Gorer PA. The genetic and antigenic basis of tumour transplantation. *J Pathol Bacteriol*. 1937 May 1;44(3):691–697.
211. Gorer PA, Lyman S, Snell GD, et al. Studies on the genetic and antigenic basis of tumour transplantation Linkage between a histocompatibility gene and "fused" in mice. *Proceedings of the Royal Society B: Biological Sciences*. 135; 1948:499–505 Dec 14.
212. Farney AC, Matas AJ, Noreen HJ, Reinsmoen N, Segall M, Schmidt WJ, et al. Does re-exposure to mismatched HLA antigens decrease renal re-transplant allograft survival? *Clin Transplant*. 1996;10(2):147–156.
213. Yu PB, Holzknecht ZE, Bruno D, Parker W, Platt JL. Modulation of natural IgM binding and complement activation by natural IgG antibodies: a role for IgG anti-Gal alpha1-3Gal antibodies. *The Journal of Immunology*. 1996;157(11):5163LP–5168LP Dec 1.
214. Nossal GJ. Kinetics of antibody formation and regulatory aspects of immunity. *Acta endocrinologica Supplementum*. 1975;194:96–116.
215. Nossal GJV. The Florey Lecture, 1986 - The regulatory biology of antibody formation. *Proceedings of the Royal Society of London Series B Biological Sciences*. 1986;228(1252):225–240 Aug 22.
216. 2nd W G C, RE T, Blatt PM, Roberts HR. Treatment of a high titer anti-factor-VIII antibody by continuous factor VIII administration: report of a case. *Blood*. 1983;62(1):141–145.
217. Chong AS, Sciammas R. Memory B cells in transplantation. *Transplantation*. 2015;99(1):21–28.
218. Zachary AA, Kopchaliiska D, Montgomery RA, Leffell MS. HLA-specific B cells: I. A method for their detection, quantification, and isolation using HLA tetramers. *Transplantation*. 2007;83(7):982–988.
219. Zachary AA, Kopchaliiska D, Montgomery RA, Melancon JK, Leffell MS. HLA-specific B cells: II. Application to transplantation. *Transplantation*. 2007;83(7):989–994.
220. Béland S, Désy O, Vallin P, Basoni C, De Serres SA. Innate immunity in solid organ transplantation: an update and therapeutic opportunities. *Expert Rev Clin Immunol*. 2015;11(3):377–389.
221. Gordon S, Taylor PR. Monocyte and macrophage heterogeneity. *Nature reviews Immunology*. 2005;5(12):953–964.

222. Tinckam KJ, Djurdjev O, Magil AB. Glomerular monocytes predict worse outcomes after acute renal allograft rejection independent of C4d status. *Kidney Int*. 2005;68(4):1866–1874.
223. Kirk AD, Hale DA, Mannon RB, Kleiner DE, Hoffmann SC, Kampen RL, et al. Results from a human renal allograft tolerance trial evaluating the humanized CD52-specific monoclonal antibody alemtuzumab (CAMPATH-1H). *Transplantation*. 2003;76(1):120–129.
224. Nathan CF. Secretory products of macrophages. *J. Clin. Invest*. 1987;79(2):319–326.
225. Ricardo SD, van Goor H, Eddy AA. Macrophage diversity in renal injury and repair. *J. Clin. Invest*. 2008;118(11):3522–3530.
226. Haniffa M, Ginhoux F, Wang X-N, Bigley V, Abel M, Dimmick I, et al. Differential rates of replacement of human dermal dendritic cells and macrophages during hematopoietic stem cell transplantation. *J. Exp. Med*. 2009;206(2):371–385.
227. Oberbarnscheidt MH, Zeng Q, Li Q, Dai H, Williams AL, Shlomchik WD, et al. Non-self recognition by monocytes initiates allograft rejection. *J. Clin. Invest*. 2014;124(8):3579–3589.
228. Liu W, Li XC. An overview on non-T cell pathways in transplant rejection and tolerance. *Curr Opin Organ Transplant*. 2010;15(4):422–426.
229. Thomson AW. Tolerogenic dendritic cells: all present and correct? *American journal of transplantation : official journal of the American Society of Transplantation and the American Society of Transplant Surgeons*. 2010;10(2):214–219.
230. Chamorro S, García-Vallejo JJ, Unger WWJ, Fernandes RJ, Bruijns SCM, Laban S, et al. TLR triggering on tolerogenic dendritic cells results in TLR2 up-regulation and a reduced proinflammatory immune program. *Journal of immunology (Baltimore, Md : 1950)*. 2009;183(5):2984–2994.
231. Darrasse-Jèze G, Deroubaix S, Mouquet H, Victora GD, Eisenreich T, Yao K, et al. Feedback control of regulatory T cell homeostasis by dendritic cells in vivo. *J. Exp. Med*. 2009;206(9):1853–1862.
232. Villard J. The role of natural killer cells in human solid organ and tissue transplantation. *J Innate Immun*. 2011;3(4):395–402.
233. Luan FL, Steffick DE, Gadegbeku C, Norman SP, Wolfe R, Ojo AO. Graft and patient survival in kidney transplant recipients selected for de novo steroid-free maintenance immunosuppression. *American journal of transplantation : official journal of the American Society of Transplantation and the American Society of Transplant Surgeons*. 2009;9(1):160–168.
234. Liu W, Xiao X, Demirci G, Madsen J, Li XC. Innate NK cells and macrophages recognize and reject allogeneic nonself in vivo via different mechanisms. *Journal of immunology (Baltimore, Md : 1950)*. 2012;188(6):2703–2711.
235. Kitchens WH, Uehara S, Chase CM, Colvin RB, Russell PS, Madsen JC. The changing role of natural killer cells in solid organ rejection and tolerance. *Transplantation*. 2006;81(6):811–817.
236. Kroemer A, Xiao X, Degauque N, Edtinger K, Wei H, Demirci G, et al. The innate NK cells, allograft rejection, and a key role for IL-15. *Journal of immunology (Baltimore, Md : 1950)*. 2008;180(12):7818–7826.
237. Vasconcellos LM, Schachter AD, Zheng XX, Vasconcellos LH, Shapiro M, Harmon WE, et al. Cytotoxic lymphocyte gene expression in peripheral blood leukocytes correlates with rejecting renal allografts. *Transplantation*. 1998;66(5):562–566.
238. Beilke JN, Kuhl NR, Van Kaer L, Gill RG. NK cells promote islet allograft tolerance via a perforin-dependent mechanism. *Nat. Med*. 2005;11(10):1059–1065.
239. Kreisel D, Nava RG, Li W, Zinselmeyer BH, Wang B, Lai J, et al. In vivo two-photon imaging reveals monocyte-dependent neutrophil extravasation during pulmonary inflammation. *Proceedings of the National Academy of Sciences of the United States of America*. 107; 2010:18073–18078.
240. Mócsai A. Diverse novel functions of neutrophils in immunity, inflammation, and beyond. *J. Exp. Med*. 2013;210(7):1283–1299.
241. Potter NS, Harding CV. Neutrophils process exogenous bacteria via an alternate class I MHC processing pathway for presentation of peptides to T lymphocytes. *Journal of immunology (Baltimore, Md : 1950)*. 2001;167(5):2538–2546.
242. Megiovanni AM, Sanchez F, Robledo-Sarmiento M, Morel C, Gluckman JC, Boudaly S. Polymorphonuclear neutrophils deliver activation signals and antigenic molecules to dendritic cells: a new link between leukocytes upstream of T lymphocytes. *J. Leukoc. Biol*. 2006;79(5):977–988.
243. Kreisel D, Sugimoto S, Zhu J, Nava R, Li W, Okazaki M, et al. Emergency granulopoiesis promotes neutrophil-dendritic cell encounters that prevent mouse lung allograft acceptance. *Blood*. 2011;118(23):6172–6182.

244. Yamamoto S, Nava RG, Zhu J, Huang HJ, Ibrahim M, Mohanakumar T, et al. Cutting edge: pseudomonas aeruginosa abolishes established lung transplant tolerance by stimulating B7 expression on neutrophils. *Journal of immunology (Baltimore, Md : 1950)*. 2012;189(9):4221–4225.
245. Leventhal JS, Schröppel B. Toll-like receptors in transplantation: sensing and reacting to injury. *Kidney Int*. 2012;81(9):826–832.
246. Chen L, Wang T, Zhou P, Ma L, Yin D, Shen J, et al. TLR engagement prevents transplantation tolerance. *American journal of transplantation : official journal of the American Society of Transplantation and the American Society of Transplant Surgeons*. 2006;6(10):2282–2291.
247. Testro AG, Visvanathan K, Skinner N, Markovska V, Crowley P, Angus PW, et al. Acute allograft rejection in human liver transplant recipients is associated with signaling through toll-like receptor 4. *J. Gastroenterol. Hepatol*. 2011;26(1):155–163.
248. Wu H, Noordmans GA, O'Brien MR, Ma J, Zhao CY, Zhang GY, et al. Absence of MyD88 signaling induces donor-specific kidney allograft tolerance. *Journal of the American Society of Nephrology : JASN*. 2012;23(10):1701–1716.
249. Ricklin D, Lambris JD. Complement in immune and inflammatory disorders: pathophysiological mechanisms. *Journal of immunology (Baltimore, Md : 1950)*. 2013;190(8):3831–3838.
250. Ricklin D, Hajishengallis G, Yang K, Lambris JD. Complement: a key system for immune surveillance and homeostasis. *Nat. Immunol*. 2010;11(9):785–797.
251. Sacks SH, Zhou W. The role of complement in the early immune response to transplantation. *Nature reviews Immunology*. 2012;12(6):431–442.
252. Møller-Kristensen M, Wang W, Ruseva M, Thiel S, Nielsen S, Takahashi K, et al. Mannan-binding lectin recognizes structures on ischaemic reperfused mouse kidneys and is implicated in tissue injury. *Scand. J. Immunol*. 2005;61(5):426–434.
253. Foreman KE, Vaporciyan AA, Bonish BK, Jones ML, Johnson KJ, Glovsky MM, et al. C5a-induced expression of P-selectin in endothelial cells. *J. Clin. Invest*. 1994;94(3):1147–1155.
254. Vieyra M, Leisman S, Raedler H, Kwan W-H, Yang M, Strainic MG, et al. Complement regulates CD4 T-cell help to CD8 T cells required for murine allograft rejection. *Am. J. Pathol*. 2011;179(2):766–774.
255. Kwan W, van der Touw W, Paz-Artal E, Li MO, Heeger PS. Signaling through C5a receptor and C3a receptor diminishes function of murine natural regulatory T cells. *J. Exp. Med*. 2013;210(2):257–268.
256. Nelson PJ, Krensky AM. Chemokines, chemokine receptors, and allograft rejection. *Immunity*. 2001;14(4):377–386.
257. Strom TB, Koulmanda M. Recently discovered T cell subsets cannot keep their commitments. *Journal of the American Society of Nephrology : JASN*. 2009;20(8):1677–1680.
258. de Menezes Neves PDM, Machado JR, dos Reis MA, Faleiros ACG, de Lima Pereira SA, Rodrigues DBR. Distinct expression of interleukin 17, tumor necrosis factor α, transforming growth factor β, and forkhead box P3 in acute rejection after kidney transplantation. *Ann Diagn Pathol*. 2013;17(1):75–79.
259. Dinarello CA. Interleukin-1 and interleukin-1 antagonism. *Blood*. 1991;77(8):1627–1652.
260. Pepper AR, Gala-Lopez B, Ziff O, Shapiro AJ. Current status of clinical islet transplantation. *World J Transplant*. 2013;3(4):48–53.
261. Mertens M, Singh JA. Anakinra for rheumatoid arthritis: a systematic review. *J. Rheumatol*. 2009;36(6):1118–1125.
262. Zhao X, Boenisch O, Yeung M, Mfarrej B, Yang S, Turka LA, et al. Critical role of proinflammatory cytokine IL-6 in allograft rejection and tolerance. *American journal of transplantation : official journal of the American Society of Transplantation and the American Society of Transplant Surgeons*. 2012;12(1):90–101.
263. Shen H, Goldstein DR. IL-6 and TNF-alpha synergistically inhibit allograft acceptance. *Journal of the American Society of Nephrology : JASN*. 2009;20(5):1032–1040.
264. Tinckam K. Histocompatibility methods. *Transplantation reviews (Orlando, Fla)*. 2009;23(2):80–93.
265. Gorer PA. The Detection of Antigenic Differences in Mouse Erythrocytes by the Employment of Immune Sera. *Br J Exp Pathol*. 1936;17:42–50.
266. Montgomery RA, Tatapudi VS, Leffell MS, Zachary AA. HLA in transplantation. *Nature reviews Nephrology*. 2018;14(9):558–570.
267. Man- B. Complete sequence and gene map of a human major histocompatibility complex. *The MHC Sequencing Consortium*. 1999;401(October):921–923.
268. Shiina T, Inoko H, Kulski JK. An update of the HLA genomic region, locus information and disease associations: 2004. *Tissue Antigens*. 2004;64(6):631–649.

269. Ascher NL, Simmons RL, Noreen H, VanHook J, Howard RJ, Sutherland DE, et al. 100 HLA-identical sibling transplants. *Prognostic factors other than histocompatibility. Annals of surgery*. 1979;189(2):209–216.
270. Williams RC, Opelz G, McGarvey CJ, Weil EJ, Chakkera HA. The Risk of Transplant Failure With HLA Mismatch in First Adult Kidney Allografts From Deceased Donors. *Transplantation*. 2016;100(5):1094–1102.
271. Tinckam K. Histocompatibility methods. *Transplantation reviews (Orlando, Fla)*. 2009;23(2):80–93.
272. Opelz G. Correlation of HLA matching with kidney graft survival in patients with or without cyclosporine treatment. *Transplantation*. 1985;40(3):240–243.
273. Lim WH, Chapman JR, Coates PT, Lewis JR, Russ GR, Watson N, et al. HLA-DQ Mismatches and Rejection in Kidney Transplant Recipients. *Clinical journal of the American Society of Nephrology : CJASN*. 2016;11(5):875–883.
274. Sethi S, Choi J, Toyoda M, Vo A, Peng A, Jordan SC. Desensitization: overcoming the Immunologic Barriers to Transplantation. *J Immunol Res*. 2017;2017:6804678.
275. Loupy A, Hill GS, Jordan SC. The impact of donor-specific anti-HLA antibodies on late kidney allograft failure. *Nature Reviews Nephrology*. 2012;8(6):348–357.
276. Wongsaroj P. Modern approaches to incompatible kidney transplantation. *World J Nephrol*. 2015;4(3):354.
277. Glotz D, Haymann JP, Sansonetti N, Francois A, Menoyo-Calonge V, Bariety J, et al. Suppression of HLA-specific alloantibodies by high-dose intravenous immunoglobulins (IVIg). A potential tool for transplantation of immunized patients. *Transplantation*. 1993;56(2):335–337.
278. Jordan SC, Pescovitz MD. Presensitization: the problem and its management. *Clinical journal of the American Society of Nephrology : CJASN*. 2006;1(3):421–432.
279. Markasz L, Vanherberghen B, Flaberg E, Otvös R, Stuber G, Gustafsson Jernberg A, et al. NK cell-mediated lysis is essential to kill Epstein-Barr virus transformed lymphoblastoid B cells when using rituximab. *Biomed. Pharmacother*. 2009;63(6):413–420.
280. Orandi BJ, Zachary AA, Dagher NN, Bagnasco SM, Garonzik-Wang JM, Van Arendonk KJ, et al. Eculizumab and splenectomy as salvage therapy for severe antibody-mediated rejection after HLA-incompatible kidney transplantation. *Transplantation*. 2014;98(8):857–863.
281. Vo AA, Lukovsky M, Toyoda M, Wang J, Reinsmoen NL, Lai C-H, et al. Rituximab and intravenous immune globulin for desensitization during renal transplantation. *The New England journal of medicine*. 2008;359(3):242–251.
282. Everly MJ, Everly JJ, Susskind B, Brailey P, Arend LJ, Alloway RR, et al. Bortezomib provides effective therapy for antibody- and cell-mediated acute rejection. *Transplantation*. 2008;86(12):1754–1761.
283. Sberro-Soussan R, Zuber J, Suberbielle-Boissel C, Candon S, Martinez F, Snanoudj R, et al. Bortezomib as the sole post-renal transplantation desensitization agent does not decrease donor-specific anti-HLA antibodies. *American journal of transplantation : official journal of the American Society of Transplantation and the American Society of Transplant Surgeons*. 2010;10(3):681–686.
284. Trivedi HL, Terasaki PI, Feroz A, Everly MJ, Vanikar AV, Shankar V, et al. Abrogation of anti-HLA antibodies via proteasome inhibition. *Transplantation*. 2009;87(10):1555–1561.
285. Walsh RC, Everly JJ, Brailey P, Rike AH, Arend LJ, Mogilishetty G, et al. Proteasome inhibitor-based primary therapy for antibody-mediated renal allograft rejection. *Transplantation*. 2010;89(3):277–284.
286. Nigos JG, Arora S, Nath P, Hussain SM, Marcus RJ, Ko TY, et al. Treatment of antibody-mediated rejection in kidney transplant recipients: a single-center experience with a bortezomib-based regimen. *Experimental and clinical transplantation : official journal of the Middle East Society for Organ Transplantation*. 2012;10(6):609–613.
287. Gibson T, Medawar PB. The fate of skin homografts in man. *J. Anat*. 1943;77(Pt 4):299–310 Jul4.
288. Billingham RE, Brent L, Medawar PB. Actively acquired tolerance" of foreign cells. *Nature*. 1953;172(4379):603–606.
289. Main JM, Prehn RT. Successful skin homografts after the administration of high dosage x radiation and homologous bone marrow. *J. Natl. Cancer Inst*. 1955;15(4):1023–1029.
290. Sharabi Y, Sachs DH. Mixed chimerism and permanent specific transplantation tolerance induced by a nonlethal preparative regimen. *Journal of Experimental Medicine*. 1989;169(2):493–502.
291. Calne RY. Prope tolerance - The future of organ transplantation from the laboratory to the clinic. *Int. Immunopharmacol*. 2005;5(1):163–167.

292. Kitchens WH, Adams AB. Nonhuman primate models of transplant tolerance: closer to the holy grail. *Curr Opin Organ Transplant*. 2016;21(1):59–65.
293. BILLINGHAM RE, BRENT L, MEDAWAR PB. Actively acquired tolerance of foreign cells. *Nature*. 1953;172(4379):603–606.
294. Calne RY. Prope tolerance–the future of organ transplantation from the laboratory to the clinic. *Int. Immunopharmacol*. 2005;5(1):163–167.
295. Hori J, Yamaguchi T, Keino H, Hamrah P, Maruyama K Immune privilege in corneal transplantation. Progress in retinal and eye research. 2019 Sep;72:100758.
296. Kawai T, Benedict Cosimi A. Induction of tolerance in clinical kidney transplantation. *Clin Transplant*. 2010;24(Suppl 2):2–5 Jul0 22.
297. Rickert CG, Markmann JF. Current state of organ transplant tolerance. *Curr Opin Organ Transplant*. 2019;24(4):441–450.
298. Oura T, Hotta K, Cosimi AB, Kawai T. Transient mixed chimerism for allograft tolerance. *Chimerism*. 2015;6(1–2):21–26.
299. Balner H. Persistence of tolerance towards donor-type antigens after temporary chimerism in rats. *Transplantation*. 1964;2(4):464–474.
300. Kawai T, Poncelet A, Sachs DH, Mauiyyedi S, Boskovic S, Wee SL, et al. Long-term outcome and alloantibody production in a non-myeloablative regimen for induction of renal allograft tolerance. *Transplantation*. 1999;68(11):1767–1775.
301. Kawai T, Cosimi AB, Spitzer TR, Tolkoff-Rubin N, Suthanthiran M, Saidman SL, et al. HLA-mismatched renal transplantation without maintenance immunosuppression. *The New England journal of medicine*. 2008;358(4):353–361.
302. Abe M, Wang Z, de Creus A, Thomson AW. Plasmacytoid dendritic cell precursors induce allogeneic T-cell hyporesponsiveness and prolong heart graft survival. *American journal of transplantation : official journal of the American Society of Transplantation and the American Society of Transplant Surgeons*. 2005;5(8):1808–1819.
303. Ke N, Su A, Huang W, Szatmary P, Zhang Z. Regulating the expression of CD80/CD86 on dendritic cells to induce immune tolerance after xeno-islet transplantation. *Immunobiology*. 2016;221(7):803–812.
304. Liu Y-J. IPC: professional type 1 interferon-producing cells and plasmacytoid dendritic cell precursors. *Annu. Rev. Immunol*. 2005;23:275–306.
305. Steinman RM, Hawiger D, Nussenzweig MC. Tolerogenic dendritic cells. *Annu. Rev. Immunol*. 2003;21:685–711.
306. Chatenoud L, Bluestone JA. CD3-specific antibodies: a portal to the treatment of autoimmunity. *Nature reviews Immunology*. 2007;7(8):622–632.
307. Chatenoud L. CD3-specific antibody-induced active tolerance: from bench to bedside. *Nature reviews Immunology*. 2003;3(2):123–132.
308. Hirshberg B, Rother KI, 3rd D B J, Lee J, Gaglia JL, Hines K, et al. Benefits and risks of solitary islet transplantation for type 1 diabetes using steroid-sparing immunosuppression: the National Institutes of Health experience. *Diabetes Care*. 2003;26(12):3288–3295.
309. Liu C, Noorchashm H, Sutter JA, Naji M, Prak EL, Boyer J, et al. B lymphocyte-directed immunotherapy promotes long-term islet allograft survival in nonhuman primates. *Nat. Med*. 2007;13(11):1295–1298.
310. Wojciechowski D, Vincenti F. Current status of costimulatory blockade in renal transplantation. *Curr. Opin. Nephrol. Hypertens*. 2016;25(6):583–590.
311. Guinan EC, Gribben JG, Boussiotis VA, Freeman GJ, Nadler LM. Pivotal role of the B7:CD28 pathway in transplantation tolerance and tumor immunity. *Blood*. 1994;84(10):3261–3282.
312. Turka LA, Linsley PS, Lin H, Brady W, Leiden JM, Wei RQ, et al. T-cell activation by the CD28 ligand B7 is required for cardiac allograft rejection in vivo. *Proceedings of the National Academy of Sciences of the United States of America*. 89; 1992:11102–11105.
313. Kenyon NS, Fernandez LA, Lehmann R, Masetti M, Ranuncoli A, Chatzipetrou M, et al. Long-term survival and function of intrahepatic islet allografts in baboons treated with humanized anti-CD154. *Diabetes*. 1999;48(7):1473–1481.

314. Azimzadeh AM, Pfeiffer S, Wu G, Schröder C, 3rd Z G L, Kelishadi SS, et al. Alloimmunity in primate heart recipients with CD154 blockade: evidence for alternative costimulation mechanisms. *Transplantation*. 2006;81(2):255–264.
315. Kirk AD, Harlan DM, Armstrong NN, Davis TA, Dong Y, Gray GS, et al. CTLA4-Ig and anti-CD40 ligand prevent renal allograft rejection in primates. *Proceedings of the National Academy of Sciences of the United States of America*. 94; 1997:8789–8794.
316. Vincenti F, Klintmalm G, Yang H, Ram Peddi V, Blahunka P, Conkle A, et al. A randomized, phase 1b study of the pharmacokinetics, pharmacodynamics, safety, and tolerability of bleselumab, a fully human, anti-CD40 monoclonal antibody, in kidney transplantation. *American journal of transplantation : official journal of the American Society of Transplantation and the American Society of Transplant Surgeons*. 2020;20(1):172–180.
317. Harland RC, Klintmalm G, Jensik S, Yang H, Bromberg J, Holman J, et al. Efficacy and safety of bleselumab in kidney transplant recipients: a phase 2, randomized, open-label, noninferiority study. *American journal of transplantation : official journal of the American Society of Transplantation and the American Society of Transplant Surgeons*. 2020;20(1):159–171.
318. Brunkow ME, Jeffery EW, Hjerrild KA, Paeper B, Clark LB, Yasayko SA, et al. Disruption of a new forkhead/winged-helix protein, scurfin, results in the fatal lymphoproliferative disorder of the scurfy mouse. *Nat. Genet*. 2001;27(1):68–73.
319. Ohue Y, Nishikawa H. Regulatory T (Treg) cells in cancer: can Treg cells be a new therapeutic target? *Cancer Sci*. 2019;110(7):2080–2089.
320. Kholodenko IV, Kholodenko RV, Lupatov AY, Yarygin KN. Cell Therapy as a Tool for Induction of Immunological Tolerance after Liver Transplantation. *Bulletin of experimental biology and medicine*. 2018;165(4):554–563.
321. Guinan EC, Cole GA, Wylie WH, Kelner RH, Janec KJ, Yuan H, et al. Ex Vivo Costimulatory Blockade to Generate Regulatory T Cells From Patients Awaiting Kidney Transplantation. *American journal of transplantation : official journal of the American Society of Transplantation and the American Society of Transplant Surgeons*. 2016;16(7):2187–2195.
322. Ochando JC, Homma C, Yang Y, Hidalgo A, Garin A, Tacke F, et al. Alloantigen-presenting plasmacytoid dendritic cells mediate tolerance to vascularized grafts. *Nat. Immunol*. 2006;7(6):652–662.
323. Kinsella FAM, Zuo J, Inman CF, Pearce H, Maggs L, Eldershaw SE, et al. Mixed chimerism established by hematopoietic stem cell transplantation is maintained by host and donor T regulatory cells. *Blood advances*. 2019;3(5):734–743.
324. Belghith M, Bluestone JA, Barriot S, Mégret J, Bach J-F, Chatenoud L. TGF-beta-dependent mechanisms mediate restoration of self-tolerance induced by antibodies to CD3 in overt autoimmune diabetes. *Nat. Med*. 2003;9(9):1202–1208.
325. Govender L, Wyss J-C, Kumar R, Pascual M, Golshayan D. IL-2-Mediated In Vivo Expansion of Regulatory T Cells Combined with CD154-CD40 Co-Stimulation Blockade but Not CTLA-4 Ig Prolongs Allograft Survival in Naive and Sensitized Mice. *Front Immunol*. 2017;8:421.
326. Zheng XX, Sánchez-Fueyo A, Sho M, Domenig C, Sayegh MH, Strom TB. Favorably Tipping the Balance between Cytopathic and Regulatory T Cells to Create Transplantation Tolerance. *Immunity*. 2003;19(4):503–514.
327. Flippe L, Bézie S, Anegon I, Guillonneau C. Future prospects for CD8(+) regulatory T cells in immune tolerance. *Immunol. Rev*. 2019;292(1):209–224.
328. Guillonneau C Ex Vivo expanded human efficiently Delay skin graft rejection and gVhD in humanized Mice. 2018;8(January).
329. Segundo DS, Ruiz JC, Izquierdo M, Fernández-Fresnedo G, Gómez-Alamillo C, Merino R, et al. Calcineurin inhibitors, but not rapamycin, reduce percentages of CD4+CD25+FOXP3+ regulatory T cells in renal transplant recipients. *Transplantation*. 2006;82(4):550–557.
330. Zeiser R, Leveson-Gower DB, Zambricki EA, Kambham N, Beilhack A, Loh J, et al. Differential impact of mammalian target of rapamycin inhibition on CD4+CD25+Foxp3+ regulatory T cells compared with conventional CD4+ T cells. *Blood*. 2008;111(1):453–462.
331. Pidala J, Kim J, Jim H, Kharfan-Dabaja MA, Nishihori T, Fernandez HF, et al. A randomized phase II study to evaluate tacrolimus in combination with sirolimus or methotrexate after allogeneic hematopoietic cell transplantation. *Haematologica*. 2012;97(12):1882–1889.

332. Ramírez E, Morales JM, Lora D, Mellado M, Cevey M, Alfaro FJ, et al. Peripheral blood regulatory T cells in long-term kidney transplant recipients. *Transplant. Proc.* 2009;41(6):2360–2362.
333. Lee KM, Stott RT, Zhao G, SooHoo J, Xiong W, Lian MM, et al. TGF-β-producing regulatory B cells induce regulatory T cells and promote transplantation tolerance. *Eur. J. Immunol.* 2014;44(6):1728–1736.
334. Zhao G, Moore DJ, Lee KM, Kim JI, Duff PE, O'Connor MR, et al. An unexpected counter-regulatory role of IL-10 in B-lymphocyte-mediated transplantation tolerance. *American journal of transplantation : official journal of the American Society of Transplantation and the American Society of Transplant Surgeons.* 2010;10(4):796–801.
335. Huang X, Moore DJ, Mohiuddin M, Lian M-M, Kim JI, Sonawane S, et al. Inhibition of ICAM-1/LFA-1 interactions prevents B-cell-dependent anti-CD45RB-induced transplantation tolerance. *Transplantation.* 2008;85(5):675–680.
336. Reichardt P, Dornbach B, Rong S, Beissert S, Gueler F, Loser K, et al. Naive B cells generate regulatory T cells in the presence of a mature immunologic synapse. *Blood.* 2007;110(5):1519–1529.
337. Schuetz C, Lee KM, Scott R, Kojima L, Washburn L, Liu L, et al. Regulatory B Cell-Dependent Islet Transplant Tolerance Is Also Natural Killer Cell Dependent. *American journal of transplantation : official journal of the American Society of Transplantation and the American Society of Transplant Surgeons.* 2017;17(6):1656–1662.
338. Deng S, Moore DJ, Huang X, Lian M-M, Mohiuddin M, Velededeoglu E, et al. Cutting edge: transplant tolerance induced by anti-CD45RB requires B lymphocytes. *Journal of immunology (Baltimore, Md : 1950).* 2007;178(10):6028–6032.
339. Lee KM, Kim JI, Stott R, Soohoo J, O'Connor MR, Yeh H, et al. Anti-CD45RB/anti-TIM-1-induced tolerance requires regulatory B cells. *American journal of transplantation : official journal of the American Society of Transplantation and the American Society of Transplant Surgeons.* 2012;12(8):2072–2078.
340. Weiden PL, Sullivan KM, Flournoy N, Storb R, Thomas ED. Antileukemic effect of chronic graft-versus-host disease: contribution to improved survival after allogeneic marrow transplantation. *The New England journal of medicine.* 1981;304(25):1529–1533.
341. Weiden PL, Flournoy N, Thomas ED, Prentice R, Fefer A, Buckner CD, et al. Antileukemic effect of graft-versus-host disease in human recipients of allogeneic-marrow grafts. *The New England journal of medicine.* 1979;300(19):1068–1073.
342. Sullivan KM, Weiden PL, Storb R, Witherspoon RP, Fefer A, Fisher L, et al. Influence of acute and chronic graft-versus-host disease on relapse and survival after bone marrow transplantation from HLA-identical siblings as treatment of acute and chronic leukemia. *Blood.* 1989;73(6):1720–1728.
343. Gorin NC, Labopin M, Fouillard L, Meloni G, Frassoni F, Iriondo A, et al. Retrospective evaluation of autologous bone marrow transplantation vs allogeneic bone marrow transplantation from an HLA identical related donor in acute myelocytic leukemia. *A study of the European Cooperative Group for Blood and Marrow Transplantation . Bone marrow transplantation.* 1996;18(1):111–117.
344. Fefer A, Sullivan KM, Weiden P, Buckner CD, Schoch G, Storb R, et al. Graft versus leukemia effect in man: the relapse rate of acute leukemia is lower after allogeneic than after syngeneic marrow transplantation. *Prog. Clin. Biol. Res.* 1987;244:401–408.
345. Horowitz MM, Gale RP, Sondel PM, Goldman JM, Kersey J, Kolb HJ, et al. Graft-versus-leukemia reactions after bone marrow transplantation. *Blood.* 1990;75(3):555–562.
346. Childs R, Clave E, Contentin N, Jayasekera D, Hensel N, Leitman S, et al. Engraftment kinetics after nonmyeloablative allogeneic peripheral blood stem cell transplantation: full donor T-cell chimerism precedes alloimmune responses. *Blood.* 1999;94(9):3234–3241.
347. Baron F, Maris MB, Storer BE, Sandmaier BM, Panse JP, Chauncey TR, et al. High doses of transplanted CD34+ cells are associated with rapid T-cell engraftment and lessened risk of graft rejection, but not more graft-versus-host disease after nonmyeloablative conditioning and unrelated hematopoietic cell transplantation. *Leukemia.* 2005;19(5):822–828.
348. Giralt S, Estey E, Albitar M, van Besien K, Rondón G, Anderlini P, et al. Engraftment of allogeneic hematopoietic progenitor cells with purine analog-containing chemotherapy: harnessing graft-versus-leukemia without myeloablative therapy. *Blood.* 1997;89(12):4531–4536.
349. Giralt S, Thall PF, Khouri I, Wang X, Braunschweig I, Ippolitti C, et al. Melphalan and purine analog-containing preparative regimens: reduced-intensity conditioning for patients with hematologic malignancies undergoing allogeneic progenitor cell transplantation. *Blood.* 2001;97(3):631–637.

350. Oran B, Giralt S, Saliba R, Hosing C, Popat U, Khouri I, et al. Allogeneic hematopoietic stem cell transplantation for the treatment of high-risk acute myelogenous leukemia and myelodysplastic syndrome using reduced-intensity conditioning with fludarabine and melphalan. *Biology of blood and marrow transplantation : journal of the American Society for Blood and Marrow Transplantation*. 2007;13(4):454–462.
351. Popat U, de Lima MJ, Saliba RM, Anderlini P, Andersson BS, Alousi AM, et al. Long-term outcome of reduced-intensity allogeneic hematopoietic SCT in patients with AML in CR. *Bone Marrow Transplant*. 2012;47(2):212–216.
352. Slavin S, Nagler A, Naparstek E, Kapelushnik Y, Aker M, Cividalli G, et al. Nonmyeloablative stem cell transplantation and cell therapy as an alternative to conventional bone marrow transplantation with lethal cytoreduction for the treatment of malignant and nonmalignant hematologic diseases. *Blood*. 1998;91(3):756–763.
353. Schmid C, Schleuning M, Ledderose G, Tischer J, Kolb H-J. Sequential regimen of chemotherapy, reduced-intensity conditioning for allogeneic stem-cell transplantation, and prophylactic donor lymphocyte transfusion in high-risk acute myeloid leukemia and myelodysplastic syndrome. *Journal of clinical oncology : official journal of the American Society of Clinical Oncology*. 2005;23(24):5675–5687.
354. Detrait M, Chevallier P, Sobh M, Guillaume T, Thomas X, Morisset S, et al. Outcome of High-Risk and Refractory AML/MDS Patients Receiving a Flamsa Sequential Chemotherapy Regimen Followed by Reduced-Intensity Conditioning (RIC) and Allogeneic Hematopoeitic Stem Cell Transplantation (allo-HSCT). *Biology of Blood and Marrow Transplantation*. 2012 Feb 1;18(2):S335–S336.
355. Kröger N, Zabelina T, Wolschke C, Lellek H, Stübig T, Lestin M, et al. Induction Chemotherapy Followed Immediately by Busulfan-Based Reduced Conditioning and Allografting in Elderly Patients with Advanced MDS or sAML. *Blood*. 2009 Nov 20;114(22):3387.
356. Chevallier P, Labopin M, Buchholz S, Ganser A, Ciceri F, Lioure B, et al. Clofarabine-containing conditioning regimen for allo-SCT in AML/ALL patients: a survey from the Acute Leukemia Working Party of EBMT. *Eur. J. Haematol*. 2012;89(3):214–219.
357. van Besien K, Stock W, Rich E, Odenike O, Godley LA, O'Donnell PH, et al. Phase I-II study of clofarabine-melphalan-alemtuzumab conditioning for allogeneic hematopoietic cell transplantation. *Biology of blood and marrow transplantation : journal of the American Society for Blood and Marrow Transplantation*. 2012;18(6):913–921.
358. McSweeney PA, Niederwieser D, Shizuru JA, Sandmaier BM, Molina AJ, Maloney DG, et al. Hematopoietic cell transplantation in older patients with hematologic malignancies: replacing high-dose cytotoxic therapy with graft-versus-tumor effects. *Blood*. 2001;97(11):3390–3400.
359. Storb R, Gyurkocza B, Storer BE, Sorror ML, Blume K, Niederwieser D, et al. Graft-versus-host disease and graft-versus-tumor effects after allogeneic hematopoietic cell transplantation. *Journal of clinical oncology : official journal of the American Society of Clinical Oncology*. 2013;31(12):1530–1538.
360. Khouri IF, McLaughlin P, Saliba RM, Hosing C, Korbling M, Lee MS, et al. Eight-year experience with allogeneic stem cell transplantation for relapsed follicular lymphoma after nonmyeloablative conditioning with fludarabine, cyclophosphamide, and rituximab. *Blood*. 2008;111(12):5530–5536.
361. Sauter CS, Barker JN, Lechner L, Zheng J, Devlin SM, Papadopoulos EB, et al. A phase II study of a nonmyeloablative allogeneic stem cell transplant with peritransplant rituximab in patients with B cell lymphoid malignancies: favorably durable event-free survival in chemosensitive patients. *Biology of blood and marrow transplantation : journal of the American Society for Blood and Marrow Transplantation*. 2014;20(3):354–360.
362. Pillai AB, George TI, Dutt S, Strober S. Host natural killer T cells induce an interleukin-4-dependent expansion of donor CD4+CD25+Foxp3+ T regulatory cells that protects against graft-versus-host disease. *Blood*. 2009;113(18):4458–4467.
363. Lowsky R, Takahashi T, Liu YP, Dejbakhsh-Jones S, Grumet FC, Shizuru JA, et al. Protective conditioning for acute graft-versus-host disease. *The New England journal of medicine*. 2005;353(13):1321–1331.
364. Lan F, Zeng D, Higuchi M, Huie P, Higgins JP, Strober S. Predominance of NK1.1+TCR alpha beta+ or DX5+TCR alpha beta+ T cells in mice conditioned with fractionated lymphoid irradiation protects against graft-versus-host disease: "natural suppressor" cells. *Journal of immunology (Baltimore, Md : 1950)*. 2001;167(4):2087–2096.

365. Petersen FB, Deeg HJ, Buckner CD, Appelbaum FR, Storb R, Clift RA, et al. Marrow transplantation following escalating doses of fractionated total body irradiation and cyclophosphamide–a phase I trial. *Int. J. Radiat. Oncol. Biol. Phys.* 1992;23(5):1027–1032.
366. Clift RA, Buckner CD, Appelbaum FR, Bearman SI, Petersen FB, Fisher LD, et al. Allogeneic marrow transplantation in patients with acute myeloid leukemia in first remission: a randomized trial of two irradiation regimens. *Blood.* 1990;76(9):1867–1871.
367. Appelbaum FR, Matthews DC, Eary JF, Badger CC, Kellogg M, Press OW, et al. The use of radiolabeled anti-CD33 antibody to augment marrow irradiation prior to marrow transplantation for acute myelogenous leukemia. *Transplantation.* 1992;54(5):829–833.
368. Press OW, Eary JF, Appelbaum FR, Martin PJ, Badger CC, Nelp WB, et al. Radiolabeled-antibody therapy of B-cell lymphoma with autologous bone marrow support. *The New England journal of medicine.* 1993;329(17):1219–1224.
369. Jurcic JG, Caron PC, Nikula TK, Papadopoulos EB, Finn RD, Gansow OA, et al. Radiolabeled anti-CD33 monoclonal antibody M195 for myeloid leukemias. *Cancer Res.* 1995;55(23 Suppl):5908s–5910s.
370. Shimoni A, Zwas ST, Oksman Y, Hardan I, Shem-Tov N, Yerushalmi R, et al. Yttrium-90-ibritumomab tiuxetan (Zevalin) combined with high-dose BEAM chemotherapy and autologous stem cell transplantation for chemo-refractory aggressive non-Hodgkin's lymphoma. *Exp. Hematol.* 2007;35(4):534–540.
371. Tositumomab I-131. (131)I-anti-B1 antibody, (131)I-tositumomab, anti-CD20 murine monoclonal antibody-I-131, B1, Bexxar, (131)I-anti-B1 antibody, iodine-131 tositumomab, iodine-131 anti-B1 antibody, tositumomab. *BioDrugs : clinical immunotherapeutics, biopharmaceuticals and gene therapy.* 2003;17(4):290–295.
372. Gopal AK, Rajendran JG, Gooley TA, Pagel JM, Fisher DR, Petersdorf SH, et al. High-dose [131I] tositumomab (anti-CD20) radioimmunotherapy and autologous hematopoietic stem-cell transplantation for adults ≥ 60 years old with relapsed or refractory B-cell lymphoma. *Journal of Clinical Oncology.* 2007;25(11):1396–1402.
373. Vose JM, Bierman PJ, Enke C, Hankins J, Bociek G, Lynch JC, et al. Phase I trial of iodine-131 tositumomab with high-dose chemotherapy and autologous stem-cell transplantation for relapsed non-Hodgkin's lymphoma. *Journal of clinical oncology : official journal of the American Society of Clinical Oncology.* 2005;23(3):461–467.
374. Vose JM, Bierman PJ, Loberiza FR, Enke C, Hankins J, Bociek RG, et al. Phase II trial of 131-Iodine tositumomab with high-dose chemotherapy and autologous stem cell transplantation for relapsed diffuse large B cell lymphoma. *Biology of blood and marrow transplantation : journal of the American Society for Blood and Marrow Transplantation.* 2013;19(1):123–128.
375. Pagel JM, Gooley TA, Rajendran J, Fisher DR, Wilson WA, Sandmaier BM, et al. Allogeneic hematopoietic cell transplantation after conditioning with 131I-anti-CD45 antibody plus fludarabine and low-dose total body irradiation for elderly patients with advanced acute myeloid leukemia or high-risk myelodysplastic syndrome. *Blood.* 2009;114(27):5444–5453.
376. Matthews DC, Appelbaum FR, Eary JF, Fisher DR, Durack LD, Bush SA, et al. Development of a marrow transplant regimen for acute leukemia using targeted hematopoietic irradiation delivered by 131I-labeled anti-CD45 antibody, combined with cyclophosphamide and total body irradiation. *Blood.* 1995;85(4):1122–1131.
377. Pagel JM, Appelbaum FR, Eary JF, Rajendran J, Fisher DR, Gooley T, et al. 131I-anti-CD45 antibody plus busulfan and cyclophosphamide before allogeneic hematopoietic cell transplantation for treatment of acute myeloid leukemia in first remission. *Blood.* 2006;107(5):2184–2191.
378. Montgomery RA, Loupy A, Segev DL. Antibody-mediated rejection: new approaches in prevention and management. *American journal of transplantation : official journal of the American Society of Transplantation and the American Society of Transplant Surgeons.* 2018;18(Suppl 3):3–17.
379. Gerlach UA, Lachmann N, Ranucci G, Sawitzki B, Schoenemann C, Pratschke J, et al. Non-HLA Antibodies May Accelerate Immune Responses After Intestinal and Multivisceral Transplantation. *Transplantation.* 2017;101(1):141–149.
380. Kenta I, Takaaki K. Molecular Mechanisms of Antibody-Mediated Rejection and Accommodation in Organ Transplantation. *Nephron.* 2020;144:2–6.

381. Levine DJ, Glanville AR, Aboyoun C, Belperio J, Benden C, Berry GJ, et al. Antibody-mediated rejection of the lung: a consensus report of the International Society for Heart and Lung Transplantation. *The Journal of heart and lung transplantation : the official publication of the International Society for Heart Transplantation*. 2016;35(4):397–406.
382. Drachenberg CB, Torrealba JR, Nankivell BJ, Rangel EB, Bajema IM, Kim DU, et al. Guidelines for the diagnosis of antibody-mediated rejection in pancreas allografts-updated Banff grading schema. *American journal of transplantation : official journal of the American Society of Transplantation and the American Society of Transplant Surgeons*. 2011;11(9):1792–1802.
383. Demetris AJ, Bellamy C, Hübscher SG, O'Leary J, Randhawa PS, Feng S, et al. 2016 Comprehensive Update of the Banff Working Group on Liver Allograft Pathology: introduction of Antibody-Mediated Rejection. *American journal of transplantation : official journal of the American Society of Transplantation and the American Society of Transplant Surgeons*. 2016;16(10):2816–2835.
384. Haas M, Sis B, Racusen LC, Solez K, Glotz D, Colvin RB, et al. Banff 2013 meeting report: inclusion of c4d-negative antibody-mediated rejection and antibody-associated arterial lesions. *American journal of transplantation : official journal of the American Society of Transplantation and the American Society of Transplant Surgeons. United States*. 2014;14:272–283.
385. Berry GJ, Burke MM, Andersen C, Bruneval P, Fedrigo M, Fishbein MC, et al. The 2013 International Society for Heart and Lung Transplantation Working Formulation for the standardization of nomenclature in the pathologic diagnosis of antibody-mediated rejection in heart transplantation. *The Journal of heart and lung transplantation : the official publication of the International Society for Heart Transplantation. United States*. 2013;32:1147–1162.
386. Mengel M, Husain S, Hidalgo L, Sis B. Phenotypes of antibody-mediated rejection in organ transplants. *Transplant International*. 2012;25(6):611–622.
387. Schinstock CA, Mannon RB, Budde K, Chong AS, Haas M, Knechtle S, et al. Recommended Treatment for Antibody-mediated Rejection After Kidney Transplantation: the 2019 Expert Consensus From the Transplantion Society Working Group. *Transplantation*. 2020;104(5):911–922.
388. Haas M, Loupy A, Lefaucheur C, Roufosse C, Glotz D, Seron D, et al. The Banff 2017 Kidney Meeting Report: revised diagnostic criteria for chronic active T cell-mediated rejection, antibody-mediated rejection, and prospects for integrative endpoints for next-generation clinical trials. *American journal of transplantation : official journal of the American Society of Transplantation and the American Society of Transplant Surgeons*. 2018;18(2):293–307.
389. Randhawa P. T-cell-mediated rejection of the kidney in the era of donor-specific antibodies: diagnostic challenges and clinical significance. *Curr Opin Organ Transplant*. 2015;20(3):325–332.
390. Venner JM, Famulski KS, Badr D, Hidalgo LG, Chang J, Halloran PF. Molecular landscape of T cell-mediated rejection in human kidney transplants: prominence of CTLA4 and PD ligands. *American journal of transplantation : official journal of the American Society of Transplantation and the American Society of Transplant Surgeons*. 2014;14(11):2565–2576.
391. Ramachandran V, Kolli SS, Strowd LC. Review of Graft-Versus-Host Disease. *Dermatol Clin*. 2019;37(4):569–582.
392. Murali AR, Chandra S, Stewart Z, Blazar BR, Farooq U, Ince MN, et al. Graft Versus Host Disease After Liver Transplantation in Adults: a Case series, Review of Literature, and an Approach to Management. *Transplantation*. 2016;100(12):2661–2670.
393. Molaro GL, De Angelis V. La malattia da "graft-versus-host" dopo trasfusione di sangue e suoi prodotti. *Riv Emoter Immunoematol*. 1984;31(2):107–123.
394. Fidler C, Klumpp T, Mangan K, Martin M, Sharma M, Emmons R, et al. Spontaneous graft versus host disease occurring in a patient with multiple myeloma after autologous stem cell transplant. *Am. J. Hematol*. 2012;87(2):219–221.
395. Weisdorf D, Haake R, Blazar B, Miller W, McGlave P, Ramsay N, et al. Treatment of moderate/severe acute graft-versus-host disease after allogeneic bone marrow transplantation: an analysis of clinical risk features and outcome. *Blood*. 1990;75(4):1024–1030.
396. Ferrara JLM, Reddy P. Pathophysiology of graft-versus-host disease. *Semin. Hematol*. 2006;43(1):3–10.
397. Couriel D, Caldera H, Champlin R, Komanduri K. Acute graft-versus-host disease: pathophysiology, clinical manifestations, and management. *Cancer*. 2004;101(9):1936–1946.

398. Pidala J, Kurland B, Chai X, Majhail N, Weisdorf DJ, Pavletic S, et al. Patient-reported quality of life is associated with severity of chronic graft-versus-host disease as measured by NIH criteria: report on baseline data from the Chronic GVHD Consortium. *Blood*. 2011;117(17):4651–4657.
399. Lee SJ. Classification systems for chronic graft-versus-host disease. *Blood*. 2017;129(1):30–37.
400. Zeiser R, Blazar BR. Pathophysiology of Chronic Graft-versus-Host Disease and Therapeutic Targets. *The New England journal of medicine*. 2017;377(26):2565–2579.
401. Jagasia MH, Greinix HT, Arora M, Williams KM, Wolff D, Cowen EW, et al. National Institutes of Health Consensus Development Project on Criteria for Clinical Trials in Chronic Graft-versus-Host Disease: I. The 2014 Diagnosis and Staging Working Group report. *Biology of blood and marrow transplantation : journal of the American Society for Blood and Marrow Transplantation*. 2015;21(3):389–401 Mare1.
402. McDonald GB, Tabellini L, Storer BE, Lawler RL, Martin PJ, Hansen JA. Plasma biomarkers of acute GVHD and nonrelapse mortality: predictive value of measurements before GVHD onset and treatment. *Blood*. 2015;126(1):113–120.
403. Ahmed SS, Wang XN, Norden J, Pearce K, El-Gezawy E, Atarod S, et al. Identification and validation of biomarkers associated with acute and chronic graft versus host disease. *Bone Marrow Transplant*. 2016;51(6):890.
404. Paczesny S, Braun TM, Levine JE, Hogan J, Crawford J, Coffing B, et al. Elafin is a biomarker of graft-versus-host disease of the skin. *Sci Transl Med*. 2010;2(13):13ra2.
405. Lin K, Stewart D, Cooper S, Davis CL. Pre-transplant cardiac testing for kidney-pancreas transplant candidates and association with cardiac outcomes. *Clin Transplant*. 2001;15(4):269–275.
406. Marks C, Stadler M, Häusermann P, Wolff D, Buchholz S, Stary G, et al. German-Austria-Swiss Consensus Conference on clinical practice in chronic graft-versus-host disease (GVHD): guidance for supportive therapy of chronic cutaneous and musculoskeletal GVHD. *Br. J. Dermatol*. 2011;165(1):18–29.
407. Dignan FL, Clark A, Amrolia P, Cornish J, Jackson G, Mahendra P, et al. Diagnosis and management of acute graft-versus-host disease. *Br. J. Haematol*. 2012;158(1):30–45.
408. Hill L, Alousi A, Kebriaei P, Mehta R, Rezvani K, Shpall E. New and emerging therapies for acute and chronic graft versus host disease. *Ther Adv Hematol*. 2018;9(1):21–46.
409. Doycheva I, Amer S, Watt KD. De Novo Malignancies After Transplantation: risk and Surveillance Strategies. *Med. Clin. North Am*. 2016;100(3):551–567.
410. Dharnidharka VR, Webster AC, Martinez OM, Preiksaitis JK, Leblond V, Choquet S. Post-transplant lymphoproliferative disorders. *Nature reviews Disease primers*. 2016;2:15088.
411. Doak PB, Montgomerie JZ, North JD, Smith F. Reticulum cell sarcoma after renal homotransplantation and azathioprine and prednisone therapy. *Br Med J*. 1968;4(5633):746–748.
412. Starzl TE, Nalesnik MA, Porter KA, Ho M, Iwatsuki S, Griffith BP, et al. Reversibility of lymphomas and lymphoproliferative lesions developing under cyclosporin-steroid therapy. *Lancet*. 1984;1(8377):583–587.
413. Babcock GJ, Decker LL, Volk M, Thorley-Lawson DA. EBV persistence in memory B cells in vivo. *Immunity*. 1998;9(3):395–404.
414. Fishman JA. Infection in Organ Transplantation. *American journal of transplantation : official journal of the American Society of Transplantation and the American Society of Transplant Surgeons*. 2017;17(4):856–879.
415. Nellore A, Fishman JA. The Microbiome, Systemic Immune Function, and Allotransplantation. *Clin. Microbiol. Rev*. 2016;29(1):191–199.
416. Kumar D, Chernenko S, Moussa G, Cobos I, Manuel O, Preiksaitis J, et al. Cell-mediated immunity to predict cytomegalovirus disease in high-risk solid organ transplant recipients. *American journal of transplantation : official journal of the American Society of Transplantation and the American Society of Transplant Surgeons*. 2009;9(5):1214–1222.
417. Westall GP, Mifsud NA, Kotsimbos T. Linking CMV serostatus to episodes of CMV reactivation following lung transplantation by measuring CMV-specific CD8+ T-cell immunity. *American journal of transplantation : official journal of the American Society of Transplantation and the American Society of Transplant Surgeons*. 2008;8(8):1749–1754.

418. van Duin D, van Delden C. Multidrug-resistant gram-negative bacteria infections in solid organ transplantation. *American journal of transplantation : official journal of the American Society of Transplantation and the American Society of Transplant Surgeons*. 2013;13(Suppl 4):31–41.
419. Fishman JA. Infection in solid-organ transplant recipients. *The New England journal of medicine*. 2007;357(25):2601–2614.
420. Kaminski H, Fishman JA. The Cell Biology of Cytomegalovirus: implications for Transplantation. *American journal of transplantation : official journal of the American Society of Transplantation and the American Society of Transplant Surgeons*. 2016;16(8):2254–2269.
421. Razonable RR, Humar A. Cytomegalovirus in solid organ transplant recipients-Guidelines of the American Society of Transplantation Infectious Diseases Community of Practice. *Clin Transplant*. 2019;33(9):e13512.
422. Allen UD, Preiksaitis JK. Post-transplant lymphoproliferative disorders, Epstein-Barr virus infection, and disease in solid organ transplantation: guidelines from the American Society of Transplantation Infectious Diseases Community of Practice. *Clin Transplant*. 2019;33(9):e13652.
423. Loren AW, Porter DL, Stadtmauer EA, Tsai DE. Post-transplant lymphoproliferative disorder: a review. *Bone Marrow Transplant*. 2003;31(3):145–155.
424. Buxbaum NP, Pavletic SZ. Autoimmunity Following Allogeneic Hematopoietic Stem Cell Transplantation. *Front Immunol*. 2020;11:2017.
425. Weber TM, Lockhart ME. Renal transplant complications. *Abdom Imaging*. 2013;38(5):1144–1154.
426. Faenza A, Spolaore R, Poggioli G, Selleri S, Roversi R, Gozzetti G. Renal artery stenosis after renal transplantation. *Kidney international Supplement*. 1983(14):S-54-9.
427. Sandhu C, Patel U. Renal Transplantation Dysfunction: the Role of Interventional Radiology. *Clin Radiol*. 2002 Sep 1;57(9):772–783.
428. Saidi R, Kawai T, Kennealey P, Tsouflas G, Elias N, Hertl M, et al. Living Donor Kidney Transplantation With Multiple Arteries: recent Increase in Modern Era of Laparoscopic Donor Nephrectomy. *Archives of Surgery*. 2009 May 18;144(5):472–475.
429. Hamper UM, DeJong MR, Caskey CI, Sheth S. Power Doppler imaging: clinical experience and correlation with color Doppler US and other imaging modalities. *RadioGraphics*. 1997 Mar 1;17(2):499–513.
430. Akbar SA, Jafri SZH, Amendola MA, Madrazo BL, Salem R, Bis KG. Complications of Renal Transplantation. *RadioGraphics*. 2005 Sep 1;25(5):1335–1356.
431. Koçak T, Nane I, Ander H, Ziylan O, Oktar T, Ozsoy C. Urological and surgical complications in 362 consecutive living related donor kidney transplantations. *Urol. Int*. 2004;72(3):252–256.
432. Park S B, Kim JK, Cho K-S. Complications of renal transplantation: ultrasonographic evaluation. *Journal of ultrasound in medicine : official journal of the American Institute of Ultrasound in Medicine*. 2007;26(5):615–633.
433. Craig EV, Heller MT. Complications of liver transplant. *Abdominal Radiology*. 2021;46(1):43–67.
434. Birati EY, Rame JE. Post-heart transplant complications. *Crit Care Clin*. 2014;30(3):629—637.
435. Legendre C, Caillat-Zucman S, Samuel D, Morelon S, Bismuth H, Bach JF, et al. Transfer of symptomatic peanut allergy to the recipient of a combined liver-and-kidney transplant. *The New England journal of medicine*. 1997;337(12):822–824.
436. Ozdemir O, Arrey-Mensah A, Sorensen RU. Development of multiple food allergies in children taking tacrolimus after heart and liver transplantation. *Pediatr Transplant*. 2006;10(3):380–383.
437. De Bruyne R, Dullaers M, Van Biervliet S, Vande Velde S, Raes A, Gevaert P, et al. Post-transplant food allergy in children is associated with liver and not with renal transplantation: a monocentric comparative study. *Eur. J. Pediatr*. 2013;172(8):1069–1075.
438. Berry A, Campsen J, Shihab F, Firszt R. Transfer of peanut IgE sensitisation after combined pancreas-kidney transplant. *Clinical and experimental allergy : journal of the British Society for Allergy and Clinical Immunology. England*. 2014;44:1020–1022.
439. Newman EN, Firszt R. Post-transplantation Development of Food Allergies. *Curr Allergy Asthma Rep*. 2018;18(1):4.
440. Coppell JA, Richardson PG, Soiffer R, Martin PL, Kernan NA, Chen A, et al. Hepatic veno-occlusive disease following stem cell transplantation: incidence, clinical course, and outcome. *Biology of blood and marrow transplantation : journal of the American Society for Blood and Marrow Transplantation*. 2010;16(2):157–168.

441. Ho VT, Revta C, Richardson PG. Hepatic veno-occlusive disease after hematopoietic stem cell transplantation: update on defibrotide and other current investigational therapies. *Bone Marrow Transplant.* 2008;41(3):229–237.
442. Dalle J-H, Giralt SA. Hepatic Veno-Occlusive Disease after Hematopoietic Stem Cell Transplantation: risk Factors and Stratification, Prophylaxis, and Treatment. *Biology of blood and marrow transplantation : journal of the American Society for Blood and Marrow Transplantation.* 2016;22(3):400–409.
443. Dhar R. Neurologic Complications of Transplantation. *Neurocrit Care.* 2018;28(1):4–11.
444. Pedroso JL, Dutra LA, Braga-Neto P, Abrahao A, De Andrade JBC, Da Silva GL, et al. Neurological complications of solid organ transplantation. *Arq Neuropsiquiatr.* 2017;75(10):736–747.
445. Lim MA, Kohli J, Bloom RD. Immunosuppression for kidney transplantation: where are we now and where are we going? *Transplantation reviews (Orlando, Fla).* 2017;31(1):10–17.
446. Starzl TE. Personal reflections in transplantation. *Surg. Clin. North Am.* 1978;58(5):879–893.
447. Calne RY, Alexandre GPJ, Murray JE. a Study of the Effects of Drugs in Prolonging Survival of Homologous Renal Transplants in Dogs. *Ann. N.Y. Acad. Sci.* 1962;99(3):743–761.
448. Moini M, Schilsky ML, Tichy EM. Review on immunosuppression in liver transplantation. *World J Hepatol.* 2015;7(10):1355–1368.
449. Pirsch JD, Miller J, Deierhoi MH, Vincenti F, Filo RS. A comparison of tacrolimus (FK506) and cyclosporine for immunosuppression after cadaveric renal transplantation. FK506 Kidney Transplant Study Group. *Transplantation.* 1997;63(7):977–983.
450. Johnson C, Ahsan N, Gonwa T, Halloran P, Stegall M, Hardy M, et al. Randomized trial of tacrolimus (Prograf) in combination with azathioprine or mycophenolate mofetil versus cyclosporine (Neoral) with mycophenolate mofetil after cadaveric kidney transplantation. *Transplantation.* 2000;69(5):834–841.
451. Ekberg H, Tedesco-Silva H, Demirbas A, Vítko S, Nashan B, Gürkan A, et al. Reduced exposure to calcineurin inhibitors in renal transplantation. *The New England journal of medicine.* 2007;357(25):2562–2575.
452. Staatz CE, Tett SE. Pharmacology and toxicology of mycophenolate in organ transplant recipients: an update. *Arch. Toxicol.* 2014;88(7):1351–1389.
453. Kim WR, Smith JM, Skeans MA, Schladt DP, Schnitzler MA, Edwards EB, et al. OPTN/SRTR 2012 Annual Data Report: liver. *American journal of transplantation : official journal of the American Society of Transplantation and the American Society of Transplant Surgeons.* 2014;14(Suppl 1):69–96.
454. Liu CL, Fan ST, Lo CM, Chan SC, Ng IO, Lai CL, et al. Interleukin-2 receptor antibody (basiliximab) for immunosuppressive induction therapy after liver transplantation: a protocol with early elimination of steroids and reduction of tacrolimus dosage. *Liver transplantation : official publication of the American Association for the Study of Liver Diseases and the International Liver Transplantation Society.* 2004;10(6):728–733.
455. Gotthardt DN, Bruns H, Weiss KH, Schemmer P. Current strategies for immunosuppression following liver transplantation. *Langenbeck's archives of surgery.* 2014;399(8):981–988.
456. Deeks ED, Keating GM. Rabbit antithymocyte globulin (thymoglobulin): a review of its use in the prevention and treatment of acute renal allograft rejection. *Drugs.* 2009;69(11):1483–1512.
457. Magliocca JF, Knechtle SJ. The evolving role of alemtuzumab (Campath-1H) for immunosuppressive therapy in organ transplantation. *Transplant international : official journal of the European Society for Organ Transplantation.* 2006;19(9):705–714.
458. Morris PJ, Russell NK. Alemtuzumab (Campath-1H): a systematic review in organ transplantation. *Transplantation.* 2006;81:1361–1367.
459. Penninga L, Wettergren A, Wilson CH, Chan A-W, Steinbrüchel DA, Gluud C. Antibody induction versus corticosteroid induction for liver transplant recipients. *Cochrane Database Syst Rev.* 2014(5):CD010252.
460. https://www.accessdata.fda.gov/drugsatfda_docs/label/2018/011153s075lbl.pdf.
461. https://www.accessdata.fda.gov/drugsatfda_docs/label/2018/210115s000,050708s047,050709s040lbl.pdf.
462. https://www.novartis.us/sites/www.novartis.us/files/sandimmune.pdf.
463. https://www.accessdata.fda.gov/drugsatfda_docs/label/2009/050722s021,050723s019,050758s019,050759s024lbl.pdf.

464. https://www.accessdata.fda.gov/drugsatfda_docs/label/2011/016324s034s035lbl.pdf.
465. https://www.accessdata.fda.gov/drugsatfda_docs/label/2020/021083s067,021110s085lbl.pdf.
466. https://www.novartis.us/sites/www.novartis.us/files/afinitor.pdf?irmasrc=ONCWB0043&source=01030.
467. Ten Berge IJ, Parlevliet KJ, Raasveld MH, Buysmann S, Bemelman FJ, Schellekens PT. Guidelines for the optimal use of muromonab CD3 in transplantation. BioDrugs. 1999;11(4):277–284. 1173-8804. doi:10.2165/00063030-199911040-00006.
468. https://www.accessdata.fda.gov/drugsatfda_docs/label/2021/103948s5182lbl.pdf.
469. https://www.fda.gov/media/78206/download#:~:text=ATGAM%20Sterile%20Solution%20contains%20lymphocyte,immunized%20with%20human%20thymus%20lymphocytes.
470. https://www.accessdata.fda.gov/drugsatfda_docs/label/2017/761029s007lbl.pdf.
471. https://www.accessdata.fda.gov/drugsatfda_docs/label/2003/basnov010203lb.htm.

# Index

Page numbers followed by "*f*" and "*t*" indicate, figures and tables respectively.

## A

## B



## C

## D



## E



## F



## G



## H

## I

## J



## K



## L



## M



## N



## O



## P

## U



## V



## W



## X



## Y



## Z